Family Practice Review

Family Practice Review

A Problem Oriented Approach
Third Edition

Richard W. Swanson, M.D., C.C.F.P., F.C.F.P.
Director of Educational Programs
National Medical School Review
Newport Beach, California

Adjunct Professor of Family Medicine
Morehouse University School of Medicine
Atlanta, Georgia

Consultant
R and S Educational Consultants, Inc.
Calgary, Alberta, Canada

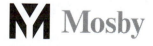 Mosby

St. Louis Baltimore Boston Carlsbad Chicago Naples New York Philadelphia Portland
London Madrid Mexico City Singapore Sydney Tokyo Toronto Wiesbaden

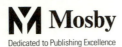
Mosby
Dedicated to Publishing Excellence

A Times Mirror
Company

Editor: Stephanie Manning
Developmental Editor: Laura Berendson
Project Manager: Linda Clarke
Associate Production Editor: Jennifer Harper
Production: Graphic World Publishing Services
Designer: Carolyn O'Brien
Manufacturing Manager: William A. Winneberger, Jr.

Third Edition
Copyright © 1996 by Mosby–Year Book, Inc.

Second edition copyrighted 1991 by B.C. Decker, Inc.

Printed in the United States of America
Composition by Graphic World, Inc.
Printing and binding by Maple Vail–Binghamton

Mosby–Year Book, Inc.
11830 Westline Industrial Drive
St. Louis, Missouri 63146

Library of Congress Cataloging-in-Publication Data

Swanson, Richard W.
    Family practice review : a problem oriented approach / Richard W.
Swanson. —3rd ed.
        p.   cm.
    Includes bibliographical references and index.
    ISBN 0-8151-8624-X (alk. paper)
    1. Family medicine—Examinations, questions, etc.   I. Title.
    [DNLM: 1. Family Practice—examination questions.   WB 18.2 S972f
1995]
RC58.S93   1996
616'.0076—dc20
DNLM/DLC
for Library of Congress   95-40824
                                                            CIP

97 98 99 00 / 9 8 7 6 5

This book is dedicated to Stella Marie Swanson—my wife, and the most wonderful woman in the world.

Preface

The world is constantly changing, and in business, we are all constantly striving to improve. The terms that are currently being used to describe this phenomenon are "Continuous Quality Improvement" and "Total Quality Management." We all have "customers." Those customers can be corporations, students, residents, practicing physicians, patients, other types of clients, or almost anyone else.

Medical students, residents, and practicing physicians who buy this third edition are customers of both myself and Mosby. You, in turn, have your patients as customers. It is my goal that all who buy this book will be able to take its contents and translate it into superior care for your patients. After all, those of us who call ourselves physicians have a *prima facie* duty to serve our patients and provide them with the best medical care available.

Keep this book beside you; take it with you; read it and re-read it. It was written in a manner that encourages you to do this. Throughout the book I have tried to explain the most important medical concepts in the simplest and most understandable manner possible. I sincerely hope you find this to be true for you.

This book can be used throughout the continuum of medical education (undergraduate, postgraduate, and continuing medical education) to significantly improve your performance on any and all medical examinations that you take. Previous readers from all levels of medical education have repeatedly told us this is true.

The third edition is significantly different from the second edition. Briefly, the significant differences are:

- The number of multiple choice questions increases from 900 to more than 2100.
- The number of chapters increases from 118 to 150.
- New chapters were determined through a "needs assessment" of users of previous editions.
- Hundreds of "SAMP" questions have been added. "SAMP" refers to "Short Answer Management Problems." This format is being used more and more in medical examinations around the world.
- We have eliminated "K-Type" multiple choice questions, which are no longer employed in board examinations. Medical research has definitely shown these questions to be less valid and less reproducible than single answer questions.
- There is increased information in the answers to all questions.
- There are increased and expanded summaries after each chapter.
- There are more comprehensive "case histories" to improve the validity of these problems as "true representations of what you will meet in practice."
- There is an increased emphasis on pathophysiology.
- There is an effort, in every problem, to be "inclusive" rather than "exclusive."

We hope you will find these changes interesting, stimulating, more useful for preparing for boards, and most importantly, of greater use to you and your patients.

Richard Swanson, M.D., C.C.F.P., F.C.F.P.

Acknowledgments

Everyone in the world needs to be recognized in positive ways; yet for some that remains an elusive goal.

I wish to acknowledge, with deep and sincere gratitude, two men who have literally changed my life—Jon and Victor Gruber, National Medical School Review, Newport Beach, California. Jon and Victor have provided me with a wonderful opportunity to do what I love so much, and that is to teach.

I wish to acknowledge two other people for whom I have a great deal of respect, and who also are not recognized for their great human qualities and attributes. First is Dr. Penny Jennett, Director of the Office of Medical Education, Faculty of Medicine, University of Calgary. Penny, thank you for your support, friendship, respect, and your academic contribution to my life. Second is Dr. Victor Sawchuk, Associate Professor, Department of Family Medicine, University of Calgary. Victor, you never let me down. Sometimes you held me up when there was no one else. A wise, old philosopher once said, "There will be one." Victor, I fully realize that few people, if any, ever believed in your ideas and your enthusiasm towards the department in general, and rural medicine in particular. I did, and I still do. You were well ahead of your time, but like so many other visionaries, you fell by the wayside. This formal acknowledgement, seen before the world, will set the record straight. Few would try, and none would succeed, in being the ideal role model that you were and continue to be. Now, Victor, you are finally recognized.

Tips on Passing the Board Examinations

This section will briefly discuss the philosophy and techniques of passing board examinations or any other type of medical examination.

First, realize that you are "playing a game." It is, of course, a very important game, but is nevertheless a game. When answering each question you must ask yourself the following: "What is it that the examiner wants from this question?" Let us turn our attention to the most common type of questions, the multiple-choice question (MCQ).

There are many pros and many cons to multiple-choice questions, and a brief review of those ideas in this chapter is in order.

The pros of multiple-choice questions are as follows:

1. An MCQ item requires the student to choose among a fixed set of alternatives. In other words, you simply have to recognize the choices, a far cry from having to memorize them.

2. An MCQ test can sample a broad range of facts and a variety of facts using specific questions requiring a choice among responses.

3. An MCQ test that is well written is more valid and more reliable than any other form of examination; this conclusion is drawn strictly from the number of questions asked.

4. An MCQ test correlates highly with short answer tests; this should turn out to be an advantage for the student.

5. An MCQ test increases the reliability or precision of the score distribution. The score distribution is not dependent on who is marking the examination.

The cons of multiple-choice questions are as follows:

1. An MCQ test lends itself to esoterica. In other words, many examiners go out of their way to ask questions that are at best questionable and at worst completely irrelevant to anything you will ever encounter in practice.

2. An MCQ test does not allow you to qualify or explain your answer.

3. In an MCQ test, the correct answer is provided for recognition, a situation not equivalent to real practice.

4. The answer to a particular question on an MCQ test is dependent not only on the facts tested but also on the manner in which the question is written.

What this book provides for you is a way to "outfox the fox." There is a story about an individual who passed five different speciality board exams while knowing nothing about the content. This individual, was, however, an expert in multiple-choice questions.

So, how do you outfox the fox? Following these rules will maximize your chances.

Rule 1: allocate your time appropriately. At the beginning of the examination divide the number of questions by the time allotted. A fair examination will allow approximately 1 minute/question. Pace yourself accordingly and check your progress every half hour.

Rule 2: do not wait until the end to transfer your answers from the question paper to the answer sheet. You may find that you have run out of time and your answer sheet is blank.

Rule 3: answer every question in order. Do not leave an answer space blank. If you do, you run the risk of unsequencing your answers and having all answers out of order.

Rule 4: do not spend more than your allotted time on any one question. If you don't know the answer and no marks are subtracted for wrong answers, simply guess.

Rule 5: even if marks are subtracted for wrong answers and you can eliminate even one choice, answer the question anyway. The laws of mathematics indicate that you will still come out ahead.

Rule 6: if there is a question in which one choice is significantly longer than the others and you do not know the answer, choose the long choice.

Rule 7: if you are faced with an "all of the above" choice, realize that it is right far more often than it is wrong. Choose all of the above.

Rule 8: become suspicious if you have more than three choices of the same letter in a row. Two of one choice in a row is common, three is less common, and four is almost unheard of. Something is probably wrong.

Rule 9: answer choices tend to be very evenly distributed. In other words, the number of correct (a) choices is close to the number of correct (b) choices, and so on. However, there may be somewhat more choice (e)'s than any other, especially if there are a fair number of "all of the above" choices. If you have time, do a quick check to provide yourself with some reassurance.

Rule 10: never, never change an answer once you have recorded it on the answer sheet unless you have an extraordinary reason for doing so. Many people taking MCQ examinations, especially if they have time on their hands after completing the examination, start second-guessing themselves and thinking of all kinds of unusual exceptions. Resist this temptation.

Rule 11: if you have absolutely no idea regarding the correct answer and marks are not subtracted for guessing, choose (c). It tends to have a slightly higher frequency of being correct.

Rule 12: before you write anything on the answer sheet, always, always read each and every choice. Do not get caught by seeing what you believe is the correct answer jump out at you. Read all of the choices.

Rule 13: read each question carefully. Be especially careful to read words such as *not, except,* and so on. Some people find it helpful to carefully underline certain parts of the question containing such words.

This author cannot guarantee success with these or any other rules. I do, however, believe that these rules will help you achieve better results on your board examinations.

Contents

Pediatrics and Adolescent Medicine

General Surgery and Surgical Specialties

Geriatric Medicine

Epidemiology and Public Health

Emergency Medicine

Family Practice Review

Internal Medicine

PROBLEM 1   A 72-YEAR-OLD MALE WITH ACUTE CHEST PAIN

A 72-year-old farmer is brought to the emergency department of his local rural hospital by his wife. Apparently he developed a "twinge of chest pain" while shoveling grain 3 hours ago. He insisted on staying home until "he collapsed on the floor." Even then, he wanted to stay home and rest, but his wife insisted he receive medical care, and she brought him to the emergency department. He states that the pain is "almost gone." He is obese, smokes two packs of cigarettes daily, drinks a "goodly amount of beer," and has been told that his serum cholesterol level is "way out of sight." He seems confused on the cholesterol issue, believing that the higher the cholesterol, the better.

He describes dull, aching, viselike pain around his chest, with radiation to the left shoulder. His wife says that she has never seen him in so much pain. He admits that when the pain was at its worst he experienced nausea and vomiting.

On physical examination, he is sweating and diaphoretic. He has vomited twice since coming to the emergency department. His blood pressure is 160/100 mm Hg, and his pulse is 120 and irregular. His abdomen is obese, and you believe you can detect an enlarged aorta by deep palpation.

His ECG reveals significant Q waves in V1 to V4 with significant ST segment elevation in the same leads. There are reciprocal ST changes (ST segment depression) in the inferior leads (II, III, avF).

SELECT THE ONE BEST ANSWER TO THE FOLLOWING QUESTIONS

1. The most likely diagnosis in this patient is:
   a) acute inferior wall myocardial infarction
   b) acute anterior wall myocardial infarction
   c) acute myocardial ischemia
   d) acute pericarditis
   e) musculoskeletal chest wall pain

2. Given the history, physical examination, and ECG, your first priority is to:
   a) call the ambulance for immediate transport to another hospital that "knows how to treat this thing"
   b) admit the patient for observation
   c) administer streptokinase or t-PA intravenously
   d) administer heparin intravenously
   e) none of the above

3. Given your attention to your first priority, you would now:
   a) call the ambulance for immediate transport to another hospital that "knows how to look after this thing"
   b) admit the patient for observation
   c) administer streptokinase or t-PA intravenously immediately
   d) administer heparin intravenously immediately
   e) none of the above

4. Which of the following criteria should be met before a patient is given thrombolytic therapy following the history, physical examination, and ECG previously described?
   a) typical chest pain suggestive of a myocardial infarction
   b) ECG changes confirming myocardial infarction
   c) the absence of other diseases that would explain the symptoms
   d) all of the above
   e) none of the above

5. Which of the following thrombolytic agents is the agent of choice for thrombolysis in acute MI?
   a) streptokinase
   b) APSAC
   c) t-PA
   d) there is no agent of choice; any of the above can be justified, depending on the circumstances
   e) I don't know

6. Which of the following statements regarding the use of heparin in patients with acute myocardial infarction is(are) true?
   a) heparin therapy is now used almost routinely with thrombolytic therapy during acute phase of myocardial infarction treatment, providing certain criteria are met
   b) heparin is recommended whenever there is echocardiographic evidence of left ventricular thrombi

c) heparin should be administered (unless contraindicated) to all patients with acute anterior wall myocardial infarction
d) heparin is contraindicated in patients with uncontrolled hypertension
e) all of the above

7. Which of the following are contraindications to the use of thrombolytic therapy in patients with acute myocardial infarction?
   a) active gastrointestinal bleeding
   b) recent surgery (<2 weeks post-op)
   c) history of cerebrovascular accident
   d) atrial fibrillation or mitral stenosis
   e) all of the above

8. Which of the following statements regarding patients admitted to the coronary care unit (CCU) following presumed myocardial infarction is(are) true?
   a) patients with suspected MIs should have the left ventricular ejection fraction measured before leaving the unit
   b) patients without additional complications (except as discussed in Problem 1) should have a submaximal exercise tolerance test with thallium-201 imaging on the fourth or fifth hospital day
   c) patients with negative submaximal stress tests should have a maximal exercise stress test performed after 4 to 6 weeks
   d) all of the above
   e) a and c

9. Which of the following is(are) significant features of the pathophysiology of myocardial infarction?
   a) endothelial cell wall damage
   b) coronary atherosclerosis
   c) thromboxane A_2 production
   d) all of the above
   e) a and b

10. Which of the following is(are) true concerning aspirin in the treatment of acute myocardial infarction?
    a) aspirin may serve as a substitute for streptokinase or t-PA
    b) aspirin may serve as a substitute for heparin
    c) aspirin may serve as a substitute for beta blockade
    d) all of the above
    e) none of the above

11. Which of the following statements regarding thrombolytic therapy is false?
    a) thrombolytic therapy limits myocardial necrosis
    b) thrombolytic therapy preserves left ventricular function
    c) thrombolytic therapy reduces mortality

d) all of the above statements are false
e) none of the above statements are false

12. In the United States today, what percentage of patients with acute myocardial infarction who would potentially qualify for thrombolytic therapy receive it?
    a) 95%
    b) 80%
    c) 60%
    d) 30%
    e) 5%

13. Which of the following statements concerning dysrhythmias and dysrhythmic drugs in patients who have sustained a myocardial infarction is(are) true?
    a) premature ventricular contractions are common and should be treated with lidocaine
    b) sustained runs of ventricular tachycardia frequently progress to ventricular fibrillation
    c) prophylactic lidocaine is recommended to prevent dysrhythmias in all patients who have sustained an MI
    d) none of the above
    e) all of the above

14. One of the major patient concerns following a myocardial infarction is the risk of a second or subsequent attack. In which of the following circumstances is the risk of reinfarction and/or mortality following myocardial infarction significantly increased?
    a) left ventricular ejection fraction <40%
    b) exercise-induced ischemia
    c) non Q-wave infarction (subendocardial infarction)
    d) a and b
    e) all of the above

15. Which of the following medications have been shown to be of benefit in some post–myocardial infarction patients?
    a) beta blockers
    b) calcium-channel blockers
    c) aspirin
    d) a and c
    e) all of the above

16. Which of the following statements concerning rehabilitation of the patient after a myocardial infarction is(are) true?
    a) sexual intercourse should not resume for at least 3 months
    b) patients who have sustained an MI should stay off work for at least 4 months
    c) patients who have sustained an MI may gradually increase activity over 6 to 8 weeks

d) no significant psychological distress regarding the myocardial infarction has been shown to occur in the patient's spouse or significant other
e) all of the above

17. The major pathophysiologic difference between (1) unstable angina and non Q-wave or nontransmural infarction and (2) transmural infarction is:
a) the presenting signs and symptoms of the attack
b) the duration and completeness of the occlusion
c) the risk factor profile
d) the male-female ratio
e) the degree of injury pattern surrounding the true ischemic area(s)

18. The best single confirmatory investigation for acute myocardial infarction is:
a) the ECG
b) the height of ST segment elevation in the affected area (in mm) plus the depth of ST segment depression in the reciprocally affected leads (in mm)
c) the creatine kinase isoenzyme MB fraction
d) the presence of dysfunctional heart muscle as demonstrated by echocardiography
e) none of the above

19. Sudden death as a result of myocardial infarction is almost always due to:
a) third-degree heart block resulting from infarction of the AV node
b) ventricular tachycardia
c) ventricular fibrillation

d) ventricular standstill
e) none of the above

20. Which of the following statements regarding shock and its treatment in acute myocardial infarction is(are) true?
a) the acute MI patient may develop shock secondary to hypovolemic hypotension
b) the acute MI patient may develop shock secondary to persistent hypotension and a poor cardiac index
c) both forms of shock respond well to treatment with IV fluids (Ringer's lactate or normal saline solution)
d) a and b only
e) all of the above

21. Coronary reperfusion with thrombolytic agents has been shown to be of benefit when the onset of the pain occurs up to how many hours (maximum) before the initial assessment?
a) 4
b) 6
c) 12
d) 24
e) 48

22. In Problem 1 there is a key finding on physical examination of the patient's abdomen that should be further assessed by:
a) an abdominal ultrasound
b) an IVP
c) a digital subtraction angiogram
d) a CT scan
e) an MRI scan

Short Answer Management Problem 1

List the adjunctive agents commonly used in the treatment of acute myocardial infarction.

ANSWERS

1. B. This patient has most likely suffered an anterior wall MI. The history suggests that he is at high risk for an infarct, and the Q waves in V1 to V4 and ST segment elevation in the anterior chest leads plus reciprocal changes in the inferior wall confirm the diagnosis.

An acute inferior wall MI would present with ST segment elevation and possibly Q waves in the inferior leads.

Acute pericarditis would present with ST segment elevation in all leads.

Musculoskeletal chest wall pain does not produce the abnormalities in the ECG that we see in this patient.

2. E. The history, physical examination, and ECG point clearly to acute anterior wall MI. First, ascertain that the patient's airway is patent (without obstruction, vomit, or any blockage) and administer 100% oxygen.

3. C. Administer streptokinase or t-PA. The recommended dose of streptokinase in acute MI is 1.5 million U IV over 30 to 60 minutes.

The two recommended regimens for administration of t-PA are the standard regimen and the front-loaded regimen. The front-loaded regimen, used in the GUSTO trial, may produce a higher early patency rate than the standard regimen.

The standard regimen for the administration of

t-PA is 10 mg IV bolus, then 50 mg IV over the first hour, followed by 40 mg IV over the next 2 hours. The front-loaded regimen used in the GUSTO trial is 15 mg IV bolus, then 50 mg IV over 30 minutes, followed by 35 mg over 1 hour for a 100 mg total dose.

A third choice is APSAC (Eminase), which is delivered with a dose of 30 mg IV bolus over 5 minutes.

4. D. Thrombolytic therapy should be administered only when the following criteria are met: (1) typical chest pain suggestive of an MI, (2) ECG changes confirming MI, and (3) the "absence" of other diseases that would explain the symptoms.

An age greater than 70 years was formerly a criterion for exclusion of patients for thrombolytic therapy; this is no longer the case. Contraindications to thrombolytic therapy include (1) active internal bleeding, (2) suspected aortic dissection, (3) prolonged or traumatic cardiopulmonary resuscitation, (4) recent head trauma or known intracranial neoplasm, (5) hemorrhagic retinopathy, (6) pregnancy, (7) systolic blood pressure over 180 mm Hg, (8) history of cerebrovascular disease, and (9) trauma or surgery within the last 2 weeks.

5. D. A large amount of attention has focused on determining the "best" thrombolytic agent. Although determining which agent saves the most lives is clearly important, the most important point to remember is to give the thrombolytic agent—not which one to give.

6. E. The role of concomitant heparin in the initial treatment of acute MI has become increasingly clear over time. The HART study has shown that early, effective anticoagulation with heparin maintains t-PA–induced coronary artery patency more effectively than aspirin alone. Subgroup analyses have shown that patients receiving therapeutic heparin, as measured by the activated partial thromboplastin time (APTT), have an extremely high patency approaching 95% following t-PA administration. Although there is some evidence to the contrary, it may be reasonable to believe that what applies to t-PA plus heparin also applies to streptokinase plus heparin.

In the GUSTO trial (t-PA vs. streptokinase) patients received 5000 U of heparin bolus followed by 1000 U/hr constant infusion, titrated every 6 hours, to maintain an APTT of 60 to 85 seconds for at least 48 hours.

The two most important indications for concomitant use of heparin are acute anterior wall MI and echocardiographic evidence of left ventricular thrombi.

7. E. The major contraindications to adjunctive heparin therapy in MI are history of major surgery with time from discharge under 14 days, history of CVAs, chronic atrial fibrillation or chronic mitral stenosis, and acute gastrointestinal hemorrhage.

8. D. Once placed in the CCU, the patient should have his left ventricular ejection fraction measured. If no other cardiac conditions are discovered, the patient should have a submaximal stress test before discharge. If this result is negative, a maximal exercise stress tolerance test should be performed after 4 to 6 weeks.

9. D. The pathophysiology of acute MI centers around the formation of significant coronary artery atherosclerosis. The progression of atherosclerosis is as follows: (1) superficial atherosclerotic fatty streaks form in the coronary arteries of children; (2) the fatty streaks progress to elevated fibrous plaques by the third and fourth decades of life; and (3) these fibrous plaques progress to complex, eccentric, ulcerated, and hemorrhagic plaques by the fifth and sixth decades, culminating in plaque rupture or intraplaque hemorrhage and coronary artery occlusion.

The endothelial injury eventually provides the basis for atherogenesis. The fragile endothelium is damaged by hypertension, elevated low-density lipoprotein (LDL) cholesterol, diabetes, smoking, and other factors.

Simple denudation exposes the vascular collagen, which triggers circulating platelet adhesion and aggregation and a cascade of growth factor release including thromboxane A_2, prostacyclin, platelet-derived growth factor (PDGF). Smooth muscle cell and monocyte proliferation, along with lipid accumulation under the influence of growth factors, leads to the ultimate end: severe atherosclerosis.

10. E. Aspirin is the only adjunctive agent that has unequivocally been shown to reduce mortality alone or in conjunction with thrombolytic agents in patients with acute MI. The ISIS-II study showed that acetylsalicylic acid (ASA) reduced mortality by 25%. However, when ASA was added to streptokinase the effect was synergistic, and mortality from MI was reduced by 42%.

Thus aspirin has been shown to reduce rethrombosis and recurrent MI. It is not, however, a substitute for anything; it should be used along with other acute agents in the treatment of MI.

11. E. The cornerstone of treatment of acute MI is thrombolytic therapy. It is an established, effective therapy that limits myocardial necrosis, preserves left ventricular function, and reduces mortality. Presently the following statement can be made: "The use of thrombolytic therapy in acute myocardial infarction has been established to the point where not to use such therapy is considered to be substandard care." (From Rakel R, ed: Conn's Current Therapy. Philadelphia: WB Saunders, 1994.)

12. D. Thrombolytic therapy currently is underutilized in the treatment of acute MI in the United States. Despite excellent data supporting thrombolytic therapy, only

approximately 30% of patients with acute MI receive it. Of the remaining 70%, only 20% have true contraindications or equivocal ECG changes that would preclude thrombolytic therapy.

13. D. PVCs occur frequently following acute MI and do not require treatment. Couplets, triplets, multifocal PVCs, and short runs of nonsustained ventricular tachycardia are effectively treated with intravenous lidocaine. In spite of the fact, however, that they are treated with intravenous lidocaine, no survival advantage has been shown with lidocaine in this setting.

Most clinicians do not treat these nonmalignant ventricular dysrhythmias because they rarely progress to life-threatening situations, and if they do they can be treated effectively with cardioversion or defibrillation.

Lidocaine is not recommended in the routine prophylaxis of acute MI. In addition, long-term prophylaxis with oral antiarrhythmics such as flecainide and encainide following acute MI have been shown to increase mortality drastically.

14. E. The risk of subsequent infarction and/or mortality following discharge from the hospital following an MI is increased in patients with (1) postinfarction angina pectoris; (2) non–Q wave infarction; (3) congestive cardiac failure; (4) left ventricular ejection fraction less than 40%; (5) exercise-induced ischemia diagnosed by ECG or by scintigraphy; and (6) ventricular ectopy (frequency >10 PVCs/min).

15. E. Beta blockers, aspirin, and calcium-channel blockers have improved the prognosis in some patients following an MI.

Beta blockers appear to reduce the risk of sudden death in patients who are at increased risk.

Antiplatelet agents, particularly aspirin, have been shown to be of benefit in patients who have had an MI. Aspirin reduces both rethrombosis and recurrent MI.

Calcium-channel blockers (particularly diltiazem) have been shown to decrease the risk of reinfarction after a non–Q wave infarction.

Anticoagulants have not been shown to improve prognosis, although they do reduce peripheral embolization in the early discharge phase.

Antiarrhythmics other than beta blockers have not been shown to be effective as prophylactic agents.

16. C. Patients who have suffered an MI should gradually increase activity levels over a period of 6 to 8 weeks. Patients can return to work by approximately 8 weeks.

Patients who have suffered an uncomplicated MI may be safely started in an activity program by 3 to 4 weeks postinfarct.

Sexual intercourse can resume within 4 to 6 weeks of the infarction. There does not seem to be any logical rea-

son for the patient to wait 3 months to resume intercourse. A good rule to follow in this case is: "If the patient can climb the stairs to the bedroom, the rest is probably okay too!"

In many patients the psychological impact of an MI outweighs the physical impact. Also, in a significant percentage of families, the spouse is affected as much as, if not more than, the patient. One of the most common errors in cardiac rehabilitation is not to involve the spouse or significant other at every stage of the program.

17. B. The pathophysiologic difference between (1) unstable angina and non–Q wave or nontransmural infarction on the one hand and (2) transmural infarction on the other is the duration and completeness of the occlusion.

There is no difference between (1) the presenting and symptoms of the attack; (2) the risk factor profile; (3) the male-female ratio; and (4) the "area of injury" surrounding the actual "area of infarction."

18. C. The single best confirmatory test for the diagnosis of acute MI is creatine kinase isoenzyme MB fraction. Elevation of the ST segment can result from either injury or infarction. It is neither sensitive nor specific enough for the diagnosis of infarction in the absence of Q waves.

For the diagnosis of acute MI, the ECG is sensitive (70%–90% with more than 1 mm of elevation in two contiguous leads); unfortunately it is less specific.

The presence of dysfunctional heart muscle on echocardiography means that there is likely to be a lowering of both the ejection fraction and the cardiac index; it says nothing about whether an MI has occurred or anything regarding the age of same.

19. C. Sudden death as a result of acute MI is almost always due to ventricular fibrillation (VF) induced by the electrical instability of the ischemic/infarction zone. VF is most common either at the immediate onset of coronary occlusion or at the time of coronary reperfusion (reperfusion arrhythmia).

20. D. Shock in the presence of an acute MI can be of two pathophysiologic varieties. Either there is hypovolemia and associated hypotension (hypovolemic shock), or there is persistent hypotension and a poor cardiac index in the presence of adequate left ventricular filling pressures.

Hypovolemic shock is best treated with volume replacement using either Ringer's lactate or normal saline solution. Care must be taken to avoid "volume overloading" which may produce pulmonary edema and congestive cardiac failure.

Cardiogenic shock is generally associated with severe left ventricular dysfunction and occurs with large infarcts that produce damage to greater than 40% of the left ventricle. Treatment is urgent and mortality is high. The treatments of choice include (1) intraaortic balloon pump placement to increase coronary flow and decrease afterload; (2) coronary reperfusion with percutaneous transluminal balloon angioplasty (PTCA) (the mainstay of treatment); and (3) pharmacologic agents including morphine, dopamine, and dobutamine.

21. C. One clinical trial has shown unequivocally that there is a significant survival advantage to patients with acute MI, even when thrombolytic agents are given up to 12 hours after the onset of the chest pain.

22. A. The finding on physical examination of the abdomen of "an enlarged aorta" should be further assessed by an abdominal ultrasound study. The patient probably has an aortic aneurysm.

Although this finding also could be assessed by CT or MRI, an abdominal ultrasound is considerably less expensive and just as sensitive.

SOLUTION TO SHORT ANSWER MANAGEMENT PROBLEM 1

The commonly used adjunctive agents in acute MI are as follows:

1. Aspirin: 160 mg at the time of infarct and 160 mg every day following. Aspirin reduces rethrombosis and recurrent myocardial infarction.
2. Beta blockade (e.g., metoprolol): 5 mg IV bolus q5min ×3, then 50 mg PO q6h for 48 hours, then 100 mg PO bid. Beta blockade is contraindicated with hypotension or bradycardia, severe left ventricular dysfunction, or AV block. It is especially effective for reflex tachycardia or hypertension.
3. Heparin: 5000 U IV bolus followed by 1000 U/hr. Heparin is begun concomitantly with thrombolytic therapy and continued for 24 to 48 hours.
4. Magnesium sulfate: 8 mmol IV over 5 minutes, then 65 mmol over 24 hours. Benign therapy has been shown to reduce mortality. Side effects include flushing and bradycardia.
5. Morphine sulfate: 2 to 5 mg IV every 5 to 30 minutes and as needed. Morphine sulfate is an excellent analgesic/anxiolytic. It decreases both preload and afterload and myocardial oxygen demand. However, morphine sulfate may cause hypotension.
6. Nitroglycerin: 0.4 mg sublingual followed by 5 to 10 μg/min by IV infusion. The infusion rate can be increased by 10-μg increments to 100 μg/min to control symptoms or to decrease mean blood pressure by 10%.
7. Oxygen: 2 to 4 L/min by nasal cannula is administered to all patients during initial hours of treatment. Higher flow rates may be necessary in patients with congestive heart failure or frank hypoxia.
8. Warfarin: 10 mg/day for 3 days, then 2.5 to 5 mg/day is indicated for severe left ventricular dysfunction to prevent mural thrombus.

SUMMARY OF THE DIAGNOSIS AND TREATMENT OF ACUTE MYOCARDIAL INFARCTION

1. **Signs and symptoms:** The pain of MI, unlike angina pectoris, usually occurs at rest. The pain is similar to angina in location and radiation but is more severe and builds up rapidly. Usually it is described as a retrosternal tightness or squeezing sensation or sometimes a dull ache. Radiation to the left shoulder is not uncommon. Other symptoms include sweating, weakness, dizziness, nausea, vomiting, and abdominal discomfort. Abdominal discomfort is especially common in inferior wall MIs.
2. **ECG changes:** The classical evolution of changes is from peaked (hyperacute) T waves, to ST segment elevation, to ST segment elevation, to Q wave development, to T wave inversion. This sequence may occur over a few hours or may take several days. (Note: If ECG changes are not present, do not assume an MI has not occurred. If signs and symptoms suggest MI, it is an MI until proved otherwise.)
3. **Confirmatory evidence:** Evidence of infarction is confirmed by elevation of the creatine kinase MB fraction for three days.
4. **Other diagnostic procedures:** Scintigraphic studies including technetium-99 and thallium-201 imaging and radionuclide angiography, as well as echocardiography, may help document the extent of the damage.
5. **Treatment of acute myocardial infarction:**
   a) Supplementary oxygen
   b) Morphine sulfate for pain relief as well as for its preload and afterload reducing properties
   c) Thrombolytic therapy: streptokinase, APSAC, or t-PA.
   d) Heparin therapy: initiate concomitantly with thrombolytic agent
   e) Beta-blockade: limits extent of infarction
   f) Nitroglycerin: ideal for pain control as well as its preload reducing properties
   g) Warfarin: consider if severe left ventricular dysfunction to prevent mural thrombosis
   h) Consider magnesium sulfate as analgesic/anxiolytic
   i) Aspirin one stat; 160 mg/day

(Note: Lidocaine prophylaxis is not indicated for the prevention of dysrhythmias.)
6. **Post-MI:**
   a) Submaximal stress ECG test before discharge
   b) Discharge medications: aspirin; beta blockers

c) Exercise program within 3 to 4 weeks
d) Return to work within 8 weeks
e) Sexual intercourse: 4 weeks
f) Involvement of the spouse or significant other is critical

SUGGESTED READING

Thompson MA, Ross AM. Acute myocardial infarction. In: Rakel R, ed. Conn's current therapy. Philadelphia: WB Saunders, 1994.

PROBLEM 2 A 55-YEAR-OLD MALE WITH CHEST PAIN

A 55-year-old male presents to your office for assessment of left-sided shoulder pain. The pain comes on after any strenuous activity, including walking. The pain is described as follows. (1) Quality: dull, aching; (2) Quantity: 8/10 when doing any activity—otherwise 0/10; (3) Chronology: began approximately 8 months ago and has been getting worse ever since; (4) Continuous/Intermittent: intermittent; (5) Aggravating factors: exercise of any kind; (6) Relieving factors: rest; (7) Associated manifestations: occasional nausea; (8) Pain history: no previous pain before 8 months ago; no other significant history of pain syndromes; (9) Radiation: appears to be radiating to the left shoulder area; (10) Location: mainly retrosternal; (11) Quality of life: definitely affecting quality of life by limiting activity.

The patient tells you that the pain seems somehow worse today. For the first time, it did not go away after he stopped walking.

The patient's blood pressure is 120/80 mm Hg; his pulse is 72 and regular. His heart sounds are normal. There are no extra sounds and no murmurs.

SELECT THE ONE BEST ANSWER TO THE FOLLOWING QUESTIONS

1. Which of the following statements regarding this patient's chest pain is(are) false?
   a) the patient may have suffered a myocardial infarction
   b) the patient's chest pain may be due to angina pectoris
   c) the patient's chest pain may be due to esophageal motor disorder
   d) the administration of sublingual nitroglycerin is a very sensitive test to distinguish angina pectoris from esophageal causes
   e) the patient should be admitted to the coronary care unit until the origin of the pain is firmly established

2. The patient is admitted for observation to the CCU. His pain subsides with intravenous nitroglycerin. His CK-MB fraction is normal.
   Which of the following investigations is(are) not indicated at this time?
   a) an exercise tolerance test
   b) coronary angiography
   c) an upper gastrointestinal series
   d) a plasma lipid profile
   e) a fasting blood sugar

3. The patient subsequently has an exercise tolerance test. This test reveals a 2.5-mm ST segment depression.
   Which of the following statements regarding this test result is(are) true?
   a) It probably indicates angina pectoris
   b) coronary angiography is indicated
   c) a hypotensive response with stress testing suggests severe ischemia and severe (probably multivessel) coronary artery disease
   d) a and b
   e) all of the above statements are true

4. Which of the following medications would not be indicated as a first-line therapy for the treatment of this patient?

   a) diltiazem
   b) propranolol
   c) isosorbide dinitrate
   d) prazosin
   e) nitroglycerin

5. A 67-year-old male with a history of angina pectoris is brought to the ER by his wife. For the past 3 days, he has been having increasing chest pain. The chest pain has been occurring at rest and while in bed at night as well as while walking (he is able to walk only very slowly). The pain has been getting progressively worse over the last 8 hours.
   On physical examination, his blood pressure is 120/70 mm Hg. His pulse is 96 and regular.
   His electrocardiogram shows ST segment depression of 1.5 mm. Flattening of the T waves is seen across the precordial leads.
   Which of the following statements regarding this patient is(are) true?
   a) this patient has unstable angina
   b) intravenous nitroglycerin is the treatment of first choice
   c) the patient probably has complex coronary artery stenosis
   d) this patient should be placed on 1 aspirin/day
   e) all of the above are true

6. A 50-year-old female presents to the ER with a sharp retrosternal chest pain that awoke her. This is the fourth episode in as many nights, and she is concerned that she is "finally having a heart attack." She was in to see her physician 3 weeks ago. At that time, he gave her a "clean bill of health." She was told that her blood pressure and her cholesterol were completely normal. She is a nonsmoker and has no family history of coronary artery disease.
   On physical examination, her blood pressure is 100/70 mm Hg. Her pulse is 96 and regular, and the remainder of the CV and respiratory exam is normal.
   Her ECG reveals a significant ST segment elevation in the anterior limb leads. Within one hour, the ST seg-

ment has returned to normal. CK-MB fraction levels done over the next three days are normal.

Which of the following statements regarding this patient is(are) true?

a) this patient probably has Prinzmetal's angina
b) calcium-channel blockers are the treatment of choice for this type of angina
c) beta blockers are contraindicated in this type of angina
d) all of the above
e) none of the above

7. Which of the following statements regarding percutaneous coronary angioplasty and mortality from coronary artery disease is(are) true?

a) percutaneous coronary angioplasty increases longevity
b) percutaneous coronary angioplasty improves both morbidity and mortality from coronary artery disease
c) percutaneous coronary angioplasty is of no proven benefit
d) the effect of percutaneous coronary angioplasty on mortality from coronary artery disease is unclear
e) nobody really knows for sure

8. In which of the following patients would percutaneous coronary angioplasty most likely be used?

a) a patient with left main stem disease
b) a patient with triple-vessel disease
c) a patient with a ventricular aneurysm
d) a patient with one-vessel disease
e) any of the above are good indications for percutaneous coronary angioplasty

9. Which of the following is least likely to be used as a combination therapy in patients with angina pectoris?

a) nitroglycerine-atenolol-nifedipine
b) nitroglycerine-enalapril-nifedipine
c) nitroglycerine-propranolol-verapamil
d) nitroglycerine-metoprolol-diltiazem
e) nitroglycerine-atenolol-nifedipine

10. Which of the following drugs is considered the most potent vasodilator?

a) nifedipine
b) verapamil
c) metoprolol
d) atenolol
e) propranolol

11. Coronary artery bypass surgery (CABG) may be indicated as the treatment of choice for angina pectoris with which of the following angina patients?

a) a patient with triple-vessel disease
b) a patient with one-vessel disease
c) a patient with two-vessel disease
d) CABG may be first line therapy in any of the above
e) b or c

12. A 65-year-old male presents to your office with a history strongly suggestive of angina pectoris. He also has a long history of hypertension.

On physical examination, his blood pressure is 170/100 mm Hg. Exercise tolerance testing reveals a 2.5-mm Hg ST segment depression, which strongly supports the suggested diagnosis.

Which of the following medications would you consider as the agent(s) of first choice in the treatment of this patient?

a) hydrochlorothiazide
b) verapamil
c) clonidine
d) propranolol
e) b and/or d

13. Which of the following investigations should be performed on a patient with possible angina pectoris?

a) CBC
b) CXR
c) complete urinalysis
d) thyroid function testing
e) all of the above

14. The pathophysiology of angina pectoris is best explained by which of the following?

a) significantly increased peripheral vascular resistance
b) a balance between oxygen supply and oxygen demand
c) an imbalance of oxygen supply and oxygen demand plus or minus coronary artery spasm
d) significant peripheral venous and arterial vasoconstriction
e) none of the above

15. Which of the following criteria indicate a diagnosis of unstable angina pectoris?

a) new onset angina (<2 months) that is either severe or frequent (>3 episodes/day) or both
b) patients with accelerating angina
c) patients with angina at rest
d) b and c
e) all of the above

Short Answer Management Problem 2

Briefly describe the phenomenon of asymptomatic coronary artery ischemia.

ANSWERS

1. D. Acute chest pain is a very common and often difficult diagnostic problem. Myocardial infarction must be assumed until proven otherwise in patients with any significant risk factors. This patient's 1-mm ST segment depression is not diagnostic of anything. Pain from esophageal motor disorder is often confused with pain from myocardial ischemia. This differential is often exceedingly difficult; many times (1) quality of pain, (2) quantity of pain, (3) radiation of pain, and (4) some aggravating factors are the same in both conditions. Although many physicians believe that relief with nitroglycerin is specific for myocardial ischemia and myocardial infarction, such is not the case. Sublingual nitroglycerin will relieve pain from esophageal motor disorder as well as it will relieve pain from myocardial ischemia and myocardial injury.

2. B. We are not yet far enough down the diagnostic pathway leading to angina pectoris to justify the invasive procedure of coronary angiography. A normal CK-MB fraction essentially rules out myocardial infarction. However, the origin of this patient's chest pain is still unclear and must be pursued in a systematic manner. At this time the following are the major diagnostic considerations:
   1. Myocardial ischemia
   2. Esophageal motor disorder
   3. Musculoskeletal chest wall pain

   Because this patient has other significant risk factors he should be assumed to have a cardiovascular cause for his pain until proven otherwise. Thus all possible testable risk factors should be checked. Because this patient has a relatively high pretest probability of having coronary artery disease (Bayes' theorem), a treadmill exercise stress test should be performed. On the other hand, an upper gastrointestinal series may determine any contribution from reflux esophagitis. It is most reasonable to do these tests in sequence.

3. E. The 2.5-mm ST segment depression quite likely represents severe coronary ischemia. Although we are not told the results of blood pressure monitoring during this patient's exercise tolerance test, it is certainly true that a "hypotensive response" indicates severe ischemia. With this information, coronary angiography should now be performed.

4. D. Medications indicated for treating angina pectoris include three classes of drugs:
   1. beta blockers
   2. nitrates
   3. calcium channel blockers

   The drugs listed include one calcium-channel blocker (diltiazem); two nitrates (isosorbide dinitrate and nitroglycerine); and one beta blocker (propranolol). The list also includes one peripheral alpha adrenergic agonist (prazosin), which is not a drug of choice for the treatment of angina pectoris.

5. E. The history given by this patient is one of unstable angina pectoris. *Unstable angina pectoris* is the term used to describe accelerating or "crescendo" angina in a patient who has previously had stable angina. Unstable angina can be diagnosed when the angina occurs with less exertion or at rest, lasts longer, and is less responsive to medication. IV nitroglycerine is the first treatment that should be given. If more pain relief is needed, IV or subcutaneous morphine may be used. One baby aspirin should also be given at this time.

   Unstable angina is often associated with complex coronary artery stenosis consisting of plaque ulceration, hemorrhage, and/or thrombosis. The unstable situation may rapidly progress to complete occlusion and infarction or may heal, with reendothelialization and a return to a stable angina, albeit most likely with a more severe pattern of ischemia.

   Nitrates are first-line therapy for the initial presentation of unstable angina. Nonparental therapy with sublingual or oral nitrates or nitroglycerin ointment may be sufficient. As a general rule, however, if there is any doubt as to the most appropriate route, use the IV preparation. IV beta blockers are an alternative.

   Once the acute episode is controlled, therapy can be initiated or changed using a combination of nitrates, beta blockers, and/or calcium-channel blockers. Also, heparin and/or thrombolytic therapy should be considered during the acute phase.

   In spite of the ECG showing only 1.5 mm of ST segment depression and no acute changes indicative of myocardial infarction, the patient should be hospitalized and placed in the coronary care unit. Serial CK-MB fractions should be done for 3 days.

6. D. Prinzmetal's angina (coronary artery vasospasm) is angina that occurs in the absence of precipitating factors. It is most common in the early morning, often awakening the patient from sleep. It is usually associated with ST segment elevation rather than ST segment depression. Coronary angiography should be performed to rule out coexisting fixed stenotic lesions. Calcium-channel blockers are probably the drugs of choice for Prinzmetal's angina. Nitrates are also effective. Beta blockers are contraindicated in patients who have vasospasm without fixed, stenotic lesions.

7. D.

8. D. Percutaneous transluminal coronary angioplasty (PTCA) as a treatment for dilating stenotic coronary arterial lesions was introduced in 1977. Today successful dilatation rates per stenosis exceed 90%, com-

plication rates have fallen to 4%, and procedure-related myocardial infarction and death remain uncommon.

Recent enthusiasm for balloon dilatation has been accompanied by its increasing application to more complex forms of coronary disease and a marked increase in the number of procedures performed annually in many American centers. In many centers PTCA is now the most commonly used invasive therapy for coronary artery disease.

The initial results of PTCA were considered acceptable, but the major concern at present is long-term stability of revascularization. Significant restenosis occurs within the first year in up to 40% of lesions, and both symptomatic recurrence and reintervention rates have been high during follow-up. In retrospective studies comparing the long-term results of PTCA and coronary artery bypass grafting (CABG), it appears that angina recurrence and event-free survival rates are significantly better in the CABG despite similar entry criteria. Thus, in summary, at this time we are unsure about the role of PTCA. There is certainly no evidence that it improves mortality. It seems appropriate that until long-term data are available, the currently accelerating enthusiasm for PTCA in complex forms of coronary disease should be held in check, and that its major application should be in (1) patients with severe symptoms from low-risk obstructions (such as single-vessel and mild double-vessel disease) that do not warrant surgical intervention for prognostic reasons, and (2) high-risk patients who would not survive a CABG.

The most likely condition of the choices listed for PTCA would be single-vessel disease. Triple-vessel disease and left ventricular aneurysms are definite contraindications to PTCA. Left main stem disease is also a contraindication.

9. B. Of the combinations listed, the least likely combination of drugs to treat angina pectoris would be nitroglycerine-enalapril-nifedipine. Enalapril is an ACE inhibitor. Unless the patient also has congestive heart failure, ACE inhibitors are generally not used as medical therapy for angina pectoris.

10. A. The most effective dilatator of those listed is nifedipine. Nifedipine and verapamil are both calcium-channel blockers; of the two, nifedipine is the more potent vasodilator. Sublingual nifedipine is also used for the treatment of hypertensive crises and hypertensive emergencies. The other three drugs (metoprolol, atenolol, and propranolol) are beta blockers.

11. D. Coronary artery bypass surgery (CABG) may be the treatment of choice in any of the choices listed: triple-vessel disease, double-vessel disease, or single-vessel disease. Although single-vessel disease may be treated with PTCA, the discussion on PTCA indicates that both angina and event-free survival are better with CABG.

12. E. A patient with both angina pectoris and hypertension should be treated with a calcium-channel blocker a beta blocker, or both. In this case the calcium-channel blocker verapamil or the beta blocker propranolol would be reasonable treatment options.

13. E. Patients suspected of having angina pectoris need (1) a CBC; (2) a complete urinalysis; (3) a chest X-ray; (4) an ECG; and (5) thyroid function testing. In addition, (1) renal function; (2) electrolytes; (3) blood glucose; and (4) a lipid profile should be performed. If the patient appears to have significant COPD, then arterial blood gas studies may also be helpful.

14. C. The basic pathophysiology in patients with angina pectoris is an imbalance between oxygen supply and oxygen demand due to atherosclerotic narrowing of the coronary arteries. Atherosclerosis, the basic pathophysiologic lesion, can be broken down into two components: (1) "atheroma" of the intima—the deposition of cholesterol/fibrin/calcium plaques on the intimal surface—and (2) "sclerosis" or "hardening" of the media. However, many patients with angina pectoris have been found to have a "coronary spasm" component to this "constricting" process, a vasospasm component that is present even in the absence of true Prinzmetal's angina or coronary artery spasm angina.

15. E. Unstable angina pectoris is characterized by (1) new onset angina (<2 months) that is severe and/or frequent (>3 episodes/day); (2) patients with accelerating angina; or (3) patients with angina at rest.

SOLUTION TO SHORT ANSWER MANAGEMENT PROBLEM 2

Obstructive coronary artery disease, acute myocardial infarction, and transient myocardial ischemia are frequently asymptomatic. The majority of patients with typical chronic angina pectoris are found to have objective evidence of myocardial ischemia (ST-segment depression). However, many of these same patients and some other patients who are always asymptomatic are at high risk for coronary events. Longitudinal studies have demonstrated an increased incidence of coronary events including sudden death, myocardial infarction, and angina pectoris in asymptomatic patients with positive exercise tests. As well, patients with asymptomatic ischemia following a myocardial infarction are at far greater risk for a secondary coronary event than symptomatic patients.

Patients who present and are found to have asymptomatic ischemia should be evaluated by both stress ECG and radionuclide scintigraphy.

The management of asymptomatic ischemia must be individualized and depends on (1) the degree of positivity of the exercise test; (2) the ECG leads showing a positive response; and (3) other factors such as (4) the patient's age, (5) the patient's occupation, and (6) the patient's general medical condition, but it is generally recommended that further testing and treatment be as follows:

1. Patients with severe ischemia on noninvasive testing should be referred for coronary arteriography. This may lead to a CABG procedure.
2. General management at this time favors aspirin and prophylactic beta blockade.

SUMMARY OF THE DIAGNOSIS AND TREATMENT OF ANGINA PECTORIS

1. **Definition:** Angina pectoris can be defined as an imbalance between myocardial requirements for oxygen and the amount of oxygen delivered through the coronary arteries. This can occur via a mechanism of increased demand, diminished delivery, or both.
2. **Symptoms:** The patient with angina pectoris frequently described the pain as either a "retrosternal tightness" or "retrosternal pain." Other descriptions include "retrosternal burning," "retrosternal pressing," "retrosternal choking," "retrosternal aching," "retrosternal gas," and "retrosternal indigestion." These symptoms are typically located in the retrosternal area or the left chest. Usual radiation to the left shoulder, left arm, or jaw occurs. Typical angina is aggravated by exercise and relieved by rest.
3. **Signs:** Physical examination is often normal, although hypertension is sometimes present.
4. **Initial laboratory evaluation:** CBC, urinalysis, electrolytes, blood glucose, blood lipids, uric acid, thyroid function tests, CXR, ECG, and stress ECG testing are basic. Radionuclide scintigraphy and coronary angiography may follow.
5. **Treatment:**
   Acute attacks:
   Mild: sublingual nitroglycerin or nitroglycerin spray
   Severe: IV nitroglycerin
   Long-term prophylaxis and treatment:
   Long-acting nitroglycerin, long-acting calcium-channel blockers, or beta blockers alone or in combination.
   Intervention/surgery:
   Percutaneous transluminal angioplasty has not demonstrated reduction in morbidity or mortality.
   Coronary artery bypass surgery (CABG) is the preferred method of intervention at this time.
6. **Angina Variants:**
   a) Prinzmetal's angina: Prinzmetal's angina is due to coronary artery spasm with or without fixed stenotic lesions. It is more common in women than in men. ST segment elevation is more common than ST segment depression. Calcium-channel blockers are the treatment of choice.
   b) Unstable angina: Unstable angina is an accelerating or "crescendo" pattern of angina. It may represent intermittent incomplete occlusion of coronary arteries. Acute treatment includes IV nitroglycerin or an IV beta blocker. All patients with unstable angina should be on 1 aspirin/day along with a combination of anti-angina agents.

SUGGESTED READING

Glasser S. Angina pectoris. In: Rakel R, ed. Conn's current therapy. Philadelphia: WB Saunders, 1994.

PROBLEM 3   A 51-YEAR-OLD MALE WITH A HIGH BLOOD CHOLESTEROL

A 51-year-old male comes to your office for his "yearly workup." He is a typical Type A personality: hard driving, and "married to my job and proud of it." He is, however, married to his wife as well, as he points out in retrospect. He has had previous problems with "high blood cholesterol" and wishes to have his cholesterol checked today.

On examination, his blood pressure is 170/100 mm Hg. His pulse is 84 and regular. His body mass index (BMI) is 31. His abdomen is obese.

His spot blood cholesterol in your office is 8.2 mmol/l (328 mg%).

SELECT THE ONE BEST ANSWER TO THE FOLLOWING QUESTIONS

1. Regarding this patient's cholesterol, which of the following statements is(are) true?
   a) this is a normal serum cholesterol for this patient
   b) this is a borderline serum cholesterol for this patient
   c) this is a high serum cholesterol for this patient, and intense dietary therapy and drug therapy should be considered
   d) although this is a high serum cholesterol, careful observation of the cholesterol is all that is required
   e) this is a high serum cholesterol; the patient should be further assessed by a fasting HDL and LDL cholesterol

2. Which of the following, according to the National Cholesterol Education Program, defines high blood cholesterol?
   a) TC = 200 mg%; LDL = 130 mg%
   b) TC = 240 mg%; LDL = 160 mg%
   c) TC = 280 mg%; LDL = 190 mg%
   d) TC = 320 mg%; LDL = 220 mg%
   e) TC = 360 mg%; LDL = 250 mg%

3. What is the single most important risk factor for coronary artery disease?
   a) an elevated HDL level
   b) an elevated triglyceride level
   c) an elevated LDL level
   d) a depressed HDL level
   e) an elevated total blood cholesterol

4. An elevated triglyceride level is most closely associated with which of the following?
   a) LDL cholesterol
   b) HDL cholesterol
   c) VLDL cholesterol
   d) total blood cholesterol
   e) MDL cholesterol

5. At what level of LDL cholesterol is treatment definitely indicated?
   a) 4.1 mmol/L (160 mg%)
   b) 3.4 mmol/L (130 mg%)
   c) 3.8 mmol/L (151 mg%)
   d) 5.2 mmol/L (206 mg%)
   e) 3.1 mmol/L (123 mg%)

6. Which of the following is the treatment of choice for hypercholesterolemia?
   a) gemfibrozil
   b) colestipol
   c) nicotinic acid
   d) lovastatin
   e) none of the above

7. What is the drug class of choice for the management of mild to moderate elevations of plasma LDL?
   a) the fibric acid derivatives
   b) the nicotinic acid derivatives
   c) the HMG coenzyme A reductase inhibitors
   d) the bile acid sequestrants
   e) any of the above

8. The patient described in the problem is taking hydrochlorothiazide and propranolol. Which of the following statements are true concerning the effect of these drugs on plasma lipoproteins?
   a) hydrochlorothiazide has no effect on plasma lipoproteins
   b) propranolol has no effect on plasma lipoproteins
   c) neither hydrochlorothiazide nor propranolol has any effect on plasma lipoproteins
   d) both hydrochlorothiazide and propranolol can adversely affect plasma lipoproteins
   e) nobody worries about plasma lipoproteins any longer

9. A 56-year-old male with hyperlipidemia needs a beta blocker to help control hypertension. Which of the following would be the agent of choice?
   a) propranolol
   b) metoprolol
   c) atenolol
   d) nadolol
   e) acebutolol

10. Which of the following is(are) independent risk factors for coronary artery disease?
    a) increased LDL concentration
    b) decreased HDL concentration
    c) increased total cholesterol concentration

d) increased triglyceride concentration
e) all of the above

11. Which of the following antihypertensive drugs do not have an adverse effect on plasma lipids?
    a) hydrochlorothiazide
    b) propranolol
    c) atenolol
    d) nifedipine
    e) metoprolol

12. The American Heart Association's Step 1 diet allows how much fat as a percentage of total daily calories?
    a) 20%
    b) 30%
    c) 10%
    d) 15%
    e) 40%

13. The American Heart Association's Step 1 diet allows how much saturated fat as a percentage of total daily calories?
    a) 10%
    b) 15%
    c) 20%
    d) 25%
    e) 30%

14. The American Heart Association's Step 1 diet allows how much total cholesterol in the daily intake?
    a) 500 mg
    b) 400 mg
    c) 350 mg
    d) 300 mg
    e) 200 mg

15. Which of the following statements is(are) true regarding fish oil supplements?
    a) fish oils have been shown to lower plasma triglyceride levels
    b) fish oils inhibit platelet aggregation
    c) fish oils have been shown to increase HDL levels
    d) fish oils may decrease blood pressure and blood viscosity
    e) all of the above are true

16. A 56-year-old physician presents to your office for a complete health assessment. When you question him about his alcohol intake he replies that he simply uses alcohol to favorably affect his apolipoprotein ratio. Which of the following statements regarding alcohol and apolipoproteins is(are) true?
    a) ingestion of alcohol decreases apolipoprotein A-1 levels
    b) ingestion of alcohol increases apolipoprotein A-1 levels
    c) ingestion of alcohol increases apolipoprotein B levels
    d) ingestion of alcohol decreases apolipoprotein B levels
    e) both b and d

17. What is the drug of choice for the treatment of hypertriglyceridemia?
    a) nicotinic acid
    b) gemfibrozil
    c) lovastatin
    d) cholestyramine
    e) none of the above

18. Which of the following is(are) secondary causes of hyperlipidemia?
    a) diabetes mellitus
    b) alcohol
    c) oral contraceptives
    d) all of the above
    e) none of the above

19. Chylomicrons are most closely associated with which of the following?
    a) LDL
    b) HDL
    c) VLDL
    d) MDL
    e) chylomicrons are associated with all of the above

20. Regarding the home monitoring of cholesterol, which of the following statements is(are) true?
    a) home monitoring is recommended for patients with very high cholesterol
    b) home cholesterol monitoring is sensitive
    c) home cholesterol monitoring is specific
    d) home cholesterol monitoring is both sensitive and specific
    e) none of the above

Short Answer Management Problem 3

List the risk factors that have been shown to increase the risk of coronary artery disease in the population.

ANSWERS

1. E. A cholesterol level of 8.2 mmol/l is a very high serum cholesterol. However, as serum cholesterol is generally checked with a random (nonfasting) blood sample, a fasting cholesterol with fractionation to LDL, HDL, and VLDL should be ordered.

    Normal serum cholesterol is under 5.2 mmol/l (200 mg%). Borderline serum cholesterol is 5.2-6.2 mmol/l (200 mg%-240 mg%). High serum cholesterol is greater than 6.2 mmol/l (240 mg%).

    The question of which patients should be screened for hypercholesterolemia continues to be debated. There are basically two approaches to screening: (1) screen all adult patients at periodic intervals, or (2) screen only patients who have a family history of coronary risk factors or who have other coronary risk factors themselves. The cost implications of mass screening and subsequent diagnosis and treatment have to be considered in making this decision. The current recommendation is to screen with a nonfasting sample.

2. B. The National Cholesterol Education Program defines a high blood cholesterol as follows: (1) Total cholesterol = 240 mg% (6.2 mmol/l); (2) Low-density lipoprotein = 160 mg% (4.1 mmol/l).

3. C. The single most important risk factor for coronary artery disease is an elevated low-density lipoprotein cholesterol (LDL). The second most important risk factor is a depressed high-density lipoprotein cholesterol (HDL).

4. C. An elevated triglyceride level is most closely associated with an elevated VLDL. A triglyceride level greater than 250 mg% is considered definitely elevated. A triglyceride level greater than 500 mg% is often seen with diabetes mellitus. Although triglycerides were not previously considered an independent risk factor for coronary artery disease, they are now felt to be so.

5. A. An LDL level is considered definitely elevated when it is above 4.1 mmol/l (160 mg%). The borderline level is between 3.4 mmol/l and 4.1 mmol/l.

6. E. The treatment of choice for hypercholesterolemia is diet therapy. The American Heart Association has produced Step 1 and Step 2 diets. The Step 1 diet includes less than 30% of total calories from fat, less than 10% of calories from saturated fat, and less than 300 mg/day cholesterol. The Step 2 diet includes less than 30% of total daily calories as fat; less than 7% of calories from saturated fat, and less than 200 mg/day of cholesterol.

    Management of hypercholesterolemia with drugs is indicated only after dietary treatment over a reasonable length of time has failed to reduce the cholesterol level to a sufficiently low level. Current recommendations suggest that diet therapy be continued for six months before drug therapy is started.

7. C. The drug class of choice for mild to moderate LDL elevation is one of the three 3-hydroxy-3-methylglutaryl-coenzyme A (HMG-CoA) reductase inhibitors on the market. These include lovastatin (Mevacor), pravastatin (Pravachol), and simvastatin (Zocor).

    All patients who are started on HMG-CoA inhibitors should have not only the plasma lipids but also the liver function tests and the creatine phosphokinase monthly for 3 months, then every 3 months for 6 months, and every 4 to 6 months thereafter. In patients with mild to moderate isolated LDL elevation (Type IIA), plasma lipids may be normalized with 10 mg to 20 mg once daily of any of the three agents. Patients with higher LDL levels may require higher doses of single agent therapy, or alternately, multidrug therapy. With such therapy, LDL cholesterol may be lowered up to 40% and TG levels lowered 10 to 15%. There appears to be little change in the HDL level. All three drugs have been known to produce hepatic and skeletal muscle toxicity as well as insomnia and weight gain. These side effects, however, are relatively uncommon, are dose related, and occur much more frequently in patients who are on multidrug therapy.

    The drug of second choice for Type IIA hyperlipoproteinemia is niacin. The total daily dose (500-mg tablets) is up to 3 g. All patients taking niacin require monitoring of liver function tests and creatine phosphokinase monthly for 3 months, then every 3 months for 6 months, and every 4 to 6 months thereafter. Niacin may lower plasma LDL by up to 35%, may lower TG levels by up to 75%, and at the same time raise the HDL by up to 100%. In addition, the apolipoprotein A level is lowered by up to 50%. In atherosclerosis regression trials, niacin has been the most effective agent in promoting stability and regression of coronary lesions.

    Unfortunately, niacin has a considerable number of significant side effects. It may (1) produce gastric irritation and gastritis; (2) activate long-dormant peptic ulcers; (3) elevate plasma uric acid levels, producing gout; (4) elevate blood glucose levels; and (5) exacerbate diabetes. As well, and most commonly, it causes cutaneous flushing, dry and even scaly skin, and in rare instances acanthosis nigricans. Fortunately, all side effects disappear when the drug is discontinued.

    Resins, including cholestyramine (Questran) and colestipol (Colestid), are the drugs of third choice for patients with Type IIA hyperlipoproteinemia. The dose ranges are 4 to 8 g once or twice daily for cholestyramine and 5 to 10 g once or twice daily for colestipol.

    Their advantages include an almost complete lack of absorption and potential for systemic toxicity that goes with it. Their disadvantages include an unpleasant grittiness and multiple gastrointestinal side effects, including abdominal bloating, abdominal pain, sometimes severe constipation, and GI bleeding. Because resins may decrease the absorption of other drugs, they and other drugs should be taken 2 hours apart.

8. D.

9. E. Both hydrochlorothiazide and propranolol can adversely affect plasma lipoproteins. Hydrochlorothiazide increases total cholesterol and triglyceride concentrations. In addition, very low-density lipoprotein (VLDL) cholesterol levels and low-density lipoprotein (LDL) levels are increased, and the high-density lipoprotein (HDL) cholesterol level changes are variable.

Propranolol increases plasma triglyceride levels but does not alter total cholesterol concentrations. However, propranolol does decrease HDL cholesterol levels. LDL cholesterol changes with propranolol are more variable.

The beta-1-selective adrenergic blockers, like the nonselective agents, increase triglyceride levels and lower HDL cholesterol levels without altering total cholesterol concentration. The adverse effects on lipoproteins tend to be less, however, than the changes observed with the nonselective agents.

Acebutolol hydrochloride, oxprenolol hydrochloride, and pindolol hydrochloride are beta-adrenergic blocking drugs that possess ISA (intrinsic sympathomimetic activity). Acebutolol is beta-1-selective, whereas the latter two are not. Oxprenolol may increase triglyceride concentrations and lower HDL cholesterol. Pindolol and acebutolol are lipid neutral.

Acebutolol hydrochloride would be the beta blocker of choice in the patient described in this question because it combines ISA activity, Beta selectivity, and a favorable side-effect profile.

10. E. Risk factors for coronary artery disease include (1) increased LDL concentration (most important lipid risk factor); (2) decreased HDL (second most important risk factor); (3) increased total cholesterol (TC); and (4) increased triglyceride concentration (TG).

11. D. Nifedipine, a calcium-channel blocker, is the only drug of the drugs listed that does not have an adverse affect on plasma lipids. The beta blockers propranolol, metoprolol, and atenolol all adversely affect plasma lipids. Hydrochlorothiazide also adversely affects plasma lipids.

12. B.

13. A.

14. D. As mentioned previously, the treatment of first choice for hyperlipidemia is diet. The American Heart Association's Step 1 diet and Step 2 diet are as follows:

	STEP 1	STEP 2
Cholesterol	300 mg	200 mg
Total fat	30% of calories	30% of calories
Saturated fat	10% of calories	7% of calories

15. E. Fish and fish oil supplements may lower plasma lipid levels (especially triglycerides), inhibit platelet aggregation, decrease blood pressure and viscosity, and increase HDL cholesterol. It is difficult to recommend fish oils for general use.

16. E. There is an inverse relationship between low to moderate alcohol consumption and coronary artery disease. This may be due to an inhibitory effect on platelet aggregation or to increased coronary artery diameter. As well, low doses of alcohol appear to increase the cardioprotective apolipoprotein A-1 and decrease the atherogenic apolipoprotein B.

In this patient, find out how much alcohol this physician actually does use to favorably influence his apolipoprotein ratio. It is a fairly safe bet that it is more than currently recommended.

17. B. The drug of choice for most hypertriglyceridemias is gemfibrozil or another fibric acid derivative. Hypertriglyceridemia may be associated with Type 2a, Type 2b, Type 3, or Type 4 hyperlipoproteinemia. The usual dose of gemfibrozil is 0.6 g bid. Gemfibrozil will decrease hypertriglyceridemia by 40% to 80% and will increase HDL by 10% to 40%.

Until very recently, combining a reductase inhibitor with gemfibrozil was not recommended. This combination should still be used with caution, but may be tolerated if a low dose of one drug is given 12 hours apart from a low dose of the other (for example, pravastatin 10 mg to 20 mg am with gemfibrozil 600 mg in the evening).

18. D. Diabetes mellitus usually produces a very significant elevation of plasma triglycerides and plasma VLDL. Triglyceride levels as high as 25,000 mg/dl have been reported in diabetes.

The daily consumption of large amounts of alcohol can produce a mild, asymptomatic elevation in the plasma triglycerides due to an elevation of VLDL. The ingestion of estrogen-containing birth control pills causes an increase in the VLDL secretion rate from the liver and subsequent elevation in the triglyceride level.

19. C. Chylomicrons are usually associated with an elevation of plasma VLDL and thus plasma triglycerides.

20. E. Unfortunately, home cholesterol monitoring is now available. This will likely result in the following: (1) increase in sales of the products available; (2) an increased proportion of the public becoming cholesterolphobic; (3) increased anxiety regarding "cardiac status"; and (4) increased costs to the health care system.

The laboratory standardization panel of the National Cholesterol Education Program has recommended that for a method of cholesterol determination to be acceptable, the number of analyses having an error of more than 8.9% compared to the standard chemical method should not exceed 5%. In a recent study of home cholesterol monitoring products, this figure was 11.9%. Thus significant error will probably occur in more than twice the number of individuals as it should.

It is very likely that the increased sales of home cholesterol monitors will result in more visits to physicians, more tests, and more anxiety. Whether it will result in any significant benefit to the patient population is highly debatable.

SOLUTION TO SHORT ANSWER MANAGEMENT PROBLEM 3

The risk factors for coronary artery disease in the population are as follows:

1. Family history of coronary artery disease
2. Male sex
3. Hypertension
4. Hypercholesterolemia: High LDL
5. Hypercholesterolemia: Low HDL
6. Hypertriglyceridemia: High VLDL
7. Cigarette smoking
8. High alcohol intake (via its effect on hypertension)
9. Lack of aerobic exercise
10. Obesity
11. Diabetes mellitus: IDDM
12. Diabetes mellitus: NIDDM

SUMMARY OF THE DIAGNOSIS AND MANAGEMENT OF HYPERLIPOPROTEINEMIA

1. **Screening:** The U.S. Preventive Services Task Force recommendation is as follows: "Periodic measurement of total serum cholesterol is most important for middle aged men, and it may also be clinically prudent in young men, women, and the elderly. All patients should receive periodic counselling regarding dietary intake of fat (especially saturated fat) and cholesterol."
2. **Normal and high cholesterol values:**
   a) Total cholesterol:
      Normal: <5.2 mmol/L (200 mg%)
      Borderline: 5.2-6.2 mmol/L (200-240 mg%)
      Elevated: >6.2 mmol/L (>240 mg%)
   b) LDL cholesterol:
      Ideal: <3.4 mmol/L (130 mg%)
      Borderline: 3.4-4.1 mmol/L (130-159 mg%)
      Elevated: >4.1 mmol/L (>159 mg%)
   c) VLDL cholesterol (triglycerides):
      Ideal: <1.4 mmol/L (125 mg%)
      Borderline: 1.4-2.8 mmol/L (125-250 mg%)
      Elevated: >2.8 mmol/L (>250 mg%)
3. **Treatment:**
   a) Hypercholesterolemia: Treat hypercholesterolemia if LDL cholesterol >4.1 mmol/L or > 3.4 mmol/L with two or more risk factors.

      Dietary management is treatment of first choice. Begin with the Step 1 Diet of the American Heart Association: (1) <300 mg cholesterol; (2) <30% total fat; (3) <10% saturated fat. Continue for at least 6 months. If cholesterol levels do not normalize, consider AHA Step 2 diet: (1) <200 mg cholesterol; (2) <30% total fat; (3) <7% saturated fat.

      The choices for drug treatment are as follows:
      Drugs of first choice: HMG Co-A reductase inhibitors
      Drug of second choice: niacin
      Drug of third choice: bile acid sequestrants
   b) Hypertriglyceridemia: Hypertriglyceridemia has been established as an independent risk factor for coronary artery disease. Look for a secondary cause of hypertriglyceridemia, such as diabetes mellitus, alcohol, or oral contraceptives.

      Treatments include the AHA Step 1 and Step 2 diets as mentioned previously, and the drug of choice for drug treatment of hyperlipoproteinemia that is mainly elevated triglycerides is gemfibrozil.

NEW INFORMATION 1995

Up to this time, cholesterol-lowering drugs have not been shown to reduce deaths from coronary artery disease and sudden cardiac death. The Scandinavian Simvastatin Survival Study, however, has changed that view. In this study the HMG-CoA reductase inhibitor Simvastatin substantially improved survival, reducing the overall risk of death by 30% and the risk of coronary death by 42%. This adds even more credibility to the recommendation that HMG-CoA reductase inhibitors be considered the drugs of first choice for the treatment of hyperlipidemia.

SUGGESTED READINGS

Lees R, Lees A. Hyperlipoproteinemia. In: Rakel R, ed. Conn's current therapy. Philadelphia: WB Saunders, 1994.

U.S. Preventive Services Task Force. Guide to clinical preventive services: An assessment of the effectiveness of 169 interventions. Baltimore: Williams and Wilkins, 1989.

PROBLEM 4   A 78-YEAR-OLD MALE WITH SHORTNESS OF BREATH

A 78-year-old male presents with a 6-month history of shortness of breath, aggravated by exertion. He has found that he has to get up at night and open the window to get air. There has not been any significant weight gain, nor has there been any swelling of his ankles and legs.

His history reveals a myocardial infarction 8 years ago. Although the shortness of breath has been a significant problem for only 6 months, he does mention having "some problems" for at least 4 years.

On physical examination, the patient's blood pressure is 140/90 mm Hg. Both S_1 and S_2 are normal; there are no extra sounds and no murmurs. There also appears to be no elevated JVP. The hepatojugular reflex is negative. Examination of the respiratory system reveals rales in both lung bases. The respiratory rate is 28/min.

SELECT THE ONE BEST ANSWER TO THE FOLLOWING QUESTIONS

1. Based on the history and physical examination, what is the most likely diagnosis?
   a) left ventricular heart failure
   b) right ventricular heart failure
   c) biventricular heart failure
   d) cor pulmonale
   e) bronchial asthma

2. The patient described above is treated with bed rest and the appropriate medication. He returns one month later complaining of dyspnea and fatigue as before, but now significant dependent edema has developed. At this time, the JVP has risen to 8 cm above the sternal angle. The hepatojugular reflex is now positive. There is +3 pitting edema. He has gained 10 lb in weight. At this time, what is the most likely diagnosis?
   a) left ventricular failure
   b) right ventricular failure
   c) biventricular heart failure
   d) cor pulmonale
   e) bronchial asthma

3. The nonpharmacologic treatments(s) of choice for this condition may include which of the following?
   a) salt restriction
   b) fat restriction
   c) water restriction
   d) all of the above
   e) none of the above

4. What is(are) the current indication(s) for the use of digitalis in this condition?
   a) a dilated left ventricle
   b) an S_3 or S_4 gallop
   c) decreased stroke volume
   d) atrial fibrillation
   e) all of the above

5. Physiologically speaking, the condition just described (as illustrated by the second presentation of this patient) has which of the following characteristics?
   a) elevated preload

   b) elevated afterload
   c) reduced preload
   d) reduced afterload
   e) a and b
   f) c and d

6. The condition described in the second presentation of the patient is significantly improved with nonpharmacologic and pharmacologic therapy. Physiologically, this is based on the following: (1) decreased cardiac work and (2) reduced end diastolic volume. Treatment is successful when increased cardiac work is performed for a given level of end-diastolic volume. How is this phenomenon best described?
   a) the Contraction-Retraction theory
   b) the "Pump Working Again" theory
   c) the Frank-Starling curve
   d) the "Heart of a 50-Year-Old syndrome"
   e) none of the above

7. Which drug(s) is(are) the first choice for the management of mild cases of this condition?
   a) a thiazide diuretic
   b) a loop diuretic
   c) a vasodilator
   d) a beta blocker
   e) an ACE inhibitor

8. Which is the drug of first choice for moderate to severe cases of the condition described?
   a) a thiazide diuretic
   b) a loop diuretic
   c) a vasodilator
   d) a beta blocker
   e) an ACE inhibitor

9. Which of the following drugs has the potential to produce the most significant toxic reaction when used in the treatment of the condition described?
   a) a thiazide diuretic
   b) a loop diuretic
   c) digoxin
   d) a venous dilator
   e) an ACE inhibitor

10. What is the single most important treatment for increasing both the quality and the quantity of remaining life for patients with severe chronic disease?
    a) a beta blocker
    b) a loop diuretic
    c) an ACE inhibitor
    d) a calcium-channel blocker
    e) any of the above

11. Which of the following drugs is(are) potassium-sparing diuretics?
    a) chlorthalidone
    b) hydrochlorothiazide
    c) ethacrynic acid
    d) spironolactone
    e) all of the above

Short Answer Management Problem 4

A major error in treating heart failure is assuming that all patients who appear to be in heart failure need furosemide. When given furosemide, some patients actually get worse. Provide an example of a practical situation in which this could occur.

ANSWERS

1. A. This patient has left ventricular failure. Dyspnea is the most common sign of left-sided congestive heart failure. Initially, the dyspnea is present only with moderate amounts of exertion, but as the severity of the heart failure increases, the shortness of breath may occur with only minimal exertion or even at rest. Other common symptoms are fatigue and lethargy.

   In a patient with left-sided cardiac failure, lying flat is often followed by increasing shortness of breath. Paroxysms of nocturnal dyspnea (PND) suggest severe left-sided failure. On careful questioning the patient describes the bouts as marked breathlessness, a "suffocating feeling," and these symptoms are often accompanied by significant anxiety. The patient has to sit upright or even stand up to breathe and may have the urge to rush to an open window to relieve the "suffocating feeling." Extra pillows are needed to reduce the number and severity of attacks. Some patients even have to resort to sleeping upright in a chair at all times.

   In severe left-sided congestive heart failure pulmonary edema occurs and is usually severe and is accompanied by cough, frothy sputum, blood-tinged secretions, and wheezing (the so-called condition of cardiac asthma).

   In this patient, the absence of (1) peripheral edema, (2) hepatic congestion/absent hepatojugular reflex, and (3) an elevated JVP indicates that right-sided heart failure has not yet developed.

2. C. At this time, the patient has developed signs of right ventricular failure secondary to left ventricular failure, hence the diagnosis of biventricular failure.

   Whereas left ventricular cardiac failure is manifested by symptoms, right ventricular cardiac failure is manifested by signs. As in this patient, enlargement of the liver, a positive hepatojugular reflex, and an elevated JVP occur.

   In severe cases of elevated right-sided atrial pressure, splanchnic engorgement may accompany anorexia, nausea, vomiting, ascites, and eventually cachexia.

3. D. Nonpharmacologic therapy for congestive heart failure involves the following in order of importance:
   1. Bed rest
   2. Salt restriction (2-3 grams sodium/day)
   3. Fluid restriction (related to sodium restriction)
   4. Fat restriction (as a reasonable approach to a healthy life-style—American Heart Association Step 1 diet: 300 mg cholesterol; 30% total calories from fat; 10% of calories from saturated fat

4. E. Digoxin has come full circle. This drug, isolated from the foxglove plant, used to be the mainstay of treatment for congestive heart failure. For various reasons, it then fell into disfavor, to the point where it was virtually never used. The completion of the circle has resulted in digoxin once again being used extensively. Its primary indications are (1) reduced stroke volume, (2) a dilated left ventricle, (3) atrial fibrillation, and (4) An S_3 or S_4 gallop (often associated with left ventricular dilatation).

5. E. Biventricular congestive cardiac failure is manifested by two components: (1) preload (or venous return) and (2) afterload (vasoconstriction). The afterload is associated with elevated left ventricular end-diastolic volume (left-sided failure); the preload is associated with elevated venous volume (right-sided failure).

6. C. The relationship between cardiac work and left-ventricular end-diastolic volume is known as the *Frank-Starling curve*. Physiologically speaking this relationship implies that for a given cardiac cell fiber length

a certain amount of cardiac work is performed. In addition, the degree of adaptation of the heart is quite remarkable; when stressed it responds by significantly increasing pump activity. Following the interpretation of the Frank-Starling curve, only when the cardiac muscle cell fiber length reaches a critical length (a length at which it can no longer function well even under the impetus of the sympathetic drive) do cardiac work and output suffer.

7. B.

8. E. In mild cases of biventricular failure the most important pharmacologic treatment is to reduce venous return to the right side of the heart; to do this requires a diuretic. The diuretic of choice is a loop diuretic such as furosemide or ethacrynic acid.

    In moderate to severe cases of biventricular failure it is still important to reduce venous return to the heart. It is, however, also important to reduce the afterload factor. This combination of requirements is best accomplished by an ACE inhibitor such as captopril or enalapril. This is most commonly used in combination with either a loop diuretic or a thiazide diuretic.

9. C. The most significant potentially toxic reaction would be produced by the digoxin. Digoxin, a positive inotropic agent, has made a comeback for treating congestive heart failure. However, in combination with a loop diuretic, digoxin has the potential to significantly decrease serum potassium. In the presence of hypokalemia, the toxic effects of digoxin (manifested usually by nausea and vomiting) may occur.

10. C. ACE inhibitor drugs such as captopril, enalapril, and lisinopril have been shown to reduce both morbidity and mortality in patients with severe heart failure.

11. D. The only potassium-sparing diuretic of those listed as diuretics is spironolactone. Spironolactone (Aldactone) may be used in combination with a loop diuretic (furosemide) or a thiazide diuretic (hydrochlorothiazide) to keep the serum potassium in the normal range.

SOLUTION TO SHORT ANSWER MANAGEMENT PROBLEM 4

A practical example of a patient becoming worse after being given furosemide is the following:

A 55-year-old uremic male with a history of congestive heart failure manifests an increasing shortness of breath and increasing edema of the extremities. You naturally assume that his CHF is worsening, and you administer furosemide. He deteriorates rapidly. The cause: uremic pericarditis. What appeared to be congestive cardiac failure was not.

Make sure the patient *has* congestive heart failure before you *treat* the congestive heart failure.

SUMMARY OF THE DIAGNOSIS AND TREATMENT OF CONGESTIVE HEART FAILURE

1. **Left-sided failure** Left-sided failure produces mainly symptoms such as increasing shortness of breath (dyspnea), shortness of breath on assuming the recumbent position (orthopnea), and having to wake up at night to catch one's breath (paroxysmal nocturnal dyspnea).
2. **Right-sided failure** Right-sided failure produces mainly signs such as increasing dependent edema and increased JVP positive hepatojugular reflex.
3. **Biventricular failure:** The most common cause of right-sided heart failure is left-sided heart failure.
4. **Pathophysiology of heart failure:** This is explained best by the Frank-Starling curve: left ventricular end diastolic volume versus cardiac work. Compensation via the sympathetic nervous system will allow normal cardiac output to be maintained to a certain point; following that the decompensation begins.
5. **Treatment:**
    a) Nonpharmacologic:
       1. Bed rest
       2. Sodium restriction
       3. Water restriction
       4. Avoidance of other risk factors: stop smoking, avoid excessive alcohol intake, avoid high-fat diet
       5. Increased aerobic exercise
    b) Pharmacologic:
       1. Use loop diuretics (furosemide) to decrease venous pressure overload.
       2. Add thiazide diuretics and/or potassium sparing diuretics to increase effectiveness of the loop diuretics.
       3. ACE inhibitors such as captopril, enalapril, or lisinopril decrease both preload and afterload and are the drugs of first choice in moderate to severe heart failure.
       4. Digoxin can be combined with the above to improve the contractility (positive inotropic effect).

SUGGESTED READING

Braunwald E. Heart failure. In: Isselbacher et al. (eds). Harrison's principles of internal medicine. 13th Ed. New York: McGraw-Hill, 1994.

PROBLEM 5   AN OBESE 47-YEAR-OLD MALE WITH HYPERTENSION

A 47-year-old male presents to your office for a yearly checkup. He weighs 250 pounds, smokes two packs of cigarettes/day, and "slams down" 12 oz whiskey/day.

On P/E, you detect a number of extrasystoles/min. His blood pressure is 180/105 mm Hg. His point of maximum impulse (PMI) is detected in the sixth intercostal space in the anterior axillary line. His fundoscopic examination is normal.

SELECT THE ONE BEST ANSWER TO THE FOLLOWING QUESTIONS

1. Which of the following statements about this patient's blood pressure is(are) false?
   a) a single blood pressure reading of diastolic 105 is satisfactory for a diagnosis of hypertension
   b) this patient's alcohol intake may be a significant contributing factor to his elevated blood pressure
   c) the patient should have his blood pressure rechecked after a period of rest in the office
   d) the patient should return for reassessment of his blood pressure in 1 week
   e) the patient should not be started on antihypertensive medication at this time

2. A single diastolic reading of what level is considered to be diagnostic of hypertension?
   a) 90 mm Hg
   b) 95 mm Hg
   c) 100 mm Hg
   d) 105 mm Hg
   e) 110 mm Hg

3. The minimum goal in hypertension therapy is to reduce his blood pressure to a level below which of the following?
   a) 150/90 mm Hg
   b) 140/90 mm Hg
   c) 130/90 mm Hg
   d) 120/80 mm Hg
   e) 110/70 mm Hg

4. What is the treatment of choice in the patient just described (presuming his other blood pressure readings are similar to the one today)?
   a) hydrochlorothiazide (a thiazide diuretic)
   b) a beta blocker
   c) a calcium-channel blocker
   d) an angiotensin converting enzyme inhibitor
   e) none of the above

5. What is the first-line pharmacological therapy now recommended for most patients with hypertension?
   a) a beta blocker
   b) a thiazide diuretic
   c) a calcium-channel blocker
   d) an angiotensin converting enzyme inhibitor
   e) a or b

6. What is the starting dosage of a thiazide diuretic in a patient with hypertension?
   a) 25 mg
   b) 50 mg
   c) 75 mg
   d) 100 mg
   e) 125 mg

7. The Joint National Consensus on the Diagnosis, Evaluation, and Treatment of Hypertension (JNCV) would recommend which of the following drugs as a drug of first choice?
   a) atenolol
   b) enalapril
   c) nifedipine
   d) prazosin
   e) captopril

8. The initial diagnostic workup of a patient with hypertension should include which of the following?
   a) electrolytes
   b) BUN
   c) creatinine
   d) 24-hour urine for VMA and metanephrines
   e) a, b, and c
   f) all of the above

9. Based on the patient's history and P/E, which of the following statements concerning hypertensive complications is(are) true?
   a) the patient is unlikely to have any hypertensive complications
   b) this patient likely has hypertensive retinopathy
   c) this patient likely has cardiac hypertrophy
   d) this patient likely has hypertensive renal failure
   e) none of the above is true

10. Which of the following statements accurately applies to *mild hypertension?*
    a) the term is no longer considered appropriate in defining hypertension
    b) mild hypertension describes a systolic level of 140-159 mm Hg
    c) mild hypertension describes a diastolic level of 90-104 mm Hg
    d) b and c
    e) none of the above

11. Which of the following drugs is(are) useful for the treatment of hypertensive emergencies and urgencies?
    a) IV labetalol
    b) oral clonidine
    c) oral or sublingual nifedipine
    d) all of the above
    e) none of the above

12. A 50-year-old male is being treated for hypertension with a low-salt diet, hydrochlorothiazide 25 mg/day, and propranolol 120 mg bid. His blood pressure at present is 180/100 mm Hg. Which of the following would be a reasonable third-line agent for the treatment of this patient's blood pressure?
    a) atenolol
    b) metoprolol
    c) labetalol
    d) furosemide
    e) enalapril

13. What is the most common side effect of angiotensin converting enzyme inhibitors?
    a) cough
    b) constipation
    c) headache
    d) skin rash
    e) depression

14. What is the most common side effect of propranolol?
    a) cough
    b) constipation
    c) headache
    d) skin rash
    e) depression

15. Based on the history and physical examination of the patient described in Problem 5, which of the following additional investigations should be undertaken?
    a) digital subtraction angiography
    b) IVP
    c) echocardiogram
    d) retinal ultrasound
    e) renal ultrasound

Short Answer Management Problem 5

Describe the individualistic approach to hypertension that still applies. Comment on (1) drugs of choice and (2) drugs to avoid in patients with the following conditions:

1. Young, hyperdynamic circulation
2. Elderly patients
3. Black patients
4. Patients with gout
5. Patients with ischemic heart disease
6. Patients with asthma
7. Patients with peripheral vascular disease
8. Patients with NIDDM
9. Patients with IDDM
10. Patients with hypercholesterolemia
11. Patients with congestive heart failure
12. Patients in pregnancy

ANSWERS

1. A.

2. E. Hypertension should not be diagnosed until a sustained, repetitive elevation of blood pressure has been documented. For diagnosis, at least three readings, averaging greater than 140 mm Hg systolic or 90 mm Hg diastolic, must be documented, preferably by the same observer using the same technique. However, if a single reading of a diastolic blood pressure reading of 110 mm Hg is documented, the probability that the blood pressure will return to normal is small enough that the diagnosis of hypertension can be made. If end-organ damage is detected, these criteria may not apply. In this patient, although his PMI is displaced, we can not necessarily assume that this is due to hypertension.

   Alcohol abuse is a significant cause of hypertension. Any patient with hypertension should be questioned regarding alcohol intake. Although a low dose of alcohol has been shown to be cardioprotective, *low* must be carefully defined. An absolute maximum of two drinks/day may be cardioprotective; any more than that will be definitely harmful and, indeed, an additional risk factor for CAD.

The patient described in this case should have his blood pressure taken again after 5 minutes of controlled rest. If his arm circumference is greater than 33 cm, obtain his blood pressure reading with the obese blood pressure cuff. Also instruct this patient to abstain from caffeine and cigarette smoking for at least 2 hours before his pressure is checked on his next visit.

A patient whose blood pressure returns to normal after a period of rest is known as a "labile hypertensive." Of labile hypertensives, approximately 50% go on to develop sustained hypertension.

It has been well established that home blood pressure readings (if done correctly and taken with a blood pressure recording device that has been calibrated against a mercury manometer) are more accurate and a more significant predictor of cardiovascular morbidity and mortality than office blood pressure readings.

The patient should not be started on antihypertensive medication at this time. First, the diagnosis must be established. Second, before considering antihypertensive medication you must consider nonpharmacologic therapy and attempt to lower his blood pressure without drugs.

3. B. The minimum goal in antihypertensive therapy is to reduce the blood pressure to a level of <140 mm Hg systolic and <90 mm Hg diastolic.

4. E. The first step in treating this patient's blood pressure is to use nondrug, or nonpharmacologic, therapy. There is no doubt that nonpharmacologic therapy has a major role to play in the management of hypertension. In this patient the following are the nonpharmacologic therapies that have been shown to make a difference:

Weight reduction
Alcohol elimination (in a person such as this, who "slams down" 12 ounces of whiskey/day, your best bet would be to attempt to eliminate the "slamming" completely)
Discontinue cigarette smoking
Aerobic exercise (4 hours/week or 1200 kcal), in this patient after an exercise tolerance test
Salt reduction
Fat reduction, following the American Heart Association's Step 1 Diet (decreasing the fat content of the diet without changing the total caloric intake will automatically begin the weight reduction process)

You need to decide which of these therapies you are going to begin with; obviously attempting to alter everything at once will not work. An alcohol rehabilitation program would be an excellent first choice.

5. E. The Fifth Report of the Joint National Committee on Detection, Evaluation, and Treatment of High Blood Pressure (JNC V) has previously recommended that first-line pharmacologic therapy could be a drug from any of the four classes: (1) thiazide diuretics, (2) beta blockers, (3) calcium-channel blockers, or (4) ACE inhibitors. However, it now recommends that first-line therapy be either a thiazide diuretic or a beta blocker. The rationale for this change is that thiazide diuretics and beta blockers are the only drugs that have been shown to reduce both morbidity and mortality.

The other (and not insignificant issue) is cost. The cost of a thiazide diuretic may be as little as $^{1}/_{25}$ of the cost of one of the newer agents.

6. A. The starting dose of a thiazide diuretic (such as hydrochlorothiazide) is 25 mg. A low dose (25 mg) has been shown in many studies to be just as efficacious as a higher dose (50 mg, 75 mg, or 100 mg). The only difference between the low dose and the high dose is the greatly increased incidence of side effects with the high doses. Thiazide diuretics may produce any of six metabolic side effects: hyperglycemia, hyperuricemia, hyperlipidemia, hypomagnesemia, hyponatremia, and hypokalemia.

7. A. The only drug in the choices provided that is either a beta blocker or a thiazide diuretic is atenolol (a non-cardioselective beta blocker). Of the other choices, (1) enalapril and captopril are ACE inhibitors, (2) prazosin is a peripherally acting alpha agonist, and (3) nifedipine is a calcium-channel blocker.

8. E. The basic (and cost-effective) hypertensive workup includes the following: (1) complete urinalysis, (2) hemoglobin and hematocrit, (3) BUN and creatinine, (4) serum calcium, (5) random cholesterol, (6) plasma glucose, (7) plasma uric acid, (8) CXR, and (9) ECG.

Other tests, including renal ultrasound, IVP, or 24-hour urine for VMA and metanephrines, are indicated only under special circumstances. A patient that is, for example, 55 years old and who develops hypertension for the first time should be suspected of having a secondary cause. (As a general rule, if essential hypertension is going to develop, it will develop before the age of 50.) In a patient > age 50, the most common secondary cause of hypertension is renal artery stenosis. This would call for investigation with an IVP and digital subtraction angiography.

Other secondary causes include pheochromocytoma (hypertension, sweating, and palpitations) and hyperthyroidism (hypertension, sweating, and palpitations).

9. C. This patient probably has cardiac hypertrophy. This is suspected from the P/E of the heart, when the point of maximal impulse is found in the sixth intercostal space–anterior axillary line. The normal apical impulse is located at or medial to the midclavicular line in the fourth or fifth intercostal space.

10. A. The term *mild hypertension* is no longer considered appropriate in defining hypertension, because

it may very well give some a false sense of security ("I've been told I have hypertension, but I've also been told it is mild; therefore, I really don't have to worry about it"). The following represents the new classification of blood pressure in patients over the age of 18 years:

1. *Normal*—Systolic: <130 mm Hg Diastolic: <85 mm Hg
2. *High normal*—Systolic: 130-139 mm Hg or Diastolic: 85-89 mm Hg
3. *Hypertension*
   Stage 1: Systolic: 140-159 mm Hg or Diastolic: 90-99 mm Hg
   Stage 2: Systolic: 160-179 mm Hg or Diastolic: 100-109 mm Hg
   Stage 3: Systolic: 180-209 mm Hg or Diastolic: 110-119 mm Hg
   Stage 4: Systolic: >210 mm Hg or Diastolic: >120 mm Hg

11. D. Hypertensive emergencies and hypertensive urgencies are defined as follows:

A *hypertensive emergency* is a clinical situation in which blood pressure must be lowered within one hour. Examples of hypertensive emergencies are malignant hypertension, acute myocardial ischemic syndromes, acute pulmonary edema, acute renal insufficiency, acute intracranial events, postoperative bleeding, eclampsia, and pheochromocytoma.

A *hypertensive urgency* is a clinical situation in which blood pressure should be lowered within 24 hours. Examples of hypertensive urgencies are accelerated hypertension, marked hypertension associated with congestive cardiac failure, stable angina pectoris, transient cerebral ischemic attacks, and perioperative hypertension.

Hypertensive emergency/urgency drug selection must be made on a pathophysiologic basis.

Summary of current recommendations:

1. Central nervous system disorder:
   Drug of choice: Sodium nitroprusside
   Alternatives: Trimethaphan camsylate, labetalol, diazoxide
2. Intracranial hemorrhage:
   Drug of choice: Sodium nitroprusside
   Alternatives: Trimethaphan camsylate, labetalol, diazoxide
3. Acute left ventricular failure:
   Drug of choice: Sodium nitroprusside
   Alternatives: Trimethaphan camsylate
   Contraindicated: Labetalol
4. Acute coronary ischemia:
   Drug of choice: Nitroglycerin
   Alternatives: Labetalol, sodium nitroprusside

5. Unstable angina:
   Drug of choice: Nitroglycerin
   Alternatives: Labetalol
6. Aortic dissection:
   Drug of choice: Trimethaphan camsylate
   Alternatives: Sodium nitroprusside and propranolol
   Contraindicated: Hydralazine
7. Eclampsia:
   Drug of choice: MgSo$_4$ (magnesium sulfate)
   Alternatives: Hydralazine
8. Pheochromocytoma:
   Drug of choice: Phentolamine
   Contraindicated: Beta-adrenoreceptor blockers
9. Stage 3 or 4 hypertension with imminent or mild target organ damage:
   Drug of choice: Nifedipine (oral short-acting preparation)
   Alternatives: Captopril, clonidine, labetalol

12. E. This patient is currently on a thiazide diuretic and a beta blocker. Therefore the most reasonable alternative as a third-line agent would be either an ACE inhibitor or a calcium-channel blocker.

Atenolol and metoprolol are also beta blockers and thus would not be reasonable choices.

Labetalol is a combination alpha-beta blocker and thus would also be a poor choice.

Furosemide is a loop diuretic and would not be a reasonable choice for the management of this patient's hypertension.

Enalapril is an ACE inhibitor and would be an excellent choice for a third-line agent.

13. A. The most common side effect of ACE inhibitors is cough. The mechanism of the cough appears to be bradykinin induced. It does not appear to be truly allergic in nature. Approximately 15% of patients on chronic ACE inhibitors develop a chronic cough.

14. E. The most common side effect of propranolol is depression. Propranolol is certainly one of the most common drugs, if not the most common depression-causing drug.

15. C. The patient's point of maximum impulse is in the sixth intercostal space in the anterior axillary line. This suggests left ventricular hypertrophy secondary to hypertension (and perhaps also due to the obesity). An echocardiogram is indicated to evaluate the thickness of the left ventricle.

SOLUTION TO SHORT ANSWER MANAGEMENT PROBLEM 5

Patient 1: A young patient with "hyperdynamic circulation"
Recommended drugs: Beta blockers
Contraindicated drugs: None

Patient 2: An elderly patient with no particular chronic diseases other than hypertension
Recommended drugs:
  First line: diuretics, with reduced drug dose
  Second line: ACE inhibitors, calcium-channel blockers
Contraindicated drugs: None

Patient 3: An African-American patient
Recommended drugs: Diuretics
Contraindicated drugs: None

Patient 4: A patient with gout
Recommended drugs: Any drug but diuretics
Contraindicated drugs: Diuretics

Patient 5: A patient with ischemic heart disease
Recommended drugs: Beta blockers, calcium-channel blockers
Contraindicated drugs: None

Patient 6: A patient with asthma
Recommended drugs: Calcium-channel blockers
Contraindicated drugs: Beta blockers

Patient 7: A patient with peripheral vascular disease
Recommended drugs: Calcium-channel blockers or other vasodilators
Contraindicated drugs: Beta blockers

Patient 8: A patient with non-insulin-dependent diabetes
Recommended drugs: ACE inhibitors
Contraindicated drugs: None

Patient 9: A patient with insulin-dependent diabetes
Recommended drugs: ACE inhibitors
Contraindicated drugs: Beta blockers

Patient 10: A patient with hypercholesterolemia
Recommended drugs: ACE inhibitors, calcium-channel blockers, alpha blockers, beta blockers with ISA
Contraindicated drugs: High dose beta blockers without ISA, high dose diuretics

Patient 11: A patient with congestive heart failure
Recommended drugs: ACE inhibitors, diuretics
Contraindicated drugs: Beta blockers

Patient 12: A patient in pregnancy
Recommended drugs: Alpha-methyl dopa, hydralazine
Contraindicated drugs: Diuretics, ACE inhibitors

SUMMARY OF THE DETECTION, EVALUATION, AND TREATMENT OF PATIENTS WITH HIGH BLOOD PRESSURE

1. **Diagnosis:** Blood pressure measurement: Three readings, separated by a time of at least 1 week where (1) after 5 minutes of controlled rest and (2) after having not consumed caffeine or smoked during the last hour, the average systolic pressure is at least 140 mm Hg and/or the average diastolic pressure is at least 90 mm Hg. A single reading of a diastolic of 110 mm Hg is probably sufficient for the diagnosis of hypertension.

2. **Evaluation:** History, P/E, and laboratory evaluation should include the evaluation of other risk factors, including family history of hypertension and other cardiovascular disease, presence of diabetes mellitus, obesity, alcohol intake, hyperlipidemia, smoking, exercise pattern, and stress.

    Look for evidence of end-organ damage: cardiac hypertrophy (may need echocardiogram), fundoscopy, renal function.

    Laboratory evaluation should include CBC, urinalysis, electrolytes, BUN, creatinine, calcium, cholesterol, glucose, uric acid, and ECG.

3. **Classification:** Staging system outlined in answer to Question 10. Stages 1, 2, 3, and 4 have replaced mild, moderate, and severe hypertension.

4. **Treatment:**
    a) Nonpharmacologic:
       1. Weight reduction
       2. Increase in aerobic exercise
       3. Restriction of sodium
       4. Restriction of saturated fat
       5. Discontinue smoking
       6. Decrease stress
    b) Pharmacologic: The Fifth Report of the Joint National Committee on Detection, Evaluation, and Treatment of High Blood Pressure (JNC V) has reversed recommendations found in the previous Report (JNC IV).

Following is a comparison of JNC III (1985), JNC IV (1988), and JNC V (1993):

JNC III:
JNC III devised the "step-care approach" to hypertension, in which Step 1 was nonpharmacologic therapy, Step 2 was therapy with a thiazide diuretic or a beta blocker, and Step 3 was the addition or substitution of a drug from a different class.

JNC IV:
JNC IV reversed this approach and indicated that after Step 1 (nonpharmacologic therapy) therapy with a drug from any of the following four classes could be added: thiazide diuretics, beta blockers, calcium-channel blockers, or ACE inhibitors.

JNC V:
JNC V has gone full circle. JNC V states that after beginning with a reasonable period of nonpharmacologic therapy, either a thiazide diuretic or a beta blocker should be used as the drug of first choice. The reason for this recommendation is that thiazide diuretics and beta blockers are the only drug

classes that have been shown to reduce mortality from cardiovascular disease.

After beginning with either a thiazide diuretic or a beta blocker and finding it to be ineffective alone, (1) the drug dose can be increased, (2) another drug may be substituted, or (3) a second drug from a different class may be added.

SUGGESTED READING

Fifth Report of the Joint National Committee on Detection, Evaluation, and Treatment of High Blood Pressure (JNC V). Archives of Internal Medicine 1993; 153: 154-208.

PROBLEM 6   A 37-YEAR-OLD MALE WITH "SKIPPING HEART BEATS"

A 37-year-old male presents to your office for assessment of "skipping heart beats." These skipped beats have been a concern for the past 8 months. The patient reports no other symptoms accompanying these skipped beats. Specifically, he reports no increased sweating, no palpitations, no weight loss, no chest pain, no pleuritic pain, and no anxiety.

On P/E, his blood pressure is 100/70 mm Hg. On auscultation of his heart you observe that S_1 and S_2 are normal—there are no extra sounds or murmurs. You hear approximately 5 premature beats/min.

SELECT THE ONE BEST ANSWER TO THE FOLLOWING QUESTIONS

1. What is the most commonly encountered "premature contraction"?
   a) a ventricular premature beat
   b) an atrial premature beat
   c) atrial flutter
   d) atrial fibrillation
   e) none of the above

2. Most atrial premature beats discovered on clinical examination are:
   a) of sinister prognosis
   b) completely benign
   c) associated with an increase in cardiovascular morbidity
   d) associated with an increase in cardiovascular mortality
   e) c and d

3. Most ventricular premature beats discovered on clinical examination are:
   a) of sinister prognosis
   b) completely benign
   c) associated with an increase in cardiovascular morbidity
   d) associated with an increase in cardiovascular mortality
   e) c and d

4. A 51-year-old male presents to the ER with an acute episode of chest pain. He has a history of atrial fibrillation. On examination, his blood pressure is 80/60 mm Hg and his ventricular rate is approximately 160 beats/min. He is in acute distress. His respiratory rate is 32/min. His ECG shows atrial fibrillation with a rapid ventricular response. What should you do at this time?
   a) digitalize the patient
   b) give the patient IV verapamil
   c) give the patient IV procainamide
   d) cardiovert the patient with a direct current
   e) do nothing; wait to see what happens next

5. The same 51-year-old male (who was fortunately successfully treated by you the last time he was in the ER) comes again 3 weeks later. At this time, he complains of the same symptom (mainly retrosternal chest pain), but he appears not to be in as much distress as he was previously.

On P/E, his blood pressure is 120/80 mm Hg and his ventricular rate is again 160 beats/minute. His ECG again confirms atrial fibrillation with a rapid ventricular response. What should you do at this time?
   a) digitalize the patient
   b) treat the patient with IV verapamil
   c) treat the patient with IV procainamide
   d) cardiovert the patient
   e) do nothing; this worked last time, even though you were told by your senior chief that it wasn't the smartest medical decision you had ever made

6. What is the recommended treatment for paroxysmal supraventricular tachycardia PSVT with hemodynamic compromise?
   a) synchronized cardioversion
   b) DC countershock
   c) IV adenosine
   d) IV verapamil
   e) IV digoxin

7. Patients with chronic atrial fibrillation are at increased risk for which of the following conditions?
   a) acute MI
   b) ventricular tachycardia
   c) sudden cardiac death
   d) cerebrovascular accident
   e) ventricular fibrillation

8. What is the drug of choice for the prevention of the appropriate complication described in Question 7?
   a) prophylactic streptokinase
   b) prophylactic warfarin
   c) prophylactic heparin
   d) prophylactic lidocaine
   e) aspirin

9. Which of the following statements regarding the medical treatment of atrial premature beats with antiarrhythmic drugs is true?
   a) the benefit outweighs the risk
   b) the risk outweighs the benefit
   c) the risk and the benefit are equal
   d) the risk and benefit depend on the patient
   e) nobody really knows for sure

10. Which of the following statements regarding the medical treatment of ventricular premature beats with antiarrhythmic drugs is true?
    a) the benefit outweighs the risk

    b) the risk outweighs the benefit
    c) the risk and the benefit are equal
    d) the risk and the benefit depend on the patient
    e) nobody really knows for sure

Short Answer Management Problem 6

Discuss the significance of the results of the CAST study with respect to the treatment of ventricular extrasystole.

ANSWERS

1. B

2. B. Atrial premature beats are the most common premature beats encountered in the adult population. They are almost always asymptomatic and are often discovered incidentally during a medical examination. Patients with atrial premature beats often complain of "palpitations" or "a feeling of skipped heart beats" during periods of emotional stress or during periods of quiet such as while resting in bed. Atrial premature beats may be associated with tachycardias that, particularly if nonsustained (less than 30 seconds), may not be perceived by the patient.

   Atrial premature beats require no treatment except reassurance of the patient. Reassurance is particularly important because the more convinced the patient is that something is seriously wrong, the more atrial premature beats he or she will sustain.

   There are obviously other causes of palpitations that must be considered, such as thyrotoxicosis, panic disorder, and pheochromocytoma. However, benign premature atrial contractions are much more common than premature atrial contractions due to thyrotoxicosis, panic disorder, or pheochromocytoma.

3. B. Most ventricular premature contractions, as with atrial premature contractions, turn out to be completely benign. As with atrial premature contractions, most patients simply need reassurance.

   As with atrial premature contractions, most ventricular premature contractions are asymptomatic and are often discovered during a medical examination. Occasionally, PVCs (in contradistinction to PACs) may be symptoms of more serious underlying heart disease. With runs of ventricular premature beats (ventricular tachycardia), the patient may develop angina, dyspnea, dizziness, syncope, and even cardiac arrest.

   If there is a serious question about the number of ventricular premature beats/min, a 24-hour Holter monitor is an excellent way to measure. Again, however, (and this will be discussed later in more detail) the risk

of placing a patient on a prophylactic antiarrhythmic drug for ventricular ectopy outweighs the benefit.

4. D. This patient presents with what appears to be an acute attack of atrial fibrillation with rapid ventricular response. The treatment of choice of this patient is synchronized cardioversion at 100 joules of energy. ACLS protocol recommends cardioversion energies of (1) 100 joules, (2) 200 joules, (3) 300 joules, and (4) 360 joules, in that order, and in succession if the previous energy level was not successful.

5. B. In this case, the patient has the same condition, atrial fibrillation. However, in this case he is hemodynamically stable instead of hemodynamically unstable. Therefore a less dramatic intervention than cardioversion can be attempted at this time.

   ACLS protocol would suggest that for rate control in this situation, both beta blockers and calcium-channel blockers are appropriate. The pharmacologic drug of choice at this time is IV verapamil 2.5-5.0 mg IV.

6. C. A patient who presents with paroxysmal supraventricular tachycardia (PSVT) should first be treated with vagal maneuvers. The term *vagal maneuvers* is commonly used, and yet few people know how many vagal maneuvers there are. Also, the character of these vagal maneuvers varies from the commonplace to the bizarre.

   The list includes carotid sinus pressure; breath holding; facial immersion in ice water; coughing; nasogastric tube placement; gag reflex stimulation by tongue blades, fingers, and oral ipecac; eyeball pressure; squatting; medical antishock trousers; Trendelenburg's position; and a circumferential digital sweep of the anus.

   The treatment of choice in this case is adenosine. The dose recommended for PSVT is 6 mg rapid IV push over 1-3 seconds.

7. D.

8. B. Patients with chronic atrial fibrillation are often left untreated for inexplicable reasons. Patients with chronic atrial fibrillation are at risk for embolic cerebrovascular

accidents. It is recommended that if there is no contraindication, they should be placed on warfarin prophylaxis.

All of the trials to date have shown that patients with chronic atrial fibrillation (whether persistent or intermittent) have a significant reduction in the incidence of strokes (0.5-2.0 strokes per year) with chronic warfarin therapy maintained with an international normalized ratio (INR) of 2.0-4.5. One of the trials has shown that the benefit of aspirin, 160-325 mg/day, is equivalent to warfarin when risk of stroke or major bleed is considered.

9. B.

10. B. In patients with either PACs or PVCs it is obvious that unless the circumstances are unusual and have been documented electrophysiologically, the risk of treatment with antiarrhythmic drugs outweighs the benefit. A number of trials have confirmed this.

SOLUTION TO SHORT ANSWER MANAGEMENT PROBLEM 6

"Treatment of potentially dangerous dysrhythmias in high-risk populations, especially following myocardial infarction, has not proven to be beneficial. The largest study, the Cardiac Arrhythmia Suppression Trial (CAST), was a multicenter study designed to determine the effects of suppression of ventricular extrasystoles in post-myocardial infarction patients with decreased left ventricular function and more than six ventricular extrasystoles per hour on a 24 hour Holter recording. After demonstration of suppression of the extrasystole by dysrhythmic therapy, patients were randomly assigned to medical therapy or placebo.

"In CAST, the two most effective drugs with the fewest noncardiac side effects, flecainide and encainide, were used. The CAST STUDY was terminated early due to an increase in mortality in the patients treated with either of these drugs" (Goldberg, in Conn's Current Therapy, 1994).

SUMMARY OF THE DIAGNOSIS AND TREATMENT OF PREMATURE BEATS AND CERTAIN SUPRAVENTRICULAR RHYTHMS

1. **Atrial premature beats:** These are benign and extremely common; reassurance the only treatment recommended.
2. **Ventricular premature beats:** The vast majority are benign, they are extremely common, and reassurance the only treatment recommended after a complete cardiovascular status is determined for the patient.

   According to the CAST study, with ventricular ectopy, even in patients at high risk (that is, following an MI), the risk of treating this dysrhythmia is greater than the risk of doing nothing.
3. **Paroxysmal supraventricular tachycardia:**
   Vagal maneuvers
   Adenosine 6 mg IV push has replaced verapamil as treatment of choice
4. **Atrial fibrillation:**
   Hemodynamically unstable: cardiovert: 100J-200J-300J-360J
   Hemodynamically stable: IV verapamil is treatment of choice
   Prophylaxis against embolic cerebrovascular accidents should be maintained with warfarin. If warfarin is contraindicated, one aspirin/day is effective.

SUGGESTED READING

Emergency Cardiac Care Committee and Subcommittees, American Heart Association. Guidelines for cardiopulmonary resuscitation and emergency cardiac care. JAMA 1992; 268:2172-2183.

Goldberg AD. Premature beats. In: Rakel R, ed. Conn's current therapy. Philadelphia: WB Saunders, 1994.

McAnulty J. Atrial fibrillation. In: Rakel R, ed. Conn's current therapy. Philadelphia: WB Saunders, 1994.

PROBLEM 7   A 45-YEAR-OLD MALE WEIGHING 320 LB AND COMPLAINING OF FATIGUE

A 320-lb, 45-year-old male comes to your office complaining of fatigue. He has been obese all his life. He tells you that his obesity has nothing to do with calorie intake and everything to do with his slow metabolic rate. He has been investigated extensively at many major centers specializing in "slow metabolic rates." The result of his encounters has been a conclusion that he is simply "eating too much" (with which he disagrees, of course). He has heard from a friend that "you are different," and has come to you for "the truth."

On examination, his body mass index is off the scale. He weighs 320 lb, and although you cannot feel his PMI, you believe it is in the region of the anterior axillary line, sixth intercostal space. S_1 and S_2 are distant, as are his breath sounds.

His abdomen is obese with striae covering the abdomen. His liver and spleen can not be felt.

You refer him to your local dietician and promise that you will "investigate his slow metabolic rate" if he will agree to adhere to a diet. The dietician puts him on a 1800 kcal/day diet and calculates his ideal weight at 170 lb.

SELECT THE ONE BEST ANSWER TO THE FOLLOWING QUESTIONS

1. Assuming that (1) you are unable to convince him to increase his exercise, (2) his total energy expenditure is 2300 kcal/day, and (3) he does, in fact, stick to his diet, how long will it take for him to reach his ideal weight?
   a) 125 days
   b) 225 days
   c) 325 days
   d) 525 days
   e) 1050 days

2. How is obesity generally defined?
   a) an increase in the ponderal index of 20% above normal
   b) a decrease in the ponderal index of 30% below normal
   c) an increase in the body mass index of 20% above normal
   d) a body mass index of 30
   e) none of the above

3. Which of the following statements is(are) true regarding obesity?
   a) obesity is associated with increased death rates from cancer
   b) obesity is associated with increased death rates from coronary artery disease
   c) obesity is associated with increased death rates from diabetes mellitus
   d) all of the above
   e) none of the above

4. What is the overall prevalence of obesity in the United States?
   a) 1%
   b) 5%
   c) 10%
   d) 20%
   e) 50%

5. Which of the following conditions is obesity most commonly associated with?
   a) alveolar hypoventilation syndrome
   b) hypertension
   c) hyperlipidemia
   d) diabetes mellitus
   e) angina pectoris

6. The use of severe calorie-restricted diets (<800 kcal/day) has been responsible for many deaths. What is the most common cause of death in these cases?
   a) sudden cardiac death (secondary to dysrhythmia)
   b) congestive cardiac failure secondary to anemia
   c) hepatic failure
   d) renal failure
   e) septicemia

7. Which of the following theories have been postulated to explain the physiology of obesity?
   a) the fat-cell theory
   b) the lipoprotein-lipase theory
   c) the thermogenesis-brown adipose tissue theory
   d) all of the above
   e) none of the above

8. Which of the following statements is(are) true regarding the use of anoretic drugs?
   a) short-term studies demonstrate that weight loss is greater with these agents at time = 1 month than with placebo agents
   b) hypertension is a documented side effect of these agents
   c) renal failure is a documented side effect of these agents
   d) long-term studies suggest that these agents are not beneficial as part of a weight-loss program
   e) all of the above

9. Which of the following is(are) advocated as part of a weight-loss program?
   a) a nutritionally balanced diet
   b) a lowering of the percentage of calories derived from fat

c) an exercise program

d) caloric restriction to approximately 500 kcal/day less than maintenance

e) all of the above

10. The practical management of weight loss by the family physician should involve which of the following?

a) multiple office visits over 8 to 12 weeks

b) changes to the act of eating

c) keeping of a daily food diary

d) all of the above

e) none of the above

11. Which one of the following statements concerning the use of echocardiography in obese patients is true?

a) echocardiography is not indicated in obese patients; it is a waste of time and money

b) echocardiography cannot predict future risk in obese patients

c) echocardiography is indicated in obese patients to document the size of the right ventricle; right ventricular hypertrophy is a major predicator of future risk

d) echocardiography may disclose the formation of "obese heart clots"

e) none of the above are true

Short Answer Management Problem 7

The vast majority of patients with obesity have *essential obesity* (analogous to essential hypertension). There are, however, secondary causes. List the potential secondary causes of obesity.

ANSWERS

1. E. One pound of fat is equal to 3500 kcal. Therefore, if his total energy expenditure is 2300 kcal/day and the patient is taking in only 1800 kcal/day (the recommended difference in a weight-loss program between energy expenditure and energy intake is 500 kcal), his energy deficit is 500 kcal/day. His excess weight above ideal body weight is 150 lb. This 150 lb is equal to 525,000 kcal. The corresponding time to lose this number of calories is 1050 days (2.87 years).

2. D. The definition of obesity is either (a) a body mass index $> 30 \text{kg/m}^2$; or (b) a body weight greater than 20% above ideal body weight.

3. D. Obesity is a major public health issue. There is a certain stigmatization to the diagnosis of obesity not present in other conditions. Some authorities suggest that as we label hypertension as essential hypertension, so we should label obesity as *essential obesity*. The comparison between hypertension and obesity does not end there. Obesity is a major risk factor for coronary artery disease and other cardiovascular conditions including hypertension, congestive heart failure, cardiomyopathy, and angina pectoris. In fact, obese individuals are 250% more likely to develop coronary artery disease than non-obese subjects.

Obesity is associated with an increased incidence of NIDDM (non-insulin dependent diabetes mellitus); this is mediated by an effective increase in insulin resistance.

Obesity has been established indirectly as a risk factor for some cancers. For example, it appears from some studies that the high-fat diet usually associated with obesity is also associated with an increased risk of colon cancer. The link between obesity, total fat intake, saturated fat intake, and cancer prevalence ratio needs to be very thoroughly documented.

Other diseases that have been shown to be directly linked to obesity include (1) thromboembolic disease, (2) endometrial carcinoma, (3) restrictive lung disease, (4) Pickwickian syndrome, (5) gout, (6) degenerative arthritis, (7) gallstone formation and gallbladder disease, (8) infertility, and (9) hyperlipoproteinemias.

4. D. The overall prevalence of obesity in the North American population is approximately 20%. In certain groups, such as the Pima Indians, the prevalence is 50%. A higher prevalence of obesity appears in those individuals in the lowest socioeconomic groups; the prevalence does, in fact, decrease as socioeconomic status increases.

5. B. Of the conditions already postulated as linked with obesity, the strongest association is between obesity and hypertension.

6. A. The most common cause of death reported among patients who are on severe calorie-restricted diets is sudden cardiac death due to ventricular arrhythmias or dysrhythmias.

7. D. Some of the theories that have been brought forward to explain essential obesity include (1) the fat cell theory, (2) the lipoprotein-lipase theory, and (3) the thermogenesis-brown fat adipose tissue theory.

Studies done on monozygotic twins have established that 70% of the variance in BMI is due to genetic factors with only 30% due to environmental factors. This puts a different light on the whole question of slow metabolizers versus fast metabolizers. This genetic information suggests that metabolism is very much a function of genetics and genetic endowment.

8. E. Most, if not all, drugs used to treat obesity are CNS stimulants. Although these agents demonstrate significantly greater efficacy in producing weight loss at T = 1 month, there is no documentation of their continuing efficacy in long-term studies. There is some evidence, in fact, that their use may impair long-term weight loss. Complications of anoretic agents include (1) hypertension, (2) psychosis, (3) seizures, (4) renal failure, (5) cardiac arrhythmias, and (6) myocardial infarction.

9. E. A structured program is essential for successful long-term weight loss. This structured program is not in any way linked to any of the fad diets promoted by "snake-oil salesman" around the world.

   The weight-loss program must contain three essential components: (1) a nutritionally balanced diet, (2) aerobic exercise, and (3) a reduction in the percentage of calories derived from fat. It has now been shown that reducing the percentage of calories derived from fat (compared to carbohydrates and proteins) by itself produces weight loss. Current recommendations suggest that the energy intake should be approximately 500 calories less than energy output in a weight-loss program.

   There is no secret to a successful weight loss program. The simple fact is that calories consumed must be less than calories expended.

10. D. The practical management of weight loss in a patient by the patient's family physician should include (1) weekly office visits over a period of 8 to 12 weeks and gradual lengthening of time between visits after that; (2) changes to the act of eating; (3) keeping a food diary; and (4) increasing aerobic exercise activity.

    Home weighing is not recommended due to significant fluxuations in body weight due to body water. If it is necessary for the patient to weigh him/herself at home, it should be done no more frequently than once every two weeks.

    The concept of changes to the act of eating is an important and interesting component of the overall plan. First, patients must begin to regard eating as a conscious activity rather than something that happens while thinking of other things. Second, the suggestion of drinking two glasses of water just before the meal to decrease appetite has validity. Third, instructing the patient to eat more slowly and chew food more thoroughly also appears to be valid.

11. E. Echocardiography is an important investigational modality in obese patients. It measures the size of the left, not the right, ventricle, and is an indicator of left ventricular hypertrophy, not right ventricular hypertrophy. Left ventricular hypertrophy is a major predicator of morbidity and mortality, and hypertrophy is significantly more common in obese than non-obese patients.

SOLUTION TO SHORT ANSWER MANAGEMENT PROBLEM 7

The most common causes of secondary obesity include:

1. Iatrogenic Disease: drugs that produce either (1) weight gain as a side effect, or (2) produce salt and water retention
2. Depression: many patients gain rather than lose weight
3. Cushing's syndrome
4. Hypothyroidism
5. Diabetes Mellitus: Type II

SUMMARY OF THE DIAGNOSIS AND MANAGEMENT OF OBESITY

1. **Pathophysiology:** Evidence suggests that the etiology of obesity is at least 70% genetic and only 30% environmental.
2. **Definition:** A BMI greater than 30 kg/m²
   Alternative definition: > 20% above suggested ideal body weight
3. **Prevalence:** 30% of North Americans
4. **Importance:** A major public health problem that is often ignored due to the social stigma attached to it
5. **Complications:** Cardiovascular morbidity and mortality; hypertension, congestive heart failure, cardiomyopathy, angina pectoris, and hyperlipidemia. Obese patients are 250% more likely to develop coronary artery disease than non-obese patients.

   Other complications include diabetes mellitus, gall bladder disease, restrictive lung disease, cancer (associated with a high-fat diet), gout, and degenerative arthritis.
6. **Treatment:**
   a) Avoid all diet fads and diet "revolutions." Avoid anoretic drugs as well.
   b) Change the composition of the diet: increase carbohydrate, increase protein, decrease fat.
   c) Multiple office visits are essential to establish a baseline and to motivate continual weight loss.
   d) Decrease caloric intake to approximately 500 kcal/day less than energy expenditure. This produces a weight loss of approximately 1 lb/wk. Basic equation for successful weight loss: calories out > calories in.
   e) Increase aerobic exercise. This is essential to long-term weight loss and maintenance of same.
   f) Receive positive reinforcement from a support group, the physician, family, and friends.

NEW INFORMATION 1995

Obesity is becoming a greater, rather than a smaller, problem in the United States.

1. Obesity is now regarded as the most important public health problem in the United States.

2. In 1970, 25% of Americans were obese; in 1995, 33% of Americans are obese.

3. Even more important is the increase in prevalence in obesity in adolescents. In 1970, 15% of adolescents in the United States were obese; in 1995, 22% of adolescents in the United States are obese (approximately a 33% increase).

4. This increase in obesity translates into increased prevalences of the following diseases:
   a) coronary heart disease
   b) myocardial infarction
   c) cerebrovascular disease
   d) left ventricular hypertrophy and congestive heart failure
   e) diabetes mellitus Type II with macrovascular complications
      1. diabetic nephropathy
      2. diabetic retinopathy
      3. diabetic neuropathy
      4. autonomic neuropathy
      5. generalized atherosclerotic vascular disease
   f) osteoarthritis
   g) cholelithiasis and cholecystitis
   h) chronic renal failure (Remember, diabetes mellitus Type II is the most common cause of chronic renal failure in the United States. This is the case because Type II diabetes is 10 times more frequent than Type I diabetes.)
   i) Obstructive sleep apnea and Pickwickian syndrome

SUGGESTED READINGS

Garrow JS. Treatment of obesity. The Lancet 1992; 340: 409-413.

Ravussin E, Swinburn B. Pathophysiology of obesity. The Lancet 1992; 340:404-408.

PROBLEM 8   A 65-YEAR-OLD FEMALE WITH CYANOSIS, SHORTNESS OF BREATH, AND SUBSTERNAL CHEST PAIN

A 65-year-old female is admitted to the ER with a 3-hour history of cyanosis, shortness of breath, and substernal chest pain. She had been discharged 5 days earlier after having a total hip replacement for severe osteoarthritis. The hip surgery was uneventful.

On P/E, the patient is in obvious acute respiratory distress. Her respiratory rate is 40/min and her breathing is labored. Her blood pressure is 100/70 mm Hg. Cyanosis is present. There appear to be decreased breath sounds in the lower lobe of the right lung, as well as adventitious breath sounds in all lobes.

SELECT THE ONE BEST ANSWER TO THE FOLLOWING QUESTIONS

1. Based on the information provided, what is the most likely diagnosis in this patient?
   a) late-onset gram-negative nosocomial pneumonia with septic shock
   b) acute myocardial infarction
   c) dissecting aortic aneurysm
   d) acute pulmonary embolism
   e) late-onset status asthmaticus

2. Which of the following scintigraphic findings is most sensitive in diagnosing the condition just described?
   a) no perfusion defects
   b) two or more medium to large perfusion defects with no ventilation-perfusion mismatch
   c) two or more medium to large perfusion defects with ventilation-perfusion mismatch
   d) a single medium or large perfusion defect with ventilation-perfusion mismatch
   e) none of the above

3. On clinical examination of a patient with the precursor condition leading to the ultimate diagnosis, as just described, which of the following statements is true?
   a) clinical examination is diagnostic in every case
   b) clinical examination is, in most cases, diagnostic
   c) clinical examination is of some value but has low sensitivity and low specificity
   d) clinical examination is of no value
   e) nobody really knows for sure

4. Which of the following blood gas combinations occur most commonly in the condition described above?
   a) decreased P_{O_2} and decreased P_{CO_2}
   b) decreased P_{O_2} and increased P_{CO_2}
   c) increased P_{O_2} and increased P_{CO_2}
   d) increased P_{O_2} and decreased P_{CO_2}
   e) none of the above

5. What is the most common cause of morbidity and mortality among hospitalized immobile patients?
   a) myocardial infarction
   b) cerebrovascular accident

   c) deep venous thrombosis/pulmonary embolism
   d) nosocomial infection
   e) none of the above

6. What is the drug of choice for patients with a documented pulmonary embolus?
   a) continuous intravenous heparin
   b) intermittent intravenous heparin
   c) intermittent subcutaneous heparin
   d) any of the above
   e) none of the above

7. Which of the following is evidence of adequate anticoagulation in patients with deep venous thrombosis/pulmonary embolism?
   a) PTT 1.2 × that of the control
   b) PTT 1.4 × that of the control
   c) PTT 1.5-2.0 × that of the control
   d) PTT 2.0-3.0 × that of the control
   e) none of the above

8. Which of the following is(are) risk factors for the condition described earlier?
   a) prolonged immobilization
   b) long leg fractures
   c) pregnancy
   d) malignancy
   e) all of the above

9. What would be the diagnostic procedure of choice for this patient in the outpatient setting?
   a) pulmonary angiography
   b) pelvic vein ultrasound
   c) impedance plethysmography
   d) V/Q scan
   e) MRI scan

10. What is the diagnostic procedure of choice for a patient who presents to the ER with "a swollen leg" and has one or more of the risk factors described in Question 8?
    a) pulmonary angiography
    b) pelvic vein ultrasound
    c) impedance plethysmography
    d) V/Q scan
    e) MRI scan

11. Which of the following is(are) specific recommendations regarding DVT prophylaxis?
    a) patients at moderate risk for any reason should receive low-dose heparin or intermittent pneumatic compression
    b) patients undergoing neurosurgical procedures should be treated with pneumatic compression
    c) patients undergoing urological procedures should be treated with pneumatic compression
    d) patients undergoing surgery for hip fracture should receive warfarin to a PT time of 1.2-1.5 × that of control
    e) all of the above

Short Answer Management Problem 8

The management of the condition described in this problem has changed significantly over the last two years. Describe the treatment of the following: (1) a patient with this condition but without "severe disease" or hypotension; and (2) a patient with this condition but with either "severe disease" or hypotension.

ANSWERS

1. D. This patient has a pulmonary embolus. Hip surgery is a common predisposing factor for PE. Symptoms of pulmonary embolism are often subtle. It is often impossible to distinguish pulmonary embolism from myocardial infarction on the basis of the symptoms alone. Chest pain, dyspnea, anxiety, hyperventilation, and syncope are common to both conditions. Signs of pulmonary embolism include adventitious breath sounds, fever, and cyanosis. Pulmonary embolism is suggested by the triad of cough, hemoptysis, and pleuritic chest pain.

    Pulmonary embolism may lead to acute cor pulmonale. This complication produces (1) distended neck veins, (2) tachycardia, (3) an accentuated and split pumonic heart sound, (4) Kussmaul's sign (distention of the jugular veins on inspiration), and (5) pulsus paradoxus (exaggerated fall in blood pressure on inspiration). Systemic hypotension and shock suggest massive pulmonary embolism.

2. C. If two or more medium or large perfusion defects on V/Q scan mismatch, there is a 90% probability of pulmonary embolism. Although a negative V/Q scan virtually excludes PE (high sensitivity), a positive scan does not confirm the diagnosis (low specificity). If only a single medium or large defect with mismatch is present, the probability of pulmonary embolism drops to under 50%. Small perfusion defects with ventilation-perfusion mismatch confer a low probability of pulmonary embolism.

3. C. The clinical diagnosis of DVT is difficult and unreliable. DVT is frequently present in the absence of clinical signs (such as pain, heat or swelling), and it is absent in 50% of patients in whom clinical signs or symptoms suggest its presence.

4. A. Massive embolism is commonly associated with arterial hypoxemia, hypocapnia, and respiratory alkalosis. In addition, the difference between the alveolar P_{O_2} and the arterial P_{O_2} ($P_{A_{CO_2}}$-$P_{a_{CO_2}}$) may be widened owing to the increase in alveolar dead space. However, a normal $P_{A_{O_2}}$ does not exclude the diagnosis.

5. C. The commonest cause of morbidity and mortality among hospitalized immobile patients is DVT and pulmonary embolism. This is directly related to the immobile state.

    In the United States the incidence of fatal plus nonfatal pulmonary emboli exceeds 500,000 annually. This overall incidence is verfieid by autopsy statistics. Evidence of recent or old embolism is detected in 25 to 30% of routine autopsies.

6. D. In DVT and pulmonary embolism, three methods of heparin administration have been advocated by various investigators: (1) continuous intravenous heparin, (2) intermittent intravenous heparin, and (3) intermittent subcutaneous heparin.

    Continuous intravenous heparin is usually given in a dose of approximately 1000 units/hr. Intermittent intravenous heparin is commonly given in a dose of 5000 units q4h or 7500 units q6h. Subcutaneous heparin has been recommended in a dose of 5000 units q4h, 10,000 units q8h, or 20,000 units q12h. It is unclear at this time which method is best. Intramuscular injection of heparin should be avoided because of hematoma development.

7. C. The value of partial thromboplastin time (PTT) or clotting time (CT) in monitoring the safety and efficacy of heparin administration remains controversial. With respect to safety, the risk of hemorrhage (the principal complication of heparin therapy) is not clearly related to coagulation test alterations; rather, it appears related to factors such as the coexis-

tence of other diseases associated with bleeding risk (gastric or duodenal ulcer, coagulopathies, uremia) and advanced age. Likewise, achievement of the desired effect of heparin (cessation of thrombus growth in vivo) has not been related consistently to coagulation tests.

Current recommendations suggest keeping the PTT measured just prior to the next intermittent dose at or above 1.5 times the control, and at 1.5-2.0 times the control with the continuous infusion regime.

8. E. The risk of deep venous thrombosis and pulmonary embolism is increased by the following risk factors:
   1. immobility (both posttraumatic and postoperative)
   2. long leg fractures
   3. a prior history of DVT
   4. a history of DVT
   5. oral contraceptive or estrogen use
   6. CVA or a history of CVA
   7. pregnancy
   8. malignancy
   9. autoimmune disease
   10. nephrotic syndrome
   11. polycythemia
   12. inflammatory bowel disease
   13. congestive heart failure
   14. obesity

9. C.

10. D. In the outpatient setting, impedance plethysmography would be the most useful and available investigational tool. Impedance plethysmography can be performed by a physician in the office and offers a fair sensitivity in the diagnosis of DVT.

   For the patient who comes to the ER with a swollen leg and one or more risk factors, the diagnostic modality of choice would be the V/Q scan.

Current knowledge regarding the investigational modalities for DVT and pulmonary embolism:

1. The chest X-ray: The chest X-ray may show a parenchymal infiltrate and evidence of a pleural effusion if pulmonary infarction has occurred.

2. Transthoracic echo-Doppler studies: Standard transthoracic echo-Doppler studies may suggest the diagnosis of pulmonary embolism by demonstrating right ventricular enlargement, thrombi "trapped" in the right atrium or ventricle; an elevated pulmonary artery pressure; or echogenic densities in the right main pulmonary artery.

3. CT/MRI scanning: The value of CT scanning with contrast and MRI scanning in the diagnosis of pulmonary embolus remains to be determined.

4. Arterial blood gases: The blood gas results in pulmonary embolism show (1) arterial hypoxemia, (2) hypocapnia, and (3) respiratory alkalosis. Blood gas results are most useful when used in conjunction with other information.

5. The ventilation/perfusion scan: The ventilation/perfusion scan is the diagnostic modality of choice in the acute care facility setting. The diagnosis of pulmonary embolism is made when there are two or more perfusion defects with no matching ventilation defects.

6. Impedance plethysmography: Impedance plethysmography is an excellent screening tool for DVT and can be used by the physician in the office either to (1) establish the diagnosis of DVT or (2) increase the index of suspicion regarding the diagnosis of DVT. IPG is highly sensitive for detecting proximal deep vein thrombi but not for detecting thrombi in the calves.

7. Pelvic vein ultrasound: Pelvic vein ultrasound, which is presently used in some centers, will evolve as time and experience are gained with the technique.

8. Radionuclide scanning: Radionuclide scanning is sensitive for detecting thrombi in the calves.

9. Pulmonary angiography: Pulmonary angiography is the "gold standard" for the diagnosis of PE in the presence of an equivocal V/Q scan.

10. Venography: Ascending venography is the "gold standard" for the diagnosis of deep venous thrombi.

11. E. Recommendations for the prevention of venous thromboembolism include the following:
   a) Patients at moderate risk of venous thromboembolism for any reason should receive preventive therapy with low-dose heparin (5000 units q12h) or with intermittent pneumatic compression.
   b) Patients undergoing neurosurgical procedures, urologic procedures, and major knee surgery should be treated with intermittent pneumatic compression.
   c) Patients undergoing elective hip surgery should receive prophylaxis with adjusted-dose heparin therapy or moderate-dose warfarin therapy.
   d) Patients who are undergoing repair of a hip fracture should receive prophylactic therapy with moderate-dose warfarin therapy.

SOLUTION TO SHORT ANSWER MANAGEMENT PROBLEM 8

1. Treatment of deep venous thrombosis/pulmonary embolism without severe cardiovascular compromise:
   a) Full anticoagulation is advised for 7-10 days
   b) Supplementary oxygen in the acute phase—3 l/min
   c) Heparin: Three treatment regimes are acceptable:
      i) Continuous infusion IV heparin: 1000 U/hr
      ii) Intermittent IV infusion: 5000 U q4h or 7500 U q6h
      iii) Subcutaneous heparin 5000 U q4h, 10,000 U q8h, or 20,000 U q12h
   d) Warfarin: Should be initiated on day 2 or day 3 of heparin therapy. Heparin should not be discontinued until the prothrombin time is 1.5-1.8 times control for at least 3 days.
   e) Option to prophylactic warfarin: Self-injected subcutaneous heparin
   f) Prophylactic treatment time: At least 3 months; 6 months is probably wiser
   g) Progress of therapy: PTT for heparin: 1.5-2.0 that of control; PT for warfarin: 1.5-1.8 that of control

2. Treatment of deep venous thrombosis/pulmonary embolism with severe cardiovascular compromise: The treatment regime just described plus a first- or second-generation thrombolytic agent (first generation = streptokinase, second generation = tPA)
   Recommended dosages:
   Streptokinase = 250,000 IV loading with 100,000 units/hr for 24 hours
   tPA = 100 mg as peripheral infusion over 2 hours

SUMMARY OF THE DIAGNOSIS AND TREATMENT OF DEEP VENOUS THROMBOSIS AND PULMONARY THROMBOEMBOLISM

1. **Diagnosis:** Most patients who develop DVT and subsequent PE have one of the previously described risk factors. Remember that DVT is often clinically silent, and the clinical diagnosis is notoriously inaccurate.

   Pulmonary embolism, however, is often heralded by the abrupt onset of dyspnea, chest pain, apprehension, hemoptysis, or syncope. When massive pulmonary embolism is present, the signs of acute cor pulmonale are evident. With pulmonary embolism, rhonchi are frequently heard in the chest.

2. **Laboratory diagnosis:** Blood: Arterial blood gases: Low PO_2, Low PCO_2, respiratory alkalosis

3. **Diagnostic imaging:** For deep venous thrombosis: Impedance plethysmography (IPG) is very sensitive in the diagnosis of proximal thrombi but lacks sensitivity with more distal thrombi. Consider radionuclide scanning in more distal thrombi. Venography is "the gold standard" for the diagnosis of DVT.

   For pulmonary thromboembolism: Ventilation/perfusion scan is 90% sensitive when there are at least two perfusion defects with no matching ventilation defects (ventilation-perfusion mismatch).

4. **Treatment:**
   a) Supplemental oxygen
   b) Heparin: continuous IV, intermittent IV, or subcutaneous
   c) Warfarin: begin warfarin on second or third day
   d) Thrombolytic therapy: consider streptokinase or tPA when the patient has significant cardiovascular compromise

5. **Length of treatment time and prophylaxis:**
   a) Treat for at least 3 months and possibly up to 6 months with warfarin
   b) Consider prophylaxis for those surgical procedures just described

SUGGESTED READING

Moser K. Pulmonary thromboembolism. In: Isselbacher et al., eds. Harrison's principles of internal medicine. 13th Ed. New York: McGraw-Hill, 1994.

PROBLEM 9   A 55-YEAR-OLD MALE WITH A CHRONIC COUGH

A 55-year-old male presents to your office for assessment of a chronic cough. He complains of "coughing for the last 10 years"; the cough has become more bothersome lately. The cough is productive of sputum that is usually mucoid; occasionally it becomes purulent.

He has a 35-year history of smoking 2 packs of cigarettes/day (70 pack/year history). He quit smoking approximately 2 years ago.

On physical examination his blood pressure is 160/85 mm Hg. His pulse is 96 and regular. He has a BMI (body mass index) of 34. He weighs 280 lb. He wheezes while he talks. On auscultation, adventitious breath sounds are heard in all lobes. His CXR reveals significant bronchial wall thickening. There are increased markings at both lung bases.

SELECT THE ONE BEST ANSWER TO THE FOLLOWING QUESTIONS

1. What is the most likely diagnosis in this patient?
   a) smoker's cough
   b) subacute bronchitis
   c) emphysema
   d) chronic bronchitis
   e) allergic bronchitis

2. What is the most likely cause of this condition?
   a) right-sided heart failure
   b) cor pulmonale
   c) cigarette smoking
   d) obstructive sleep apnea
   e) hypercarbia

3. Which of the following statements regarding this condition is(are) true?
   a) the disease develops in 10-15% of cigarette smokers
   b) cigarette smokers in whom this disease develops usually report the onset of cough with expectoration 10 to 12 years after smoking began
   c) dyspnea is noted initially only on extreme exertion; as the condition progresses it becomes more severe and occurs with mild activity
   d) pneumonia, pulmonary hypertension, cor pulmonale, and chronic respiratory failure characterize the late stages of the disease
   e) all of the above are true

4. Which of the following regarding the patient described above is(are) true?
   a) this patient is a "pink puffer"
   b) this patient's blood gases will likely show a decreased P_{CO_2}
   c) this patient's CXR will demonstrate hyperinflation
   d) this patient's disease is a disease of the large airways
   e) all of the above are true

5. Which of the following pulmonary function results is *not* associated with the condition described above?
   a) reduced FEV_1
   b) reduced FEV_1/FVC
   c) reduced FEF_{25-75}

d) decreased residual volume
   e) none of the above are associated with this disease state

6. Regarding the pathophysiology of chronic bronchitis, which of the following statements is(are) false?
   a) most histologic studies in patients with chronic bronchitis have shown an increase in the size of mucus-secreting glands as measured by the Reid index (a ratio of gland : bronchial wall thickness)
   b) smooth muscle hyperplasia occurs in patients with chronic bronchitis
   c) chronic bronchitis is characterized by chronic, excessive secretion of mucus
   d) in chronic bronchitis, there is a clear relationship between smooth muscle hyperplasia and bronchodilator responsiveness or methacholine sensitivity
   e) none of the above are false

7. Which of the following is(are) established risk factors for COPD?
   a) smoking
   b) atopy
   c) elevated levels of IgE
   d) bronchial hyperresponsiveness
   e) all of the above

8. Which of the following is(are) accurate statements regarding the role of bacteria in chronic bronchitis?
   a) the delay in mucociliary clearance allows inhaled bacteria to colonize the normally sterile airways and to multiply, leading to further infectious exacerbations
   b) *Haemophilus infuenzae* is present in the sputum of about 60% of patients with stable chronic bronchitis
   c) *Haemophilus influenzae* may act synergistically with tobacco smoke to impede mucociliary clearance and allow the organism to colonize the airways further
   d) nicotine stimulates the growth of *Haemophilus influenzae*
   e) a, b, and c
   f) all of the above

9. Which of the following is(are) considerations in the diagnosis of chronic bronchitis?
   a) asthma
   b) postnasal drip
   c) chronic ACE inhibitor therapy
   d) a and b
   e) all of the above

10. Which of the following statements regarding smoking cessation and COPD is(are) true?
    a) cessation of smoking dramatically reduces symptoms in established COPD patients
    b) coughing stops in 80% of patients with COPD who stop smoking
    c) coughing stops in over 50% of patients with COPD within 4 weeks
    d) all of the above
    e) none of the above

11. Which of the following drugs is(are) the most effective for long-term pharmacologic management in a patient with chronic bronchitis?
    a) an inhaled beta agonist
    b) an inhaled anticholinergic
    c) an inhaled corticosteroid
    d) oral prednisone
    e) a, b, and c are considered to be equally efficacious

12. Which of the following drugs is(are) recommended as routine pharmacologic management for a patient with chronic bronchitis?
    a) an inhaled beta agonist
    b) an inhaled anticholinergic
    c) an inhaled corticosteroid
    d) a and b
    e) all of the above

13. Long-term home oxygen therapy is indicated in which of the patients with chronic bronchitis?
    a) all patients who have established chronic bronchitis and who have met the criteria of symptoms for at least 5 years
    b) all patients who have a resting arterial partial pressure of oxygen of 55 mm Hg or less
    c) all patients who have a resting arterial partial pressure of oxygen of 60 mm Hg or less with evidence of chronic tissue hypoxia as demonstrated by cor pulmonale or polycythemia
    d) b and c
    e) all of the above

14. The patient described in the problem above is stabilized on long-term therapy. Unfortunately, over the Christmas holidays, he travels to his son's home in a distant state and finds himself in an environment where 6 packs of cigarettes/day are being smoked by his son and his son's wife (4 packs for the son and 2 packs for his wife). There is a

layer of definite haze that hangs approximately 1 ft below all the ceilings in the house. As he sits around the house one day (unable to go outside or walk any distance at all because of significantly increased shortness of breath since arriving) he counts the number of ashtrays (47). As he gets worse and worse he wonders whether the "ashtray count" may be a possible entry into the *Guinness Book of World Records*. His son, through the haze of smoke, finally notices that his dad is out of breath and his lips appear very blue. He takes him to the nearest ER.

The ER doctor diagnoses his condition as an acute exacerbation of chronic bronchitis. His major symptoms at this time include dyspnea, increased sputum production, and purulence. The patient's PaO_2 when measured in the ER is 44 mm Hg. Which of the following should be instituted as therapy for this condition?
   a) low-flow oxygen
   b) intravenous corticosteroids
   c) oral or IV amoxicillin
   d) a and b only
   e) all of the above

15. Which of the following organisms have been implicated in the pathogenesis of acute exacerbations of chronic bronchitis?
    a) Haemophilus influenzae
    b) Streptococcus pneumoniae
    c) Moraxella catarrhalis
    d) a and b only
    e) all of the above

16. A 23-year-old male presents to your office for assessment of a 10-day cough which has "now gone into my lungs." He complains of sputum production, which was initially clear but has now turned "yellow." He said that he called your partner last night and your partner told him to "get in here today and we will prescribe an antibiotic and clear this thing up quick." This patient has no history of other respiratory illnesses. On examination, the patient's lungs are clear. His temperature is normal (98.6° C). No other positive physical findings are present.
    What would you do?
    a) reach for the "good old prescription pad" and scribble down the first reasonable thing that comes to mind
    b) reach for the "good old prescription pad" but think briefly about which antibiotic you wish to prescribe before you prescribe it
    c) reach for the "good old prescription pad" but think quite a bit before deciding which antibiotic you wish to prescribe
    d) auscultate the patient's lung through his shirt, sweater, and winter jacket, and then reach for the prescription pad
    e) take the Fifth Amendment on this question
    f) none of the above

Short Answer Management Problem 9

Describe the difference between the two major types of COPD in terms of the following:

A. Part of airway affected
B. Color of lips in severely affected individual
C. Definition of both types
D. Pathophysiology

ANSWERS

1. D.

2. C. This patient has chronic bronchitis. Chronic bronchitis is defined as cough and sputum production on most days for at least 3 months of the year for at least 2 years. Chronic bronchitis is most commonly caused by cigarette smoking.

   Acute bronchitis is an inflammation of the bronchi caused by an infectious agent or acute exposure to a nonspecific irritant. Acute bronchitis is most often caused by a viral infection. Acute bronchitis may occur as a complication of chronic bronchitis.

   Emphysema is a destructive process involving the lung parenchyma. It is defined as abnormal permanent enlargement of air spaces distal to the terminal bronchioles accompanied by destruction of alveolar walls.

   Right-sided heart failure and cor pulmonale may result from chronic bronchitis and/or emphysema. Obstructive sleep apnea is often a complication of COPD. Hypercarbia (increased Pco_2 level) is a valuable prognostic sign in chronic bronchitis and allows the prediction of when certain therapies, especially home oxygen, should be used.

3. E. Chronic bronchitis usually develops in cigarette smokers 10 to 12 years after smoking began. Patients with chronic bronchitis have an increased susceptibility to recurrent respiratory tract infections.

   Chronic obstructive lung disease develops in 10%-15% of patients who are cigarette smokers. In these patients, airflow obstruction worsens over time if cigarette smoking is continued.

   Dyspnea is initially noted only on extreme exertion, but as the COPD progresses, it becomes more severe and occurs with mild activity. In severe disease, dyspnea may occur at rest.

   Complications of COPD include pneumonia, pulmonary hypertension, cor pulmonale, and chronic respiratory failure.

4. D. Chronic obstructive pulmonary disease patients are divided into two basic types: Type A COPD patients, or "pink puffers," and Type B COPD patients, or "blue bloaters." The patient described in this question is a typical blue bloater.

   Blue bloaters are (1) often stocky or obese, (2) often have cough and sputum production, (3) have normal or increased lung markings, (4) usually have a markedly reduced Po_2 and an elevated Pco_2, and (5) often develop pulmonary hypertension and/or cor pulmonale. Blue bloaters = Chronic bronchitis.

   Pink puffers are (1) usually thin, (2) usually have dyspnea, (3) have hyperinflated lungs on CXR, (4) have a slightly decreased Po_2 and a normal or slightly decreased Pco_2. Pink puffers = Emphysema.

5. D. Chronic bronchitis is characterized by several abnormalities observed on pulmonary function testing. Abnormalities noted most frequently include (1) an increased (not decreased) residual volume, (2) a decrease in FEV_1 (the forced vital capacity in 1 second), (3) a decrease in FEV_1/FVC, and (4) a decrease in FEF_{25-75}.

6. D. Most mucus is secreted by subepithelial glands in the large airways. It follows that chronic bronchitis, a disorder characterized by chronic, excessive secretion of mucus, is a disease of the large airways. Most histologic studies of chronic bronchitis have shown an increase in the size of the mucus-secreting glands as measured by the Reid Index (a ratio of gland to bronchial wall thickness), although no clear-cut relation between this index and the degree of airflow obstruction has been established. Patients with chronic bronchitis also have smooth muscle hyperplasia; however, unlike the situation in asthma, there is no clear-cut relationship between their responsiveness or methacholine sensitivity. Bronchial hyperresponsiveness, which is present in at least 50% of patients with COPD, may lead to dyspnea and hypoxemia.

7. E. It is commonly thought that cigarette smoking is the only risk factor for COPD. In fact, a number of other risk factors are implicated: (1) exposure to tobacco smoke; (2) domestic and occupational pollutants and recurrent respiratory tract infections, particularly in infancy; (3) atopy, which is characterized by eosinophilia or an increased level of serum immunoglobulin E (IgE); (4) the presence of bronchial hyperresponsiveness; (5) a

family history of COPD; and (6) certain protease deficiencies such as alpha$_1$-antitrypsin deficiency.

8. F. Cigarette smoking, as the most common cause of chronic bronchitis, leads to loss of ciliated epithelium and more viscous secretions, compromising the local defenses of the respiratory tract. The delay in mucociliary clearance allows inhaled bacteria to colonize the normally sterile airways and to multiply, leading to further infectious exacerbations. *Haemophilus influenzae* is present in the sputum of about 60% of patients with stable chronic bronchitis. This organism may act synergistically with tobacco smoke to impede mucociliary clearance and allow further multiplication and colonization of the airway. Byproducts of *H. influenzae* have been shown to cause further impairment of ciliated cells in vitro, stimulate mucus production, and secrete IgA protease that may further impair host defenses. In addition, nicotine has been shown to stimulate the growth of this organism; and *H. influenzae* has been shown to engender an immune reaction in the airways.

9. E. The diagnosis of chronic bronchitis rests on clinical criteria that have already been described. There are no characteristic physical findings and no specific radiographic changes or laboratory features diagnostic of this disease.

    The differential diagnosis of chronic cough, however, must be considered. This includes (1) asthma, (2) postnasal drip, (3) gastroesophageal reflux, (4) foreign body aspiration, (5) congestive heart failure, (6) bronchiectasis, and (7) chronic ACE inhibitor therapy (15% of patients on ACE inhibitors develop a chronic cough).

10. D. The cessation of smoking produces dramatic symptomatic benefits for patients with chronic bronchitis. Coughing stops in up to 77% of quitters and improves in 17%. When coughing stops, it does so within 4 weeks in 54% of patients.

    Influenza virus can worsen the epithelial damage induced by cigarette smoke and predispose the airways to subsequent bacterial proliferation, leading to excessive mucus hypersecretion and greater airflow obstruction. Annual influenza vaccination reduces morbidity and mortality caused by influenza in patients with COPD, although its role in this disease has not been assessed in large-scale clinical trials.

11. B.

12. D.

13. D. Symptomatic therapy for patients with chronic bronchitis includes the use of (1) inhaled bronchodilators, (2) oral bronchodilators, (3) inhaled corticosteroids, (4) oral corticosteroids, (5) inhaled anticholinergics, (6)

home oxygen therapy, and (7) rehabilitation programs.

    The use of inhaled bronchodilators by patients with airflow obstruction may increase flow rates and reduce dyspnea. Inhaled anticholinergic agents appear to produce greater bronchodilatation than inhaled beta 2 agonists in COPD, with fewer side effects. This may be related to increased cholinergic tone in the airways as the degree of obstruction progresses. Combination therapy with agents from both groups may have an additive effect in some patients. Patients who demonstrate symptomatic or physiologic improvement, or both, with these medications should be maintained on the inhaled drugs indefinitely. In patients who remain symptomatic on inhaled bronchodilators, a trial of an oral theophylline medication is warranted. These medications are weaker bronchodilators than inhaled anticholinergics or beta-agonist drugs but may have additional beneficial effects in chronic bronchitis by increasing respiratory muscle strength and endurance, improving mucociliary clearance, and increasing central respiratory drive, all of which may lead to a symptomatic improvement in patients with the disease.

    At present, regular use of oral or inhaled corticosteroids cannot be recommended as routine therapy for all patients with chronic bronchitis. Although steroids have clear anti-inflammatory effects and decrease mucus hypersecretion, a beneficial effect can be shown in only 10% to 20% of patients.

    The benefits of home oxygen therapy have been clearly demonstrated in major clinical trials. To be considered candidates for treatment, patients must be (1) in a stable clinical state, (2) have a resting arterial partial pressure of oxygen Pa$_{O_2}$ of 55 mm Hg or less, or (3) have a Pa$_{O_2}$ of 60 mm Hg with evidence of chronic tissue hypoxia as demonstrated by cor pulmonale or polycythemia. In properly selected patients, the use of home oxygen for more than 18 hr/day may increase the life span of the COPD patient by 6 or 7 years.

14. E.

15. E. Treatment of an acute exacerbation of chronic bronchitis provides symptomatic relief and prevents any transient decline in pulmonary function. Low-flow oxygen should be instituted if hypoxemia is present (as in this case). The goal of oxygen therapy in this case is to get the Pa$_{O_2}$ above 60 mm Hg. In addition, oral or IV corticosteroids should be given, as they have been shown to hasten the resolution of patients in the acute exacerbation phase of chronic bronchitis.

    Patients with all three of the following "acute exacerbative symptoms" have been shown to benefit from antibiotic therapy: (1) increasing dyspnea, (2) increased sputum production, and (3) purulence of sputum.

    In patients with two or less of the three symptoms, the case is less clear. The following antibiotics have been found to be equally effective in cases as just described: (1) trimethoprim-sulfamethoxazole, (2) amoxicillin, and (3) doxycycline.

Antibiotic choices should obviously be based on both host and pathogen factors. The latter relate to resistance problems. The three most common isolates associated with acute exacerbations of chronic bronchitis are (1) *Haemophilus influenzae*, (2) *Streptococcus pneumoniae*, and (3) *Moraxella catarrhalis*.

16. **F.** This patient has acute bronchitis and is a healthy young man with no concomitant illnesses. The cause of acute bronchitis in a patient like this is almost always a viral infection (adenovirus, influenza virus, or rhinovirus). It has only been present for 24 hours, and at this time there is *no good reason* for prescribing an antibiotic. What your partner says or what your patient expects are not satisfactory reasons for doing something that, on the basis of probability, is likely to do no good whatsoever.

A reasonable treatment protocol to follow for the treatment of acute bronchitis follows:
1. Healthy middle-aged adult; no other respiratory problems; cough and purulent sputum production of short duration: no culture; no antibiotic
2. Healthy middle-aged adult; no other respiratory problems; cough and purulent sputum production persists for longer than one week: no culture; macrolide antibiotic (to cover mycoplasma)
3. Healthy elderly adult; no other respiratory problems; cough and purulent sputum production of short duration: no culture; no antibiotic.
4. Healthy elderly adult; no other respiratory problems, cough and purulent sputum production for greater than 1 week: no culture; septra or amoxicillin
5. Elderly adult with chronic disease; cough and sputum production: no culture initially; septra no matter how long symptoms have persisted

SOLUTION TO SHORT ANSWER MANAGEMENT PROBLEM 9

The two forms of COPD are (1) chronic bronchitis and (2) emphysema.

A. Chronic bronchitis affects the large airways of the lung
Emphysema affects the terminal bronchi.

B. Color of lips in severely affected individuals:
Chronic bronchitis: Blue; the "blue bloater"
Emphysema: Pink; the "pink puffer"

C. Definitions:
Chronic bronchitis: Excessive cough, productive of sputum on most days, for at least 3 months a year, during at least 2 consecutive years

Emphysema: Defined histologically by abnormal permanent enlargement, without obvious fibrosis, of the airspaces distal to the terminal bronchi, accompanied by destruction of their walls.

D. Pathophysiology:
Chronic bronchitis: (1) Chronic, excessive secretion of mucus; (2) increase in the size of the mucus-secreting cells; (3) smooth muscle hyperplasia; and (4) bronchial airway hyperresponsiveness
Emphysema: (1) Distal airspace enlargement; (2) no significant fibrosis; (3) loss of alveolar attachments; (4) decrease in elastic recoil; (5) increase in lung compliance; (6) hyperinflation; and (7) ventilation-perfusion mismatching
Cause: Most cases of both chronic bronchitis and emphysema are due to cigarette smoking; alpha-1-antitrypsin deficiency is a factor in some cases of emphysema.

SUMMARY OF THE DIAGNOSIS AND MANAGEMENT OF CHRONIC OBSTRUCTIVE PULMONARY DISEASE

1. **Definitions:** See the short answer management problem.
2. **Pathophysiology:** See the short answer management problem.
3. **Differentiation of disease entities in COPD:** See the short answer management problem.
4. **Signs and symptoms:**
   a) Symptoms: Dyspnea, cough, sputum production, and sputum purulence. When cor pulmonale and right-sided heart failure present—extremity swelling
   b) Signs: Increased respiratory rate, respiratory distress, cyanosis, barrel chest, distant heart sounds, increased JVP
   c) Three most important signs/symptoms indicating deterioration: (1) Increasing dyspnea; (2) increased sputum volume; and (3) increased purulence
5. **Pulmonary function test abnormalities:**
   a) Decreased FEV_1
   b) Decreased ratio of FEV_1/FVC
   c) Decreased FEF_{25-75}
   d) Increased residual volume
   e) Normal to increased functional residual capacity
   f) Decreased diffusion capacity
6. **Pathologic organisms associated with infection in COPD:**
   a) *Haemophilus influenzae*
   b) *Streptococcus pneumoniae*
   c) *Moraxella catarrhalis*
7. **Treatment:**
   a) Bronchodilators:
      1. Best single agent for long-term treatment in chronic bronchitis is an inhaled anticholinergic-ipratropium (Atrovent).
      2. Beta agonists should be combined with (1).

b) Corticosteroids: Routine use of inhaled corticosteroids cannot be recommended in chronic care. Corticosteroids (both inhaled and IV/oral) are most helpful in acute exacerbations.

c) Antibiotics: Routine prophylactic use of antibiotics cannot be recommended. Most useful in acute exacerbations if all three of the following are present: (i) increasing dyspnea; (ii) increasing sputum production; and (iii) increasing sputum purulence. Antibiotics of choice include (i) TMP-SMX; (ii) amoxicillin; and (iii) doxycycline.

d) Home oxygen: Home oxygen indicated if (1) $PaO_2 < 55$ mm Hg or less at rest or (2) $PaO_2 < 60$ mm Hg with evidence of chronic tissue hypoxia as demonstrated by cor pulmonale or polycythemia.

e) Diuretics: Use indicated only for treatment of cor pulmonale and right-sided heart failure

f) Smoking cessation: At any time in the course of COPD smoking cessation can be and is of benefit. Do not accept "I've smoked too long and I am too old to quit."

g) Counseling/support groups: Group therapy with other COPD patients is often helpful in helping the patient come to terms with the disease.

SUGGESTED READING

Proceedings from the Canadian Bronchitis Symposium, Toronto, Canada, February, 1994. Recommendations on the management of chronic bronchitis: A practical guide for Canadian physicians. Supplement, CMAJ 1994; 151(10).

PROBLEM 10   A 22-YEAR-OLD MALE WITH A CHRONIC COUGH

A 22-year-old male presents to your office for assessment of a chronic cough. He has just moved to your city and will be attending the university there. He has moved into a bachelor apartment in the basement of a house.

As soon as he moved in, he began to notice a chronic, nonproductive cough associated with shortness of breath. He has never had these symptoms before, and he has no known allergies. When he leaves for school for the day, the symptoms disappear. The symptoms are definitely worse at night.

His landlady, however, has three cats. He didn't think he was allergic to cats, but now he thinks that might, in fact, be the case.

On examination, his respiratory rate is 16 and regular. He is in no distress at the present time. There are a few expiratory rhonchi heard in all lobes. His blood pressure is 120/70, and his pulse is 72 and regular.

SELECT THE ONE BEST ANSWER TO THE FOLLOWING QUESTIONS

1. What is the most likely diagnosis in this patient?
   a) paroxysmal nocturnal cough syndrome
   b) hyporesponsive airways disease
   c) cough variant asthma
   d) bronchial asthma: nonwheezing variant
   e) allergic bronchitis

2. In children, which of the following statements is(are) true?
   a) it is often difficult to differentiate bronchial asthma from bronchiolitis
   b) children with bronchiolitis who do not develop asthma may be inappropriately labeled with the "stigma" of asthma
   c) the relationship between bronchiolitis, ongoing bronchial hyperactivity, and bronchial asthma is unclear; it appears that bronchiolitis may precipitate bronchial asthma
   d) all of the above
   e) none of the above

3. Which of the following is(are) included in the working definition of bronchial asthma?
   a) reversible airway obstruction
   b) bronchial airway inflammation
   c) bronchial airway hyperresponsiveness to a variety of stimuli
   d) expiratory rhonchi
   e) a, b, and c
   f) all of the above

4. Which of the following statements regarding health care costs and mortality regarding bronchial asthma is(are) false?
   a) the mortality from bronchial asthma is decreasing (presumably because of improved therapies)
   b) more cases of bronchial asthma are being associated with environmental pollutants than was the case previously
   c) in the United States in 1990, the estimated health care costs associated with bronchial asthma was approximately $3.4 million

   d) all of the above statements are false
   e) none of the above statements are false

5. Bronchial asthma, on a pathophysiologic basis, is primarily:
   a) a bronchoconstricting process
   b) an allergenic stimulus process
   c) an inflammatory process
   d) a bronchial hyperreactivity process
   e) an IgE-mediated antigen-antibody reaction

6. Following antigenic stimulation of the bronchial airway, which cell is most responsible for the beginning of the airway's response?
   a) the basophil
   b) the mast cell
   c) the eosinophil
   d) the bronchial epithelial cell
   e) the bronchial mucous-producing goblet cells

7. What are the substances released by the cell mentioned in Question 6?
   a) histamine
   b) proteolytic enzymes
   c) heparin
   d) chemotactic factors
   e) all of the above

8. The substance(s) described in Question 7 produce which of the following?
   a) bronchoconstriction of the airway
   b) inflammation of the airway
   c) bronchodilation of the airway
   d) all of the above
   e) none of the above

9. The event described in Question 6 leads to activation of which of the following?
   a) neutrophils
   b) eosinophils
   c) mononuclear cells
   d) b and c
   e) all of the above

10. The recruitment of the cells described above results primarily in which of the following?
    a) bronchoconstriction
    b) inflammation of the airways
    c) mucous cell hyperplasia and hypertrophy
    d) b and c
    e) all of the above

11. What is the classic hallmark of bronchial asthma?
    a) bronchial hyperresponsiveness
    b) bronchial hyporesponsiveness
    c) wheezing
    d) shortness of breath
    e) nocturnal dyspnea

12. A 24-year-old woman patient develops wheezing and shortness of breath when exposed to cold air or when exercising. These symptoms are getting worse. Which of the following is the prophylactic agent of choice for the treatment of bronchial asthma in these circumstances?
    a) inhaled beta-2 agonists
    b) oral aminophylline
    c) inhaled anticholinergics
    d) inhaled sodium cromoglycate
    e) oral corticosteroids

13. What is the mechanism of action of the agent of choice in Question 12?
    a) mast cell stabilizer
    b) inhibitor of early-phase reaction
    c) inhibitor of late-phase reaction
    d) all of the above
    e) none of the above

14. What is the treatment of choice for immediate bronchodilation?
    a) an inhaled beta-2 agonist
    b) oral aminophylline
    c) an inhaled anticholinergic
    d) an inhaled sodium cromoglycate
    e) oral corticosteroids

15. Which of the following statements regarding inhaled beta-2 agonists is(are) true?
    a) inhaled beta-2 agonists are completely safe agents
    b) inhaled beta-2 agonists have been associated with increased mortality in asthma
    c) inhaled beta-2 agonists can be used as often as needed during the day
    d) a and c
    e) b and c

16. Which of the following beta-2 agonists has been most commonly implicated in side effects?
    a) metaproterenol
    b) terbutaline
    c) albuterol
    d) pirbuterol
    e) none of the above

17. Which of the following most accurately describes the preferred treatment of chronic bronchial asthma in patients with moderately severe disease?
    a) inhaled sodium cromoglycate alone
    b) inhaled beta-2 agonists alone
    c) inhaled corticosteroids alone
    d) inhaled corticosteroids continually plus intermittent inhaled beta-2 agonists
    e) inhaled sodium cromoglycate continually plus intermittent inhaled beta-2 agonists

18. The early phase of bronchial asthma bronchoconstriction is associated with which of the following drugs as the drug's only mediating effect?
    a) an inhaled beta agonist
    b) inhaled sodium cromoglycate
    c) an inhaled corticosteroid
    d) all of the above
    e) none of the above

19. Which of the following agents affect the previously described late-phase reaction of asthma only?
    a) an inhaled beta-2 agonist
    b) inhaled sodium cromoglycate
    c) an inhaled corticosteroid
    d) all of the above
    e) none of the above

20. Which of the following agents affect the previously described early-phase reaction plus the late-phase reaction of asthma?
    a) an inhaled beta-2 agonist
    b) inhaled sodium cromoglycate
    c) an inhaled corticosteroid
    d) all of the above
    e) none of the above

21. Which of the following pulmonary function tests is the most useful for diagnosis of bronchial asthma?
    a) decreased forced vital capacity
    b) increased residual volume
    c) a ratio of $FEV_1/FVC < 75\%$
    d) increased functional residual capacity
    e) increased total lung capacity

22. Which of the following pulmonary function tests is most easily carried out at home?
    a) FEV_1/FVC ratio
    c) forced vital capacity
    c) mid-expiratory flow rate
    d) peak expiratory flow rate
    e) residual volume

23. Which of the following is the most common abnormality observed on the chest X-ray in a patient with asthma?
    a) hyperinflation
    b) increased bronchial markings
    c) atelectasis
    d) flattening of the diaphragm
    e) all of the above are equally common

24. What is the most common abnormality seen on physical examination of an asthmatic patient?
    a) use of the accessory muscles of respiration
    b) inspiratory rales
    c) inspiratory rhonchi
    d) expiratory rales
    e) expiratory rhonchi

25. Asthma in children is often worse than asthma in adults due to the smaller diameter of the airway. The diameter of a child's airway is 6 mm at a certain point in the airway. This is reduced to 4 mm during an acute attack of bronchial asthma. Previously, he had an airflow of 81 air flow units (AFUs). What will this child's airflow be through that particular section of the bronchial tree during the acute attack of asthma?
    a) 64 AFUs
    b) 48 AFUs
    c) 32 AFUs
    d) 24 AFUs
    e) 16 AFUs

26. Pure cough variant asthma has which of the following characteristics?
    a) patients often have to go from doctor to doctor until someone makes the diagnosis
    b) patients are treated in the same manner as non-cough variant asthma
    c) cough variant asthma is very uncommon
    d) a and b
    e) all of the above

27. Which of the following statements regarding extrinsic asthma and intrinsic asthma is(are) true?
    a) intrinsic asthma is more common in asthmatic children than in asthmatic adults
    b) extrinsic asthma is more common in asthmatic adults than in asthmatic children
    c) extrinsic asthma more often leads to chronic obstructive pulmonary disease than does intrinsic asthma
    d) intrinsic asthma is more easily treated than extrinsic asthma
    e) none of the above are true

28. A patient who presents to the ER in acute respiratory distress due to a severe attack of asthma should be treated with all of the following *except:*
    a) warm, humidified, high-flow-rate oxygen
    b) constant bedside monitoring
    c) intravenous corticosteroids
    d) epinephrine subcutaneously
    e) discharge of the patient the same day if his condition is stable

29. Which of the following statements regarding childhood asthma is(are) false?
    a) there is a very significant hereditary component to the probability of a child acquiring asthma
    b) asthma in children is associated with parental smoking
    c) asthmatic children are often allergic to ASA (aspirin)
    d) inhaled corticosteroids, administered properly, do not pose a major risk or hazard to childhood growth
    e) many children who are asthmatic go on to outgrow it

30. Which of the following viral agents has been implicated as a cause of bronchial asthma?
    a) respiratory syncytial virus
    b) parainfluenza virus
    c) adenovirus
    d) rhinovirus
    e) influenza virus

Short Answer Management Problem 10

Clinical Puzzle

A rural family physician has noticed an interesting phenomenon. This summer, there have been two very severe lightning storms. In the first instance, approximately 1 hour after the storm subsided, six children displayed signs and symptoms of bronchial asthma. In the second instance, eight children displayed signs and symptoms of bronchial asthma an hour after the storm. (Only three children appeared on both occasions.)

 Can you explain this?

ANSWERS

1. C. This patient has cough variant asthma. Physicians should be aware that cough variant asthma is particularly common in children but can occur, as in this case, in adults as well. The diagnosis is often missed because in many cases there is no wheezing.

2. D. First, it is sometimes difficult to differentiate on the basis of symptoms, signs, and laboratory findings between bronchial asthma and bronchiolitis. Second, a physician may, in fact, make an inappropriate diagnosis of bronchial asthma that may "stick for life." Third, the relationship between bronchiolitis and bronchial asthma is unclear. There is good evidence at this time that bronchiolitis is a very significant risk factor for bronchial asthma and may predispose to bronchial asthma.

3. E. The current working definition of bronchial asthma is as follows:
   A. A lung disease with airway obstruction that is usually reversible
   B. A lung disease that is characterized by airway inflammation
   C. A lung disease that is characterized by increased bronchial hyperresponsiveness to various stimuli

4. A. The morbidity and mortality from bronchial asthma are increasing, not decreasing. It is associated with staggering health care costs: It is estimated that the direct cost in 1990 dollars in health expenditure for asthma was approximately $3.4 billion, and the indirect costs were estimated to be another $2.5 billion.

   These costs are almost certainly going to continue to increase in the future. Despite the vast sums of money invested in both direct and indirect health care for asthma prevention and management, the mortality from asthma continues to rise.

5. C. The pathophysiology of bronchial asthma has undergone considerable change in the past few years. This has had a substantial impact on treatment. The pathophysiology of bronchial asthma has changed from that of a noninflammatory disorder to an inflammatory disorder. Although bronchoconstriction and bronchial hyperreactivity are characteristics of bronchial asthma, the basic underlying pathophysiologic process is inflammation of the bronchial wall.

6. B.

7. E.

8. A.

9. E.

10. B.

11. A.

The Pathophysiology of Bronchial Asthma

Questions 6-11 describe the pathophysiology of bronchial asthma. The order of events is outlined as follows:

Event 1: Beginning of the response of the bronchial wall to the particular antigenic stimulation
Event 2: Antigenic stimulation leads to mast cell degranulation
Event 3: Mast cell degranulation leads to:
   A. Immediate release of performed mediators from granules
   B. Release of secondary mediators, including:
      1. Histamine
      2. Chemotactic factors
      3. Proteolytic enzymes
      4. Heparin
Event 4: The release of these mediators leads to significant smooth muscle bronchoconstriction.
Event 5: The initial bronchial constriction leads to recruitment of other inflammatory cells, including the following:
   1. Neutrophils
   2. Eosinophils
   3. Mononuclear cells
Event 6: The recruitment of these "secondary mediator cells" has demonstrated the release of the following:
   1. Cytokines
   2. Vasoactive factors
   3. Arachidonic acid metabolites
Event 7: Activation of epithelial and endothelial cells occurs, enhancing inflammatory responses.
Event 8: Release of interleukins 3 to 6, tumor necrosis factor, and interferon-gamma has been demonstrated in the inflammatory response.

Importance of These Series of Events:
   1. The early-phase reaction of asthma is mediated by the "primary mediators": neutrophils, eosinophils, and mononuclear cells.
   2. The late-phase reaction of asthma is mediated by the "secondary mediators": cytokines, vasoactive factors, and arachidonic acid metabolites.

Important Summary Points
   1. The mast cell begins the process.
   2. Bronchoconstriction is the primary event.
   3. Bronchial wall inflammation is the secondary event.
   4. Bronchial wall hyperresponsiveness is the hallmark of asthma.

12. D.

13. D. The prophylactic agent of choice for exercise-induced or cold-air-induced bronchial asthma is sodium cromoglycate. Sodium cromoglycate is a mast cell stabilizer that affects the early-phase and the late-phase reactions.

14. A. The treatment of choice for immediate and intermediate bronchodilation in patients with bronchial asthma is an inhaled beta-2 agonist.

15. B.

16. B.

17. D. The mortality from asthma is increasing. The reasons for that increase are unclear. However, there appears to be a possible association between the increased use of beta-2 agonists and that increase in mortality.

    Of the beta-2 agonists, the agent that has been implicated more often than the others is terbutaline. The long-term treatment of bronchial asthma (pharmacologic treatment) should include the following:
    1. Liberal use of sodium cromoglycate to prevent both exercise-induced and cold-induced asthma
    2. Long-term use of inhaled corticosteroids to decrease airway inflammation
    3. Intermittent and cautious use of inhaled beta-2 agonists (no more than 4 times/day)

18. A.

19. C.

20. B. First, sodium cromoglycate prevents both early and late bronchorestrictive phases of asthma. That is why it is so valuable in the treatment of asthma that comes on after exercise. Second, the early phase of bronchorestriction are prevented by administration of a beta-2 agonist. Third, the late phase of bronchorestriction is prevented by the administration of a corticosteroid.

21. C.

22. C.

23. B.

24. E. Following is an overview of pulmonary function tests and their importance in asthma.

Overview of Physical Examination Findings, Chest X-Ray Findings, and Pulmonary Function Tests in Asthma

I. Physical Examination Signs and Symptoms
   A. Increased respiratory rate
   B. Use of accessory muscles of respiration (intercostals, sternocleidomastoid, scalene muscles)
   C. Dyspnea and anxiety
   D. The most characteristic lung finding on auscultation is expiratory rhonchi; rhonchi are high-pitched sounds that occur when air has to travel through a constricted or inflamed passageway
   E. Nasal flaring
   F. Cyanosis in severe cases (lips)
   G. Paroxysmal cough

II. Chest X-Ray Findings
   A. The most characteristic CXR abnormality in bronchial asthma is the presence of increased bronchial wall markings. This is most prominent when viewed from the end-on position.

      This finding is due to (1) increase in the thickness of the bronchial wall and (2) changes in the epithelium that are associated with inflammation. These changes are translated into increased radio-opacity.
   B. There is also flattening of the diaphragm in some cases due to chronic inflammation and use of the accessory muscles of respiration.

III. Most Useful Pulmonary Function Tests
   A. FEV_1/FVC in percentage: (normal $> 80\%$). This measures the amount of air volume that can be expressed in one second over the total amount of lung air volume that can be expressed. It is by far the most important test done in a spirometry laboratory for the diagnosis and management of bronchial asthma.
   B. MEF_{25-75} in percentage: (normal $> 75\%$). This is the maximum expiratory flow that occurs between 25% and 75% of the vital capacity.
   C. Mid-expiratory flow rate: This test is done using a peak flow meter at home, and once a baseline is established it can certainly predict worsening asthma. The most important aspects of these tests are as follows:
      1. They allow pulmonary function measurement at home.
      2. They provide an early-warning system for the possibility of a severe asthma attack, especially in a child. The reading in this case would be very worrisome if it has decreased significantly and abruptly after a long period of stability.

25. E. The relationship between vessel radius and airflow is very important. For a very small change in the diameter of the airway, there is a very large change in airflow. The airflow in the bronchial tubes is proportional to the inverse of the fourth power of the radius.

    Therefore, in this Question,
    Original situation:
    A. Diameter = 6 MM
    B. Therefore, radius = 3 MM

C. A radius of 3 MM in this section of the airway produces an airway of 81 AFUs (airflow units) (3 × 3 × 3 × 3 = 81 AFUs)

Following the decrease in diameter of the airway:

A. Diameter = 4 MM

B. Therefore, radius = 2 MM

C. (2 × 2 × 2 × 2 = 16 AFUs)

26. D. The following features of cough variant asthma should be borne in mind:

1. Cough variant asthma is very common. At least 33% of children with asthma will have only the cough, no wheezing.

2. Adults, as with the patient described, may also present with cough variant asthma.

27. E. This is an important distinguishing point. Following is a comparison of the two varieties of asthma.

I. Extrinsic asthma:

1. Extrinsic asthma is associated with a precipitating factor that is almost always an allergen.

2. Extrinsic asthma is much more common in children than in adults.

3. If age is used as a variable, the following applies: extrinsic asthma—onset before age 40.

4. The most important aspects of treatment are (1) trying to find out what the allergen is and (2) how to get rid of it.

5. The most common extrinsic allergens in children are house dust and house dust mites.

II. Intrinsic asthma:

1. Intrinsic asthma is usually associated with a non-allergic etiology.

2. Intrinsic asthma is much more common in adults than in children.

3. If age is used as a variable, the following applies: extrinsic asthma—onset before age 40; intrinsic asthma—onset after age 40.

4. Treatment: most important treatment is (as in intrinsic asthma) to identify and eliminate the cause; this, however, is often very difficult.

5. The basic treatment of intrinsic asthma is corticosteroid therapy.

28. E. An acute, severe asthmatic attack is an emergency. The basic elements of treatment are as follows:

Treatment of severe, acute asthma:

1. Epinephrine 0.3 cc subcut (this can be repeated every 5 minutes).

2. The patient should be sitting up.

3. Immediately give the patient warm, humidified 100% oxygen via a venturi mask.

4. Start two intravenous lines.

5. Begin an IV corticosteroid (such as solucortef) immediately.

6. Draw blood gases and electrolytes.

7. Mix a beta-2 agonist and an anticholinergic in neb-mix solution and add that to the oxygen delivery system (this neb-mix solution can be administered for five minutes every 15 to 20 minutes).

8. Monitor vital signs continuously (with an ECG hooked into the main computer at the nurses' desk).

9. Once the patient is stable, transfer him or her to an observation unit ward: if this has been a severe attack and you have had trouble controlling it, do not discharge the patient.

29. E. First, there is a very significant heredity component to bronchial asthma. If one parent has it, the child may have up to a 25% risk. If two parents have it, the child's risk may be up to 50%.

Second, there is a very strong association between parental smoking and bronchial asthma in children.

Third, many children who have bronchial asthma are allergic to aspirin and other nonsteroidal antiinflammatory drugs.

Remember that: asthma + nasal polyps + aspirin allergy is a recognized triad.

Finally, patients do not "outgrow" asthma. Children who have asthma may, in fact, experience less severe attacks as adults, or they may never experience problems. They have not, however, outgrown it.

30. A. There appears to be a very strong association between respiratory syncytial virus (the cause of bronchiolitis) and bronchial asthma. Although it is difficult to say that the relationship is cause and effect, there is enough good evidence to suggest that it might be.

SOLUTION TO SHORT ANSWER MANAGEMENT PROBLEM 10

Indeed, this is a fascinating situation. The town in which the physician practices is, by the way, very small. It has only 3200 people.

An environmentalist she knew suggested the possibility of ozone production as a side effect of the lightning strikes. In fact, ozone has been shown to be associated with bronchial asthma, and it appears that this is the most probable explanation.

SUMMARY OF THE DIAGNOSIS AND TREATMENT OF BRONCHIAL ASTHMA

1. All that wheezes is not asthma, and all asthma does not wheeze.

2. A moderately severe to severe attack of bronchial asthma is an emergency. Do not discharge the patient unless you are very sure that the asthma attack is completely resolved.

3. Bronchial asthma is an inflammatory disease.

4. The mortality from asthma is rising, not falling.
5. There is effective prophylaxis for exercise-induced asthma.
6. Cough variant asthma is very common.
7. Beta-2 agonists (especially terbutaline) have been tentatively linked to the increase in asthma mortality. If they have to be used more than four times/day, your patient's asthma is out of control.
8. There is nothing wrong with a short course of oral steroids (prednisone 20 mg to 30 mg/day) for a severe case of asthma. It works, and it will keep the patient out of the hospital and out of danger.
9. Suggest peak flow meters to all of your asthmatic patients for home monitoring.
10. Bronchial hyperresponsiveness is the hallmark of bronchial asthma.
11. Drugs of choice for chronic asthma:
    First choice: inhaled corticosteroids
    Second choice: inhaled Beta-2 agonisis
    Drug of choice for prophylaxis of exercise-induced asthma: sodium chromoglycate

SUGGESTED READING

Khan D, Li J. Asthma in adolescents and adults. In: Rakel R, ed. Conn's current therapy. Philadelphia: WB Saunders, 1994.

PROBLEM 11   A 24-YEAR-OLD UNIVERSITY STUDENT WITH A PNEUMONIA

A 24-year-old university student presents to the Student Health Service with a 3-day history of a dry, hacking cough that was initially nonproductive but has become productive of scant, white sputum. The patient also complains of malaise, headache, fever, and muscle aches and pains. The patient did not have any other upper respiratory tract symptoms before this illness began (no rhinorrhea, no sore throat, no conjunctivitis, and so on).

The patient has had no episodes like this in the past; however, her roommate developed the same symptoms 2 days ago.

On examination, the patient has a temperature of 39° C. You hear a few scattered rales in the left lung base. No other abnormalities are found.

SELECT THE ONE BEST ANSWER TO THE FOLLOWING QUESTIONS

1. Which of the following is the most cost-effective strategy at the present time?
   a) order no laboratory tests or imaging investigations; assume that it is viral and will clear up on its own
   b) order no laboratory tests or imaging investigations; treat with ampicillin just to be on the safe side
   c) order the complete workup: every possible test; no matter what the patient has, you are not the one who is going to get sued
   d) order a chest X-ray on the basis of your clinical findings
   e) forget the tests; just treat her with "big gun therapy," guaranteed to kill anything that vaguely resembles a bug

2. What is the most likely diagnosis in this patient?
   a) viral pneumonia
   b) *Mycoplasma pneumoniae*
   c) *Streptococcus pneumoniae*
   d) *Klebsiella pneumoniae*
   e) no pneumonia of any kind; a case of simple acute bronchitis

3. If you ordered a chest X-ray, what would be the most likely finding?
   a) nothing: clear and normal
   b) left lower lobe pneumonia
   c) left lower lobe interstitial pneumonia
   d) bilateral lower lobe infiltrates
   e) bilateral upper lobe infiltrates

4. What is the treatment of choice for the patient described in Question 1?
   a) symptomatic treatment only
   b) ribavirin for respiratory syncytial virus
   c) erythromycin
   d) ampicillin
   e) penicillin G

5. A 55-year-old female, previously healthy and recovering from an episode of bronchitis, suddenly develops a "shaking chill" followed by the onset of a high fever—40° C; pleuritic chest pain, and cough productive of purulent, rust-colored sputum.

   On examination, the patient appears ill. Her respiratory rate is 30/minute, and chest splinting is heard. Bronchial breath sounds are heard in the left lower lobe. Chest X-ray reveals consolidation present in the left lower lobe.

   On the basis of the history, the physical examination, and the chest X-ray, what is the most likely organism responsible for this patient's illness?
   a) gram-negative rod
   b) gram-negative cocci
   c) gram-positive rod
   d) gram-positive cocci (lancet-shaped)
   e) no growth on aerobic growth media

6. What is the most likely organism responsible for this patient's illness?
   a) *Streptococcus pneumoniae*
   b) *Klebsiella pneumoniae*
   c) *Mycoplasma pneumoniae*
   d) influenza A
   e) *Haemophilus influenzae*

7. What is the definitive treatment of choice for the patient described in Question 5?
   a) penicillin G
   b) erythromycin
   c) ampicillin
   d) gentamicin
   e) c and d

8. A 35-year-old male patient with chronic renal failure who had a renal transplant 6 months ago and is being treated with corticosteroids and cyclosporine has failed to respond to the following antibiotics for treatment of a pneumonia: (1) ampicillin and gentamicin, (2) ceftriaxone, and (3) cefazolin. On the basis of his immunocompromised status and his failure to respond to the antibiotics listed, what is the most likely organism causing his pneumonia?
   a) *Pneumocystitis carinii*
   b) *Legionella*
   c) Mycobacterium tuberculosis
   d) *Mycobacterium avium intracellulare*
   e) Cytomegalovirus

9. What is the drug of first choice for the patient described in Question 8?
   a) erythromycin (EES)
   b) clarithromycin
   c) ciprofloxacin
   d) trimethoprim-sulfamethoxazole
   e) doxycycline

10. A 75-year-old alcoholic with a history of congestive heart failure is admitted to hospital suffering from fever, shortness of breath, chest pain, and cough productive of purulent sputum and blood.

    On physical examination, the patient has a temperature of 39°C, a respiratory rate of 28/minute, and bronchial breath sounds in the right upper lobe.

    A chest X-ray confirms the diagnosis of a right upper lobe pneumonia. What is the most likely organism responsible for this patient's illness?
    a) *Streptococcus pneumoniae*
    b) *Klebsiella pneumoniae*
    c) *Mycoplasma pneumoniae*
    d) influenza A pneumonia
    e) *Haemophilus influenzae pneumoniae*

11. What is(are) the treatment(s) of choice for the patient described in Question 10?
    a) erythromycin
    b) cefuroxine plus clarithromycin
    c) penicillin G
    d) ampicillin
    e) ampicillin plus gentamicin

12. A 55-year-old male with a 60 pack/year history of smoking and documented COPD presents with a high fever, chills, a productive cough (yellowish-green sputum) and shortness of breath.

    On examination, there are decreased breath sounds in the right middle lobe and right lower lobe. You suspect a pneumonia.

    A chest X-ray confirms right middle lobe and right lower lobe pneumonia.

    A Gram stain reveals gram-negative rods in abundance.

Based on his 60 pack/year history of smoking, the Gram stain result, and his history of chronic bronchitis, what is the most likely organism in this patient?
a) *Moraxella catarrhalis*
b) *Legionella sp.*
c) *Haemophilus influenzae*
d) *Mycoplasma pneumoniae*
e) *Streptococcus pneumoniae*

13. What is(are) treatment(s) of choice for this patient?
    a) erythromycin
    b) cefuroxine plus clarithromycin
    c) penicillin G
    d) ampicillin
    e) ampicillin plus gentamicin

14. An elderly patient in a long-term care facility develops influenza A pneumonia in spite of both vaccination and amantadine prophylaxis. What is the organism most likely to complicate influenza pneumonia?
    a) *Streptococcus pneumoniae*
    b) *Haemophilus influenzae*
    c) *Chlamydia trachomatis*
    d) *Staphylococcus aureus*
    e) *Mycoplasma pneumoniae*

15. What is the most common cause of community-acquired pneumonia?
    a) *Mycoplasma pneumoniae*
    b) *Haemophilus influenzae*
    c) *Streptococcus pneumoniae*
    d) *Staphylococcus aureus*
    e) a viral pneumonia

16. What is the most common cause of nosocomial pneumonia?
    a) *Mycoplasma pneumoniae*
    b) aerobic gram-negative bacteria
    c) *Streptococcus pneumoniae*
    d) *Haemophilus influenza*
    e) viral pneumonia

Short Answer Management Problem 11

Discuss the characteristics of a satisfactory sputum specimen (satisfactory for Gram stain and for culture).

ANSWERS

1. D.

2. B.

3. D.

4. C. This patient most likely has a *Mycoplasma* pneumonia. *Mycoplasma* pneumonia is a common respiratory tract illness in young adults. The most common respira-

tory symptom is a dry, hacking, usually nonproductive cough. Systemic symptoms include malaise, headache, and fever. Rash, serous otitis media, and joint symptoms occasionally accompany the respiratory symptoms.

Physical findings are usually either minimal or unremarkable. Auscultation of the chest usually reveals only scattered rhonchi or fine, localized rales. The chest X-ray, on the other hand, often reveals fine or patchy lower lobe or perihilar infiltrates. The WBC is often elevated (10,000 to 15,000/mm³). Cold agglutinins are nonspecific and negative in 33% of cases. The diagnosis is confirmed by acute and convalescent mycoplasma complement fixation titers.

Clinically and radiographically, pneumonia caused by adenovirus is often difficult to differentiate from mycoplasma pneumonia. The clinical picture does not fit that of *Streptococcal pneumoniae,* and the patient has no risk factors that should produce a *Klebsiella pneumonia.*

Mycoplasma pneumonia is the favored diagnosis over viral pneumonia (adenovirus) because of age, the absence of other upper respiratory tract symptoms, the prevalence of mycoplasma pneumonia in students of colleges and universities, and the disparity of findings on auscultation relative to the findings on chest X-ray.

Certainly the most reasonable course of action following the history and physical examination is to perform a chest X-ray, especially if you are suspicious that it may be mycoplasma. The treatment of choice is either erythromycin or tetracycline for a period of 10 days.

5. D.

6. A. This patient has a classical history of pneumococcal pneumonia. *Streptococcus pneumoniae* (Pneumococcus) is the most common cause of pneumonia in the adult population.

Pneumococcal pneumonia usually presents with a "shaking rigor" (as in this patient, followed by fever), pleuritic chest pain, and cough with purulent or rust-colored sputum. Viral upper or lower respiratory tract infections may precede pneumococcal pneumonia.

In elderly or debilitated patients, the presentation may be atypical. Fever may be low grade, behavior disturbances may seem more significant than respiratory symptoms, and cough may not be prominent. Patients appear acutely ill, frequently with dyspnea and chest splinting. Signs of consolidation are frequently present.

An elevated WBC with left shift is common. Chest X-ray usually shows disease confined to one lobe (frequently a lower lobe), but several lobes may be involved with either consolidation or bronchopneumonia. Gram stain of the sputum shows polymorphonuclear leukocytes and lancet-shaped gram-positive diplococci.

Sputum cultures should be obtained, but up to 40% of patients with bacteremic pneumococcal pneumonia

will have negative sputum cultures. Therefore blood cultures should be obtained in these patients.

7. A. The treatment of choice for this patient is penicillin G. With the patient's clinical picture including a respiratory rate of 30/minute and chest splinting, IV penicillin is indicated. As well, the patient should receive warm, humidified 100% oxygen. It may be more appropriate to start with a drug combination such as ampicillin/gentamicin until either sputum cultures or blood culture confirms the diagnosis of pneumococcal pneumonia.

8. B.

9. A. The combination of a pneumonia in an immuno-compromised host plus failure to respond to certain potent antibiotics such as (1) ampicillin plus gentamicin, (2) ceftriaxone, or (3) cefazolin point to the diagnosis of Legionella.

Legionella is best treated by erythromycin (EES) plus/minus rifampin. Second-line choices include azithromycin, clarithromycin, ciprofloxacin, doxycycline plus/minus rifampin, or trimethoprim-sulfamethoxazole (TMP-SMX).

10. B.

11. B. The most likely cause of pneumonia in an elderly, debilitated alcoholic is a gram-negative organism, most commonly in alcoholics the organism *Klebsiella pneumoniae.* It is frequently nosocomial.

Although the presentation may be similar to pneumococcal pneumonia, the upper lobes are more frequently involved than the lower lobes. Sudden onset is common. Pleuritic chest pain and hemoptysis are common features. Sputum is thick and often bloody. Other important causes of pneumonia in elderly patients include other gram-negative organisms such as *E. coli, H. influenzae* and gram-positive organisms such as *Streptococcus pneumoniae* and *Staphylococcus aureus.*

The treatment of first choice for this patient is the cephalosporin cefuroxime plus clarithromycin. This drug combination is effective against all the pathogens listed.

12. C.

13. B. In a patient with a pneumonia-complicating chronic bronchitis, the most likely organisms are *Haemophilus influenzae* and *Moraxella catarrhalis.* The treatment of choice is the same as for the last patient: a second-generation cephalosporin plus the new macrolide antibiotic clarithromycin (Biaxin).

14. A.

15. C.

16. B. The most likely organism to complicate influenza pneumonia is *Streptococcus pneumoniae*. The most common cause of community-acquired pneumonia is *Streptococcus pneumoniae*. The most common cause of nosocomial pneumonia is aerobic gram-negative bacteria.

SOLUTION TO SHORT ANSWER MANAGEMENT PROBLEM 11

Sputum cytology is essential to make an accurate diagnosis of pneumonia. Saliva or nasopharyngeal secretions are of little value in determining the etiology of pneumonia, because colonization with gram-negative bacilli and other organisms is frequent.

If more than 25 squamous epithelial cells are seen/LPM field, the specimen is considered inadequate for culture. The ideal sputum specimen contains fewer than 10 squamous epithelial cells/LPM and many polymorphonuclear leukocytes.

SUMMARY OF THE DIAGNOSIS AND MANAGEMENT OF PNEUMONIA IN THE ADULT

1. Young adults:

   Mycoplasma pneumoniae: Mycoplasma pneumonia is most common. In mycoplasma pneumonia, there is often a difference between the signs/symptoms as elicited on history and physical examination and the findings on chest X-ray.

   Diagnostic clues to mycoplasma pneumoniae are a harsh, nonproductive, constant cough with little evidence of the shaking chills and high fever seen in streptococcal pneumonia. The major differential diagnosis is adenoviral pneumonia.

2. Middle-aged adults (non-immunocompromised):

   Streptococcal pneumoniae: Streptococcal pneumonia is the most common cause of community-acquired pneumonia and the most common complicating pneumonia following influenza. Streptococcal pneumonia begins usually with a "shaking chill," followed by high fever, pleuritic chest pain, purulent sputum, tachypnea, tachycardia, and bronchial breath sounds.

3. Middle-aged adults (with COPD):

   Haemophilus influenzae: Haemophilus influenzae pneumonia is the most common pneumonia-complicating chronic obstructive pulmonary disease. The second most common cause is *Moraxella catarrhalis.*

4. Immunocompromised individuals who have failed to respond to conventional therapy and individuals with COPD:

   Legionella Pneumonia: The signs and symptoms of *Legionella* pneumonia include (a) malaise, (b) headache, (c) myalgia, (d) weakness, (e) fever and intermittent rigors 24 hours after a–d, and nonproductive or minimally productive cough. Scant hemoptysis and pleuritic chest pain are common.

5. Elderly patients with immune compromise secondary to alcohol:

   Klebsiella Pneumonia: *Klebsiella* pneumonia has much the same signs and symptoms as other bacterial pneumonias (see the following section).

6. Bacterial versus viral pneumonia:

   a) Bacterial pneumonia: fever, chills (sudden onset of shaking chills in pneumococcal Pneumonia), pleuritic chest pain, productive cough, purulent sputum, tachycardia, tachypnea, bronchial breath sounds.

   b) Viral pneumonia: gradual onset, general malaise, headache, prominent cough (often nonproductive), sometimes few abnormalities on examination of the lung (auscultation). Chest X-ray findings more prominent.

   c) Mycoplasma pneumonia: As in viral pneumonia, except cough can be almost constant, and harsh, nonproductive, and irritative.

7. Treatment:

   a) Mycoplasma pneumonia: erythromycin, tetracyline, or doxycycline

   b) Streptococcal pneumonia: penicillin G

   c) *Legionella* pneumonia: erythromycin plus/minus rifampin

   d) *Klebsiella* pneumonia: cefuroxime plus clarithromycin

   e) *Haemophilus influenzae* pneumonia: cefuroxime plus clarithromycin

8. Prevention:

   a) pneumococcal vaccine (once): All patients at high risk

   b) Influenza vaccine (annually): All patients and health care workers at high risk

SUGGESTED READING

Isselbacher KJ et al., eds. Harrison's principles of internal medicine, part six: infectious disease. 13th Ed. New York: McGraw Hill, 1994.

PROBLEM 12   A 53-YEAR-OLD MALE WITH BURNING SUBSTERNAL AND RETROSTERNAL PAIN

A 53-year-old male presents to your office with a 3-month history of intermittent burning substernal and retrosternal pain radiating to his neck. The burning is usually relieved quickly with antacids. There is no relationship of these symptoms to exercise or exertion.

On P/E, his blood pressure is 140/85 mm Hg and his pulse is 96 and regular. His heart sounds are normal. His lungs are clear. His abdomen is soft; no masses and no tenderness are felt.

SELECT THE ONE BEST ANSWER TO THE FOLLOWING QUESTIONS

1. Which of the following must be considered in the differential diagnosis of this patient's problem?
   a) acid-reflux disease
   b) myocardial ischemia
   c) peptic ulcer disease
   d) panic disorder
   e) a, b, and c only
   f) all of the above

2. Given the history and physical examination, which one of the following conditions is the most likely diagnosis?
   a) acid-reflux disease
   b) peptic ulcer disease
   c) myocardial ischemia
   d) panic disorder
   e) it is difficult to say

3. What is the major pathophysiologic mechanism involved in the condition described?
   a) transient relaxation of the lower esophageal sphincter
   b) decreased resting pressure of the lower esophageal sphincter
   c) coronary artery thrombosis
   d) excess production of hydrogen (H+) ions in the stomach
   e) decreased levels of serotonin in the brain

4. At this time, what would you do?
   a) send the patient ASAP to a psychiatrist and end the consultation
   b) perform an ECG
   c) perform an ECG and if normal prescribe definitive therapy
   d) perform an ECG and serial CPK enzyme levels
   e) call the cardiologist and have a thrombolytic agent injected as quickly as possible

5. What are the pharmacologic drugs of first and second choice (in order) in this patient?
   a) Tums (calcium carbonate) and Maalox
   b) streptokinase and heparin
   c) imipramine and fluoxetine
   d) an H_2 receptor blocker and omeprazole
   e) omeprazole and an H_2 receptor blocker

6. What is the most common cause of dysphagia?
   a) achalasia
   b) esophageal spasm
   c) a lower esophageal ring (Schatzki ring)
   d) nonspecific motor disorders
   e) an esophageal stricture

7. What is malignant dysphagia usually related to?
   a) a squamous cell carcinoma related to Barrett's esophagus
   b) an adenocarcinoma related to Barrett's esophagus
   c) a squamous cell carcinoma unrelated to Barrett's esophagus
   d) an adenocarcinoma unrelated to Barrett's esophagus
   e) none of the above

8. What is the drug of choice in the treatment of achalasia?
   a) a nitroglycerine derivative
   b) a calcium-channel blocker
   c) a benzodiazepine
   d) an antacid
   e) any of the above

9. Achalasia is characterized by which of the following?
   a) transient relaxation of the lower esophageal sphincter
   b) decreased resting pressure of the lower esophageal sphincter
   c) abnormal production of H+ ions in the stomach leading to acid-induced damage in the lower and middle esophagus
   d) loss of peristalsis and relaxation of the lower esophageal sphincter
   e) none of the above

10. Esophageal spasm is best characterized by which of the following?
    a) a loss of peristalsis and relaxation of the lower esophageal sphincter
    b) increased resting pressure of the lower esophageal sphincter
    c) an increased percentage of simultaneous waves with some discoordinated peristalsis
    d) transient contraction of the lower esophageal sphincter
    e) none of the above

Short Answer Management Problem 12

Provide (a) a differential diagnosis of the common causes of dysphagia, (b) the definition of each, and (c) the treatment of each. (This will serve as the summary of the diagnosis and treatment of dysphagia.)

ANSWERS

1. E.

2. A. The differential diagnosis in this patient lies between (a) acid-reflux disease (or heartburn), (b) peptic ulcer disease with associated acid-reflux disease, (c) esophageal motility disorders, and (d) myocardial ischemia/injury/infarction. The most likely diagnosis is acid-reflux disease.

    Although it is often difficult to differentiate acid-reflux disease from myocardial ischemia, there are two clues in this patient that point to acid-reflux disease:
    1. No relationship of the symptoms to exercise
    2. Relief of the symptoms quickly with the administration of calcium carbonate

    Esophageal motility disease is subdivided into (a) achalasia, (b) esophageal spasm, (c) nonspecific motor disorders, and (d) systemic sclerosis. The two most common disorders are achalasia and esophageal spasm. The pain of esophageal motility disease is much more likely to produce a spasmodic type of pain rather than a heartburn-like type of pain.

    Although chest discomfort is often present in panic disorder, the absence of other symptoms makes the diagnosis likely.

3. A. For the past 20 years, it has been assumed that decreased pressure in the lower esophageal sphincter was the primary determinant of acid reflux. It is now recognized, however, that transient relaxation as opposed to decreased pressure of the lower esophageal sphincter is the most important determinant of reflux.

4. C.

5. D. At this time you should (1) perform an ECG to rule out myocardial ischemia or injury, and (2) prescribe a mixture of (a) magnesium and aluminum hydroxide and (b) viscous lidocaine (known as the "pink lady") as an acute diagnostic and therapeutic test. Finally, prescribe an H_2 receptor blocker such as cimetidine or ranitidine. If after a few weeks the therapy is ineffective, then omeprazole should be prescribed.

    Cisapride (a prokinetic motility agent) is now the drug of choice to prevent relapse of the disorder.

6. C. The most common cause of dysphagia is an esophageal ring, or Schatzki ring, at the border of the esophagus and stomach. It is almost always associated with a hiatal hernia, as the ring is just proximal to the hernia. Most commonly, the dysphagia is intermittent and applies to solid foods only. Once the diagnosis is confirmed by radiographic or endoscopic means (or both), the treatment of choice is rupture of the ring by dilatation.

7. B. Malignant dysphagia is usually related to squamous cell carcinoma or adenocarcinoma, the latter of which is often secondary to Barrett's esophagus. Barrett's esophagus is an acquired metaphasia that replaces the normal squamous epithelium of the distal esophagus. The change is thought to be induced by chronic gastroesophageal reflux and is of major clinical significance because of its unequivocal association with adenocarcinoma. Adenocarcinoma of the esophagus is found in 10% of patients with Barrett's esophagus at first endoscopic examination.

8. B.

9. D. Achalasia is characterized by a loss of normal peristalsis and by relaxation of the lower esophageal sphincter in response to swallowing. All treatments are designed to reduce the functional obstruction of the sphincter.

    The treatment of first choice is a calcium-channel blocker, especially nifedipine. This agent reduces the resting lower esophageal sphincter pressure. The usual recommendation is to bite a 10-mg nifedipine capsule and then swallow the capsule (approximately 30 minutes before meals).

    Most patients with achalasia should undergo pneumatic dilatation of the esophagus. Various dilators have been used, but currently the most commonly used is the Microvasive Rigiflex achalasia dilator.

10. C. Esophageal spasm is a disorder in which there is an increased percentage of simultaneous waves, with some preserved peristalsis. No drug has been found to be effective. However, sublingual or oral nitrates, sublingual or oral anxiolytics, and calcium-channel blockers have been used with some success. The other treatment that appears to many experts to be the treatment of choice is dilatation of the esophagus with a bougienage.

SOLUTION TO SHORT ANSWER MANAGEMENT PROBLEM 12 (AND CHAPTER SUMMARY)

A differential diagnosis of the common causes of dysphagia is listed below:

1. **Primary esophageal disorders:**
   a) Achalasia:
   Definition: Achalasia is characterized by the loss of peristalsis and constriction of the lower esophageal sphincter.
   Diagnosis and treatment:
   1. Esophageal manometry: measures intraluminal pressure, pH, and transit time
   2. Pneumatic dilatation of the esophagus with the Microvasive Rigiflex achalasia dilatator
   3. Nifedipine (sublingual)
   b) Esophageal spasm:
   Definition: Esophageal spasm is a disorder in which there is an increased percentage of simultaneous waves with some preserved peristalsis.
   Diagnosis and treatment:
   1. Esophageal manometry
   2. Treatment with bougienage
   3. Drug treatment: (i) calcium-channel blockers, (ii) nitrates, and (iii) anxiolytics
   c) Systemic sclerosis:
   Definition: A disease characterized by progressive muscle atrophy and fibrosis leading to loss of peristalsis as well as reduction of sphincter. This disease may lead to substantial gastroesophageal reflux disease and its complications.
   Diagnosis and treatment:
   1. Chew food well and drink adequate liquids with food.
   2. Use H_2 receptor blockers or proton pump inhibitors
   d) Mechanical obstruction: esophageal rings
   Definition: A constriction of the lower esophageal sphincter that leads to dysphagia for solids only. Almost always associated with a hiatal hernia. Because of the pathophysiology, the dysphagia is intermittent and for solid food only.
   Diagnosis and treatment:
   1. Confirmation of diagnosis by barium swallow or by endoscopy.
   2. Dilatation of the ring is the treatment of choice.
   e) Mechanical obstruction: esophageal stricture:
   Definition: A narrowing in one or more parts of the esophagus: most often caused by ingestion of toxic liquids or solids
   Diagnosis and treatment:
   1. Diagnosis by barium swallow or endoscopy
   2. Treatment of choice is progressive dilatation
   f) Neoplasms: benign and malignant:
   Characteristics of malignant tumors:
   1. Adenocarcinoma of the esophagus is the most common cancer. It usually occurs secondary to Barrett's esophagus.
   2. Squamous cell carcinoma can also occur.
   Diagnosis and treatment:
   1. Endoscopy with biopsy is preferable.
   2. Surgical resection is procedure of choice.
   3. Radiotherapy can be used for palliation.
   g) Gastroesophageal reflux:
   Definition: Patients with gastroesophageal reflux disease have a transient relaxation of the lower esophageal sphincter.
   Diagnosis and treatment:
   1. Therapeutic challenge: magnesium and aluminum hydroxide and viscous lidocaine; if symptoms improve, the diagnosis is confirmed.
   2. H_2 blockers and omeprazole (in that order) for treatment.
   3. Consider cisapride (motility prokinetic agent) as long-term prophylactic therapy.
   h) Miscellaneous disorders:
   1. AIDS candidal esophagitis
   2. AIDS herpes simplex esophagitis
   3. Acute obstruction and foreign body (especially in children)
   4. Cerebrovascular accidents and other neurological disorders

SUGGESTED READING

Traube M. Dysphagia and esophageal obstruction. In: Rakel R, ed. Conn's current therapy. Philadelphia: WB Saunders, 1994.

PROBLEM 13   A 32-YEAR-OLD FEMALE WITH FEVER, WEIGHT LOSS, AND CHRONIC DIARRHEA

A 32-year-old female presents to your office with a 6-month history of loose bowel movements, approximately 8/day. Blood has been present in many of them. She has lost 30 lb. For the past six weeks she has had an intermittent fever. She has had no previous GI problems, nor is there any family history.

On examination, the patient looks ill. Her blood pressure is 130/70 mm Hg. Her pulse is 108 and regular. There is generalized abdominal tenderness with no rebound. A sigmoidoscopy reveals a friable rectal mucosa with multiple bleeding points.

SELECT THE ONE BEST ANSWER TO THE FOLLOWING QUESTIONS:

1. What is the most likely diagnosis in this patient?
   a) irritable bowel syndrome
   b) Crohn's disease
   c) ulcerative colitis
   d) Crohn's colitis
   e) bacterial dysentery

2. The investigations at this time should include which of the following?
   a) colonoscopy
   b) barium enema
   c) upper GI series and follow-through
   d) a and b
   e) all of the above

3. Which of the following may be indicated in the management of the acute phase of the condition described?
   a) hydrocortisone enemas
   b) oral corticosteroids
   c) parenteral corticosteroids
   d) a and b
   e) all of the above

4. Which of the following statements regarding the use of sulfasalazine in the condition described above is(are) false?
   a) sulfasalazine is structurally related to both aspirin and to sulfa drugs
   b) sulfasalazine is effective in maintaining remission in this condition as well as in the acute treatment of mild disease
   c) sulfasalazine may impair folic acid metabolism
   d) all of the above are false
   e) none of the above statements are false

5. Which of the following statements regarding the long-term prognosis of the patient described in the case history is false?
   a) following an initial attack, 10% of patients go into remission lasting up to 15 years
   b) following an initial attack, 75% of patients experience intermittent exacerbations for many years
   c) following an initial attack, 10% of patients continue to have active disease until surgical intervention is undertaken

   d) following an initial attack, 5% of patients die within a year
   e) none of the above are false

6. Which of the following is(are) complications of the disease described?
   a) toxic megacolon
   b) colonic cancer
   c) colonic strictures
   d) iritis
   e) a, b, and c
   f) all of the above

7. A 25-year-old male presents with an 18-month history of chronic abdominal pain. The patient has seen several physicians, and has been diagnosed as having "nervous stomach," irritable bowel syndrome, and "depression." Associated with this abdominal pain for the last three months has been nonbloody diarrhea, anorexia, and a weight loss of 20 lb. He has developed a painful area around the anus.

   On examination, the patient has diffuse abdominal tenderness. He looks thin and unwell. He has a tender, erythematous area in the right perirectal area. What is the most likely diagnosis?
   a) irritable bowel syndrome
   b) Crohn's disease
   c) ulcerative colitis
   d) bacterial dysentery
   e) amebiasis

8. Pathologically, what is the difference between the patient in question seven and the patient described in Problem 13?
   a) inflammation in this case involves all layers of the bowel; the former involves only the mucosa
   b) inflammation in the former case involves all layers of the bowel; the latter involves only the mucosa
   c) inflammation in the former case involves the first two layers of the bowel (mucosa and submucosa); the latter involves only the mucosa
   d) inflammation in this case involves the first two layers of the bowel (mucosa and submucosa); the former involves only the mucosa
   e) the two diseases are identical on a pathophysiologic basis

9. Which of the following investigations is the most sensitive test for confirming the diagnosis in this patient?

a) sigmoidoscopy
b) colonoscopy
c) barium enema
d) CT scan of the abdomen
e) MRI scan of the abdomen

10. Which of the following drugs is the most appropriate initial therapy in the acute phase of the condition described in Question 7?
a) prednisone
b) sulfasalazine
c) metronidazole
d) 6-mercaptopurine
e) azaathiopurine

11. Sulfasalazine is effective in which of the following subtypes of Crohn's disease?
a) Crohn's colitis
b) Crohn's ileocolitis
c) Crohn's disease of the small bowel
d) a and b
e) all of the above

12. Which of the following is(are) associated with Crohn's disease?
a) skip lesions on X-ray
b) thumbprinting on X-ray
c) ineffective surgical treatment
d) none of the above
e) all of the above

13. Which of the following statements regarding complications of the condition described in Question 7 is(are) false?
a) rectal fissures, rectocutaneous fistulas, and perirectal abscesses are common complications of this condition
b) arthritis is sometimes seen as a complication of this condition
c) erythema nodosum and pyoderma gangrenosum are sometimes found with this condition
d) patients with this condition are not at increased risk of colorectal cancer
e) none of the above statements are false

14. A 31-year-old female presents to your office with a 6-month history of gastrointestinal complaints including abdominal distention, excessive flatus, foul-smelling stools, weight loss, and nonspecific complaints of weakness and fatigue. The patient describes the symptoms as being especially severe after the intake of cereal grains and bread of any kind.

The patient has not travelled to any specific area in the recent past. She has not left the country.

Examination of the patient reveals that she is in semi-acute distress. She is thin and looks anemic.

On the basis of this information, what is the most likely diagnosis in this patient?
a) lactase deficiency
b) acute pancreatitis
c) celiac sprue
d) tropical sprue
e) bacterial overgrowth syndrome

15. What is the pathophysiology of this disease?
a) an immunological disorder of the small bowel mucosa
b) a disaccharide deficiency of the small intestinal mucosa
c) a deficiency of pancreatic exocrine
d) secondary contamination of the small intestine by coliform bacteria
e) none of the above

16. A 15-year-old female presents to your office with a 1-month history of abdominal cramping, abdominal bloating, and increased flatulence following the ingestion of milk or milk products. The patient drank three glasses of milk 2 hours ago.

On examination, the abdomen is tympanic and appears to be slightly distended. No other abnormalities are found on examination.

What is the most likely diagnosis in this patient?
a) tropical sprue
b) celiac sprue
c) lactase deficiency
d) regional enteritis
e) chronic pancreatitis

Short Answer Management Problem 13

Discuss the relationship between inflammatory bowel disease (ulcerative colitis and Crohn's disease) and carcinoma of the colon.

ANSWERS

1. C.

2. D. This patient almost certainly has ulcerative colitis. Ulcerative colitis usually presents with (a) abdominal pain, (b) diarrhea, (c) passage of blood/rectum, (d) tenesmus,

(e) fever, (f) chills, (g) malaise and fatigue, and (h) weight loss. Sigmoidoscopy usually reveals friability (with easy bleeding) and granularity.

Crohn's disease (regional enteritis) is usually not associated with rectal bleeding, although it may be. Crohn's disease will be discussed in a subsequent question.

Bacterial dysentery would not be as long-lasting as this illness.

Irritable bowel syndrome is a diagnosis of exclusion and does not present with systemic symptoms.

Barium enema and colonoscopy should be performed in this patient. Sigmoidoscopy has already been done. Barium enema findings include the following: (a) loss of haustral pattern, (b) foreshortening of the colon in certain places, and (c) the presence of gross ulcers at the mucosal margin. Although the rectum and the distal colon are the most common sites of involvement, patients with more severe disease may have involvement of the entire colon.

Colonoscopy identifies the extent of disease and at the same time allows biopsies to be taken. A GI series and follow-through would not add any useful information to the investigation of a patient strongly suspected of having ulcerative colitis.

3. E. The initial therapy of ulcerative colitis depends upon the severity of the disease and the site of the disease.
    1. Mild to moderate disease:
        a) Sulfasalazine remains the initial therapy of choice in the treatment of patients with mild to moderate disease and in the maintenance of remission.
        b) Mesalamine, which has fewer side effects than sulfasalazine, is indicated as the drug of first choice in some patients. In addition, mesalamine can be given in an enema preparation and achieves a high local concentration.
    2. Moderate to Severe Disease: Corticosteroids remain the cornerstone of management of patients with acute ulcerative colitis. They are not, however, efficacious in the maintenance of remission.
        i) Topical corticosteroids: Local corticosteroid therapy may be useful in the treatment of patients with active left-sided disease. They can be given as a retention enema, hydrocortisone 100 mg once or twice/day.
        ii) Oral corticosteroids: For moderate to severe acute ulcerative colitis, oral corticosteroids are indicated. They are usually given as prednisone in the range of 20 to 60 mg/day as a single oral dose for 2 weeks to 4 weeks. When the relief of symptoms has been attained, the dose can be tapered gradually.
        iii) Parenteral corticosteroids: IV corticosteroids should be considered in patients with severe to fulminant ulcerative colitis. These patients are usually severely ill and require hospitalization.

They also need to be closely monitored for the development of toxic megacolon and silent perforation.
        iv) Refractory ulcerative colitis: The purine analogues, azathioprine (Imuran) and 6-mercaptopurine, have corticosteroid-sparing effects and may be useful in the induction and maintenance of remission in patients with refractory ulcerative colitis.
        v) Cyclosporine: A preliminary report suggests that this drug, an immunosuppressant that suppresses the immune response by inhibiting the production of cytokine by helper T cells, may have a role to play in patients that have very severe disease refractory to IV.

4. E. Sulfasalazine has a proven efficacy in the management of patients with ulcerative colitis. It is the therapy of choice in the treatment of patients with mild to moderate severe active disease. It is the treatment of choice for the maintenance of remission in patients with established ulcerative colitis.

Sulfasalazine is structurally related both to aspirin and to sulfa drugs. It inhibits folic acid, and patients taking it thus need a supplement of at least 1 mg of folic acid/day.

5. E. All of the statements are true. Following an initial attack of ulcerative colitis, 10% of patients go into remission lasting up to 15 years. Seventy-five percent of patients have continually active disease, and 5% of patients die within 1 year of the initial attack.

Of all patients with ulcerative colitis of any severity, 25% of patients will undergo total proctocolectomy within 5 years of the first attack. The risk of colonic cancer increases with time. By 15 years post-initial diagnosis, patients with colonic disease are at a risk significant enough to consider prophylactic hemicolectomy.

6. F. Complications of ulcerative colitis include (a) toxic megacolon, (b) perforation, (c) colorectal carcinoma, (d) colonic stricture, and (e) hemorrhage. Extracolonic complications include (a) skin disease—erythema nodosum and pyoderma gangrenosum, (b) aphthous ulcers, (c) iritis, (d) arthritis, and (e) hepatic disease.

7. B.

8. A. This patient has Crohn's disease (regional enteritis). Pathologically, Crohn's disease involves an inflammation of all layers of the bowel, in contradistinction to ulcerative colitis, which involves just the mucosa.

Associated anorectal complications include (a) fistulas, (b) fissures, and (c) perirectal abscesses. The peak incidence of Crohn's disease is at 30 years of age; most cases occur between ages of 20 and 40 years.

Crohn's disease may follow an indolent course resulting in diagnostic delay. The signs and symptoms include (a) mild chronic abdominal pain, (b) mild non-bloody diarrhea, (c) anorexia, (d) weight loss, and (e) fatigue. Pain is often confined to the lower abdomen and is "aching" or "cramping." A misdiagnosis of irritable bowel syndrome is often made.

9. C. An air-contrast barium enema is the most important single diagnostic procedure in the confirmation of the diagnosis of Crohn's disease in this patient. Crohn's disease often presents as segmental involvement of two or more colonic areas; between these areas the colon is normal. The transmural involvement is often suggested by radiologic features including the protrusion of a defect into the lumen (thumbprinting).

Sigmoidoscopy will miss Crohn's disease in 30% to 50% of patients. Colonoscopy is more sensitive than sigmoidoscopy but will not show the transmural involvement.

CT scanning and MRI scanning are not commonly employed in Crohn's disease.

10. A. The drug of choice for the induction of remission in patients with Crohn's disease is prednisone. The initial dose is between 20 mg and 40 mg/day. As in ulcerative colitis, this dosage can often be tapered after a few weeks of therapy. Metronidazole, azathioprine, and 6-mercaptopurine are used when prednisone is not effective or is contraindicated. The use of sulfasalazine will be discussed later.

11. D. Sulfasalazine is effective in the management of Crohn's colitis and Crohn's ileocolitis. It is not, however, effective in the treatment of Crohn's disease of the small bowel.

12. E. Radiographic manifestations of Crohn's disease include skip lesions of X-ray (normal and abnormal alternating sections of bowel) and thumbprinting (characteristic defect protruding into the lumen). In addition, surgical treatment appears to be relatively ineffective. If an area of bowel affected by Crohn's disease is removed, the disease often recurs in other unaffected segments.

13. D. Rectal fissures, rectocutaneous fistulas, or perirectal abscesses occur in up to 50% of patients with Crohn's disease at some time during their illness. Extracolonic manifestations of Crohn's disease occur in 10% of patients with the disease. These include arthritis (which in fact may precede the gastrointestinal symptoms), iritis, erythema nodosum, pyoderma gangrenosum, and aphthous ulcers.

The risk of colorectal cancer is less in patients with Crohn's disease than in patients with ulcerative colitis. Patients who have had the disease for more than 15 years are still, however, at increased risk of a malignancy.

14. C.

15. A. This patient has celiac sprue (gluten enteropathy). Gluten enteropathy is an immunologic disorder of the small bowel observed in both children and adults. Exposure of the small intestine to antigenic components of certain cereal grains in susceptible persons causes subtotal or total villous atrophy with reactive crypt hyperplasia.

Common gastrointestinal complaints include (a) abdominal distention, (b) excessive flatus, (c) large, bulky, foul-smelling stools, and (d) weight loss. Other nonspecific complaints that commonly occur are weakness or fatigue. Patients may present with anemia from either an iron deficiency anemia or a megaloblastic anemia (folic acid deficiency). Other patients suffer from deficiency of a fat-soluble vitamin or vitamin B_{12}.

Therapy consists of a gluten-free diet (avoiding any products containing wheat, rye, barley, or oats). Cereals such as corn, rice, buckwheat, sorghum, and millet are not pathogenic and may be substituted. Clinical improvement is generally seen after several days on a gluten-free diet. Restoration of normal histologic architecture takes weeks to months.

16. C. This patient has a lactase enzyme deficiency in the small intestine. Thus symptoms characteristic of malabsorption (bloating, diarrhea, crampy abdominal pain, foul-smelling stools) occur when milk or milk products are absorbed. The treatment of choice for these patients is replacement of the enzyme deficiency with an enzyme supplement such as Lactaid tablets.

SOLUTION TO SHORT ANSWER MANAGEMENT PROBLEM 13

Inflammatory bowel disease, which includes ulcerative colitis and Crohn's disease, is directly related to the risk of acquiring carcinoma of the colon. The risk is related to the following:
1. Which disease: Ulcerative colitis has a greater risk than Crohn's disease.
2. Severity of the disease: The more severe the disease, the greater is the risk of carcinoma of the colon.
3. The length of the disease: The longer the patient has had the disease, the greater the risk.
4. The site of the disease: The risk of cancer of the colon is much higher in patients who have ulcerative colitis than ulcerative proctitis.

Patients with ulcerative proctitis, ulcerative colitis, and Crohn's colitis should be screened by endoscopy (colonoscopy) every 1 to 2 years depending on the factors just listed. For ulcerative colitis, the screening process may indicate the appropriate time for a prophylactic hemicolectomy (average 15 years since disease onset).

SUMMARY OF DIAGNOSIS AND TREATMENT OF INFLAMMATORY BOWEL DISEASE

1. **Ulcerative colitis:**
   a) Pathophysiology involves the mucosa only.
   b) Local symptoms include (1) diarrhea (bloody), (2) mucus/rectum, (3) tenesmus, (4) constipation (may alternate with diarrhea), and (5) abdominal pain. Complications such as toxic megacolon and perforation are uncommon.
   c) Systemic symptoms include (1) fever, (2) chills, (3) anorexia, (4) weight loss, (5) malaise, (6) fatigue, (7) erythema nodosum, (8) pyoderma gangrenosum, (9) aphthous ulcers, (10) iritis, (11) arthritis, and (12) hepatic disease
   d) Investigations include (1) sigmoidoscopy, (2) colonoscopy, and (3) air-contrast barium enema. If there is danger of perforation (megacolon), barium enema is contraindicated.
   e) Treatment:
      1. Acute disease:
         i) Mild disease: sulfasalazine or mesalamine
         ii) Local disease (proctitis): hydrocortisone enemas
         iii) Moderate to severe disease: oral corticosteroids (prednisone 40 mg-60 mg/day), parenteral corticosteroids, azathioprine/6-mercaptopurine
         iv) Nutritional support: total parenteral nutrition may be necessary for some very ill patients.
      2. Maintenance of remission:
         i) Sulfasalazine
         ii) Mesalamine

2. **Crohn's disease:**
   a) Pathophysiology: involves all layers of the bowel wall
   b) Local symptoms: (1) abdominal pain, (2) nonbloody diarrhea, (3) mucus/rectum
   c) Systemic symptoms: (1) fever, (2) chills, (3) anorexia, (4) malaise, (5) fatigue, (6) weight loss, (7) erythema nodosum, (8) pyoderma gangrenosum, (9) aphthous ulcers, (10) arthritis, and (11) iritis

   d) Other features: (1) rectal fistulas, (2) rectal fissures, and (3) perirectal abscesses
   e) Investigations: (1) barium enema and (2) GI series and follow-through
   f) Treatment:
      1. Acute disease:
         i) Oral corticosteroids (prednisone 20 mg-40 mg/day)
         ii) Azathioprine, 6-mercaptopurine
         iii) Nutritional support with TPN in severe cases
         iv) Metronidazole when other treatments ineffective
      2. Remissions:
         i) Sulfasalazine and mesalamine are useful for Crohn's colitis and Crohn's ileocolitis only, not for Crohn's disease of the small bowel.
         ii) Metronidazole
         iii) Surgery: Results are disappointing; when the diseased area is removed, other areas assume disease profile.

3. **Other diseases that may resemble inflammatory bowel disease:**
   a) Celiac sprue:
      1. Pathophysiology: gluten-sensitive enteropathy. It is an immunologic reaction of the small bowel wall that causes villous atrophy and crypt hyperplasia.
      2. Symptoms: bloating, diarrhea, foul-smelling stools, and weight loss, especially after eating gluten-containing products (breads, etc.)
      3. Treatment: elimination of gluten from the diet
   b) Lactase deficiency:
      1. Pathophysiology: deficiency of the disaccharide enzyme *lactase*
      2. Symptoms: (i) crampy abdominal pain, (ii) bloating, (iii) foul-smelling stools, and (iv) diarrhea after the ingestion of milk or milk products
      3. Treatment: replacement enzymes, such as lactase supplements before ingesting milk and milk products

SUGGESTED READINGS

Choi PM, Targan SR. Ulcerative colitis. In: Rakel R, ed. Conn's current therapy. Philadelphia: WB Saunders, 1994.

Ives CW, Hines C. Crohn's disease. In: Rakel R, ed. Conn's current therapy. Philadelphia: WB Saunders, 1994.

PROBLEM 14 A 51-YEAR-OLD MALE WITH EPIGASTRIC PAIN

A 51-year-old male with a 4-month history of epigastric pain presents to your office. The characterization of the pain is as follows: (1) location: epigastrium; (2) quality: dull ache; (3) quantity: baseline 6/10, intermittent increases of 8/10, intermittent decreases to 0/10; (4) constant/intermittent: intermittent; (5) radiation: none; (6) aggravating factors: coffee only; (7) relieving factors: milk, most meals; (8) chronology: began 4 months ago; intensity, location, and other factors have stayed the same; (9) previous pain history: no significant pain syndromes in the past, including no history of this type of pain; (10) provocative maneuver: palpation in the epigastric area; (11) associated manifestations: heartburn; (11) quality of life: some effect, although not marked.

In terms of other important history, the patient has not been on any medication (specifically aspirin or NSAIDs). He describes his profession as a "high-powered executive." He admits to being a "workaholic."

On examination, the patient has epigastric tenderness. No other abnormalities are found.

SELECT THE ONE BEST ANSWER TO THE FOLLOWING QUESTIONS

1. What is the most likely diagnosis in this patient?
   a) gastric carcinoma
   b) gastric ulcer
   c) duodenal ulcer
   d) cholecystitis/cholelithiasis
   e) irritable bowel syndrome

2. Which of the following statements regarding the patient described is(are) false?
   a) if you are going to investigate this patient at this time, either a gastrointestinal series or a gastroscopy is the investigation of choice
   b) cigarette smoking may aggravate the condition
   c) alcohol does not aggravate the condition
   d) this patient should be treated with a bland diet
   e) this condition may be aggravated by the ingestion of certain medications

3. The patient described is placed on a combination of ranitidine and amoxicillin for his condition. His symptoms improve rapidly, and he is essentially pain free in 2 weeks. Which of the following statements is(are) true about this treatment?
   a) amoxicillin was prescribed because of a high probability of sepsis in his condition
   b) amoxicillin was prescribed because of the association between this condition and *Helicobacter pylori*
   c) ranitidine is an H_1 receptor antagonist
   d) b and c
   e) a and c

4. Which of the following drugs have been shown to be effective against *Helicobacter pylori*?
   a) bismuth subsalicylate
   b) metronidazole
   c) amoxicillin
   d) b and c
   e) all of the above

5. What is the agent known as *omeprazole?*
   a) an H_1 receptor antagonist
   b) an H_2 receptor antagonist
   c) a NA+:K+:ATPase agent
   d) a cytoprotective agent
   e) an anticholinergic agent

6. The condition described should respond to treatment with complete healing within a maximum of how many weeks?
   a) 1-2 weeks
   b) 3-6 weeks
   c) 8-12 weeks
   d) 16-20 weeks
   e) 26-52 weeks

7. Which of the following drugs is(are) classified as H_2 receptor antagonists?
   a) cimetidine
   b) ranitidine
   c) famotidine
   d) a and b
   e) all of the above

8. Which of the following statements regarding the role of drugs and alcohol in the condition described above is(are) true?
   a) the incidence of this condition in patients taking indomethacin or other NSAIDs is increased
   b) the use of dexamethasone is a risk factor for this condition
   c) aspirin may precipitate this condition
   d) some NSAIDs seem more likely to precipitate this condition than others
   e) all of the above are true

9. Which of the following statements regarding cimetidine is(are) true?
   a) cimetidine is an H_2 receptor antagonist
   b) cimetidine plus antacids are no more effective than cimetidine alone in the treatment of the condition described
   c) recurrence of the condition described is common
   d) cimetidine may interfere with warfarin metabolism
   e) all of the above are true

10. Which of the following combinations of drugs may decrease recurrence risk of this condition?
    a) misoprostol plus amoxicillin
    b) omeprazole plus amoxicillin
    c) ranitidine plus amoxicillin
    d) b or c
    e) all of the above

11. Which of the following statements regarding the diagnosis and treatment of gastric ulcers is(are) true?

a) the pain of gastric ulcers, in contrast with duodenal ulcers, is sometimes aggravated rather than relieved by food
b) anorexia, nausea, and vomiting are more common in patients with gastric ulcer than duodenal ulcer
c) endoscopy should follow the identification of a gastric ulcer on a GI series
d) the healing rate and the time to heal for gastric ulcers is generally longer than for duodenal ulcers
e) all of the above

Short Answer Management Problem 14

Describe the pathophysiologic differences between duodenal ulcer related to NSAIDs and duodenal ulcer not related to NSAIDs.

ANSWERS

1. C. This patient has a duodenal ulcer. Duodenal ulcer pain is characterized by a deep, aching, recurrent pain located in the mid-epigastrium. It is often relieved by food or antacids and aggravated by aspirin, coffee, or other irritants. Nocturnal pain is common.

   Anorexia, weight loss, and vomiting are infrequent associated symptoms of duodenal ulcer. The occurrence of these symptoms should lead one to suspect a gastric ulcer.

   Irritable bowel syndrome and acute cholecystitis are described elsewhere in this book. Nervous stomach is not a diagnosis.

2. D. The diagnostic procedures of choice in this patient are a gastroscopy plus/minus a GI series. It is reasonable and safe, however, to treat patients with typical duodenal ulcer symptoms for 6 weeks before investigating. If the symptoms improve during that time, then no investigation is needed. If they do not, investigation with a gastroscopy should proceed.

   Cigarette smoking has been shown to aggravate peptic ulcer disease and delay healing of peptic ulcers. Patients who smoke also have an increased probability of recurrence.

   Aspirin and other nonsteroidal antiinflammatory drugs may aggravate or produce a peptic ulcer. Alcohol has not been shown for certain to predispose to peptic ulcer.

   Bland diets or other special diets should not be prescribed; they may actually increase acid production.

3. B.

4. E. Amoxicillin is prescribed because of the recently proven association between active peptic ulcers (not re-

lated to NSAIDs) and infection with *Helicobacter pylori*. Therefore these patients should be treated with "triple therapy" plus omeprazole. Regimen 1 is: amoxicillin 500 mg qid; plus metronidazole 250 mg tid; plus bismuth subsalicylate 2 tablets qid; plus omeprazole 20 mg bid. Regimen 2 substitutes tetracycline 500 mg qid for amoxicillin. Regimen 1 or 2 should be given for at least 2 weeks. Omeprazole should be given for at least 4-6 weeks.

   The use of amoxicillin in the treatment of peptic ulcers has nothing to do with sepsis.

   Ranitidine is an H_2 receptor antagonist, not an H_1 receptor antagonist.

5. C. Omeprazole binds to the proton pump of the parietal cell, inhibiting secretion of hydrogen ions into the gastric lumen. In doses of 20 mg to 40 mg/day, it inhibits more than 90% of total 24-hour gastric acid secretion, a significant improvement when compared with the 50% to 80% inhibition achieved with a H_2 blocker. This greater inhibition of gastric acid secretion is translated into an increase in pain relief, and a decrease in healing time for the peptic ulcer.

6. B. A duodenal ulcer, treated appropriately, should respond to treatment and heal completely within 3 to 6 weeks.

7. E. Ranitidine, famotidine, and cimetidine are all H_2 receptor antagonists. H_2 receptor antagonists inhibit the action of histamine at the histamine H_2 receptor of the parietal cell, decreasing both basal and food-stimulated acid secretion. All H_2 receptor antagonists are equally efficacious.

   At this time, the treatment of choice for peptic ulcer disease is either (1) the proton-pump inhibitor (omeprazole) or (2) the H_2 receptor antagonists.

Omeprazole has the advantage of a shorter healing time and a lower chance of recurrence.

8. E. Nonsteroidal antiinflammatory drugs including indomethacin are well known to be causative agents in both gastritis and peptic ulcer disease. Thus, the prevalence of peptic ulcer disease is higher in patients taking NSAIDs, especially in elderly patients.

   Dexamethasone (a potent corticosteroid) is extensively used in palliative care to reduce cerebral edema and inhibit centrally mediated nausea and/or vomiting. It is, however, a potent producer of gastric acid secretion and must be used with an H_2 receptor antagonist or omeprazole to prevent gastritis or septic ulcer formation.

9. E. Cimetidine is an H_2 receptor antagonist. Other H_2 receptor antagonists have fewer side effects and thus have become the H_2 receptor antagonists of choice (like famotidine or rantidine). Warfarin ametidine specifically (1) can lead to confusion in the elderly and (2) interferes with anticoagulant activity.

   An H_2 receptor antagonist, used in combination with an antacid, is no more effective than an H_2 receptor antagonist alone for either treatment or maintenance.

   The 1-year recurrence rate for duodenal ulcer is at least 60% in nonsmokers and greater than 75% in smokers. The endoscopic recurrence rate is 20% higher in both cases. Controversy exists regarding which patients should be offered prophylactic therapy. A reasonable approach appears to be the offering of prophylactic therapy to those with frequent recurrences. Omeprazole has lowered this one-year recurrence rate substantially.

10. B. The treatment of choice for non-NSAID-associated peptic ulcer is omeprazole for 4 to 6 weeks plus either of the following regimens (to eliminate *Helicobacter pylori*): (1) amoxicillin 500 mg qid; metronidazole 250 mg tid; bismuth subsalicylate 2 tablets qid; *or* (2) tetracycline 500 mg qid; metronidazole 250 mg tid; bismuth subsalicylate 2 tablets qid.

11. E. A gastric ulcer identified endoscopically must be followed by another endoscopy to confirm that healing has occurred. The pain of gastric ulcer is aggravated rather than relieved by food. Anorexia, nausea, and vomiting are more common in patients with gastric ulcer than patients with duodenal ulcer. The healing rate for gastric ulcers are generally slower than with duodenal ulcers.

SOLUTION TO SHORT ANSWER MANAGEMENT PROBLEM 14

The pathophysiologic difference between NSAID-related peptic ulcer and non-NSAID-related peptic ulcer reflects the direct gastric irritative effect of NSAID drugs. NSAIDs may produce an acute or chronic gastritis, a reflux esophagitis, or a peptic ulcer. NSAID-related peptic ulcer is not associated with *Helicobacter pylori*, whereas non-NSAID-related ulcers are.

The significance of this pathologic difference is reflected in treatment. Patients with NSAID-related peptic ulcer must receive the treatment protocol (that includes treatment for *Helicobacter pylori*); non-NSAID-related peptic ulcer patients should not.

SUMMARY OF THE DIAGNOSIS AND MANAGEMENT OF PEPTIC ULCER DISEASE

1. **Symptoms:**
   Duodenal ulcer: mid-epigastric pain, relieved by ingestion of food or antacids. Nocturnal pain is present.
   Gastric ulcer: midepigastric pain, relieved by antacids but often aggravated by food. Anorexia, weight loss, nausea, and vomiting are frequently associated.

2. **Differential diagnosis:** Cholecystitis, pancreatitis, appendicitis, carcinoma of the stomach, ischemic bowel disease in the elderly, inflammatory bowel disease

3. **Investigations:**
   a) No investigation may be appropriate if the symptoms suggest duodenal ulcer and healing takes place within a maximum of 6 weeks.
   b) Gastroscopy must be used for both the assessment and the reassessment of gastric ulcers; a GI series and follow-through may be sufficient for duodenal ulcers.

4. **Treatment:**
   a) NSAID-associated peptic ulcer:
      1. H_2 receptor antagonist
      2. proton pump inhibitor (omeprazole)
   b) non-NSAID-associated peptic ulcer: omeprazole or H_2 receptor antagonist and treatment for *Helicobacter pylori*:
      1. omeprazole for 4-6 weeks
      2. regime 1 or 2 for two weeks (see question 10)
   c) limited role at this time for antacid therapy, sulcrafate, misoprostol, which has as its chief function, the possible prevention of gastric ulcers

SUGGESTED READINGS

Achord J. Peptic ulcer disease. In: Rakel R, ed. Conn's current therapy. Philadelphia: WB Saunders, 1994.

Drugs for treatment of peptic ulcers. Medical Letter 1994; 36: 927-928.

PROBLEM 15 A 25-YEAR-OLD COLLEGE STUDENT WITH A FEVER AND A SORE THROAT

A 25-year-old college student presents to your office with a 3-week history of fatigue, malaise, fever, chills, and a sore throat. She was well prior to the onset of this illness and was taking part in many activities. She finds at this time that she has no energy and is barely able to make her university classes in the mornings. She also describes aches and pains all over.

On P/E, the patient's temperature is 39° C. There is pharyngeal hyperemia, and edema and marked exudates are present in both tonsillar areas. There is significant cervical lymphadenopathy present.

On abdominal examination, there is dullness over Trobe's space, and you can just feel the tip of the spleen. There is no hepatic enlargement.

SELECT THE ONE BEST ANSWER TO THE FOLLOWING QUESTIONS

1. Based on the history and the physical examination described, what is the most likely diagnosis?
   a) infectious hepatitis
   b) infectious mononucleosis
   c) chronic fatigue syndrome
   d) fibromyalgia
   e) 20th-century disease

2. Of the following clinical features of the disorder, what is the least common?
   a) splenomegaly
   b) hepatomegaly
   c) fever
   d) exudative tonsillitis
   e) generalized lymphadenopathy

3. Which of the following statements regarding this condition is false?
   a) this condition is caused by the Epstein-Barr virus
   b) kissing is thought to be the most common mode of transmission
   c) greater than 90% of all adults are carriers of the virus that causes the disease
   d) in young children, fever and pharyngitis may be clinically indistinguishable from upper respiratory tract infections caused by other viral agents
   e) bacterial throat culture is not necessary in patients suspected of having this disease

4. Which of the following statements concerning the serologic testing for the condition described is false?
   a) the rapid heterophile antibody test is 95% sensitive in diagnosis
   b) the rapid heterophile antibody test is 95% specific in diagnosis
   c) in acute primary infections, anti-EA (early antigen) titers are usually low
   d) in acute primary infections, IgM-VCA (IgM viral capsid antigen) titers are high
   e) after several months, the anti-EBNA (Epstein-Barr nuclear antigen) titers become high

5. The infectious agent that causes most of the cases of this disease has been associated with another condition. In fact, infection with the condition described could lead to this complication. What is this complication?
   a) fibromyalgia
   b) 20th-century disease
   c) chronic fatigue syndrome
   d) acute lymphocytic leukemia
   e) none of the above

6. Of the following clinical features of the acute infection described, which is most common?
   a) fever
   b) hepatomegaly
   c) periorbital edema
   d) palatine petechiae
   e) splenomegaly

7. What is the treatment of choice for an uncomplicated episode of this condition?
   a) penicillin
   b) prednisone
   c) penicillin plus prednisone
   d) penicillin plus high-dose aspirin
   e) none of the above

8. Which of the following is(are) complications of this condition?
   a) pneumonitis
   b) pericarditis
   c) meningoencephalitis
   d) Bell's palsy
   e) all of the above

9. Which of the following findings in this condition is so specific that serologic testing becomes unnecessary?
   a) a combination of fever, tonsillitis, and generalized lymphadenopathy
   b) splenomegaly
   c) lymphocytosis
   d) lymphocyte atypia of more than 40%
   e) none of the above

10. The patient described in the initial presentation presents 1 week later with great difficulty swallowing (solids and liquids). You notice a significant increase in the erythema of the pharynx, an increase in tonsillar hypertrophy, and increased exudates on the tonsils. What should you do at this time?
    a) repeat the throat culture
    b) start the patient on ampicillin
    c) start the patient on penicillin
    d) start the patient on prednisone
    e) start the patient on high-dose ASA

11. The disease is an infection of which of the following?

    a) T-cell lymphocytes
    b) B-cell lymphocytes
    c) neutrophils
    d) basophils
    e) none of the above

12. What is the most common age group affected with this condition?
    a) children < 15
    b) young adults 15-30
    c) middle aged females 30-45
    d) middle aged males 30-45
    e) the elderly (>65)

Short Answer Management Problem 15

Describe the possible connection between acute infectious mononucleosis and chronic fatigue syndrome.

ANSWERS

1. B. This patient has infectious mononucleosis. Infectious mononucleosis is caused by the Epstein-Barr virus and is most commonly seen in young adults, particularly college students and military recruits.

   The major symptoms of infectious mononucleosis are an extremely sore throat, profound fatigue, malaise, severe myalgias, fever, and sometimes chills.

   The major signs of infectious mononucleosis include pharyngeal erythema, pharyngeal edema, significant tonsillar exudates, swollen and tender generalized lymphadenopathy, splenomegaly in some patients, palatine petechiae, periorbital edema and hepatomegaly.

   Fibromyalgia, although most characteristic for its description of "pain all over" is characterized by multiple trigger points on examination. 20th-century disease is also known as chronic candidiasis and is thought by most authorities not to exist.

   Infectious hepatitis, although it presents with fatigue and malaise, also presents with abdominal pain, jaundice, and an aversion to cigarettes.

   Chronic fatigue syndrome shares certain features with infectious mononucleosis. In fact, the Epstein-Barr virus, as the cause of infectious mononucleosis, may (over a period of time) become a trigger factor for chronic fatigue syndrome.

2. B. The least common clinical feature is hepatomegaly. The major clinical features are discussed in the previous answer.

3. E. Infectious mononucleosis is caused by the Epstein-Barr virus. The usual mode of transmission of the virus is through infected saliva (kissing). Most adults (>90%) have been infected with Epstein-Barr virus and are carriers.

   Infectious mononucleosis is usually distinguishable from other viral infections in older children and adults. In younger children and adults, however, it may be difficult to distinguish from other respiratory tract infections including those caused by other viruses, mycoplasma, or streptococci.

   Bacterial throat culture should be done in patients with significant pharyngitis to exclude coexisting Group A beta-hemolytic streptococcal infection.

4. C. The heterophil antibody test is 95% sensitive and 95% specific for the diagnosis of infectious mononucleosis. If this test does not support your clinical impression, further testing may be necessary.

   Serologic testing for EBV infection includes determining antibody titers to latently infected (anti-EBNA) viral proteins and determining antibody titers to early-replication-cycle (anti-EA) viral proteins, or determining antibody titers to late-replication-cycle (anti-VCA) viral proteins.

   Acute infectious mononucleosis produces high anti-EA and anti-IgM VCA titers and low anti-IgG-VCA and anti-EBNA titers. In recovering patients, the anti-IgG-VCA titer is high and the anti-EA, anti-IgM, and anti-EBNA titers are low. With time, the anti-EBNA titer also becomes high.

5. C. The Epstein-Barr virus is not only associated with infectious mononucleosis. The possible link to chronic fatigue syndrome is presented in the answer to Question 11.

6. A. The following are the major clinical features of acute symptomatic infectious mononucleosis:

	PERCENTAGE OF PATIENTS
Fever	98-100
Exudative tonsillitis	98-100
Generalized lymphadenopathy	98-100
Splenomegaly	75
Palatine petechiae	50
Periorbital edema	33
Hepatomegaly	20

7. E. Symptomatic treatment including bed rest, avoidance of strenuous exercise (due to the potential complication of splenic rupture), and analgesics are the only treatments necessary in acute uncomplicated infectious mononucleosis.

   Antibiotics are unnecessary unless a streptococcal pharyngitis coexists. Antibiotics (especially ampicillin) will produce a skin rash in approximately 90% of patients with infectious mononucleosis.

8. E. The complications of acute infectious mononucleosis include meningoencephalitis, Guillain-Barre syndrome, Bell's palsy, pneumonitis, pericarditis, myocarditis, and inappropriate ADH (antidiuretic hormone) secretion.

9. D. A lymphocyte count in which more than 40% of lymphocytes are atypical is so specific for infectious mononucleosis that further serologic testing (including either a heterophil antibody titer or a monospot test for heterophil antibodies) is unnecessary.

10. D. At this time, the single most important maneuver is to begin the patient on a corticosteroid to decrease the swelling and inflammation present in the airway. In severe cases of infectious mononucleosis the swelling and inflammation of the airway may be so significant that airway compromise and respiratory distress may occur. A reasonable starting dose would be in the range of 30 mg to 50 mg of prednisone/day with gradual tapering of the dose over 10 to 14 days.

11. B. The Epstein-Barr virus, which causes infectious mononucleosis, is a B-cell lymphotropic human herpes virus. EBV is a ubiquitous agent that has been found in all population groups surveyed to date.

12. B. The peak incidence of infectious mononucleosis occurs between 14 and 16 years of age for girls and between 16 and 18 years of age for boys.

SOLUTION TO SHORT ANSWER MANAGEMENT PROBLEM 15

The connection between acute infectious mononucleosis and chronic fatigue syndrome is in the viral agent itself. The agent that causes infectious mononucleosis, the Epstein-Barr virus (EBV), has been studied as a possible major cause of chronic fatigue syndrome.

We do know that one of the causes of chronic fatigue syndrome is a persistent postviral state. EBV and cytomegalovirus are the two viruses that appear to be most closely linked to chronic fatigue syndrome.

SUMMARY OF THE DIAGNOSIS AND MANAGEMENT OF INFECTIOUS MONONUCLEOSIS

1. **Identification:** Epstein-Barr virus is the causative agent.
2. **Incubation period:** 2-5 weeks
3. **Symptoms:** malaise, fatigue, fever, chills, myalgias, and severe sore throat
4. **Signs:** pharyngeal erythema and edema, exudative tonsillitis, generalized lymphadenopathy, splenomegaly, and hepatomegaly
5. **Laboratory diagnosis:** lymphocyte atypia > 40%, positive heterophil antibody titer, and antibodies to EBV antigens:
   1. Acute phase antibodies: anti-EA, anti-IgM VCA
   2. Convalescent antibody: anti-IgG VCA
   3. Recovered state: anti-IgG VCA, anti-EBNA
6. **Treatment:**
   a) Symptomatic treatment: rest, fluids, mild analgesics
   b) Treatment of severe odynophagia and airway compromise: oral prednisone
7. **Connection to other conditions:**
   a) Chronic fatigue syndrome: EBV (same viral agent)
   b) Fibromyalgia: description of "hurts all over" may occur in both conditions

SUGGESTED READING

D'Angelo L. Infectious mononucleosis. In Rakel R, ed. Conn's current therapy. Philadelphia: WB Saunders, 1994.

PROBLEM 16   A 50-YEAR-OLD MALE WITH ASCITES

A 50-year-old male is brought into your office by his wife. His wife states that for the past several months he has experienced extreme weakness and fatigue. In addition, he has gained 20 pounds during the past 3 weeks. During the last few weeks the patient has eaten nothing. When you question the patient he states that his wife is overreacting. The patient's wife is extremely concerned about his alcohol intake. When you question the patient, he states that he is a social drinker. When you pursue this line of questioning further and ask him what he means by being a social drinker, you find out that he means that he drinks a few drinks before and after most meals plus a few drinks before he goes to bed.

You decide to pursue the question of drinking even further. When you ask him what he drinks, he says vodka. When you ask him if he drinks two 26-oz bottles/day he says, "Heck, no! I would never put away more than a bottle a day."

On physical examination, the patient has a significantly enlarged abdominal girth. There is a level of shifting dullness present. The patient's liver edge is felt 6 cm below the right costal margin. It has a nodular edge. In addition, spider nevi are present over the upper part of the patient's body. Palmar erythema is noted, and a flapping tremor is elicited.

SELECT THE ONE BEST ANSWER TO THE FOLLOWING QUESTIONS

1. Which of the following statements regarding this patient's condition is false?
   a) the most likely diagnosis is cirrhosis of the liver
   b) this condition is probably associated with alcohol abuse
   c) jaundice is an uncommon sign in the disorder described
   d) approximately 33% of patients with a history of alcohol abuse will go on to develop alcoholic hepatitis
   e) approximately 50% of patients with this condition (in an advanced stage) will die within 2 years

2. A 25-year-old male with a history of heavy alcohol intake presents to your office for a periodic health assessment. He states that his appetite has been off and he has had generalized abdominal pain for the past 3 weeks.

   On examination, there is no clinical jaundice. There is tenderness present in the right upper quadrant of the abdomen. The liver edge is palpable 5 cm below the right costal margin. You suspect alcoholic hepatitis.

   Which of the following statements regarding alcoholic hepatitis is false?
   a) alcoholic cirrhosis develops in approximately 10% of patients with alcoholic hepatitis
   b) serum bilirubin may often be 10 to 20 times normal in this condition
   c) serum ALT is almost always lower than serum AST
   d) hepatomegaly is seen in 80-90% of patients with alcoholic hepatitis
   e) a mortality rate of 10 to 15% is seen in acute alcoholic hepatitis

3. What is the most common cause of cirrhosis?
   a) hepatitis A
   b) hepatitis B
   c) non-A, non-B hepatitis
   d) alcoholic hepatitis
   e) cytomegalovirus hepatitis

4. The ascites associated with cirrhosis should generally be treated by which of the following?
   a) sodium restriction
   b) water restriction
   c) spironolactone
   d) a and c
   e) a, b, and c

5. A 25-year-old schoolteacher presents with nausea, vomiting, anorexia, aversion to her usual 2 packs/day habit, and right upper quadrant pain. She has been sick for the past 3 days. Two of the students in her class have come down with similar symptoms. She has had no exposure to blood products, and has no other significant risk factors for sexually transmitted disease.

   On examination, her sclera are icteric and her liver edge is tender. She looks acutely ill.

   What is the most likely diagnosis in this patient?
   a) hepatitis A
   b) hepatitis B
   c) non-A, non-B hepatitis
   d) atypical infectious mononucleosis
   e) none of the above

6. Which of the following tests is the most sensitive in confirming the diagnosis suspected in the patient presenting in the preceding question?
   a) anti-HAV-IgG
   b) anti-HAV-IgM
   c) hepatitis A core antigen
   d) anti-HB core antigen
   e) anti-non-A, non-B hepatitis antigen

7. Initial screening for hepatitis B should include which of the following?
   a) anti-HBs and anti-HBc
   b) HBeAg and anti-HBe
   c) HBsAg and anti-HBs
   d) HBsAg and anti-HBc
   e) anti-HBe and anti-HBc

8. Which of the following laboratory tests is(are) usually abnormal in a patient with acute viral hepatitis?
   a) serum AST
   b) serum bilirubin
   c) serum ALT
   d) serum alkaline phosphatase
   e) all of the above

9. Clinical manifestations of cirrhosis include which of the following?
   a) fatigue
   b) jaundice
   c) splenomegaly
   d) hypoalbuminemia
   e) all of the above

10. Indications for the use of hepatitis B vaccine include which of the following?
    a) health care personnel
    b) hemodialysis patients
    c) normal newborns
    d) a and b only
    e) all of the above

11. Which of the following types of viral hepatitis is(are) associated with the development of chronic active hepatitis?
    a) hepatitis B
    b) non-A, non-B hepatitis
    c) hepatitis A
    d) a and b only
    e) all of the above

12. The pathophysiology of alcoholic cirrhosis includes which of the following?
    a) macronodular and micronodular fibrosis
    b) nodular regeneration
    c) increased portal vein pressure
    d) increase in hepatic size followed by a decrease
    e) all of the above

13. Which of the following has been suggested as treatment for complications of cirrhosis of the liver?
    a) prednisone
    b) α-interferon
    c) colchicine and probenecid
    d) propylthiouracil
    e) all of the above

14. Which of the following is(are) complications of alcoholic cirrhosis?
    a) hypersplenism
    b) hepatic encephalopathy
    c) congestive gastropathy
    d) spontaneous bacterial peritonitis
    e) all of the above

15. Treatment of the ascites accompanying cirrhosis includes which of the following?
    a) spironolactone
    b) hydrochlorothiazide
    c) furosemide
    d) all of the above
    e) a and b only

Short Answer Management Problem 16

Describe the pathophysiology of cirrhosis of the liver and the relationship between cirrhosis of the liver and right-sided heart failure.

ANSWERS

1. C. This patient has cirrhosis of the liver and alcoholism. Most cases of cirrhosis of the liver are directly attributable to alcohol abuse.

   Cirrhosis is an irreversible inflammatory disease that disrupts liver structure and function. It is the fifth leading cause of death in the United States. Cirrhosis is the disorganization of hepatic tissues caused by diffuse fibrosis and nodular regeneration. Nodules of regenerated tissue form between fibrous bands, giving the liver a cobbly appearance.

   Symptoms of early cirrhotic liver disease include weakness, fatigue, and weight loss. In advanced disease the patient develops the following: anorexia, nausea and vomiting, swelling of the abdomen and the lower extremities, and central nervous system symptoms related to the cirrhotic liver disease. Other symptoms that may occur include loss of libido, gynecomastia, and menstrual irregularities in women.

   The liver is usually enlarged, palpable, and firm. In advanced cirrhosis, the liver may actually shrink. Dermatologic manifestations include spider nevi, palmar erythema, telangiectases on exposed areas, and occasional evidence of vitamin deficiencies.

   Although jaundice is rarely an initial sign, it usually develops later. Other later developing signs include ascites, lower extremity edema, pleural effusion, purpuric lesions, asterixis, tremor, delirium, coma, fever, splenomegaly, and superficial venous dilatation on the abdomen and thorax.

   Approximately 33% of chronic alcoholics will go on

to develop alcoholic hepatitis. Many of these will then develop cirrhosis of the liver. There appears to be a genetic predisposition to the development of these complications.

Fifty percent of patients with advanced cirrhosis will be dead in a period of 2 years; 65% will be dead in 5 years. Hematemesis, jaundice, and ascites are unfavorable signs.

2. A. The first clinical stage of alcoholic liver disease is termed alcoholic hepatitis. Alcoholic hepatitis is a precursor of cirrhosis that is characterized by inflammation, degeneration, and necrosis of hepatocytes and infiltration of polymorphonuclear leukocytes and lymphocytes.

Over the last 10 years in the United States deaths from alcohol-related liver disease have increased. The incidence is greatest in the middle-aged males and mortality from cirrhosis is higher in blacks than in whites. Although alcoholic cirrhosis is the most prevalent type of cirrhosis, only about 25% of alcoholics actually develop the disease. There appears to be a genetic predisposition to its development. The amount and duration of alcohol consumption are correlated directly with the extent of damage to the liver.

The symptoms of alcoholic hepatitis include anorexia, nausea, vomiting, weight loss, emesis, fever, and generalized abdominal pain.

Hepatomegaly is found in 80% to 90% of these patients. Other signs include jaundice, ascites, splenomegaly, and spider angiomas.

Laboratory abnormalities in alcoholic hepatitis include hyperbilirubinemia and elevated serum transaminase. The ratio of serum AST/serum ALT is often 2/1 or greater. This can help differentiate alcoholic hepatitis from viral hepatitis. Other laboratory abnormalities include elevated alkaline phosphatase, hypoalbuminemia, and a prolonged prothrombin time.

The prognosis of alcoholic hepatitis is variable; many patients develop only a mild illness. There is, however, a 10% to 15% mortality from the acute event.

The treatment of alcoholic hepatitis involves cessation of alcohol consumption, increased caloric and increased protein intake, and vitamin supplementation (especially thiamine).

Alcoholic cirrhosis develops in approximately 50% of patients surviving alcoholic hepatitis. In the other 50% various degrees of hepatic fibrosis develop.

3. D. The most common type of cirrhosis is alcoholic cirrhosis, and the most common cause of alcoholic cirrhosis is alcoholic hepatitis (see the preceding answer). Hepatitis A does not progress to chronic active hepatitis. Hepatitis B progresses to chronic active hepatitis and subsequently to cirrhosis in approximately 10% of cases. Patients with non-A, non-B hepatitis go on to develop chronic active hepatitis and subsequent cirrhosis in approximately 40% of cases.

Cytomegalovirus infection does not produce cirrhosis.

4. D. The treatment of the ascites and the edema associated with ascites includes the following:
1. Sodium restriction to 250-500 mg/day
2. Spironolactone (Aldactone) 25mg-50 mg tid or qid (effective in 40-75% of cases)
3. Paracentesis
4. Combination diuretic therapy in those patients who do not respond: (a) spironolactone plus hydrochlorothiazide; (b) spironolactone plus furosemide
5. Paracentesis with albumin (or dextran) infusion in refractory cases

Fluid restriction is usually not necessary unless the serum sodium level is <125 mEq per liter.

5. A. This patient most likely has hepatitis A. Hepatitis A occurs either spontaneously or in epidemics. Transmission is via the oral-fecal route. The presenting signs and symptoms of hepatitis A include the following:
1. General malaise and fatigue
2. General myalgias
3. Arthralgias
4. Abdominal pain
5. Nausea and vomiting
6. Severe anorexia out of proportion to the degree of illness
7. Aversion to smoking

Hepatitis B and non-A, non-B hepatitis are unlikely in this case as risk factors are absent. Although infectious mononucleosis may involve the liver and present with some of the same signs and symptoms, hepatitis A is much more likely.

6. B. Acute infection with hepatitis A is confirmed by the demonstration of IgM antibodies to hepatitis A virus (IgM-anti-HAV). These antibodies persist for approximately 12 weeks after appearance. IgG antibodies to hepatitis A virus follow and simply indicate exposure at some time in the past.

Hepatitis A does not possess a recognizable core or surface antigen; these tests apply to hepatitis B only. Antibodies to HB core antigen have nothing to do with hepatitis A. Anti-non-A, non-B hepatitis antigen does not exist.

7. D. There are so many antigens and antibodies associated with hepatitis virology that it is difficult to figure out what is what. However, it can be simplified considerably.

Initial screening for hepatitis B should include HBsAg (hepatitis B surface antigen) and anti-HBc (the antibody to the core antigen). These two tests will identify most cases of acute hepatitis B.

There is a window period between the clearance of HBsAg and the appearance of anti-HBs. This period lasts for 4-6 weeks, and during this time the only marker

for hepatitis B that can predict the infection with any certainty is anti-HBc. If acute hepatitis B is suggested from the initial screening, then further laboratory tests should be ordered. These include the following:
1. HBeAg: the E antigen indicates the presence of a highly infectious or contagious state or a chronic infection.
2. anti-HBe (the antibody to the antigen above): the presence of this antibody indicates low infectivity and predicts the later seroconversion or resolution of hepatitis B.
3. anti-HBs (the antibody to the surface antigen): the presence of this antibody indicates past hepatitis B infection and current immunity.

8. E. In acute viral hepatitis, the serum transaminase (serum AST) and serum ALT are elevated, along with serum bilirubin and serum alkaline phosphatase.

9. E. The clinical manifestations of cirrhosis were discussed earlier. Another common finding in cirrhosis is hypoalbuminemia due to accumulation of ascitic fluid in the abdomen.

10. E. Hepatitis B vaccine should be offered to persons at high risk and those with continued exposure to hepatitis B infection. Hepatitis B vaccines manufactured using DNA-recombinant technology are now the vaccines of choice. Persons at high risk for acquiring hepatitis B include (1) all health care personnel, (2) hemodialysis patients, (3) patients requiring frequent blood transfusions, (4) employees and residents of institutions for people with developmental disabilities, (5) male homosexuals and all of their contacts, (6) intravenous drug users, and (7) sexual contacts of chronic HBsAg carriers. In addition, the Center for Disease Control now recommends that all newborns be immunized with Hepatitis B vaccine. Newborn immunization should take place at birth, 2 months, and 4 or 6 months.

11. D. Chronic active hepatitis (which may lead to cirrhosis of the liver, liver failure, and hepatocellular carcinoma), is associated with hepatitis B, hepatitis C, hepatitis D (delta hepatitis, which occurs only in patients who are also infected with hepatitis B, and non-A, non-B hepatitis; which is largely due to infection with hepatitis C, parenterally transmitted), and enterically transmitted hepatitis E.

Chronic active hepatitis is not associated with hepatitis A.

12. E. Cirrhosis is an irreversible inflammatory condition of disordered and disrupted liver structure and function. Cirrhosis results from the disorganization of hepatic tissues caused by diffuse fibrosis and nodular regeneration. Micronodular and macronodular fibrosis occur.

Nodules of regenerated tissue form between the fibrous bands, giving the liver a cobbly appearance. The liver is initially larger than normal in size and then usually becomes smaller than normal. The changes in the liver result in increased portal vein pressure, which leads to the formation of ascites as well as to esophageal varices.

13. E. Treatments that have been suggested as possibly beneficial for cirrhosis of the liver include the following:
1. Penicillamine (inhibiting the formation of cross-linkages of collagen)
2. Colchicine and probenecid (interference with microtubular function and transcellular movement of collagens and increased collagenase production)
3. Propylthiouracil (reduces hepatic hypermetabolism)
4. Corticosteroids (reduces hepatic hypermetabolism)
4. Corticosteroids (reduces inflammation)
5. Actigall (replacement of hydrophobic and potentially hepatotoxic bile acids by the more hydrophilic ursodiol, Actigall)
6. Alpha interferon (inhibits fibrogenic activity in the liver)

Other treatments for cirrhosis include lactulose for hepatic encephalopathy and Laveen shunt placement.

14. E. Complications of cirrhosis include the following:
1. Portal hypertension, leading to esophageal varices, congestive gastropathy, and hypersplenism
2. Hepatic encephalopathy
3. Ascites, leading to spontaneously bacterial peritonitis and umbilical hernia (spontaneous rupture)
4. Hepatorenal syndrome
5. Coagulation abnormalities
6. Hepatocellular carcinoma
7. Pulmonary dysfunction
8. Hepatic osteodystrophy
9. Cholelithiasis
10. Pericardial effusion
11. Impaired reticuloendothelial system function

15. D. The management of ascites in cirrhotic patients is complicated.

Paracentesis should be performed in any cirrhotic patient who undergoes clinical deterioration. Defined indications for the treatment of ascites include significant patient discomfort, respiratory compromise, a large umbilical hernia, and recurrent bacterial peritonitis.

Sodium restriction is considered the cornerstone of therapy for ascites. Cirrhotic patients require significant curtailment of sodium intake (250 to 500 mg/day) to obtain clinical benefit. Approximately 10% to 20% of patients who maintain a strict low-salt diet achieve complete resolution of ascites without additional therapy.

Spironolactone (Aldactone), an aldosterone antagonist, is the first-line diuretic of choice in the treatment of cirrhotic ascites. It is effective in controlling 40% to

75% of cirrhotics. Other potassium-sparing diuretics may be substituted for spironolactone, including triamterene (Dyrenium) and amiloride (Midamor). Sometimes either a thiazide diuretic (such as hydrochlorothiazide) or a loop diuretic (such as furosemide) have to be added to achieve maximum benefit.

SOLUTION TO SHORT ANSWER MANAGEMENT PROBLEM 16

The pathophysiology of cirrhosis has already been discussed. Briefly, micronodular fibrosis, macronodular fibrosis, and nodular regeneration eventually lead to portal hypertension with all of its complications. The development of ascites and dependent edema may lead to both right-sided valvular disease and constrictive pericarditis. In most cases right-sided heart failure is a direct result of left-sided heart failure; however, when it occurs because of cirrhosis it is not.

SUMMARY OF THE DIAGNOSIS AND TREATMENT OF HEPATITIS AND CIRRHOSIS

1. **Infectious forms of hepatitis:**
   a) Hepatitis A:
      1. Symptoms: anorexia, nausea, vomiting, malaise, aversion to smoking
      2. Signs: fever, enlarged liver, tender liver, jaundice
      3. Laboratory findings: normal to low white blood cell count; abnormal ALT, AST, bilirubin, and alkaline phosphatase
      4. Epidemiology: sporadic infection or epidemic, spread by oral-fecal route
      5. Diagnostic clues: transaminase elevations, IgM Anti-HAV
      6. Treatment: symptomatic; rest; immunoglobulin in severe cases
      7. Prevention: because oral-fecal route is the main route of spread, meticulous handwashing is essential. Gamma-globulin is also useful.
   b) Hepatitis B:
      1. Epidemiology: usually transmitted by blood or blood products; particularly common in intravenous drug users and in patients with AIDS
      2. Treatment: symptomatic; hepatitis B hyperimmunoglobulin
      3. Diagnosis: transaminase elevation, HBsAg, anti-HBc
      4. Prevention: hepatitis B hyperimmunoglobulin after exposure, hepatitis B vaccine
   c) Non-A, non-B hepatitis:
      1. Epidemiology: usually associated with either hepatitis C or hepatitis E
      2. Transmission: blood or blood products most common form of post-transfusion hepatitis
   d) Hepatitis C:
      1. Epidemiology: transmission by blood or blood products; sexual exposure or needle stick injury less effective in transmitting the infection
   e) Delta hepatitis (hepatitis D):
      1. Epidemiology: found only in association with hepatitis B. It is particularly likely to lead to chronic active hepatitis and its complications, including cirrhosis, liver cell failure, and hepatocellular carcinoma. These complications can also occur with hepatitis B, hepatitis C, and hepatitis E.
   f) Hepatitis E:
      1. Definition: the enterically transmitted form of non-A, non-B hepatitis
2. **Alcoholic hepatitis and cirrhosis:**
   a) Alcoholic hepatitis:
      1. Signs and symptoms: the symptoms of alcoholic hepatitis closely resemble the symptoms of viral hepatitis. In alcoholic hepatitis, the ratio of AST to ALT is usually 2:1. Patients who develop alcoholic hepatitis are at high risk for developing cirrhosis of the liver.
   b) Cirrhosis of the liver:
      1. Symptoms and signs: weakness, fatigue, weight loss, anorexia, hepatomegaly, spider nevi, palmar erythema, asterixis, tremor, and ascites. Patients often develop portal hypertension with its complications and hepatic encephalopathy.
      2. Treatment: try penicillamine, propylthiouracil, Actigall, colchicine and probenecid, and interferon-α to treat the cirrhosis itself. Treatments for complications of cirrhosis include paracentesis for ascites, sodium restriction, diuretics (especially spironolactone) with/without thiazides or loop diuretics, and Laveen shunt.
      3. Complications: upper gastrointestinal bleeding from varices, hemorrhagic gastritis, or gastroduodenal ulcers; liver failure, hepatic encephalopathy, hepatorenal syndrome, and hepatocellular carcinoma

SUGGESTED READINGS

Sievert W. Acute and chronic hepatitis. In: Rakel R, ed. Conn's current therapy. Philadelphia: WB Saunders, 1994.

Zucker S, Gollan J. Cirrhosis. In: Rakel R, ed. Conn's current therapy. Philadelphia: WB Saunders, 1994.

PROBLEM 17   A 38-YEAR-OLD FEMALE WITH LOWER ABDOMINAL PAIN AND CONSTIPATION

A 38-year-old female presents to your office with a 1-year history of lower abdominal pain associated with constipation (one hard bowel movement every 3 days) and the passage of mucus per rectum on a regular basis. She has never passed blood/rectum to her knowledge. She describes no fever, chills, weight loss, jaundice, or any other symptoms. There is no relationship between the abdominal pain and food intake.

On P/E, the abdomen is scaphoid, and no hepatosplenomegaly or other masses are palpated. There is a very mild generalized abdominal tenderness, but it does not localize.

SELECT THE ONE BEST ANSWER TO THE FOLLOWING QUESTIONS

1. What is the most likely diagnosis in this patient?
   a) psychosocial abdomen
   b) Crohn's disease
   c) ulcerative colitis
   d) lactose intolerance
   e) none of the above

2. Which of the following statements regarding the condition described is(are) false?
   a) the typical location of the abdominal pain is the lower abdomen
   b) defecation frequently relieves the pain
   c) there is often a perception of incomplete emptying of the rectum
   d) bowel action is often irregular
   e) very severe abdominal tenderness is a hallmark of the disease

3. What is the most likely cause of the disorder described?
   a) a mass lesion in the area of the sigmoid colon
   b) a low-grade chronic inflammation of the entire small and large bowel
   c) an autoimmune phenomenon
   d) a decreased ability to digest certain foods
   e) none of the above

4. Which of the following would be most unlikely in a patient with the above condition?
   a) alternating diarrhea and constipation
   b) increased pain at times of stress
   c) pain upon awakening from sleep
   d) abdominal bloating
   e) increased passage of flatus

5. Which of the following investigations is not indicated in the condition described?
   a) a complete blood count
   b) an ESR
   c) electrolytes
   d) abdominal ultrasound
   e) thyroid function studies

6. Which of the following may have to be considered in the differential diagnosis of the condition described above?
   a) colonic adenocarcinoma
   b) fecal impaction
   c) celiac disease
   d) endometriosis
   e) all of the above

7. Which of the following conditions (symptoms) is not associated with the condition?
   a) gastroesophageal reflux disease
   b) cholelithiasis
   c) noncardiac chest pain
   d) depression
   e) fatigue

8. Which of the following statements concerning the condition described is(are) true?
   a) this condition is the most common reason for referral from a family physician to a gastroenterologist
   b) this condition is slightly more common in men
   c) the symptoms associated with this condition are more common in young adults than in older adults
   d) this condition has been associated with a specific biochemical abnormality in some patients
   e) all of the above statements are true

9. Which of the following is the most important component of management of the condition described?
   a) single-agent pharmacologic therapy
   b) multiple-agent pharmacologic therapy
   c) a therapeutic physician-patient relationship
   d) a focused diet
   e) a diet elimination trial: eliminating one food at a time until the responsible food is found

10. Which of the following medications should not be used in the treatment of the condition described above?
    a) psyllium
    b) loperamide
    c) cholestyramine
    d) codeine phosphate
    e) desipramine

11. Recent initial research suggests a significant correlation between IBS and which of the following?
    a) hypochondriasis
    b) history of sexual abuse
    c) somatoform disease
    d) early ulcerative colitis
    e) none of the above

Short Answer Management Problem 17

A 32-year-old female with chronic abdominal pain that has been fully investigated and diagnosed as irritable bowel syndrome (IBS) presents to your office as a new patient. She has seen two family physicians and two gastroenterologists. Although she has been told the same thing by all physicians, she seeks another opinion from you. Discuss what you would and would not do in your consultation with this patient.

ANSWERS

1. E. The most likely diagnosis is irritable bowel syndrome (IBS). IBS is characterized by the following:
   a. Abdominal pain or discomfort, relieved with defecation or associated with a change in frequency or consistency of stools
   b. An irregular pattern of defecation at least 25% of the time, consisting of three or more of the following:
      i) altered stool frequency
      ii) altered stool form (hard or loose and watery)
      iii) altered stool passage (straining or urgency), feeling of incomplete evacuation
      iv) passage of mucus
      v) bloating or a feeling of abdominal distention
   Psychosocial abdomen is not a diagnosis.

   Crohn's disease is unlikely in the absence of systemic symptoms including nonbloody diarrhea, anorexia, weight loss, fever, and fatigue.

   Ulcerative colitis is unlikely in the absence of weight loss, tenesmus, and the passage of bright red blood/rectum.

   Lactose intolerance is specifically linked to the intake of milk and milk products.

   Although many consider IBS to be a diagnosis of exclusion, the diagnostic criteria given in this answer suggest very specific inclusive clues. This suggests that in a field as complicated as medicine and oriented toward the biopsychosocial model of illness, it is rather dangerous to suggest the following: if not (A), not (B), and if not (C), then (D).

2. E. The perception of incomplete emptying of the rectum, the irregular bowel action, and the relief of the abdominal pain with defecation have already been discussed. In IBS, the abdominal pain is confined to the lower abdomen, with the commonest location being in the area of the sigmoid colon. Although abdominal tenderness may be present, it is usually not very severe, and it certainly is not a hallmark of the disease.

3. E. The cause of irritable bowel syndrome is unknown, except for a likely association with either altered motility or altered visceral sensation. IBS may be associated with significant psychosocial dysfunction or psychological (psychiatric) disorders. Spousal abuse, a history of sexual abuse, or depression should be considered.

4. C. Pain upon awakening from sleep is suggestive of an organic etiology. In addition to this symptom, pain that interferes with normal sleep patterns, diarrhea that awakens the patient from sleep, visible or occult blood in the stool, weight loss, and fever suggest organic disease.

5. D. The investigations that are recommended in a patient with IBS include CBC, ESR, a chemistry panel, a flexible sigmoidoscopy, stool for ova/parasites/fecal leukocytes, and thyroid function studies.

6. E. Diagnoses that may need to be considered in patients with symptoms of IBS include colonic adenocarcinoma, ulcerative colitis, Crohn's disease, abdominal angina, ischemic colitis, drugs, pseudo-obstruction, intermittent sigmoid volvulus, megacolon, celiac disease, bacterial overgrowth syndrome, giardiasis, endometriosis, depression, somatization, and panic disorder.

7. B. Conditions that are more common in patients with IBS include gastroesophageal reflux disease with heartburn, dysphagia, globus hystericus, noncardiac chest pain, urologic dysfunction, fatigue, and gynecologic problems. Cholelithiasis is not associated with irritable bowel syndrome.

8. A. IBS is the most common reason for referral by a family physician to a GI specialist.

   IBS is slightly more common in women than in men. Although symptoms typically begin in young adulthood, the prevalence is similar in elderly and younger adults.

   IBS is one of a group of disorders that includes chest pain of unexplained origin, non-ulcer dyspepsia, and biliary dyskinesia. These chronic disorders are frequently considered functional, because no specific structural or biochemical causes have been found.

9. C. The most important component of treatment in IBS is establishing a therapeutic, communicative, and trusting physician-patient relationship and educating the patent regarding the benign nature of the condition and favorable long-term prognosis.

   The important components of doctor-patient relationship that should be emphasized include a nonjudgmental attitude, concern regarding the patient's understanding of the illness, expectations and consistent limits, and involvement of the patient in treatment decisions. Because of the long-term nature of IBS, primary management by a family physician is essential. Although consultants may be needed in some cases for both patient and family physician reassurance, this should be the exception rather than the rule.

Diet therapy and pharmacologic therapy will be discussed in a subsequent question.

10. D. Treatment of irritable bowel syndrome includes the following:
   1. The elimination of certain foods including gas-forming foods such as legumes or dairy products
   2. Supplements with high-fiber foods such as bran
   Other agents recommended in the treatment of IBS include the following:
   1. psyllium (another bulking agent)
   2. antispasmodic or anticholinergic agents such as belladonna and dicyclomine when abdominal spasm is the predominant symptom
   3. antidiarrheal agents such as diphenoxylate, loperamide, or cholestyramine where diarrhea is the predominant symptom
   4. tricyclic antidepressants such as amitriptyline or desipramine where pain (or a chronic pain syndrome) is the predominant symptom
   5. prokinetic agents such as cisapride for patients when constipation is the predominant symptom
   Long-term benzodiazepines are not recommended, although treatment for short periods may be indicated. Codeine phosphate or other narcotic agents are contraindicated in the treatment of IBS because of the potential for abuse or tolerance.

11. B. A disturbing correlation between IBS and a previous history of sexual abuse in the patient has recently been established. Although the results need to be verified, this should alert the clinician to ask about sexual abuse in anyone who presents with or is diagnosed as having IBS. Thus a history of sexual abuse joins the questions associated with depression as lead questions required to be asked by the family physician.

SOLUTION TO SHORT ANSWER MANAGEMENT PROBLEM 17

In the management of this patient, you, the new family physician, should consider doing and not doing the following:

You Should:
1. Do a complete history including a psychosocial history, a family history, and a marital history.

2. Attempt to ascertain the patient's understanding and concerns about the condition.
3. Establish a strong, trusting family physician-patient relationship. This forms the basis for the therapy (supportive psychotherapy) that follows
4. Have the patient ask all of his or her questions in an unhurried atmosphere.
5. Perform a complete or relatively complete physical examination for two reasons: to reassure yourself that nothing significant has been missed, and to reassure the patient that you are truly interested in the problem.
6. Ascertain what dietary and drug therapies have been tried, and decide on those therapies that may be indicated at this time.

You Should Not:
1. Repeat investigations, nor should you order other, more costly investigations.
2. Criticize your colleagues for failure to completely investigate this problem until a cause was found; you will find yourself in the same situation someday.
3. Promise what you cannot deliver: a cure for IBS. Also, do not let the patient transfer ownership of the problem to you. It is the patient's problem, and your job is not to solve it; your job is to provide the empathic support necessary to help the patient understand and deal with the illness.
4. Rely on a polypharmacy approach to achieve a better result. Use the suggested drugs with prudence and caution.
5. Use narcotic analgesics as a treatment for IBS.

SUMMARY

1. IBS is extremely common; prevalence estimates suggest that 10%-22% of the population have symptoms compatible with this diagnosis at some time in their lives.
2. IBS is the most common condition that gastroenterologists see in referral or consultation practice.
3. Consider IBS as a diagnosis of inclusion rather than exclusion. Base your diagnosis on the positive criteria discussed previously.
4. Consider the minimal investigations that have been suggested as sufficient; do not overinvestigate. Remember the definition of a "normal" person: a normal person is someone who has not been sufficiently investigated.
5. After establishing a strong doctor-patient relationship, consider dietary manipulation as primary therapy.
6. Antispasmodics, anticholinergics, tricyclic antidepressants, antidiarrheal agents, and prokinetic agents are drugs that can be used for the treatment of IBS. Use caution combining them.
7. Reassurance regarding the benign nature of the condition and the provision of hope for eventual reso-

lution of the symptoms are likely the most important therapy for this condition (supportive psychotheapy).

8. Identification and treatment of psychosocial stressors (stressors of some kind are almost invariably associated with this condition) are paramount.

9. Recent research suggests strong correlation between IBS and a history of sexual abuse.

SUGGESTED READINGS

Gwyther RE, et al. Validity of the family APGAR in patients with irritable bowel syndrome. Family Medicine 1993; 25:21-25.

Lynn RB, Friedman LS. Irritable bowel syndrome. N Engl J Med 1993; 329(26):1940-1945.

PROBLEM 18   A 75-YEAR-OLD MALE WITH METASTATIC BONE PAIN SECONDARY TO ADVANCED PROSTATE CANCER

A 75-year-old male diagnosed with stage D cancer of the prostate 6 months ago presents to your office. He has been asymptomatic for the past 6 months, but last week he began to develop severe pain in the lower lumbar spine. He also appears quite pale.

On examination his prostate is rock-hard. He has tender lumbar vertebrae L2 to L5.

Your suspicions of metastatic bone disease are confirmed when a technetium-99 bone scan shows increased uptake of radionuclide in L2-5 and in both femurs, both tibias, and both humeri.

SELECT THE ONE BEST ANSWER TO THE FOLLOWING QUESTIONS

1. What is the treatment of first choice at this time?
   a) high-dose morphine sulfate
   b) high-dose hydromorphone
   c) transdermal fentanyl
   d) palliative radiotherapy to the lumbar spine
   e) acetaminophen-hydrocodone

2. You institute appropriate therapy for this patient. He quickly becomes pain free and remains that way for 6 months. He then returns with cervical, thoracic, and lumbar back pain; bilateral thigh pain; bilateral knee and leg pain; and pain in both shoulders and both arms (diffuse). Therapeutic options at this time include which of the following?
   a) IV clodrinate
   b) IV radioactive strontium
   c) morphine sulfate
   d) hydromorphone
   e) naproxen
   f) all of the above

3. Which of the following pharmacologic agents is the drug of first choice for the treatment of mild metastatic bone pain?
   a) morphine sulfate
   b) hydromorphone
   c) fentanyl
   d) an NSAID
   e) carbamazepine

4. Which of the following drug(s) should not be used in the management of chronic pain?
   a) codeine
   b) meperidine
   c) levorphanol
   d) methadone
   e) a and b
   f) b and d

5. A 52-year-old male with metastatic renal cell carcinoma presents for assessment of a pain beginning in the buttocks and traveling down the left leg. It has a sharp, stabbing, burning, or "zinger-like" quality, according to the patient. The patient indicates that the baseline pain is 5 on a 10-point scale increasing up to 7/10 and decreasing down to 3/10. What is(are) the drug(s) of first choice for the management of this patient's cancer pain?
   a) carbamazepine
   b) hydromorphone
   c) morphine sulfate
   d) amitriptyline
   e) desipramine

6. Another patient with metastatic renal cell carcinoma presents for assessment of a pain also beginning in the buttocks and traveling down the left leg. The only difference between the two patients is that this patient describes his pain as dull and throbbing. The baseline level is 4/10 increasing up to 8/10 and decreasing down to 2/10. What is(are) the drug(s) of first choice for the management of this patient's cancer pain?
   a) carbamazepine
   b) hydromorphone
   c) morphine sulfate
   d) desipramine
   e) valproic acid

7. The location of the lesions described in the two patients presented in Questions 5 and 6 is best portrayed as which of the following?
   a) retroperitoneal
   b) lumbar-sacral plexopathy
   c) intraabdominal-visceral
   d) a and b
   e) b and c

8. What percentage of patients with cancer pain respond well to first-line analgesic therapy such as acetaminophen or NSAIDs?
   a) 1%
   b) 5%
   c) 10%
   d) 15%
   e) 20%

9. Which of the following agents would be classified as second-line analgesic therapy for the management of cancer pain?

a) hydrocodone
b) acetaminophen
c) morphine sulfate
d) levorphanol
e) hydromorphone

10. Which of the following agents is not classified as third-line pharmacological agents in the management of cancer pain?
    a) methadone
    b) morphine sulfate
    c) hydromorphone
    d) fentanyl
    e) codeine

11. A patient presents to your office with moderately severe cancer pain. You prescribe the third-line agent (due to the description of the pain as moderately severe). Which of the following best describes the preferred approach to managing this patient's cancer pain?
    a) begin with a twice daily PO dose of long-acting morphine
    b) begin with a twice daily PO dose of long-acting morphine plus short-acting PO morphine for breakthrough pain
    c) begin with a q4h dose of short-acting PO morphine
    d) begin with a transdermal fentanyl analgesic patch
    e) begin with a dose of 200 mg morphine/day in any form

12. A patient who is maintained on long-acting morphine with short-acting morphine for breakthrough presents with a 1-week history of an increasing need for short-acting morphine. He is now taking three times the number of short-acting tablets as previously. What should you do at this time?
    a) prescribe more short-acting morphine; keep the amount of long-acting morphine the same
    b) transfer the increased requirement into long-acting morphine and maintain a supply of short-acting morphine
    c) transfer the increased requirement into both increasing amounts of long-acting morphine and increased amounts of short-acting morphine
    d) switch to another third-line oral agent
    e) switch to a transdermal delivery system

13. What is the average starting daily dose of morphine sulfate in the treatment of a patient with moderately severe cancer pain?
    a) 10 mg–15 mg
    b) 15 mg–30 mg
    c) 30 mg–60 mg
    d) 60 mg–120 mg
    e) 120 mg–240 mg

14. Which of the following statements regarding the use of morphine in the treatment of cancer pain is(are) true?
    a) morphine produces rapid tolerance
    b) morphine produces euphoria
    c) morphine produces addiction
    d) morphine produces respiratory depression
    e) none of the above

15. When starting a patient on a narcotic analgesic, what is the single most important agent that should be started at the same time?
    a) an agent to prevent constipation
    b) an agent to prevent nausea and vomiting
    c) an agent to enhance sedation
    d) an agent to prevent drowsiness
    e) an antidepressant

16. Which of the following is(are) essential elements of cancer pain management?
    a) a collaborative, interdisciplinary approach to care
    b) an individualized pain-control plan developed and agreed on by the patient
    c) ongoing assessment and reassessment of the patient's pain
    d) the use of both pharmacologic and nonpharmacologic therapies to prevent or control pain
    e) all of the above

17. Which of the following is(are) aims of pain management in palliative care?
    a) to identify the cause of the pain
    b) to prevent the pain from recurring
    c) to maintain a clear sensorium
    d) to maintain a normal effect
    e) all of the above

18. Which of the following is the most effective (quality of life years effect) strategy for reversing the confusion and drowsiness caused by the administration of narcotic analgesics?
    a) decrease the amount of the analgesic given
    b) switch to another oral narcotic analgesic
    c) add methylphenidate to the treatment plan
    d) switch to a transdermal delivery system
    e) switch specifically to oral methadone

19. Which of the following factors modify the pain threshold in patients with cancer pain?
    a) insomnia
    b) fear
    c) anxiety
    d) sadness
    e) all of the above

20. Which of the following statements concerning the use of narcotic analgesics in the treatment of cancer pain is(are) true?
    a) most patients with cancer pain can be effectively treated with oral agents
    b) narcotic analgesics may be effectively administered by the rectal route
    c) the subcutaneous infusion of narcotic analgesics has become the delivery method of choice in patients who cannot, for whatever reason, tolerate oral analgesics any longer
    d) intramuscular narcotic administration on a regular basis is a reasonable alternative for pain control in terminally ill cancer patients
    e) all of the above
    f) a, b, and c only

21. A patient develops severe nausea and vomiting as the dose of morphine being used for terminal cancer pain (endometrial) is increased. The patient is on triple antinauseant therapy. Triple antinauseant therapy includes dimenhydrinate, metoclopramide, and prochlorperazine. Which of the following statements regarding this situation is(are) true?
    a) you should add a fourth antinauseant to the regime at this time, preferably a corticosteroid or ondansetron
    b) you should put an IV in place and make sure the input equals the output; do not change drugs
    c) decrease the dose of the morphine by 10% for 24 hours
    d) switch to another narcotic analgesic; no further investigations necessary or desired
    e) none of the above

22. A patient is switched from morphine sulfate to hydromorphone. You are aware that the oral equianalgesic equivalent dose is 6/1 (6 parts morphine = 1 part hydromorphone). What should you do at this time?
    a) start oral hydromorphone at the equianalgesic dose
    b) start oral hydromorphone at $\frac{1}{5}$ of the equianalgesic dose
    c) start oral hydromorphone at twice the equianalgesic dose

d) start oral hydromorphone at $\frac{1}{2}$ the equianalgesic dose
e) start oral hydromorphone at $\frac{1}{3}$ the equianalgesic dose

23. A patient who is being treated for terminal cancer pain (esophageal adenocarcinoma) with oral morphine is requiring increased morphine doses daily. Six weeks ago his morphine dose was 180 mg/day; it is 600 mg/day now. Which of the following statements regarding this increased dose of morphine is(are) true?
    a) the dosage increase most likely represents tolerance to the morphine
    b) the dosage increase most likely represents increased requirements due to tumor growth
    c) both of the above statements are true
    d) either a or b could be true, but not both
    e) neither a nor b

24. A patient is being treated for breast cancer with adjuvant chemotherapy following a lumpectomy. One of the drugs she is taking is cisplatin. She develops intractable nausea and vomiting while on this drug. Which of the following antiemetics is the drug of first choice for this patient?
    a) prochlorperazine
    b) ondansetron
    c) dimenhydrinate
    d) metoclopramide
    e) dexamethasone

25. A patient develops intractable nausea and vomiting secondary to carcinoma of the colon with partial bowel obstruction. She has been on both morphine and hydromorphone by mouth but is having great difficulty keeping anything down. What would you do at this time?
    a) switch to levorphanol for the pain
    b) switch to methadone for the pain
    c) switch from the oral medication route to a subcutaneous infusion
    d) switch from the oral route to the suppository route
    e) switch from the oral route to the intravenous route

Short Answer Management Problem 18

Discuss the following statement: "Overdosing cancer patients with narcotic analgesics is much more of a problem than underdosing cancer patients with narcotic analgesics."

ANSWERS

1. D. This patient, who was diagnosed as stage D cancer of the prostate 6 months ago, was treated in a responsible way. When a man with metastatic cancer has no symptoms, it is probably better to wait and save the limited weapons available until needed.

   A very important point in this case is that although

his bone scan shows more diffuse skeletal disease, his clinical status suggests symptoms only in the lumbar spine. Thus, radiation therapy to the lumbar spine is the most reasonable course of action. Again, the reasoning is that local symptoms should receive local therapy. (This applies to palliative situations only.)

Although it wouldn't be wrong to start with morphine sulfate or hydromorphone, it would be wrong to start high-dose morphine sulfate or high-dose hydromorphone. These narcotics will be discussed in great length in subsequent questions.

2. F. The therapeutic options for the treatment of metastatic bone disease are rapidly increasing. The following treatment options have been shown to be effective: Clodrinate (a biphosphatate derivative), radioactive strontium, nonsteroidal antiinflammatory drugs, and narcotic analgesics.

A reasonable treatment plan at this time would be the following: begin with a nonsteroidal antiinflammatory agent (naproxen) plus short-acting morphine sulfate or short-acting hydromorphone for breakthrough pain.

Ask the patient to call you within 24 hours to ensure the beginning of pain decrease. On his next visit (in perhaps a week if you are beginning to get his pain under control) you could switch him to (1) a long-acting morphine preparation or a longer-acting hydromorphone preparation, plus (2) continue the nonsteroidal antiinflammatory agent, plus (3) continue to supply him with short-acting narcotics for breakthrough pain, plus (4) decide on either Clodrinate or radioactive strontium as adjuvant therapy.

3. D. The drug class of first choice for the management of mild to moderate metastatic bone pain is the NSAID agents. The most commonly used NSAIDs for bone pain include diclofenac, and naproxen.

4. B. Meperidine (Demerol) is contraindicated in the management of chronic pain (both malignant and nonmalignant). The reasons for its contraindication are its relatively short half-life and its lack of efficacy.

The other drugs, fentanyl (transdermal, SC, or IV), levorphanol (oral), and methadone (oral), are all very reasonable agents to use in the management of chronic cancer pain. Note the words cancer pain. From experience and the opinions of world authorities on this issue, it is best (in almost all cases) not to use narcotic analgesics to manage chronic nonmalignant pain.

5. A.

6. D.

7. D. These questions illustrate the use of adjuvant analgesics in the treatment of neuropathic pain. Neuropathic pain is the most common type of cancer pain and presents diagnostic and therapeutic challenges.

We have determined the following about neuropathic pain:
A. There are basically two descriptions of the pain:
   1. Sharp, stabbing, burning, or "zinger-like"
   2. Dull, aching pain
B. Both types of neuropathic pain respond better to adjuvant analgesics than to narcotic analgesics.
C. The two pain types that respond better to different adjuvant agents are as follows:
   1. The sharp, stabbing, burning, or "zinger-like" pain (responds better to anticonvulsant medications):
      First choice: carbamazepine
      Second choice: valproic acid
   2. The dull, "aching" pain (responds better to two tricyclic antidepressants):
      First choice: desipramine
      Second choice: amitriptyline (unless sedation also would be of benefit to the patient)

The greatest number of neuropathic pains seen in cancer pain management result from retroperitoneal lesions either infiltrating or pressing on the lumbar-sacral plexus.

8. E.

9. A.

10. E. The World Health Organization has developed an analgesic ladder for the treatment of cancer pain. Although it is not necessarily always in the patient's best interest to start with a first-line agent (the pain may be too severe), many patients can be managed with first-line agents such as acetaminophen or NSAIDs. In fact, 20-25% of patients with cancer pain can have their pain totally or almost totally controlled with these agents.

The World Health Organization's analgesic ladder is summarized as follows:
I. First-line agents:
   A. ASA
   B. NSAIDs
   C. Acetaminophen
II. Second-line agents:
   A. Hydrocodone
   B. Codeine
III. Third-line agents:
   A. Morphine sulfate
   B. Hydromorphone
   C. Fentanyl
   D. Levorphaneol
   E. Leritine
   F. Methadone

11. C. The best approach to the management of moderately severe cancer pain is to begin with an every-4-hour dose of short-acting morphine sulfate (the drug of first choice in the third-line group) and have the patient use the analgesic as needed to attain complete pain control. Once the dose is established you may switch to a longer-acting preparation (bid) and maintain for the patient a supply of short-acting morphine for breakthrough pain.

12. B. What the patient needs at this time is an increased supply of long-acting morphine as well as the maintenance of a supply of short-acting morphine for breakthrough pain.

13. C. The average daily starting dose of morphine sulfate (oral) in a patient with moderately severe cancer pain is 30 to 60 mg.

14. E. All of the above statements regarding morphine are false. These statements are known as the "morphine myths" and do not apply to patients who are in the terminal or palliative phase of illness.

    There is no maximum morphine or other analgesic equivalent dose. Each patient requires the dose to be individualized. This should be done by starting at lower doses and increasing the dose until you have achieved total pain control and are able to prevent further pain.

15. A. Any patient who is started on a narcotic analgesic should also be started on a regime to prevent constipation. The drugs most commonly used at this time include lactulose, an osmotic agent; and a combination of a stool softener and a peristaltic stimulant (such as docusate sodium and senna). An antiemetic such as dimenhydrinate, prochlorperazine, or metoclopramide may be indicated for the first 2 or 3 weeks to prevent nausea and vomiting that sometimes accompanies the initiation of a narcotic.

16. E. New clinical-practice guidelines have been issued by the Agency for Health Care Policy and Research, a branch of the Department of Health and Human Services. The purpose of these guidelines is to correct the problem of inadequate treatment (or underdosing) pain treatment for cancer.

    These guidelines call for the following:
    1. A collaborative, interdisciplinary approach to the care of patients with cancer pain
    2. An individualized pain-control plan developed and agreed on by the patient. The patient must be regarded as the head of the health care team.
    3. Ongoing assessment and reassessment of the patient's pain
    4. The use of both nonpharmacologic and pharmacologic therapies to prevent or control pain

    5. Explicit institutional policies on the management of cancer pain, with clear lines of responsibility for pain management and for monitoring its effectiveness

17. E. The aims of pain management in palliative care are as follows:
    1. To identify the cause of the pain
    2. To prevent the pain from occurring again
    3. To erase the memory of the pain
    4. To maintain a clear sensorium and a normal effect

    Remember that palliative care is active treatment, not passive treatment.

18. C. The most effective strategy for reversing the confusion and drowsiness caused by the administration of narcotic analgesics is to add the drug methylphenidate to the treatment regime. To decrease the amount of analgesic given will only increase the patient's pain.

    The switching to another oral agent will not solve the problem; the patient will most likely develop drowsiness and confusion on that agent as well.

    A transdermal delivery system should not be used until the patient's cancer pain is very well controlled.

19. E. Cancer pain is a complex entity that requires treatment of not only the somatic source(s) but also the other aspects including depression, anxiety, anger, and isolation. Pain threshold is raised by relief of symptoms, sleep, rest, empathy, understanding, diversion, elevation of mood, effective analgesic therapy, anxiolytic therapy, and antidepressant therapy.

    Pain threshold is lowered by discomfort, insomnia, fatigue, anxiety, fear, anger, sadness, depression, mental isolation, introversion, and past painful experiences.

    Cancer pain should be considered as a complex consisting of a physical component, a psychological component, a social component, and a spiritual component. Unless each one of these areas is addressed in the overall cancer pain management strategy, therapy will not be effective.

20. F. The following facts/treatments should be considered in cancer pain management:
    A. Cancer pain can be controlled in 90% of patients with oral medication.
    B. The subcutaneous infusion of opioid analgesics by a programmed subcutaneous pump is the treatment of choice in patients who, for whatever reason, cannot tolerate the oral route.
    C. The rectal route is an acceptable alternative in patients who cannot tolerate the oral route.
    D. Regular intramuscular injections to control cancer pain should be absolutely discouraged. There is no valid reason for their use.

21. E. At this time, the first priority is to determine the cause of the nausea. The narcotic analgesic may not be the cause. A thorough search for all other serious and potential causes of the nausea must be undertaken. In this case, a likely cause is hypercalcemia. Another common cause is the production by the tumor of emetic substances. Once causes such as these are ruled out, it is then reasonable to switch to another narcotic analgesic (such as hydromorphone) and/or to institute effective anti-emetic therapy.

22. B. When a patient is switched from one narcotic analgesic to another, a major adjustment has to be made in equianalgesic dose. A common mistake made is to begin the patient on the exact equivalent (in mg) of the previously used narcotic. An equianalgesic dose no greater than one-fifth should be the starting dose of the next opioid. This is due to different types of opioid receptors in the brain.

    For example, the switch from oral morphine to oral hydromorphone should be as follows:
    1. The patient is currently on 120 mg of oral morphine/day.
    2. The equianalgesic dose is 120 mg/6 (conversion factor) = 20 mg hydromorphone.
    3. Starting the patient at one fifth of the equianalgesic dose will be 20 mg/5 = 4 mg hydromorphone.

    The pain control should be assessed frequently and the dose increased as needed.

23. C. The increase in the dose of morphine over the 6-week period most likely represents a combination of tolerance to morphine and increased requirements due to growth of the tumor. As pointed out earlier, rapid tolerance is not usually seen when the patient is being given a narcotic for cancer pain. However, tolerance does develop and must be considered. That is another reason for the answer that was given to Question 22.

24. B. Chemotherapy that includes the drug cisplatin is very likely to produce very severe nausea and vomiting. It is mandatory, therefore, to treat this aggressively. Ondansetron, a new serotonin antagonist, has been found to be extremely useful for the control of chemotherapy-induced nausea and is recommended. In other cases in which control is difficult despite combination antinauseant therapy, ondansetron should be used.

25. C. Cancer pain can be controlled by oral medications in the vast majority of cases (90%). When control, with oral medications becomes impossible, however, it is necessary to switch to another route. Three possible routes are available: the suppository route, the intravenous route, and the subcutaneous route.

    With a patient in severe discomfort, the subcutaneous route is the route of choice. This is best accomplished with the use of a computer-controlled subcutaneous infusion pump. This provides a constant infusion rate and boluses whenever needed.

SOLUTION TO SHORT ANSWER MANAGEMENT PROBLEM 18

This statement is completely false. Exactly the opposite is true. Patients with cancer pain are often very ineffectively treated. The ineffectiveness of treatment equates to significant undertreatment. It is estimated that 50% of patients with cancer pain die in significant pain. The major reasons for this appear to be the following:
1. Fear on the part of physicians of using "too much" narcotic
2. Fear on the part of physicians that the cancer patients will become addicted to the narcotics
3. Fear on the part of physicians that they will personally get in trouble with their state medical board for prescribing strong narcotics to anyone
4. A lack of knowledge regarding cancer pain management, the drugs that need to be used, and the doses of those drugs

All of these contribute to the significant undertreatment described. Consequently, many patients suffer needless pain in the final stages of life.

SUMMARY OF THE DIAGNOSIS AND TREATMENT OF CANCER PAIN

1. **The Ten Commandments of Cancer Pain Management:**
    1. Thou shalt not assume that the patient's pain is due to the malignant process. Always begin with steps aimed at making a specific, anatomic, and pathologic diagnosis.
    2. Thou shalt consider the patient's feelings. Pain threshold varies with mood and morale. Given the opportunity to express fears, the patient should experience less pain.
    3. Thou shalt not use the abbreviation PRN. Achieving balanced pain control means avoiding the return of pain due to gaps in medication administration. Less medication will be required if given around the clock.
    4. Thou shalt prescribe adequate amounts of medication. The right dose of medication is not dictated by recommendations from a book, but rather by the patient's level of pain. Use what it takes to relieve the pain, titrating for effect.
    5. Thou shalt always try nonnarcotic medications as the first step unless your clinical judgment deems the patient to be in moderately severe or severe pain. Mild to moderate pain in many cases will respond to acetaminophen or NSAIDs. NSAIDs are particularly useful for bony metastases.
    6. Thou shalt not be afraid of narcotic analgesics. When nonnarcotic agents fail, move to a narcotic agent quickly.

7. Thou shalt not limit thyself to using only drug therapies. Nondrug therapies such as hypnosis, imagery techniques, biofeedback, physiotherapy, individual psychotherapy, group psychotherapy, and family psychotherapy are very beneficial.

8. Thou shalt not be reluctant to seek a colleague's advice. When you have exhausted your skills or run out of ideas, ask someone else to evaluate your patient.

9. Thou shalt provide support for the entire family. Treatment of anticipatory grief experienced by the family will help to prevent isolation and loneliness. Be able to intervene quickly when a crisis arises.

10. Thou shalt maintain an air of quiet confidence and cautious optimism. Aim for "graded relief," choosing small goals that can be accomplished to build the patient's trust and hope. Exhibit a determination to succeed.

2. **The World Health Organization Analgesic Ladder:**
   Step 3
   a) Morphine sulfate
   b) Hydromorphone
   c) Fentanyl
   d) Levorphanol
   e) Methadone
   Step 2
   a) Codeine (with or without acetaminophen)
   b) Hydrodocone (with or without acetaminophen or ASA)
   Step 1
   a) Acetaminophen
   b) ASA
   c) NSAIDs

3. **Classification of cancer pain:**
   a) Somatic pain (including bone pain)
   b) Neuropathic pain:
      1. Sharp, stabbing, burning, "zinger" = Type I
      2. Dull, aching = Type II
   c) Visceral pain

4. **Adjuvant analgesics:**
   a) Corticosteroids: Adjuvant analgesics used especially in visceral pain where there is swelling around a visceral capsule (for example, the hepatic capsule)
   b) Tricyclic antidepressants: Adjuvant analgesic used for neuropathic pain of the dull, aching pain (amitriptyline, desipramine)
   c) Anticonvulsant medications: Adjuvant analgesics for neuropathic pain of the sharp, stabbing, burning, "zinger-like" type
   d) Nonsteroidal antiinflammatory drugs: Adjuvant analgesics for somatic pain (metastatic bone)

5. **Pathophysiology of cancer pain:**
   a) Physical (biologic) component: 25%
   b) Psychological (emotional) component: 25%
   c) Social component: 25%
   d) Spiritual component: 25%
   Unless all four components are addressed, the treatment of cancer pain will be unsuccessful.

6. **Routes of administration:**
   a) Oral (90% of cancer cases)
   b) Subcutaneous (5% of cancer cases)
   c) Rectal (5% of cancer cases)

7. **Conversion of one narcotic analgesic to another:**
   a) Calculate equianalgesic doses between drug 1 (the drug about to be discontinued) and drug 2 (the drug to be started).
   b) Begin drug 2 at no more than 20% of equianalgesic dose. The reasons for this are that there is tolerance built up to the first drug, and that different narcotics react on different receptors in the brain.

8. **Method of beginning narcotic analgesic for moderate to severe cancer pain:**
   a) Choice drug: usually morphine sulfate
   b) Begin morphine sulfate with short-acting morphine (morphine 5- or 10-mg tabs)
   c) Daily starting dose: 30 mg-60 mg/day
   d) In one week, switch total daily dose to long-acting morphine; continue short-acting morphine for breakthrough
   e) Begin bowel regime at same time as narcotic is begun: (1) lactulose or (2) stool softener (Colace) plus peristaltic stimulant (senna alkaloid)
   f) Consider antiemetic therapy for the first few weeks of narcotic therapy (prochlorperazine, dimenhydrinate, metoclopramide)

9. **Cancer pain:** optimal management combines pharmacologic management with nonpharmacologic management:
   Nonpharmacologic therapies:
   a) Relaxation techniques
   b) Support groups
   c) Biofeedback
   d) Mental imagery
   e) Physiotherapy
   f) Transcutaneous electrical nerve stimulation (TENS)
   g) Physical activity
   h) Individual psychotherapy
   i) Group psychotherapy
   j) Family psychotherapy

10. **Other forms of palliative cancer pain therapy:**
    a) Palliative radiotherapy: especially useful for metastatic bone pain and neuropathic pain (lumbo-sacral plexopathy and brachial plexopathy)
    b) Palliative surgery
    c) Palliative chemotherapy

SUGGESTED READINGS

Doyle D, Hanks G, MacDonald N, eds. Oxford textbook of palliative medicine. Oxford: Oxford University Press, 1993.

Twycross R. Principles and practice of pain relief in terminal cancer. In: Corr C, Corr D, eds. Hospice care: Principles and practice. New York: Springer, 1983.

PROBLEM 19   A 51-YEAR-OLD FEMALE WITH SEVERE NAUSEA, VOMITING, AND ANOREXIA IN SEVERE, ADVANCED OVARIAN CANCER

A 51-year-old female patient with advanced ovarian cancer has terminal disease. She is constantly nauseated, vomiting, and anorexic. You are called to see her at home. In addition to the symptoms mentioned, the patient complains of a "sore abdomen" and is having significant difficulty breathing. She also has a "sore mouth."

The patient has gone through chemotherapy with cisplatinum. This therapy ended 8 months ago. Her ovarian cancer was first discovered 12 months ago. Since that time her condition has deteriorated to the point where she has lost 40 pounds and is feeling "weaker and weaker" every day.

On examination, the patient's breathing is labored. Her respiratory rate is 28/minute. The breath sounds heard in both lungs are normal.

Her mouth is dry, and there are whitish lesions that rub off with a tongue depressor. She looks significantly cachetic. Her abdomen is significantly enlarged.

There is a level of shifting dullness as well as the presence of a large abdominal mass that is approximately 8 cm × 5 cm.

SELECT THE ONE BEST ANSWER TO THE FOLLOWING QUESTIONS

1. What is(are) the drug(s) of choice for the management of cancer-associated cachexia and anorexia?
   a) prednisone
   b) prochlorperazine
   c) megestrol acetate
   d) cyproheptadine
   e) a or c

2. The nausea and vomiting that this patient has developed may be treated with various measures or drugs. Which of the following could be recommended as first-line agents for this patient's nausea and vomiting?
   a) prochlorperazine
   b) dimenhydrinate
   c) metoclopramide
   d) all of the above
   e) none of the above

3. The drug that you selected for the treatment of the nausea and vomiting unfortunately was not effective. What would you do at this time?
   a) forget drugs and use an NG tube
   b) combine two or three of the above drugs
   c) forget treatment and attempt hydration with IV fluids
   d) select ondansetron as an antiemetic
   e) b or d

4. Based on the history of her "sore mouth" and white lesions that scrape off with a tongue depressor, what would you recommend treatment with?
   a) ketoconazole
   b) penicillin
   c) amphotericin B
   d) chloramphenicol
   e) methotrexate

5. The patient described undergoes palliative radiotherapy for severe bone pain that develops 1 month after the problems described. Following this, significant diarrhea develops. Which of the following agents may be helpful in the treatment of this problem?
   a) diphenoxylate hydrochloride
   b) loperamide
   c) codeine
   d) all of the above
   e) none of the above

6. What is the most prevalent symptom in patients with cancer?
   a) anorexia
   b) asthenia
   c) pain
   d) nausea
   e) constipation

7. What is the most frequent cause of chronic nausea and vomiting in advanced cancer?
   a) bowel obstruction
   b) raised intracranial pressure
   c) narcotic bowel syndrome
   d) hypercalcemia
   e) autonomic failure

8. The patient described in the question becomes increasingly short of breath. You suspect a pleural effusion. A chest X-ray confirms the diagnosis of a left pleural effusion. Which of the following is the treatment of first choice for the treatment of this complication?
   a) a thoracocentesis
   b) home oxygen
   c) a hospital bed that is elevated at the head
   d) decreased fluid intake
   e) prochlorperazine

9. Which of the following treatments may also be useful in treating this symptom?

a) palliative radiotherapy
b) prednisone
c) morphine sulfate
d) dexamethasone
e) all of the above

10. You treat the patient's pleural effusion effectively. One week later she develops increasing abdominal distention, nausea, and vomiting. You suspect a partial bowel obstruction.

    On examination, there are increased bowel sounds. A plain film of the abdomen confirms a diagnosis of partial bowel obstruction. Which of the following is(are) generally recommended as palliative measures for this symptom?
    a) decreased fluid intake
    b) metoclopramide
    c) chlorpromazine
    d) all of the above
    e) none of the above

11. A 53-year-old male presents to the ER with the sudden onset of left-sided weakness. He has a history of COPD from chronic bronchitis. He describes himself as "healthy as a horse" even though he smokes three packs of cigarettes/day.

    On examination, the patient has a left-sided hemiplegia. A chest X-ray shows a left-sided mass lesion and prominent hilar lymphadenopathy. You suspect a bronchogenic carcinoma.

    Which of the following statements regarding this patient is(are) true?
    a) there is likely no relationship between the hemiplegia and the chest X-ray findings
    b) the chances of recovery from the hemiplegia are essentially zero
    c) the cause of the hemiplegia is likely a cerebral embolus
    d) dexamethasone may be used both as a diagnostic test and a therapeutic maneuver in this patient
    e) none of the above are true

12. You are called to the home of a 42-year-old female with disseminated breast cancer. She has a fungating breast carcinoma that is emitting a very offensive odor. Her friends have stopped coming to see her because of the odor. The patient and her family have tried numerous remedies without success.

    Which of the following may be useful in the treatment of the odor associated with this fungating growth?
    a) frequent cleansings with saline
    b) application of yogurt dressings
    c) application of buttermilk dressings
    d) charcoal briquettes strategically placed throughout the house
    e) all of the above

13. You are called to the home of a 51-year-old patient with terminal colon cancer. He has become increasingly depressed and agitated and now is unable to sleep at night.

    As you talk to the patient and review in your head the DSM-IV criteria for depression, you realize that this patient has an agitated depression.

    Which of the following may be indicated in the treatment of this patient's condition?
    a) a sedating tricyclic antidepressant in the evening
    b) an anxiolytic agent given on a PRN basis
    c) fluoxetine
    d) a and/or b
    e) all of the above

14. With regard to narcotic-induced nausea and vomiting, which of the following statements is(are) true?
    a) nausea and/or vomiting is common in the initial narcotic administration period
    b) nausea and/or vomiting associated with narcotic analgesics usually subsides within 2 weeks of beginning therapy
    c) nausea and/or vomiting associated with narcotic administration can usually be prevented by the prophylactic use of medication
    d) all of the above are true
    e) none of the above are true

15. What is the drug of choice for the medical management of malignant ascites?
    a) hydrochlorothiazide
    b) spironolactone
    c) prednisone
    d) dexamethasone
    e) none of the above

16. What is the most common metabolic derangement associated with advanced malignancy?
    a) hyponatremia
    b) hypokalemia
    c) hypercalcemia
    d) hypomagnesemia
    e) hyperkalemia

17. What is the drug of choice for the management of narcotic-induced constipation?
    a) a senna preparation
    b) a psyllium compound
    c) sodium docusate
    d) lactulose
    e) Metamucil

18. Which of the following statements regarding the use of combination antinauseant therapy in cancer is true?
    a) combination antinauseants should not be used

b) the combination of any two drugs is just as effective as the combination of any other two

c) combination drugs should have affinity for different therapeutic receptors

d) oral antinauseants, especially when given together, are rarely effective for resistant nausea and or vomiting

e) none of the above are true

Short Answer Management Problem 19

Asthenia is the most commonly encountered symptom in terminally ill patients. Describe what the term *asthenia* means to you.

ANSWERS

1. E. Prednisone (a corticosteroid) and megestrol acetate (a progestational agent) are the pharmacological treatments of choice in patients with advanced cancer who have significant anorexia.

   In patients with anorexia, oral nutrition should be the first priority, with particular attention being paid to the timing of meals in relation to medical and nursing procedures and to the administration of drugs. Selected patients in whom oral nutrition or hydration is not possible may benefit from enteral nutrition or hypodermoclysis. Parenteral nutrition has shown no significant benefit in terms of improving survival or comfort, and its routine use is not indicated in palliative care.

   Megestrol acetate in a dosage of 460 mg/day is rapidly becoming the pharmacologic agent of choice in the treatment of anorexia.

   An alternative to progestational agents is prednisone. Prednisone may be given in doses of approximately 10 mg-15 mg/day. This may be increased if necessary.

   With anorexia, particular attention must be paid to the mouth to prevent candidiasis and other problems.

   Other potential choices for the pharmacologic treatment of anorexia include cyproheptadine, hydrazine sulfate, and cannabinoids.

2. D. The nonpharmacologic treatment of nausea and vomiting should include (1) attempting to find the cause, (2) the avoidance of a supine position to prevent the dangers of aspiration of vomit, (3) a general assessment of the environment of the patient and how it could be improved, (4) attention to body odors, (5) small, frequent meals (that the patient likes—not a bland diet), and (6) attractive food presentation.

   Antiemetics can be divided into several classes: (1) anticholinergics such as hyoscine and atropine, (2) pheothiazines such as prochlorperazine and chlorpromazine, (3) butyrophenones such as haloperidol and droperidol, (4) antihistamines such as cyclizine and promethazine, (5) gastrokinetic agents such as domperidone and metoclopramide, (6) 5-HT$_3$ receptor antagonists such as ondansetron, (7) corticosteroids such as prednisone and dexamethasone, and (8) miscellaneous agents such as ibuprofen, tricyclic antidepressants, benzodiazepines, and nabilone.

   There are some specific indications for certain antinauseants, such as the treatment of a partial bowel obstruction with a gastrokinetic agent, cyclizine for vestibular associated emesis, and ondansetron for chemotherapy-induced emesis. In most cases, however, an antinauseant from any of the classes can be tried for any cancer-associated nausea.

   Three general rules should be followed when prescribing antinauseants in cancer and palliative care management:

   1. Before prescribing an antinauseant on a long-term basis, conduct a vigorous search for the underlying cause.
   2. If you are using combination antinauseant therapy, do not combine antinauseants from the same class of drugs.
   3. If you are using combination antinauseant therapy, remember that antinauseants that work on the same neurotransmitter (dopamine, muscarinic/cholinergic, histamine) tend to be less effective when combined than antinauseants that work on different receptors.

   Although a discussion of the receptors involved in each antinauseant is too detailed for this book, the following approach to treating the nausea and vomiting associated with cancer and palliative care is suggested:

   1. Always consider nonpharmacologic therapy first; small, frequent meals; appropriate food presentation; and foods that the patient likes.
   2. Begin with prochloroperazine, dimenhydrinate, or metoclopramide.
   3. Combine any two of the above or all three for resistant nausea.
   4. Consider adding a corticosteroid such as prednisone or dexamethasone to the treatment regime.
   5. Consider ondansetron for chemotherapy-induced nausea and vomiting.
   6. If emesis continues in spite of the above, try the rectal, subcutaneous, or suppository route.

3. E. As mentioned, a combination of two or three of the antinauseants discussed in the choices in Question 2 would be very appropriate. Surprisingly, few significant problems with extrapyramidal side effects occur with combination therapy.

Ondansetron, the newest antiemetic, is a 5-HT receptor antagonist. However, it is very expensive ($15.00 per tablet), and this should certainly be considered when selecting between this and a combination of older agents.

Try to avoid an NG tube in palliative care patients whenever possible. Nasogastric tubes are uncomfortable and thus tend to have a negative, rather than a positive, impact on symptom control in cancer patients.

4. A. White lesions that scrape off with a tongue depressor are almost certainly oral thrush. Oral thrush is extremely common in palliative cancer patients, even with good mouth care. Treatment with mycostatin, nystatin, or a newer agent such as ketoconazole is recommended.

5. D. The diarrhea in this case is likely due to the effect of the radiotherapy on the bowel. Diphenoxylate, loperamide, and codeine are all good treatment choices. In most patients, the diarrhea will settle down 1-2 weeks after the completion of the course of radiotherapy.

6. B. Asthenia (fatigue) is the most prevalent symptom in advanced cancer patients. The prevalence of symptoms in advanced cancer patients is as follows: (a) asthenia, 90%; (b) anorexia, 85%; (c) pain, 76%; (d) nausea, 68%; (e) constipation, 65%; (f) sedation confusion, 60%; and (g) dyspnea, 12%.

7. A. Although autonomic failure, hypercalcemia, narcotic bowel syndrome, and raised intracranial pressure can cause nausea and vomiting, the most frequent cause is bowel obstruction due to pressure of an intraabdominal tumor on the bowel itself, involvement of the bowel in the tumor process, associated gastric stasis, or other causes.

8. A.

9. E. A large pleural effusion should initially be treated by thoracocentesis. If it recurs at infrequent intervals, this technique can be used repeatedly. However, if it recurs frequently, you may decide to use other symptom-relieving measures, including elevating the head of the bed, oxygen, fresh air, decreased fluid intake, prednisone or dexamethasone, morphine, and palliative radiotherapy.

10. D. A partial bowel obstruction may be treated effectively by any of the following: gastrokinetic agents such as metoclopramide or domperidone; decreased fluid intake; antiemetic agents such as prochlorperazine, dimenhydrinate, metoclopramide, or ondansetron; or corticosteroids such as prednisone.

11. D. This patient most likely has a primary lung carcinoma with metastatic disease to the brain. The metastatic disease has produced increased intracranial pressure, which has resulted in the neurological symptoms.

The use of dexamethasone in this case can be both diagnostic and therapeutic. If the symptoms improve with dexamethasone, your suspicion of increased intracranial pressure as a cause of the symptoms is confirmed. An H_2 receptor antagonist such as ranitidine should always be used when a palliative care patient is being treated with dexamethasone.

12. E. Fungating growths, particularly carcinomas of the breast, can produce very unsightly lesions, as well as very offensive odors that have psychological and social implications as well as medical implications. Often friends of the patient will stop coming because of the odor.

The most important aspects of treatment include: proper cleaning of the fungating growth with saline compresses (not Dakin's solution or other solutions that may actually make it worse, not better), the application of yogurt (not fruit flavored) or buttermilk dressings, and the placement of charcoal briquettes strategically throughout the patient's room. The latter are very effective in weakening the odor of the fungating growth.

13. D. An agitated depression is best treated by a combination of a sedating tricyclic antidepressant, and/or an anxiolytic agent given on a PRN basis.

Fluoxetine, in this case, may actually make the situation worse. Although fluoxetine and other selective serotonin reuptake inhibitors (SSRIs) have turned out to be a very important advance in the treatment of depressive disorders, fluoxetine has the potential to make an agitated depression worse. In this case, thus, it is safer to stick to the older, proven reliable tricyclic antidepressants, especially a TCA with sedating properties.

14. D. When starting a patient on a narcotic analgesic, it is wise also to begin the patient on an antiemetic agent. Nausea and/or vomiting is an extremely common initial side effect that quickly (within 2-3 weeks) disappears. The antiemetic can then be discontinued. A good initial choice is prochlorperazine or dimenhydrinate.

15. B. The drug of choice for the management of malignant ascites is the aldosterone antagonist spironolactone. Spironolactone has been shown to be effective in both malignant ascites and in the ascites associated with cirrhotic liver disease. Paracentesis may provide significant relief from malignant ascites and should be considered a method of first choice for the acute relief.

16. C. Hypercalcemia is the most common life-threatening metabolic disorder associated with cancer. It usually occurs in the context of advanced disseminated malignancy and produces a number of distressing symptoms. These include general symptoms such as dehydration, polydipsia, polyuria, and pruritus; gastrointestinal symptoms such as anorexia, weight loss, nausea, vomiting, constipation, and ileus; neurological symptoms such as fatigue, lethargy, confusion, myopathy, hyporeflexia, seizures, psychosis, and coma; and cardiovascular symptoms such as bradycardia, atrial dysrhythmias, ventricular dysrhythmias; prolonged PR intervals, QT interval reductions; and wide T waves.

The primary treatment of hypercalcemia is IV fluid therapy. Other important treatments include corticosteroids, biphosphonates, and calcitonin.

17. D. The treatment of choice for narcotic-induced constipation is lactulose. Lactulose is an osmotic agent that has also been shown to be extremely useful in the management of hepatic encephalopathy.

A very reasonable alternative would be a combiantion of a stool softener such as docusate sodium and a peristaltic stimulant such as senna.

The advantages of lactulose appear to be greater efficacy, especially in patients who are on high-dose narcotics; and that it is a liquid rather than a pill.

Metamucil is contraindicated in the treatment of constipation in patients on narcotic analgesics. Metamucil appears, in many cases, to make things worse by absorbing water and actually increasing the mass of stool that has to be evacuated.

Always attempt to find out why the patient is constipated—do not assume that it is due to narcotic analgesics.

18. C. Antinauseants have been discussed previously. It was also mentioned that there are various neurotransmitter receptor sites that have been identified for antiemetic drugs. These neurotransmitters include dopamine, muscarinic/cholinergic receptors, and histamine receptors. In brief, some of the common antiemetics and their predominant neurotransmitter receptor sites include the following:

ANTIEMETIC	RECEPTOR SITE
Dimenhydrinate	Dopamine
Prochlorperazine	Muscarinic/cholinergic
Chlorpromazine	Muscarinic/cholinergic
Metoclopramide	Muscarinic/cholinergic
Hycosine	Dopamine/muscarinic/cholinergic

SOLUTION TO SHORT ANSWER MANAGEMENT PROBLEM 19

Asthenia is the most prevalent symptom in patients with advanced cancer. Two symptoms are usually included in the term asthenia: (1) fatigue or lassitude, defined as easy tiring and decreased capacity to maintain adequate performance; and (2) generalized weakness, defined as the anticipatory subjective sensation of difficulty in initiating a certain activity.

SUMMARY OF SYMPTOM MANAGEMENT IN PALLIATIVE CARE

1. **Nausea and vomiting:**
   a) Small, frequent meals
   b) Avoid bland foods. Give patient what he or she wants to eat.
   c) Antiemetics:
      1. Prochlorperazine
      2. Dimenhydrinate
      3. Metoclopramide
      4. Prednisone
      5. Hyocosine/atropine
      6. Ondansetron
   d) Consider combination of antiemetics if one is not sufficient.
   e) If vomiting continues, consider suppository or subcutaneous route.
2. **Constipation:**
   a) Attempt to find the cause—don't automatically assume it is due to narcotics.
   b) Lactulose appears to be the agent of choice for the treatment of constipation in palliative care. A combination of a stool softener and a peristaltic stimulant is a good alternative.
3. **Anorexia:**
   a) Small, frequent meals
   b) Avoid blended, pulverized foods; give the patient what he or she wants to eat.
   c) Megestrol acetate is most the most effective agent for treating anorexia and cachexia in terminally ill patients. Prednisone is a good alternative.
4. **Dry mouth/oral thrush:**
   a) Mouth care is very important.
   b) Avoid drying agents such as lemon-glycerine swabs.
   c) Hydrogen peroxide at $\frac{1}{4}$ strength, lemon drops, pineapple chunks, tart juices
   d) Look for oral thrush every day; treat with nystatin, mycostatin, or, if treatment resistant, ketoconazole.
5. **Dehydration:** Dehydration is usually not symptomatic; that is, usually does not have to be treated. Always base your decision to use fluids on whether or not you think it will make the patient feel better and improve the patient's quality of life. Remember, the most common occurrence from treating palliative care patients with IV fluids is iatrogenic pulmonary edema.
6. **Diarrhea:**
   a) Try to identify the cause.
   b) Diphenoxylate, loperamide, and codeine are equally effective.

7. **Dyspnea and pleural effusion:** Open windows, supplementary oxygen, semi-Fowler's position, bronchodilators, prednisone, narcotic analgesics, anxiolytics, diuretics, and palliative radiotherapy may all be of help with recurrent pleural effusions. Treat first occurrence of thoracocentesis. How often you repeat this procedure depends on the patient's comfort level and also how quickly the fluid reaccumulates.

8. **Partial bowel obstruction:**
   a) Restrict fluids.
   b) Antiemetics: consider prokinetic agents such as metoclopramide first.
   c) Corticosteroids: prednisone
   d) Narcotic analgesics
   e) Try to avoid the use of a NG tube if possible.

9. **Malignant ascites:**
   a) Paracentesis is often effective: how often you perform this procedure is again dependent on the reaccumulation of fluid.
   b) Spironolactone alone or with thiazide and/or loop diuretics may be helpful.

10. **Cerebral edema:**
    a) Dexamethasone with an H_2 receptor antagonist is both diagnostic and therapeutic.

11. **Fungating growths:**
    a) Frequent dressing changes; normal saline or hydrogen peroxide
    b) Yogurt or buttermilk dressings
    c) Charcoal briquettes around the house
    d) Fresh air

12. **Depression and anxiety:**
    a) Remember bio-psycho-social-spiritual model of pain and symptom control.
    b) Psychotherapy: "be there, be sensitive, be silent."
    c) Tricyclic antidepressants/serotonin reuptake inhibitors
    d) Anxiolytics (sublingual especially effective)

13. **Hypercalcemia:**
    a) Most common serious metabolic abnormality in palliative care
    b) Think about the diagnosis: otherwise, you won't make it.
    c) Fluids will effectively treat hypercalcemia in most cases.

SUGGESTED READING

Doyle D, Hanks G, MacDonald N. Oxford textbook of palliative medicine. Oxford: Oxford University Press, 1993.

PROBLEM 20   A 17-YEAR-OLD FEMALE WITH WEIGHT LOSS, POLYURIA, AND POLYDYPSIA

A 17-year-old female presents to your office with her mother. Her mother tells you that her daughter has lost 20 lb in the last 6 months. As well, she has been increasingly thirsty and has been experiencing a significantly increased frequency of urination. The patient has been feeling generally well, but she complains that her breath smells "funny."

On examination, the patient is well below the 5th percentile for weight. She looks thin and pale. Her blood pressure is 100/70 mm Hg. She has a few anterior cervical and axillary nodes measuring 1.0 cm. Her abdomen is slightly tender. No other abnormalities are found.

There appears to be an excessive amount of gas in the stomach on her KUB.

SELECT THE ONE BEST ANSWER TO THE FOLLOWING QUESTIONS

1. If you could order only one test, which would it be?
   a) urine for protein and glucose
   b) spot blood sugar
   c) serum electrolytes
   d) blood gases
   e) CBC

2. You perform your one test. The result is 250 mg%. Which of the following statements is(are) false?
   a) the diagnosis of the above disorder should be confirmed with a 3-hour test
   b) the diet used to manage this condition is based on exchanges
   c) a special diet is an essential component of treatment of this disorder
   d) insulin will likely be required to manage this patient's illness
   e) hospital inpatient management may not be necessary to begin treatment of this disorder

3. Which of the following statements regarding the diagnosis of the above disorder is(are) true?
   a) this disorder is confirmed if the fasting level of the particular substance exceeds 140 mg% on two occasions
   b) this disorder is confirmed if the venous plasma level of the particular substance exceeds 200 mg% on one occasion in the presence of symptoms
   c) this disorder is confirmed if, following a 3-hour test, two values measuring the particular substance exceed 200 mg%
   d) all of the above
   e) none of the above

4. Which of the following conditions is most closely associated with the described disorder?
   a) hypercholesterolemia
   b) hypothyroidism
   c) hypertriglyceridemia
   d) obesity
   e) cholelithiasis

5. What is(are) the best measure(s) of long-term control of the disease described?
   a) urine sugar levels
   b) daily blood sugar levels ($\times 4$/day)
   c) hemoglobin A_{1C}
   d) hemoglobin F
   e) no microvascular or macrovascular complications

6. The Hemoglobin A_{1C} should be below what value to be of use in predicting the development of microvascular and macrovascular complications?
   a) <3.5%
   b) <5.0%
   c) <7.2%
   d) <9.0%
   e) <10.0%

7. Which of the following statements is true?
   a) microvascular complications are associated with type I diabetes; macrovascular complications are associated with type II diabetes
   b) macrovascular complications are associated with type I diabetes; microvascular complications are associated with type II diabetes
   c) microvascular and macrovascular complications are associated with type I diabetes; neither is associated with type II diabetes
   d) microvascular and macrovascular complications are associated with both type I and type II diabetes
   e) none of the above

8. Type II diabetics develop diabetic retinopathy in what percentage of cases?
   a) 80%
   b) 60%
   c) 40%
   d) 20%
   e) 5%

9. Type I diabetics develop diabetic retinopathy in what percentage of cases?
   a) 80%
   b) 60%
   c) 40%

d) 20%

e) 10%

10. Type II diabetics develop diabetic nephropathy in what percentage of cases?
    a) 80%
    b) 60%
    c) 40%
    d) 20%
    e) 5%

11. Type I diabetics develop diabetic nephropathy in what percentage of cases?
    a) 80%
    b) 60%
    c) 40%
    d) 20%
    e) 5%

12. Which one of the following statements is true regarding diabetic nephropathy in the United States?
    a) the prevalence of diabetic nephropathy is mainly contributed to by type I diabetics
    b) the prevalence of diabetic nephropathy is mainly contributed to by type II diabetics
    c) the ratio of type II diabetics to type I diabetics in the United States is 10 to 1
    d) the ratio of type I diabetics to type II diabetics in the United States is 2 to 1
    e) a and d
    f) b and c

13. A 27-year-old type I diabetic presents to your office for her regular 3-month checkup. Your urine dipstick shows proteinuria +1. A 24-hour urine produces a protein reading of 150 mg. What would you do now?
    a) nothing—this is microalbuminuria
    b) nothing—this is still considered normal
    c) start the patient on an ACE inhibitor
    d) change the patient's diet—decrease protein by 10%/day
    e) Refer the patient to a diabetologist—you are a family doctor and are in no position to make these decisions

14. Which one of the following statements regarding diet and diabetes is(are) false?
    a) diet is basic in the treatment of all diabetics
    b) new evidence suggests that diabetics do not have to avoid sweets and foods that contain simple carbohydrates
    c) the diabetic on insulin therapy must have three meals at fixed times each day
    d) the diabetic on insulin therapy should have frequent snacks
    e) the diabetic on insulin should have a fixed caloric distribution

15. What is the average starting insulin dose for a newly diagnosed diabetic?
    a) 2-4 units
    b) 6-8 units
    c) 10-12 units
    d) 15-20 units
    e) 20-30 units

16. Which of the following best explains the Somogyi effect?
    a) the Somogyi effect is due to rebound hyperglycemia
    b) the Somogyi effect is due to relative insulin deficiency in the morning
    c) the Somogyi effect is due to rebound hypoglycemia
    d) the Somogyi effect is due to relative insulin excess due to administration of excessive insulin in the evening
    e) a and d

17. Which of the following best explains the dawn phenomenon?
    a) the dawn phenomenon is due to relative insulin deficiency in the morning
    b) the dawn phenomenon is due to rebound hyperglycemia
    c) the dawn phenomenon is due to rebound hypoglycemia
    d) the dawn phenomenon is due to the wrong mixture of insulins
    e) none of the above

18. A newly diagnosed type I diabetic is diagnosed and placed on a total insulin dose of 18 units. What is the correct morning/evening: AM/PM: regular/intermediate insulin dose?
    a) morning: total 12 units: regular 6 units, intermediate 6 units
       evening: total 6 units: regular 3 units, intermediate 3 units
    b) morning: total 9 units: regular 6 units, intermediate 3 units
       evening: total 9 units: regular 6 units, intermediate 6 units
    c) morning: total 12 units: regular 4 units, intermediate 8 units
       evening: total 6 units: regular 2 units, intermediate 4 units
    d) morning: total 6 units: regular 4 units, intermediate 2 units
       evening: total 12 units: regular 4 units, intermediate 8 units
    e) morning: total 6 units: regular 3 units, intermediate 3 units
       evening: total 12 units: regular 8 units, intermediate 4 units

19. What is the most likely explanation for the "abnormal gas in the stomach" described in the case presentation?

a) gastroparesis due to diabetic autonomic neuropathy
b) gastroparesis due to sympathetic dysfunction
c) associated with diabetic ketoacidosis
d) associated with hyperosmolar coma
e) none of the above

20. Regarding the pathophysiology of the disorder described, which of the following statements is(are) true?
    a) environmental factors are likely involved in the pathology of this condition
    b) HLA-DR4 is strongly associated with this condition
    c) this disorder may be associated with other autoimmune disorders
    d) all of the above
    e) none of the above

21. A 65-year-old asymptomatic obese female has a routine fasting sugar drawn at the time of her annual physical examination. The level comes back at 240 mg%. Her urine is negative for ketones. The test is repeated the following day and comes back at the same level. Which of the following statements about this patient is(are) incorrect?
    a) the patient has non–insulin-dependent diabetes mellitus (NIDDM)
    b) insulin is the agent of first choice in the management of this condition
    c) a diabetic diet forms the cornerstone of therapy in this condition
    d) insulin and oral hypoglycemic may be used together in the treatment of this condition
    e) monitoring of this condition is best done by home glucose monitoring

22. The pathophysiology of type II diabetes is associated with all of the following except:
    a) increased insulin resistance

b) decreased serum insulin levels
c) abnormal glucagon secretion
d) a decrease in B-cell mass, abnormal function of B cells, or both
e) amyloid of the islet cells

23. Gestational diabetes mellitus of pregnancy is screened by a 50-g glucose load, with blood drawn 1 hour after administration of the load. What is the usual value considered the upper limit of normal for this test?
    a) 110 mg%
    b) 140 mg%
    c) 160 mg%
    d) 180 mg%
    e) 200 mg%

24. Which of the following statements regarding type II diabetes mellitus is(are) true?
    a) most patients present to their physicians with symptoms
    b) most patients are essentially asymptomatic at diagnosis (apart from being obese)
    c) most patients can control the diabetes by diet and exercise
    d) most patients will not manifest complications
    e) most patients are under the age of 40

25. Which of the following statements regarding individuals with type II diabetes of onset during youth (MODY) is(are) true?
    a) these patients are usually normal weight to underweight
    b) this is an autosomal dominant condition
    c) this type of diabetes is present in 50% of the siblings of the parents with this disease
    d) all of the above
    e) none of the above

Short Answer Management Problem 20

List the macrovascular and microvascular complications of diabetes mellitus.

ANSWERS

1. A.

2. A.

3. D. This patient has *diabetes mellitus type I*. Diabetes mellitus type I is also known as insulin-dependent diabetes and must be managed with a combination of a diabetic diet using "exchanges" and human insulin. Unless

the patient has diabetic ketoacidosis, there is no reason that both diagnosis and initial management cannot take place on an outpatient basis.

The diagnosis of diabetes mellitus type I is very important. The criteria that have been adopted by the National Diabetes Study Group are as follows:
1. Two fasting plasma glucose values exceeding 140 mg%, or
2. One random plasma glucose value exceeding 200 mg% in the presence of symptoms, or

3. Two values exceeding 200 mg% in a 3-hour 75-g glucose tolerance test with one of the two values being at T = 2 hours

   In the patient described, Criterion 2 can be used to make the diagnosis of diabetes mellitus.

4. C. The disease of those listed that is most closely associated with diabetes mellitus is hypertriglyceridemia. Triglyceride levels of two to three times normal are often the first sign of undiagnosed diabetes mellitus. All individuals with a significantly elevated serum triglyceride level should be screened for diabetes mellitus.

5. C.

6. C. The best measure of long-term control of diabetes mellitus (type I and type II) is hemoglobin A_{1c}. Recent studies have shown that "tight control" (Mean plasma glucose < 155 mg% and HgB A_{1c} < 7.2%) produces at least a 60% reduction in microvascular and macrovascular complications.

7. D. One very important and underappreciated fact is that both macrovascular (atherosclerotic heart disease, coronary artery disease, peripheral vascular disease, cerebrovascular disease) and microvascular disease (retinopathy, nephropathy, peripheral neuropathy) are associated with both types of diabetes. Type II diabetics are not immune to diabetic complications; quite the contrary is true.

8. D.

9. D.

10. D.

11. C.

12. F. Complications (macrovascular and microvascular) in type I diabetes and type II diabetes are as follows:
    1. Type I diabetes:
       A. Retinopathy: 20% of patients
       B. Nephropathy: 40% of patients
    2. Type II diabetes:
       A. Retinopathy: 20% of patients
       B. Nephropathy: 20% of patients

13. C. The diabetic patient who presents with microalbuminuria already has a problem. The probability of this individual's going on to overt nephropathy is quite high. It has now been demonstrated that progression to overt nephropathy can be prevented by the prophylactic administration of an ACE inhibitor. The drugs of choice are captopril, or enalapril.

14. B. Diet is an essential component of treatment in all diabetic patients. It is especially important, however, for the insulin-dependent type I diabetic. In the diabetic the rate at which insulin enters the blood from an injection site is fixed, and the diabetic must match meals to the pattern of insulin absorption. The diabetic's diet should be the same as the diet suggested for a nondiabetic of the same age.

    During the past several years the avoidance of sweets and foods that contain simple carbohydrates has been challenged, but until further information is presented it seems reasonable to instruct diabetics to avoid beverages with sucrose and desserts that are highly sweetened.

    The diabetic on insulin therapy must have three meals at fixed times each day, with a fixed distribution of calories. Frequent snacks, also with a fixed distribution of calories, are recommended as well.

    If a diabetic patient is overweight, a weight-reducing program should be initiated. This may be facilitated by substituting complex carbohydrates with high residue for simple sugars. As well, saturated animal fats should be replaced with polyunsaturated vegetable fats. One-fifth of the daily caloric intake should be consumed at breakfast and about two-fifths at each of lunch and supper. These percentages may be reduced to allow for small snacks, such as crackers or fruit, in midafternoon and bedtime.

15. D. The average starting dose of insulin is 15-20 units. The obese individual may need 25-30 units/day. The dose, however, must be individualized; some persons require more, some persons require less. In addition, patients who are initially placed on insulin in the hospital may end up with very different insulin requirements when they are at home and more active; usually the insulin requirement will be significantly smaller.

16. E.

17. A. Morning hyperglycemia in a diabetic on insulin may be due to relative insulin deficiency (the dawn phenomenon) or to rebound hyperglycemia (the Somogyi phenomenon). Because the treatment of these two conditions is completely opposite, they must be distinguished.

    The dawn phenomenon, a relative insulin deficiency due to a waning-off of insulin action in the early morning hours, is most likely mediated by an increased nocturnal output of growth hormone (which has anti-insulin activity). It is treated by increasing the dose of evening insulin.

    The Somogyi effect, a rebound hyperglycemia following a hypoglycemic reaction, is treated by decreasing, not increasing, the dosage of evening insulin.

The dawn phenomenon can be distinguished from the Somogyi effect by determination of the 3:00 AM glucose. Therefore all diabetic patients should periodically measure their 3:00 AM blood sugar in addition to regularly measuring their blood sugars four times/day.

18. C. The starting dose of insulin should be begun as follows:
    1. Morning: $\frac{2}{3}$ of total daily dose
    2. Evening: $\frac{1}{3}$ of total daily dose
    3. Morning: $\frac{2}{3}$ intermediate, $\frac{1}{3}$ regular
    4. Evening: $\frac{2}{3}$ intermediate, $\frac{1}{3}$ regular

19. A. The "abnormal gas in the stomach" is most likely due to diabetic gastroparesis. This is a very common complaint, and it is best treated by a prokinetic agent such as metoclopramide, domperidone, or cisapride.

20. D. Two distinct types of type I diabetes have been identified. In type IA, the environmental factors combined with genetic factors are thought to result in cell-mediated destruction of pancreatic beta cells. Human leukocyte antigen (HLA-DR4) is strongly associated with this phenomenon.

    Type IB is an uncommon primary autoimmune condition that occurs in individuals with other autoimmune conditions, such as Hashimoto's disease, Graves' disease, pernicious anemia, and myasthenia gravis. This condition is associated with histocompatibility antigen HLA-DR3 and occurs later in life, typically between the ages of 30 and 50.

    Specific environmental factors linked to type I diabetes mellitus are the following:
    1. Drugs and chemicals: streptozocin and pentamidine
    2. Viruses: mumps, coxsackie, rubella (40% of patients with congenital rubella develop type I diabetes late), and cytomegalovirus

21. B. This patient has *non–insulin-dependent diabetes mellitus (NIDDM)*. NIDDM accounts for 90% of all cases of diabetes. NIDDM is characterized by both an impairment of beta-cell function and a decreased sensitivity to insulin.

    NIDDM is often discovered in asymptomatic patients by finding an elevated blood sugar. It may also present with nonspecific symptoms including fatigue, weakness, blurred vision, vaginal and perineal pruritus, impotence, and paresthesias. Weight loss is uncommon in these patients. The majority of patients with NIDDM are obese; many have a strong family history of obesity and diabetes.

    A diabetic diet plus weight management plus exercise should be pushed to the maximum. If these are not effective, an oral hypoglycemic agent should be the next step.

    All oral hypoglycemic agents currently available are sulfonylurea agents. The first-generation agents include tolbutamide, chlorporamide, acetohexamide, and tolazamide. The second-generation agents include glyburide and glipizide. At this time there is no conclusive evidence that the second generation agents are more effective, have fewer side effects, or produce fewer interactions with other drugs than first-generation agents.

    Oral hypoglycemic therapy should begin with the lowest effective dose; this should then be increased every few days to achieve maximal control. Self-monitoring of blood glucose is the key to the evaluation of efficacy of an oral hypoglycemic mediated treatment program.

    About 25% to 30% of NIDDM patients fail to respond to sulfonylurea drugs. These patients are called *primary failures*. In addition, about 5% of patients who initially responded to these drugs will lose their responsiveness. These patients are termed *secondary failures*. Sometimes a combination of a morning oral hypoglycemic and an evening intermediate-acting insulin can be beneficial in lowering blood sugar to normal.

    Home glucose monitoring is the method of choice for monitoring blood sugars in diabetic patients. It is recommended that blood sugars initially be checked 4 times/day until they revert toward normal; the frequency of monitoring can be decreased to two or three times weekly (3-4 times/day). Also, the 3:00 AM sugar should be occasionally checked.

22. B. The cause of type II diabetes mellitus is unknown. Although it is thought to be autosomal recessive, it mainly affects obese people over the age of 40. Subsequent insulin resistance (secondary to obesity) is a factor in 60% to 80% of type II diabetics. Decreased beta-cell responsiveness to glucose is noted; abnormal glucagon secretion accompanies this. The islet cell dysfunction may be caused by a decrease in beta-cell mass, abnormal function of the beta cells, or some other combination.

    Amyloid of the islet cells occurs in up to 40% of type II diabetics. Fatty infiltration, ischemia caused by vascular sclerosis, and pancreatic fibrosis occur in up to 66% of type II diabetics; this contributes to pancreatic atrophy.

23. B. The screening test for gestational diabetes mellitus is as follows:
    1. Time: 24-28 weeks
    2. Glucose load: 50 g
    3. Time sample drawn: 1 hour
    4. Screening cut-off: 140 mg%

24. B. Patients with type II diabetes demonstrate the following:
    1. Most patients are asymptomatic; identification most often occurs by screening.
    2. Most patients are over the age of 40.

3. Most patients develop the same complications (microvascular and macrovascular complications) as type I diabetics.
4. Most patients have motivational difficulties in relation to diet and exercise.

25. D. Type II diabetes of youth (maturity onset diabetes of youth), also known as MODY, has the following characteristics:
1. Most patients are normal weight to underweight.
2. Most patients are younger than age 40.
3. Fifty percent of patients have parents with the disorder.
4. The disorder is autosomal dominant.

SOLUTION TO SHORT ANSWER MANAGEMENT PROBLEM 20

Macrovascular complications:
1. Atherosclerotic vascular disease:
   A. Coronary artery disease
   B. Myocardial infarction: sudden cardiac death
   C. Cerebrovascular disease and stroke
   D. Peripheral vascular disease
   E. Intestinal ischemia
   F. Renal artery stenosis
Microvascular complications:
1. Renal disease:
   A. Diabetic nephropathy
2. Peripheral neuropathy:
   A. Parasthesias
   B. "Glove and stocking" neuropathy
3. Autonomic neuropathy:
   A. Gastroparesis
   B. Impotence
4. Diabetic retinopathy:
   A. Cotton-wool exudates
   B. Neovascularization

SUMMARY OF THE DIAGNOSIS AND TREATMENT OF DIABETES MELLITUS:

1. **Type I diabetes:**
   a) Epidemiology: 10% of all cases of diabetes
   b) Signs/symptoms: polyuria, polydipsia, nocturia, weight loss
   c) Etiology: genetics plus environment
      1. Most common: HLA-DR4 plus viral exposure
      2. Less common: associated with other autoimmune diseases
   d) Diagnosis:
      1. Two values of 140 mg%, or
      2. One random blood sugar > 200 mg% plus symptoms, or
      3. Two blood sugars > 200 mg% in 3-hour 75-g GTT (one value at 2-hour)

   e) Self-monitoring: home blood sugar monitoring
      1. 4 values $\times$ 3 times/week
      2. Strict control reduces complications
   f) Long-term control: Hemoglobin A_{1c} < 7.2%
   g) Treatment:
      1. Diet (based on exchanges)
      2. Exercise
      3. Insulin (regular intermediate)
      4. Total initial dose: 15-20 units
         i) $\frac{2}{3}$ total dose AM (split 2:1 regular:intermediate)
         ii) $\frac{1}{3}$ total dose PM (split 2:1 regular:intermediate) "The Rule of $\frac{2}{3}$'s"
   h) Complications:
      1. Macrovascular
      2. Microvascular
         Both in type I and type II diabetes mellitus are macrovascular and microvascular complications present. Because the ratio of type II/type I diabetics is 10/1, of 100 cases of diabetic nephropathy, 80 are due to type II diabetes.

2. **Type II diabetes mellitus:**
   a) Epidemiology: 90% of all cases of diabetes mellitus are type II.
   b) Signs/symptoms:
      1. Most patients are discovered when undergoing screening in a medical setting.
      2. The minority of type II diabetes present symptoms.
   c) Etiology:
      1. Race (such as North American Indian)
      2. Genetic factor
      3. Obesity
   d) Diagnosis: diagnosis of type II diabetes is the same as type I.
   e) Self-monitoring: Same as type I
   f) Long-term control: Same as type I
   g) Treatment:
      1. Weight control absolutely essential
      2. Exercise (regular: 3 times/week)
      3. Oral hypoglycemics: second- or first-degree oral agents
      4. A small percentage (15% to 20%) of type I diabetics need insulin in the evening in addition to oral hypoglycemics (Glyburide/Glipizide) in the morning.
   h) Complications: same as type I diabetes mellitus

SUGGESTED READINGS

Anderson JW, DeAngulo MO. Diabetes mellitus in adults. In: Rakel R, ed. Conn's current therapy. Philadelphia: WB Saunders, 1994.

Beymer PL, Huether SE, Gray DP. Alterations of hormonal regulation. In: McCance KL, Huether SE, eds. Pathophysiology: The biologic basis for disease in adults and children. St. Louis: Mosby, 1994.

PROBLEM 21   A 45-YEAR-OLD MALE WITH "VISUAL PROBLEMS," HEADACHES, WEIGHT GAIN, SWEATING, AND "HANDS AND FEET THAT ARE CHANGING"

A 45-year-old male presents to your office with his wife. He is very concerned about some "bizarre symptoms" that he has been experiencing. He is the CEO of a major manufacturing company and is "really embarrassed to go out in public any longer."

He tells you that about 6 months ago he began to experience the following symptoms: headaches, visual spots or defects, weight gain, an appearance of his forehead growing, enlarging hands and feet (he could no longer get his gloves and shoes on), and increased sweating.

On examination, the apical impulse is felt in the 5th intercostal space, midclavicular line. His blood pressure is 170/105 mm Hg. He does have a protruding brow, and three discrete visual field defects are noted (two in the left eye and one in the right eye). His tongue appears enlarged and he is sweating profusely.

SELECT THE ONE BEST ANSWER TO THE FOLLOWING QUESTIONS

1. What is the most likely diagnosis in this patient?
   a) ACTH excess
   b) acromegaly
   c) prolactinoma
   d) primary hypopituitarism
   e) primary hyperparathyroidism

2. The pathophysiologic lesion resides in which of the following?
   a) adrenal gland: adenoma
   b) hyperparathyroid glands: adenoma in one or more of the four glands
   c) pituitary gland: adenoma
   d) gastrointestinal ectopic tumor: adenoma
   e) none of the above

3. The treatment(s) for this patient may include which of the following?
   a) surgery: transsphenoidal
   b) radiation
   c) bromocriptine
   d) heavy-particle pituitary radiation
   e) all of the above
   f) none of the above

4. A 24-year-old male presents to your office with the following symptoms: an extreme feeling of weakness, a 20-pound weight loss, a change in the color of his skin (his skin has become very hyperpigmented), and light-headedness and dizziness.

   On examination, the patient has a definite change in skin color since you last saw him 9 months ago. His blood pressure is 90/70 mm Hg. He looks acutely ill.

   On laboratory examination, his serum Na+ is low (115 mEq/L); his serum potassium is high (6.2 mEq/L); his urea is elevated at 9.0 mg/dl; and his serum calcium is elevated (12.0 mg/dl).

   On this basis of the above history, physical examination, and laboratory findings, what is the most likely diagnosis in this patient?
   a) Conn's syndrome
   b) Cushing's syndrome
   c) Addison's syndrome
   d) primary hyperparathyroidism
   e) primary pituitary failure

5. What is the most likely cause for this patient's symptoms?
   a) overstimulation of the adrenal gland
   b) an adrenal adenoma
   c) autoimmune destruction of the hyperparathyroid glands
   d) autoimmune destruction of the adrenal gland
   e) a pituitary adenoma

6. What is the acute treatment of choice for this patient?
   a) prednisone orally
   b) dexamethasone orally
   c) cortisol IV
   d) ACTH IV
   e) depoprovera IM

7. This patient will need chronic treatment with which of the following?
   a) hydrocortisone
   b) fludrocortisone acetate
   c) a or b
   d) a and b
   e) none of the above

8. A 25-year-old female presents with the sudden onset of increased thirst and increased urination. This began abruptly 1 week ago and has not abated since. She states that since that time she has been thirsty all the time. The only significant illness in her life has been the recent diagnosis of bipolar affective illness—subtype I that was made 6 weeks ago. She was started on lithium carbonate and is currently taking 1200 mg/day. Her serum lithium levels have been normal since the beginning.

   On examination, her blood pressure is 110/70 mm Hg. She has lost 5 lb during the last week and looks somewhat dehydrated.

What is the most likely diagnosis in this patient?
a) psychogenic polydipsia
b) diabetes mellitus type I
c) central diabetes insipidus
d) nephrogenic diabetes insipidus
e) adverse drug reaction to lithium

9. What is the treatment of choice in this patient?
a) hospitalization and complete psychiatric assessment
b) insulin: beginning at 10-20 units/day
c) glyburide
d) discontinuation of lithium carbonate
e) substitution of carbamazepine for lithium carbonate

10. A 37-year-old female presents to your office because she was found to be "hypertensive" by a nurse in a shopping mall screening program. She tells you that when she thinks about it, she really has not felt well for a couple of months. Her major complaint has been profound generalized fatigue and weakness. She has also been increasingly thirsty, urinating more frequently, and having to urinate frequently at night.

On P/E, her blood pressure is 190/110 mm Hg. Laboratory abnormalities include a mildly increased serum Na^+ (150 mEq/L), hypokalemic metabolic alkalosis, a low renin level, and increased urine potassium.

What is the most likely diagnosis with the information you have available?
a) Conn's syndrome
b) Cushing's syndrome
c) Addison's syndrome
d) Bartter's syndrome
e) diabetes insipidus

11. What is the most likely pathophysiologic cause of this syndrome?
a) benign adenoma of the adrenal gland
b) malignant adenoma of the adrenal gland
c) pituitary adenoma
d) bilateral hyperplasia of the adrenal gland
e) none of the above

12. What is the treatment of choice for the condition described?
a) bromocriptine
b) transsphenoidal surgery
c) clomiphene
d) spironolactone
e) surgical removal of the adenoma

13. A 22-year-old female, married for 18 months, has been trying to get pregnant without success. Approximately 9 months ago, she developed breast secretions, amenorrhea, and decreased libido. No other symptoms are present.

On examination, there is definite galactorrhea present. Her blood pressure is 140/80 mm Hg. No abnormalities are found on P/E.

From the information provided, what is the most likely diagnosis?
a) anorexia nervosa
b) stress-induced amenorrhea
c) "I want to have a baby but can't" syndrome
d) prolactinoma
e) hypopituitarism

14. If you could order only one test, what would that test be?
a) serum estrogen
b) serum progesterone
c) serum LH
d) serum FSH
e) serum prolactin

15. What is the treatment of choice for this condition?
a) transsphenoidal resection
b) bromocriptine
c) clomiphene
d) lithium carbonate
e) thyroxine

16. A 42-year-old female presents to your office with the following signs and symptoms: obesity (she has gained 40 pounds in the last 6 months), elevated blood pressure at her last walk-in clinic visit, increased body hair, purple streaks on her abdomen, "a fat face" (her description), and pains in her bones and joints.

She is on no medication at present, nor has she been on any medication for the past year.

On examination, her BMI (body mass index) is 35. Her blood pressure is 160/110 mm Hg; she has obvious hirsutism over her entire body, and her abdomen (which is obese) has purple stria. Her face is not only plethoric but also demonstrates a double chin. Her thoracic spine shows evidence of what is known as a buffalo hump.

Based on the information provided, what is the most likely diagnosis in this patient?
a) Conn's syndrome
b) Cushing's syndrome
c) Addison's syndrome
d) primary hyperparathyroidism
e) prolactinoma

17. Of all possible causes for the condition in this patient, which of the following is the most common?
a) adenoma of the adrenal gland
b) adenoma of the pituitary gland
c) hyperplasia of the adrenal gland
d) corticosteroid therapy for suppression of inflammation
e) small cell carcinoma of the lung

18. Which of the following tests is(are) appropriate screening tests for the patient diagnosed in Question 16?
    a) serum cortisol
    b) low-dose dexamethasone (cortisol analogue) suppression test
    c) 24-hour urine for free cortisol
    d) all of the above
    e) none of the above

19. Due to the likely pathophysiology of the condition described in the patient in Question 16, which of the following is the recommended treatment?
    a) surgery to remove the adenoma of the pituitary gland
    b) surgery to remove the adenoma of the adrenal gland
    c) surgery to remove the carcinoma of the adrenal gland
    d) chemotherapy to kill as much abnormal tissue as possible
    e) none of the above

20. Which of the following conditions is metastatic malignancy most likely to mimic?
    a) Cushing's syndrome
    b) primary hyperparathyroidism
    c) Conn's syndrome
    d) Addison's syndrome
    e) Nelson's syndrome

Short Answer Management Problem 21

For the condition Hyperparathyroidism:
1. Define the condition.
2. Provide sex predilection.
3. Provide the age predilection.
4. Explain pathogenesis.
5. Provide the clinical symptoms.
6. Explain the mnemonic "stones, bones, abdominal groans, and psychic moans"
7. Explain the changes in blood and serum levels that characterize the condition.
8. Discuss treatment.
9. Identify the most characteristic laboratory abnormality.

ANSWERS

1. B.

2. C.

3. E. This patient has a growth hormone excess caused by a pituitary adenoma. The condition is acromegaly, and often goes undiagnosed for many years. Acromegaly produces many signs and symptoms, including the following:
   I. General symptoms:
      A. Fatigue
      B. Increased sweating
      C. Heat intolerance
      D. Weight gain
   II. Skin and subcutaneous tissues:
      A. Enlarging hands and feet
      B. Coarsening facial features
      C. Oily skin
      D. Hypertrichosis
   III. Head
      A. Headaches
      B. Parotid enlargement
      C. Frontal bossing
   IV. Nose-throat:
      A. Sinus congestion
      B. Voice change
      C. Obstructive sleep apnea
      D. Goiter
   V. Cardiovascular system:
      A. Hypertension
      B. Congestive cardiac failure
      C. Left ventricular hypertrophy
   VI. Genitourinary system:
      A. Kidney stones
      B. Decreased libido/impotence
      C. Infertility
      D. Oligomenorrhea
   VII. Neurologic system:
      A. Paresthesias
      B. Hypersomnolence
      C. Carpel tunnel syndrome
   VIII. Musculoskeletal system:
      A. Weakness
      B. Proximal myopathy
   IX. Skeletal system:
      A. Joint pains
      B. Osteoarthritis
   Treatments include transsphenoidal surgery, heavy-

particle pituitary radiation, conventional pituitary radiation, bromocriptine, and the somatostatin analogue octreotide.

4. C.

5. D.

6. C.

7. D. This patient has *Addison's disease* or *primary adrenocortical insufficiency.* Most commonly, Addison's disease results from an autoimmune destruction of the adrenal gland. At least 50% of patients with Addison's disease have antiadrenal antibodies. Other potential causes of adrenocortical insufficiency include tuberculosis, disseminated meningococcemia, and metastatic cancer.

The prominent clinical features of Addison's disease include weakness (100%), weight loss (100%), hyperpigmentation (95%), and hypotension.

The pertinent laboratory findings include hyponatremia, hyperkalemia, increased BUN, hypercalcemia, increased plasma ACTH, and decreased serum cortisol level.

In Addison's disease both the short ACTH stimulation test and the prolonged ACTH stimulation test yield no cortical response.

Because of the acutely ill state of this patient, cortisol as a phosphate or succinate ester should be given in a 100-mg bolus IV and infused at a rate of 50 mg/hr until physiologic parameters are restored (especially normotension).

The chronic treatment of Addison's disease is a combination of hydrocortisone (10 mg to 30 mg/day) and 9-alpha-fluorocortisol (50 μg-100 μg/day). This combination is based on the need for a combination of glucocorticoid replacement and mineralocorticoid replacement.

8. D.

9. E. This patient has *nephrogenic diabetes insipidus.* This has resulted from the lack of antidiuretic hormone (ADH); in this case the diabetes insipidus is of the nephrogenic subtype and caused by the drug lithium carbonate.

There are two basic types of diabetes insipidus:
1. Central: the central type is usually idiopathic.
2. Nephrogenic: the collecting tubules of the kidney are not responsive to the ADH that is produced.

The nephrogenic type of diabetes is usually due to either a drug (lithium carbonate, amphotericin B) or severe hypokalemia (which makes the renal tubules resistant to ADH).

The treatment for central diabetes insipidus is intra-

muscular ADH; nephrogenic diabetes insipidus is best treated by discontinuation of the offending drug (if the drug is the cause, as is the most common scenario). In the case of this patient, who was put on lithium carbonate to treat bipolar affective disorder, a switch to carbamazepine would be most appropriate.

10. A.

11. A.

12. E. This patient has *Conn's syndrome.* Conn's syndrome is primary aldosteronism that results from an excess mineralocorticoid production from (in most cases) an adenoma of the adrenal cortex. If not due to an adenoma, hyperplasia of the adrenal cortex is found. The benign adenoma is usually present in the zona glomerulosa.

The clinical signs/symptoms of Conn's syndrome are weakness (due to the effect of hypokalemia); hypertension; carbohydrate intolerance (due to increased insulin release from hypokalemia); and polyuria, polydipsia, and nocturia due to either hypokalemic nephropathy or nephrogenic diabetes insipidus.

Laboratory abnormalities include mild hypernatremia, hypokalemic metabolic alkalosis, low renin, increased urine potassium, and an inability to suppress aldosterone with isotonic saline load, captopril, or use of another mineralocorticoid.

The treatment of choice for Conn's syndrome is, for a benign adenoma, surgical removal of the adenoma, and for bilateral hyperplasia of the adrenal glands, spironolactone.

13. D.

14. E.

15. B. This patient has *hyperprolactinemia,* most likely due to a pituitary adenoma. The combination of galactorrhea, amenorrhea, infertility, and decreased libido is almost certainly due to a prolactinoma.

A prolactinoma can be confirmed by performing a serum prolactin level (a level of serum prolactin > 300 ng/ml is always due (in the absence of pregnancy) to a pituitary adenoma.

A CT scan of the pituitary gland will confirm the diagnosis. It should be mentioned that a prolactinoma is the most common overall pituitary tumor in women.

Treatment is controversial, but due to a high rate of recurrence with surgery, initial therapy with bromocriptine is the best choice. Treatment with bromocriptine is not curative; it does, however, reduce the prolactin level, reduce the tumor mass, and increase fertility. Side effects include nausea and vomiting, increase in liver enzymes, and increase in serum uric acid.

16. B.

17. B.

18. D.

19. A. This patient has *Cushing's disease*. The definition of *Cushing's syndrome* is "a manifestation of hypercorticalism due to any cause." The most common cause of *Cushing's syndrome* is corticosteroid therapy. If steroids are excluded, the three major causes are as follows:
    1. Pituitary Cushing's (60%-70%): an adenoma
    2. Adrenal Cushing's (15%): adenoma, hyperplasia, or malignancy
    3. Ectopic Cushing's (15%): malignancy (small cell carcinoma of the lung)

    Thus the most likely cause of *Cushing's syndrome* in the patient described is a pituitary adenoma. The most common cause, as mentioned, is exogenous steroids.

    The clinical features of *Cushing's disease* consist of the following:
    Truncal obesity (90%)
    Hypertension (85%)
    Decreased glucose tolerance (80%)
    Hirsutism (70%)
    Wide, purple, abdominal stria (65%)
    Osteoporosis (55%)
    Plethoric face
    Easy bruising
    Mental aberrations
    Myopathy

    In terms of laboratory tests, the best overall screening tests are serum cortisol level, low-dose (1 mg) dexamethasone suppression test (in *Cushing's syndrome* there is no suppression), and 24-hour urine for free cortisol. Confirmation tests include high-dose (8 mg) dexamethasone suppression test (suppresses pituitary Cushing's but will not suppress adrenal or ectopic Cushing's), and plasma ACTH (normal to slightly increased in pituitary Cushing's, markedly increased in ectopic Cushing's, and very low in adrenal Cushing's; suppressed by cortisol).

    Because of the very high possibility of this being a pituitary *Cushing's syndrome*, the correct answer is surgery to remove the pituitary adenoma.

20. B. Metastatic malignancy is most likely to produce hypercalcemia. Hypercalcemia is most likely to mimic primary hyperparathyroidism. (Hyperparathyroidism will be discussed in the Short Answer Management Problem.)

SOLUTION TO SHORT ANSWER MANAGEMENT PROBLEM 21

Hyperparathyroidism:
1. Definition: Overactivity of the parathyroid glands (1 or more of the 4 glands)
2. Sex predilection: females > males
3. Age predilection: age 40-age 70
4. Pathology:
   a) 82% of cases of hyperparathyroidism are due to adenomas
   b) 15% of cases of hyperparathyroidism are due to hyperplasia of the glands
   c) 3% are malignant
5. Clinical symptoms:
   a) Renal stones (calcium oxalate): most common symptomatic presentation
   b) Peptic ulcer disease: calcium stimulates gastrin release
   c) Acute pancreatitis: calcium activates phospholipases
   d) Constipation: most common GI complaint
   e) Band keratopathy: metastatic calcification in the limbus of the eye
   f) Nephrocalcinosis: polyuria, loss of concentrating ability, and diluting capability due to metastatic calcification of the renal tubules
   g) Pruritus: metastatic calcification in the skin
   h) Short QT interval; bradycardia
   i) Hypertension: calcium increases muscular contraction in the resistance vessels.
   j) Osteitis fibrosa cystica: late finding, commonly found in jaw, called "brown tumor" due to hemorrhage into cysts
   k) Pseudogout: calcium pyrophosphate; positively birefringement crystals
   l) Mental changes: personality changes, psychosis, depression
   m) X-ray changes:
      1. "Salt and pepper skull" on X-ray
      2. Subperiosteal resorption of bone from the second and third middle phalanges and lamina dura around the teeth
      3. Distal resorption of clavicle
6. The mnemonic "stones, bones, abdominal groans, and psychic moans"
   a) Stones: calcium oxalate renal stones
   b) Bones: osteitis fibrosa cystica, salt and pepper skull, resorption of clavicle, subperiosteal resorption of bone from the second and third phalanges and the lamina dura around the teeth
   c) Abdominal pain: due to acute pancreatitis
   d) Psychic moans: psychosis, depression
7. Changes in blood and serum:
   a) Hypercalcemia (most common characteristic)
   b) Hypercalciuria
   c) Hypophosphatemia
   d) Hyperphosphaturia
   e) Normal anion gap metabolic acidosis
8. Treatment:
   a) Adenoma: surgery to locate and remove adenoma (biopsy second gland to see if atrophic)
   b) Hyperplasia: remove 3½ glands and autotransplant some tissue into the muscle of the arm
9. Most common laboratory abnormality: hypercalcemia

SUMMARY OF THE DIAGNOSIS AND SOME FEATURES OF CERTAIN ENDOCRINE DISEASES

1. **Acromegaly:**
   a) Signs/symptoms: enlarged hands, feet, and head; hypertension; cardiomegaly; weight gain
   b) Pathology: due to pituitary adenoma, growth hormone
   c) Treatment: transsphenoidal surgery, radiation, bromocriptine
2. **Addison's disease:**
   a) Signs/symptoms: weakness, hypotension, hyperpigmentation
   b) Pathology: autoimmune destruction of adrenal glands
   c) Acute treatment: acutely ill: IV cortisol
   d) Chronic treatment: Replacement with glucocorticoid (hydrocortisone) plus mineralocorticoid (9-alpha-fluorocortisol)
   e) Results: adrenocortical insufficiency
3. **Diabetes insipidus:**
   a) Signs/symptoms: polyuria, polydypsia due to deficiency of antidiuretic hormone
   b) Subtypes: central and nephrogenic
   c) Differential diagnosis: psychogenic polydypsia
   d) Most common cause: nephrogenic subtype most commonly due to lithium
   e) Treatment: IM ADH for treatment of central subtype
4. **Prolactinoma:**
   a) Signs/symptoms: galactorrhea, amenorrhea, infertility, decreased libido
   b) Frequency: most common pituitary tumor
   c) Investigation and confirmation: serum prolactin >300
   d) Differential diagnosis: rule out pregnancy, drugs (major tranquilizers, OCPS, hypothyroidism, IV cimetidine, opiates)
   e) Treatment: transsphenoidal surgery, bromocriptine for treatment
5. **Conn's syndrome:**
   a) Signs/symptoms: weakness (due to hypokalemia), hypertension, carbohydrate intolerance (polyuria, polydypsia)
   b) Most common cause: adenoma of the adrenal
   c) Pathology: excess mineralocorticoid production
   d) Laboratory investigations: mild hypernatremia, hypokalemic metabolic alkalosis
   e) Treatment: adenoma removal; hyperplasia-spironolactone

6. **Cushing's syndrome:**
   a) Signs/symptoms: truncal obesity, CHO intolerance, moon face, buffalo hump, abdominal stria, osteoporosis, psychic changes (depression and euphoria), easy bruising, myopathy, plethoric face
   b) Pathology: pituitary adenoma, adrenal adenoma, steroid therapy
   c) Most common cause: corticosteroid therapy
   d) Laboratory investigation: lab tests (screen): serum cortisol; 24-hour urine for cortisol; dexamethasone suppression test (1 mg). Confirmation and differentiation between pituitary Cushing's, adrenal Cushing's, and ectopic Cushing's; plasma ACTH; high-dose dexamethasone (8 mg) suppression test
   e) Treatment:
      1. Exogenous Cushing's: stop steroids, decrease dose, or every other day steroids with a drug holiday
      2. Endogenous Cushing's: removal of adenoma in pituitary and adrenal Cushing's syndrome.
7. **Primary hyperparathyroidism:**
   a) Signs/symptoms: mnemonic: stones, bones, abdominal groans, psychic moans; renal colic (Ca oxal); acute pancreatitis; constipation; X-ray: bone resorption, salt and pepper skull
   b) Pathology: most commonly adenoma of the parathyroid gland
   c) Laboratory abnormalities: hypercalcemia, hypophosphatemia, hypocalciuria, hyperphosphaturia. Hypercalcemia is most common metabolic abnormality; may also occur in metastatic carcinoma.
   d) Treatment: adenoma: removal; hyperplasia: removal of 3½ glands

SUGGESTED READINGS

Azar ST, Melby JC. Primary aldosteronism. In: Rakel R, ed. Conn's current therapy. Philadelphia: WB Saunders, 1994.

Frantz AG. Hyperprolactinemia. In: Rakel R, ed. Conn's current therapy. Philadelphia: WB Saunders, 1994.

Lester LB, McClung MR. Hyperparathyroidism. In: Rakel R, ed. Conn's current therapy. Philadelphia: WB Saunders, 1994.

Melby JC. Adrenocortical insufficiency. In: Rakel R, ed. Conn's current therapy. Philadelphia: WB Saunders, 1994.

Trainer PJ, Besser GM. Cushing's syndrome. In: Rakel R, ed. Conn's current therapy. Philadelphia: WB Saunders, 1994.

Vance ML. Acromegaly. In: Rakel R, ed. Conn's current therapy. Philadelphia: WB Saunders, 1994.

Verbalis JG, Greenberg A. Diabetes insipidus. In: Rakel R, ed. Conn's current therapy. Philadelphia: WB Saunders, 1994.

PROBLEM 22   A 38-YEAR-OLD FEMALE WITH SWEATING, PALPITATIONS, NERVOUSNESS, IRRITABILITY, AND TREMOR

A 38-year-old female presents with a 3-month history of sweating, palpitations, weight loss, nervousness, irritability, insomnia, hand tremors, and diarrhea.

She has had no significant past personal illnesses. One of her sisters has rheumatoid arthritis. The patient, a teacher, is finding it harder and harder to perform her job due to profound fatigue and inability to concentrate.

On examination, her blood pressure is 160/70 mm Hg. Her pulse is 120 and regular. She demonstrates mild proptosis; you feel a smooth, diffusely enlarged and nontender thyroid gland. CV examination reveals a loud S_1 and a loud S_2 with an ejection systolic murmur heard loudest along the left sternal edge. This murmur does not radiate. No other abnormalities are noted.

SELECT THE ONE BEST ANSWER TO THE FOLLOWING QUESTIONS

1. What is the most likely diagnosis in this patient?
   a) toxic multinodular goiter
   b) Graves' disease
   c) Hashimoto's thyroiditis
   d) atypical pheochromocytoma
   e) panic disorder

2. What is the etiology of the disorder described?
   a) idiopathic
   b) an autoimmune disease
   c) a hereditary disease
   d) due to an as-yet-undetermined interaction between genetic and environmental factors
   e) iatrogenic in most cases

3. What is(are) the laboratory test(s) of choice in this patient at this time?
   a) 24-hour radioiodine uptake test
   b) thyroid scan
   c) free serum T_4 (directly measured)
   d) serum TSH
   e) c and d
   f) b and c

4. What is the treatment of choice for the patient presented in Question 1?
   a) propylthiouracil
   b) methimazole
   c) radioactive iodine
   d) subtotal thyroidectomy
   e) a or b

5. The recommended treatment of choice is undertaken in this patient. Which of the following will be the end result of this treatment?
   a) complete cure: no further medication or other treatments necessary
   b) complete cure: no hyperthyroid or hypothyroid medication necessary

   c) complete cure: hypothyroid medication needed for lifetime use
   d) partial cure: hypothyroid medication needed for 5 years
   e) partial cure: hyperthyroid medication needed for 5 years

6. A 25-year-old female is seen for her periodic health examination. Her past history is unremarkable; she is feeling well at present and is currently taking the oral contraceptive pill.

   On P/E, her blood pressure is 130/75 mm Hg. Examination reveals that the head and neck are completely normal; specifically, no abnormalities of the thyroid gland are noted. A routine serum T_4 level done is elevated at 13 μg/dl (169 nmol/l). What is the most likely explanation for the elevated T_4 level?
   a) Graves' disease
   b) thyrotoxicosis
   c) toxic nodular goiter
   d) an elevated thyroid binding globulin (TBG) secondary to the oral contraceptive pill
   e) laboratory error

7. To confirm your diagnosis in the patient just described, which of the following would you order?
   a) the all-out, all-inclusive, miss nothing workup
   b) serum T_3
   c) serum TBG
   d) serum free T_4
   e) serum TSH
   f) d or e

8. Which of the following statements about the category of disorders labeled as thyroiditis is(are) true?
   a) thyroiditis represents a diverse group of conditions
   b) inflammation of the thyroid gland is the prominent clinical feature in thyroiditis
   c) thyroiditis can be acute, subacute, or chronic
   d) thyroiditis may be either symptomatic or asymptomatic
   e) all of the above

9. A 28-year-old female is seen in your office for a complete baseline health assessment. You have never seen this patient before. She feels well and tells you that she is "wonderfully healthy." She has had no weight loss or gain; no sweating, no tremors, no diarrhea or constipation; no anxiety or depression; no irritability; and no other symptoms.

   On examination she is found to have a 3-cm nodule in the left lobe of the thyroid gland. Her blood pressure is 130/70 mm Hg. Her pulse is 96 and regular.

   What is the most important investigation to be carried out on a patient with this finding?
   a) a serum T_4
   b) a serum free T_4
   c) a thyroid scan
   d) a thyroid ultrasound
   e) a CT scan of the thyroid

10. Which of the following statements regarding "warm (hot) nodules" and "cold nodules" is(are) true?
    a) cold nodules are more likely to be benign than warm nodules
    b) cold nodules need not be investigated any further
    c) cold nodules are more likely to be associated with signs and symptoms of hyperthyroidism than warm nodules
    d) cold nodules require further investigation to differentiate benign from malignant status
    e) none of the above statements are true

11. Following the initial investigation of a cold nodule, what should be the next investigation?
    a) a CT scan of the thyroid gland
    b) an MRI scan of the thyroid gland
    c) an ultrasound examination of the thyroid gland
    d) a repeat thyroid scan
    e) none of the above

12. The correct investigation is chosen in Question 11. From that investigation you now know that the cold nodule is a solid but not cystic mass. What would you do now?
    a) obtain a CT scan of the head and neck to look for metastatic disease
    b) obtain an MRI scan of the head and neck to look for metastatic disease
    c) perform a fine-needle aspiration of the thyroid mass
    d) perform an excisional biopsy of the thyroid mass
    e) none of the above

13. What is the most common cause of hypothyroidism in the United States?

    a) autoimmune thyroiditis
    b) post ^{131}I hypothyroidism
    c) iodine deficiency
    d) idiopathic hypothyroidism
    e) post-thyroidectomy hypothyroidism

14. Which of the following statements is(are) true regarding Hashimoto's thyroiditis?
    a) Hashimoto's thyroiditis is more common in females than in males
    b) antithyroid antibodies are found in 80% of individuals with this condition
    c) this condition is also known as chronic lymphocytic thyroiditis
    d) symptoms of hyperthyroidism often precede symptoms of hypothyroidism
    e) a, b, and c
    f) all of the above

15. A 65-year-old male presents with a 6-month history of lethargy, weakness, psychomotor retardation, cold intolerance, constipation, hair loss, and weight gain. You suspect hypothyroidism. Which of the following investigations will provide the most useful information for diagnosing hypothyroidism in this patient?
    a) serum T_4
    b) serum T_3
    c) free serum T_4
    d) serum TSH
    e) serum TBG

16. Which of the following statements regarding the treatment of the patient described in Question 15 is(are) false?
    a) optimal therapy for this condition can be determined by measurement of the serum TSH level
    b) until the serum TSH is normal, full replacement has not been established
    c) patients with significant cardiac disease and elderly patients should be treated cautiously
    d) desiccated thyroid is the treatment of choice
    e) none of the above statements are false

17. Which of the following statements concerning thyroid carcinoma is(are) true?
    a) papillary carcinoma is the most common type of thyroid cancer
    b) papillary carcinoma is the thyroid cancer with the best prognosis
    c) papillary carcinoma, even when metastatic to lymph nodes, may not adversely influence prognosis
    d) a and b
    e) all of the above

Short Answer Management Problem 22

List the most common causes of each of the following thyroid conditions:
1. Hyperthyroidism
2. Hypothyroidism
3. Thyroid-antibody-associated condition
4. Thyroid carcinoma
5. Elevated total serum T_4; elevated TBG

ANSWERS

1. B.

2. B. This patient has *Graves' disease.* Graves' disease is the most common cause of hyperthyroidism. It usually presents with symptoms of sweating, palpitations, nervousness, irritability, tremor, diarrhea, heat intolerance, and weight loss.

   Physical signs of Graves' disease include a diffuse, nontender thyroid gland enlargement (goiter); tachycardia; systolic hypertension; loud heart sounds; and a cardiac murmur. A *bruit* is sometimes heard over the thyroid gland itself. Proptosis, with a straight-ahead stare and lid lag, are frequently seen. Occasionally patients present with severe exophthalmos accompanied by ophthalmoplegia, follicular conjunctivitis, chemosis, and even loss of vision.

   Graves' disease is thought to be due to an autoimmune process, and antibodies are present in the serum.

   Toxic nodular goiter and toxic adenoma are other causes of hyperthyroidism. Their presentation, however, is usually significantly more subtle than the presentation of Graves' disease and are generally not confused with this condition.

   Hashimoto's thyroiditis is a cause of hypothyroidism rather than hyperthyroidism. Its presentation will be discussed in a subsequent question.

   Atypical pheochromocytoma and panic disorder are not really serious considerations with this presentation history.

3. E. The methods of measuring thyroid hormone have changed considerably in the last two years, and the serum TSH level is now being used to measure and detect hyperthyroidism as well as hypothyroidism. Indeed, the sine quo non of hyperthyroidism at this time is a low serum TSH level. That, along with a directly measured free T_4, are the screening tests that should be used. If the free T_4 comes back normal, then a serum T_3 should be ordered; 10% to 15% of the cases of hyperthyroidism are actually due to a T_3 toxicosis rather than a T_4 problem.

4. C.

5. C. The two basic treatments for Graves' disease are antithyroid drugs (propylthiouracil or methimazole) and radioiodine therapy.

   Antithyroid drugs
   1. Advantage: These drugs provide the opportunity for the patient to experience a spontaneous remission and require lifelong medication.
   2. Disadvantages:
      a) Remissions are attained in fewer than 50% of patients.
      b) Continuous or repeated courses of drug therapy are usually necessary.

   Radioiodine therapy
   1. Advantages:
      a) Radioiodine is curative.
      b) Managing post-radiation hypothyroidism is simpler than managing most patients on long-term antithyroid drug therapy.
   2. Disadvantage: Iatrogenic hypothyroidism is produced in all patients.

   On the basis of weighing advantages versus disadvantages for both, the recommendation has been made that radioiodine is the treatment of choice for adult patients. In children and adolescents, the antithyroid drug therapy remains first-line treatment, with radioiodine being second-line treatment.

6. D.

7. F. The most likely explanation for the elevated serum T_4 in this patient is an elevated thyroid binding globulin secondary to the estrogen component of the OCP.

   TBG is increased in the following patients:
   1. Patients on the OCP
   2. Patients taking estrogen supplementation
   3. Patients with infectious hepatitis

   TBG is decreased in the following patients:
   1. Patients with chronic liver disease
   2. Patients with nephrotic syndrome
   3. Patients with hypoproteinemia from other causes
   4. Patients on androgen therapy

   In order to confirm your diagnosis of the patient described in Question 6, you would order either a serum free T_4 level or a TSH level. As stated before, the serum

TSH level is now being used to diagnose hyperthyroidism as well as hypothyroidism. Thus, in this patient, you would expect to find a normal TSH level as opposed to a low TSH level.

8. E. The group of disorders labeled as thyroiditis encompasses a diverse group of thyroid disorders of various causes; inflammation of the thyroid gland is a prominent and consistent histologic feature. These may be relatively asymptomatic or self-limited disorders, or they can be accompanied by long-term abnormalities of thyroid growth including goiter formation and nodularity. Thyroiditis can also be classified as acute, subacute, or chronic.

9. C.

10. D.

11. C.

12. C. The most important investigation to be carried out in this patient is a radioactive thyroid scan to determine whether this is a hot nodule or a cold nodule. With hot nodules, no further testing is warranted unless the patient is hyperthyroid. If the nodule is a cold nodule, then an ultrasound should be done to differentiate a cystic lesion from a mixed or solid lesion. Cystic lesions can be treated by simple drainage; mixed lesions or solid lesions should be further investigated by aspiration cytology and fine-needle biopsy. Aspiration cytology and fine-needle biopsy will sharply decrease surgical intervention rates. Cold nodules are much more likely to be malignant than warm or hot nodules. In the final diagnosis, however, most cold nodules are benign as well.

13. A.

14. F. The most common cause of hypothyroidism is autoimmune thyroiditis or Hashimoto's thyroiditis. The patient with Hashimoto's thyroiditis may be initially hyperthyroid but always progresses to a hypothyroid state. Symptoms of hypothyroidism include fatigue, lethargy, constipation, cold intolerance, dry skin, hair loss, weight gain, edema, headache, arthralgias, hoarseness, amenorrhea, bradycardia, and hypotension.

Hashimoto's thyroiditis is also known as chronic lymphocytic thyroiditis. It is much more common in females than in males. Antithyroid antibodies are present in up to 80% of patients. In the acute thyroiditis stage of the disease, symptoms of hyperthyroidism precede symptoms of hypothyroidism.

15. D.

16. D. The most useful test for diagnosing hypothyroidism is the serum TSH level. Serum TSH is elevated in almost all cases of primary hypothyroidism. If hypothyroidism is suspected, the serum TSH will provide definite proof for or against the condition.

The serum TSH level will determine optimal thyroid replacement therapy. With adequate replacement, the serum TSH should return to normal.

Thyroxine is the preferred therapeutic agent, although both desiccated thyroid and triiodothyronine can return the TSH to normal.

17. E. The following features of thyroid papillary carcinoma have been found to be true:
    1. It is the most common type of thyroid cancer.
    2. It is the thyroid cancer with the best prognosis.
    3. Spread to regional lymph nodes does not necessarily influence the prognosis.

SOLUTION TO SHORT ANSWER MANAGEMENT PROBLEM 22

The most common causes of thyroid conditions are as follows:
1. Hyperthyroidism: Graves' disease
2. Hypothyroidism: Hashimoto's thyroiditis
3. Thyroid-antibody-associated condition: Hashimoto's thyroiditis
4. Thyroid carcinoma: papillary carcinoma
5. Elevated total serum T_4 plus elevated TBG: oral contraceptive pill

SUMMARY OF THE DIAGNOSIS AND TREATMENT OF THYROID DISORDERS

1. **Important epidemiology:**
   a) Hypothyroidism is one of the most commonly underdiagnosed conditions, particularly in the elderly.
   b) Hypothyroidism is significantly more common than hyperthyroidism. All elderly patients admitted to a long-term care facility or nursing home should probably have a serum TSH performed.
2. **Hyperthyroidism:**
   a) Causes:
      1. Graves' disease: most common cause
      2. Toxic nodular goiter
      3. Toxic adenoma
   b) Signs/symptoms: most common signs/symptoms include the following:
      1. Tremor
      2. Anxiety/nervousness/irritability
      3. Diarrhea
      4. Weight loss
      5. Sweating
      6. Palpitations
      7. Insomnia
      8. Proptosis/exopthalmosis

9. Systolic hypertension
10. Loud cardiac sounds/cardiac murmur
c) Investigations: a simplified initial investigation approach would be the following:
   1. Directly measured free serum T$_4$
   2. Serum TSH (Note: This is becoming more important in diagnosis of hyperthyroidism as well as hypothyroidism.)
   3. If directly measured free serum T$_4$ is normal, serum T$_3$ should be measured as well.
   4. A thyroid scan followed by a thyroid ultrasound to identify and categorize thyroid nodules (cold/warm)
d) Treatment:
   1. Radiation is the treatment of choice for Graves' disease in adults.
   2. Antithyroid drugs are the treatment of choice in children and adolescents.
   3. Surgery: subtotal thyroidectomy may be the most appropriate treatment for a toxic or solitary adenoma (nonmalignant). Radiation may sometimes be a reasonable alternative.
   4. Antithyroid drugs of choice are propylthiouracil and methimazole.
3. **Hypothyroidism:**
   a) Most common cause:
      1. Hashimoto's thyroiditis, or chronic lymphocytic thyroiditis, is the most common cause.
      2. Other common causes include hypothyroidism induced by thyroid surgery or radiation ablation.
   b) Investigations: Serum TSH is the most sensitive test in diagnosing primary hypothyroidism.
      For the elderly patient who has become depressed and is losing interest in life in general: think of hypothyroidism and screen for it. Screen all elderly patients entering a long-term care facility for clinical hypothyroidism.
   c) Treatment: Levothyroxine 50 μg-200 μg/day (start at 50 μg and work up)
4. **Thyroid carcinoma:** most common cause: papillary carcinoma. Minimally invasive even after it has spread to regional lymph nodes.

SUGGESTED READINGS

Cooper DS. Hyperthyroidism. In: Rakel R, ed. Conn's current therapy. Philadelphia: WB Saunders, 1994.

Kinder BK. Thyroid cancer. In: Rakel R, ed. Conn's current therapy. Philadelphia: WB Saunders, 1994.

Magner JA. Hypothyroidism. In: Rakel R, ed. Conn's current therapy. Philadelphia: WB Saunders, 1994.

PROBLEM 23   A 27-YEAR-OLD FEMALE WITH WEAKNESS, VISUAL LOSS, ATAXIA, AND SENSORY LOSS

A 27-year-old female presents to your office for assessment of symptoms including weakness, visual loss, bladder incontinence, sharp, shooting pain in the lower back, clumsiness when walking, and sensory loss. These symptoms have occurred during three episodes (different combinations of symptoms each time) approximately 3 months apart, and each episode lasted approximately 3 days.

The first episode consisted of weakness, bladder incontinence, and sharp shooting pains in the lower back (in both hip girdles). The second episode consisted of visual loss, clumsiness when walking, and sensory loss. The third episode (last week) consisted of sharp, shooting pains in the lower back and sensory loss (bilateral) in the upper extremities.

On neurologic examination, you find the following: swelling of the optic disc on fundoscopy, inability to walk heel to toe, and slight objective weakness of both hip girdles. She has no symptoms today.

SELECT THE ONE BEST ANSWER TO THE FOLLOWING QUESTIONS

1. Given this information, what is the most likely diagnosis in this patient?
   a) amyotrophic lateral sclerosis
   b) multiple sclerosis
   c) subacute combined degeneration of the cord—vitamin B_{12} deficiency
   d) hysterical conversion reaction
   e) tertiary syphilis

2. There are three subtypes of the disease. Which of the following subtypes does the patient presented in Question 1 fit into?
   a) definite disease
   b) probable disease
   c) at risk of disease
   d) b or c
   e) none of the above

3. If you had the opportunity to do only one diagnostic test, which of the following would you choose?
   a) CT scan of the head/spinal cord
   b) MRI scan of the brain/spinal cord
   c) serum vitamin B_{12} levels
   d) Beck's Depression scale
   e) VDRL test for syphilis

4. The disease described is most correctly described as which of the following?
   a) an uncommon neurological disease that can be corrected by the administration of subcutaneous vitamin B_{12}
   b) the number-one cause of disabling disease of young adults in the United States
   c) a very common psychiatric condition in which psychological symptoms are manifested by physical symptoms
   d) a fatal neurological condition that results in continual deterioration to the point of respiratory depression and the cessation of respiration
   e) none of the above

5. The disease described is associated with which of the following?
   a) racial predilection: whites > blacks
   b) sex predilection: females > males
   c) high socioeconomic status
   d) environmental exposure
   e) all of the above

6. Which of the following statements regarding the behavior of the disease described above is(are) true?
   a) in 90% of all cases, the first episode is followed by a cycle of relapses and remissions
   b) in 60% of the group labeled "definite disease," the relapsing/remitting pattern converts to a progressive course after 5 years
   c) ten percent of patients have progressive disease from the onset of symptom
   d) up to 20% of patients with this disease have a subtype labeled "benign"
   e) all of the above

7. The disease, if diagnosed as a central nervous system disease, has to involve how many different areas of the central nervous system?
   a) one
   b) two
   c) three
   d) four
   e) not applicable: not primarily a neurologic disease

8. Which of the following clinical findings support the diagnosis made above?
   a) a CSF mononuclear cell pleocytosis
   b) an increase in CSF IgG
   c) oligoclonal banding of CSF IgG (two or more bands)
   d) abnormalities in evoked response testing (any type)
   e) all of the above

9. The target of this disease process is an attack on which of the following?
   a) the neurotransmitter balance in the CNS
   b) the "oligodendrocytes" of the CNS

c) the peripheral nerves in the posterior columns of the spinal cord
d) the cerebral hemispheres
e) the cerebellum

10. What is(are) the treatment(s) of choice for arresting the disease process described?
a) ACTH
b) corticosteroids
c) cytotoxic immunosuppressive agents
d) a and b
e) all of the above

11. Symptomatic treatments that have been suggested for treatment for the disease process described include which of the following?
a) hydrotherapy
b) aerobic exercise
c) low-fat/high-fiber diet

d) extra antioxidants (β-carotene, vitamin C, vitamin E)
e) a, b, and c
f) all of the above

12. Which of the following symptoms is the most common symptom in this disorder?
a) optic neuritis
b) ataxia
c) vertigo
d) loss of bladder control
e) impotence

13. Of the symptoms described in Question 12, which is the least common symptom?
a) optic neuritis
b) ataxia
c) vertigo
d) loss of bladder control
e) impotence

Short Answer Management Problem 23

Describe the pathophysiology of the disease process and how it produces its signs and symptoms.

ANSWERS

1. B.

2. A. This patient has multiple sclerosis. The patient also meets the criteria for the subtype "definite multiple sclerosis," which is discussed later.

The important diagnostic criteria for multiple sclerosis include the following:
A. Examination must reveal objective abnormalities of the CNS.
B. Involvement must reflect predominantly the white matter long tracts including the pyramidal pathways, the cerebellar pathways, the medial longitudinal fasciculus (MLF), the optic nerve (optic neuritis), and the posterior columns.
C. Examination or history must implicate involvement of two more areas of the central nervous system.
D. Age 15-60 years
E. There must be two or more separate episodes of "clusters of symptoms" involving different sites of the CNS, or gradual or stepwise progression over at least 6 months.
F. There can be no other explanation for the CNS symptoms.

Multiple sclerosis is further subdivided into three subtypes:
Subtype I, definite multiple sclerosis: all criteria are fulfilled.
Subtype II, probable multiple sclerosis: all criteria are

fulfilled except (a) only one objective abnormality despite two symptomatic episodes or (b) one symptomatic episode and unrelated signs detected on examination.
Subtype III, at risk for multiple sclerosis: all criteria are fulfilled except that there is only one symptomatic episode and corresponding signs are detected on examination.

3. B. The most sensitive and specific investigation for this disorder is an MRI of the brain and/or spinal cord scan. The MRI scan will reveal the following abnormalities in a patient with multiple sclerosis:
A. Plaque formation (a subsequent stage that results from the loss of the myelin sheath in different parts of the CNS)
B. Spotty and irregular demyelination in the affected areas

4. B. Multiple sclerosis is the number-one disabling disease of young adults; 250,000-350,000 persons in the United States in 1990 were at the time documented victims of the disease. It is more common at northern latitudes than at southern latitudes. Other risk factors will be addressed in subsequent questions.

5. E. The documented risk factors for multiple sclerosis are as follows:
A. White race > black race
B. Female > male (2:1)

C. Environmental influence
1. Latitude (north > south)
2. Other unidentified environmental toxins (suspected)
D. Genetic: HLA histocompatibility antigens
E. Viral infections: no specific virus has been identified, but suspicion exists.
F. High socioeconomic status

6. E. Almost all patients fall into one of the following courses based on symptoms and signs:
A. Ninety percent of all cases after the first symptom have relapses followed by remissions.
B. Sixty percent (of the 90%) have relapsing/remitting cases that switch to a progressive course approximately 5 years after the onset of the first symptoms.
C. Ten percent have progressive disease from the onset.
D. Twenty percent are benign. These patients have one or two relapses and then recover. This 20% have multifocal plaques at autopsy without evidence of an inflammatory demyelinating reaction.
E. There is a very rare type termed *acute multiple sclerosis of the Marburg type* with rapid progression of symptoms.

7. B. For a patient to be diagnosed as having multiple sclerosis, two separate areas of the central nervous system must be involved.

8. E. The following are laboratory findings that support the diagnosis of multiple sclerosis:
A. CSF mononuclear cell pleocytosis (> 5 cells/microliter)
B. CSF IgG is increased in the absence of a normal concentration of total protein.
C. Oligoclonal banding of CSF IgG is detected by agarose gel electrophoresis techniques. Two or more oligoclonal bands are found in 75% to 90% of MS patients.
D. Metabolites from myelin breakdown may be detected in the CSF.
E. Evoked response testing may detect slowed or abnormal conduction in visual, auditory, somatosensory, or motor pathways. One or more evoked potentials are abnormal in 80% to 90% of patients with MS.
F. CT scanning of the brain is abnormal in a proportion of patients with MS and may reveal any of the following: ventricular enlargement, low-density periventricular abnormalities, and focal regions of enhancement following injection of a contrast agent.
G. MRI imaging is the most useful imaging method available, and abnormal MRI scans are seen in > 90% of patients with definite multiple sclerosis.

9. B. The target of the MS disease process are the oligodendrocytes of the CNS. These cells fabricate and maintain the myelin sheaths, the material covering the axons that is necessary for the normal conduction of nerve impulses. Destruction of oligodendrocytes occurs in clusters and is accompanied by loss of oligodendrocytes as well as their myelin sheath appendages with axon sparing (primary demyelination).

The cluster destruction of oligodendrocytes-myelin sheaths form multifocal plaques, the pathologic hallmark of the disease. The majority of these plaques are in the white matter.

10. D. The treatments of choice for acute attacks of multiple sclerosis are as follows:
A. ACTH:
1. Aqueous ACTH (20 U/ml), 80 U is given IV in 500 mls of dextrose in water over 6-8 hours for 3 days.
2. ACTH gel (40 U/ml) is then given IM in a dose of 40 units every 12 hours for 7 days. The dose is then reduced every 3 days.
B. Methylprednisolone:
1. Methylprednisolone is mixed in 500 ml D5W and administered slowly, over 4 to 6 hours, preferably in the morning:
   i) 1000 mg daily for 3 days
   ii) 500 mg daily for 3 days
   iii) 250 mg daily for 3 days
C. Methylprednisone-prednisone:
1. Methylprednisolone, 1000 mg IV daily for 3 days, followed by oral prednisone (1 mg/kg per day) for 14 days

11. F. The symptomatic treatment of multiple sclerosis has many aspects. The following have been suggested:
1. Keeping cool: It has been reported that a "cool suit" that lowers the normal eardrum temperature 1°F (brain temperature) in 1 hour used twice/day for 1-2 months combined with an exercise prescription can improve neurologic function in some patients.
2. A regular exercise program: A regular exercise program has special benefits for patients with MS. A regular exercise prescription helps overcome fatigue, enhances endurance, induces a feeling of well-being, and benefits every organ.
3. Pursuit of wellness and a positive attitude: Health maintenance to combat the aging process should be emphasized as almost all patients' longevity with MS is minimally affected. This includes regular visits to the neurologist and family doctor for a thorough checkup with appropriate screening tests and treatments. It is further recommended that a low-fat, high-fiber diet, daily cranberry juice, multivitamins with extra antioxidants (β-carotene, vitamin C, and vitamin E), calcium daily, low-dose ASA daily (81 mg), ideal weight maintenance, regular sleep, and naps be a regular part of the program.
4. Education: be "multiple sclerosis smart:" Patients should become experts in MS. They should learn

medical terminology, the hypotheses about the disease process, the symptoms/signs, and the complications in an attempt to better understand their condition.

5. Support: The therapy for MS patients starts with self-help. Patients benefit greatly where goals are committed to and met.

12. A.

13. E. The initial symptoms of multiple sclerosis and their frequency are as follows:

SYMPTOM	PERCENTAGE OF CASES
1. Sensory loss	37%
2. Optic neuritis	36%
3. Weakness	35%
4. Paresthesias	24%
5. Diplopia	15%
6. Ataxia	11%
7. Vertigo	6%
8. Paroxysmal symptoms	4%
9. Bladder disorders	4%
10. Lhermitte sign	3%
11. Pain	3%
12. Dementia	2%
13. Visual loss	2%
14. Facial palsy	1%
15. Impotence	1%
16. Myokymia	1%
17. Epilepsy	1%
18. Falling	1%

Thus, of the symptoms listed in the question, the most common is optic neuritis, and the least common is impotence/other sexual dysfunction

SOLUTION TO SHORT ANSWER MANAGEMENT PROBLEM 23

The etiologic agent(s) producing multiple sclerosis is(are) unknown. There is reasonable evidence that it results from an interaction between the individual (immunology) and his(her) environment. The basic target of multiple sclerosis is the oligodendrocyte, the cell that fabricates and maintains myelin. Destruction of oligodendrocytes occurs in clusters and is accompanied by loss of not only the oligodendrocyte but, more importantly, their myelin sheaths. The cluster destruction of oligodendrocytes-myelin sheaths produces plaques, the pathologic hallmark of MS. This destruction of oligodendrocytes and myelin is patchy, leaving more areas unaffected. The axons are invariably spared.

SUMMARY OF THE DIAGNOSIS AND TREATMENT OF MULTIPLE SCLEROSIS

1. **Prevalence:** Number-one disabling condition of young adults in the United States; 250,000 to 350,000 persons in the United States in 1990 had physician-diagnosed multiple sclerosis.

2. **Epidemiology:**
   a) Almost all patients fit into one or more of the following categories:
      1. 90% of patients have after their first symptom a cycle of relapses and remissions.
      2. 60% of the 90% switch to a progressive course about 5 years after the first symptom.
      3. 10% of patients have progressive disease from the onset.
      4. Up to 20% are benign, with one or two relapses and then a good recovery.
   b) Risk factors for multiple sclerosis:
      1. Race: white > black
      2. Sex: females > males (2:1)
      3. High socioeconomic status
      4. Northern latitudes
      5. Other environmental factors as yet not identified:
         i) toxins
         ii) viruses seem to be implicated in relapses.
      6. HLA histocompatible antigens

3. **Symptoms:** most common symptoms are the following:
   a) Sensory loss
   b) Optic neuritis
   c) Weakness
   d) Paraesthesias

4. **Diagnosis:** criteria given previously:
   a) Two episodes, or attacks, of symptoms
   b) Two different areas of the CNS involved

5. **Testing for multiple sclerosis:**
   a) MRI scan of the brain: This will show the areas of demyelination better than any other test.
   b) CSF pleocytosis
   c) Increased CSF IgG
   d) Oligoclonal banding of IgG in the CSF
   e) Evoked potentials: visual, auditory, somatosensory, and motor

6. **Treatment:**
   a) Treatment for acute attacks:
      1. ACTH
      2. Methylprednisolone
      3. Prednisone
   b) General supportive treatments:
      1. Keeping cool
      2. A regular exercise program
      3. The pursuit of wellness and a positive attitude
      4. Education regarding the disease
      5. Support: family/support groups

SUGGESTED READINGS

Hauser SL. Multiple sclerosis and other demyelinating diseases. In: Isselbacher K et al., eds. Harrison's principles of internal medicine. 13th Ed. New York: McGraw-Hill, 1994.

Tourtellotte WW, Baumhefner RW. Multiple sclerosis. In: Rakel R, ed. Conn's current therapy. Philadelphia: WB Saunders, 1994.

PROBLEM 24   A 45-YEAR-OLD MALE WITH A HEADACHE

A 45-year-old male presents with a 4-week history of recurrent headaches that wake him up in the middle of the night. The headaches have been occurring every night and have been lasting approximately 1 hour. The headaches are described as a deep burning sensation centered behind the left orbit. The headaches are excruciating (he rates them as a 15 on a 10 point scale) and are associated with watery eyes, "a sensation of heat and warmth in my face," nasal discharge, and redness of the left eye.

Before the onset of these headaches 4 weeks ago, the patient describes no more than the occasional tension headache. Headaches were certainly never a problem.

The patient describes no recent life changes and no major life stresses. He is happily married, has three children, and has a secure job that he enjoys.

On examination, his blood pressure is 120/70 mm Hg. His pulse is 96 and regular.

SELECT THE ONE BEST ANSWER TO THE FOLLOWING QUESTIONS

1. What is the most likely cause of this patient's headache?
   a) subarachnoid hemorrhage
   b) tension-migraine syndrome
   c) atypical migraine headache
   d) cluster headache
   e) classic migraine headache

2. Which one of the following statements concerning this patient's headaches is false?
   a) oxygen may be useful in the treatment of the acute attack
   b) ergotamine may be used as a prophylactic drug in the condition
   c) methysergide may be used as a prophylactic agent in the condition
   d) lithium carbonate may be used as a prophylactic agent
   e) none of the above statements are false

3. A 32-year-old female presents with a 2-year history of recurrent headaches. These headaches occur between three and four times per month and last 12-24 hours. The headaches are almost always confined to the left side of the head and are associated with malaise, nausea, vomiting, photophobia, and phonophobia.

   The patient has been using acetaminophen (up to 6 g in a 12-hour period) without significant relief.

   On examination, the patient's blood pressure is 100/70 mm Hg. Her neurological examination is within normal limits. The optic fundi is normal, as is the rest of the neurological examination.

   What is the most likely headache in this patient?
   a) migraine headaches without aura (common migraine)
   b) migraine headaches with aura (classic migraine)
   c) complicated migraine
   d) tension-migraine syndrome
   e) nervous headache

4. A 38-year-old female presents with a 6-year history of recurrent headaches. These headaches occur approximately once per week. In contradiction to the patient discussed in Question 3, this patient has an unusual set of symptoms prior to both the prodromal phase and the headache itself. The symptoms are actually a "type of odd visual feeling or sight—flashing lights, almost like a pattern in front of my eyes." With respect to the headache itself, it usually lasts for 24-36 hours. It is throbbing in nature and often "switches from one side to the other" during the acute attack.

   On physical examination, the patient's blood pressure is 140/70 mm Hg. Examination of the optic fundi is completely normal as is the rest of the neurological examination.

   What is the most likely type of headache in this patient?
   a) migraine headache with aura (classic migraine)
   b) migraine headache without aura (common migraine)
   c) basilar migraine
   d) tension-migraine syndrome
   e) complicated migraine headache

5. A 24-year-old patient presents to your office for assessment of headache. She describes the onset of, characteristics of, duration of, and associated features of a migraine headache that is preceded by nausea and vomiting; that is confined to the left side of the head; and that is characterized by a throbbing pain lasting approximately 48 hours. The unusual feature of this headache is that it always begins approximately 2 days before menstruation, and it always ends with the onset of menstruation.

   On physical examination, the patient's blood pressure is 120/70 mm Hg. Her optic fundi are clear and her neurological examination is completely normal.

   What is the most likely type of headache in this patient?
   a) migraine without aura: premenstrual syndrome
   b) menstrual migraine
   c) migraine without aura: premenstrual dysphoric disorder

d) migraine-tension syndrome: premenstrual symptom complex

e) complicated migraine syndrome

6. Which of the following statements regarding migraine headaches is(are) true?
   a) migraine headache is more common in men than in women
   b) migraine headache is more common in patients who have a family history of migraine headache
   c) migraine headache is more common in patients in lower socioeconomic groups than in higher socioeconomic groups
   d) migraine headache is more common in urban dwellers than in rural dwellers
   e) all of the above

7. What is the prevalence of migraine headache in adult women?
   a) 1%
   b) 4%
   c) 14%
   d) 19%
   e) 31%

8. Regarding the pathogenesis of migraine headache, which of the following theories best explains the symptomatology?
   a) migraine headache is produced by spasm of the cerebral blood vessels (the aura and the prodrome) followed by spasmodic rebound producing vasodilatation and the accompanying headache
   b) migraine headache is produced by spasmodic rebound of the cerebral blood vessels (the aura and the prodrome) followed by spasm producing vasodilatation and the accompanying headache
   c) migraine headache is produced by an imbalance of the neurotransmitters dopamine and acetylcholine producing first spasm and then relaxation
   d) migraine headache is produced by a complex physiologic process involving platelet aggregation and the release of serotonin in the brain that is accompanied by a cycle of increase/decrease in blood brain catecholamines
   e) migraine headache is produced by a complex physiologic process involving platelet decrease, the depletion of serotonin, and a cycle of increase/decrease in blood brain catecholamines

9. Which of the following is(are) recognized triggers of migraine headache?
   a) stress, worry, and anxiety
   b) excessive sleep
   c) certain foods and alcohol
   d) weather changes
   e) all of the above

10. What is(are) the drug(s) of first choice for the abortive treatment of moderate severe to very severe migraine headache?
    a) sumatriptan
    b) dihydroergotamine mesylate
    c) ergotamine
    d) chlorpromazine
    e) all of the above

11. The abortive treatment of migraine headache is enhanced by the use of antiemetics. Which of the following antiemetics is the agent of first choice for use in conjunction with an abortive agent?
    a) prochlorperazine
    b) dimenhydrinate
    c) metoclopramide
    d) ondansetron
    e) prednisone

12. Which of the following has not been recommended as a prophylactic agent for the prevention of migraine headache?
    a) naproxen
    b) propranolol
    c) amitriptyline
    d) fluoxetine
    e) methysergide

13. A 35-year-old male presents to your office with a 6-month history of recurrent daily headaches, usually in the late afternoon. The headaches are described by the patient as "a vice around my head."

    The headaches are not associated with nausea, vomiting, or malaise. The patient does, however, describe some dizziness and light-headedness with these headaches.

    On examination, the patient's blood pressure is 100/70 mm Hg. His optic fundi are normal. There are no neurological abnormalities.

    What is the likely type of headache in this patient?
    a) chronic daily headache: tension type
    b) episodic tension-type headache
    c) migraine without aura
    d) migraine tension-type headache complex (missed or combined headache)
    e) cluster headache

14. What is(are) the treatment(s) of first choice for the patient described in Question 13?
    a) a prostaglandin synthetase inhibitor
    b) acetaminophen
    c) codeine
    d) a tricyclic antidepressant
    e) all of the above
    f) a, b, and/or d

15. Consider the patient described in Question 3. You note that the patient is taking 6 g of acetaminophen within a 12-hour period when the acute headache is present.

    Which of the following statements best represents the recommendation about this drug and this dose?
    a) given that this is an infrequent occurrence (once per week to once every 2 weeks), it is unlikely to produce any serious pathology
    b) given that this is an infrequent occurrence (once per week to once every 2 weeks) and the dose used is 6 g/12 hours, it would be prudent to allow the patient to continue this dose under careful monitoring
    c) given the dose of acetaminophen used in the very short time interval, it would be wise to check her liver function and suggest a decrease in the dose
    d) given the dose of acetaminophen used, the syndrome of analgesic rebound is a definite consideration
    e) b and d
    f) c and d

16. A 75-year-old female presents to your office with a severe left-sided temporal headache. She describes a tender area in the left temple. She also describes pain in the area of the jaw while chewing her food. This headache has been present for the past 3 days.

    On physical examination, the patient's blood pressure is 170/100 mm Hg. Her neurologic examination is normal. There is moderate tenderness in the area of the left temple.

    Which of the following statements regarding this patient's symptoms is(are) true?
    a) this probably represents a late-onset migraine syndrome
    b) simple analgesics should be prescribed before embarking on any extensive investigation of these symptoms
    c) this headache is unlikely to be associated with any significant complications
    d) an ESR should be ordered on this patient
    e) all of the above

17. Which of the following statements regarding the investigation of headaches is(are) true?
    a) patients with migraine with aura or migraine without aura rarely require more than a careful history and physical examination
    b) patients with episodic tension-type headaches rarely require more than a careful history and physical examination
    c) the EEG rarely is useful in the diagnosis of headache (other than when headache may indicate a CNS brain tumor)
    d) radioisotope brain scanning is no longer indicated

in the investigation of a patient with a headache syndrome
    e) all of the above

18. A 35-year-old female presents to the ER with another "migraine headache." She has had migraine headaches for the past 20 years, and during the last 4 years they have been almost constant.

    Her headaches have required IM Demerol and Gravol injections approximately twice per week for the last 3 years. She has made 157 trips to the ER with the same symptoms during the past year.

    This patient categorically tells you that she has "tried every abortive agent and every prophylactic agent and nothing has worked."

    Which of the following statements regarding this patient's headaches is(are) true?
    a) this headache most likely is an example of status migrainosus
    b) the major component of this headache is likely an analgesic rebound headache
    c) the scenario presented here is uncommon
    d) the majority of the patients with this headache type are female
    e) all of the above

19. What is the treatment of choice for the headache described in Question 18?
    a) continue the present treatment plan: repeated injections of Demerol and Gravol
    b) change the treatment plan to regular injections of dihydroergotamine and metoclopramide
    c) seek immediate psychiatric consultation
    d) change the treatment plan to one that employs non-narcotic analgesics (in fairly large doses) in place of the narcotic analgesics
    e) none of the above

20. A 62-year-old patient presents to the ER with headaches that have been getting progressively worse over the last 7 days. He has not had previous problems with headache, and his only significant illness was a lobectomy and radiation therapy for carcinoma of the lung 3 years ago. He has not had any recurrence and is feeling well.

    The significant features of this headache include the following: the headache appears to be significantly worse every day; the headache is absolutely constant: it never goes away and never decreases in severity to any extent; and the headache is described as a "terrible pressure within my head."

    What is the most likely cause of this patient's headache?
    a) migraine without aura: status migrainosus type
    b) migraine without aura: complex etiology
    c) secondary headache: cerebral edema

d) secondary headache: primary brain tumor due to previous radiation therapy

e) none of the above

21. What is the drug of choice for this patient at this time?

a) sumatriptan

b) ergotamine

c) meperidine and Gravol

d) dexamethasone

e) chlorpromazine

22. A 17-year-old male presents to the ER with "a headache like I've never had before." He is brought to the ER by his mother. The patient has been completely well, healthy, and active prior to this episode (which began last night). Nausea and vomiting began shortly after the headache onset.

   On examination, there is significant neck stiffness. The patient is unable to move his neck without extreme pain. You are just about to continue with the neurolog-ical examination when a patient with a cardiac arrest is wheeled through the ER doors.

   At this time, with this information you have to this point, what is the most likely diagnosis?

a) acute subdural hematoma

b) acute epidural hematoma

c) subarachnoid hemorrhage

d) migraine headache without aura: severe

e) glioblastoma multiforme

23. With the provisional diagnosis you have made on the patient in Question 22, what should you do now?

a) perform a lumbar puncture

b) perform a CT or MRI of the brain

c) observe the patient for 12 hours before doing anything

d) sedate and medicate the patient in an effort to alleviate the headache, sort things out later

e) none of the above

Short Answer Management Problem 24

Discuss the classification of primary headache disorders that has recently been proposed by the International Headache Society. Distinguish between primary headache and secondary headache.

ANSWERS

1. D.

2. E. This patient has developed a typical cluster headache. Although we can diagnose with considerable confidence, it is too early to predict which of the two subtypes of cluster headache the patient will ultimately develop. These subtypes are episodic cluster headache and chronic cluster headache.

   The typical cluster headache awakens a patient from sleep, although both daytime clusters and nighttime clusters are well described. Multiple daily episodes usually lasting between 45 minutes and 1 hour may occur on a regular basis for periods of 2 to 3 minutes. Remissions may last from several months to several years. Episodic cluster headaches constitute 90% of cases. In the other 10% of patients, the headaches do not remit (chronic cluster headache). The typical description of cluster headache is a headache that has the properties of a "deep, burning, or stabbing pain." It is very often described by the patient as "excruciating," "the worst pain I have ever had." It is almost exclusively unilateral in nature. The pain may become so bad that the patient actually becomes suicidal. Cluster headache is associated with lacrimation, facial flushing, and nasal discharge. The affected eye often becomes red, conjunctival vessels become dilated, and a Horner's-type syndrome including both ptosis and pupillary constriction develops.

   Cluster headache is thought by many authorities to be a migraine variant. Sumatriptan (imitrex) is the drug of choice for acute episodes of cluster headache. As well, oxygen inhalation is very beneficial in an acute cluster attack. Ergotamine preparations have also been shown to be effective. Prophylactic medications that are indicated in the treatment of cluster headache include verapamil, ergotamine, lithium, methysergide, prednisone and other corticosteroids, indomethacin, beta blockers, tricyclic antidepressants, and selective serotonin reuptake inhibitors (SSRIs).

3. A. This patient has migraine headache without aura (common migraine headache).

   Migraine headache is a type of headache that is typically episodic, usually occurring 1 or 2 times/month. More frequent episodes of migraine, such as migraine headache every day, second day, or third day, should make you suspicious regarding the true diagnosis. The most common alternative diagnosis would be rebound analgesic headaches, and many patients who are labeled as having migraine headaches actually have analgesic rebound headaches.

The prodromal phase of migraine consists of symptoms of excitation or inhibition of the CNS, including elation; excitability; irritability; increased appetite and craving for certain foods, especially sweets; depression; sleepiness; and fatigue. This phase occurs in approximately 30% of patients. These symptoms may precede the migraine attack by up to 24 hours. The headache phase of the cycle is certainly the most prominent. Migraine headache is unilateral in more than 50% of patients, but bilateral migraine is more common than previously thought. In addition, it is not uncommon for a migraine headache to begin on one side and switch to the other. The character of the pain is also much more variable than previously thought: "pulsating or throbbing" in only 50% of cases, and a "dull, achy" pain in the other 50%. The headache phase itself usually lasts between 4 and 72 hours but is occasionally longer. Migraine headache is almost invariably associated with other symptoms including nausea, vomiting, and diarrhea. Heightened sensory perceptions such as photophobia, phonophobia, and increased sensitivity to smell occur during the attacks.

Although a mixed headache syndrome (mixed migraine and tension headaches) and tension headaches themselves are often confused with migraine, pure migraine headache can usually be distinguished by moderate to severe intensity and aggravation by activities including coughing, running, or bending down. Those two characteristics, plus one of nausea, vomiting, photophobia, or phonophobia, establish the diagnosis as migraine headache.

4. A. This patient has migraine headache with aura.

The visual symptoms that this patient describes follow the classical description for what is called an *aura*. An aura is usually visual, although neurological auras consisting of hemisensory disturbances, hemiparesis, dysphasia, and change in memory or state of consciousness can occasionally occur.

Only approximately 20% of migraine headaches can be classified as migraine with aura. Also, it is quite frequent for a patient to alternate between migraine with aura and migraine without aura. Migraine with aura and migraine without aura are, other than the aura itself, quite similar in characteristic features.

5. B. Although migraine headache without aura can occur at any time during the menstrual cycle, this patient's description of a cyclical repeatable headache that occurs between 2 days prior to menstruation and the last day of menses clearly establishes this headache as what is referred to as menstrual migraine.

The important therapeutic difference between menstrual migraine and migraine headaches with or without aura is that true menstrual migraine is less responsive to prophylactic medication. The recommended treatment for menstrual migraine that begins before the menses is a combination of ergotamine (one tab bid) and naproxen 500 mg bid starting 3 days before the expected first day of flow and continued until menses is finished.

6. B.

7. D. Migraine headache is more common in women than in men. In the general population the prevalence of migraine headache is approximately 19% in women. Migraine headache is significantly more common in women who have a family history of migraine headache, particularly women who had a mother with migraine headache.

Migraine headache prevalence does not vary among the populations of the world; the prevalence is the same in rural Nigeria as it is in cosmopolitan Los Angeles. As well, contrary to what is commonly believed, migraine headache is not more common among lower socioeconomic groups than among higher socioeconomic groups unless there are triggering factors (see the answer to Question 9) that may be more common in a certain segment of the population.

8. D. There has been a significant increase in the understanding of the pathophysiology and pathogenesis of migraine headache since the second edition of this textbook was published. The pathophysiology is best summarized as an orderly process that involves the following events in this order:
   1. Platelet aggregation occurs in the CNS.
   2. There is a release of serotonin from the synaptic nerve endings.
   3. At the same time or following the release of serotonin, there is an increase and then a decrease in the levels of the blood brain catecholamines norepinephrine and epinephrine.

   This is significantly different from previous ideas of spasm followed by rebound vasodilation that was purported to explain the vasoconstriction (aura), and vasodilatation (headache).

9. E. The triggers of migraine are as follows:
   Common factors:
   1. Stress, worry, anxiety
   2. Menstruation
   3. Oral contraceptives
   4. Certain foods (aged cheese, chocolate)
   5. Alcohol
   6. Lack of sleep
   7. Glare, dazzle
   8. Weather or ambient temperature changes
   9. Physical exertion
   10. Fatigue

11. Head trauma
Less common factors:
1. High humidity
2. Excessive sleep
3. High altitude
4. Excessive vitamin A
5. Drugs: nitroglycerine, reserpine, estrogens, hydralazine, ranitidine
6. Pungent odors
7. Fluorescent lighting
8. Allergic reactions
9. Cold foods
10. Refractory errors

10. A.

11. C. The drug of first choice for the abortive treatment of acute severe to very severe migraine headache is sumatriptan (Imitrex). Sumatriptan is one of the most exciting new drugs (in all classes) to be released in the last 5 years.

Sumatriptan is a 5-hydrotryptophan (5-HT) agonist. Oral and subcutaneous preparations are available. It is extremely effective in over 80% of cases. The dosage is 6 mg subcutaneously initially that may be repeated within 24 hours, or a 100-mg oral tablet initially repeated within 24 hours.

As well, dihydroergotamine mesylate (DHE) given intravenously (1 mg iv) and ergotamine (rectal suppositories, sublingual tablets, and oral tablets) are also used to abort acute migraine headache in moderately severe cases of migraine.

Phenothiazines (such as chlorpromazine) and nonsteroidal antiinflammatory agents are useful as alternative agents in the treatment of migraine headaches and can be thought of as an alternative to the abortive agents just mentioned.

It is good idea to use an antiemetic drug in conjunction with the abortive agent. The most commonly used and effective antiemetic agent is metoclopramide.

12. A. Prophylactic pharmacotherapy for migraine headaches includes drugs from the following classes:
Beta-adrenergic blocking agents: propranolol, metoprolol, atenolol, and the like
Antidepressants:
1. Tricyclic antidepressants: amitriptyline, doxepin, desipramine
2. Selective serotonin reuptake inhibitors: fluoxetine, sertraline
3. Monamine oxidase inhibitors: phenelzine, isocarboxazid
4. Calcium-channel blockers: verapamil, flunarizine
5. Serotonin antagonists: methysergide, pizotifen
6. Anticonvulsants: valproate, phenytoin
7. Alpha-adrenergic agonists: clonidine

13. A. This patient has chronic tension-type headache. Chronic tension-type headaches are often described as a steady, aching, "vise-like" sensation that encircles the entire head. Chronic tension-type headaches are often accompanied by tight and tender muscles at the site of maximal pain, often in the posterior cervical, frontal, or temporal muscles. Tension headaches are recurrent and are often brought on by stress.

The pathogenesis of tension-type headaches is unclear. It may be related to the release of vasoactive substances that also explain migraine headaches. Often it is very difficult to separate the two syndromes. In this case the diagnosis is chronic daily headache: migraine tension-type headache complex (mixed or combined headache).

14. F. Chronic daily headaches (either tension type or migraine tension type) are usually related to causal factors that include the following: stress and worry, depression, overwork, lack of sleep, incorrect posture, and marital and family dysfunction.

Treatment approaches for the relief of tension-type headaches should center on the following principles:
1. Attempt to identify the causal factor(s).
2. Attempt to modify or eliminate the stressor with behavior modification, biofeedback, relaxation therapy, yoga, and so on.
3. Consider the use of mild analgesics such as acetaminophen, nonsteroidal antiinflammatory agents, aspirin, tricyclic antidepressants, and selective serotonin reuptake inhibitors.
Codeine or other narcotic agents should be avoided.

15. F. The total daily recommended dose of acetaminophen is 4000 mg/day. Even though this is a sporadic event, it would be wise to suggest a decrease to no more than 4 g/day, check her liver function now and (if she continues taking acetaminophen) continue checking it, and discuss the concept of analgesic rebound headaches with her.

16. D. This patient has temporal arteritis (giant cell arteritis) until proven otherwise. When an elderly patient presents with a new-onset headache, temporal arteritis must be excluded. This patient presents with a unilateral headache although a tender temporal area. This probably represents the inflamed temporal artery.

The most significant complication of temporal arteritis is sudden unilateral blindness due to occlusion of the terminal branches of the opthalmic artery. This is a completely preventable complication.

Temporal arteritis is often associated with polymyalgia rheumatica. Hypothyroidism may also be associated with temporal arteritis.

The ESR is a highly sensitive test in a patient you suspect of having temporal arteritis. The ESR is usually elevated above 50 mm/hr and may exceed 100 mm/hr.

The treatment of choice for a patient with temporal arteritis is high-dose prednisone. When cranial arteritis is diagnosed or even suspected, treatment should be started immediately with at least 50 mg of prednisone. If the diagnosis is confirmed, treatment should be continued for at least 4 weeks before any gradual reduction is instituted. If ocular complications have occurred, treatment should continue for 1 to 2 years.

17. E. As headache is such a common disorder, and the excessive application of expensive and highly technical laboratory procedures to the diagnosis and management of benign headache is expensive and epidemiologically unsound, the following principles should apply to the investigation of headache:

1. Patients with migraine headache with or without aura or tension-type headache rarely require more than a careful history and physical examination.
2. Headaches of recent origin or progression deserve investigation. This is especially true of headaches that have a consistently focal distribution, headaches that follow trauma, or headaches that begin after the age of 40 years. CT or MRI scanning is recommended.
3. The EEG is almost never helpful in the diagnosis of primary headache.
4. Skull X-rays are useful only when abnormalities involving the base of the brain are suspected, or immediately following head trauma.
5. Diagnostic lumbar puncture should be performed in any patient with a headache that is accompanied by fever or is explosive in nature. Lumbar puncture, should, if possible, be deferred until after CT scanning in other forms of acute headache, especially if the patient has a stiff neck.
6. CT scanning and MRI scanning are the diagnostic modalities of choice in the evaluation of acute headache in which serious pathology is suspected.

18. B.

19. E. This is an extremely common scenario that is repeated thousands of times daily in ERs across North America. When these patients come through the ER doors we all feel like "heading for the nearest exit."

This patient is an excellent example of the mistakes made in treating this type of headache pattern.

1. These patients should not be started on narcotic analgesics in the first place. Although there is a place in the rare patient for a one- or two-time dose of Demerol, that should be the limit.
2. When a patient with migraine headache tells you that "no abortive or prophylactic agent has ever worked," they are essentially telling you that they do not have a migraine headache. We now realize the importance of the neurotransmitter *serotonin* in the pathogenesis of migraine headache. If none of the abortive prophylactic agents work, then you can draw the reasonable conclusion that the major headache component is not dependent on serotonin. In this patient, there is no doubt that migraine headache was the beginning of the problem, but now rebound analgesic headache with migraine underlay is the most likely diagnosis and the treatment problem to be faced.
3. The treatment of this patient must include both an empathic physician who takes the time to explain what is happening to the patient, and a physician who is prepared to do what needs to be done: gradual reduction (suggested 10%/week) of the total narcotic dosage.
4. It would be very unwise to use large doses of non-narcotic analgesics in this patient. The most common cause of rebound analgesic headaches is, in fact, acetaminophen.

Status migrainosus indicates a prolonged migraine attack usually lasting for more than 72 hours associated with nausea, vomiting, and dehydration. Often, these patients are extremely sick and need to be hospitalized and rehydrated. By the time they arrive in the ER they almost always have already tried large quantities of analgesic medications and/or ergotamine with no benefit.

20. C. This patient has a secondary headache (a headache due to a secondary disease or process). The description is a classic presentation of the headache of cerebral edema. In this case, the cerebral edema is due to metastatic deposits related to the carcinoma of the lung that was previously resected and radiated. The classic symptoms in this case are fairly acute onset, constant headache, pressure-like sensation, and a progressively more severe headache every day.

The treatment of choice for this patient is dexamethasone. The correct starting dose is 4 mg qid with ranitidine or omeprazole to protect the gastric mucosa and prevent peptic or stress ulceration.

21. D.

22. C. This patient has the classic description of a subarachnoid hemorrhage ("headache like I've never had before" and acute onset). This is subarachnoid hemorrhage until proven otherwise.

This patient should have an immediate CT scan or MRI scan, and this should be followed by angiography or special MRI technique imaging to localize the blood vessel. The most common pathogenesis of subarachnoid hemorrhage is rupture of a berry aneurysm in the circle of Willis.

23. B.

SOLUTION TO SHORT ANSWER MANAGEMENT PROBLEM 24

The reclassification of primary headache disorders (according to the International Headache Society) is as follows:

A. Migraine:
   1. Migraine without aura (common migraine)
   2. Migraine with aura (classic migraine)
   3. Complicated migraine (migraine with prominent neurologic symptoms)
   4. Basilar migraine
   5. Hemiplegic migraine
   6. Ophthalmoplegic migraine
B. Cluster headache:
   1. Episodic
   2. Chronic
C. Episodic tension-type headache
D. Chronic daily headache:
   1. Chronic tension-type headache
   2. Migrane tension-type headache complex (mixed or combined headache); usually evolved from migraine
   3. Analgesic/ergotamine rebound headache

Secondary headache is defined as a headache that is due to a disease or condition that is initially unrelated to the headache. The most common cause of secondary headache is probably related to side effects or adverse reactions produced by any number of pharmaceutical products.

SUMMARY OF THE DIAGNOSIS AND TREATMENT OF HEADACHE

This chapter has completely outlined the important points of the diagnosis and treatment of headache; the summary will take the form of a list of do's and don'ts in headache diagnosis and management.

1. Do take a complete history and perform a complete physical (especially neurological) examination.
2. Don't rely on CT scans or MRI scans to make the majority of your headache diagnoses.
3. Do recognize that migraine headache in the same patient may have different presentations on different occasions.
4. Don't label a headache as tension headache unless the criteria for its diagnosis are met.
5. Do attempt to discover the triggers or stresses that bring on both migraine-type headache and tension-type headaches.
6. Do remember that the pathophysiology of migraine is related to serotonin depletion: utilize this powerful knowledge in its sumatriptan (Imitrex) preparation.
7. Do recognize the contraindications to sumatriptan:
   a) Ischemic heart disease/angina pectoris
   b) Previous myocardial infarction
   c) Uncontrolled hypertension
   d) Basilar artery migraine
   e) Hemiplegic migraine
   f) Patients on MAOs, SSRIs, or lithium
8. Don't begin the Demerol/Gravol injection cycle for the treatment of migraine headaches.
9. Do recognize the underdiagnosis of rebound analgesia headache.
10. Do beware of the patient with "migraine headache" for whom no abortive agent and no prophylactic agent works. The probability of that patient having migraine headache as the primary headache diagnosis is very low.

SUGGESTED READING

Mathew N. Headache. In: Rakel R, ed. Conn's current therapy. Philadelphia: WB Saunders, 1994.

PROBLEM 25   A 65-YEAR-OLD MALE WITH A NEW-ONSET SEIZURE

A 65-year-old male is brought to the ER after suffering a seizure while eating a meal in a restaurant. His wife states that he has never had anything like this before. Apparently, the patient developed convulsive jerking in his right arm and leg that lasted approximately 5 minutes. As well, the patient lost consciousness for a short interval.

This patient's past history includes a history of 80 packs/year of cigarette smoking and chronic bronchitis.

On examination, the neurologic examination is completely normal. His blood pressure is 150/100 mm Hg. His pulse is 96 and regular.

SELECT THE ONE BEST ANSWER TO THE FOLLOWING QUESTIONS

1. Regarding problem 1, (the seizure) and problem 2 (chronic bronchitis and the 80 pack/year history of smoking), which of the following statements is true?
   a) there is no association between problem 1 and problem 2
   b) there is a small probability of association between problem 1 and problem 2
   c) there is a moderate probability of association between problem 1 and problem 2
   d) there is a high probability of association between problem 1 and problem 2
   e) there is no way of estimating association between problem 1 and problem 2

2. What is the seizure described in this patient?
   a) a simple partial seizure
   b) a complex partial seizure
   c) an absence seizure
   d) a tonic-clonic (grand mal) seizure
   e) a myoclonic seizure

3. What is the most common cause of a new-onset seizure in a patient of this age?
   a) idiopathic
   b) iatrogenic
   c) head trauma
   d) brain tumor
   e) an old stroke

4. Which of the following medications would not be a drug of first choice for the prevention of further seizures in this patient?
   a) phenytoin
   b) carbamazepine
   c) phenobarbital
   d) valproic acid
   e) ethosuximide

5. Which of the following investigations is the most important investigation in this patient at this time?
   a) an MRI of the brain
   b) an EEG of the brain
   c) angiography of the cerebral vessels
   d) a brain scan
   e) a CT scan of the chest

6. A 22-year-old male is brought to the ER by his wife. While he was raking leaves in the backyard, he suddenly lost consciousness, became rigid, and fell to the ground. His respirations temporarily ceased. This lasted for approximately 45 seconds and was followed by a period of jerking of all four limbs lasting 2 to 3 minutes. The patient then became unconscious for 3 to 4 minutes.

   On examination, the patient is drowsy. There is a large laceration present on his tongue and a small laceration present on his lip. The neurological examination is otherwise normal. The vital signs are normal.

   What is the seizure described in this patient?
   a) simple partial seizure
   b) complex partial seizure
   c) absence seizure
   d) grand-mal (tonic-clonic) seizure
   e) myoclonic seizure

7. Which of the following medications would not be a drug of first choice for the prevention of further seizures in the patient described in Question 6?
   a) phenytoin
   b) carbamazepine
   c) phenobarbital
   d) primidone
   e) ethosuximide

8. A mother presents to your office with her 12-year-old daughter. The mother states that for the past 6 months she (and the girl's teacher) have frequently noted the child staring into space. This lack of concentration usually lasts only 30 to 45 seconds. Sometimes there appears to be brief twitching of all limbs during this time.

   The child's neurological examination is normal.

   What is the most likely cause of this patient's symptoms?
   a) simple partial seizures
   b) complex partial seizures
   c) absence seizures
   d) myoclonic seizures
   e) none of the above

9. All of the following may be useful in the treatment of the patient's condition described in Question 7 except:
   a) valproic acid
   b) clonazepam
   c) ethosuximide
   d) phenytoin
   e) all of the above are useful

10. Which of the following statements regarding beginning and stopping antiepileptic therapy is(are) true?
    a) antiepileptic therapy can safely be discontinued after a seizure-free interval of one year
    b) antiepileptic medication should be started on every patient who has a seizure
    c) antiepileptic medication should be started with a combination of two or more antiepileptic agents
    d) the decision to stop antiepileptic medication should be guided by the results of the EEG
    e) none of the above are true

11. Which of the following investigations is(are) useful in the evaluation of a patient with seizures?
    a) EEG
    b) MRI scan of the brain
    c) CT scan of the brain
    d) Skull X-ray
    e) a, b, and c
    f) all of the above

12. Which of the following statements regarding the diagnosis and treatment of status epilepticus is(are) true?
    a) poor compliance with the anticonvulsant drug regimen is the most common cause of tonic-clonic status epilepticus
    b) the mortality rate of status epilepticus may be as high as 20%
    c) the establishment of an airway is the first priority in the management of status epilepticus

    d) intravenous diazepam is the drug of first choice in the immediate management of status epilepticus
    e) all of the above statements are true

13. Which of the following is(are) causes of nonepileptic seizures?
    a) hypocalcemia
    b) hypomagnesemia
    c) pyridoxine deficiency
    d) thyrotoxic storm
    e) a, b, and c
    f) all of the above

14. Which of the following is most often confused with petit mal seizures (absence seizures) in adults?
    a) benign rolandic epilepsy
    b) complex partial seizures
    c) myoclonic seizures
    d) simple partial seizures
    e) clonic seizures

15. Which of the following is the most common neurologic disorder?
    a) epilepsy
    b) multiple sclerosis
    c) stroke
    d) myasthenia gravis
    e) Bell's palsy

16. Which of the following primary brain tumors is most likely responsible for a new-onset seizure in a 68-year-old male?
    a) meningioma
    b) schwannoma
    c) ependymoma
    d) glioblastoma
    e) pituitary adenoma

Short Answer Management Problem 25

Discuss the pathophysiology and treatment of febrile seizures in children.

ANSWERS

1. D. There is a high probability of association between problem 1 and problem 2. The association is the following:

   Problem 1: In a patient greater than 40 years of age the most common cause of a new-onset seizure is a brain tumor (primary or secondary).

   Problem 2: The history of chronic bronchitis and an 80 pack/year history of cigarette smoking suggests a significant probability of bronchogenic carcinoma.

   Seizure + cigarette smoking = probability of primary bronchogenic CA with secondary metastases to the brain

2. A. The seizure described in this patient is a complex seizure. The symptoms of simple seizures include

focal motor symptoms and somatosensory symptoms that spread or "march" to other parts of the body. Other symptoms include special sensory symptoms that involve visual, auditory, olfactory, or gustatory regions of the brain, and autonomic symptoms or signs. Psychologic symptoms, often accompanied by impaired level of consciousness, can also occur.

The other types of seizures will be considered in other questions in this chapter.

3. D. The most common cause of a new-onset seizure in this patient is a brain tumor. A primary bronchogenic carcinoma with secondary brain metastases would be the most likely cause of a new-onset seizure in a 65-year-old heavy cigarette smoker with COPD. The common causes of new onset seizures by age are as follows:
   a) Less than 10 years:
      i) Idiopathic
      ii) Congenital
      iii) Birth injury
      iv) Metabolic
   b) 10 to 40 years of age:
      i) Idiopathic
      ii) Head trauma
      iii) Preexisting focal brain disease
      iv) Drug withdrawal
   c) Greater than 40 years:
      i) Brain tumor
      ii) Old stroke
      iii) Trauma

4. E. Partial seizures can be treated effectively with phenytoin, carbamazepine, phenobarbital, primidone, and valproic acid. Treatment with one drug is preferable to combination therapy.
   Ethosuximide is not a good choice for the treatment of partial seizures. It is primarily indicated in petit mal (or absence) seizures.

5. A. The most important investigation in this patient at this time is an MRI scan of the brain. An MRI scan of the brain will identify an intracerebral or leptomeningeal mass that may be associated with the new-onset seizure. A CT scan would be a reasonable alternative. An electroencephalogram will identify the type of abnormal discharge and the location of same. It would, however, be a poor second choice.

6. D.

7. E. This patient has had a grand mal (tonic-clonic) seizure. Tonic-clonic seizures are often associated with a sudden loss of consciousness. The tonic phase is followed by a clonic phase characterized by generalized body musculature jerking. Following this is a stage of flaccid coma.
   Associated manifestations include tongue or lip biting, urinary or fecal incontinence, and other injuries.
   An aura may precede a generalized seizure.
   As in partial (focal) seizures, the drugs of choice are phenytoin, carbamazepine, phenobarbital, primidone, and valproic acid. Ethosuximide is not an effective drug in the treatment of grand mal seizures.

8. C.

9. D. This patient presents with typical absence (petit mal) seizures. Petit mal seizures may present with impairment of consciousness, sometimes accompanied by mild clonic, tonic, atonic, or autonomic symptoms. These seizures, often very brief in duration, interrupt the current activity and are characterized by a description of the patient "staring into space."
   Petit mal seizures that begin in childhood are terminated by the beginning of the third decade of life.
   A bilaterally synchronous and symmetric 3-Hz "spike-and-wave" pattern is seen.
   Petit mal seizures can be effectively treated with ethosuximide, valproic acid, or clonazepam. Phenytoin is not an effective treatment for petit mal seizures.

10. D. The criteria for decision to treat or not to treat an initial seizure should include details of the seizure; adequate laboratory data including measurement of glucose, electrolytes, alcohol, and other toxins; and the presence of EEG evidence of epileptic activity at least 2 weeks after the seizure. Careful reevaluation and monitoring are essential.
    A consideration of discontinuation of medication can be made after a seizure-free period of 4 years. This decision should be confirmed by a lack of seizure activity on EEG.

11. E. Laboratory investigations for a patient with an initial seizure should include a complete blood count, blood glucose determination, liver and renal function tests, and a serological test for syphilis.
    Initial and periodic electroencephalography is mandatory. CT scanning or MRI scanning should be performed in patients with focal neurological symptoms and/or signs, focal seizures, or EEG findings indicating a focal disturbance.
    A chest X-ray should be performed in all patients who are cigarette smokers; a primary lung neoplasm with secondary brain metastases producing cerebral edema and seizures is not uncommon.
    A plain X-ray of the skull or a skull series is unlikely to produce any useful diagnostic information.

12. E. Status epilepticus is a medical emergency, with a mortality rate of up to 20% and a high incidence of neurologic and mental sequelae in survivors.

Status epilepticus may be caused by poor compliance with medication, alcohol withdrawal, intracranial infection, neoplasm, a metabolic disorder, or a drug overdose. Prognosis depends on the length of time from the onset of the seizure activity to effective treatment.

The management of status epilepticus includes establishing an airway, giving 50% dextrose in case of hypoglycemia, giving IV diazepam, giving IV phenytoin, and treating resistant cases with IV phenobarbital.

13. F. There are many causes of nonepileptic seizures. These are divided into the following categories:
   A. Cardiogenic:
      1. Simple syncope
      2. Transient ischemic attacks
      3. Arrhythmias
      4. Sick sinus syndrome
   B. Electrolyte imbalance:
      1. Hypocalcemia
      2. Hyponatremia and water intoxication
      3. Hypomagnesemia
   C. Metabolic:
      1. Hypoglycemia
      2. Hyperglycemia
      3. Thyrotoxic storm
      4. Pyridoxine deficiency
   D. Acute drug withdrawal:
      1. Alcohol
      2. Benzodiazepines
      3. Cocaine
      4. Barbiturates
      5. Meperidine
   E. Drug intoxication:
      1. Cocaine
      2. Dextroamphetamine
      3. Theophylline
      4. Isoniazid
      5. Lithium
      6. Nitrous oxide anesthesia
      7. Acetylcholinesterase inhibitors
   F. Metals:
      1. Mercury
      2. Lead
   G. Infections:
      1. Gram-negative septicemia with shock
      2. Viral meningitis
      3. Bacterial meningitis (gram-negative or syphilitic)
   H. Hyperthermia
   I. Pseudoseizures (psychogenic)
   J. Malignancies
   K. Idiopathic (isolated unprovoked seizure)

14. B. Absence (petit mal) seizures are often confused with CPS (complex partial seizures) in adolescents and adults. An accurate diagnosis can often be made on the basis of history, the duration of the seizure, the presence of an aura and/or postictal confusion, the pattern of autonomic behavior, and the EEG.

In absence seizures, minor clonic activity (eye blinks or head nodding) is present in up to 45% of cases; the mean duration is seconds; and the EEG shows the typical bilateral symmetrical 3 cycle second spike and wave that may be easily provided by hyperventilation. There is no aura or posticital confusion.

In contrast, complex partial seizures may be preceded by an aura, are followed by postical confusion, last longer (1 to 3 minutes), and are associated with more complex automatisms and less frequent clonic components. The EEG tends to show focal slow or sharp and slow wave activity. The differentiation between these two types of seizures is important. Absence seizures tend to disappear in adulthood, but CPS seizures do not. Furthermore, phenytoin (Dilantin) and carbamazepine (Tegretol) are effective in treating complex partial seizures but not absence attacks.

15. C. The most common neurologic disorder is stroke. Epilepsy is the second most common disorder, with the prevalence ranging anywhere between 0.6% and 3.4% in the general population.

16. D. The most common primary brain tumor in elderly patients is a glioma. Of the gliomas, the glioblastomas and the astrocytomas are by far the most common.

SOLUTION TO SHORT ANSWER MANAGEMENT PROBLEM 25

Febrile seizures in children:
1. Age of risk: age 6 months to age 5 years
2. Risk factors for febrile convulsions:
   A. Previous febrile convulsion: the risk of a subsequent febrile convulsion is 30% when the first seizure occurred between the ages of 1 and 3 years; 50% when it occurred first at other ages; and 50% after a second febrile seizure.
   B. Family history of febrile convulsion (25%)
3. Prognosis: The prognosis for normal school progress and for seizure remission is excellent in children with febrile seizures.
4. Chances of progression of febrile seizures to epilepsy:
   A. Very small: 98% of children with febrile seizures will have no further seizures after 5 years of age.
5. Factors that increase the chance of progression of febrile seizures to epilepsy:
   A. Presence of developmental delay
   B. Cerebral palsy
   C. Abnormal neurologic development
   D. History of epilepsy in a parent or sibling
   E. A seizure that has a focal onset, lasts more than 15 minutes, or recurs in the same febrile illness.

6. Treatment: prophylactic anticonvulsants
   A. Usually not indicated. If you do use prophylactic anticonvulsants it will only be to treat the febrile seizure, not to prevent later epilepsy.
   B. Drug of choice when indicated: rectal or oral diazepam—5 mg every 8 hours when the rectal temperature is raised to greater than 38.5° C. The use of rectal diazepam at home to stop a febrile seizure not only increases the chance of preventing a prolonged febrile seizure but also gives the parent a sense of control over the situation.

SUMMARY OF THE DIAGNOSIS AND TREATMENT OF SEIZURES

1. **Absolute rules concerning seizures:**
   Not all that seizes is epilepsy.
   Not all epilepsy seizes.
   Many "seizures" are associated with other systemic disorders.
2. **Major classification causes of nonepileptic seizures:**
   a) Metastases to the brain
   b) Cardiogenic
   c) Electrolyte imbalance
   d) Metabolic causes
   e) Acute drug withdrawal
   f) Drug intoxication
   g) Heavy metal poisoning
   h) Infections
   i) Hyperthermia
   j) Pseudoseizures
3. **Greatly simplified classification of epileptic seizures:**
   a) Partial seizures:
      1. Simple partial seizures
      2. Complex partial seizures
   b) Generalized seizures:
      1. Petit mal (absence seizures)
      2. Tonic-clonic (grand mal) seizures
      3. Myoclonic seizures
      4. Tonic, clonic, or atonic seizures

4. **Diagnosis and investigations:**
   a) history (from a relative or bystander)
   b) Physical examination
   c) EEG
   d) CT and/or MRI
   e) Blood profile including CBC, blood glucose, liver function tests, renal function tests, HIV serology (in high-risk groups), serum calcium, serologic test for syphilis.
5. **Treatment:**
   a) Carefully evaluate whether or not the patient needs treatment after the first seizure.
   b) Drugs for generalized tonic-clonic (grand-mal) seizures or partial seizures include the following:
      1. Phenytoin (drug of choice)
      2. Carbamazepine
      3. Phenobarbital
      4. Primidone
      5. Valproic acid
   c) Once antiepileptic drug therapy is initiated, it should be maintained for a time period measured in years, not months. Patients must be carefully considered for discontinuation of therapy
   d) Febrile seizures: rectal suppository of diazepam 5 mg or oral diazepam every 8 hours is treatment of choice for prevention of subsequent seizures, if that has been carefully evaluated.
   e) Status epilepticus: treatment is 50 mg dextrose, IV diazepam, IV phenytoin, and IV phenobarbital

SUGGESTED READINGS

Farrell KF, Connolly MB. Epilepsy in infants and children. In: Rakel R, ed. Conn's current therapy. Philadelphia: WB Saunders, 1994.

Uthman BM, Wilder BJ. Epilepsy in adolescents and adults. In: Rakel R, ed. Conn's current therapy. Philadelphia: WB Saunders, 1994.

PROBLEM 26   A 67-YEAR-OLD MALE WITH A SUDDEN-ONSET LEFT-SIDED HEMIPLEGIA, DYSPHAGIA, AND A "VISUAL PROBLEM"

A 67-year-old male is brought to the ER by ambulance following the gradual onset of the following: inability to move his right leg, followed by his right arm; speech impairment; and a "visual problem."

On examination, the patient has a flaccid paralysis of the muscles of the right leg and the muscles (excluding the deltoid) of the right arm, a homonymous hemianopia, and dysphagia. In addition, he "does not recognize" that he is paralyzed, nor can he turn his eyes toward the right side. His deep tendon reflexes are hyperflexic on the right side. His right great toe is up-going.

It is now 6 hours since the symptoms began. It appears from talking to his wife that they are "still changing."

SELECT THE ONE BEST ANSWER TO THE FOLLOWING QUESTIONS

1. What is the most likely diagnosis at this time?
   a) transient ischemic attack
   b) completed stroke
   c) stroke-in-evolution
   d) subarachnoid hemorrhage
   e) complicated migraine

2. The location of symptoms correlates the site of the lesion to which of the following?
   a) left middle cerebral artery
   b) right middle cerebral artery
   c) left anterior cerebral artery
   d) right anterior cerebral artery
   e) left posterior cerebral artery

3. What is the most likely pathophysiologic process involved at this time?
   a) a thrombotic stroke
   b) an embolic stroke
   c) a hemorrhagic stroke
   d) a lacunar stroke
   e) a subarachnoid hemorrhage

4. What is the most common pathophysiologic process in patients who have suffered a cerebrovascular accident (CVA)?
   a) a thrombotic stroke
   b) an embolic stroke
   c) a hemorrhagic stroke
   d) a lacunar stroke
   e) a subarachnoid hemorrhage

5. In which of the following conditions would you most likely find an embolic phenomena as the pathophysiology of a CVA?
   a) hypertension
   b) atrial fibrillation
   c) ventricular fibrillation
   d) a young woman on the oral contraceptive pill
   e) b and d

6. What is the number one risk factor for cerebrovascular accidents?
   a) cigarette smoking
   b) hypertension
   c) hypercholesterolemia
   d) hypertriglyceridemia
   e) hypothyroidism

7. Lacunar strokes (lacunar infarcts) are most closely associated with which of the following?
   a) thrombosis
   b) embolization
   c) hypertension
   d) subarachnoid bleeding
   e) cerebral infarction

8. A 47-year-old patient develops the following symptoms and signs: impaired mental status, including confusion, amnesia, perseveration, and personality changes; footdrop; apraxia on the affected side; left-sided hemiplegia; left-sided numbness (both muscle power and sensation retained to some degree in left upper extremity). This patient most likely has had a cerebrovascular accident affecting which of the following arteries?
   a) right middle cerebral artery
   b) posterior cerebral artery
   c) vertebral-basilar artery
   d) right anterior cerebral artery
   e) posterior/inferior cerebellar artery

9. A 77-year-old female presents to the ER with the following signs/symptoms: dysarthria and dysphagia, vertigo, nausea, and syncope, memory loss and disorientation, and ataxic gait.

   On P/E, the patient has nystagmus, homonymous hemianopia, numbness in the area of the XIIth cranial nerve, and facial weakness. You suspect a cerebrovascular accident. Which of the following arteries is most likely to be involved?
   a) middle cerebral artery
   b) posterior cerebral artery
   c) vertebral-basilar artery

d) anterior cerebral artery

e) posterior inferior cerebellar artery

10. A 67-year-old female presents to the ER with the following signs/symptoms: lack of depth perception, perseveration, failure to see objects not centered in the field of vision, dyslexia, intentional tremor, and diffuse "numbness."

    On examination, the patient has homonymous hemianopia, cortical blindness, loss of muscle movement innervated by the oculomotor—third cranial nerve.

    You suspect a cerebrovascular accident. With the information available, which of the following arteries is most likely to be involved?

    a) middle cerebral artery

    b) posterior cerebral artery

    c) vertebral-basilar artery

    d) anterior cerebral artery

    e) posterior inferior cerebellar artery

11. An 80-year-old female presents to the ER with the following signs/symptoms: dysarthria, dysphagia, and dysphonia; vertigo, nystagmus, and unsteady gait; left pupil constriction/left eyelid drooping/left sided lack of perspiration; "ringing in the ears"; hiccoughs and vomiting; no sense of pain and temperature on the right side; and no sense of pain and temperature on the left side of the face.

    You are certain that this is a cerebrovascular accident. Which of the following arteries is most likely involved?

    a) middle cerebral artery

    b) posterior cerebral artery

    c) vertebral-basilar artery

    d) anterior cerebral artery

    e) posterior inferior cerebellar artery

12. The patient described in Question 11 has which of the following syndromes?

    a) subclavian steal syndrome

    b) Horner's syndrome

    c) Wallenberg's syndrome

    d) a and b

    e) b and c

13. A transient ischemic attack is most closely associated with which of the following?

    a) amaurosis fugax

    b) subarachnoid hemorrhage

    c) lacunar hemorrhage

    d) intracranial aneurysm

    e) fusiform aneurysm

14. A ruptured berry aneurysm is usually located in which of the following?

a) anterior cerebral artery distribution

b) posterior cerebral artery distribution

c) circle of Willis

d) middle cerebral artery distribution

e) none of the above

15. A patient is suspected of having a thrombotic stroke. If you had the opportunity of ordering only one investigation, what investigation would that be?

    a) a regular angiogram of the cerebral circulation

    b) a CT scan of the brain

    c) an MRI angiogram of the brain

    d) a digital subtraction angiogram of the brain

    e) an immediate lumbar puncture

16. Considering the pathophysiology of stroke, which of the following substances makes the most therapeutic sense in terms of inclusion in a treatment protocol?

    a) labetalol IV

    b) dextromethorphan IV

    c) diazoxide IV

    d) dexamethasone orally

    e) prednisone orally

17. Which of the following is not a risk factor for the development of a cerebrovascular accident?

    a) diabetes mellitus type I

    b) diabetes mellitus type II

    c) black race

    d) cigarette smoking

    e) diabetes insipidus

18. The incidence of stroke in the United States over the last 15 years has

    a) increased significantly

    b) increased slightly

    c) decreased significantly

    d) decreased slightly

    e) nobody really knows for sure

19. A 29-year-old male presents to your office and gives the following description: "Like, Doc, something really weird happened—man, I tell you: the lights went out—completely, Doc—no jive, total blackout." You are somewhat unsure what "lights" he is talking about. You briefly consider referring him to an electrician.

    You ask him to describe everything; the following highlights are revealed: Family history: early cardiovascular death, both sides of the family; father: dead at age 28, MI; mother: dead at age 31, stroke. Description of "lights out": "like a curtain coming down in front of my eyes." Complicating factors: he was using cocaine at the time.

    If you could order only one test, which would you choose?

a) ultrasound of the carotid arteries
b) CT scan of the brain
c) MRI scan of the brain
d) fluorescein angiography of the fundi
e) lumbar puncture

20. Which of the following statements regarding carotid endarterectomy is(are) true?
   a) carotid endarterectomy is indicated in the presence of a completed stroke
   b) carotid endarterectomy is indicated in the presence of a complete arterial occlusion
   c) randomized, controlled trials have established the benefit of carotid endarterectomy over standard medical therapy for the treatment of carotid artery stenosis
   d) carotid endarterectomy has been established as the treatment of choice in patients with a documented TIA and a tightly stenotic lesion (>70% stenosis)
   e) nobody really knows for sure

Short Answer Management Problem 26

Define the following terms:
   1. Transient ischemic attack
   2. Stroke-in-evolution
   3. Completed stroke

ANSWERS

1. C. At this time, the most likely diagnosis is stroke-in-evolution. The typical development of thrombotic stroke causes a clinical syndrome known as stroke-in-evolution. An intermittent or slow progression over hours to days is characteristic of stroke-in-evolution or slow hemorrhage.

2. A. The symptoms that this patient is currently experiencing suggest a lesion of the left middle cerebral artery. The signs/symptoms of middle cerebral artery occlusion are as follows:
   Dysphagia (left hemisphere involvement), dyslexia, dysgraphia
   Contralateral hemiparesis or hemiplegia
   Contralateral hemisensory disturbances
   Rapid deterioration in consciousness from confusion to coma
   Vomiting
   Homonymous hemianopia
   Denial of or lack of recognition of a paralyzed extremity
   Inability to turn the eyes toward the affected side

3. A. Because of the slow and continuing progression of the CNS symptomatology, this is much more characteristic of a thrombotic stroke rather than an embolic stroke.

4. A. The pathophysiology of stroke in order of frequency is as follows:
   Most common: thrombotic stroke

   Second most common: embolic stroke
   Third most common: hemorrhagic stroke
   Fourth most common: lacunar stroke (lacunar infarct)
   Fifth most common: subarachnoid hemorrhage

5. B. An *embolic stroke* involves fragments that break from a thrombus formed outside the brain in the heart, aorta, common carotid, or thorax. Emboli infrequently arise from the ascending aorta or the common carotid artery. The embolus usually involves small vessels and obstructs at a bifurcation or other point of narrowing, thus enabling ischemia to develop and extend. An embolus may completely occlude the lumen of the vessel, or it may remain in place or break into fragments and move up the vessel.

   Conditions associated with the onset of an embolic stroke include the following:
   1. Atrial fibrillation
   2. Myocardial infarction
   3. Endocarditis
   4. Rheumatic heart disease
   5. Valvular prostheses
   6. Atrial septal defect
   7. Disorders of the aorta
   8. Disorders of the carotids
   9. Disorders of the vertebral-basilar system
   10. Other embolic phenomena: air, fat, and tumor

6. B. Cerebrovascular accidents or strokes remain the third-leading cause of death in North America. The single most important risk factor for stroke is hypertension. The decrease in the incidence of stroke is largely due to

the successful, aggressive, and ideal treatment of hypertension in North America.

Other factors that are important in the etiology of stroke include the following:

Age (the older the patient, the greater the risk)

Other heart disease (valvular, conductive, infective, atherosclerotic)

Cigarette smoking

Diabetes mellitus (type I and type II)

The oral contraceptive pill when combined with smoking and older age

Race: African-Americans are more prone than white Americans

Family history (of lipid disorders or cardiovascular diseases in general)

Sex: strokes are more common in females than in males

7. C. Lacunar strokes (lacunar infarcts) are infarcts smaller than 1 cc in size and involve the small perforating arteries predominately in the basal ganglia, internal capsule, and the brainstem. Lacunar infarcts are primarily associated with hypertension. Because of the subcortical location and small area of infarction, these strokes may have pure motor and sensory deficits.

8. D. This patient most likely has a lesion in the territory of the right anterior cerebral artery. Signs and symptoms of a cerebrovascular accident in the territory of the anterior cerebral artery are as follows:
   1. Mental status impairments
      a) Confusion
      b) Amnesia
      c) Perseveration
      d) Personality changes: flat affect, apathy
      e) Cognitive changes:
         i) Short attention span
         ii) Slowness
      f) Deterioration of intellectual function
   2. Urinary continence (long duration)
   3. Contralateral hemiparesis or hemiplegia
   4. Sensory impairments (contralateral)
   5. Foot and leg deficits (more frequent than arm deficits)
   6. Footdrop
   7. Apraxia on affected side
   8. Expressive aphasia (for left hemisphere only)
   9. Deviation of the eyes and head toward the affected side
   10. Abulia (inability to make decisions or perform voluntary acts)
   11. Gait dysfunction

9. C. This patient has had a cerebrovascular accident involving the vertebral-basilar system. The signs/symptoms of vertebral-basilar stroke are as follows:
   1. Dysarthria, dysphagia

   2. Vertigo, nausea, and syncope
   3. Memory loss, disorientation
   4. Ataxic gait
   5. Visual symptoms: double vision, homonymous hemianopia
   6. Tinnitus, hearing loss
   7. Ocular signs: nystagmus, conjugate gaze paralysis, ophthalmoplegia
   8. Akinetic mutism (locked-in syndrome when basilar artery occlusion occurs)
   9. Numbness of the tongue
   10. Facial weakness, alternating motor paresis
   11. Drop attacks

10. B. This patient has had a cerebrovascular accident of the posterior cerebral artery. The signs/symptoms of a CVA of the PCA are as follows:
    I. Peripheral signs:
       A. Visual disturbances
          i) Homonymous hemianopia
          ii) Cortical blindness
          iii) Lack of depth perception
          iv) Failure to see objects not centered in the field of vision
          v) Visual hallucinations
       B. Memory deficits
       C. Perseveration
       D. Dyslexia
    II. Central signs:
       A. Thalamic or subthalamic nuclei involvement: diffuse sensory loss, mild hemiparesis, intentional tremor
       B. Cerebral peduncle involvement: contralateral hemiplegia, oculomotor nerve deficits
       C. Brainstem involvement: pupillary dysfunction, nystagmus, loss of conjugate gaze

11. E.

12. E. This patient has had a CVA involving the posterior inferior cerebellar artery, of which one subtype is known as *Wallenberg syndrome*. The signs/symptoms of a CVA of the posterior/inferior cerebellar artery as follows:
    1. Dysarthria, dysphagia, dysphonia
    2. Vertigo, nystagmus, unsteady gait
    3. Ipsilateral Horner's syndrome
    4. Sensory changes: ipsilateral face and contralateral body

    The true Wallenberg syndrome consists of the following:
    1. Vertigo, horizontal nystagmus, ataxia
    2. Nausea and vomiting
    3. Dysphagia
    4. Horner's syndrome (ipsilateral)
    5. Pain and temperature loss on trunk and limbs (contralateral)

6. Balance loss on affected side
7. Pain and temperature loss on face (ipsilateral)

Because the Wallenberg syndrome has, as a component, Horner's syndrome, the answer to Question 12 is E.

13. A. A transient ischemic attack probably represents thrombotic particles causing an intermittent blockage of circulation or spasm. *Amaurosis fugax*, which is described by patients as "a curtain coming down in front of my eyes—a blackout," is really a TIA of the ophthalmic artery.

14. C. Intracranial aneurysms may result from arteriosclerosis, congenital abnormality, trauma, inflammation, infection. Cocaine has recently been linked to aneurysm formation. The size may vary from 2 mm to 2 or 3 cm. Most aneurysms are located at bifurcations in or near the circle of Willis in the vertebrobasilar artery system. Aneurysm may be single, but in 20% to 25% of cases, more than one aneurysm is present. The peak incidence occurs between age 35 and age 60. Berry aneurysms are also known as saccular aneurysms.

15. C (acceptable alternative answer: B).

The diagnostic test of choice for a thrombotic stroke (if the technology is available) is an MRI angiogram, which will indicate the exact location of the thrombus, the size of the thrombus, the area of infarction or hemorrhage, while differentiating between the two, and the area of ischemia surrounding the area of infarction or hemorrhage.

If this technology is not available, a CT scan of the brain is the next-best alternative.

16. A. Labetalol, an alpha-beta blocker, is the drug of choice for the treatment of hypertensive urgencies and hypertensive emergencies. One of the most important ways to limit the damage (in a stroke-in-evolution) is to reduce the blood pressure to a point where its elevation no longer does any damage, but not to a point where cerebral perfusion is adversely affected. This follows a J-curve phenomenon.

17. E. The risk factors for cerebrovascular accidents include the following:
1. Hypertension (single most important risk factor)
2. Hypercholesterolemia
3. Hypertriglyceridemia (because it has been found to be an independent risk factor for vascular disease)
4. African-American race: probably due to increased risk of hypertension
5. Obesity: also related to increased risk of hypertension
6. Sedentary life style (related to 5)
7. Cigarette smoking

8. A woman in her final reproductive years (37-45) who is a heavy cigarette smoker and who for some reason is on the oral contraceptive pill
9. Family history of cerebrovascular accidents
10. Family history of hyperlipidemia
11. Age: > 65 years
12. Female > male
13. Diabetes mellitus type I
14. Diabetes mellitus type II
15. Hypothyroidism (related to hyperlipidemia)

Diabetes insipidus has nothing to do with CVA (with the possible exception of Sheenan's syndrome—postpartum pituitary necrosis).

18. C. Estimates vary widely. However, the incidence of stroke in the United States has declined dramatically in the last 15 years due to the relative success of the "Treatment of Hypertension" campaign.

19. A. This patient has had a transient ischemic attack. With this patient's terrible family history, his classic description of amaurosis fugax, and his cocaine use (obviously causing intense vasospasm)* there is little wonder that "the lights went out." One may speculate that the lights never were on in the first place.

Therefore the answer is A. This patient needs an ultrasound of his carotid arteries and he needs it soon.

20. D. There is still a great deal of debate about carotid endarterectomy (when to do/when not to do). One definite indication is as follows: a documented TIA plus a highly stenotic lesion (>70%) = carotid endarterectomy.

SOLUTION TO SHORT ANSWER MANAGEMENT PROBLEM 26

Definitions:
1. *Transient ischemic attack:* A disturbance of cerebrovascular system in which neurologic symptoms both appear and then disappear within 24 hours. At time = 24 hours, there are no neurologic symptoms remaining.
2. *Stroke-in-evolution:* The typical course of a thrombotic stroke. This is also known as a *progressive stroke.* It is best defined as an intermittent progression of a neurologic deficit over hours to days.
3. *Completed stroke:* A cerebrovascular accident that has reached its maximum destructiveness in producing neurologic deficits, although cerebral edema may not have reached its maximum.

SUMMARY OF THE DIAGNOSIS AND TREATMENT OF CEREBROVASCULAR ACCIDENTS

1. **Incidence:** very significant decrease over last 15 years; Reason (probable): hypertension control

*Cocaine is an intensely powerful vasoconstrictor, much more powerful than either angiotensin II or thrombohoxane (a prostoglandin).

2. **Pathologic classification** (in order of frequency):
   a) Thrombotic stroke
   b) Embolic stroke
   c) Hemorrhagic stroke
   d) Lacunar stroke
   e) Subarachnoid hemorrhage
3. **Risk factors for CVA:**
   a) Hypertension is the single most important risk factor.
   b) There is no such entity as mild hypertension any longer.
      See also the answer to Question 17.
4. **Classification of CVAs:** See Short Answer Management Problem.
   a) Transient ischemic attack
   b) Stroke-in-evolution
   c) Completed stroke
      Don't just forget about a TIA if it is over; do something! Especially carotid ultrasound: indication for endarterectomy:
   a) At least one TIA
   b) At least 70% stenosis
5. **Signs/symptoms:** see details on every artery in earlier question
6. **Investigations/treatment:**
   a) History
   b) Physical exam
   c) MRI angio or CT stat!
   d) If not hemorrhagic and if not a completed stroke, consider heparin followed by warfarin. If it is already complete, do not follow this approach.
   e) Cerebral edema may become a major problem. Be very careful with the use of IV mannitol, but when you have demonstrated edema, treat it with IV mannitol.
   f) Unless contraindicated, all patients with TIAs, history of stroke, and risk factors for stroke (major) should be on aspirin prophylaxis.
   g) Rehabilitation: aggressive, early, and forceful
7. **Concomitant conditions:** depression is the single most important coexisting or concomitant condition. Remember also that this applies to both the patient and the patient's caregiver (see the next item).
8. **The biopsychosocial model of illness:** Few diseases are as devastating to a patient and a patient's family as stroke. Often the person that really gets lost in this whole ordeal is the spouse. Please remember the spouse.
9. **Prevention:**
   a) Treat hypertension aggressively
   b) Treat obesity and sedentary lifestyle aggressively
   c) Stop smoking
   d) Remember, an aspirin a day keeps the neurologist away.

SUGGESTED READINGS

Boss BJ, Sunderland PM, Heath J. Alterations of neurologic function. In: McCance KL, Huether SE, eds. Pathophysiology: The biologic basis for disease in adults and children. 2nd Ed. St. Louis: Mosby Year Book, 1994.

Kneisl CR, Ames SA. Adult health nursing: A biopsychosocial approach to illness. Reading, MA: Addison-Wesley, 1986.

PROBLEM 27   A 35-YEAR-OLD FEMALE WITH FATIGUE

A 35-year-old female presents with a 4-month history of fatigue. Her history is unremarkable; she has had no major medical illnesses. She has noticed that during the past 12 months her menstrual periods have become heavier and longer; instead of lasting for only 4 days with bleeding that was "light to moderate," she now has a 7 to 9 day period with "very heavy flow." She is the mother of three healthy children.

On examination, the patient appears pale. Her lower eyelids are pale and so is her skin. Her blood pressure is 100/70 mm Hg.

Her blood smear reads as follows: RBCs are microcytic and appear to be hypochromic. Her platelet count is 175,000. Her hemoglobin is 9.5 grams/dl.

SELECT THE ONE BEST ANSWER TO THE FOLLOWING QUESTIONS

1. What is the most likely cause of this patient's anemia?
   a) iron deficiency anemia
   b) hemolytic anemia
   c) folic acid deficiency anemia
   d) pernicious anemia
   e) anemia of chronic disease

2. What is(are) the treatment(s) of choice to prevent this condition in this patient?
   a) naproxen 375 mg bid (or a similar NSAID) during the last 2 weeks of the menstrual cycle
   b) a low-dose OCP given either continuously or in a cyclical manner
   c) ferrous sulfate 300 mg od to 300 mg tid
   d) a or b
   e) any of the above
   f) none of the above

3. What is(are) the acute treatment(s) of choice to improve this patient's symptoms?
   a) naproxen 375 mg bid (or a similar NSAID) during the last 2 weeks of the menstrual cycle
   b) a low-dose OCP given either continuously or in a cyclical manner
   c) ferrous sulfate 300 mg od to 300 mg tid
   d) a or b
   e) any of the above
   f) none of the above

4. In a patient who presents with *very severe menorrhagia* (menorrhagia that has the capacity to produce a hypovolemic shock-like state), what is the recommended first-line treatment?
   a) IM medroxyprogesterone acetate
   b) IV premarin
   c) cryoprecipitate
   d) fresh frozen plasma
   e) high-dose OCPs given every hour

5. Which of the following disorders is(are) possible secondary causes of the disorder just described?
   a) uterine fibroids
   b) endometriosis

   c) von Willebrand's disease
   d) intrinsic factor deficiency
   e) a, b, or c
   f) any of the above

6. Which of the following investigations should be performed in this patient to rule out a secondary cause?
   a) pelvic ultrasound plus/minus pelvic laparoscopy
   b) coagulation profile
   c) CT scan of the abdomen/pelvis
   d) a and b
   e) all of the above
   f) none of the above

7. What is the most sensitive test for the detection of the disorder described?
   a) serum iron
   b) serum iron binding capacity
   c) serum ferritin
   d) serum transferrin
   e) reticulocyte count

8. A pregnant woman at 22 weeks' gestation presents for her regular checkup. Her hemoglobin level is 10.8 g/dl. Which of the following statements regarding this patient's hemoglobin is(are) true?
   a) this patient has, by definition, an iron-deficient anemia
   b) the reason for this hemoglobin level in this trimester is the relative expansion of the plasma volume relative to the red blood cell mass
   c) this patient should be treated with ferrous sulfate on a once or twice daily basis
   d) all of the above
   e) none of the above

9. A 55-year-old male presents for a periodic health assessment. His only complaint is that he has been feeling quite fatigued during the last 3 months.

   On P/E, the patient appears pale. His blood pressure is 100/80 mm Hg. His pulse is 96 and regular. No other abnormalities are found.

   A CBC reveals a hemoglobin of 10.0 grams/dl. His blood smear also shows a decreased MCHC and a decreased MCV.

Until proven otherwise, what is the most likely cause of this blood pressure?
a) lymphoma
b) gastrointestinal malignancy
c) lack of intrinsic factor
d) dietary deficiency of folic acid
e) dietary lack of iron

10. A 78-year-old female presents to your office complaining of a "lack of energy" that began 8 months ago.

    On examination, the patient has marked pallor. Her hemoglobin level is 7.5 grams/dl at this time. A peripheral blood smear reveals hypochromasia and microcytosis. One year ago her hemoglobin was 13.0 grams/dl.

    What is the most likely cause of this patient's anemia?
    a) malnutrition
    b) pernicious anemia
    c) folic acid deficiency
    d) gastrointestinal bleeding
    e) hypothyroidism

11. The anemia of chronic disease is most often which of the following?
    a) hypochromic and normocytic
    b) hypochromic and microcytic
    c) normochromic and macrocytic
    d) normochromic and normocytic
    e) hyperchromic and macrocytic

12. What is the most common cause of anemia of chronic disease?
    a) chronic hepatic failure
    b) chronic renal failure
    c) congestive cardiac failure
    d) autoimmune disease
    e) chronic neurologic disease

13. Which of the following disorders is(are) associated with the anemia of chronic disease?
    a) rheumatoid arthritis
    b) non-Hodgkin's lymphoma
    c) chronic renal failure
    d) chronic hepatic failure
    e) all of the above

14. Which of the following is the most common type of anemia in the North American population?
    a) anemia of chronic disease
    b) iron deficiency anemia
    c) macrocytic anemia
    d) autoimmune hemolytic anemia
    e) iatrogenic anemia

15. A 75-year-old female presents to your office with a 4-month history of fatigue, paresthesias, weakness, and an unsteady gait. These are new symptoms.

On examination, her skin is pale, as are her lower conjunctival lids. She has a number of interesting neurological findings on physical examination, including patchy impairment of the sensations of touch and temperature, loss of both vibration and position sense, a positive Romberg sign, hyperreflexia, and bilateral upgoing Babinski signs. Her hemoglobin is 6.8 grams/dl.

Which of the following statements regarding this patient's condition is(are) true?
a) this patient has a hemolytic anemia
b) a CT scan of the brain should be performed
c) hyposegmented neutrophils will be seen on the blood smear
d) the MCV value will be $> 100 \ \mu m^3$
e) all of the above

16. If you could choose only one next investigation, what would it be in this patient?
    a) reticulocyte count
    b) serum folate
    c) serum vitamin B_{12} level
    d) gastroscopy
    e) bone marrow biopsy

17. The one next investigation confirms your suspicions. You now need to confirm the presence or absence of which of the following?
    a) megakaryocytes in the bone marrow
    b) hypersegmented neutrophils on the blood smear
    c) intrinsic factor produced by the gastric parietal cells
    d) extrinsic factor produced by the gastric secretin cells
    e) folic acid synthesis precursors

18. During the first 2 weeks of therapy for the condition described in Question 15, which of the following is the most reasonable treatment regime?
    a) folic acid 5 mg/day orally
    b) vitamin B_{12} 100 μg/day orally
    c) vitamin B_{12} 1000 μg BOD (every other day) subcutaneous
    d) ferrous sulfate 300 mg/day + folic acid 5 mg/day + Vitamin B_{12} 100 mg/day (all orally)
    e) none of the above

19. The condition described above, when diagnosed by bone marrow biopsy, will most likely show which of the following?
    a) neutropenia
    b) thrombocytopenia
    c) anemia
    d) pancytopenia
    e) leukopenia plus anemia

20. Which of the following statements regarding folic acid deficiency is(are) false?
    a) folic acid deficiency demonstrates a macrocytic anemia

b) hypersegmented neutrophils are often seen on the peripheral blood smear
c) the most common cause of folic acid deficiency is an inadequate dietary intake of folic acid

d) folic acid deficiency is uncommon in patients who demonstrate alcohol abuse
e) reduced folate levels are usually seen in red blood cells and in the serum

Short Answer Management Problem 27

Distinguish between the terms *macrocytosis* and *megaloblastosis*.

ANSWERS

1. A.

2. D.

3. C.

4. B.

5. E.

6. D.

7. C. This patient has an iron deficiency anemia. This is the most common cause of anemia. In this patient, the most likely cause of the anemia is excessive blood during her menstrual periods.

Pernicious anemia, folic acid deficiency, hemolytic anemia, and hypothyroidism are all associated with anemia; however, they are not associated with hypochromic, microcytic changes that are characteristic of iron deficiency anemia only.

It is very important to rule out secondary causes of this iron deficiency anemia, especially because this patient's menstrual periods were normal until a very short time ago. The most common secondary causes of iron deficiency anemia in menstruating women would be two major gynecologic causes: uterine fibroids and endometriosis. Von Willebrand's disease is certainly less common; it is, however, the most common inherited bleeding disorder and may often present as menorrhagia, metrorrhagia, or menometrorrhagia.

Thus the most appropriate investigations in this patient are pelvic ultrasound, laparoscopy, and a coagulation profile.

A CT scan of the abdomen/pelvis is not indicated.

An NSAID drug such as naproxen can have a profound effect on decreasing the menstrual blood flow; in many cases NSAIDs decrease menstrual flow from 75 cc/period to 15 cc/period. The OCP will accomplish the same. These two drug classes are thus prophylactic; that is, they prevent the recurrence of heavy bleeding.

The acute treatment for this patient to build up her iron stores is ferrous sulfate or ferrous gluconate. The initial dose of ferrous sulfate should be 300 mg tid. It may only be necessary to use ferrous sulfate for 1 to 2 months; at that time the patient can be taken off iron and remain on either the NSAID or the OCP.

In a patient with severe menorrhagia with hemodynamic compromise or potential hemodynamic compromise, the treatment of choice is IV premarin, 25 mg repeated very 4 hours until the menorrhagia subsides.

The most sensitive test for the diagnosis of iron deficiency anemia is the serum ferritin level. In iron deficiency anemia, the serum ferritin level usually falls first. Thereafter, total iron binding capacity (TIBC) increases and serum iron levels gradually decrease. The transferrin saturation will also decrease at this time. The reticulocyte count is not useful in assessing the degree of iron deficiency anemia.

8. B. Extensive hematological measurements have been made in healthy nonpregnant women, none of whom were either iron deficient or folate deficient. Anemia in nonpregnant women is defined as a hemoglobin concentration <12 g/dl and < than 10 g/dl during pregnancy or the puerperium. The hemoglobin concentration is lower in midpregnancy. In early pregnancy and again near term the hemoglobin level of most healthy women with adequate iron stores is 11.0 g/dl. For these reasons, the Center for Disease Control in Atlanta has defined anemia as less than 11.0 g/dl in the first and third trimesters and less than 10.5 g/dl in the second trimester.

9. B. Until proven otherwise, iron deficiency anemia in a middle-aged or elderly male is due to gastrointestinal blood loss, the most sinister cause of which is a gastrointestinal malignancy; carcinoma of the colon or rectum are the most important and most common malignancies found in this situation. This patient should have fecal occult blood testing followed by colonoscopy. Air-contrast barium enema may or may not be indicated for further elucidation. If all of the investigations are normal, the upper GI tract should be investigated by gastroscopy.

Dietary iron deficiency or dietary folic acid deficiency is extremely unusual in a male.

A lymphoma is more likely to produce a normochromic-normocytic blood smear rather than a hypochromic-microcytic picture.

Bleeding hemorrhoids may also produce iron deficiency anemia in middle-aged males.

Vitamin B_{12} deficiency due to lack of intrinsic factor would present as a macrocytic rather than a microcytic anemia.

10. D. This patient's hypochromic-microcytic blood picture, coupled with a drop in hemoglobin from 13.0-7.5 g/dl in 1 year, is almost certainly due to blood loss from a gastrointestinal malignancy or other bleeding source. The discussion in Question 9 regarding the iron deficiency anemia in males also applies to females past the menopause. The other common cause of iron deficiency in the anemia in elderly patients is malnutrition.

In contradistinction to hypochromic-microcytic anemia, the most common cause of megaloblastic anemia is folic acid deficiency.

11. D.

12. B.

13. E. The anemia of chronic disease is most often normochromic and normocytic, and it is most frequently associated with the following diseases:
A. Anemia of chronic inflammation:
   1. Infection
   2. Connective tissue disorders
   3. Malignancy (excluding malignancies where blood loss is a major factor, as in Ca colon)
B. Anemia due to chronic renal failure
C. Anemia due to endocrine failure
D. Anemia of hepatic disease

14. B. In North America the most common category of anemia is iron deficiency anemia. In order of frequency, anemia prevalence is as follows:
Number 1: Iron Deficiency Anemia
a) Blood loss due to excessive menstrual flow
b) Blood loss from the GIO tract
Number 2: Anemia of chronic disease
a) Chronic renal failure
b) Anemia due to connective tissue disorders
Number 3: Macrocytic anemia
a) Pernicious anemia
b) Folic acid deficiency anemia
Number 4: Hemolytic anemia
a) Autoimmune hemolytic anemias
b) Non-autoimmune hemolytic anemias

15. D.

16. C.

17. C.

18. C.

19. D. This patient has pernicious anemia. The signs and symptoms of pernicious anemia can be remembered well by the following mnemonic:
A. Pancytopenia
B. Peripheral neuropathy
C. Posterior spinal column neuropathy
D. Pyramidal tract signs
E. Papillary (tongue) atrophy

The blood smear of a patient with pernicious anemia will show the following: megaloblastic anemia as demonstrated by MCV > 100 μm^3, hyper (not hypo) segmented neutrophils, and oval macrocytes.

Pernicious anemia is defined as a deficiency of Vitamin B_{12} due to lack of production of intrinsic factor by the gastric parietal cells (remember that Vitamin B_{12} deficiency can also be produced by other causes such as a vegetarian diet). The deficiency of intrinsic factor is measured by the Schilling test. The Schilling test uses radiolabeled Vitamin B_{12} and follows excretion with and without intrinsic factor.

The acute treatment of pernicious anemia that is recommended is 1000 μg/day for 1 week followed by 1000 μg/week for 4 weeks and then followed by maintenance therapy of 1000 μg/month.

20. D. Folic acid deficiency is most commonly seen in alcoholics, patients with a malignancy, elderly patients, patients on a vegan diet, and pregnant patients.

The most common cause of folic acid deficiency is inadequate intake.

Folic acid deficiency anemia is also a megaloblastic anemia. Patients with folic acid deficiency usually have normal Vitamin B_{12} levels.

Patients with folic acid deficiency anemia should be given 1-5 mg of folic acid/day.

SOLUTION TO SHORT ANSWER MANAGEMENT PROBLEM 27

The difference between macrocytosis and megaloblastosis is as follows:
Megaloblastosis: The macrocytes are oval shaped.
Macrocytosis: The macrocytes are round shaped.
Megaloblastic anemias are only one cause of macrocytosis.
The differential diagnosis of macrocytosis is as follows:
1. Megaloblastic anemias
2. Liver disease
3. Reticulocytosis

4. Myeloproliferative diseases (leukemia, myelofibrosis)
5. Multiple myeloma
6. Metastatic disease of bone marrow
7. Hypothyroidism
8. Aplastic anemia
9. Drugs (cytotoxic agents, alcohol)
10. Autoagglutination/cold agglutination disease

SUMMARY OF THE DIAGNOSIS AND TREATMENT OF ANEMIAS

1. **Normal hemoglobin levels:**
   a) Males: 14.0-18.0 g/dl
   b) Females: 12.0-16.0 g/dl
2. **Iron deficiency anemia:**
   a) Most common cause of anemia
   b) Most common cause in premenopausal women is excessive menstrual flow. Iron deficiency anemia in males or in postmenopausal females should be considered to be from GIO blood loss until proven otherwise. Most common cause is GIO malignancy.
   c) Iron deficiency anemia is hypochromic-microcytic: microcytosis comes first; hypochromasia is seen in advanced cases.
   d) Serum ferritin level is usually less than 12 μg/L and is the most sensitive test for iron deficiency.
   e) Most pregnant women with decreased hemoglobin are not truly anemic; they simply have a greater increase in plasma volume than in RBC mass. True anemia in pregnancy has been defined by the CDC-Atlanta: hemoglobin in first and third trimester is less than 12.0 g/dl; hemoglobin in second trimester is less than 10.5 g/dl.
   f) Investigations in women with excessive menstrual flow include pelvic ultrasound/laparoscopy (uterine fibroids, endometriosis) and coagulation disorders (von Willebrand's disease).
   g) Treatment for iron deficiency anemia:
      1. Find the cause and correct if possible.
      2. Ferrous sulfate 300 mg od or tid
      3. Menorrhagia: prophylaxis: NSAID or OCP
         Severe: IV premarin
3. **Anemia of chronic disease:**
   a) Anemia of chronic disease is normochromic-normocytic.
   b) Causes of anemia of chronic disease:
      1. Chronic renal failure (most common)
      2. Connective tissue disorders (autoimmune diseases)
      3. Malignancies (except GIO blood loss) such as multiple myeloma or lymphomas
      4. Inflammatory diseases
      5. Chronic hepatic disease
   c) Make the diagnosis (find the cause) and treat the cause.

4. **Megaloblastic anemias:**
   a) Pernicious anemia:
      1. Pernicious anemia is most common: Vitamin B_{12} deficiency due to lack of intrinsic factor
      2. Blood smear: i) MCV > 100 μm^3; ii) hypersegmented neutrophils; and iii) oval macrocytes. Confirmed by i) serum Vitamin B_{12} level and ii) Schilling test
      3. Pernicious anemia = The Five P's:
         i) Pancytopenia
         ii) Peripheral neuropathy
         iii) Posterior spinal column neuropathy
         iv) Papillary (tongue) atrophy
         v) Pyramidal tract signs
      4. Treatment: i) vitamin B_{12} sc 1000 μg BOD every second day; ii) vitamin B_{12} sc 1000 μg once/week; iii) vitamin B_{12} sc 1000 μg/month
      5. Other causes of pernicious anemia are total or subtotal gastrectomy and vegan diet.
   b) Folic acid deficiency:
      1. Diagnosis: blood smear with hypersegmented neutrophils and macro-ovalocytes
         Confirmation: serum folate or RBC folate
      2. Most common cause of folic acid deficiency: dietary deficiency
      3. Associated with alcoholism, vegan diet, medications such as methotrexate and OCP, pregnancy, malignancy, and elderly patients on a "tea and toast" diet
      4. Folic acid supplementation is recommended for all pregnant women (1 mg).
5. **Hemolytic anemias:**
   a) Classification:
      1. Autoimmune hemolytic anemias
      2. Nonautoimmune hemolytic anemias
   b) Most common causes (all autoimmune in classification):
      1. Lymphoproliferative disorders: (CLL, non-Hodgkin's lymphoma)
         i) Most common cause of hemolytic anemia: drugs (iatrogenic disease)
         ii) Other causes: lymphoproliferative disorders
      2. Connective tissue disorders: SLE, rheumatoid arthritis
      3. Infections: EB virus, cytomegalovirus, mycoplasma pneumoniae
      4. Drug induced
      5. Paroxysmal cold hemoglobinuria
   c) Diagnosis:
      1. Coombs test: direct and indirect
      2. Reticulocyte count (elevated)
   d) Treatment:
      1. Corticosteroids
      2. Splenectomy (in those who do not respond)
      3. Intravenous immunoglobulin

6. **Miscellaneous disorders:**
   a) Aplastic anemias
   b) Thalassemia
   c) Sickle cell disease
   d) Hemophilia
   e) Platelet-associated bleeding disorders
   f) Disseminated intravascular coagulation

SUGGESTED READING

Rakel R. Section 5: The blood and spleen. In Rakel R, ed. Conn's current therapy. Philadelphia: WB Saunders, 1994.

PROBLEM 28   A 16-YEAR-OLD MALE WITH A MASS IN THE LEFT SUPRACLAVICULAR AREA

A 16-year-old male is brought to your office by his mother. He has noticed a significant swelling in the area of the left supra-clavicular area that has been present for approximately 4 months. It has, according to the patient, not changed significantly in size over that time.

The patient has no fever, chills, nausea, vomiting, fatigue/malaise, weight loss, or other symptoms.

On examination, the abdomen is soft. No hepatomegaly or splenomegaly is present. No significant lymph node enlargement is present in the axillary chain, the cervical chain, or the inguinal chain.

A mass measuring 2.5 cm × 1.5 cm is felt to be attached to the muscular area above the left scapula.

SELECT THE ONE BEST ANSWER TO THE FOLLOWING QUESTIONS

1. What is the first step in the evaluation of this patient?
   a) a complete blood workup
   b) an incisional biopsy
   c) an excisional biopsy
   d) a radical neck dissection
   e) none of the above

2. The evaluation produces a report that reads as follows: "Reed-Sternberg cells present." What is the most likely diagnosis?
   a) solitary lymph node enlargement
   b) AIDS
   c) metastatic carcinoma
   d) Hodgkin's disease
   e) non-Hodgkin's lymphoma

3. What is the next step in the investigation of this patient?
   a) staging of the disease
   b) radiation therapy
   c) combination chemotherapy
   d) bone scan
   e) CT scan of the abdomen

4. In the staging of the disease described, there are two distinct categories, A and B. To what do these two categories refer?
   a) the presence or absence of metastases
   b) the presence or absence of symptoms
   c) the presence or absence of bone marrow involvement
   d) the possibility or nonpossibility of cure
   e) the presence or absence or intraabdominal disease

5. Staging of the disease includes all of the following except:
   a) CT scan of the abdomen
   b) CT scan of the brain
   c) lower lymphangiography
   d) bone marrow biopsy
   e) liver and spleen scan

6. The stage of the disease in the patient described is Stage IA. At this time, what would you do?

   a) do nothing; wait for further symptoms
   b) combination chemotherapy
   c) localized radiotherapy
   d) combination chemotherapy plus localized radio-therapy
   e) radical surgery

7. With respect to the histologic pathology of this disease, which of the following patterns of disease is most common in North America?
   a) lymphocyte predominance type
   b) nodular sclerosis type
   c) mixed cellularity type
   d) lymphocyte depletion type
   e) none of the above

8. A 52-year-old male comes to your office to reassure himself about "some swellings in my neck, elbows, as well as some chest pain." The other symptom is profound fatigue (for the last 3 months).

   On examination, the patient has multiple enlarged cervical lymph nodes (as well as bilateral epitrochlear nodes). They measure anywhere from 1.0 cm to 2.0 cm in diameter. His liver edge is palpated approximately 3 cm below the left costal edge, and the tip of the spleen can be felt when he lies on his side.

   If you could select only one test to perform, which of the following would you select?
   a) ELISA HIV screening test
   b) IgG-VCA antibody titer for cytomegalovirus
   c) IgG-VCA antibody titer for toxoplasmosis
   d) CT scan of the chest
   e) excisional lymph node biopsy

9. The test you ordered is performed. The result is which one of the following?
   a) diffuse small cleaved cell (Diffuse Poorly Differentiated Lymphocytic) Histology
   b) nodular sclerosis histology: Reed-Sternberg cells present
   c) Hilar mass seen on CT scan (measuring 6 cm × 3 cm)
   d) ELISA HIV test inconclusive
   e) IgG-VCA antibodies absent

10. Based on what you know at present, what is the most likely diagnosis?
    a) non-Hodgkin's lymphoma
    b) Hodgkin's disease
    c) systemic toxoplasmosis: systemic immune deficiency
    d) systemic cytomegalovirus: systemic immune deficiency
    e) AIDS

11. The treatment of choice based on all of your assumptions is which of the following?
    a) AZT
    b) intensive chemotherapy and bone marrow transplantation
    c) interferon-α
    d) intensive chemotherapy only
    e) intensive therapy with ribavirin and acyclovir

12. A 75-year-old male presents with a chief complaint of "bone pain" in "my breast bone and my head, Doc." He tells you that he is sure he is OK but is here only because "the wife kept bugging me until I gave in."

    The patient also appears somewhat pale and does tell you that he has been feeling tired lately, and a bit "weak, depressed, and maybe confused, Doc."

    He had a "touch of the flu" a few months ago. His wife tells you that this "touch of the flu" was actually bacterial pneumonia-organism: *Streptococcus pneumoniae.* On examination, the patient has a tender sternum, tender occipital area of the skull, and a pale conjunctiva.

    With this information, if you could perform only one of the following initial tests, which one would you choose?
    a) electrolytes/BUN/creatinine
    b) complete blood count
    c) ESR

    d) serum calcium
    e) platelet count

13. The laboratory test results come back as follows:
    1) hemoglobin = 8.5 grams/dl: normochromic/normocytic anemia
    2) ESR = 55 mm/hr
    3) platelets = 15,000
    4) serum calcium = 14 mg/dl
    5) electrolytes: Na+ = 115 mEq/L; serum creatinine = 330 μmol/L

    Based on the information you now have, what is the most likely diagnosis?
    a) metastatic carcinoma: metasatic to bone
    b) chronic lymphocytic leukemia
    c) multiple myeloma
    d) chronic renal failure: secondary to macroglobulinemia
    e) chronic myelogenous leukemia

14. Further investigations substantiate your findings. What is the treatment of choice at this time?
    a) bone marrow transplantation
    b) total body radiotherapy
    c) adjuvant combination chemotherapy: Adriamycin, vincristine, bleomycin
    d) melphalan plus prednisone
    e) none of the above

15. The disease described in Question 12 is due to a proliferation of which of the following?
    a) myeloblasts
    b) lymphoblasts
    c) metastatic cancer cells
    d) plasma cells
    e) none of the above

Short Answer Management Problem 28

Matching Question

In Part A certain hematologic disorders are listed. Match each numbered question with an appropriate disease. Each disease may be used once, twice, three times, or not at all.

In part B the characteristics of certain hematologic disorders are described.

Part A: Diseases

A. aplastic anemia
B. secondary polycythemia
C. hemolytic anemia
D. drug-induced thrombocytopenia
E. idiopathic thrombocytopenia purpura
F. sickle cell disease
G. sickle cell trait
H. preleukemia
I. acute lymphocytic leukemia

J. disseminated intravascular coagulation
K. hemophilia
L. multiple myeloma
M. chronic lymphocytic leukemia
N. hemochromatosis
O. acute myelogenous leukemia
P. chronic myelogenous leukemia
Q. cutaneous T-cell leukemia

R. neutrophilia
S. von Willebrand's disease
T. thalassemia
U. hairy cell leukemia
V. acute intermittent porphyria
W. polycythemia rubra vera
X. secondary thrombocytopenia
Y. transfusion reaction
Z. myelofibrosis

Part B:

1. Clinical case 1:   Choice _____
   1. Disease is associated with excessive proliferation of erythroid, granulocytic, and megakaryocytic precursors.
   2. Splenomegaly is almost universal in this disease.
   3. Disease has significantly elevated red blood cell mass.
   4. Patient presents with plethora.
   5. Disease characteristically has thrombocytosis.

2. Clinical case 2:   Choice _____
   1. Disease produces a major disorder of the bone marrow.
   2. Splenomegaly is present in all patients.
   3. As the disease progresses, patients experience weight loss; skin and mucous membrane bleeding; and bone pain, jaundice, and lymphadenopathy.
   4. Bone marrow tap is almost always unsuccessful: it is known as a "dry tap."
   5. Bone marrow biopsy reveals fibrosis of marrow spaces and osteosclerosis.

3. Clinical case 3:   Choice _____
   1. This disease has the presence of the Philadelphia chromosome.
   2. When this disease is diagnosed, the total WBC often exceeds 200,000 cells/mm³.
   3. This disease usually follows the following course: (a) chronic phase of variable duration; (b) blastic transformation; with (c) some patients experiencing a distinct intermediate accelerated phase.
   4. The most consistent physical finding is splenomegaly.
   5. This is the most common serious hematologic disorder diagnosed in patients who survived the atomic bombs of Hiroshima and Nagasaki.

4. Clinical case 4:   Choice _____
   1. This form of leukemia is the most common form of leukemia in the United States.
   2. The disease is usually seen in patients greater than 50 years of age.
   3. The abnormal cells morphologically resemble mature, small lymphocytes of the peripheral blood, and accumulate in the bone marrow, blood, lymph nodes, and spleen in large numbers.
   4. This disease has an "indolent nature."
   5. Median survival exceeds 10 years, and many patients require no treatment.

Continued

Short Answer Management Problem 28—*cont'd*

5. Clinical case 5:   Choice _____
   1. This disease has characteristic cells that exhibit cytoplasmic projections on their surfaces.
   2. This disease is due to an expansion of neoplastic type B lymphocytes.
   3. This disease usually presents in male patients over the age of 40 years.
   4. Approximately 30% of patients with this disease have a vasculitis-like disorder.
   5. The treatment of choice for this disease is very characteristic of the disease: interferon-α.

6. Clinical case 6:   Choice _____
   1. This disease is a disease of children and young adults.
   2. This disease is characterized by the clonal proliferation of immature hematopoietic cells.
   3. The most common abnormal cells seen on bone marrow biopsy are immature lymphoblasts.
   4. Infection is a nearly universal complication.
   5. Approximately 50% of patients are either cured or characterized as being in long-term remission.

7. Clinical case 7:   Choice: _____
   1. The incidence of this disease increases with increasing age.
   2. The most common abnormal cells seen on bone marrow biopsy are immature myeloblasts or immature promyelocyte.
   3. Some patients with this disease develop the disease after either a preleukemia syndrome or a myelodysplastic syndrome.
   4. Between 10% and 30% of patients with this disease survive 5 years; most of these patients are probably cured.
   5. Bone marrow transplantation from either an identical twin or HLA-identical sibling is a very important part of treatment.

8. Clinical case 8:   Choice: _____
   1. This disease usually follows recovery from either a viral exanthem or a viral upper respiratory tract illness.
   2. The acute form of this disease is caused by immune complexes containing viral antigens that bind to platelet receptors.
   3. This disease produces a profound rapid decrease in the cell line in question.
   4. Corticosteroids are the agents of choice in the treatment of this disease.
   5. In severe cases of this disease, splenectomy may need to be performed.

9. Clinical case 9:   Choice: _____
   1. This is the most common inherited bleeding disorder.
   2. The factor that is missing in this disease is responsible for platelet adhesion.
   3. The factor that is missing in this disease also serves as a plasma carrier for factor VIII.
   4. Women with this disorder may be initially diagnosed because of severe menorrhagia.
   5. The treatment of choice for this disease is cryoprecipitate.

10. Clinical case 10:   Choice: _____
    1. This disease is most frequently associated with obstetrical catastrophes.
    2. Other major causes of this disease are major trauma, metastatic malignancies, and bacterial sepsis.
    3. In this disease, the combination of potent thrombogenic stimuli causes the deposition of small thrombi and small emboli throughout the microvasculature.
    4. Most patients with this disease have extensive skin and mucous membrane bleeding and hemorrhage from multiple sites.
    5. Patients with bleeding as a major symptom should receive fresh frozen plasma as therapy for the disorder.

ANSWERS

1. C.

2. D.

3. A.

4. B.

5. B.

6. D.

7. B. This patient should have an excisional biopsy of the mass performed as soon as possible. Although a piece of tissue could be removed (an incisional biopsy), an excisional biopsy makes more sense.

   The anatomic pathology report of Reed-Sternberg cells present (these are large binucleate cells with a single distinct nucleoli) is pathognomonic of Hodgkin's disease. Hodgkin's disease is one of the most important success stories of medical oncology. It is a disease that used to be uniformly fatal; at this time, the vast majority of patients are cured.

   After an anatomic diagnosis is made, the disease must be staged. Staging of Hodgkin's disease includes the following:
   A. Chest X-ray
   B. Bipedal lower extremity lymphangiography
   C. Liver scan
   D. Spleen scan
   E. CBC/platelet count/differential count
   F. Bone marrow aspiration and biopsy
   G. Serum liver enzymes including alkaline phosphatase and 5'-nucleotidase
   H. ESR
   I. CT scan of the abdomen

   The Ann Arbor Staging Classification of Hodgkin's disease is as follows:

   Stage I: single lymph node (I) or single extralymphatic organ

   Stage II: two or more lymph nodes on the same side of the diaphragm

   Stage III: lymph nodes involved on both sides of the diaphragm or localized involvement of spleen or extralymphatic organ or both

   Stage IV: diffuse or disseminated disease or involvement of the liver or bone marrow

   The staging is further added to by the presence or absence of the following symptoms: fever, night sweats and weight loss > 10% in the last 6 months. The presence of any of the symptoms indicates that the stage of the disease should be labeled B. The absence of any of the above symptoms indicates that the stage of the disease should be labeled A.

   The histologic typing of Hodgkin's disease and the significance of some of the histologic types are as follows:
   A. Nodular sclerosis: most common histologic type in North America and Western Europe
   B. Mixed cellularity:
      1. Second most common histologic type in North America
      2. More frequent in poorer parts of the world and in older patients
   C. Lymphocyte predominance:
      1. Abundance of Reed-Sternberg cells
      2. Associated with a favorable prognosis
   D. Lymphocyte depletion:
      1. Paucity of cellular elements
      2. Rarest histologic type
      3. Associated with advanced age, systemic symptoms, retroperitoneal nodes, and extranodal involvement
      4. Worst prognosis

   The current treatment recommendations for more localized disease (Stages I, II, and III) are as follows:
   A. Combination chemotherapy (ABVD regime):
      1. Adriamycin
      2. Bleomycin
      3. Vinblastine
      4. Dacarbazine (six cycles of ABVD at 28-day intervals) plus
   B. Involved region radiotherapy: This aggressive treatment regime provides the best chance of cure.

   One or two enlarged lymph nodes in a young person indicates Hodgkin's disease until proven otherwise. Excisional biopsy should always be undertaken.

8. E.

9. A.

10. A.

11. B. This patient has a non-Hodgkin's lymphoma. The characteristics that suggest this diagnosis over Hodgkin's disease are the presence of lymph nodes draining Waldeyer's ring, the presence of epitrochlear lymph nodes, and the presence of chest pain suggesting involvement of lung tissue.

    The lymph node histology involving non-Hodgkin's lymphoma will not be discussed in detail. However, the lymph node pathology of diffuse small cleaved cell (diffuse poorly differentiated lymphocytic) suggests a high-grade lymphoma with extensive involvement including the liver, the spleen, and the bone marrow. Your physical examination confirms the possibility of the former two.

    Staging is similar (although not identical) to the staging for Hodgkin's disease.

Treatment of this stage (Stage IV) includes intensive multiple drug chemotherapy, bone marrow transplantation, and CNS prophylactic treatment.

12. D.

13. C.

14. D.

15. D. The critical elements of this patient's history/ physical/laboratory data are as follows:
    A. Signs of bone pain (sternum and skull) and anemia
    B. Symptoms of weakness, depression, fatigue, and confusion
    C. Recent history of bacterial pneumonia; possible immune suppression
    D. Laboratory evidence of the following:
       1. Anemia
       2. Hypercalcemia
       3. Renal failure
       4. Thrombocytopenia
       5. Hyponatremia
       6. Elevated ESR

The combination of bone pain (Location Specific), hypercalcemia, normochromic/normocytic anemia, renal failure, weakness/depression/confusion, and history of bacterial pneumonia points to the diagnosis of multiple myeloma.

The diagnosis will be substantiated by skull X-ray (showing punched-out lesions), serum electrophoresis with monoclonal peak, and demonstration of Bence-Jones protein in the urine.

Although you were asked to select only one laboratory test, you were given the results from all of the tests. In selection, the one best test to perform of the tests listed is probably the serum calcium level.

Multiple myeloma is a disease of older patients, with the mean age being 68 years. It appears to be more common than average in farmers, petroleum workers, woodworkers, and leather workers.

Pathologically, multiple myeloma is a plasma cell malignancy or proliferation.

The treatment of choice is a combination of melphalan and prednisone administered for 4 to 7 days every 4 to 6 weeks for 1 to 2 years. The disease is almost invariably fatal, but patients may live significantly long periods with virtually no symptoms once stablized on therapy.

SOLUTION TO SHORT ANSWER MANAGEMENT PROBLEM 28

1. W.
2. Z.
3. P.
4. M.
5. U.
6. I.
7. O.
8. E.
9. S.
10. J.

SUMMARY OF THE DIAGNOSIS AND MANAGEMENT OF CERTAIN HEMATOLOGIC CONDITIONS

1. **Most common solid hematologic malignancies: lymphomas**
   a) Disorders and their prevalence:
      1. Non-Hodgkin's lymphoma: most common (40,000 new cases/year in the United States)
      2. Hodgkin's lymphoma: second most common (7500 new cases/year in the United States)
   b) Signs and symptoms:
      1. Most common sign/symptom is solitary or non-solitary lymph node enlargement.
      2. The presence or absence of systemic symptoms not only is a staging phenomenon (A or B) but is also prognostic.
      3. Most common systemic symptoms include weight loss, night sweats, fevers, and pain.
      4. Differentiation of Hodgkin's from non-Hodgkin's:
         i) Systemic symptoms more common in Hodgkin's lymphoma
         ii) Location of lymph node enlargement:
            a) Hodgkin's supraclavicular area very common
            b) Non-Hodgkin's: lymph nodes draining Waldeyer's ring and epitroclear nodes most common
         iii) Non-Hodgkin's lymphoma often presents with mediastinal, abdominal, and extranodal symptomatology.
      5. Prognosis:
         i) Hodgkin's lymphoma has a better prognosis than non-Hodgkin's lymphoma, primarily because of less spread at the time of diagnosis.
         ii) Prognosis depends on accurate staging.
      6. Treatment: combination chemotherapy plus radiotherapy
2. **Multiple myeloma:**
   a) Prevalence: multiple myeloma is mainly a disease of the elderly.
   b) Pathology: plasma cell malignancy/plasma cell proliferation
   c) Signs and symptoms:
      1. Bone pain (sternum, skull, ribs, and back)
      2. Anemia: normochromic/normocytic

3. Immune suppression (history of bacterial infections)
4. Renal failure
5. Hypercalcemia
6. Weakness/confusion/depression/fatigue

d) Diagnosis:
1. Serum protein electrophoresis
2. Bone marrow biopsy
3. Urine: Bence-Jones protein

3. **Miscellaneous important hematologic conditions**

a) Polycythemia rubra vera:
Plethora, sometimes cyanosis
Proliferation of all hematopoietic cell lines
Elevated hemoglobin, RBC mass, thrombocytosis

b) Myelofibrosis:
Weight loss, bleeding from skin and mucous membranes
Bone marrow biopsy: dry tap
Normal bone marrow replaced by fibrotic material

c) Chronic myelogenous leukemia:
Atomic bomb survivors
Philadelphia chromosome
WBC at diagnosis often > 200,000
Chronic phase followed by blastic phase

d) Chronic lymphocytic leukemia:
Most common leukemia in United States
Disease of older patients
Indolent nature; no treatment needed in many patients; median survival > 10 years

e) Hairy cell leukemia:
Cytoplasmic projections give disorder its name.
Proliferation of B lymphocytes
Remarkably effective treatment with α-interferon

f) Acute lymphocytic leukemia:
Disease of children
Immature lymphoblasts
Infections very common
50% cure rate at present

g) Acute myeloblastic leukemia:
Most common acute leukemia of adults
Immature myeloblasts on smear
Infections very common
Bone marrow transplantation essential for survival (10%-30%)
May follow myelodysplastic disorder or preleukemia

h) Idiopathic thrombocytopenic purpura:
Acute onset after viral exanthem or viral infection
Rapid drop in platelet count
Corticosteroids are treatment of choice: splenectomy in resistant cases

i) Von Willebrand's disease:
Most common inherited bleeding disorder
Results in factor VIII deficiency
Often presents as severe menorrhagia in women
Cryoprecipitate is treatment of choice.

j) Disseminated intravascular coagulation:
Follows obstetrical catastrophes, major trauma, metastatic malignancies, bacterial sepsis
Microemboli or microthrombi in vasculature
Profuse bleeding from many sites
Treatment: fresh frozen plasma

SUGGESTED READING

Isselbacher KJ et al., ed. Harrison's principles of internal medicine. 13th Ed. New York: McGraw-Hill, 1994.

PROBLEM 29   A 35-YEAR-OLD FEMALE WITH MALAISE, WEIGHT LOSS, VASOMOTOR DISTURBANCE, AND VAGUE PERIARTICULAR PAIN AND STIFFNESS

A 35-year-old female presents with a 6-month history of malaise, paraesthesias in both hands, and vague pain in both hands and wrists. She has also felt extremely fatigued. She tells you that the pains in her joints are much worse in the morning. She is also beginning to notice pain and swelling in both knees.

The patient has a normal family history, with no significant diseases noted. The patient is taking no drugs and has no allergies.

On examination, there is a sensation of "bogginess" and slight swelling in both hands, both wrists, and in the small bones of her hands. Both knees also feel somewhat "swollen and boggy." There are no other joint abnormalities, and the rest of the physical examination is normal.

SELECT THE ONE BEST ANSWER TO THE FOLLOWING QUESTIONS

1. What is the most likely diagnosis in this patient?
   a) nonarticular rheumatism
   b) synovitis
   c) gonococcal arthritis
   d) rheumatoid arthritis
   e) systemic lupus erythematosis

2. What is the most characteristic symptom of this disease?
   a) early-morning joint stiffness
   b) progressive joint pain
   c) predilection for the small joints
   d) joint swelling
   e) normal cartilage in spite of joint pain

3. What is the most characteristic sign of this disease?
   a) joint swelling
   b) bilateral (symmetrical) joint involvement
   c) erythema surrounding the affected joints
   d) joint bogginess
   e) involvement of the glenohumeral joint in all cases

4. Upon what is the pathophysiology of this disease based?
   a) bone destruction
   b) bone spur formation
   c) bone sclerosis
   d) symmetrical joint involvement
   e) synovial inflammation

5. In the course of the pathophysiology of this disease, which of the following is most characteristic of the disease?
   a) synovial proliferation with cartilage erosion stimulated by cytokines
   b) cartilage destruction stimulated by the proliferation of proteoglycans
   c) cartilage destruction stimulated by the enzymatic action of proteoglycans
   d) loss of the synovial membrane
   e) none of the above; the pathophysiology of the disease is not known with any certainty

6. The disease described affects one particular part of the spine. What is the affected part, and what are the affected vertebrae?
   a) cervical: C6-C7
   b) cervical: C1-C2
   c) thoracic: T7-T9
   d) lumbar: L1-L3
   e) lumbar: L4-L5

7. Which anemia usually accompanies this disease process?
   a) microcytic: hypochromic
   b) microcytic: normochromic
   c) normocytic: noromochromic
   d) macrocytic: hyperchromic
   e) normocytic: hypochromic

8. Which of the following is(are) systemic complications of the disease process?
   a) vasculitis
   b) pericarditis
   c) pleural effusion
   d) diffuse interstitial fibrosis of the lung
   e) all of the above

9. Felty's syndrome is a complication of the described disorder. Which of the following is(are) part of Felty's syndrome?
   a) splenomegaly
   b) neutropenia
   c) positive rheumatoid factor
   d) a and b
   e) all of the above

10. What is the drug of choice for inducing remission in patients with signs and symptoms of the disease described?
    a) auranofin
    b) hydroxychloroquine
    c) methotrexate
    d) D-penicillamine
    e) cyclophosphamide

11. The patient develops a local flare-up in her right knee. Her left knee is affected to a small degree, but not nearly

as severely as the right knee. Up to this time, remission had been induced and she was taking antiinflammatory agents for suppression of inflammation.

What is the treatment of choice for this local flare-up?
a) methotrexate
b) hydroxychloroquine
c) intraarticular corticosteroid injection
d) oral prednisone
e) auranofin

12. What is the drug of choice for the suppression of inflammation in a patient with this disease?

a) auranofin
b) methotrexate
c) oral prednisone
d) naproxen
e) D-penicillamine

13. Which of the following is not a classical radiologic feature of rheumatoid arthritis?
a) loss of juxta-articular bone mass
b) narrowing of the joint space
c) bony erosions
d) subarticular sclerosis
e) all of the above are radiologic manifestations

Short Answer Management Problem 29

Matching Question 14–25
Part A lists a number of different types of arthritis or diseases in which arthritis is a major component. Part B lists characteristics of a number of different types of arthritis. Match the characteristic in Part B with the type of arthritis in Part A.

Part A:
1. ankylosing spondylitis: _____
2. gonocococcal arthritis _____
3. systemic lupus erythematosis _____
4. lyme disease _____
5. rheumatic fever _____
6. gouty arthritis _____
7. juvenile rheumatoid arthritis _____
8. reiter's disease _____
9. psoriatic arthritis _____
10. IBD (inflammatory bowel disease) arthritis _____
11. CPPD (calcium pyrophosphate) arthritis _____
12. tuberculous arthritis _____

Part B:
A. Positively birefrigent under the polarizing microscope
B. Negatively birefrigent under the polarizing microscope
C. Most common cause of infective arthritis in young adults
D. Conjunctivitis and urethritis are other features.
E. Erythema chronicum migrans
F. Bamboo spine
G. Streptococcal pharyngitis usually occurs first.
H. Arthritis may precede abdominal symptoms.
I. Renal failure is major cause of death in this disease.
J. Arthritis may appear before classical "silver-scaled" skin lesions.
K. Major cause of arthritis in children
L. Lung disease is major manifestation of this disease in most patients.

ANSWERS

1. D.

2. A.

3. B. Rheumatoid arthritis is a disease that has the following features:
   A. Morning stiffness (characteristic symptom)
   B. Pain on motion of joints

C. Tenderness in joints
D. Swelling (soft-tissue inflammation of fluid, not bony overgrowth)
E. Symmetrical joint involvement
F. Subcutaneous nodules
G. Positive agglutination (rheumatoid arthritis) factor
H. Characteristic histiologic changes in the synovial membrane

The most characteristic symptom of rheumatoid arthritis is early-morning stiffness. The most characteristic sign of rheumatoid arthritis is symmetrical joint involvement.

In most patients, rheumatoid arthritis starts out with a whimper and not a bang. The disease has an insidious start with nonspecific symptoms, such as fatigue and malaise, accompanied by arthralgias and low-grade fever. Later, polyarticular, symmetrical joint swelling begins (usually with the proximal interphalangeal, metacarpophalangeal, wrist, elbow, shoulder, knee, ankle, and metatarsophalangeal joints involved) but sparing the distal interphalangeal joints. Cervical spine involvement is common at the region C1-C2, but the remainder of the spine is usually spared.

4. E.

5. A. The pathophysiology of rheumatoid arthritis begins with synovial membrane swelling and synovial membrane proliferation. The synovium, which is normally only two cell layers thick, proliferates and erodes adjacent cartilage and adjacent bone. Cytokines, particularly interleukin-1 and tumor necrosis factor alpha, that are secreted by macrophages produce the following:
   A. Chondrocyte and osteoclast stimulation
   B. Prostaglandin secretion and endothelial activation
   C. CD4 + helper cells promote the inflammation early in the disease and are abundant in the synovium and the synovial fluid.
   D. Systemic effects such as fever and anemia are also effects of the macrophage/cytokine system.

6. B. Instability of the cervical spine is a life-threatening complication of rheumatoid arthritis. The instability results from a cervical ligament synovitis in the region of the first two cervical vertebrae. This complication occurs in 30% to 40% of patients who develop rheumatoid arthritis. Five percent of RA patients eventually develop a myelopathy or cord injury as a result of this instability.

7. C. The anemia that most often accompanies rheumatoid arthritis is characterized as mild, normochromic: normocytic.
   The characteristics at the cellular level of the anemia include the following: low to normal iron, low to normal iron-binding protein, and normal to high erythropoietin.

8. E. Rheumatoid arthritis is a systemic disease. Some of the more important complications are as follows:
   A. Vasculitis: from the very beginning of the synovial membrane thickening process, a microvascular vasculitis process is involved. This can progress to mesenteric vasculitis, polyarthritis nodosa, or other vascular syndromes.
   B. Pericarditis: fibrinous pericarditis is present in 40% of patients with rheumatoid arthritis at autopsy. Al-

though infrequent, this pericarditis can occasionally be of the constricting type with life-threatening tamponade.
   C. Pleural effusions: rheumatic pleural effusions are extremely common.
   D. Rheumatic nodules in the heart (affecting the conducting system): rheumatic nodules may frequently lead to conducting disturbances including heart block and bundle-branch blocks.
   E. Rheumatic nodules in the lung can cavitate or become infected.
   F. Diffuse interstitial fibrosis with a restrictive pattern on pulmonary function tests and with a honeycomb pattern on chest X-ray may occur.

9. E. Felty's syndrome usually occurs fairly late in the disease process. Felty's syndrome is manifested by splenomegaly, neutropenia, and a positive rheumatoid factor.

10. C. The drug of first choice for inducing remission in patients with rheumatoid arthritis is methotrexate. Methotrexate, based on the benefit/risk ratio, is considered superior to second-line drugs such as auranofin (oral gold), D-penicillamine, hydroxychloroquine, cyclophosphamide, and oral corticosteroids.

11. A. Because the flare-up is limited to one joint, it seems perfectly reasonable to treat it with a localized approach. An intraarticular corticosteroid injection would seem to be the place to start. An injection of DepoMedrol or SoluCortef mixed with lidocaine would be considered a treatment of first choice.

12. D. The drug(s) of choice for the suppression of inflammation in a patient with rheumatoid arthritis are the NSAIDs. Although aspirin (ASA) is still theoretically the agent of first choice, patients are more likely to take 1-2 pills/day than the 10-12 required with aspirin therapy. Thus the answer to this question is naproxen. If a NSAID from a certain class does not work when given up to maximum dose, then try an agent from a second or different class. For example, naproxen (a proprionic acid derivative) may be changed to tolmetin (a heterocyclic acetic acid derivative).

13. D. In early rheumatoid arthritis, few radiologic findings are seen. Soft-tissue changes in synovial fluid or capsular thickening may occasionally be seen on the radiograph but are more readily detected by P/E. Loss of juxtaarticular bone mass (osteoporosis) is often detected near the finger joints and may be seen early in the disease. Narrowing of the joint space, due to thinning of the articular cartilage, is usually seen late in the disease. Bony erosions are seen best at the margins of the joint. Subarticular sclerosis is a feature of osteoarthritis, not rheumatoid arthritis.

SOLUTION TO SHORT ANSWER MANAGEMENT PROBLEM 29

1. F.
2. C.
3. I.
4. E.
5. G.
6. B.
7. K.
8. D.
9. J.
10. H.
11. A.
12. L.

SUMMARY OF THE DIAGNOSIS AND MANAGEMENT OF RHEUMATOID ARTHRITIS

1. **Prevalence:** rheumatoid arthritis occurs in 1% of the population.
2. **Signs/symptoms** (most common and others):
   a) Early morning stiffness is most common symptom.
   b) Symmetrical joint swelling is most common sign. Other signs/symptoms:
   c) Tenderness, swelling, and "bogginess of joints"
   d) Characteristic changes in the synovial membrane including microvascular changes
   e) Positive rheumatoid factor
   f) Subcutaneous nodules
   g) Radiographic changes:
      1. Loss of juxtaarticular bone mass
      2. Joint space narrowing
      3. Bony erosions
3. **Pathophysiology:**
   Sequence and order of changes:
   a) Macrophage activation
   b) Product(s) of activation are production of cytokines: interleukin and tumor necrosis factor
   c) Synovial membrane thickening, proliferation, and local "microvasculitis"
   d) Chondrocyte, osteoclast, CD4+ helper cells, endothelial proliferation
   e) Joint space narrowing
   f) Cytokines are also responsible for extraarticular symptoms such as fever and anemia.

4. **Systemic manifestations:**
   a) Normochromic-normocytic anemia
   b) Fever
   c) Pericarditis
   d) Pleural effusion
   e) Rheumatoid nodules in lung
   f) Diffuse interstitial disease
   g) Felty's syndrome
   h) Rheumatoid nodules in heart causing heart block and bundle-branch block
   i) Systemic vasculitis
5. **Treatment:**
   a) Nonpharmacologic treatment:
      1. Systemic rest
      2. Articular rest
      3. Physiotherapy including heat, cold, and active-assistive exercises
   b) Remittive agents:
      First-choice: methotrexate
      Second choice:
      1. Auranofin
      2. Prednisone
      3. D-penicillamine
      4. Hydroxychloroquine
      5. Cyclophosphasmide
   c) Local remittive agents:
      First choice: injected corticosteroids (maximum = twice)
   d) Suppression of inflammation:
      1. First choice:
         i) NSAID: class: proprionic acids (naproxen, ibuprofen, fenoprofen)
         ii) NSAID: class: Heterocyclic acidic acids (tolmetin, suldinac)
         iii) NSAID: class: oxicams/indole acidic acids (piroxicam/indomethacin)
      2. Alternative first choice: aspirin
      3. Second choice: nonacetylated salicylates (trilisate, salsalate)

SUGGESTED READING

Kandanoff RD. Rheumatoid arthritis. In Rakel R, ed. Conn's current therapy. Philadelphia: WB Saunders, 1994.

PROBLEM 30   AN 80-YEAR-OLD FEMALE WITH PAINFUL FINGER JOINTS

An 80-year-old female presents with a 6-month history of stiffness in her hands bilaterally. This stiffness is at its worst in the morning and subsides thereafter. She has also noticed increasing (but not severe) pain in the lower back, both hips, and both knees.

On examination, the patient is obese. She has significant swellings of both the proximal interphalangeal joints and the distal interphalangeal joints. There is also deformity of both knees on examination. The rest of her P/E is within normal limits.

SELECT THE ONE BEST ANSWER TO THE FOLLOWING QUESTIONS

1. Which of the following statements regarding this patient's condition is(are) true?
   a) the swellings present at the DIP may represent Bouchard's nodes
   b) the swellings present at the PIP may represent Heberden's nodes
   c) this patient will most likely demonstrate an elevated ESR and a positive rheumatoid factor
   d) synovial fluid analysis will probably demonstrate a low viscosity and normal mucin clotting
   e) none of the above are true

2. Which of the following statements regarding the symptomatology of the condition described is(are) false?
   a) pain is the chief symptom of osteoarthritis and is usually deep and aching in character
   b) stiffness of the involved joint is common but of relatively brief duration
   c) the pain of osteoarthritis is characteristically dull and aching
   d) the major physical finding in osteoarthritis is bony crepitus
   e) the presence of osteophytes is sufficient for the diagnosis of osteoarthritis

3. Which of the following statements concerning the condition described is(are) false?
   a) this condition is the most common form of joint disease in the North American population
   b) 80% of the population have radiographic features of this condition in weight-bearing joints before the age of 65 years
   c) this condition has both primary and secondary forms
   d) narrowing of the joint space is unusual
   e) pathologically, the articular cartilage is first roughened and then finally worn away

4. A 65-year-old female with moderately severe osteoarthritis of her left hip presents to your office requesting an exercise prescription. She wishes to "get into shape."

   Which of the following would you recommend to this patient at this time?
   a) exercise is not good for osteoarthritis; rest is much more appropriate
   b) a graded exercise program consisting of brisk walking gradually increasing the distance to 3-4 miles/day will probably not cause pain and will be good for her.
   c) a passive isotonic exercise program is preferable to an active isometric exercise program
   d) any exercise program will probably hasten her need for total hip replacements
   e) swimming is the best exercise prescription you can give her; it promotes cardiovascular fitness and at the same time keeps pressure off the weight-bearing joints

5. Which of the following radiographic features is(are) usually seen with the condition just described?
   a) narrowing of the joint spaces
   b) bony sclerosis
   c) osteophyte formation
   d) subchondral cyst formation
   e) all of the above

6. Which of the following is(are) useful treatment modalities in the treatment of the condition just described?
   a) weight loss in obese patients
   b) canes, crutches, and walkers
   c) the application of heat to involved joints
   d) NSAIDs
   e) all of the above

7. Which of the following statements concerning the incidence of the condition described above is(are) true?
   a) one-third of adults aged 25 to 75 have radiographic evidence of osteoarthritis
   b) cartilaginous fraying is common
   c) mild synovitis may develop in response to crystals or cartilaginous debris
   d) the most common sites for this disease are in the small joints of the hand, the foot, and the knees and/or hips
   e) all of the above are true

8. What is(are) the major goal(s) of therapy in the disease just described?
   a) minimize pain
   b) prevent disability
   c) delay progression
   d) a and b only
   e) all of the above

9. Which of the following statements regarding the use of NSAIDs in the condition described and as given to an elderly patient is(are) true?
   a) NSAIDs are generally very safe for the treatment of the condition described in elderly patients
   b) NSAID toxicity in elderly patients is uncommon
   c) NSAID toxicity in elderly patients is unlikely to be associated with renal insufficiency
   d) the most common NSAID toxicity in elderly patients is gastrointestinal
   e) none of the above are true

10. What is(are) the drug(s) of choice for the treatment of primary osteoarthritis?
   a) acetaminophen
   b) naproxen sodium
   c) diclofenac
   d) indomethacin
   e) any of the above

Short Answer Management Problem 30

Describe the nonpharmacologic and the pharamcologic management of the condition described.

ANSWERS

1. E. This patient has obvious osteoarthritis. However, the location of Bouchard's nodes represents both overgrowth and significant osteoarthritic changes at the PIP joints (not the distal interphalangeal joints), whereas Heberden's nodes represent bony overgrowth and significant osteoarthritic changes at the distal (not the proximal) interphalangeal joints.

   A significantly elevated ESR is seldom seen with osteoarthritis (except in the unusual cases in which there is a significant inflammatory component).

   Synovial fluid analysis will most likely reveal a high (not low) viscosity and normal mucin clotting. The total leukocyte count in the synovial fluid will likely be less than 1000 cells/mm³.

2. E. The most common symptom in osteoarthritis is pain. The pain is described as deep, aching, aggravated by joint use, and relieved by joint rest. Joint stiffness in weight-bearing joints is common but usually is a very transient finding (especially in the morning). It also occurs after prolonged rest.

   Osteoarthritis pain is due to movement of one joint surface against another with both joint surfaces exhibiting characteristic articular cartilate damage including fraying and, ultimately, complete lack of cartilage. In addition, there are subchondral bone microfractures, irritation of the periosteal nerve endings, ligamentous stress, muscular strain, and soft tissue inflammation such as bursitis and tendinitis.

   Bony crepitus is the most common physical finding in osteoarthritis. Osteophytes are a common radiologic finding, especially with advanced age. The diagnosis of osteoarthritis, however, is clinical, and the mere presence of osteophytes on an X-ray is not sufficient for the diagnosis itself.

3. D. Joint space narrowing is common. It is almost always associated with osteoarthritis. The pathological process involved in osteoarthritis is as follows:
   1) The primary defect in primary osteoarthritis and secondary osteoarthritis (secondary meaning due to acute or chronic trauma, congenital deformities), and endocrine disorders such as acromegaly, obesity, and diabetes) is loss of articular cartilage.
   2) Cartilage changes progress as follows:
      a) Glistening appearance is lost.
      b) Surface areas of the articular cartilage flake off.
      c) Deeper layers of the articular cartilage develop longitudinal fissures (fibrillation).
      d) The cartilage becomes thin and eventually absent in some areas, leaving the underlying subchondral bone unprotected.
      e) The unprotected subchondral bone becomes sclerotic (dense and hard).
      f) Cysts develop within the subchondral bone and communicate with the longitudinal fissures in the cartilage.
      g) Pressure builds up in the cysts until the cystic contents are forced into the synovial cavity, breaking through the articular cartilage on the way.
      h) As the articular cartilage erodes, cartilage-coated osteophytes may grow outward from the underlying bone and alter the bone contours and joint anatomy. These spurlike bony projections enlarge until small pieces, called joint mice, break off into the synovial cavity.
      i) The process of loss of articular cartilage probably takes place through the enzymatic breakdown of the cartilage matrix—the proteoglycans, glycosaminoglycans, and collagen are involved.

4. E. Muscle spasm and muscle atrophy can be prevented in osteoarthritis by a graded exercise program. Active

exercises are preferred to passive exercises; isometric exercises are preferred to isotonic exercises.

Because of minimal involvement of the weight-bearing joints, swimming can be recommended as an ideal exercise.

A graded exercise program that includes walking 3-4 miles/day will result in trauma to the joints and should be discouraged. It may very well hasten the need for total hip or knee replacement. When walking is used as an exercise for osteoarthritis it is best to keep the pressure off the involved joint by the use of a cane.

5. E. Radiographic changes in osteoarthritis include narrowing of the joint space due to loss of articular cartilage, bony sclerosis due to thickening of subchondral bone, subchondral bone cysts, and osteophyte (bone spur) formation.

6. E. The treatment of osteoarthritis includes nonpharmacologic measures and pharmacologic measures.

Nonpharmacologic measures include rest; the avoidance of overuse of the affected joint; walking aids such as canes, crutches, and walkers; weight loss; the application of heat; and other physiotherapy techniques.

Pharmacologic measures include simple analgesics such as acetaminophen, NSAIDs, and local steroid injections.

Orthopedic surgery (the option utilized in severe cases) is most effective for osteoarthritis of the hips. Knee replacement, although common and effective for relieving pain, has a lower success rate in terms of a lasting solution to the problem.

7. E. At least 33% of adults between the ages of 25 and 75 have radiographic evidence of osteoarthritis. There are some studies that suggest that osteoarthritis begins as early as 15 or 16 years.

The cartilaginous fraying that is associated with cartilage degeneration has been described. Associated with this may be a mild synovitis that develops in response to cartilaginous fragments (joint mice) in the joint space itself.

The most common sites for osteoarthritis to develop are the small joints of the hands, the small joints of the feet, the hips, the knees, and the vertebral column where the cartilaginous degeneration is of a somewhat different type (the intervertebral discs) but nevertheless is the same basic pathologic process.

8. E. The goals for the patient with osteoarthritis are to minimize pain, prevent disability, and delay progression.

Some would argue that it is not possible to delay progression in osteoarthritis. However, this is false. If a patient is obese, weight loss will certainly delay the progression of osteoarthritis. The same holds true for diabetes mellitus.

9. D. The most common type of toxicity associated with NSAIDs in elderly patients is gastrointestinal. This may take the form of an acute or chronic gastritis, a peptic ulcer, or a perforated duodenal ulcer. This may result in secondary anemia and other complications.

10. A. NSAIDs (even though a mainstay of treatment for osteoarthritis) have very significant toxicity, especially when used in elderly patients with renal impairment or any other disease. Thus ordinary acetaminophen is safer and must be considered a drug of first choice.

If a NSAID is used for the treatment of osteoarthritis in elderly patients it is suggested that
1) The dose be kept as low as possible.
2) The drug be given with food and preferably with a cytoprotective agent such as misoprostol. In Canada a combination drug known as Arthotec supplies diclofenac and misoprostol together in a single tablet. This may become the preferred method of giving a NSAID to an elderly patient.
3) Avoid NSAIDs with greater propensity to produce side effects (indomethacin, phenylbutazone, and the like).

SOLUTION TO SHORT ANSWER MANAGEMENT PROBLEM 30

Nonpharmacologic treatment:
1. Weight loss
2. Exercise prescription: gentle; gradual; of the following character: gentle regular stretching/mild aerobic/active/isometric
3. Work modification (limiting walking with significant hip or knee osteoarthritis)
4. Regular physiotherapy (heat, cold, ultrasound)
5. TENS (transcutaneous electric nerve stimulation)
6. Walking aids (if a cane, then use on the side opposite the most severely affected side)

Pharmacologic treatment:
1. Acetaminophen for analgesia: drug of first choice
2. NSAIDs (with cytoprotection if possible)
3. Intraarticular steroid injection (limit to easily injectable joints and limit number of injections to 2 to 3/joint)

SUMMARY OF THE DIAGNOSIS AND TREATMENT OF OSTEOARTHRITIS

1. **Diagnosis:** a noninflammatory joint disease characterized by its lack of inflammatory signs and symptoms and characterized by the loss of articular cartilage and degeneration in synovial joints
2. **Prevalence:** most common rheumatologic condition. Eventually everyone develops at least X-rays of this disorder.

3. **Pathology:** proteolytic enzymes (proteoglycans, glycosaminoglycans) produce the characteristic changes in the articular cartilage just described.

4. **Subtypes:** idiopathic and secondary. Secondary osteoarthritis is related to acute or chronic trauma, congenital abnormalities, and certain common conditions including obesity and diabetes mellitus.

5. **Treatment:** divided into nonpharmacologic and pharmacologic. The keys of nonpharmacologic treatment include weight loss; physiotherapy; stretching leading up to a mild aerobic, active, isometric exercise program (swimming is the single best exercise); work modification to limit weight bearing on affected joints; and use of aids such as canes and walkers.

The most important key of pharmacologic therapy is *primum non nocere*—first do no harm. Acetaminophen is the drug of choice because of its relative lack of toxicity in the elderly; if using NSAIDs, use cytoprotection at all times in elderly patients. Limit intraarticular corticosteroid injections to large joints that fail to respond to other measures. Limit the number of injections to any one joint to two or three.

Consider surgery (hip or knee replacement) if all therapies fail and/or osteoarthritis is very severe.

SUGGESTED READINGS

Mourad L, Hoare K, Donohoe K. Alterations in musculoskeletal function. In: McCance KL, Huether SF, eds. Pathophysiology: The biologic basis for disease in adults and children. St. Louis: Mosby, 1994.

Sack K. Osteoarthritis. In Rakel R, ed. Conn's current therapy. Philadelphia: WB Saunders, 1994.

PROBLEM 31   A 35-YEAR-OLD FEMALE WITH TOTAL BODY MUSCLE PAIN

A 35-year-old female presents to your office with a 1-year history of "aching and hurting all over." As well, she complains of a chronic headache, difficulty sleeping, and generalized fatigue. When questioned carefully, she describes "muscle areas tender to touch." Although the pain is "worse in the back," there really is no place where "it doesn't exist."

She also describes headaches, generalized abdomen pains, and some constipation.

On examination, the most striking finding is the presence of 13 discrete "trigger points" (tender muscle areas when palpated). These include the trapezius muscle, the sternomastoid, the masseter muscle, the levator scapulae, the muscles inserting into the area of the greater trochanter, the muscles inserting into the upper border of the patellae, and six areas on the back that together cover almost the entire back area.

The rest of the physical examination is normal. Her blood pressure is 120/70 mm Hg and her CV, respiratory, and abdomen exams are normal.

SELECT THE ONE BEST ANSWER TO THE FOLLOWING QUESTIONS

1. What is the most likely diagnosis in this patient?
   a) polymyalgia rheumatica
   b) masked depression
   c) fibromyalgia
   d) diffuse musculoskeletal pain NYD
   e) early rheumatoid arthritis

2. Which one of the following is not usually a site of tenderness in the disorder described?
   a) the rectus abdominis muscle
   b) the supraspinatus tendon
   c) the lateral epicondyle of the humerus
   d) the trapezius muscle
   e) the middle gluteus muscle

3. The differential diagnosis of the condition described above includes which of the following?
   a) chronic fatigue syndrome
   b) hypothyroidism
   c) masked depression
   d) myofascial pain syndrome
   e) all of the above

4. The diagnostic criteria of the disorder described includes tenderness at how many of 18 specific sites?
   a) 5
   b) 7
   c) 9
   d) 11
   e) 13

5. What is the most characteristic symptom of the condition described?
   a) pain in at least three or four body quadrants
   b) "pain all over my body"
   c) pain in specific bursa and tendons
   d) pain in specific joints
   e) pain in both arms, the posterior neck, and the upper back

6. What is the most important condition that must be considered in the differential diagnosis of the condition described?
   a) generalized anxiety disorder
   b) panic disorder
   c) major depression
   d) rheumatoid arthritis
   e) osteoarthritis

7. What is the cause of this disorder?
   a) an autoimmune process
   b) a chronic inflammatory process
   c) an acute inflammatory process
   d) a slow or chronic virus infection
   e) idiopathic

8. Which of the following statements regarding sleep disorders and the condition described is true?
   a) there is no association between this condition and sleep disorders
   b) patients with this disorder have an abnormal (alpha-delta) sleep
   c) patients with this disorder have difficult sleep induction, early-morning wakening, and nightmares
   d) patients with this disorder have profound insomnia
   e) patients with this disorder usually have profound hypersomnia

9. Regarding therapy for this disorder, which of the following statements is(are) true?
   a) NSAIDs have demonstrated a significant advantage over placebo
   b) antidepressants are superior to placebo
   c) muscle relaxants are superior to placebo
   d) b and c
   e) all of the above are true

10. Regarding the use of corticosteroids in the condition described, which of the following statements is(are) true?
   a) repetitive local injections with corticosteroids/lidocaine should be considered a first-line treatment option

b) oral prednisone has been shown to be effective
c) local injection of steroids/lidocaine should be reserved for resistant cases of this disorder

d) no benefit from oral steroids has been demonstrated
e) none of the above are true

Short Answer Management Problem 31

Review the criteria established by the American Rheumatologic Society for the diagnosis of this condition.

ANSWERS

1. C. This patient has fibromyalgia. Fibromyalgia is characterized by widespread musculoskeletal pain (defined
as pain in three or more qudrants of the body plus axial
pain) and the presence of 11 out of 18 specifically designated tender points or trigger points.

   These musculoskeletal symptoms are often associated with total body pain, severe fatigue, nonrestorative
sleep (alpha-delta sleep), post-exertional increase in
muscle pain, reduced functional ability, recurrent
headaches, irritable bowel syndrome, atypical paraes-
thesia, cold sensitivity (Raynaud's phenomena), aerobic
deconditioning, restless leg syndrome, sleep apnea, and
nocturnal myoclonus.

   Fibromyalgia is much more common in women than
in men and is usually diagnosed between the ages of
35 and 65.

   Rheumatoid arthritis is unlikely because of the lack
of objective evidence of joint warmth, swelling, or deformity, and the multiple soft-tissue areas. Laboratory
evaluation, however, is necessary to exclude this inflammatory condition.

   Polymyalgia rheumatica occurs in an older age group
and will be discussed in another section of this book.

   Diffuse musculoskeletal pain NYD is not a diagnosis.

   A primary diagnosis of masked depression or a somatoform disorder should always be considered when
vague, somatic complaints are accompanied by sleep
disturbance and fatigue. The multiple tender areas,
however, are not usually seen in masked depression.

2. A. Fibromyalgia is associated with tender points, or trigger points, at multiple characteristic locations. These locations include (1) the supraspinatus tendon, (2) the
costochondral junction, (3) the lateral epicondyle of the
humerus, (4) the iliac crest, (5) the greater trochanteric
bursa of the femur, (6) the medial fat pad of the knee,
(7) the suboccipital region of the head, (8) the nuchal
ligament, (9) the trapezius muscle, (10) the infraspina-
tus tendon, (11) the rhomboid muscle, (12) the erector
spinae of the lumbar spine, (13) the middle gluteus
muscle, and (14) the piriformis muscle. An additional
four less anatomically descriptive areas are also included. The rectus abdominous muscle is not included.

The sensitivity of the trigger points can be assessed
by measuring the exact amount of pressure applied over
a certain anatomic site. This can be measured by a do-
lorimeter.

3. E. Fibromyalgia certainly has some vague symtoms, and
the trigger points are the most objective evidence of the
disorder. Many health care professionals, however, still
doubt its authenticity.

   Hypothyroidism and chronic fatigue syndrome present with severe fatigue and share this major symptom
with fibromyalgia.

   Myofascial pain syndrome shares the symptom of
trigger points with fibromyalgia and should be considered in the differential diagnosis.

4. D. The number of trigger points identified by the American College of Rheumatology as being diagnostic of fibromyalgia is 11.

5. B. The most characteristic symptom of fibromyalgia is
the symptom described by patients as "total body muscle
pain." This is a symptom that from clinical experience
appears to have reasonable sensitivity and specificity.

6. C. The most important differential diagnosis of fibromyalgia is major depression or a somatoform disorder. Depression is a very common correlate with fibromyalgia, and it appears that many patients actually
meet the criteria for both disorders. In addition, the
TCAs are recommended for both conditions. In many
cases, the major depression that accompanies fibromyalgia is a masked depression, with many of the
symptoms being somatic in origin.

7. E. The cause of fibromyalgia is unknown. There is no
significant evidence that the process is an autoimmune
process, due to a true acute or chronic inflammatory
process (although this is a possibility), or due to any
type of viral infection.

8. B. The many nonrheumatological features of fibromyalgia include a pattern that is best described as a disorder
of nonrestorative sleep (alpha-delta sleep). Although
other sleep disorders including sleep apnea in a small

minority of patients, nocturnal myoclonus, and restless leg syndrome are associated with fibromyalgia, a disorder of nonrestorative sleep (alpha-delta disorder) is the most common and the most diagnostic.

9. E. There is certainly considerable controversy regarding what pharmacologic medications (if any) work and which do not. Results have been mixed, but it is fair to say that at least some studies have demonstrated favorable results for NSAIDs, tricyclics, and muscle relaxants.

    Because of the sleep disturbances that are often associated with fibromyalgia, it is not recommended that the serotonin reuptake inhibitors (particularly fluoxetine) be used in the treatment of this condition.

10. C. It is currently recommended that local injections of corticosteroid/lidocaine combination be reserved for resistant trigger points because the risk/benefit ratio (especially for repeated injections) is questionable. Muscle atrophy, overlying skin atrophy, fibrosis, infection, abscess formation, and other complications may certainly arise from repeated steroid injections.

SOLUTION TO SHORT ANSWER MANAGEMENT PROBLEM 31

American College of Rheumatology Diagnosis of fibromyalgia:

1. Widespread musculoskeletal pain in three or more quadrants of the body plus axial pain; typically described by patient as "total body muscle pain" or "I hurt all over."
2. The presence of 11 out of a total of 18 specifically designated tender points or trigger points. The major clinical features of fibromyalgia include the following:
    i) Total body pain
    ii) Multiple tender points on examination
    iii) Severe fatigue
    iv) Nonrestorative sleep (alpha-delta sleep)
    v) Post-exertional increase in muscle pain
    vi) Reduced functional ability
    vii) Recurrent headaches
    viii) Irritable bowel syndrome
    ix) Atypical paresthesia
    x) Cold sensitivity (often Raynaud's phenomenon)
    xi) Restless leg syndrome
    xii) Aerobic deconditioning

SUMMARY OF THE DIAGNOSIS AND TREATMENT OF FIBROMYALGIA

1. **Diagnosis:** See the previous section.
2. **Treatment:**
    a) Nonpharmacologic:
        1. Physical therapy (heat, cold, ultrasound, TENS)
        2. Massage therapy
        3. Psychological counseling
        4. Biofeedback
        5. Maximize exercise
    b) Pharmacologic
        1. Tricyclic antidepressants (low dose); prefer the following:
            i) Amitriptyline
            ii) Doxepin
            iii) Nortriptyline
            iv) Trazodone
                Avoid fluoxetine due to exacerbation of insomnia and agitation.
        2. Nonsteroidal antiinflammatory drugs: controversial efficacy
        3. Muscle relaxants: controversial efficacy and controversial appropriateness

SUGGESTED READING

Bennett R. Bursitis, tendinitis, myofascial pain and fibromyalgia. In: Rakel R, ed. Conn's current therapy. Philadelphia: WB Saunders, 1994.

PROBLEM 32   A 25-YEAR-OLD FEMALE WITH CHRONIC FATIGUE

A 25-year-old female presents to your office with a 9-month history of "unbearable fatigue." Before the fatigue began 9 months ago, she worked as a high school chemistry teacher. Since the fatigue began she has been unable to work at all. She tells you that "one day it just hit me—I literally could not get out of bed."

Her past history is unremarkable. She has a husband and two children who have been very supportive during her 9-month illness. She has no history of any significant illnesses, including no history of any psychiatric disease. There is no family history of psychiatric disease.

The other symptoms that the patient describes are difficulty concentrating, headache, sore throat, tender lymph nodes, muscle aches, joint aches, feverishness, difficulty sleeping, abdominal cramps, chest pain, and night sweats.

On physical examination, the patient has a low-grade fever (38.6°), nonexudative pharyngitis, and palpable and tender anterior and posterior cervical and axillary lymph nodes.

SELECT THE ONE BEST ANSWER TO THE FOLLOWING QUESTIONS

1. What is the most likely diagnosis in this patient?
   a) major depressive illness
   b) masked depression
   c) chronic fatigue syndrome
   d) fibromyalgia
   e) malingering

2. What is the etiology of the condition presented here?
   a) unequivocally related to a viral infection
   b) associated with an imbalance of neurotransmitters in the brain
   c) a factitious illness
   d) associated with major psychiatric pathology in almost all cases
   e) unknown

3. In spite of your answer to Question 2, you may wish to reconsider when the question is asked in a somewhat different manner. Which viral agent is more closely linked to this condition than any other viral agent?
   a) influenza A
   b) influenza B
   c) Epstein-Barr virus
   d) parainfluenza virus
   e) polio virus

4. Which of the following statements regarding the condition described is(are) false?
   a) this condition is relatively new
   b) this condition is also known as epidemic neuromyasthenia
   c) this condition is also known as myalgic encephalomyelitis
   d) this condition is also known as multiple chemical sensitivity syndrome
   e) none of the above are false

5. Which of the following statements concerning the epidemiology of the condition described is(are) true?

   a) patients with this condition are twice as likely to be women as to be men
   b) the patients with this condition are likely to be in the 25-to-45 age bracket
   c) clusters of outbreaks of this condition have occurred in many countries over the last 60 years
   d) the primary symptom of this condition may be found in up to 20% of patients attending a general medical clinic
   e) all of the above are true

6. Which of the following best describes the onset of the condition described in the majority of patients?
   a) gradually increasing symptoms over a 3-month period
   b) gradually increasing symptoms over a 6-month period
   c) acute onset of symptoms in a previously healthy, well-functioning patient
   d) chronic onset of symptoms over 1-2 years
   e) the onset of symptoms is extremely variable; it is impossible to predict them with any degree of certainty

7. Which of the following is not a "minor criterion" in the diagnosis of the condition described?
   a) sore throat
   b) mild fever
   c) prolonged generalized fatigue following previously tolerable levels of exercise
   d) sleep disturbance
   e) anxiety or panic attacks

8. Which of the following must be present for the diagnosis of the condition described to be made with certainty?
   a) persisting or relapsing fatigue that does not resolve with bed rest
   b) satisfactory exclusion of other criteria, including preexisting psychiatric conditions
   c) two of (1) low-grade fever, (2) nonexudate pharyngitis, and (3) palpable or tender anterior or posterior cervical lymph nodes

d) a and b only

e) all of the above

9. Regarding the laboratory diagnosis of the condition, which of the following statements is true?
   a) no laboratory test, however esoteric or exotic, can diagnose this condition or measure its severity
   b) a well-defined laboratory test that is sensitive but not specific exists for diagnostic purposes
   c) a well-defined laboratory test that is specific but not sensitive exists for diagnostic purposes
   d) a well-defined laboratory test that is both sensitive and specific exists for diagnostic purposes
   e) a number of laboratory tests in combination are used for definite confirmation of the condition

10. Which of the following has been shown to be the most effective therapy for the condition described?
    a) a tricyclic antidepressant
    b) an NSAID
    c) a sensitive, empathetic physician who is willing to listen
    d) cognitive psychotherapy
    e) none of the above

11. The disorder described is associated with all of the following except:
    a) hypothalamic dysfunction
    b) conversion disorder
    c) alpha-intrusion sleep disorder
    d) chronic immune activation
    e) myofascial pain

12. The disorder described is associated with which of the following symptoms?
    a) sleep disruption
    b) cognitive dysfunction
    c) anxiety and/or depression
    d) neurologic symptoms
    e) all of the above

13. Some evidence suggests that symptoms of the disorder can be induced in healthy individuals through which of the following?
    a) three nights of sleep deprivation
    b) chronic pain resulting from a motor vehicle accident

c) leakage from silicon breast implants

d) *Mycoplasma pneumoniae* infections

e) all of the above

14. Empirical evidence suggests that the best drug(s) to treat symptoms of the disorder is(are) which of the following?
    a) dimenhydrinate
    b) lorazepam
    c) clarithromycin
    d) tryptophan
    e) c and d

15. When using antidepressant medications to treat either the sleep disorder or the mood disorder associated with this condition, what should the dose be?
    a) the usual dose given to treat depression
    b) 1 ½ times the usual dose given to treat depression
    c) ½ the usual dose given to treat depression
    d) ¼ or less of the usual dose given to treat depression
    e) twice the usual dose given to treat depression

16. What is the main therapeutic strategy used to reduce the symptoms of the disorder described?
    a) correct the sleep disorder
    b) provide psychotherapy for the conversion disorder
    c) encourage the development of a support network
    d) encourage the patient to return to work and full activity as soon as possible
    e) none of the above

17. Most patients with the disorder:
    a) fully recover with 2 years
    b) partially recover with 2 years
    c) never recover
    d) are at risk for relapse following recovery
    e) b and d

18. Risk factors for the development of the condition above include which of the following?
    a) a family member with the condition
    b) a recent motor vehicle accident
    c) recurrent immune activation
    d) a spouse with the disorder
    e) all of the above

Short Answer Management Problem 32

Describe the relationship between the described disorder and fibromyalgia.

ANSWERS

1. C. This patient has the clinical manifestations that support a diagnosis of chronic fatigue syndrome. The Center for Disease Control in Atlanta has established a working definition of chronic fatigue syndrome. It consists of major and minor criteria. To make the diagnosis of chronic fatigue syndrome the patient must exhibit the following: both major criteria and either (a) at least six minor symptom criteria plus at least two minor physical criteria or (b) no fewer than eight symptom criteria.

  I. Major criteria:
    1. Persistent or relapsing fatigue or easy fatigability that does not resolve with bed rest and is severe enough to reduce average daily activity by greater than or equal to 50%
    2. Satisfactory exclusion of other chronic conditions, including preexisting psychiatric diseases

  II. Minor criteria:
  Symptoms:
    1. Mild fever (37.5-38.6° C) or chills
    2. Sore throat
    3. Lymph node pain in anterior or posterior cervical or axillary lymph chains
    4. Unexplained generalized muscle weakness
    5. Muscle discomfort, myalgias
    6. Prolonged (>24 hours) generalized fatigue following previously tolerable levels of exercise
    7. New, generalized headaches
    8. Migratory noninflammatory arthralgia
    9. Neuropsychological symptoms: photophobia, transient visual scotomata, forgetfulness, excessive irritability, confusion, difficulty thinking, inability to concentrate, or depression
    10. Sleep disturbance
    11. Patient's description of initial onset of symptoms as acute or subacute
  Physical findings (documented by a physician on at least two occasions at least one month apart):
    1. Low-grade fever (37.6-38.6° oral or 37.8-38.8° rectal)
    2. Nonexudative pharyngitis
    3. Palpable or tender anterior or posterior cervical or axillary lymph nodes (<2 cm in diameter)

2. E.

3. C. The etiology of chronic fatigue syndrome is unknown. There are several common themes underlying attempts to understand the disorder. It is often postinfectious, is often accompanied by immunologic disturbances, and is commonly accompanied by depression.

Among the viral agents that have been implicated as causative agents of chronic fatigue syndrome include the lymphotropic herpesviruses, the retroviruses, and the enteroviruses. The viral agent that is most commonly associated with chronic fatigue syndrome is, however, the Epstein-Barr virus.

4. A. Chronic fatigue syndrome is not a new disease; it has been around for centuries. Certain individuals in the past have been labeled with a variety of diagnoses such as neurasthenia, effort syndrome, hyperventilation syndrome, chronic brucellosis, epidemic neuromyasthenia, myalgic encephalomyelitis, hypoglycemia, multiple chemical sensitivity syndrome, chronic candidiasis, chronic mononucleosis, chronic Epstein-Barr virus infection, and postviral fatigue syndrome.

5. E. Patients with chronic fatigue syndrome are twice as likely to be women as men and are generally 25 to 45 years of age.

Cases are recognized in many developed countries. Most arise sporadically, but over 30 clusters of similar illnesses have been reported.

The most famous of such outbreaks occurred in Los Angeles County Hospital in 1934; in Akureyri, Iceland, in 1948; in the Royal Free Hospital, London, in 1955; in Punta Gorda, Florida, in 1945; and in Incline Village, Nevada, in 1985.

The prevalence of chronic fatigue syndrome is difficult to estimate because this is entirely dependent on case definition. Chronic fatigue itself is a ubiquitous symptom, occurring in as many as 20% of patients attending a general medical clinic; the syndrome itself is much less common.

6. C. The typical case of chronic fatigue syndrome arises suddenly in a previously active and healthy individual. An otherwise unremarkable flu-like illness or some other acute stress is recalled with great clarity as the triggering event. Unbearable exhaustion is left in the wake of the incident. Other symptoms, such as headache, sore throat, tender lymph nodes, muscle and joint aches, and frequent feverishness lead to the belief that an infection persists. Then, over several weeks, the impact of reassurances offered during the initial evaluation fades as other features of the syndrome become evident such as disturbed sleep, difficulty in concentration, and depression.

7. E. Panic attacks and anxiety are not minor criteria as defined by the CDC definition given.

8. D. The only criteria that must be present to make the diagnosis of chronic fatigue syndrome are the major criteria as outlined in the case definition. The diagnosis can be made by eight or more symptom criteria being present.

9. A. No laboratory test, however exotic or esoteric, can make the diagnosis of chronic fatigue syndrome. Elabo-

rate, expensive laboratory workups should be avoided; they only make an already complicated picture even more so.

10. C. A sensitive, empathetic physician who is willing to listen is the most effective intervention that can be offered for chronic fatigue syndrome.

Nonsteroidal antiinflammatory agents alleviate headache and diffuse pain and feverishness. Nonsedating antidepressants improve mood and disordered sleep and thereby attenuate the fatigue to some degree.

The ingestion of caffeine and alcohol at night makes it harder to sleep, compounding fatigue, and should be avoided. Nothing, however, takes the place of an empathetic physician.

In terms of psychotherapy, the most effective therapy appears to be behavior-oriented therapy, not cognitive psychotherapy.

11. B. Chronic fatigue syndrome is not a conversion disorder, nor is it a psychosomatic illness. Current research describes immune dysfunction in which T cells are chronically activated and hypothalamic dysfunction presumably due to cytokine penetration of the blood-brain barrier. Alpha-intrusion sleep disorder is also probably due to cytokine penetration and may be worsened by myofascial pain, if present.

12. E. Chronic fatigue syndrome may be classified as mild, moderate, or severe, depending on the number of symptoms present. Severe chronic fatigue syndrome may include not only fatigue, myofascial pain, and sleep disruption but also numerous neurologic complaints such as blurred vision, migrating paresthesias, and tinnitus. Mood disruption may be present; either depression or anxiety or both are often endogenous, reflecting neurochemical dysequilibrium. Cognitive dysfunction may be severe, with complaints of poor memory, poor concentration, and the inability to read.

13. E. The symptoms of chronic fatigue syndrome can be induced in healthy individuals after only three nights of sleep disruption. This reduces stage 3, stage 4, or REM sleep. Individuals who develop significant post-MVA back pain to the degree that it causes sleep disruption may also develop chronic fatigue syndrome. If immune activation is the initial trigger for the disease, it may be the result of many pathogens, not just Epstein-Barr virus (parvovirus and *Mycoplasma pneumoniae* are other pathogens implicated).

There is an initial suggestion that the chronic immune activation caused by macroscopic and microscopic leakage of silicon from breast implants may be also associated with chronic fatigue syndrome symptoms.

14. E. The effectiveness of NSAIDs in treating some of the symptoms of chronic fatigue syndrome and the use of tricyclic antidepressants to treat the anxiety and depression sometimes associated with the disorder have already been discussed.

However, empirical evidence suggests that the best drugs to treat chronic fatigue syndrome may be tryptophan (an amino acid) and clarithromycin (an erythromycin derivative). Tryptophan is a precursor of serotonin and promotes deep sleep. Clarithromycin is an antibiotic that will treat many infective agents, among them *Mycoplasma pneumoniae*.

15. D. Empirical evidence suggests that patients with chronic fatigue syndrome lose their tolerance to many agents, including toxins such as secondhand cigarette smoke, certain fumes, alcohol, and medications. Antidepressants, such as amitriptyline, should be initially given to chronic fatigue patients in a dose approximately 1/4 of the usual dose, although gradual tolerance may develop. When higher doses are used, physicians should carefully watch for symptoms of neurological toxicity, which may, according to some, leave permanent deficits.

16. A. The main therapeutic strategy in treating chronic fatigue syndrome should be to correct the sleep disorder. If the sleep disorder can be reduced and a period with more stage 3, stage 4, or REM sleep attained, the number of symptoms and their severity may be greatly reduced. This includes not only the symptoms of fatigue and pain but also the neurologic and mood/cognitive complaints. Patients required to return to work early when still symptomatic tend to suffer relapses and actually prolong their illness.

17. E. Most patients with chronic fatigue syndrome recover within 2 years, often to the extent that they can return to work and resume most of the normal activities of their previous life. They are, however, at risk for relapse at any time (especially at times where they experience immune activation or sleep disruption).

18. E. Risk factors for the development of chronic fatigue syndrome include a family member (especially a spouse) with the disorder, recurrent immune activation, and a recent MVA.

SOLUTION TO SHORT ANSWER MANAGEMENT PROBLEM 32

The relationship between chronic fatigue syndrome and fibromyalgia is fascinating. There certainly seems to be some connection between the two disorders. Some authorities believe that fibromyalgia and chronic fatigue syndrome are actually the same illness with different presentations. Clinicians see patients with more pain than fatigue, with more fatigue than pain, or with both fatigue and pain. Both fibromyalgia and chronic fatigue syndrome appear to share the alpha-intrusion sleep disorder.

SUMMARY OF THE DIAGNOSIS AND MANAGEMENT OF CHRONIC FATIGUE SYNDROME

1. **Prevalence:** difficult to establish: one study suggests a prevalence of 37 cases/100,000 people.

   Chronic fatigue syndrome is not a new disease; it has been present for centuries. Most evidence for the disorder comes from outbreaks of the disorder, discussed earlier.

2. **Etiology:** the etiology of chronic fatigue syndrome is unknown. Chronic fatigue syndrome, does, however, appear to be related to infectious agents (especially the Epstein-Barr virus and perhaps *Mycoplasma pneumoniae*) and immunologic disturbances; T-cell activation may play a prominent role. Cytokines also appear to be involved. Alpha-intrusion sleep disorder appears to be related to cytokine involvement.

3. **Signs and symptoms:** the best diagnostic criteria at present have been set by the CDC in Atlanta. These criteria are listed in the answer to Question 1. It is important to diagnose and treat other syndromes, including major depressive disorder, which may complicate the picture.

4. **Course:** most patients partially recover within 2 years. All, however, are prone to relapse.

5. **Treatment:**
   a) Nonpharmacologic: an understanding physician who is prepared to spend time with the patient and listen and counsel in an empathetic fashion
   b) Pharmacologic: empiric evidence suggests that the treatments of choice are L-tryptophan and clarithromycin. Please note that this is empiric evidence.

      Other pharmacologic agents that have been shown to be effective include NSAIDs and the tricyclic antidepressants. Select the dose carefully and begin at $\frac{1}{4}$ of the useful dose for healthy patients.

SUGGESTED READING

Straus S. Chronic fatigue syndrome. In: Isselbacher K et al., ed. Harrison's principles of internal medicine. 13th Ed. New York: McGraw-Hill, 1994.

PROBLEM 33   A 45-YEAR-OLD MALE WITH EXCRUCIATING PAIN IN HIS LEFT FOOT

A 45-year-old obese male presents to the ER in the middle of the night screaming and holding his left foot. He tells you that he thinks he has an "acute blood vessel blockage" in his left toe. He wakes up the entire ER observation unit with his screams.

His past history is significant for essential hypertension, for which he has been treated with a thiazide diuretic for the past 5 years. He categorically relates to you that he has never had the symptoms that he is experiencing now (and further adds that instead of all these questions he would prefer if you just got on with treatment).

On examination the patient's temperature is 38° C and his blood pressure is 170/110 mm Hg. He has an inflamed, tender, swollen left great toe. There is extensive swelling and erythema of the left foot, and his whole foot is tender. No other joints are swollen. No other abnormalities are found on P/E.

SELECT THE ONE BEST ANSWER TO THE FOLLOWING QUESTIONS

1. What is the most likely diagnosis?
   a) acute cellulitis
   b) acute gouty arthritis
   c) acute rheumatoid arthritis
   d) acute septic arthritis
   e) acute vasculitis

2. Which of the following statements regarding this man's condition is(are) false?
   a) the disease is more common in males than in females
   b) fever is unusual
   c) more than 50% of the initial attacks of this condition are confined to the first metatarsophalangeal joint
   d) peripheral leukocytosis can occur
   e) involvement is usually asymmetric

3. What is the definitive diagnostic test of choice for this patient's condition?
   a) a plasma level
   b) a random urine determination
   c) a 24-hour urine determination
   d) a synovial fluid analysis
   e) a Gram stain plus culture and sensitivity

4. What is the most common metabolic abnormality found in the condition described in this patient?
   a) increased production of uric acid
   b) decreased renal excretion of uric acid
   c) increased production of uric acid metabolites
   d) decreased renal excretion of uric acid metabolites
   e) none of the above

5. What is the pharmacologic agent of choice for the initial managemet of this patient's condition?
   a) indomethacin
   b) colchicine
   c) acetaminophen
   d) aspirin
   e) phenylbutazone

6. Regarding the prophylaxis recommended for the prevention of future attacks of the condition described in the patient, which of the following would most accurately describe the current recommendation (as applied)?
   a) this patient probably should not be treated with a prophylactic agent
   b) this patient should be treated with a uricosuric agent as prophylaxis against future attacks of this condition
   c) this patient should be treated with a xanthine oxidase inhibitor as prophylaxis against future attacks of this condition
   d) this patient could be treated with either a uricosuric agent or a xanthine oxidase inhibitor as prophylaxis against future attacks of this condition
   e) none of the above

7. The determination of the agent of choice for the prophylaxis of the condition described is made by which of the following?
   a) a serum blood level
   b) a joint fluid aspiration
   c) a 24-hour urine determination
   d) a joint X-ray
   e) none of the above

8. Which of the following drugs increase(s) the excretion of uric acid?
   a) sulfinpyrazone
   b) probenecid
   c) allopurinol
   d) a and b only
   e) all of the above

9. In patients started on prophylactic therapy, which of the following statements regarding the use of prophylactic agents is(are) true?
   a) the patient who is begun on a prophylactic agent should also be started on colchicine
   b) colchicine should be added and maintained for 3-6 mo
   c) indomethacin can replace colchicine in this instance
   d) none of the above statements are true
   e) all of the above statements are true

10. Which of the following drugs would be most likely to provide significant relief in the case of an acute attack of the condition described?
    a) oral prednisone
    b) oral decadron
    c) IV SoluCortef
    d) IV SoluMedrol
    e) intraarticular triamcinolone hexacetonide

11. Which of the following classes of drugs is most likely to precipitate the condition described?
    a) thiazide diuretics
    b) calcium-channel blockers
    c) ACE inhibitors
    d) beta blockers
    e) alpha blockers

12. The condition described is associated with an elevated blood level of a certain metabolite. Which of the following statements concerning this association is true?
    a) the blood level of the metabolite referred to is elevated
    b) the blood level of the metabolite referred to is depressed
    c) if the blood level of the metabolite referred to is abnormal, treatment should be considered to prevent the condition described even if there are no symptoms
    d) a and c are true
    e) b and c are true

Short Answer Management Problem 33

Discuss the indications for the use of prophylactic agents in hyperuricemic states.

ANSWERS

1. B. This patient has acute gouty arthritis. This actually is a very typical presentation for gout.

   With acute gout, the patient usually develops an acute pain in a joint of the lower extremity, with the most common joint by far being the metatarsophalangeal joint of the big toe. The pain of acute gout often wakes the patient from sleep, and the patient ends up in the ER with a pain that is described as crushing or excruciating.

   The joint rapidly becomes erythematous, swollen, warm, and extremely tender. The skin surrounding the joint is usually tense and shiny. The swelling in acute gout often extends well beyond the joint itself and may involve the entire foot (or other part of the extremity). This swelling, due to periarticular edema, makes the differentiation from septic arthritis particularly difficult. Often the patient is unable to bear weight on the affected foot.

2. B. Fever may occur in patients with gout, especially in patients with polyarticular disease. The temperature may reach 39.5° C (103-104° F).

   The metatarsophalangeal joint is the location of the acute gouty attack in over 50% of patients experiencing their first attack. Most first attacks are asymmetric. If untreated, involvement of other joints of the foot may occur simultaneously or follow rapidly. Acute gout may also involve the bursae or the tendon sheaths.

   Leukocytosis may also be seen. Tophi are occasionally seen with the first attack. Usually, however, there is a time interval (often 10 years or more) between the initial attack and the appearance of the complication of a gouty tophi.

   Gout is more common in men than in women. In women it most often occurs following menopause.

3. D. The ultimate diagnosis of gout is made by demonstrating negatively birefringent, needle-shaped crystals under a polarizing microscope. This examination should be attempted in all patients suspected of having gout. Although an elevated serum uric acid concentration is usually seen with acute gout, it is neither as sensitive nor as specific a test as the demonstration of uric acid crystals under the microscope from the synovial fluid.

   The diagnosis of septic arthritis can be ruled out by appropriate Gram stains and cultures of the same specimen of synovial fluid as obtained for examination with the polarizing microscope.

4. B. The most common metabolic abnormality associated with gout is decreased renal excretion of uric acid. This may be a primary or a secondary event. Secondary causes such as chronic renal disease, acute ethanol ingestion, and diuretic (especially thiazide diuretic) therapy are associated with the development of elevated serum uric acid levels and subsequent gout. The most common cause of overproduction of uric acid is a myeloproliferative or lymphoproliferative disorder. In addition, when a patient is undergoing cancer chemotherapy there is a very significant liberation of uric acid from dying cells. The greater the responsiveness of

the tumor to chemotherapy or radiotherapy, the quicker is the tumor breakdown and the more extensive the breakdown of uric acid.

5. A. Until recently, colchicine was the drug of choice for the treatment of acute gout. This agent, however, has many gastrointestinal side effects that limit its usefulness, especially with the frequency and dose needed in acute gout (hourly).

NSAIDs such as indomethacin 50 mg tid are now the drugs of choice in most settings. The NSAIDs should ideally be given for a 1- to 2-week period until treatment aimed at decreasing the uric acid pool is begun.

Aspirin taken in small doses can actually aggravate the problem. Acetaminophen has no antiinflammatory activity and is not indicated in the acute treatment of gout. Phenylbutazone is an excellent antiinflammatory agent but has been associated with bone marrow suppression and aplastic anemia.

Prednisone or other corticosteroids can be used to treat patients with acute gout who have not responded to other therapies and in patients in whom other therapies are contraindicated.

6. A. From the history, you gather that this is the first attack of acute gout in this patient. The current recommendation suggests that it is not advisable to begin prophylactic therapy until the patient has had at least two attacks, or perhaps three. This recommendation is made for two reasons: (1) if there is a precipitating secondary cause (as in this patient the treatment of hypertension with a thiazide diuretic), it may very well be able to be eliminated; and (2) because a second attack may not occur for years (if at all), the risk/benefit ratio for prophylactic medication is not favorable.

7. C.

8. D. The choice of a prophylactic agent (if one is going to be used) is made by determining the 24-hour secretion of uric acid. The normal uric acid excretion in 24 hours is 250-750 mg/24 hours (1.5-4/4 mmol/day). If the patient excretes significantly more uric acid than 750 mg/24 hours, he is producing too much uric acid, and the production should be slowed by treatment with a drug that inhibits production. The rate determining step in the synthetic pathway depends on the enzyme xanthine oxidase. Allopurinol, the usual drug given, is an inhibitor of xanthine oxidase. If the patient excretes less than 250 mg/24 hours of uric acid, then the metabolic problem rests with the failure to excrete the uric acid once it is produced. In this case, drugs that increase the excretion rate, known as uricosuric agents, should be used. The two most common drugs in this class are probenecid and sulfinpyrazone.

9. E. As previously discussed, the prophylactic agents for the prevention of gouty arthritis fall into two classes: the xanthine oxidase inhibitors (which inhibit the formation of uric acid) and the uricosuric agents (which increase the excretion of uric acid).

When prophylaxis against recurrent attacks is begun, either colchicine (in low dose—0.6 mg bid) or a NSAID such as indomethacin (in low dose—25 mg bid) should be added to the choice of the prophylactic agent for 3 to 6 months. The cholchicine or indomethacin can then be discontinued, and the patient can remain on the uricosuric agent or the xanthine oxidase inhibitor indefinitely.

If the uricosuric agent is the preferred treatment because of the 24-hour urine uric acid determination, the following rules should be followed:
1) Uricosuric agents should be used only in patients under the age of 60 years.
2) Uricosuric agents should be used only in patients with normal renal function.
3) Uricosuric agents should be used only in patients who have no history of renal stone formation.
4) Uricosuric agents should be used only in patients who are not overproducers of uric acid.

The preferred dosage of a uricosuric agent such as probenecid is a starting dose of 250 mg bid with increases as necessary up to 1500 mg bid. Sulfapyrazine is usually begun at a dosage of 50 mg bid with gradual increases up to 100 mg bid.

Allopurinol is indicated in patients with urate overproduction, history of renal stones, renal impairment, and age greater than 60.

Interestingly enough, there is significant evidence that allopurinol is also effective in patients who are underexcreters of uric acid (in spite of what has been said about the 24-hour urine acid production).

10. E. A local injection of a corticosteroid such as triamcinolone hexacetonide, 20 mg, into an inflamed gouty joint reliably produces a resolution of the acute gouty condition. This treatment appears to be most beneficial in patients with acute gouty monarthritis of a large joint (which may receive injections reliably) and in patients with resistant attacks in whom coexistent infection has been excluded.

11. A. Diuretics in general, and thiazide diuretics in particular, elevate the serum uric acid level. Although the vast majority of patients who are receiving thiazide diuretics do not develop gout, those that do tend to be on relatively high doses of thiazide (anything greater than 25 mg) and have other coexistent reasons for the development of gout (such as acute ethanol intake).

It has been conclusively shown that increasing the dosage of a thiazide diuretic past 12.5-25 mg/day will not improve hypertension control; instead it will simply increase the probability of significantly elevated uric acid levels.

The six metabolic side effects of thiazide diuretics are as follows: hyperuricemia, hyperglycemia, hyperlipidemia, hypokalemia, hyponatremia, and hypomagnesemia.

12. A. The condition being discussed in this question is asymptomatic hyperuricemia. The question that arises from this condition is, "Should it be treated?" The answer is no.

Asymptomatic hyperuricemia is most commonly due to a pharmacologic agent; that pharmacologic agent is most commonly a thiazide diuretic. Even though a thiazide diuretic (especially in high dose) can produce a very significant increase in the serum uric acid level, well over 95% of patients with asymptomatic hyperuricemia remain asymptomatic. Thus the treatment of asymptomatic hyperuricemia is not recommended.

SOLUTION TO SHORT ANSWER MANAGEMENT PROBLEM 33

The prophylactic agents used in the prevention of recurrence of acute gout have been discussed in detail. In brief review, prophylactic agents should be used only if the patient has had more than one attack of gout, a gouty tophi develops, there is X-ray evidence of joint destruction from the gouty arthritis, or there is a history of urolithiasis.

SUMMARY OF THE DIAGNOSIS AND TREATMENT OF ACUTE GOUT

1. **Diagnosis:** firmly established by examination of joint aspirate under a polarizing microscope (negatively birefringent uric acid crystals)

2. **Symptoms:** acute onset of pain in a joint of the lower extremity; most commonly the first metatarsophalangeal joint. Along with the pain there are associated tenderness, erythema, and swelling of the surrounding tissues.

3. **Differential diagnosis:** the most important differential diagnosis in acute gout is septic arthritis.

4. **Pathophysiology:** acute gout is most often associated with a decreased renal excretion of uric acid (rather than an overproduction of uric acid).

5. **Treatment:**
   a) Acute attack:
      1) Indomethacin 50 mg tid or qid for 2-3 days and 25 mg tid or qid for an additional 4 or 5 days
      2) Colchicine: an alternative agent (0.5-0.6 mg orally every hour until joint symptoms improve or there is the onset of toxicity)
   b) Prophylactic treatment:
      1) Not given after only one attack
      2) Choose either a uricosuric agent or a xanthine oxidase inhibitor. Choice is based on the results of the 24-hour urine uric acid determination plus other factors previously discussed.
      3) If prophylaxis is given, then use either indomethacin or colchicine in low dose in addition to your prophylactic agent for 3 to 6 months.
      4) Do not treat asymptomatic hyperuricemia.

SUGGESTED READING

Yood R. Hyperuricemia and gout. In: Rakel R, ed. Conn's current therapy. Philadelphia: WB Saunders, 1994.

PROBLEM 34   A 61-YEAR-OLD FEMALE WITH SEVERE BACK PAIN

A 61-year-old female presents to your office for assessment of severe back pain, which she has had for the past 2 years and has been getting progressively worse. The pain is described in the following manner:

1. Location: mid-thoracic area ("on the spine itself")
2. Quality: basically a dull "background pain" with sharp, shooting exacerbations
3. Quantity: baseline quantity 7/10; incremental increase to 9/10; incremental decrease to 6/10
4. Chronology: began 2 years ago when she slipped, fell, and injured her back on a newly waxed floor in her home. Since that time, the pain has been getting progressively worse.
5. Constant/intermittent: The dull pain is relatively constant, whereas the sharp pain comes and goes.
6. Aggravating factors: movement of any kind; lateral rotation of the spine
7. Alleviating factors: rest and acetaminophen
8. Pain history: no previous significant chronic pain syndromes until this pain began 2 years ago
9. Treatments employed:
   A. Nonpharmacologic: "the chiropractor has helped."
   B. Pharmacologic: acetaminophen 500 mg tid
10. Provocative maneuver: physical exam: pain elicited on pressing on T7 and T8
11. Quality of life: before the pain began, the patient was active in her garden and social activities; at this time, however, she is severely limited. Before pain began: quality of life 10/10; since pain began: quality of life 3/10.

On examination, the patient has an obvious kyphosis. As mentioned, she is tender at both T7 and T8 on the midpoint of the vertebrae. The patient has a body mass index of 19. No other abnormalities are found on P/E.

SELECT THE ONE BEST ANSWER TO THE FOLLOWING QUESTIONS

1. The patient's pain as described is most likely due to which of the following:
   a) degenerative arthritis
   b) vertebral compression fractures secondary to osteoporosis
   c) osteoarthritis
   d) an intervertebral disc that has been dislocated
   e) spinal stenosis

2. What is the most likely pathology of the condition described?
   a) osteoporosis type I
   b) osteoporosis type II
   c) osteoarthritis type I
   d) osteoarthritis type II
   e) nerve root impingement secondary to spinal stenosis

3. How is osteoporosis defined?
   a) an increased turnover of calcium in newly formed bone
   b) a failure to deposit inorganic mineral in newly formed organic bone matrix
   c) a lack of calcium in newly formed bone
   d) a decrease in bone mass in the absence of a mineralization defect
   e) a decrease in both bone mass and matrix in trabecular and cortical bone

4. How is osteomalacia defined?
   a) an increased calcium turnover
   b) a failure to deposit inorganic mineral in newly formed organic bone matrix
   c) a lack of calcium in newly formed bone
   d) a decrease in bone mass in the absence of a mineralization defect
   e) a decrease in both bone mass and matrix in trabecular and cortical bone

5. Osteoporosis can be subdivided into types I and II. Which of the following bone sites is not associated with type II osteoporosis?
   a) the vertebral column
   b) the femoral neck
   c) the proximal humerus
   d) the proximal tibia
   e) the pelvis

6. Which of the following is(are) not an established risk factor for osteoporosis?
   a) postmenopausal status
   b) sedentary lifestyle
   c) cigarette smoking
   d) obesity
   e) alcohol intake

7. What is the most common presenting condition of osteoporosis?
   a) wrist fracture (Colles' fracture)
   b) vertebral compression fracture
   c) fracture of the neck of the femur
   d) fracture of the head of the femur
   e) the proximal tibia

8. What is the most common site for type I osteoporotic fractures?
   a) the distal radius
   b) the thoracic vertebra
   c) the lumbar vertebra
   d) head of the femur
   e) the neck of the femur

9. What is the most common site for type II osteoporotic fractures?
   a) the neck of the femur
   b) the head of the femur
   c) the thoracic vertebrae
   d) the lumbar vertebrae
   e) the pelvis

10. Which of the following sites of osteoporosis is most commonly associated with morbidity and mortality?
   a) the head of the femur
   b) the neck of the femur
   c) the thoracic vertebrae
   d) the lumbar vertebrae
   e) the distal radius

11. What is the treatment of first choice for the prevention of osteoporosis?
   a) conjugated estrogen 0.625 mg/day plus medroxy-progesterone acetate 10 mg/day on days 1-13 of the calendar month
   b) conjugated estrogen 1.25 mg/day plus medroxy-progesterone acetate 10 mg/day on days 1-13 of the calendar month
   c) calcium carbonate 1000 mg-1500 mg/day
   d) conjugated estrogen 1.25 mg/day
   e) etidronate (Didronel) 16 mg/day

12. Which of the following statements regarding the use of calcium carbonate in the treatment of osteoporosis is true?
   a) calcium carbonate (1000 mg-1500 mg/day) should be begun at menopause
   b) calcium carbonate (1000 mg-1500 mg/day) should be begun within 2 years of the onset of menopause
   c) calcium carbonate (1000 mg-1500 mg/day) should be begun between 35 and 40 years of age
   d) calcium carbonate has not been shown to be beneficial in the prevention or treatment of osteoporosis
   e) calcium carbonate is contraindicated in the management of osteoporosis

13. Which of the following is(are) recommended treatments for established osteoporosis?
   a) calcitonin
   b) calcium carbonate
   c) estrogen
   d) diphosphonate etidronate
   e) all of the above

Short Answer Management Problem 34

Discuss the relationship between the treatment of osteoporosis and the prevention of cardiovascular disease in postmenopausal women.

ANSWERS

1. B. This patient has one or more vertebral compression fracture(s) at midthoracic sites. This is a common cause of back pain in this age group, especially among women, and especially among women who also have kyphosis, another manifestation of osteoporosis. The pain associated with vertebral compression fractures can be severe and should be treated accordingly.

   The 11-point pain history described was purposefully put into the question. This can serve as a valuable tool in the evaluation of patients with any pain syndrome.

2. A. Osteoporosis can be divided into two subtypes as follows:
   Type I osteoporosis:
      Population: primarily occurs in postmenopausal women

   Pathology: decrease in trabecular bone mass
   Primary locations: trabecular bone is primarily located in the vertebral bodies and in the distal forearm; associated with fractures in both areas.
   Type II osteoporosis:
      Population: occurs in both sexes in the seventh decade of life or later.
      Pathology: decrease in both trabecular and cortical bone mass
      Primary locations: include the femoral neck, the proximal humerus, the proximal tibia, and the pelvis

3. D. Osteoporosis is defined as a decrease in bone mass in the absence of a mineralization defect.

4. B. Osteomalacia is defined as a failure to deposit inorganic mineral in newly formed organic bone matrix.

5. A. Type II osteoporosis is not associated with osteoporosis in the vertebral column (see the detailed explanation for this in Question 2).

6. D. The established risk factors for osteoporosis include the following:
Female sex
Postmenopausal status
Low skeletal mass
Poor musculature
Sedentary lifestyle
Cigarette smoking
Caucasian race
Excessive alcohol intake
Fair skin
Low calcium intake
Diabetes mellitus
Anorexia nervosa
Pernicious anemia
Excessive activity with associated secondary amenorrhea
   Obesity, one of the choices listed, appears to be protective against osteoporosis.

7. B. Vertebral compression fracture is the most common presenting condition of Type I (postmenopausal) osteoporosis. Wrist fracture (Colles' fracture) is the second most common presenting condition.

8. B. The most common site for type I osteoporosis is thoracic vertebrae (usually around T7-T9).

9. A.

10. B. The most common site for type II osteopororis is the neck of the femur. In addition to being the most common site for type II osteopororis, it is also the most common cause of osteoporosis-related morbidity and mortality due to fracture of the neck of the femur.

11. A. The recommended treatment for the prevention of osteoporosis is conjugated estrogens 0.625 mg/day continually plus medroxyprogesterone acetate 10 mg from days 1-13 of the calendar month.

12. C. Calcium carbonate, as a means of preventing osteoporosis, is recommended to begin at age 35 to age 40.

13. E. Following is a summary of the treatment of established osteoporosis:
   1) Calcitonin (Calcimar, Miacalcin), 50-100 IU subcutaneously/day
   2) Estrogen 0.625 mg/day throughout the month; Provera 10 mg on days 1-13 of calendar month
   3) Calcium carbonate 1500 mg/day (note: begin calcium carbonate as preventative therapy)
   4) Vitamin D 400 IU/day—questionable
   5) Diphosphonate etidronate (Didronel) 400 mg/day for 2 weeks, followed by vitamin D for an additional 8 to 10 weeks. The cycle is repeated every 10-12 weeks. Sodium fluoride has not been found to be effective in the treatment of established osteoporosis.

SOLUTION TO SHORT ANSWER MANAGEMENT PROBLEM 34

The relationship between the treatment of osteoporosis in postmenopausal women and the prevention of cardiovascular disease is estrogen. Estrogen (usually given in the form of Premarin 0.625 mg/day or alternatively as an Estraderm patch 50 μg/twice/week) has been found to be protective against the development of all forms of atherosclerotic vascular disease in postmenopausal women. The relative risk of a postmenopausal woman on estrogen replacement therapy developing CV compared to a woman who is not is approximately 50%. Having stated this, however, there still is not enough evidence to recommend that all woman in the postmenopausal period be treated with estrogen replacement; rather, it should be on the basis of a risk factor analysis.

SUMMARY OF THE DIAGNOSIS AND TREATMENT OF OSTEOPOROSIS

1. **Definition:** decrease in bone mass in absence of mineralization defect. Differentiate osteoporosis from osteomalacia, the latter being a group of diseases characterized by failure to deposit the inorganic mineral phase in newly formed bone.
2. **Classification:**
Type I: vertebra, distal forearm
Type II: femoral neck, proximal humerus, proximal tibia, pelvis
3. **Pathology:**
Type I: trabecular bone only
Type II: trabecular and cortical bone
4. **Treatment:** estrogen/progesterone, calcitonin, calcium carbonate, diphosphonate etidronate, vitamin D (controversial).

SUGGESTED READING

Barzel U. Osteoporosis. In: Rakel R, ed. Conn's current therapy. Philadelphia: WB Saunders, 1994.

PROBLEM 35   A 29-YEAR-OLD FEMALE WITH FATIGUE, ANOREXIA, AND BLOODY URINE

A 29-year-old female presents to your office with symptoms of extreme fatigue, no appetite, and bloody urine. She developed a very sore throat 3 weeks ago, but she did not have it examined or treated. Her 6-year-old daughter had the same sore throat 1 week before her. Her doctor (over the phone) said, "Viral infection, Mother; don't worry about it."

Three days ago she began to have bloody urine, and swelling of her hands and feet, and she felt terrible.

Her past health has been excellent. There is no family history of significant illness. She has no allergies.

On examination, she has significant edema of both lower extremities. Her blood pressure is 170/105 mm Hg. Her blood pressure was last checked 1 year ago; at that time it was normal.

SELECT THE ONE BEST ANSWER TO THE FOLLOWING QUESTIONS

1. What is the most likely diagnosis in this patient at this time?
   a) hemorrhagic pyelonephritis
   b) IgA nephropathy (Berger's disease)
   c) poststreptococcal glomerulonephritis
   d) hemorrhagic cystitis
   e) membranous glomerulonephritis

2. Which of the following is(are) pathognomonic of the disorder described?
   a) macroscopic hematuria
   b) microscopic hematuria
   c) macroscopic or microscopic hematuria
   d) red blood cell casts
   e) protein >1.0 g/24 h

3. Approximately 4 weeks after the mother develops her symptoms, her daughter comes down with an illness characterized by swelling of a number of joints with erythema and pain, bumps on both of her elbows, significant fatigue, fever, and a skin rash covering her body.

   On examination, the daughter has a grade III/VI pansystolic murmur. Her blood pressure is 100/70 mm Hg.

   What is the most likely diagnosis in her daughter's case?
   a) juvenile rheumatoid arthritis
   b) Still's disease
   c) Postviral arthritis syndrome
   d) rheumatic fever
   e) autoimmune complex disease

4. Which of the following statements regarding the prevention of the two conditions (the mother's condition and the daughter's condition) is true (assume a 10-day course of penicillin in all of the choices)?
   a) the mother's condition is preventable by penicillin; the daughter's condition is not
   b) the mother's condition is not preventable by penicillin; the daughter's condition is
   c) both the mother's condition and the daughter's condition are preventable by treatment with penicillin

   d) neither the mother's condition nor the daughter's condition is preventable by treatment with penicillin
   e) prevention is variable with both conditions: penicillin can prevent both conditions, but it may not prevent either

5. What is the treatment of choice for the condition described in the mother?
   a) penicillin
   b) gentamicin
   c) prednisone
   d) a and b
   e) none of the above

6. Which of the following statements concerning prognosis of the condition described in the mother is(are) true?
   a) most patients with this disorder eventually develop end-stage renal failure
   b) the prognosis in the mother depends on how aggressively the antecedent streptococcal infection is treated
   c) most patients with the acute disease recover completely within 1 to 2 years
   d) 5% to 20% of patients with this acute disease end up with progressive renal disease
   e) c and d

7. Which of the following is(are) complications of the general disease process described in the mother?
   a) hypertensive encephalopathy
   b) congestive cardiac failure
   c) acute renal failure
   d) a and b
   e) all of the above

8. Which of the following subtypes of the disease presented in the mother is(are) associated with group A beta-hemolytic streptococcus?
   a) minimal change
   b) focal segmental sclerosis
   c) membranous
   d) diffuse proliferative
   e) crescentic

9. Which of the following subtypes of the disease presented in the mother is most closely associated with nephrotic syndrome?
    a) minimal change
    b) focal segmental sclerosis
    c) membranous
    d) diffuse proliferative
    e) crescentic

10. What is the most common cause of chronic renal failure?
    a) glomerulonephritis (acute to chronic)
    b) chronic pyelonephritis
    c) diabetes mellitus
    d) hypertensive renal disease
    e) congenital anomalies

11. What is the least common cause of chronic renal failure among the following causes?
    a) glomerulonephritis (acute to chronic)
    b) chronic pyelonephritis
    c) hypertensive renal disease
    d) diabetes mellitus
    e) congenital anomalies

12. Which of the following antihypertensive agents is contraindicated in patients with chronic renal disease?
    a) hydrochlorothiazide-triamterene
    b) furosemide
    c) prazosin
    d) nifedipine
    e) alpha-methyldopa

13. What is the major cause of death in patients with chronic renal failure?
    a) uremia
    b) malignant hypertension
    c) hyperkalemia-induced arrhythmias
    d) myocardial infarction
    e) subarachnoid hemorrhage

14. What is the anemia usually associated with chronic renal failure?
    a) hypochromic
    b) macrocytic
    c) normochromic-normocytic
    d) microcytic
    e) hypochromic-microcytic

15. Which of the following may be indicated in the treatment of a patient with chronic renal failure?
    a) limitation of dietary protein
    b) sodium supplementation
    c) calcium supplementation
    d) a and b
    e) all of the above

16. Which of the following is/are associated with nephrotic syndrome?
    a) proteinuria > 3.5 g/day
    b) edema
    c) hypoalbuminemia
    d) hypercholesterolemia
    e) all of the above

17. Which of the following statements regarding nephrotic syndrome is(are) false?
    a) most patients with nephrotic syndrome progress to chronic renal failure
    b) some cases of nephrotic syndrome are drug induced
    c) Hodgkin's disease may lead to nephrotic syndrome
    d) preeclamptic toxemia may lead to nephrotic syndrome
    e) none of the above statements are false

18. Which of the following statements regarding diabetes mellitus and chronic renal failure is(are) true?
    a) diabetes mellitus is an uncommon cause of chronic renal failure
    b) diabetes mellitus type I is a more common cause of chronic renal failure than diabetes mellitus type II
    c) diabetes mellitus type II is a more common cause of chronic renal failure than diabetes mellitus type I
    d) diabetes mellitus type II does not lead to chronic renal failure
    e) diabetes mellitus type I does not lead to chronic renal failure

19. The treatment of nephrotic syndrome includes which of the following?
    a) corticosteroids
    b) loop diuretics
    c) thiazide diuretics
    d) protein restriction
    e) all of the above

20. What percentage of patients with any of the primary glomerulonephropathies present with a nephrotic syndrome–like picture?
    a) 10%
    b) 20%
    c) 40%
    d) 50%
    e) 75%

21. Comparing the recommended treatment of poststreptococcal glomerulonephritis with the recommended treatment on nonpoststreptococcal glomerulonephritis, which of the following statements is most accurate?
    a) the treatment protocols are the same
    b) corticosteroid treatment is indicated in both PSGN and NPSGN

c) corticosteroid treatment is generally indicated in NPSGN but not in PSGN
d) corticosteroid treatment is generally indicated in PSGN but not in NPSGN

e) the prognosis of neither PSGN nor NPSGN depends on the presence or absence of treatment

---

Short Answer Management Problem 35

Discuss the importance of the use of NSAIDs as a cause of renal dysfunction in elderly patients.

ANSWERS

1. C.

2. D. This patient has poststreptococcal glomerulonephritis. Poststreptococcal glomerulonephritis is the most common cause of acute glomerulonephritis. The syndrome may begin as early as 2 weeks after the initial streptococcal infection. In patients with mild disease, there may be no signs of symptoms. In more severe disease, the symptoms of malaise, headache, mild fever, flank pain, edema, hypertension, and pulmonary edema may occur. Oliguria is common. The urine is often described as bloody, coffee colored, or smoky.

   The red blood cell casts are found in the urine of patients with acute glomerulonephritis and are pathognomonic for this condition. Other notable abnormalities include an elevated ESR and an elevated ASO titer.

3. D. In this case, the daughter of the patient has developed rheumatic fever. The Jones criteria for the diagnosis of rheumatic fever include the following:

MAJOR CRITERIA:	MINOR CRITERIA:
1. Carditis	1. Arthralgias
2. Polyarthritis	2. Fever
3. Chorea	3. Elevated ESR
4. Erythema marginatum	4. Elevated C-reactive protein
5. Subcutaneous nodules	5. Prolonged PR interval on ECQ

   Two major criteria or one major criterion and two minor criteria are virtually diagnostic of rheumatic fever.

   It is important to realize that in some parts of the United States, the incidence of rheumatic fever is rising, not falling. This has been a relatively recent phenomenon and is a cause for concern in terms of the treatment (or lack of treatment) of *streptococcal pharyngitis*.

4. B. Poststreptococcal glomerulonephritis is not preventable by penicillin; rheumatic fever, on the other hand, is preventable. In both conditions, the cause of complications is group A beta-hemolytic streptococcus. Once the clinical or laboratory diagnosis of streptococcal pharyngitis is made, therapy with penicillin should be instituted and continued for a period of 10 days.

5. E. The primary treatment of acute glomerulonephritis associated with streptococcal infection is symptomatic. Although penicillin will eradicate the carrier state of group A beta-hemolytic streptococci, it will not influence the course of the glomerulonephritis.

   Symptomatic treatment should include bed rest and protein restriction (if the BUN or creatinine level is elevated). Fluid overload should be treated with loop diuretics such as furosemide or ethacrynic acid. If acute renal insufficiency develops and volume overload is unresponsive to diuretics, hemodialysis should be considered.

6. E. Most patients with acute glomerulonephritis recover completely within 1 to 2 years. On the other hand, 5% to 20% of patients with end up with progressive renal damage. The treatment of the antecedent streptococcal infection has no bearing on the prognosis (as has been indicated).

7. E. Complications of acute post-streptococcal glomerulonephritis include hypertensive encephalopathy, congestive cardiac failure, acute renal failure, chronic renal failure (5%-20%), and nephrotic syndrome.

8. D.

9. A. Poststreptococcal glomerulonephritis usually presents as a diffuse proliferative glomerulonephritis. Nephrotic syndrome, on the other hand, usually presents as minimal change glomerulonephritis.

10. C. The most common cause of chronic renal failure is diabetes mellitus, not glomerulonephritis. Forty percent of patients with type I diabetes mellitus eventually develop diabetic nephropathy chronic renal failure. Twenty percent of patients with type II diabetes mellitus develop diabetic nephropathy and subsequent chronic renal failure.

11. B. Chronic pyelonephritis is the least likely cause of chronic renal failure of those listed. Chronic pyelonephritis rarely leads to chronic renal failure in the absence of obstruction.

12. A. Potassium-sparing diuretics such as the Triamterene component of a mixed thiazide-potassium-sparing diuretic combination. This is due to the production of hyperkalemia. All of the other agents, including hydrochlorothiazide (alone), furosemide, prazosin, nifedipine, and alpha-methyldopa are safe to use in chronic renal failure. The dosage of all of these agents, however, should be reduced when renal failure supervenes.

    In addition to the potassium-sparing diuretics, the ACE inhibitors can also significantly raise the serum potassium level. Thus they must never be used in patients with chronic renal failure who are receiving any kind of potassium-sparing diuretic or other potassium supplement for any reason. Second, they are at least relatively contraindicated when patients develop the degree of renal insufficiency necessary to produce chronic renal failure.

13. D. The major causes of death in patients with chronic renal failure are myocardial infarction and CVAs, secondary to atherosclerosis and arteriolosclerosis. Uremia itself can be controlled by dialysis or renal transplantation. Hypertension is usually controllable by individualized antihypertensive therapy. Arrhythmias, although they do occur in these patients, are not the major cause of death. Subarachnoid hemorrhage, as a subset of a CVA, does occur but is less common as a cause of death than myocardial infarction.

14. C. The anemia of chronic renal failure is usually normochromic-normocytic. Hematocrit often starts to decrease when the serum creatinine reaches 200-300 umol/L (2-3 mg/dl) or when the glomerular filtration rate has decreased to about 20-30 ml/min. The etiology of the normochromic-normocytic anemia is probably a decreased synthesis of erythropoietin by the kidney.

15. E. Treatment of chronic renal failure may include any of the following:
    a) Limitation of dietary protein
    b) Careful control of water balance: fluid intake should be sufficient to maintain adequate urine volume, but no attempt should be made to force diuresis. If edema is present, a cautious trial of furosemide or ethacrynic acid is indicated, with careful monitoring of serum electrolytes.
    c) Electrolyte supplementation/restriction: sodium supplements may be required to restore sodium losses. Potassium intake may have to be restricted or supplemented. In severe hyperkalemia, acute measures to remove potassium may be required.
    d) Mineral supplementation/restriction: in the presence of bone disease (renal osteodystrophy), treatment with phosphate binders and supplemental calcium may be necessary.

16. E. Nephrotic syndrome, as previously mentioned, is most closely associated with minimal change glomerulonephritis.

    Nephrotic syndrome is characterized by albuminuria (>3.5 g/day), hypoalbuminemia, hyperlipidemia, edema, hypertension, and renal insufficiency.

17. A. Most cases of nephrotic syndrome do not in fact lead to chronic renal failure. It depends entirely on the etiology. The causes of nephrotic syndrome are as follows:
    I. Primary glomerular diseases (all subtypes)
    II. Secondary to infections (including post-streptococcal glomerulonephritis)
    III. Drugs (such as penicillamine and gold)
    IV. Neoplasia (as in Hodgkin's disease)
    V. Multisystem disease (SLE Goodpasture's syndrome)
    VI. Endocrine diseases (diabetes mellitus)
    VII. Miscellaneous (preeclamptic toxemia)

18. C. As stated before, diabetes mellitus is the most common cause of chronic renal failure. Although the prevalence is less common in type II (20%) as opposed to type I (40%) diabetes, the prevalence of type II diabetes is actually 10 times the prevalence of type I diabetes. The logical conclusion from this consideration is that type II diabetes mellitus is a more common cause of chronic renal failure than type I diabetes mellitus.

19. E.

20. B. Nephrotic syndrome is treated with nonpharmacologic symptomatic therapies such as protein restriction and excessive fluid restriction, pharmacologic symptomatic therapies such as thiazide and loop diuretics, and antiinflammatory/immunosuppressive therapies (prednisone and cytotoxic drugs). It has certainly been demonstrated that antiinflammatory drugs such as prednisone enhance the potential for the disorder to attain remission. The usual protocol includes high-dose corticosteroid therapy followed by a gradual reduction to the point where alternate-day therapy with prednisone is introduced.

    The natural history proposed for nephrotic syndrome suggests that approximately 20% of patients who present with a primary glomerulonephropathy of some kind will develop nephrotic syndrome.

21. C. The most important difference in therapy between post-streptococcal glomerulonephritis and non–post-streptococcal glomerulonephritis is corticosteroid therapy (useful in NPSGN but not in PSGN). In NPSGN corticosteroids can be used both in the primary presentation and in recurrences.

SOLUTION TO SHORT ANSWER MANAGEMENT PROBLEM 35

Nonsteroidal antiinflammatory drugs (NSAIDs) are a major concern due to their ability to induce nephrotoxicity, especially in elderly patients. Nephrotoxicity as a potential problem when beginning or maintaining elders on NSAIDs is frequently either not thought of or ignored. The NSAID Suldinac has been suggested as a possible exception to this problem as the one NSAID that will not cause nephrotoxicity, but extreme caution is still required. NSAID use is the most common cause of renal insufficiency in the elderly. When considering prescribing an NSAID to an elderly patient, it is wise to follow clinical practice guidelines that resemble the following:

Clinical Practice Guidelines

1. Establish a definitive diagnosis.
2. Ask yourself this question: is this an inflammatory condition? If yes, an NSAID is reasonable (as in rheumatoid arthritis). If no (as in osteoarthritis), is there an alternative medication that will provide relief with minimal adverse effects, such as acetaminophen plain or acetaminophen with a small amount of codeine (8 mg)?
3. If you decide to start an elderly patient on an NSAID, perform baseline renal function including a 24-hour urine for creatinine clearance and protein.
4. Consider choosing an NSAID with a favorable efficacy/renal toxicity profile (such as Suldinac).
5. Begin with the lowest dose.
6. Consider gastric protection to avoid gastric problems: gastritis, peptic ulcer, and reflux esophagitis. If you decide to use an H_2 receptor block, consider one demonstrated to have a favorable efficacy/side effect profile in the elderly (such as ranitidine).
7. Recheck the patient's renal function in 3 months.
8. Continue to monitor the efficacy/side effect profile at all times and always ask yourself this question: are you doing more good than harm?
9. Never combine an NSAID and a potassium-sparing diuretic, or an NSAID and an ACE inhibitor in an elderly patient. This can and will produce rapid and potentially fatal hyperkalemia.

Remember, first do no harm.

SUMMARY OF THE DIAGNOSIS AND TREATMENT OF RENAL DISEASES

1. **Glomerulonephritis:**
   a) Classification (simplified):
      1. Streptococcal glomerulonephritis (PSGN)
      2. Non–post-streptococcal glomerulonephritis(many subtypes) (NPSGN)
   b) Symptoms and signs:
      1. Malaise
      2. Headache
      3. Anorexia
      4. Low-grade fever
      5. Edema
      6. Hypertension
      7. Gross hematuria with red blood cell casts
      8. Proteinuria
      9. Impaired renal function
      Remember: Not all that appears to be congestive heart failure actually is. For example, uremic pericarditis is often diagnosed as congestive heart failure and mistreated with diuretic therapy. Increased JVP does not always equal congestive heart failure.
   c) Treatment:
      1. PSGN = symptomatic: protein restriction, fluid restriction, thiazide and loop diuretics
      2. NPSGN = symptomatic (as described) plus corticosteroids: initially high dose with gradual tapering; alternate-day therapy suggested as ideal
2. **Nephrotic syndrome:**
   a) Etiology and prevalence:
      1. Many and diverse causes
      2. Twenty percent of primary glomerulonephropathies develop into nephrotic syndrome.
   b) Signs/symptoms:
      1. Edema
      2. Hypoalbuminemia
      3. Hyperalbuminuria (greater than 3.5 g/day)
      4. Hypertension
      5. Hyperlipidemia
      6. Renal insufficiency
   c) Treatment: Symptomatic:
      1. Protein restriction
      2. Fluid restriction
      3. Thiazide and loop diuretics
      4. Prednisone
      5. Cytotoxic agents
3. **Chronic Renal Failure:**
   a) Causation: Most common cause = diabetes mellitus; Most common type of DM = type II
   b) Symptoms/signs/laboratory findings:
      1. Weakness
      2. Fatigability
      3. Headaches
      4. Anorexia
      5. Nausea and vomiting
      6. Pruritus
      7. Polyuria
      8. Nocturia
      9. Hypertension
      10. Congestive heart failure
      11. Pericarditis
      12. Anemia
      13. Azotemia

14. Acidosis
15. Elevated serum potassium
16. Decreased serum potassium
17. Decreased serum protein

c) Treatment:
    1. Protein restriction
    2. Careful fluid balance
    3. Potassium restriction or supplementation
    4. Calcium supplementation
    5. Phosphate removal

6. Hypertension control
7. Hemodialysis or peritoneal dialysis
8. Renal transplantation

SUGGESTED READINGS

Cattran DC. Primary glomerular diseases. In: Rakel R, ed. Conn's current therapy. Philadelphia: WB Saunders, 1994.

Palmer BF. Chronic renal failure. In: Rakel R, ed. Conn's current therapy. Philadelphia: WB Saunders, 1994.

PROBLEM 36   A 27-YEAR-OLD FEMALE WITH SPINA BIFIDA AND BILATERAL CVA ANGLE PAIN

A 27-year-old female presents to the ER with a 4-day history of fever, chills, and bilateral CVA (costovertebral angle) pain. She has an indwelling urinary catheter and describes to you "at least 12 of these episodes before this current one." She has been seeing the same family physician since birth and has been diagnosed as having "nervous bladder and kidney syndrome." He has prescribed some OTC "kidney pills" in the past for these symptoms. She tells you that they "never really worked," and she has often found herself bedbound with symptoms for several weeks before the fever broke.

You, the ER doctor on shift, are somewhat skeptical about the nervous bladder and kidney syndrome.

On examination, the patient is flushed. Her temperature is 40° C. She has intermittent shaking rigors. She has a CVA tenderness bilaterally. Her abdomen is somewhat tender to palpation.

There is blood in the catheter collection bag.

SELECT THE ONE BEST ANSWER TO THE FOLLOWING QUESTIONS

1. What is the most likely diagnosis in this patient?
   a) nervous bladder and kidney syndrome
   b) acute hemorrhagic cystitis
   c) acute urethritis
   d) acute pyelonephritis
   e) SBBSS (the newly named spina bifida bladder spasm syndrome)

2. What would be the most likely organism in this patient?
   a) a gram-positive coccus
   b) a gram-positive rod
   c) an anaerobic organism
   d) a fungal organism
   e) a gram-negative organism

3. Which of the following bacteria would not likely be considered as highly probable of causing this problem?
   a) *Pseudomonas* sp.
   b) *Klebsiella pneumoniae*
   c) *Enterobacter*
   d) group A beta-hemolytic streptococcus
   e) *Proteus*

4. Following a urinalysis and a urine specimen for C and S, you should now treat the patient with which of the following?
   a) the OTC kidney pills
   b) ciprofloxacin 500 mg tid po (outpatient)
   c) Septra DS two tabs bid po (outpatient)
   d) IV antibiotics in hospital
   e) IM antibiotics

5. What is the antibiotic of first choice for this patient?
   a) IV cephalosporin (third generation)
   b) IV gentamicin
   c) IV ciprofloxacin
   d) IV ampicillin
   e) IV Septra

6. The investigations that should be performed on this patient at this time include which of the following?
   a) serum BUN/creatinine
   b) renal ultrasound
   c) blood cultures
   d) CBC/diff
   e) all of the above

7. What is the most likely diagnosis in this patient?
   a) chronic pyelonephritis
   b) uterovesical reflux
   c) hydronephrosis
   d) vesicular diverticuli
   e) none of the above

8. Which of the following statements regarding chronic prophylaxis in this patient is(are) true?
   a) chronic prophylaxis is not indicated
   b) chronic prophylaxis is unlikely to be of any benefit
   c) chronic prophylaxis may make a significant difference in the preservation of this patient's renal function
   d) chronic prophylaxis will be difficult due to resistant organisms
   e) none of the above are true

9. A 34-year-old female presents with a 3-day history of hematuria, dysuria, increased urinary frequency, and nocturia. She has had no fever, no chills, no CVA tenderness, and no back pain.
   On examination, she does not look ill. Her temperature is 37.5° C. Her abdomen is nontender. There is no costovertebral angle tenderness.
   What is the most likely diagnosis?
   a) Berger's disease (IgA nephropathy)
   b) acute hemorrhagic cystitis
   c) acute hemorrhagic urethritis
   d) acute glomerulonephritis
   e) acute cystitis with concomitant coagulation disorder

10. What is the treatment of choice for the patient described in Question 9?
   a) a 10-day course of ampicillin and probenecid
   b) a 7-day course of ampicillin and probenecid

c) a 3-day course of TMP-SMX
d) a 1-day course of TMP-SMX
e) a single dose of ampicillin 3.5 g + probenecid 1 g

11. You have now decided on your therapeutic plan for the patient described in Question 10. At what time would you implement this plan?
a) right away: forget about the cultures—you likely have a big enough "gun" to kill everything in sight anyway
b) right away: start therapy immediately after taking the urine specimen for C and S
c) tomorrow: send the urine culture stat and order the pathologist to call you with the result personally
d) tomorrow: send the urine culture and ask the pathology department for a report as soon as possible without aggravating the pathologist
e) whenever: send the urine culture and when you get it back call the patient. if the symptoms have not cleared up then consider starting the antibiotic

12. What is the most likely organism involved in the infection that has developed in the patient in Question 10?
a) *Pseudomonas*
b) *Providencia*
c) *E. coli*
d) *Klebsiella*
e) *Enterococcus*

13. The Quinolone antibiotics (such as ciprofloxacin and norfloxacin) are a very significant advance in antimicrobial treatment. They also work by a unique mechanism. The mechanism(s) of action is(are):
a) bactericidal mode of action
b) inhibition of DNA gyrase
c) blocks resealing of the nicks on the DNA strands induced by the alpha subunit
d) degradation of the DNA by exonucleases
e) all of the above

Short Answer Management Problem 36

Discuss a classification of urinary tract infections in adult males and adult females.

ANSWERS:

1. D. This patient has acute pyelonephritis. First, she has very significant predisposing factors for urinary tract infections, including an indwelling urinary catheter and a neurologic condition that increases the probability of same. Second, she seems to have had some less than optimal medical diagnoses. Third, she almost certainly has had recurrent episodes of pyelonephritis. This raises the possibilities of chronic pyelonephritis, reflux kidney damage, and resistant organisms.

Fourth, the symptoms fit. Fever, chills, and CVA pain in a patient with a neurologic predisposing condition and an indwelling catheter = acute pyelonephritis.

2. E. First, this patient is classified as having a complicated urinary tract infection. A complicated urinary tract infection occurs when any of the following are present in the patient: obstruction (stones), indwelling urinary catheter, high postvoid residual urine volume, anatomic or functional genitourinary abnormalities, renal impairment, and renal transplantation.

Although the most common organism is a gram-negative organism, it is frequently an organism that would not occur in patients without urinary tract disease. Examples include *Proteus, Providencia, Serratia, Pseudomonas,* and *Klebsiella.* Overall, *E. coli* (one of many serotypes and one most likely to be resistant to many antibiotics) is probably still the most common organism.

3. D. The only organism listed that is an unlikely candidate is group A beta-hemolytic streptococcus.

4. D. This patient has not had any of the following at any time in the past:
A. A proper assessment
B. An accurate diagnosis
C. Proper treatment

At this time, she should be hospitalized, with IV fluids, IV antibiotics, and a complete assessment of both urinary tract function and urinary tract damage. In addition, ways of preventing future infections should be considered.

5. C. At this time, the drug of choice would probably be IV ciprofloxacin. Ciprofloxacin is certainly indicated for complicated urinary tract infections and will cover most if not all gram-negative organisms including *Proteus* and *Pseudomonas.* It would also be reasonable to use a combination of ampicillin and gentamicin or a third-generation cephalosporin and gentamicin. As you were asked to choose one antibiotic, Ciprofloxacin would probably be the best choice.

6. E. At this time, a complete workup should be done. This should include the following (as a minimum):
   A. Blood
      1. CBC/diff
      2. Serum BUN/creatinine
      3. Electrolytes
      4. Blood cultures if temp >39.5°
   B. Urine:
      1. Complete urinalysis
      2. Urine for C and S
      3. Urine for WBC casts and RBC casts
      4. 24-hour urine for creatinine clearance and protein
   C. Diagnostic imaging:
      1. Renal and abdominal ultrasound
      2. IVP

7. A. This patient's abnormal ultrasound (confirmed by an IVP) is likely to show small, shrunken kidneys secondary to repeated urinary tract infections that have gone untreated. It is important from this time onward to measure renal function regularly and do everything possible to preserve this patient's renal function.

8. C. First, repeated urine cultures must be done to determine the dominant organisms growing. Next, the susceptibility/resistance of these organisms needs to be determined to guide prophylactic therapy. It is difficult to say at this time what that therapy should be; it all depends on the results, but it certainly needs to be done.

9. B. This patient has acute hemorrhagic cystitis. Acute hemorrhagic cystitis is simply a variant of acute cystitis, and it is no more difficult to treat and does not have any more complications than other forms of acute cystitis.

10. C. Patients with uncomplicated UTIs respond well to a 3-day treatment regime. This abbreviated course of management is a good compromise between a 1-day course of therapy and the conventional 7- to 14-day regimes. The relapse rate with the 3-day regime is comparable to longer courses of therapy. An abbreviated therapy is also more cost-effective and is associated with fewer adverse drug effects than the more prolonged courses of therapy.

    Trimethoprim-sulfamethoxazole (TMP-SMX) is certainly a drug of first choice for uncomplicated urinary tract infections at the present time. The other drug of first choice would be a quinolone derivative such as norfloxacin.

11. B. You should not wait to begin therapy. Start immediately after you obtain the urine specimen for culture. Ask for the result as soon as possible, but don't aggravate the pathologist.

12. C. This is a case of uncomplicated urinary tract infection. Hemorrhagic cystitis cannot really be considered a complication. With an uncomplicated infection, you are likely going to be dealing with an uncomplicated organism. Therefore, *E. coli* is the most likely organism involved in the infection.

    There are many serotypes of *E. coli* that can produce urinary tract infection; some serotypes are more likely to produce hemorrhagic cystitis; others are more likely to produce nonhemorrhagic cystitis.

13. E. The quinolone antibiotics are a significant advance in antimicrobial therapy. They use a totally unique mechanism of action. These antibiotics are extremely effective against many gram-positive and especially gram-negative organisms. The quinolone antibiotics work essentially at a molecular genetic level.

    The quinolone antibiotics are bactericidal in action. Action is achieved mainly by inhibition of the DNA gyrase. This is an essential component of the bacterial DNA replication system. The inhibition of the alpha subunit of the DNA gyrase blocks the resealing of the nicks on the DNA strands induced by this alpha subunit, leading to the degradation of the DNA by exonucleases.

SOLUTION TO SHORT ANSWER MANAGEMENT PROBLEM 36

1. Females:
   A. Uncomplicated lower tract infections:
      1. Acute cystitis
      2. Acute hemorrhagic cystitis
   B. Complicated upper tract infections:
      1. Acute pyelitis
      2. Acute pyelonephritis
   C. Conditions likely to increase the risk of acquiring a complicated urinary tract infection:
      1. Diabetes mellitus
      2. Stone disease
      3. Chronic indwelling catheterization
      4. Immunosuppression
      5. Pregnancy
      6. Neuropathic bladder
      7. Congenital anomalies (reflux)
      8. Urethral stenosis
      9. Urinary tract obstruction
   D. Sexually transmitted urinary tract infections:
      1. Acute urethritis
         a) *Chlamydiae trachomatis*
         b) *Mycoplasma hominis*
         c) *Ureaplasma urealyticum*
         d) *Neisseria gonorrhea*

2. Males:
   A. Uncomplicated urinary tract infection: very rare in the absence of obstruction except for acute prostatitis
   B. Complicated urinary tract infections:
      1. Acute cystitis: needs to be investigated with renal ultrasound
      2. Acute pyelitis
      3. Acute pyelonephritis
      4. Chronic prostatitis

   The most common complicating factor in males is obstruction caused by benign prostatic hypertrophy/hyperplasia. However, all males with a urinary tract infection not due to an STD need to be investigated. The minimal investigation is a renal ultrasound.
   C. Sexually transmitted diseases:
      1. Acute urethritis:
         a) *Chlamydiae trachomatis* (NGU)
         b) *Mycoplasma hominis* (NGU)
         c) *Ureaplasma urealyticum* (NGU)
         d) *Neisseria gonorrhea* (GU)
      2. Acute epididymo-orchitis: *Chlamydiae trachomatis*

SUMMARY OF THE DIAGNOSIS AND TREATMENT OF URINARY TRACT INFECTION

1. **Classification:** see the short answer management problem.
2. **Signs/symptoms:**
   a) Lower tract: Dysuria, frequency, nocturia, hematuria, terminal dribbling, discharge (STDs)
   b) Upper tract: same as lower tract plus fever, chills, costovertebral angle pain/tenderness

3. **Laboratory:**
   a) Urinalysis, urinalysis for C and S (lower tract)
   b) CBC, blood cultures, 24-hour urine for creatinine clearance and protein, renal ultrasound, IVP
4. **Complications:**
   a) Evaluate each patient in terms of risk factors.
   b) Avoid indwelling catheterization whenever possible.
5. **Treatment:**
   a) Lower tract (females):
      1. Three-day course of trimethoprim-sulfamethoxazole
      2. Pyridium for analgesia
   b) Upper tract:
      1. Ciprofloxacin
      2. Ampicillin plus gentamicin
      3. Third-generation cephalosporin
   c) Inpatient versus outpatient: Acute pyelonephritis: hospitalize those with complications or complicating diseases; otherwise outpatient IV port therapy daily or high-dose oral therapy
   d) Prophylaxis: consider for high-risk patients: first choice, quinolones or macrodantin
   e) Sexually transmitted diseases:
      1. Gonorrhea: Rocephin IM (250 mg) + doxycycline for 10-14 days
      2. Nongonococcal urethritis: Doxycycline for 10-14 days

SUGGESTED READING

Arsdalen K. The urogenital tract. In: Rakel R, ed. Conn's current therapy. Philadelphia: WB Saunders, 1994.

PROBLEM 37   A 15-YEAR-OLD DISTRESSED ADOLESCENT WITH "THE ZITS"

A 15-year-old female presents to your office with a complaint of the "zits." She has been attempting to treat these with frequent washings and avoidance of cosmetics and other facial products. She is very distressed and breaks down crying. She is afraid that "no boys will ever be interested in me with such an ugly face."

Her past history is unremarkable. She is on no medications at present. She has no allergies. Her family history is unremarkable.

On physical examination the patient has multiple maculo-papular-pustular lesions with comedones on her face and back. No other abnormalities are found on examination.

SELECT THE ONE BEST ANSWER TO THE FOLLOWING QUESTIONS

1. What is the diagnosis in this patient?
   a) zits type IIb comedome syndrome
   b) zits type IIa comedome class B syndrome
   c) acne vulgaris
   d) rosacea
   e) propionibacterium acne class II

2. What is the treatment of first choice in this patient at this time?
   a) topical tretinoin
   b) intralesional corticosteroids
   c) topical benzoyl peroxide
   d) topical erythromycin
   e) oil-based antiacne moisturizers

3. The patient returns. There has been an improvement of about 20% in the skin lesions since her first visit. She has gradually increased the strength of the preparation you gave her.
   What would you do at this time?
   a) D/C the first agent and treat her with topical benzoyl peroxide
   b) D/C the first agent and treat her with topical tretinoin
   c) continue the first agent and add topical tretinoin
   d) D/C the first agent and treat her with topical erythromycin
   e) continue the first agent and add topical erythromycin

4. The patient returns again in another 4 weeks. She has now sustained an improvement of about 35% in the lesions since her first visit, and continues to execute your instructions faithfully. However, she is still not satisfied, and neither are you.
   What would you do at this time?
   a) D/C the first and second agents and substitute a systemic antibiotic
   b) continue the first and second agents and add a systemic antibiotic
   c) continue the first and second agents and add topical clindamycin or erythromycin
   d) continue the first and second agents and add oral 13-*cis*-retinoic acid
   e) continue the first and second agents, and add a new "oil-free" product that through your local pharmaceutical detail man you have learned "kills acne bugs dead"

5. The patient, as instructed, returns again in 1 month. She has now sustained an improvement of about 50% but is still not satisfied.
   What would you do at this time?
   a) throw up your hands in disgust and say "I give up"
   b) refer her to the first dermatologist who comes to mind
   c) tell her to "hang in there" for a little longer
   d) stop all the medication you have started her on and try something else
   e) continue all three agents you have started her on and add a systemic antibiotic

6. An 18-year-old male presents with moderately severe nodular-pustular acne on his face and back. What would be your agent of first choice in this case?
   a) topical benzoyl peroxide
   b) topical tretinoin
   c) systemic tetracycline
   d) systemic erythromycin
   e) 13-*cis*-retinoic acid

7. The patient described in Question 6 returns in 6 weeks with only moderate improvement.
   What would you now prescribe?
   a) systemic tetracycline
   b) systemic erythromycin
   c) cyproterone acetate
   d) 13-*cis*-retinoic acid
   e) none of the above

8. Closed comedomes are associated with the condition described. What is a closed comedome also known as?
   a) a whitehead
   b) a blackhead
   c) a pustule
   d) a maculo-papule
   e) a carbuncle

9. Open comedomes are associated with the condition described. What is an open comedome also known as?
   a) a whitehead
   b) a blackhead
   c) a pustule
   d) a maculo-papule
   e) a carbuncle

10. Which of the following statements concerning the association of certain foods with certain diseases and health care outcomes is/are true?
    a) chocolate can exacerbate acne vulgaris
    b) shellfish can exacerbate acne vulgaris
    c) nuts can exacerbate acne vulgaris
    d) shellfish and nuts, although not associated with acne, are associated with certain other important public health outcomes
    e) none of the above

11. Which of the following bacteria is associated with the condition described above?
    a) *Staphylococcus aureus*
    b) *Streptococcus viridans*
    c) *Propionibacterium acnes*
    d) all of the above
    e) none of the above

12. Which of the following is(are) essential for a good skin-care program specifically designed for patients with the described disorder?
    a) oil-free products
    b) frequent skin washings
    c) manual manipulation of skin lesions
    d) a and b
    e) all of the above

13. On further questioning you learn that the patient described in Question 1 has just stopped the oral contraceptive pill (last month). Which of the following statements regarding the possible use of oral/topical antibiotics in the patient above is(are) true?
    a) if the patient goes back on the pill, oral tetracycline is the systemic agent of choice for her acne
    b) if the patient goes back on the pill, oral tetracycline (for acne) is unlikely to have any effect on the OCP's efficacy
    c) if the patient goes back on the pill, because of the potential interaction with certain antibiotics, a very low-dose OCP should be used
    d) all of the above
    e) none of the above

14. What is(are) the absolute contraindication(s) to the use of oral isotretinoin for the treatment of acne vulgaris?
    a) children under the age of 14

b) women of childbearing potential who are not adequately protected against pregnancy
c) allergy to topical tretinoin
d) all of the above
e) none of the above

15. Which of the following is(are) true concerning rosacea?
    a) rosacea occurs in middle-aged individuals
    b) rosacea consists of papules and pustules on the face
    c) rosacea produces a background erythema and telangiectasias on the face
    d) all of the above
    e) none of the above

16. What is the first-line treatment of rosacea?
    a) topical benzoyl peroxide
    b) topical tretinoin
    c) topical erythromycin or clindamycin
    d) topical metronidazole
    e) none of the above

17. What is the second-line treatment of rosacea?
    a) topical metronidazole
    b) oral metronidazole
    c) oral tetracycline
    d) oral 13-*cis*-retinoic acid
    e) oral erythromycin

18. Which of the following conditions is(are) sometimes associated with rosacea?
    a) rhinophyma
    b) cellulitis
    c) multiple carbuncle formation
    d) cavernous sinus thrombosis
    e) anaerobic septicemia

19. Which of the following is a disease associated with the complication suggested in Question 18?
    a) immune deficiency: T-cell lymphopenia
    b) immune deficiency: B-cell lymphopenia
    c) alcoholism
    d) septic arthritis
    e) erysipelas

20. To decrease the inflammatory reaction that is typically produced by the application of topical tretinoin, you should consider which of the following?
    a) using lower percentages of tretinoin only
    b) applying tretinoin only every second day
    c) limit the application of tretinoin to every second week
    d) ask the pharmacist to mix one part tretinoin to one part hydrocortisone in a cream base
    e) none of the above

Short Answer Management Problem 37

Describe the pathophysiology of acne vulgaris.

ANSWERS

1. C.

2. C.

3. C.

4. C.

5. E.

6. C.

7. D. This patient has acne vulgaris. Acne vulgaris affects most teenagers and continues to affect many patients into their twenties and their thirties.

   The treatment of choice for acne can take many forms, but a commonsense approach is outlined below. In this approach, only one drug is added at a time; this allows you to evaluate clearly the efficacy of that agent.

   This approach may need to be amended if the patient presents with a nodular-pustular acne in the beginning (as in Questions 6 and 7).

   Treatment regimen for acne vulgaris:

   1. Acne washes: Acne wash agents such as chlorhexidine are somewhat effective if used regularly.
   2. Treatment protocol for mild to moderate acne:
      1. Begin with topical benzoyl peroxide 2.5%. Increase to 5% and 10% rapidly. This product is preferably given in gel form because it is less drying. Benzoyl peroxide is best given in the morning.
      2. Add topical tretinoin. This is a vitamin A derivative and comes in strengths of 0.025% and 0.050% cream and 0.01% gel. The delivery system of choice again is the gel form because it is less drying. Topical tretinoin is best given at night. Remember to tell your patient to expect redness and irritation of the face, especially in the initial period. Urge them not to discontinue the product because of this side effect.
      3. Add topical erythromycin or topical clindamycin. This should be used in combination with 1 and 2. If there are significant lesions on the back that are difficult to get at for the patient (even at the beginning of treatment) you may need to prescribe a systemic antibiotic from the beginning.

      4. Add systemic tetracycline to the topical benzoyl peroxide and topical tretinoin. Continue the topical antibiotic.
   3. Moderate to severe nodular pustular acne:
      1. Begin with systemic tetracycline. The starting dose is 500 mg bid. An alternative is systemic erythromycin.
      2. Add 13-cis-retinoic acid systemically. Use 1 mg/kg/day for a total of 20 weeks.

   In Question 1, choices a, b, and e do not exist.

8. A.

9. B. Acne is either obstructive or inflammatory. Obstructive acne is manifested by closed comedomes, or whiteheads. Inflammatory acne is manifested by papules, pustules, nodules, cysts, and ultimately, in some cases, scars.

10. D. There is no indication that the intake of certain foods is associated with acne. This includes chocolate, nuts, and shellfish. Shellfish and nuts have important public health consequences related to food allergies and anaphylaxis. Many Americans die each year due to anaphylaxis and subsequent angioneurotic edema and shock. For individuals allergic to shellfish and nuts, eating out is extremely dangerous; the word of a waiter cannot necessarily be trusted. In some patients, even the smell or odor is enough to cause an allergic reaction.

11. C. Acne vulgaris is associated with the bacterium *Propionibacterium acnes*.

12. D. A good skin-care program contains the following: frequent skin washings, the use of oil-free products, antibacterial skin wash products, and leaving the skin lesions alone.

13. E. Antibiotics in general, and tetracycline in particular, have been shown to reduce the theoretical effectiveness of the OCP in some cases. Thus consideration should be given to either using an OCP with 50 μg of ethinyl estradiol as a first choice OCP agent or supplementing the low-dose OCP with additional ethinyl estradiol (20 μg/tablet) for the few days before and after midcycle (perhaps for one week).

14. D. The single most important absolute contraindication to the use of 13-*cis*-retinoic acid (Accutane) is women in the reproductive years. Accutane is teratogenic and should never be used in this age group. Children under the age of 14 years and individuals with allergic reactions (not the redness that is characteristic of topical isotretinoin) should also not be given Accutane.

15. D.

16. D.

17. C.

18. A.

19. C. Rosacea is an acneiform condition that affects middle-aged patients. It is characterized by papules and pustules occurring on a background of erythema and telangiectasia of facial skin. The main area affected is the middle third of the face, from the forehead to the chin. With rosacea, comedones are typically absent. There is, however, a tendency for the facial skin of patients affected by rosacea to become thickened and to produce enlarged sebaceous glands. When this happens in the area of the nose, the condition is known as rhinophyma.

The first-line treatment for rosacea is a topical antibiotic. The antibiotic of choice is metronidazole (MetroGel) applied twice daily. Topical tretinoin and topical benzoyl peroxide preparations aggravate the erythema and are usually not helpful.

The second-line treatment for rosacea is a systemic antibiotic. Tetracycline is the drug of choice and the dosage of choice is 250 mg bid. After the first month, the dosage can often be lowered and then ultimately discontinued. Recurrences are common, however, and repeated courses of antibiotics are often needed. Systemic antibiotics are also useful in treating the associated keratitis and blepharitis that are occasionally associated with rosacea.

Erythromycin is an alternative antibiotic to tetracycline and may produce good results in cases where tetracycline has failed.

Rosacea that fails to respond to the treatment alternatives just outlined may respond to Accutane (in a 20-week course).

The rhinophyma has been thought to be associated with alcohol abuse and alcoholism. It is unclear how strong this connection is, but it does bear consideration when evaluating a patient (especially a middle-aged male to elderly male) with rhinophyma.

20. D. Tretinoin (vitamin A) in its topical form can be very irritating to the skin. Many patients are not told of this, and when they begin to develop significant facial erythema they discontinue the medication. The erythema gradually improves in most cases, but it is both unsightly (in some cases) and irritating. An excellent way to avoid the irritation is to have the patient's pharmacist dispense the following prescription:

Sig: Vitamin A cream 0.025% (1 part)//Hydrocortisone cream 1% (1 part) to be applied HS to affected areas of the face. Dispense: 50 grams

SOLUTION TO SHORT ANSWER MANAGEMENT PROBLEM 37

The pathophysiology of acne vulgaris involves the following six steps:

1. The androgen stimulation of sebum production
2. Keratinous obstruction of the sebaceous follicle outlet
3. Accumulation of keratin and sebum with the formation of open and closed comedomes (blackheads and whiteheads)
4. Bacterial colonization of the trapped sebum with *Propionibacterium acnes*
5. Inflammatory reaction to the colonization of the trapped sebum
6. Production of inflammatory papules, pustules, nodules, and cysts

SUMMARY OF THE DIAGNOSIS AND TREATMENT OF ACNE VULGARIS AND ROSACEA

1. **Acne vulgaris:**
   a) Prevalence: 75% of teenagers and young adults (up to and including patients in their twenties and thirties)
   b) Pathophysiology: see the short answer management problem.
   c) Causative organism: *Propionibacterium acnes*
   d) Classification of acne vulgaris.
      1. Obstructive acne:
         i) Closed comedomes (whiteheads)
         ii) Open comedomes (blackheads)
      2. Inflammatory acne:
         Formation of lesions generally follows the following order:
         i) Papules
         ii) Pustules
         iii) Nodules
         iv) Cysts
         v) Scars
   e) Treatment measures:
      1. Nonpharmacologic:
         i) Gentle face washing
         ii) Avoidance of manipulation of acne lesions
         iii) Using water-based cosmetics only
         iv) Using oil-free moisturizers only
      2. Pharmacologic: The treatment of acne vulgaris can be seen as a series of discrete steps:

Step 1: begin with benzoyl peroxide gel (2.5%, 5%, 10%)

Step 2: add tretinoin cream or gel (0.025%, 0.05%, 0.1% cream)(0.01%, 0.025% gel)

Consider using step 1 in the AM and step 2 in the PM.

Consider mixing tretinoin cream and hydrocortisone cream 50/50 to decrease irritation caused by tretinoin.

Step 3: add topical antibiotic (erythromycin, clindamycin)

Consider using step 3 along with a combination of steps 1 and 2.

Step 4: systemic antibiotics
1. Tetracycline is drug of first choice (250 mg bid).
2. Erythromycin is drug of second choice (250 mg bid).

Consider using combination of steps 1, 2, and 3 along with step 4.

Suggested: tretinoin/topical clindamycin/oral tetracycline

Step 5: For nodular-cystic acne only: Accutane 1 mg/kg for 20 weeks

Women of childbearing age are an absolute contraindication to Accutane.

2. **Rosacea:**
  a) Definition: acneiform eruption that affects middle-aged patients. Characterized by papules and pustules occurring on a background of erythema and telangiectasia of facial skin.
  b) Complications: Thick skin forms on face (especially on nose). This condition is called rhinophyma.
  c) Association with other diseases: Some association between rhinophyma and alcohol abuse and alcoholism.
  d) Treatment:
    Step 1: topical metronidazole
    Step 2: oral tetracycline or erythromycin in same dose as for acne vulgaris.

SUGGESTED READING

Lookingbill DP. Acne vulgaris and rosacea. In: Rakel R, ed. Conn's current therapy. Philadelphia: WB Saunders, 1994.

Obstetrics and Gynecology

PROBLEM 38   A 26-YEAR-OLD PRIMIGRAVIDA WHO PRESENTS TO YOUR OFFICE WITH HER HUSBAND TO DISCUSS A BIRTH PLAN

A 26-year-old female presents to your office at 14 weeks' gestation for her initial prenatal visit. She has heard that "you are an excellent physician" from her friends and would like you to assume her prenatal care and deliver her child.

Her uterus feels 14 weeks by size and her blood pressure is 100/70 mm Hg. All other aspects of the initial complete physical examination are normal.

SELECT THE ONE BEST ANSWER TO THE FOLLOWING QUESTIONS

1. The patient asks you about birth plans during this initial visit and inquires as to your acceptance of pregnant couples making their own decisions. At this time, how would you respond?
   a) by stating that you believe that birth plans are not a good idea; more often than not something goes wrong and everyone ends up disappointed
   b) birth plans are not a good idea; they frequently lead to unresolved guilt
   c) birth plans should be avoided; couples who draw up a birth plan usually have deliveries with high perinatal morbidity and mortality
   d) birth plans are an excellent idea; everything usually goes according to plan
   e) birth plans are a good idea; they involve the couple in the planning for their baby's delivery and can be a very important part of the prenatal, postnatal, and postpartum care

2. On the next prenatal visit, the couple wishes to discuss your feelings concerning a number of issues. The first issue is electronic fetal monitoring. The couple is aware that in some hospitals and with some physicians, routine continuous electronic fetal monitoring is standard procedure.

   Regarding continuous routine electronic fetal monitoring and risk management, which of the following statements is true?
   a) the perinatal mortality rate in laboring patients who undergo continuous electronic fetal monitoring (CFM) is lower than in those who do not
   b) the perinatal morbidity rate in laboring patients who undergo CFM is lower than in those who do not
   c) the incidence of C-section in laboring patients undergoing CFM is not statistically different from those who do not

   d) there is no significant difference in perinatal outcomes between those patients who undergo CFM and those patients who do not
   e) the incidence of admission to the intensive care nursery is greater in those patients whose fetuses do not undergo CFM

3. The couple then asks you about the use of routine ultrasound in pregnancy. Which of the following statements regarding the use of routine ultrasound in pregnancy is(are) false?
   a) the safety of diagnostic ultrasound in pregnancy has been established
   b) a recent well-designed study suggests an association between ultrasound in pregnancy and delayed speech
   c) estimation of gestational age by ultrasound for pregnant patients who are scheduled for elective repeat C-section should be preformed
   d) vaginal bleeding in pregnancy should be assessed by ultrasound examination
   e) a significant uterine size difference comparing symphysis pubis height with gestational age by dates is an absolute indication for obstetrical ultrasound

4. The couple is concerned about the routine administration of IV fluids during labor. Concerning this issue, which of the following statements is(are) false?
   a) the use of routine IV fluids does not limit ambulation in the first stage of labor
   b) if an epidural anesthetic is to be administered, an IV line must be in place
   c) if there is a long first stage of labor (with ketones present in the urine) an IV line should be in place
   d) if a patient has a history of a severe postpartum hemorrhage, an IV line should be established
   e) none of the above statements are false

5. When you mention the words "epidural anaesthesia," the couple becomes quite agitated. They state quite empathically that they do not wish, under any circumstances, to discuss having an epidural anesthetic.

   What should your response to this request be?
   a) "you really have to leave it up to me to decide that"
   b) "epidural anaesthesia is simply used as a method to relieve your pain. It is in no way mandatory or compulsory"
   c) "you better track down another doctor"
   d) "epidurals have no complications; you should really reconsider your position"
   e) none of the above

6. Which of the following statements regarding epidural anaesthesia is(are) true?
   a) epidural anaesthesia may increase the first stage of labor
   b) epidural anaesthesia may increase the second stage of labor
   c) epidural anaesthesia may increase the latent phase of labor
   d) a and b
   e) all of the above

7. The couple just described have registered in Lamaze classes. Lamaze can best be described as which of the following?
   a) a method emphasizing the psychoprophylaxis of labor
   b) a method describing how to keep away from physicians at all costs
   c) a method concentrating on the difficulties physicians cause in obstetrics
   d) a method emphasizing the importance of "toughing things out"
   e) all of the above

8. The couple's final question concerns "routine episiotomy." They have been told that the medical profession is "cut-happy" and that the vast majority of episiotomies are unnecessary. Which of the following statements regarding routine episiotomy is(are) true?
   a) episiotomy pain may be more severe and more long-lasting than the pain of vaginal and perineal lacerations resulting from perineal tears
   b) healing of episiotomy repairs is more rapid than healing of vaginal and perineal tears
   c) dyspareunia is more common after vaginal lacerations and perineal tear than after episiotomy
   d) episiotomy reduces the rate of subsequent pelvic relaxation problems
   e) all of the above are true

9. Which of the following are definite indications for the performance of an episiotomy?
   a) fetal distress in the second stage of labor
   b) significant maternal cardiac disease
   c) the application of forceps
   d) a prolonged second stage of labor with no other abnormalities
   e) a, b, and c

10. Which of the following statements regarding the presence or absence of a supportive person (or coach) in labor is true?
    a) the presence of a support person or coach decreases the need for analgesia in labor
    b) the presence of a support person or coach decreases the need for operative interventions such as forceps or vacuum extraction
    c) the presence of a support person or coach decreases the C-section rate
    d) all of the above are true
    e) none of the above are true

Short Answer Management Problem 38

A 28-year-old primigravida presents at 16 weeks gestation for her first prenatal visit. She is accompanied by her husband. As you begin to discuss your routine with respect to prenatal care, the couple presents you with a "list of demands." These demands include the right to decide whether an IV will be inserted, when the fetal heart can be auscultated, when the physician can "interfere" with the natural birth process, and how the infant is to be resuscitated. Describe how you would deal with this problem.

ANSWERS

1. E. Birth plans are an integral component of what has become known as family-centered maternity care (FCMC). Family-centered maternity care allows pregnant couples the opportunity of going through labor and delivery in an informal setting, preferably with as little medical intervention as possible. Family-centered maternity care involves the husband or significant other as a coach in labor and allows for immediate bonding of infant to both parents.

   Breastfeeding is encouraged, and rooming-in is available. A trusting doctor-patient relationship is essential to family-centered maternity care. If the couple is confident in their doctor, they feel secure that any intervention that is considered will obviously be discussed with them. If the couple is involved in the decision-making process throughout labor and delivery, any unresolved guilt related to the birth process will be resolved.

2. D. A definitive prospective comparison of elective and universal CFM has shown that CFM in low-risk pregnancies offers no advantages in terms of decreased morbidity and/or mortality. Universal CFM is associated with a small but significant increase in the incidence of delivery by C-section due to "presumed fetal distress." Perinatal outcomes as assessed by intrapartum stillbirths, low Apgar scores, need for assisted ventilation of the newborn, admission to NICU, and/or the onset of neonatal seizures is similar in both groups.

   This study concluded that pregnancies considered to be low risk do not need to be continuously assessed by electronic fetal monitoring.

3. A. Not only has routine obstetrical ultrasound not been shown to be unequivocally safe, but a recent case-control study of prenatal ultrasound exposure has suggested a link between this procedure and the later development of delayed speech in the child. The use of diagnostic obstetrical ultrasound on an as-needed basis has been supported by the American College of Obstetricians and Gynecologists.

4. A. An IV line can, in fact, limit ambulation in the first stage of labor. IV solutions are indicated when:
   1) An epidural anesthetic is about to be administered.
   2) There is a long first stage of labor, with ketones present in the urine.
   3) The patient has a history of severe postpartum hemorrhage.

5. B. Epidural anaesthesia should be viewed as an option and only as an option. It is highly effective at significantly reducing or completely eliminating pain in the second stage of labor. There is some evidence that severe pain in labor may cause maternal vasoconstriction and subsequent decreased oxygen flow to the fetus; however, this has not been established.

6. D. Epidurals have been said to play, in some patients, a very significant role in increasing the total length of labor. Although some patients appear to cope much better with an epidural than without one, this is a situation in which patient choice is paramount.

7. A. Patients who utilize the Lamaze technique have been schooled in the psychoprophylaxis of labor. It is fair to say that some people regard Lamaze as "anti-physician," "anti-all-intervention," and "anti-everything else." This is somewhat unfair. The Lamaze technique, if properly utilized, certainly has its place in the management of labor.

8. A.

9. E. Episiotomy pain may be more severe and long-lasting than the pain of vaginal and perineal lacerations. Healing time for vaginal and perineal lacerations is generally shorter than the healing time for episiotomy. Dyspareunia is more common after episiotomy than after vaginal and perineal tears. It appears that routine episiotomy neither increases or decreases the incidence of subsequent pelvic relaxation.

   Indications for episiotomy include fetal distress in the second stage of labor, significant maternal cardiac disease, prophylactic forceps, premature birth, or infants in the breech presentation when vaginal delivery is anticipated.

   Contraindications to episiotomy include inflammatory bowel disease, lymphogranuloma venereum, or severe perineal scarring or malformation. Complications of episiotomy include excessive blood loss and infection.

   Episiotomy rates can be reduced by following these indications and contraindications and avoiding regarding and using it routinely. Vaginal and perineal tears can be avoided by perineal massage and stretching exercises before delivery. Communication with the patient during perineal stretching will help reduce the degree and number of tears during childbirth. Also, if professional urgency to delivery the baby rapidly is controlled, the extra time that the fetal head is on the perineum provides enough time for a great deal of stretching and the greater possibility of an intact perineum as a result.

   Episiotomy does shorten the second stage of labor. That in itself is not a reason for its performance.

10. A. The presence of a support person or coach decreases the need for subsequent analgesia in labor. This does not, however, apply to subsequent operative interventions including forceps delivery, vacuum extraction, or C-section.

SOLUTION TO SHORT ANSWER MANAGEMENT PROBLEM 38

This particular scenario, which is not uncommon, can be described in one way only: bad news. It is reasonable to attempt to talk to this couple in an effort to try and discover why they feel the way they do about the medical profession. Have they had a bad experience? Do they have any trust in you, whom they have come to seeking prenatal care? These issues in this case can be quite easily summarized as follows:

1) Is the couple prepared to accept your decisions regarding when medical intervention is necessary provided you consult and explain your position to them?
2) Is the couple prepared to let you, the physician, perform your duly responsible medical functions in this case?
3) Is the couple willing to trust you providing that you earn their trust?

If the answers to all three questions can be eventually negotiated to yes, then I would proceed with the care of this patient's pregnancy. If, however, the answer to one or more of the questions is no, the best and safest course of action would be to inform the patient and her husband that in all good conscience you cannot look after their pregnancy. You, as a physician, have that ethical right except in the event of an emergency. In many cases it would be better for all concerned if the physician were to suggest that another care provider be sought. You must, however, continue to look after the patient until the time that care provider is identified.

The patient should be sent a registered letter to that effect and a copy sent to the College of Physicians and Surgeons in the state or province in which you practice.

SUMMARY OF SOME OF THE ISSUES CONCERNED WITH NATURAL CHILDBIRTH

1. Birth plans, if prudently developed and open to negotiation and change, may be of benefit in a couple's pregnancy. They have the potential to foster good doctor-patient communication.

2. Continuous electronic fetal monitoring is no more effective than regular auscultation in lowering perinatal morbidity and mortality in low-risk pregnancies.
3. Routine obstetrical ultrasound cannot be recommended in low-risk pregnancies. The first evidence of adverse effects (delayed speech) has been reported.
4. Intravenous therapy: specific indications include long labor with ketones, epidural, history of severe postpartum hemorrhage; not routinely needed in low-risk pregnancies.
5. Anaesthesia: epidural is analgesic of choice. It should be offered only if needed. Lamaze classes may decrease need.
6. Episiotomy: does not heal more quickly; is more painful; has greater incidence of dyspareunia; does not decrease the incidence of third-degree tear and does not increase or decrease incidence of later pelvic relaxation. Although it does shorten the second stage of labor, that shortening in itself offers no definitive benefit to either mother or baby.

SUGGESTED READINGS

Banta D, Thacker S. The risks and benefits of episiotomy: a review. Birth 1982; 9: 25-30.

Campbell J, Elford RW, Brant R. A case-control study of prenatal ultrasound exposure in children with delayed speech. Canadian Medical Association Journal, Nov 15, 1993.

Cunningham FG, MacDonald P, Gant N, Leveno K, Gilstrap L. Williams obstetrics. 19th Ed. Norwalk, CT: Appleton and Lange, 1993.

Hoult IJ, MacLennan AH, Carrier LE. Lumber epidural analgesia in labor: relation to fetal malposition and instrument delivery. Br Med J 1977; 1:14-16.

Klein M. Controversies in obstetrical management and maternal care. Government of Quebec, 1988.

Leveno K et al. A prospective comparison of selective and universal fetal monitoring in 34,995 pregnancies. N Engl J Med 1986; 315: 10-16.

PROBLEM 39   A 23-YEAR-OLD PRIMIGRAVIDA WITH MANY PHYSICAL COMPLAINTS OF PREGNANCY

A 23-year-old primigravida presents for her second prenatal visit. You first saw her 4 weeks ago at 7 weeks' gestation. At that time, you performed a complete history, a complete physical examination, and all necessary blood work.

At this time, she has gained 3 lb in the last 4 weeks. She has been nauseated every day. Fortunately, she has not been vomiting more than once a day at the most.

On examination, her blood pressure is 110/70 mm Hg. No other abnormalities are found on P/E.

SELECT THE ONE BEST ANSWER TO THE FOLLOWING QUESTIONS

1. Nausea and/or vomiting in pregnancy affects approximately 80 percent of women at some time during pregnancy. Current theory suggests that these symptoms are due to which of the following?
   a) increased levels of circulating estrogen
   b) increased levels of circulating progesterone
   c) increased levels of circulating human chorionic gonadotrophin
   d) all of the above
   e) none of the above

2. Which of the following should not be part of your initial advice or treatment of this patient?
   a) reassurance that this is a self-limiting condition
   b) small, frequent meals
   c) discontinuation of iron therapy if it has been previously prescribed
   d) avoidance of contact with cooking odors
   e) the prescription of an antinauseant

3. What is the drug of choice for severe hyperemesis gravidum in pregnancy?
   a) prochlorperazine
   b) promethazine
   c) chlorpromazine
   d) metoclopramide
   e) Odansetron

4. A 26-year-old multigravida (para 4/gravida 5) presents to your office at 36 weeks' gestation with the following complaint: "I've had the worst backache in my life in the last 10 days. I've put heat on it, I've put cold on it, and I've tried rest. Nothing helps, Doctor."

   On examination, the patient has no CVA tenderness. There is moderate paralumbar tenderness. She tells you that she does not recall injuring it in any way. She has had no urinary tract symptoms that would suggest UTI. Flexion, extension, lateral rotation, and lateral bending all aggravate it.

   The only other significant event in the last two weeks is that the onset of the backache appeared to correspond with the baby dropping into her pelvis. She has not had any problems with her back in other pregnancies.

   The patient describes the pain as dull, constant, and centered in the L2-L5 area, with no radiation to either the right leg or the left leg. It is aggravated by walking, moving, and bending. It is relieved somewhat by rest.

   What is the most likely reason for the back pain?
   a) motion of the symphysis pubis
   b) motion of the lumbosacral joints
   c) general relaxation of the pelvic ligaments
   d) any of the above
   e) b or c

5. What is the management of choice for this condition in this patient?
   a) nonpharmacologic therapy: massage, physiotherapy
   b) acetaminophen
   c) acetaminophen plus codeine
   d) any of the above
   e) a or b only

6. A 37-year-old multigravida presents with severe varicosities of both legs. They are present from the hips to the feet. The varicosities began approximately 4 weeks ago and have been gradually increasing in severity. The patient continues to work full-time as a family physician. The varicosities are not only unsightly, but are causing her severe pain, especially as the day goes on. The worst varicosities are her vulvar varicosities.

   What would you do at this time?
   a) advise her to discontinue the practice of medicine until after pregnancy
   b) inject the most severe veins
   c) advise her to elevate her legs and purchase support hose
   d) a and c
   e) all of the above

7. What is(are) the most common complication(s) of the disorder described in Question 6?
   a) deep venous thrombosis
   b) pulmonary embolism
   c) superficial thrombophlebitis
   d) superficial extensive thrombosis
   e) any of the above

8. A 25-year-old primigravida presents with severe rectal discomfort of 3 weeks' duration. At the present time, she is at 36 weeks' gestation.

   On examination, you notice several hemorrhoids that are 1 cm in diameter.

   Which of the following statements about hemorrhoids in pregnancy is(are) true?
   a) hemorrhoids are varicosities of the rectal veins
   b) the tendency toward constipation in pregnancy aggravates the formation and symptomatology of hemorrhoids
   c) hemorrhoids in pregnancy are related to increased pressure in the rectal veins caused by obstruction of venous return by the large uterus
   d) bleeding from rectal veins occasionally may result in sufficient loss of blood to cause iron-deficiency anemia
   e) a, b, and c
   f) all of the above are true

9. A 28-year-old multigravida presents to your office with heartburn. The heartburn that this patient is experiencing is causing severe discomfort, severe enough that the patient is in pain for the majority of the day.

   On examination, the abdomen is soft. The patient's blood pressure is 110/70 mm Hg. There is no evidence of other conditions that may have precipitated this.

   Which of the following statements regarding heartburn in pregnancy is(are) true?
   a) the increased frequency of regurgitation during pregnancy most likely results from the upward displacement and compression of the stomach by the uterus combined with decreased gastrointestinal motility
   b) in most pregnant women symptoms are mild and can be relieved by small, frequent meals and avoiding bending over
   c) aluminum hydroxide and magnesium hydroxide are excellent first-line choices
   d) sodium bicarbonate is an equally good first choice
   e) a, b, and c
   f) all of the above are true

10. Bizarre cravings for strange foods develop during pregnancy, sometimes to the point that foods considered hardly edible or unedible are consumed in great quantities. This condition is known as and is associated with which of the following?
    a) condition: pica—associated with macrocytic anemia
    b) condition: pica—associated with iron-deficiency anemia
    c) condition: amylophagia—associated with iron-deficiency anemia
    d) condition: geophagia—associated with macrocytic anemia
    e) condition: pica—associated with none of the above

11. A patient presents at 32 weeks' gestation with increased swelling in both lower extremities. She went to another physician 1 week ago with swelling from the knees down. He prescribed both a thiazide diuretic and a loop diuretic. She has come to see you.

    What would you do at this time?
    a) tell her to continue the thiazide diuretic but stop the loop diuretic
    b) tell her to continue the thiazide diuretic and the loop diuretic, and add a potassium-sparing diuretic
    c) tell her to continue the thiazide diuretic and the loop diuretic, and in addition begin slow K
    d) tell her to stop both the thiazide diuretic and the loop diuretic
    e) tell her to wait a few minutes, warm up the big office computer, and try to obtain the information from a data bank

12. A 29-year-old primigravida presents to your office complaining of increased vaginal discharge. She is 33 weeks' pregnant.

    On examination, there is considerable vaginal discharge. There is no significant odor, a wet prep is normal, and culture results are negative.

    Which of the following statements regarding increased vaginal discharge during pregnancy is(are) true?
    a) in most cases, the discharge is physiologic
    b) physiologic discharge in pregnancy is caused by increased formation of mucus by cervical glands under the influence of estrogen
    c) monilia may be cultured in up to 25% of pregnant women
    d) monilia should be treated in both symptomatic women and asymptomatic women
    e) a, b, and c
    f) all of the above

13. A 29-year-old multigravida at 22 weeks presents to your office with a chief complaint of constipation. When you ask her to define constipation, she states that she is having only one bowel movement every 5 days.

    With regard to this complaint, which of the following statements is(are) true?
    a) constipation is uncommon in pregnancy
    b) constipation is more common in early pregnancy than in late pregnancy
    c) constipation does not need to be treated in pregnancy
    d) all of the above are true
    e) none of the above are true

14. Which of the following has(have) been implicated in the pathogenesis of constipation in pregnancy?
    a) reduced gut motility
    b) mechanical obstruction by the uterus
    c) increased water resorption

d) increased estrogen levels
e) a, b, and c
f) all of the above

15. The treatment(s) of choice for the treatment of constipation in pregnancy include which of the following?
a) discontinuing iron supplements

b) increasing the amount of fiber in her diet
c) increasing her physical activity
d) addition of a bulk-forming agent
e) all of the above

Short Answer Management Problem 39

List three other complaints of pregnant women and their causes.

ANSWERS

1. C.

2. E.

3. D. Nausea and vomiting in pregnancy are common complaints, especially during the first trimester. Nausea, vomiting, or other gastrointestinal symptoms may occur in up to 50% of pregnant women. Although the etiology has not been definitely established, increased levels of human chorionic gonadotrophin appear to be the most likely explanation.

Nausea in pregnancy should be treated with conservative management whenever possible. Small, frequent meals, the avoidance of foods with a high fat content, an intake of dry foods, and reassurance may be all that is necessary. If iron therapy has been started, it should be discontinued. Avoidance of contact with situations that may induce nausea (such as cooking odors) is also recommended.

If persistent vomiting leads to weight loss, ketonuria, or electrolyte imbalance, hospitalization is necessary.

If conservative therapy fails, antinauseants are indicated. The category B drug that is used in severe hyperemesis gravidum is metoclopramide. The category C drugs include promethazine, prochlorperazine, and chlorpromazine. These drugs are used in moderately severe hyperemesis gravidum.

Categories B and C basically refer to risk of using the drug in pregnancy. With drugs that are either category B or category C, the benefit often outweighs the risk.

Odansetron is a new serotonin antagonist that is being used for severe nausea, particularly the nausea induced by cancer chemotherapy.

No experience with pregnant patients is available yet.

4. D.

5. E. Backache occurs to some extent in most pregnant women, to minor degrees following excessive strain or fatigue and excessive bending, lifting, or walking. Mild backache usually requires little more than elimination of the strain.

In some pregnant women, as in this patient, motion of the symphysis pubis and lumbosacral joints, as well as general relaxation of pelvic ligaments, may be demonstrated. The most important disease to rule out is urinary tract (especially ascending) infection.

Treatment of this condition involves education regarding back pain in pregnancy, rest for much of the remaining pregnancy as possible, massage and physiotherapy, and acetaminophen. Codeine should be avoided; it could cause an addiction problem and will certainly aggravate constipation as well.

6. D.

7. C. Varicosities, generally resulting from congenital predisposition, are certainly exaggerated by prolonged standing and advanced age in pregnancy. Femoral venous pressure increases very significantly as pregnancy advances. The symptoms produced by varicosities vary from cosmetic blemishes on the lower extremity and mild pain to quite severe pain, tenderness, discomfort, and prominence.

The suggested treatment is daily, frequent periods of rest and elevation of the lower extremities.

The most common complication of superficial varicosities is superficial thrombophlebitis. This should be treated with cold packs and rest. Fortunately, there is very little relationship between superficial thrombophlebitis and either deep venous thrombosis or pulmonary embolism.

8. F. Hemorrhoids are varicosities of the rectal veins that are most often related to increased pressure on the rectal veins caused by obstruction of venous return by the

large uterus, and by the tendency to constipation in pregnancy.

Pain and swelling can usually be relieved by topically applied anesthetics, warm soaks, and agents that soften the stool. Thrombosis of a rectal vein can cause considerable pain, and when this happens (usually related to an external rectal vein) the clot should be evacuated (as described in the chapter on office surgery).

Bleeding from the rectal veins can occasionally result in the loss of sufficient blood to cause an iron-deficiency anemia. The loss of only 15 ml of blood results in the loss of 6 mg to 7 mg of iron, an amount that is equal to the daily requirements during latter pregnancy.

9. E. Heartburn, an extremely common complaint in pregnancy, is caused by the reflux of gastric contents into the lower esophagus. The increased frequency of regurgitation during pregnancy most likely results from the upward displacement and compression of the stomach by the uterus combined with decreased gastrointestinal motility. In most pregnant women, the symptoms are mild and are relieved by a regimen of small, frequent meals and avoidance of bending over.

Antacid preparations may provide considerable relief, and most are completely safe. Aluminum hydroxide, magnesium hydroxide, and magnesium trisilicate, alone or in combination, should be used in preference to sodium bicarbonate. The pregnant woman who tends to retain sodium can become edematous as the result of ingestion of excessive amounts of sodium bicarbonate.

10. B. Occasionally during pregnancy, bizarre cravings for strange foods develop, at times for materials hardly considered edible. Some of those substances have included laundry starch, baking powder, baking soda, clay, baked dirt, powered bricks, and frost scraped from the refrigerator.

Ingestion of starch (amylophagia) or clay (geophagia) or related items is practiced more often by socioeconomically less-privileged pregnant women. The desire for dry lump starch, chopped ice, or even refrigerator frost has been considered by some to be triggered by severe iron deficiency. Although women with severe iron deficiency sometimes crave these items, and although craving is usually ameliorated after correction of the iron deficiency, not all pregnant women with pica are iron deficient.

11. D. Edema, a common complication of late pregnancy, occurs because of occlusion of the pelvic veins and inferior vena cava as a result of the pressure from the enlarging uterus. Treatment consists of avoiding prolonged standing, elevating the lower extremities, and wearing support hose. Thiazide diuretics reduce intravascular volume, as do loop diuretics. Both classes are contraindicated in pregnancy. In this patient, you should do the following:
A. Discontinue the thiazide
B. Discontinue the loop diuretic
C. Suggest elevation of extremities for 1 hour × tid
D. Suggest that she stay off her feet as much as possible

Warming up the big computer is never a bad idea. This would be a good second choice.

12. E. The most common vaginal discharge in pregnancy is a physiologic discharge. The discharge is caused by increased formation of mucus by the cervical glands under the influence of estrogen.

Monilia may be cultured from the vagina in up to 25% of women in late pregnancy; trichomonas vaginalis may be cultured in up to 20%. If symptomatic with either of these organisms, the patient should be treated. If she is not symptomatic, cultures should not be taken. Treatment required for trichomonas metronidazole should be avoided, particularly early in pregnancy. The drugs of choice for the treatment of symptomatic vaginal infections in pregnancy are clotrimazole for trichomonas and clotrimazole or miconazole for monilia.

13. E.

14. F.

15. E. The etiology of constipation in pregnancy is multifactorial. Potential causes include hormonally mediated smooth muscle relaxation and mechanical pressure from the enlarging uterus. Increasing the intake of fluids, increasing the intake of fiber, and increasing the amount of exercise (especially walking) should be encouraged. If these measures are not effective, then a bulk-forming agent such as psyllium or methylcellulose may be added. Laxatives should be used with caution.

SOLUTION TO SHORT ANSWER MANAGEMENT PROBLEM 39

Three other common complaints of pregnancy are the following:
1. Ptyalism: profuse salivation
   Cause: stimulation of the salivary glands by the ingestion of starch
   Treatment: the cause should be looked for and eradicated if possible.
2. Fatigue: in early pregnancy, most pregnant women complain of fatigue and desire excessive periods of sleep.
3. Headache: headache early in pregnancy is a frequent complaint.
   Cause: a few cases may result from sinusitis or ocular strain caused by refractive errors. In the vast majority, however, no cause can be demonstrated.

Treatment: largely symptomatic; by midpregnancy, most of these headaches decrease in severity or disappear. Pregnancy-induced hypertension is a potential cause in later pregnancy; at this stage any woman who presents with a headache should be assessed for pre-eclampsia.

SUMMARY OF THE DIAGNOSIS AND TREATMENT OF COMMON COMPLAINTS IN PREGNANCY

1. **Nausea and vomiting:**
   Pathophysiology: increased levels of circulating human chorionic gonadotrophin
   Treatments:
   a) Reassurance
   b) Small, frequent meals/dry food
   c) Discontinuation of iron therapy (if patient is on supplemental iron)
   d) Antinauseants if moderately severe:
      1. Promethazine
      2. Chlorpromazine
      3. Prochlorperazine
      If severe, metoclopramide

2. **Constipation:**
   Pathophysiology: reduced gut motility, mechanical obstruction of the uterus, increased water resorption, increased estrogen levels
   Treatments:
   1. Discontinuation of iron therapy (if patient is on iron)
   2. Increasing amount of fiber in the diet
   3. Increasing the amount of total fluid intake
   4. Increasing the amount of physical activity

3. **Back Pain:**
   Pathophysiology: motion of the symphysis pubis and lumbosacral ligaments, relaxation of the pelvic ligaments and the round ligament of the uterus
   Treatment: Symptomatic: heat, ice, acetaminophen, avoidance of activities that aggravate the problem

4. **Hemorrhoids:**
   Pathophysiology: increased pressure in the rectal vein system secondary to increased intravascular volume
   Treatment:
   1. Recumbent position
   2. TUCKS—witch hazel pads
   3. Hemorrhoidal cream plus hydrocortisone cream
   4. Excision of external thrombosed hemorrhoid

5. **Varicosities:**
   Pathophysiology: congenital predisposition in weakness of vein valves, increased pressure secondary to increased intravascular volume
   Treatment: rest, elevation, compression stockings
   Complication: superficial thrombophlebitis most common

6. **Heartburn:**
   Pathophysiology: displacement of uterus upward, exerting pressure on the diaphragm; and decreased pressure in lower esophageal sphincter
   Treatment: antacids: magnesium hydroxide/aluminum hydroxide

7. **Edema:**
   Pathophysiology: increased intravascular volume (increased by 50%), gravity
   Treatment: avoid diuretics: they will further reduce the intravascular volume.
   Rest, recumbency

8. **Increased vaginal discharge:**
   Pathophysiology: almost always normal; due to increased hormone levels, especially estrogen
   Treatment:
   1. Rule out vaginitis/cervicitis
   2. Reassurance

SUGGESTED READING

Cunningham F, ed. Williams obstetrics. 19th Ed. Norwalk, CT: Appleton and Lange, 1993.

PROBLEM 40 A 24-YEAR-OLD PRIMIGRAVIDA AT 8 WEEKS' GESTATION

A 24-year-old primigravida presents at 8 weeks' gestation for her first prenatal visit. She has asked you to be her family doctor and to look after her during the entire pregnancy. You will, and during your first visit you explain your general philosophy regarding prenatal care and perinatal care.

SELECT THE ONE BEST ANSWER TO THE FOLLOWING QUESTIONS

1. The American College of Obstetricians and Gynecologists has recommended which of the following in its latest recommendations regarding routine prenatal care?
   a) the number of routine office visits can be significantly reduced for women at low risk
   b) there should be an emphasis on prenatal care that provides an opportunity to focus on the total health and well-being of the family including medical, psychological, social, and environmental barriers affecting health
   c) systematic health care beginning long before pregnancy proves very beneficial to the physical and emotional well-being of the prospective mother and child
   d) all of the above are true
   e) b and c only

2. The American College of Obstetricians and Gynecologists has recommended that office visits be limited to visits for specific purposes during the first how many months of pregnancy?
   a) 4 months
   b) 6 months
   c) 2 months
   d) 5 months
   e) none of the above

3. A 26-yr.-old primigravida conceived on Sept. 9, 1992. According to Naegele's rule, what is the patient's estimated date of confinement (assume a normal 28-day cycle)?
   a) June 2, 1993
   b) June 16, 1993
   c) July 2, 1993
   d) July 9, 1993
   e) June 23, 1993

4. The American College of Obstetricians and Gynecologists has recommended intervals for routine and indicated tests in the prenatal period. Which of the intervals shown below is(are) recommended?
   a) initial visit: as early as possible (first visit)
   b) obstetrical ultrasound: 8-18 weeks
   c) screening for gestational diabetes: 26-28 weeks
   d) hepatitis B virus screen: as early as possible (first visit)
   e) all of the above

5. What is the recommended entire weight gain recommended by the American College of Obstetricians and Gynecologists?
   a) 22-27 lb
   b) 15-20 lb
   c) 29-34 lb
   d) 16-20 lb
   e) 10-15 lb

6. The number of calories recommended for women in pregnancy is approximately how many calories greater than for nonpregnant women?
   a) 200
   b) 300
   c) 500
   d) 750
   e) 900

7. Which of the following statements would be regarded as reasonable nutritional advice standards in pregnancy?
   a) supplementation with 30 to 60 mg of iron daily after the first 4 months
   b) supplementation with folic acid 1 mg daily throughout pregnancy
   c) a regular diet with salt added to taste
   d) weight gain of 22 to 27 lb
   e) all of the above

8. Which of the following statements regarding smoking in pregnancy is(are) true?
   a) mothers who smoke during pregnancy have infants whose birthweights are significantly lower than infants of mothers who do not smoke
   b) mothers who smoke have an elevated perinatal death rate
   c) pathophysiology of a and b may include carbon monoxide and its functional inactivation of fetal and maternal hemoglobin or vasoconstrictor action of nicotine, causing reduced placental perfusion
   d) all of the above are true
   e) none of the above are true

9. Which of the following statements regarding alcohol consumption in pregnancy and fetal alcohol syndrome is(are) true?
    a) the wisest policy is to limit alcohol intake to a glass of wine or two on very special occasions
    b) the wisest policy is to abstain completely from alcohol; even one or two drinks have not been shown to be safe
    c) fetal alcohol syndrome is decreasing in incidence in the United States
    d) a and c
    e) b and c

10. Which of the following Caldwell-Moloy classification of pelvic shapes is both the most common and the most functional in terms of delivery?
    a) the gynecoid pelvis
    b) the android pelvis
    c) the anthropoid pelvis
    d) the platypelloid pelvis
    e) a and c are equally common and equally functional

11. Which of the following pelvic size measurements is the most important measurement?
    a) the obstetrical conjugate
    b) the diagonal conjugate
    c) the pelvic inlet
    d) the midpelvis
    e) the pelvic outlet

12. When is the fetal head said to be engaged?
    a) when the frontal diameter has passed through the pelvic inlet
    b) when the occipital diameter has passed through the pelvic inlet
    c) when the biparietal diameter has passed through the pelvic inlet
    d) when the biparietal diameter has passed through the midpelvis
    e) when the occipital diameter has passed through the midpelvis

13. The uterine phases of parturition are a very important way of measuring parturition. The active phase of labor is known as which of the following?
    a) phase 0
    b) phase 1
    c) phase 2
    d) phase 3
    e) phase 4

14. The second stage of labor (the active phase) in a nullipara according to the Friedman curve should produce cervical dilatation of how many cm/hr?
    a) 0.5 cm
    b) 1.0 cm
    c) 1.5 cm
    d) 2.0 cm
    e) 2.5 cm

15. The third stage of labor begins when the baby is delivered. What is the single greatest mistake made by physicians in this phase?
    a) allowing the third stage to progress at a very slow pace
    b) allowing the third stage to progress on its own
    c) attempting to pull or tug at the umbilical cord
    d) attempting to stop the "gush of blood" that normally accompanies the third stage of labor
    e) massaging the uterus and injecting Syntocinon into the uterus

16. Which of the following statements regarding the procedure of amniotomy has(have) been shown to be true?
    a) amniotomy has been shown to shorten labor
    b) the shorter labor that may be induced by amniotomy has been shown to be helpful to the mother
    c) the shorter labor that may be induced by amniotomy has been shown to be helpful to the fetus
    d) none of the above statements are true
    e) all of the above statements are true

17. Which of the following must be demonstrated to be of benefit in decreasing the risk of postpartum hemorrhage following the delivery of the placenta?
    a) massage of the fundus of the uterus
    b) injection of IV or IM oxytocin (Syntocinon)
    c) injection of IV or IM ergonovine maleate
    d) gentle traction on the umbilical cord
    e) a, b, and c
    f) all of the above

18. What are the average duration of the first stage of labor in a nullipara and the average duration of the first stage of labor in a multipara?
    a) 10 hours (Nullipara), 7 hours (Multipara)
    b) 8 hours (Nullipara), 5 hours (Multipara)
    c) 12 hours (Nullipara), 6 hours (Multipara)
    d) 14 hours (Nullipara), 8 hours (Multipara)
    e) 9 hours (Nullipara), 6 hours (Multipara)

19. What are the average durations of the second stage of labor in a nullipara and of the second stage of labor in a multipara?
    a) 1 hour 40 minutes (Nullipara), 55 minutes (Multipara)
    b) 1 hour 20 minutes (Nullipara), 45 minutes (Multipara)
    c) 50 minutes (Nullipara), 20 minutes (Multipara)

d) 40 minutes (Nullipara), 10 minutes (Multipara)

e) 1 hour 30 minutes (Nullipara), 1 hour (Multipara)

20. Regarding screening for group B streptococcus in pregnant women, which of the following statements is true?

a) no routine screening needs to be implemented

b) routine screening should be planned for high-risk patients only

c) all pregnant women should be screened at 36 weeks' gestation

d) all pregnant women should be screened at 32 weeks' gestation

e) routine screening is so controversial that it should not be performed

Short Answer Management Problem 40

Matching Problem

Part A lists eight drugs that may be useful in pregnancy. Part B lists eight indications for treatment with those drugs. Match the numbered drug with the proper lettered condition in each case.

PART A:	PART B:
1. Aspirin	A. Severe hypertension in pregnancy
2. Zidovudine	B. Prophylaxis against group B streptococcus
3. Ergonovine	C. Drug of choice: preeclamptic toxemia
4. Aldomet	D. Possibly useful in the prevention of preeclampsia
5. Magnesium sulfate	E. Postpartum agent for uterine contractions
6. Hydralazine	F. May prevent HIV infection in the infant of an infected mother
7. Penicillin	G. Teratogenic drug
8. Ritodrine	H. No possible use in normal pregnancy
9. Hydrochlorothiazide	I. Treatment of choice in chronic hypertension
10. Captopril	J. Treatment of choice for preterm labor

ANSWERS

1. D.

2. B. The American College of Obstetricians and Gynecologists has suggested that women at low risk can reduce the number of prenatal visits significantly. Detailed recommendations have also been made regarding preconceptional care beginning within a year of a planned pregnancy. This is a marked deviation from standard practice, but there is no difference in demonstrated quality of care between low-risk women who had regular "4 weekly" office visits and women who had prenatal visits at the time of recommended intervals for indicated tests and procedures (this will be discussed in detail in another question).

There should certainly be an emphasis on prenatal care that provides an opportunity to focus on the total health and well-being of the family, including medical, psychological, social, and environmental barriers affecting health.

Systematic health care beginning long before pregnancy proves very beneficial to the prospective mother and infant.

The ACOG has recommended that this recommendation (office visits limited to those visits necessary for indicated procedures and intervals) be in effect for the first six months of pregnancy.

3. A. Naegele's rule identifies the estimated date of confinement for women that have normal menstrual periods. The mean duration of pregnancy calculated from the first day of the last normal menstrual period for a large number of healthy women has been identified as to be very close to 280 days, or 40 weeks. Naegele's rule estimates the expected date of delivery by adding 7 days to the date of the first day of the last normal menstrual period and counting back 3 months.

4. E. The American College of Obstetricians and Gynecologists suggests that the pregnant patient not only present to her physician at the first indication that she is pregnant but also take special care during the year before she plans to get pregnant to ensure the healthiest possible outcome. Exercise, diet, and other healthy lifestyles should be encouraged many months before attempting to conceive.

On the first prenatal visit, the following investigations should be performed: hemoglobin and hematocrit; urinalysis; blood group, Rh type, antibody screen, rubella antibody titer, syphilis screen, and hepatitis B virus screen; and cervical cytology.

Obstetrical ultrasound should be performed for dating of the pregnancy (accurate dating) at 18 weeks. At that time also, a maternal alpha-fetoprotein may be performed as a screen for neural tube defects.

At 26-28 weeks, the patient should have the following procedures performed: routine screen for diabetes mellitus, repeat hemoglobin or hematocrit, and repeat antibody test for unsensitized Rh-negative patients. At that time also, prophylactic administration of Rho(d) immunoglobin can be administered to patients who are Rh negative.

At 32-36 weeks, testing for sexually transmitted diseases and repeat hemoglobin or hematocrit should be performed.

5. A. The American College of Obstetricians and Gynecologists and other organizations have recommended that pregnant women gain 22-27 lb (10-12 kg) during pregnancy. Of the recommended weight gain, approximately 9 kg comprise the normal physiologic events and features of pregnancy. These include the fetus, placenta, amniotic fluid, uterine hypertrophy, increase in maternal blood volume, breast enlargement, and dependent maternal edema as the consequence of mechanical factors. The remaining 1 to 3 kg is mostly fat.

It is essential to make sure that pregnant women gain an adequate amount of weight. Failure to do so may result in intrauterine growth retardation. Thus weight gain needs to be watched carefully, especially in the last trimester.

6. B. The recommended National Research Council Recommended Daily Dietary Allowances for women before, during pregnancy, and during lactation are as follows:

	NONPREGNANT	PREGNANT	LACTATING
Kilocalories	2200	2500	2600
Protein (g)	55	60	65

7. E. In general, the pregnant woman should eat what she wants to eat in amounts she desires and with salt added to taste.

Care should be taken to make sure there is enough food to eat, especially in the case of the socioeconomically deprived woman.

As stated before, make sure, by serial weighing every expectant mother, that she is gaining weight, with a goal of about 22 to 27 lb.

Periodically explore the food intake by dietary recall to uncover the ingestion of any bizarre foods. In this way, the occasional nutritionally absurd diet (pica) will be discovered.

Give tablets of simple iron salts to pregnant women that provide between 30 mg and 60 mg of iron/day. Supplement the pregnant patient's diet with 1 mg of folic acid/day.

Recheck the hematocrit or hemoglobin concentration at 28 to 32 weeks to detect any significant decrease.

8. D. There is no question that women who smoke have an increase in perinatal deaths (4600 infants died in the United States in 1993 because of maternal smoking), and mothers who smoke during pregnancy have infants whose birthweights average less than infants of nonsmokers by a significant amount. This is also associated with intrauterine growth retardation. Other conditions linked with maternal smoking include abruptio placentae, placenta praevia, prematurity, premature rupture of the membranes, chorioamnionitis, and placental calcifications and placental hypoxia.

The pathophysiology of maternal smoking includes the following:
1. Carbon monoxide and its functional inactivation of fetal and maternal hemoglobin
2. Vasoconstrictor action of nicotine, causing reduced placental perfusion
3. Reduced appetite, and, in turn, reduced caloric intake
4. Decreased maternal plasma volume
5. An unexplained predisposition in certain women that persists even when they quit smoking

9. B. The safest policy for maternal alcohol use is no use. Even a few drinks at a critical time in organogenesis can be teratogenic. The incidence of fetal alcohol syndrome in the United States is increasing, not decreasing.

10. A. The Caldwell-Moloy classification of four parent pelvis types has allowed physicians to accurately determine in some cases how much difficulty there is going to be in the actual delivery of the infant. The CM classification that is both most common and most suited for delivery is the gynecoid pelvis.

The android pelvis has convergent sidewalls, ischial spines that are prominent, and a subpubic arch that is narrow.

The anthropoid pelvis is a pelvis in which the ischial spines are narrow. This type of pelvis is much more common in black women; the android pelvis is more common in white women.

The platypelloid pelvis has a flattened gynecoid shape. It is quite rare; only 3% of women have this type of pelvis.

11. B. The diagonal conjugate is the most important measurement. Every practitioner of obstetrics should be thoroughly familiar with the technique of its measurement and the interpretation of the information gained from its use. It is the distance from the sacral promontory to the lower margin of the symphysis pubis. It is the measurement that directly determines the measurement of the pelvic inlet. The obstetrical conjugate is determined by adding 1.5 to 2.0 cm to the diagonal conjugate. If the diagonal conjugate is greater than 11.5 cm, it is reasonable to assume that the pelvic inlet is of adequate size.

12. C. The fetal head is said to be engaged when the biparietal diameter of the fetal head has passed through the pelvic inlet. Although engagement of the fetal head is usually regarded as a phenomenon of labor, in nulliparas it often does not occur until the final few weeks of pregnancy.

13. C. The uterine phases of parturition are as follows:
    1. Phase 0: phase 0 is the prelude to parturition, the time of uterine smooth muscle contractile tranquility and cervical rigidity; this phase is normally maintained from before implantation until late in gestation.
    2. Phase 1: phase 1 is the interval of uterine preparedness for labor when functional changes in myometrium and cervix, which are required for labor, are implemented. This phase is commonly identifiable clinically during the last days of pregnancy by distinctive signs: ripening of the cervix, increasing frequency of reasonably painless uterine contractions, the development of the lower uterine segment, and myometrial irritability.
    3. Phase 2: phase 2 is the period of active labor, that is, the uterine contractions that bring about progressive cervical dilation, fetal descent, and delivery of the conceptus. This phase of partipurtion is customarily further divided into the three phases of labor.
    4. Phase 3: during phase 3 parturient recovery takes place, which culminates in uterine involution and restored fertility. Four to six weeks are required to complete uterine recovery (involution); but the duration of phase 3 is dependent on the duration of breast feeding. Generally, so long as breast feeding is continued, infertility persists because of lactation-induced anovulation and amenorrhea.

14. B. The Friedman curve is a graphic representation of cervical dilatation versus time. In a primigravida, the average dilatation during the first stage of labor is 1.0 cm/hr; in multiparas the average cervical dilatation is 1.5 cm/hr.

15. C. The biggest single mistake that can be made in the third stage of labor is for undue and unnecessary tension to be put on the umbilical cord. This can cause premature separation of the placenta from the uterus and breaking or tearing of the umbilical cord, and it may cause an inversion of the uterus, a life-threatening problem that is associated with severe postpartum hemorrhage.

16. D. If the membranes are intact and bulging, there is a fairly major temptation in many cases to rupture them. The presumed benefits of amniotomy are thought to be a more rapid labor, earlier detection of instances of meconium staining of amniotic fluid, and the opportunity to put on an internal scalp monitor and insert a pressure catheter into the uterine cavity.

There is a major controversy at the present time regarding amniotomy. It is discussed in one other chapter on the active management of labor. The answer to this question is not meant to confuse, but it is important to point out that some studies have shown that the spontaneous rupture of the membranes during labor was followed by a shorter duration of labor when compared with artificial rupture of the membranes or no rupture of the membranes. Other studies have indicated that when membranes were artificially ruptured, there was a slightly shorter labor than recorded with intact membranes. Amniotomy may shorten the length of labor slightly, but there is no evidence that shorter labor is necessarily beneficial to the fetus or to the mother.

17. E. The third stage of labor is best managed by the following:
    A. As soon as the placenta is delivered, massage of the uterine fundus is indicated.
    B. As soon as the placenta is delivered, an IV or IM injection of either oxytocin (Syntocinon) or ergonovine maleate is used to contract the uterus.
    C. Traction (even gentle traction) on the umbilical cord will increase, not decrease, the risk of postpartum hemorrhage (including massive postpartum hemorrhage caused by uterine inversion).

18. B.

19. C.

	NULLIPARA	MULTIPARA
Average Time:		
1st Stage	8 hours	5 hours
2nd Stage	50 minutes	20 minutes

20. C. Although not part of the 1992 American College of Obstetricians and Gynecologists protocol, it is now thought that screening for group B streptococcus should take place routinely at 36 weeks in all pregnant women. Women who test positive should be treated with penicillin.

SOLUTION TO SHORT ANSWER MANAGEMENT PROBLEM 40

Matching Question Answers
1. D.
2. F.
3. E.
4. I.

5. C.
6. A.
7. B.
8. J.
9. H.
10. G.

SUMMARY OF CERTAIN ANTEPARTUM AND PERIPARTUM EVENTS

1. **Routine checkups in pregnancy:** not indicated nearly as frequently as commonly practiced; especially in the first trimester

2. **Recommended screening:**
   Initial screen (as soon as possible after diagnosis):
   a) CBC
   b) Blood group and screen
   c) Rh
   d) Rubella
   e) Syphilis
   f) HIV (high risk)
   g) Hepatitis B virus
   18-week screen:
   a) Obstetrical ultrasound 1
   b) Alpha-fetoprotein
   28-week screen:
   a) Gestational diabetes—50 grams: If >140 mg%: then 3 h GTT
   b) Repeat screen for Rh
   c) Administer WhnRho if necessary
   d) Repeat CBC
   36-week screen: Group B streptococcal culture

3. **Prenatal surveillance** (every prenatal visit):
   a) Fetal:
   1. Fetal heart rate
   2. Size of fetus(es) and rate of change: Symphysis-fundal height: 1 cm = 1 week
   3. Amount of amniotic fluid
   4. Presenting part and station (late in pregnancy)
   5. Fetal activity
   b) Maternal:
   1. Blood pressure, actual and extent of change
   2. Weight, actual and amount of change
   3. Symptoms, including headache and altered vision

4. **Other prenatal factors:**
   a) Naegele's rule: first day LNMP + 7 days − 3 months = Estimated date of confinement
   b) Weight gain: ideal 22-27 lb
   c) Calories: 300 extra in pregnancy; 400 extra in lactation
   d) Supplementation: iron 30-60 mg after 4 months; folic acid 1 mg
   e) Smoking: stop; 4600 perinatal deaths/year in United States due to smoking
   f) Alcohol: none

5. **Perinatal summary:**
   a) Friedman's curve: active stage of labor: 2nd Stage 1.0 cm/hr for Nullipara; 1.5 cm/hr for Multipara
   b) Third stage of labor: 50 minutes for Nullipara; 20 minutes for Multipara
   Syntocinon, ergonovine; don't pull on the cord.
   c) Engagement: when the biparietal diameter passes the pelvic inlet
   d) Conjugates and pelvis:
   1. Diagonal conjugate: most important. This is the measurement from the sacral promontory to the symphysis pubis. If >11.5 cm, then the pelvic inlet is adequate.
   2. Most favorable pelvis: gynecoid: 50% of women

SUGGESTED READING

Cunningham FG. Antepartum care. In: Williams obstetrics. 19th Ed. Norwalk: Appleton and Lange, 1993.

PROBLEM 41   A 28-YEAR-OLD PRIMIGRAVIDA IN LABOR

A 28-year-old primigravida at term is admitted to the delivery suite with 5-minute contractions. She is found to be 3 cm dilated and is 50% effaced. When examined 5 hours later she has progressed to 4 cm dilated and is 75% effaced. The station is zero (0). Her contractions are mild to moderate and have become more irregular during the past 3 hours. She has been walking around but has not found that movement has increased either the strength or the frequency of her contractions. Her membranes are intact and bulging. The fetal heart rate tracing is reactive.

SELECT THE ONE BEST ANSWER TO THE FOLLOWING QUESTIONS

1. What is the most appropriate course of action at this time?
   a) perform an amniotomy
   b) begin oxytocin stimulation for hypotonic labor
   c) call the anesthesiologist to administer an epidural anesthetic
   d) reassure the patient that her contractions will eventually pick up
   e) none of the above

2. The appropriate action is taken. After 4 further hours, her contractions are still mild to moderate and irregular in frequency. The cervix is now 5 cm dilated and 90% effaced. The intrapartum fetal monitor strip is reactive.

   What would be the most appropriate course of action at this time?
   a) perform an amniotomy
   b) begin oxytocin stimulation for hypotonic labor
   c) call the anesthesiologist to administer an epidural anesthetic and prepare the patient for C-section
   d) tell the patient and the nursing staff to relax; everything takes time
   e) none of the above

3. With the appropriate intervention the patient progresses to full cervical dilatation. After 1/2 hour in the second stage of labor the patient is exhausted. The head is visible on the perineum. The head is occiput anterior. The fetal heart rate tracing is reactive. Her contractions are strong and 2 minutes apart.

   What would you do at this time?
   a) increase the oxytocin
   b) explain to the patient that the second stage of labor is usually a long, difficult stage and that she'll just have to try a little harder
   c) deliver the baby with outlet forceps
   d) deliver the baby with a vacuum extractor
   e) either c or d

4. Which of the following statements concerning the use of the vacuum extractor and/or outlet forceps in the second stage of labor is(are) true?
   a) the perinatal morbidity of infants delivered with outlet forceps is higher than the perinatal morbidity of infants delivered with the vacuum extractor

   b) the perinatal morbidity of infants delivered with the vacuum extractor is higher than infants delivered with the outlet forceps
   c) intracranial compression with the vacuum extractor is higher than intracranial compression with outlet forceps
   d) the Apgar scores of infants delivered by the vacuum extractor are higher than the Apgar scores of infants delivered by outlet forceps
   e) the perinatal morbidity and Apgar scores of infants delivered by outlet forceps and vacuum extractor are similar

5. Which of the following is(are) essential before a forceps delivery can be referred to as *outlet forceps*?
   a) the scalp is or has been visible at the introitus (without the need to separate the labia)
   b) the skull has reached the pelvic floor
   c) the sagittal suture is in the anteroposterior diameter of the pelvis
   d) a and b
   e) all of the above

6. Which of the following is(are) maternal indications for forceps delivery?
   a) maternal exhaustion
   b) severe cardiac or pulmonary problems accompanied by maternal dyspnea
   c) intercurrent debilitating illness
   d) all of the above
   e) none of the above

7. Which of the following is(are) fetal indications for forceps delivery if all other criteria have been met?
   a) fetal heart tones (FHT) with a persistent rate of less than 100 beats/minute or more than 160 beats/minute
   b) passage of meconium-stained amniotic fluid in a fetus who presents with a cephalic presentation
   c) presence of variable decelerations on the fetal monitor strip
   d) a and b
   e) all of the above

8. Which of the following conditions must be met before a forceps delivery is attempted?
   a) the cervix must be fully dilated
   b) the membranes must be ruptured

c) the head must be engaged
d) the bladder must be empty
e) all of the above

9. Which of the following statements regarding induction of labor by stripping the membranes is(are) true?
   a) stripping of the membranes has been firmly established as a safe and efficient method to induce labor
   b) stripping of the membranes has not been associated with infection
   c) stripping of the membranes has not been associated with subsequent vaginal bleeding

d) stripping of the membranes appears to induce labor through a prostaglandin stimulation/mediation
e) all of the above are true

10. Which of the following is(are) risks of administering oxytocin for the induction of labor?
   a) uterine rupture
   b) fetal hypoxia
   c) uterine hypertonia
   d) all of the above
   e) none of the above

Short Answer Management Problem 41

Discuss the major issues when considering the use of oxytocin for the induction of labor.

ANSWERS

1. A. This patient has hypotonic labor. Once the diagnosis of active labor followed by hypotonic uterine dysfunction has been made and the head is engaged, it probably is reasonable to perform an amniotomy. Although controversial (the issue is addressed at length in another chapter), amniotomy may augment and shorten labor. The patient should be kept in the Fowler's position after amniotomy to facilitate drainage of the amniotic fluid. Because of the disagreement among physicians of the value of this procedure, it is reasonable to suggest that it be performed only if all three of the following apply: (1) the patient has documented hypotonic labor; (2) the baby's head is fully engaged; and (3) the conditions under which the procedure are performed are absolutely sterile. There is no indication for an epidural anesthetic at this time.

2. B. In this patient, amniotomy has not been of much help. Oxytocin stimulation for hypotonic labor should now be considered. The following criteria should be adhered to before and during oxytocin administration for hypotonic labor.
   a) The patient must be in true labor, with cervical effacement and dilatation. It is suggested that cervical dilatation be at least 3 cm.
   b) There must be no evidence of a mechanical obstruction to a safe delivery.
   c) The fetus should be in a normal vertex presentation.
   d) The fetus should be singleton.
   e) There should be no gross hydramnios.
   f) The patient should be parity less than or equal to 5.
   g) The patient should not have a previous uterine scar.
   h) The fetal condition should be good.

   i) There should be no evidence of tetanic contractions following the initiation of oxytocin.
   j) There should be continuous electronic monitoring of the fetal heart and uterine activity.

3. E. The mother is exhausted. Her contractions are strong and 2 minutes apart and are therefore not hypotonic. It would be inappropriate to increase the rate of Syntocinon infusion.

   The head is on the perineum. Therefore delivery of the infant by either an outlet forceps or a vacuum extractor would be appropriate.

   When a mother has been pushing for 1/2 hour and is exhausted, it is inappropriate to advise her to "try."

4. E. The perinatal morbidity rates and Apgar scores on infants delivered by outlet forceps and vacuum extractor are similar.

   The vacuum extractor is commonly used in Europe and Canada but is less common in the United States. The Silastic vacuum extractor has the advantage over older models of being able to be applied immediately to the fetal head. The pressure should be completely released between contractions. There is lower intracranial compression with the vacuum extractor, but there is no significant difference in perinatal morbidity or Apgar scores between infants delivered by the vacuum extractor and infants delivered by outlet forceps.

   In the hands of experienced operators, both instruments are effective and safe.

5. E. Forceps deliveries are classified as follows:
   A. Outlet forceps: outlet forceps refers to the application of forceps when the scalp is or has been visible at the introitus (without the need to separate the

labia), the skull has reached the pelvic floor, and the sagittal suture is in the anteroposterior diameter of the pelvis.

  B. Low forceps: Low forceps refers to the application of forceps when the skull has reached a station of +3 (at or immediately above the pelvic floor) and the sagittal suture is in the anteroposterior or oblique diameter of the pelvis.

  C. Midforceps: Midforceps refers to the application of forceps when the head is engaged but has not reached a station of +3 or the occiput has not rotated as far as the anterior oblique diameter.

  D. High forceps: High forceps refers to the application of forceps at any time prior to engagement of the head. There are few, if any, indications for high forceps deliveries in present-day obstetric practice.

  E. Prophylactic forceps: Prophylactic forceps is the use of outlet forceps (not low or midforceps) and episiotomy in order to prevent injury to the fetal head and to reduce maternal stress.

6. D. Maternal indications for outlet forceps include maternal exhaustion, severe cardiac or pulmonary problems accompanied by dyspnea, and intercurrent debilitating illness.

7. D. The major fetal indication for termination of the second stage of labor is fetal distress. This fetal distress may be manifested by (1) fetal heart rate <100 or >160 beats/minute; (2) late deceleration patterns; (3) a grossly irregular fetal monitor pattern; (4) excessive fetal movements; or (5) the passage of meconium-stained amniotic fluid in cephalic presentation.

   Variable decelerations (cord compressions) are not necessarily an indication for termination of the second stage of labor. This is especially true if there is quick recovery to baseline after the deceleration.

   Early decelerations (head compressions) are not an indication for the termination of the second stage of labor.

   When faced with fetal distress, one must decide which method of delivery is preferable for the mother and baby at that time, considering the condition of both. In many cases C-section is preferable to a forceps delivery.

8. E. The use of forceps is permissible only when all of the following conditions prevail, regardless of the urgent need for delivery:
   a) The cervix must be fully dilated.
   b) The membranes must be ruptured.
   c) The head must be engaged (preferably deeply engaged) to a station below +2.
   d) The head must present in either vertex or face presentation with chin anterior.
   e) Cephalopelvic disproportion must have been ruled out.
   f) The bladder must be empty.

9. D. Induction of labor by stripping the membranes is a relatively common practice, although few reports documenting its efficacy and safety have been published. The potential for infection and bleeding from a previously undiagnosed placenta previa or from a low-lying placenta, as well as accidental rupture of the membranes, should be considered. Only one randomized study involving 180 pregnancies has demonstrated that membrane stripping is safe and associated with a decreased incidence of postterm gestation. If it is effective, the mechanism of action is likely to be mediated by the stimulation of prostaglandins located in the membrane itself.

10. D. Oxytocin is a powerful drug and has been associated with uterine rupture, hypertonic uterine contractions, and fetal hypoxia resulting from uterine hypertonia.

    Oxytocin must be administered on a risk-benefit basis. The risks have been previously discussed. The benefits include decreased risk of maternal exhaustion, decreased risk of intrapartum infection, and decreased risk of traumatic operative delivery. As well, failure to treat uterine dysfunction may expose the fetus to an appreciably higher risk of death.

SOLUTION TO SHORT ANSWER MANAGEMENT PROBLEM 41

Approximately 22% of labors are induced or augmented using oxytocin. The following protocol should be observed:
1) Continuous observation
2) Continuous FHR monitoring
3) Uterine activity monitoring
4) Parity ≤5
5) Reactive fetal heart
6) Thick meconium completely absent

   Oxytocin is infused initially at 1 mU/min. The dosage is titrated against uterine contractions using 1 mU/min increments but to 8 mU/min. Thereafter the infusion in increased in 2 mU/min increments up to a 20 mU/min dosage.

SUMMARY OF ACTIVE MANAGEMENT OF THE FIRST AND SECOND STAGES OF LABOR

1. **Hypotonic labor:**
   a) Establish that the patient is in true labor.
   b) If true labor is established and is not progressing, consider amniotomy.
   c) If amniotomy is performed or membranes have ruptured spontaneously and labor is not progressing,

consider oxytocin augmentation (adherence to protocol is very important).

d) Consider stripping of the membranes.

2. **Operative vaginal delivery:**

   a) Forceps and vacuum are equally effective and safe if properly used.

   b) Follow maternal and fetal indications for operative delivery.

   c) If considering operative vaginal delivery for fetal distress or other emergency situations, weigh carefully the risks and benefits of both vaginal and abdominal delivery before making a decision.

SUGGESTED READINGS

Cunningham F, MacDonald P, Gant N. Williams obstetrics. 19th Ed. Norwalk, CT: Appleton and Lange, 1993.

Danforth D. Operative delivery. In: Pernoll M, Beson R, eds. Current obstetric and gynecologic diagnosis and treatment. 6th Ed. Norwalk, CT: Appleton and Lange, 1987: 481-495.

Fall O, Ryden G, Finnstrom K, Finnstrom O, Leijon I. Forceps or vacuum extraction? A comparison of effects on the newborn infant. Acta Obstet Gynecol Scand 1986; 65(1):75-80.

PROBLEM 42   A 35-YEAR-OLD PRIMIGRAVIDA WITH HYPERTENSION

A 35-year-old primigravida presents to your office at 16 weeks' gestation. She is a new patient. She presents a negative medical history. She denies a history of hypertension although she has not had her blood pressure measured for 5 years.

She is excited about her new pregnancy and asks you to be her primary care physician who will deliver her baby. Her husband accompanies her to the visit and appears to be equally excited.

On physical examination her blood pressure after 5 minutes of rest is 160/100 mm Hg. A repeat measurement 1 week later is 154/98 mm Hg. Fundoscopy is normal, and no other abnormalities are determined.

SELECT THE ONE BEST ANSWER TO THE FOLLOWING QUESTIONS

1. What is the most likely diagnosis in this patient?
   a) preeclampsia
   b) chronic hypertension
   c) chronic hypertension with superimposed preeclampsia
   d) transient hypertension
   e) labile hypertension

2. The patient described is followed on a weekly basis. Her blood pressure remains at or around 155/98 until the 26th week of gestation. At that time, it increases to 170/106 mm Hg. At that time she also had proteinuria +2. This was quantitated to 300 mg/day. At this time, what is the most likely diagnosis?
   a) preeclampsia
   b) pregnancy-aggravated hypertension with superimposed eclampsia
   c) pregnancy-aggravated hypertension with superimposed preeclampsia
   d) coincidental hypertension
   e) none of the above

3. What is the treatment of choice in the patient described in Question 2?
   a) increase rest at home; increase office visits to twice weekly
   b) admit to hospital for bed rest and further evaluation
   c) admit to hospital; begin pharmacologic therapy
   d) institute pharmacologic therapy as an outpatient; see in the office twice/week
   e) admit to hospital for bed rest and pharmacologic therapy

4. The patient's blood pressure settles down to a level of 140/90 mm Hg on strict bed rest and stays at that level for 8 weeks (34 weeks' gestation). However, in spite of bed rest, the proteinuria increases to 2 g/day. Biophysical profile testing reveals evidence of oligohydramnios. What is the treatment of choice at this time?
   a) begin pharmacologic therapy with a thiazide diuretic
   b) begin pharmacologic therapy with a beta blocker
   c) begin pharmacologic therapy with a calcium-channel blocker
   d) begin pharmacologic therapy with a direct vasodilator
   e) none of the above

5. A 25-year-old primigravida is a known hypertensive who is presently on a thiazide diuretic. On examination at 8 weeks' gestation her blood pressure is 120/85 mm Hg. What should you do at this time?
   a) discontinue the thiazide diuretic and substitute atenolol
   b) discontinue the thiazide diuretic and substitute methyldopa
   c) discontinue the thiazide diuretic and substitute nothing
   d) continue the thiazide diuretic and see the patient every 2 weeks
   e) none of the above

6. The patient described in Question 5 has her blood pressure well controlled until 18 weeks' gestation. At that time her blood pressure rises to 160/102 mm Hg. What should you do at this time?
   a) reinstitute the thiazide diuretic if you had stopped it or increase the dosage if you had not stopped it
   b) start the patient on an ACE inhibitor
   c) start the patient on a calcium-channel blocker
   d) start the patient on α-methyldopa
   e) start the patient on a β-adrenergic blocker

7. What is the pharmacologic agent of choice for the treatment of chronic hypertension in pregnancy?
   a) atenolol
   b) propranolol
   c) alpha methyldopa
   d) nifedipine
   e) captopril

8. Which of the following antihypertensive drug classes is(are) contraindicated for use in pregnancy?
   a) thiazide diuretics
   b) ACE inhibitors
   c) calcium-channel blockers
   d) a and b only
   e) all of the above

9. What is the drug of choice for the management and control of the seizures associated with eclampsia?
   a) IV labetalol
   b) IV hydralazine
   c) IV methyldopa
   d) IV clonidine
   e) none of the above

10. Regarding the use of aspirin to prevent or treat preeclampsia, which of the following statements is true?
    a) aspirin has been conclusively shown to provide a reduction in maternal morbidity from preeclampsia
    b) aspirin has been conclusively shown to provide a reduction in maternal mortality from preeclampsia
    c) aspirin has been conclusively shown to provide an improved fetal outcome in preeclampsia
    d) aspirin has been conclusively shown to lower morbidity in preeclampsia
    e) none of the above

11. What is the etiology of preeclampsia currently thought to be?
    a) due to a deficiency of endothelin-1
    b) due to a deficiency of endothelium-derived relaxing factor
    c) due to a change in the ratio of two prostaglandins: prostacyclin (vasodilating) and thromboxane (vaso-constricting)
    d) due to an increase in free radical formation
    e) none of the above

12. The pathophysiology of preeclampsia is due primarily to which of the following?
    a) vascular endothelial cell proliferation
    b) vascular vasospasm
    c) glomerular cell hypertrophy
    d) placental vessel hyperplasia
    e) none of the above

Short Answer Management Problem 42

Discuss the risk factors for pregnancy-induced hypertension.

ANSWERS:

1. B. This patient most likely has chronic hypertension. Chronic hypertension is defined as a blood pressure of greater than or equal to 140 mm Hg systolic or 90 mm Hg diastolic either predating pregnancy or occurring before the 20th gestational week.

   Pregnancy-induced hypertension or pre-eclampsia is defined as a sustained rise in arterial blood pressure after the 20th week of gestation to a level greater than or equal to 140 mm Hg systolic or 90 mm Hg diastolic, or an increase of 30 mm Hg in systolic pressure or an increase of 15 mm Hg diastolic. Associated with this is proteinuria >300 mg/24 h. Weight gain and edema are frequently present; they are not, however, necessary to make the diagnosis of preeclampsia.

   Eclampsia and the presence of generalized or grand mal seizures is the major complication of preeclampsia.

   A patient who has chronic hypertension with superimposed preeclampsia is defined as a patient who, having preexisting hypertension, has a further increase in blood pressure or worsening of proteinuria after 20 weeks' gestation.

   The "New Classification of Hypertensive Disorders Complicating Pregnancy" proposed by the American College of Obstetricians and Gynecologists is as follows:
   1. *Pregnancy-induced hypertension:* hypertension that develops as a consequence of pregnancy and regresses postpartum.
      a) Hypertension without proteinuria or pathological edema
      b) Preeclampsia with proteinuria and/or pathological edema
         i) mild
         ii) severe
      c) Eclampsia-proteinuria and/or pathological edema along with convulsions
   2. *Pregnancy-aggravated hypertension:* underlying hypertension worsened by pregnancy
      a) Superimposed preeclampsia
      b) Superimposed eclampsia
   3. *Coincidental hypertension:* Chronic underlying hypertension that antecedes pregnancy or persists postpartum

2. C. At this time, the patient has developed pregnancy-aggravated hypertension with superimposed preeclampsia.

   This condition is associated with significant fetal morbidity and mortality and the fetus should therefore be monitored extremely closely for the duration of the pregnancy.

3. B. This patient has developed pregnancy-aggravated hypertension with superimposed preeclampsia. She

should be admitted to hospital for bed rest and for further investigation and evaluation.

Bed rest and reduced activity are essential.

The patient should be placed in the left lateral position. This position results in the following:
(1) Lower blood pressure readings
(2) Mobilization of extravascular fluid
(3) Decreased endogenous excretion of catecholamines
(4) Increased renal perfusion and diuresis
(5) Improvement in uterine blood flow

Further investigation and evaluation should include the evaluation of renal function (including 24-hour urine for protein and creatinine clearance) and clotting parameters (including platelets, PT, PTT, fibrinogen, fibrin degradation products, liver function tests, and uric acid levels).

Pharmacologic therapy should not be instituted unless the blood pressure remains significantly elevated (diastolic pressure 100-110 mm Hg depending on the authority) in spite of bed rest.

Rest at home and institution of outpatient pharmacologic therapy would not be appropriate at this time.

4. E. The treatment of choice for this patient at this time is delivery. This patient now has pregnancy-aggravated hypertension with severe preeclampsia. When the blood pressure reaches a mean arterial pressure of greater than or equal to 130 mm Hg or a diastolic pressure of greater than or equal to 110 mm Hg, intravenous hypertensives should be instituted to avoid or limit end-organ damage, particularly cerebral hemorrhage.

Intravenous preparation of alpha methyldopa, hydralazine, nitroglycerine, labetalol, or sodium nitroprusside all are potentially useful in a situation like this.

The fetus is in trouble. In general, lung maturity should be confirmed before delivery is contemplated. In the presence of fetal distress or clinical deterioration in the maternal condition, delivery should not be delayed.

5. C. Patients who become pregnant while on antihypertensives and are well controlled should probably have their medications discontinued. Therapy should be reinstituted if the mean arterial pressure (MAP) increases to greater than or equal to 117 mm Hg, the diastolic pressure rises to greater than or equal to 100 mm Hg during the second trimester, the MAP increases to greater than or equal to 127 mm Hg, or the diastolic pressure rises to greater than or equal to 110 mm Hg during the third trimester.

6. D.

7. C.

8. D. The best option of the drugs listed is α-methyldopa. Although a beta blocker could be used (these drugs have now been used to a considerable degree in pregnancy), the drug of choice still is α-methyldopa. We have more experience with this drug than with any other antihypertensive drug in pregnancy and we consider it safe. The only potential concern with beta blockers is a reported association with IUGR. This seems to have been confined to propranolol, but due to our striving for maximum-quality care we believe α-methyldopa to be a better choice.

Thiazide diuretics should not be used in pregnancy; they tend to decrease intravascular volume.

Angiotensin-converting enzyme inhibitors are contraindicated at this time because of a reported association between them and birth defects in pregnant animals.

Calcium-channel blockers, although not contraindicated in pregnancy, have a relatively short track record compared with drugs such as α-methyldopa and can currently not be routinely recommended as drugs of first or second choice.

9. E. The drug of choice for the control of seizures associated with eclampsia is magnesium sulfate. A commonly used regime is as follows:
1. Control of convulsions with magnesium sulfate. An IV loading dose is administered and then periodic intramuscular injections standardized in dose and frequency of administration are given.
2. Intermittent IV injections of hydralazine to lower blood pressure whenever the diastolic pressure is 110 mm Hg or greater
3. Avoidance of diuretics and hyperosmotic agents
4. Limitation of IV fluids administration unless fluid loss is excessive
5. Delivery

10. E. Aspirin, in some studies, has certainly been shown in low doses (60 mg/day) to prevent the development of pregnancy-induced hypertension and fetal growth retardation. Unfortunately, other studies have contradicted that conclusion. At this time, no specific conclusive recommendation can be made about aspirin and its ability to prevent preeclampsia. If this were put into recommendations of the U.S. Preventive Services Task Force on the Periodic Health Examination, it would be a Class C recommendation at this time. That is, there is not enough evidence to either support or refute its use. The wisest course of action is a consultation with a specialist in fetal-maternal medicine.

11. E.

12. B. The pathophysiology at the cellular level and the pathologic process that begins preeclampsia are still unknown. What is known, however, is that there are many possible factors that may play a role. These in-

clude endothelins (which are potent vasoconstrictors), endothelium-derived relaxing factor (EDRF), and the ratio of two particular prostaglandins that have opposite actions—the vasodilating prostacyclin and the vasoconstricting thromboxane.

In terms of the actual pathophysiology, there is little doubt that the major contributing factor that gives rise to all of the complications of preeclampsia and eclampsia is an intense vasospasm or vasoconstriction.

SOLUTION TO SHORT ANSWER MANAGEMENT PROBLEM 42

The established risk factors for preeclampsia include the following:

1. Nulliparous status
2. History of preeclampsia in the patient's mother
3. Chronic hypertension from any cause:
   a) Essential familial hypertension
   b) Secondary hypertension
4. Diabetes mellitus
5. Renal disease
6. Multiple pregnancies
7. Young nulliparous teenagers
8. "Elderly" pregnant women
9. Hydatidiform mole
10. Previous preeclampsia in the patient

SUMMARY OF THE DIAGNOSIS AND TREATMENT OF HYPERTENSION IN PREGNANCY

1. **Diagnosis/classification:**
   a) Pregnancy-induced hypertension:
      1. Hypertension without proteinuria or edema
      2. Preeclampsia
         i) Mild
         ii) Severe
      3. Eclampsia
   b) Pregnancy-aggravated hypertension:
      1. Superimposed preeclampsia
      2. Superimposed eclampsia
   c) Coincidental hypertension
2. **Definition of hypertensive disorders:**
   a) Preeclampsia: either blood pressure greater than or equal to 140 mm Hg systolic or 90 mm Hg diastolic; or an increase of 30 mm Hg systolic or an increase of 15 mm Hg diastolic after the 20th week of pregnancy
   b) Coincidental hypertension: a blood pressure of greater than 140 mm Hg systolic or 90 mm Hg diastolic either predating pregnancy or occurring before the 20th week of gestation or that persists postpartum
   c) Pregnancy-aggravated hypertension with superimposed preeclampsia: A further increase in blood pressure or a worsening of proteinuria after 20 weeks' gestation in a patient with established hypertension
   d) Pregnancy-induced hypertension without proteinuria or pathological edema: this used to be called "transient of late hypertension." It is defined as an elevation of arterial pressure to a level of systolic pressure greater than 140 mm Hg or an increase in diastolic pressure to a level greater than 90 mm Hg in the immediate puerperium with a rapid return to normal pressure no later than the 10th postpartum day.
3. **Treatment of hypertensive disorders in pregnancy:**
   a) Patients with coincidental hypertension on medication who become pregnant should discontinue all antihypertensive agents in early pregnancy if the arterial pressure is normal. The reason for this is that perinatal outcome and the incidence of pregnancy-aggravated hypertension with superimposed preeclampsia are not altered by drug treatment.
   b) Reinstitute therapy if the MAP is greater than or equal to 117 mm Hg, or the diastolic pressure is greater than or equal to 100 mm Hg during the second trimester, or the MAP is greater than or equal to 127 mm Hg, or the diastolic pressure is greater than or equal to 110 mm Hg during the third trimester.
   c) Drugs of choice in the treatment of hypertension in pregnancy:
      1. Coincidental hypertension:
         1st choice: α-methyldopa
         2nd choices: atenolol, metoprolol, labetalol
      2. Pregnancy-induced hypertension with preeclampsia:
         Mild to Moderate: no drug treatment
         Severe: intravenous antihypertensives (1st choice: IV labetalol to keep diastolic pressure less than 110 mm Hg to avoid end-organ damage, particularly cerebral hemorrhage)
         Deliver the fetus once the fetal lung maturity is established, in the presence of IUGR or fetal distress, or if there is further deterioration in the maternal condition.
4. **Pathophysiology of pregnancy-induced hypertension with preeclampsia or eclampsia:** unknown, but consideration is being given to endothelins, endothelium-derived relaxing factor, and the ratio of vasodilating prostaglandins (prostacyclin) to vasoconstricting prostaglandins (thromboxane). Vasospasm is the major pathophysiologic process responsible.

SUGGESTED READINGS

Cunningham FG, MacDonald P, Gant N, Leveno K, Gilstrap L. Williams obstetrics. 19th Ed. Norwalk, CT: Appleton and Lange, 1993.

Kramer W, Kirshon B. Hypertensive disorders in pregnancy. In: Rakel R, ed. Conn's current therapy. Philadelphia: WB Saunders, 1994.

PROBLEM 43 A 19-YEAR-OLD PRIMIGRAVIDA WITH A SMALL BABY

A 19-year-old nulliparous female with preeclampsia is being followed for intrauterine growth retardation. She is presently at 34 weeks' gestation. She has noticed decreased fetal movements for the past 2 days.

On examination in the office her blood pressure is 170/100 mm Hg. She has +3 pitting edema. Her symphysis-fundal height is 28 cm. The baby is in a vertex presentation and appears to be in a left occiput anterior position. The fetal heart is 110 beats/minute.

SELECT THE ONE BEST ANSWER TO THE FOLLOWING QUESTIONS

1. In this patient, what is the most appropriate action at this time?
   a) have the patient return in 1 week instead of 2 weeks for her next appointment
   b) have her return tomorrow for another assessment of her blood pressure and fetal heart rate
   c) instruct her carefully in the manner of fetal movement counting and have her report back in 24 hours
   d) perform a biophysical profile as an outpatient; if the score is 8/10 or 10/10, allow her to go home
   e) none of the above

2. Following your action in Question 1, what would you do now?
   a) maintain the present course of assessment
   b) increase the frequency of office visits to twice weekly
   c) book her for a nonstress test in 3 or 4 days
   d) perform a biophysical profile urgently
   e) give her a Cardiff Kick-to-Ten chart

3. A 41-year-old female, para 4 gravida 5, is hospitalized at 38 weeks' gestation due to preeclampsia and probably fetal intrauterine growth retardation. Her blood pressure is 160/108 mm Hg. The biophysical profile is 2/10. (There is virtually no amniotic fluid, and the nonstress test shows late decelerations.) At this time, what is the correct course of action?
   a) give the patient magnesium sulfate and book her for induction tomorrow
   b) give the patient magnesium sulfate and begin induction now
   c) give the patient magnesium sulfate and perform a stat C-section
   d) give the patient ritodrine and perform a stat C-section
   e) relax; things will likely improve if everybody just calms down

4. What is the leading cause of perinatal death in intrauterine growth retarded infants?
   a) intrauterine asphyxia
   b) preeclampsia in the mother
   c) diabetes in the mother
   d) meconium aspiration
   e) none of the above

5. What is the single most preventable cause of intrauterine growth retardation in pregnancy?
   a) maternal alcohol abuse
   b) maternal malnutrition
   c) maternal cigarette smoking
   d) maternal hypertension
   e) maternal illicit drug abuse

6. What is the most common maternal complication causing intrauterine growth retardation?
   a) maternal hypertension
   b) maternal anemia
   c) maternal renal disease
   d) maternal inflammatory bowel disease
   e) maternal valvular heart disease

7. What is the most common reason for suspecting intrauterine growth retardation?
   a) maternal socioeconomic status
   b) inaccurate gestational age
   c) adolescent age
   d) chronic maternal disease
   e) presentation late in pregnancy with no previous prenatal care

8. What is the most common cause of asymmetrical intrauterine growth retardation?
   a) maternal hypertension
   b) maternal diabetes mellitus
   c) maternal renal disease
   d) maternal systemic lupus erythematosus (SLE)
   e) maternal anemia

9. Which of the following is not a cause of symmetrical intrauterine growth retardation?
   a) congenital abnormalities
   b) chromosomal abnormalities
   c) teratogenic agents
   d) maternal malnutrition
   e) maternal preeclampsia

10. Which of the following is not a cause of asymmetrical intrauterine growth retardation?
   a) maternal collagen vascular disease
   b) maternal preeclampsia
   c) intrauterine infection
   d) maternal type I diabetes mellitus
   e) maternal gestational diabetes

11. Which of the following statements concerning fetal alcohol syndrome is(are) false?
    a) fetal alcohol syndrome will lead to symmetrical intrauterine growth retardation
    b) fetal alcohol syndrome is unlikely to occur in any women taking only the recommended 1-2 drinks/ day (to provide protection against cardiovascular disease)
    c) the prevalence of fetal alcohol syndrome is extremely high in many parts of the United States
    d) all of the above are false
    e) none of the above are false

12. Which of the following statements regarding cigarette smoking in pregnancy is(are) false?
    a) cigarette smoking impairs fetal growth by a direct relationship with number of cigarettes smoked: the higher the number, the greater the risk
    b) cigarette smoking in pregnancy is associated with many other complications, including preterm birth, placenta previa, and placenta abruptio
    c) presentation of the dangers of cigarette smoking in pregnancy almost always is enough to get the pregnant patient to stop smoking
    d) cigarette smoking produces symmetrical intrauterine growth retardation
    e) none of the above are false

13. Which of the following maternal drugs poses the greatest danger in terms of fetal growth retardation and other fetal and newborn problems?
    a) phenytoin
    b) propranolol
    c) verapamil
    d) atenolol
    e) diltiazem

14. Which of the following diagnostic tests offers the most sensitive evaluation of intrauterine growth retardation and subsequent fetal distress?
    a) fetal movement charts
    b) biophysical profile testing
    c) contraction stress testing
    d) nonstress testing
    e) routine obstetrical ultrasound

15. Which of the following parameters define a reactive nonstress test?
    a) the absence of late decelerations
    b) the absence of variable decelerations
    c) the absence of early decelerations
    d) all of the above
    e) none of the above

16. Which of the following does the Rule of 15's apply to?
    a) biophysical profile testing
    b) contraction stress testing
    c) nonstress testing

    d) fetal movement monitoring
    e) routine obstetrical ultrasound

17. Which of the following is(are) components of biophysical profile testing?
    a) gross fetal movements
    b) fetal breathing movements
    c) fetal tone
    d) amniotic fluid volume and amniotic fluid pockets
    e) all of the above

18. Of the components of the biophysical profile, which is the most sensitive for the detection of fetal intrauterine growth retardation?
    a) gross fetal movements
    b) fetal breathing movements
    c) fetal tone
    d) reactive nonstress test
    e) amniotic fluid volume

19. The presence of decelerations on an electronic fetal monitor strip during labor are variably important depending on the type of deceleration in relation to its occurrence relative to the uterine contraction. Each type of deceleration conveys a certain interpretation or a certain meaning. Which of the following pairs of deceleration type and deceleration meaning is(are) correct?
    a) early deceleration = head compression
    b) variable deceleration = cord compression
    c) late deceleration = fetal distress
    d) all of the above are correct
    e) none of the above are correct

20. What is the major difference between asymmetrical intrauterine growth retardation and symmetrical intrauterine growth retardation?
    a) the relationship of the growth of the upper limbs to the growth of the lower limbs
    b) the relationship of the growth of the limbs to the growth of the abdomen
    c) the relationship of the growth of the head to the growth of the rest of the body
    d) the relationship of the growth of the head to the growth of the limbs
    e) none of the above

21. What is the single best clinical indicator of a possible IUGR fetus?
    a) inadequate maternal weight gain
    b) symphysis-fundal height
    c) maternal blood pressure
    d) maternal fetal risk status
    e) none of the above

22. Intrauterine growth retardation is associated with which of the following neonatal conditions?
    a) hypothermia

b) hypoglycemia
c) hypothyroidism

d) a and b
e) all of the above

Short Answer Management Problem 43

The terminology related to decreased growth of the fetus in utero is confusing. There are two basic nomenclatures:
1. The small for gestational age nomenclature
2. The asymmetric/symmetric intrauterine growth retardation nomenclature
Define these two nomenclatures and select the one considered most appropriate.

ANSWERS

1. E. The only reasonable course of action at this time is to hospitalize the patient. The reasoning is twofold. First, this patient has preeclampsia and could possibly progress to eclampsia in a very short time. Second, the fetus shows enough evidence of intrauterine growth retardation (symphysis-fundal height and fetal bradycardia on auscultation) to consider at least urgent assessment and quite possibly urgent delivery.

2. D. This fetus needs urgent assessment with a biophysical profile score. With any score less than 8/10 delivery should be immediate; even with 8/10 or higher delivery should be contemplated if you are unable to settle her blood pressure on bed rest and magnesium sulfate.

3. C. This fetus is in grave danger and needs to be delivered now. The mother could also easily develop eclamptic convulsions within minutes. Thus a stat C-section is the only logical and reasonable course of action. As well, the patient should be started on magnesium sulfate to prevent her preeclampsia from progressing to full-blown eclampsia.

4. A. The leading cause of perinatal death in intrauterine growth retardation is intrauterine asphyxia.

    Diminished placental function is the most common causative factor in intrauterine growth retardation. This is most frequently due to abnormal function of a normal placenta (such as cigarette smoking, diminished perfusion, placental infarction, and intrauterine infection).

    The intrauterine growth retarded fetus is at risk for in utero complications including hypoxia and metabolic acidosis, which may occur at any time but are particularly likely to occur during labor.

5. C. Cigarette smoking is the single most common preventable cause of intrauterine growth retardation in North America today. Cigarette smoking is much more common among women of childbearing age than is alcoholism or illicit drug abuse. Birth weight is reduced by an average of 200 g in infants of smoking mothers. The amount of reduction is related to the number of cigarettes smoked per day. Infants of smoking mothers are also shorter in length, and there is a greater risk of perinatal death or compromise in labor.

6. A. Numerous maternal diseases are associated with suboptimal fetal growth via various mechanisms, including any that interfere with uptake or delivery of nutrients or oxygen to the fetus. Most of these diseases can be described by the acronym HARM. This acronym stands for the following:

    H = hypertension
    A = anemia
    R = renal disease
    M = malabsorption

    Hypertension is the single most common maternal complication causing intrauterine growth retardation in pregnancy. Hypertension results in decreased blood flow through the spiral arteries of the placenta, resulting in decreased delivery of oxygen and nutrients to the placenta and to the fetus. Hypertension may also be associated with placental infarction. Other maternal diseases associated with intrauterine growth retardation include maternal anemia, severe maternal malnutrition, maternal renal disease, maternal malabsorption, multiple pregnancy, extrauterine pregnancy, and maternal valvular disease.

7. B. The most common reason for suspecting intrauterine growth retardation is inaccurate gestational age. In the majority of these cases a significant discrepancy is found between gestational age and symphysis-fundal height. When a careful history is taken, it is often discovered that the last period was not a normal period but rather a shortened period, or even just spotting. Even though this does, in fact, represent a period, the first day of the last period will be calculated from the period before, thus accounting for the discrepancy between estimated gestation and true gestation of 4+ weeks.

    The date of quickening should be established. The first perception of fetal movement occurs at 18-20 weeks in primigravidas and at 14-16 weeks in multigravidas.

If dates are in doubt, obstetric ultrasound should be performed, preferably prior to 20 weeks' gestation. Obstetric ultrasound can also measure estimated fetal weight, and serial measurements of this parameter may be very useful.

8. A. The most common cause of asymmetrical intrauterine growth retardation is maternal hypertension, causing placental insufficiency due to hypertensive complications of pregnancy. The second most common cause is maternal diabetes mellitus causing impaired uteroplacental perfusion.

9. E.

10. C. Causes of symmetrical intrauterine growth retardation include the following:
    A. Congenital malformations
    B. Chromosomal abnormalities
    C. Dwarf syndromes
    D. Teratogens and drugs
    E. Severe malnutrition
    F. Maternal smoking
    G. Maternal anemia
    H. Multiple fetuses
    I. Extrauterine pregnancy

    Causes of asymmetrical intrauterine growth retardation include the following:
    A. Maternal preeclampsia
    B. Maternal eclampsia
    C. Maternal chronic hypertension in pregnancy
    D. Maternal diabetes mellitus
    E. Maternal collagen vascular disease (with the collagen vascular disease affecting the uteroplacental blood flow and causing uteroplacental insufficiency)

11. B. Fetal alcohol syndrome has a very high prevalence in some areas of the United States. Prevalence rates in some populations are up to 50% of all children born. Fetal alcohol syndrome leads to symmetrical intrauterine growth retardation. Contrary to public opinion, no amount of alcohol is a safe amount of alcohol for a pregnant woman. The prevalence of fetal alcohol syndrome in pregnant women who have an average of 1-2 drinks/day may be as high as 10%.

12. C. Cigarette smoking and its dangers increase proportionally with the number of cigarettes smoked. Cigarette smoking produces asymmetrical intrauterine growth retardation. Cigarette smoking is also associated with many other abnormal conditions in pregnancy including placenta abruptio, placenta previa, and preterm labor.

    It is difficult to get pregnant women to quit smoking, although your success rate is likely to be greater than among nonpregnant women.

    If a woman does stop smoking in pregnancy, she is very likely to start again following the end of pregnancy.

When pregnant women are told of the risks to their babies, the most common response is, "It won't happen to me."

13. A. Certain anticonvulsants, especially phenytoin and trimethadione, may produce specific and characteristic syndromes that include intrauterine fetal growth retardation (symmetrical) and other fetal problems.

    Although propranolol was thought, at one time, to produce intrauterine growth retardation, this has subsequently been shown to be false.

    Atenolol is frequently used to control the blood pressure of pregnant women with chronic hypertension. Verapamil, diltiazem, and other calcium-channel blockers will likely become more commonly used in pregnancy in the future.

14. B. The parameters that are useful for evaluating intrauterine fetal growth include the following:
    A. Maternal weight gain
    B. Symphysis-fundal height (expect 3 cm or less variation from dates: 1 cm = 1 week)
    C. Nonstress testing in pregnancy
    D. Fetal movement charting
    E. Ultrasound examination with estimated fetal weight
    F. Biophysical profile testing
    G. Contraction stress testing

    Of these evaluative measures, the most sensitive measure is the measure of the biophysical profile.

15. E.

16. C. A reactive nonstress test is defined by the Rule of 15's. There are at least three accelerations of the fetal heart:

    | Of at least: | 15 beats/minute |
    | Lasting: | 15-second duration/acceleration |
    | During a: | 15-minute measurement period |

    A reactive nonstress test is not defined by, nor does it bear any relationship to, uterine decelerations. The significance of decelerations will be discussed in a later question.

17. E. The biophysical profile has five components:
    A. The nonstress test
    B. Fetal breathing movements
    C. Fetal gross body movements
    D. Fetal muscle tone
    E. Quantitative analysis of amniotic fluid volume

    Each of these five parameters is assigned a maximum value of two points. Thus a perfect biophysical profile is 10/10. Biophysical profile scores of 8/10 and 10/10 suggest normal intrauterine fetal health, or fetuses at low risk for chronic fetal hypoxia or asphyxia. Scores of less than 8/10 suggest the possibility of chronic hypoxia to the fetus and should be reevaluated within a very short period of time (maximum = hours). If the biophysical profile continues to be low, or was very low to begin with (<4/10), immediate action is probably indicated.

18. E. The most sensitive component of the biophysical profile score is the amniotic fluid volume. More specifically, if one 3-cm pocket of amniotic fluid cannot be found, or if the fetus appears to have little or no amniotic fluid surrounding it, fetal distress should be strongly suspected.

19. D. The meaning and significance of fetal heart rate decelerations during labor are as follows:
Early decelerations:
A. Deceleration type: early in relation to the onset of the accompanying uterine contraction
B. Meaning: early fetal heart rate decelerations simply indicate compression of the fetal head by the force of uterine contractions.
C. Significance: virtually none; no cause for concern
Variable decelerations:
A. Deceleration type: variable in relation to the onset of the accompanying uterine contraction
B. Meaning: variable fetal heart rate decelerations indicate compression of the fetal umbilical cord by the contracting uterus.
C. Significance: variable decelerations have variable meaning. Sometimes, especially if the deceleration is deep (fetal heart rate goes down to a very low level and/or lasts for a long time), it may signify the need for intervention. Oxygen, laying the patient on her side, and so on usually is all that is needed to rectify this pattern.
Late decelerations:
A. Deceleration type: late in relation to the onset of the accompanying uterine contraction
B. Meaning: late fetal heart rate decelerations indicate, until proven otherwise, fetal distress or fetal hypoxia.
C. Significance: late decelerations tend to be less dramatic on the recording paper and can actually be missed if the recording paper is not turned to a vertical position to read the strip. If persistent (and this is key), late decelerations necessitate immediate intervention to correct the fetal hypoxia/asphyxia.

20. C. Asymmetrical intrauterine growth retardation essentially means head-sparing IUGR. Although the growth of the rest of the body is retarded, the head is spared. This is not the case in symmetrical intrauterine growth retardation, a situation in which the head is as affected by diminished growth as is the rest of the body. The Short Answer Management Problem answer provides significant detail regarding this difference.

21. A. Symphysis-fundal height, maternal blood pressure, maternal risk status, and especially a history of a previous IUGR fetus are all very important with respect to fe-

tal IUGR. The most important clinical measurement, and one that is not subject to change due to position or observer bias, is an inadequate maternal weight gain.

22. D. Intrauterine growth-retarded fetuses must be observed very carefully during the first few hours of life. A blood sugar level should be drawn immediately and the infant should be wrapped up in layers of more blankets. These maneuvers are necessary because IUGR babies are very prone to both hypoglycemia and hypothermia.

SOLUTION TO SHORT ANSWER MANAGEMENT PROBLEM 43

1. The small for gestational age nomenclature
   A. Definition: a small for gestational age fetus/neonate is defined as one below the 10th percentile of the mean.
   B. Problems with definition:
      1. Definition of the 10% depends on many factors. The standard was determined in Denver, Colorado, which because of its elevation above sea level, will have a lower 10th percentile than a 10th percentile at sea level.
      2. i) Although all growth-retarded infants are small for gestational age, not all small for gestational age infants are growth retarded.
         ii) A percentage of small for gestational age infants are small due to constitutional factors in the mother. These latter factors include maternal ethnic group, maternal parity, maternal weight, and maternal height.

2. The asymmetrical intrauterine growth retarded fetus versus the symmetrical intrauterine growth retarded fetus
   A. Definition: the definition of asymmetrical versus symmetrical basically defines the relationship between the size of the fetal head versus the size of the rest of the fetal body.
   B. Explanation: head size is the last fetal dimension to be affected by growth retardation, if it is affected at all. Muscle mass is also reduced, as are subcutaneous tissue fat stores. Asymmetrical fetal growth retardation is attributed to placental insufficiency due to a variety of hypertensive complications of pregnancy as well as advanced diabetes mellitus with impaired uteroplacental perfusion.

3. The terminology of choice: Previously, the terminology of choice was small for gestational age. At this time, the terminology of choice is asymmetrical/symmetrical intrauterine growth retardation because it more accurately portrays at a physiologic level what is going on.
   1) All fetuses with IUGR are also SGA fetuses.
   2) Not all fetuses who are SGA fetuses are IUGR fetuses. Thus normality of growth is more appropriately defined with this terminology.

SUMMARY OF THE DIAGNOSIS AND MANAGEMENT OF INTRAUTERINE GROWTH RETARDATION:

1. **Definitions:**
   a) Covered in Short Answer Management Problem. Preferred term at this time: intrauterine growth retardation
      1. Subtype symmetrical
      2. Subtype asymmetrical
2. **Prevalence:** the true prevalence of IUGR among all pregnant women is estimated at approximately 5%.
3. **Differentiation:** the importance of differentiating the various types of IUGR is that it allows you to propose a management plan that is based on the pathology involved. It is especially important, based on the old terminology, to separate normal from abnormal: using the old terminology, a fetus who had a mother who was of a particular ethnic group, of a certain parity, of a certain weight, or of a certain height would be considered small for gestational age and the baby probably labeled as IUGR when in fact this was not the case.
4. **Risk status:** true IUGR babies are at extremely high risk for perinatal morbidity and mortality.
5. **Important connections:**
   a) Asymmetrical IUGR: most commonly associated with either some form of maternal hypertensive process or collagen vascular process or maternal diabetes mellitus leading to placental insufficiency.
   b) Symmetrical IUGR: most commonly associated with the following:
      1. Chromosomal abnormalities
      2. Cigarette smoking
      3. Fetal alcohol syndrome
      4. Intrauterine infections
6. **Clinical clues/investigations:**
   a) Physical examination/clinical correlates:
      1. Failure to gain an adequate amount of weight in pregnancy
      2. Symphysis-fundal height
      3. Fetal movement counting
   b) Investigations:
      1. Biophysical profile testing (best indicator)
      2. Nonstress test
      3. Obstetrical ultrasound (estimated fetal weight)
      4. Contraction stress test
7. **Management strategy in third trimester:**
   a) Depends on the clinical situation, but deliver a fetus with IUGR (most types) as soon as possible (relative to fetal lung maturity).
8. **Complications in neonates:**
   a) Hypoglycemia
   b) Hypothermia

SUGGESTED READING

Cunningham FG et al., eds. Williams obstetrics. 19th Ed. Norwalk, CT: Appleton and Lange, 1993.

PROBLEM 44   A 24-YEAR-OLD FEMALE WHO HAS GONE PAST HER DUE DATE

A 24-year-old female presents to you as a new patient. She has suddenly moved to your community with her 2-year-old daughter. She has been recommended to you by a friend. She tells you that she is 43 weeks by dates. She regrets that she lost her prenatal sheet when packing. When you ask her who her previous doctor was she tells you that she only went to her doctor three or four times because she didn't have time. She even forgets the doctor's name.

She has not been keeping a "fetal kick chart," but she says the baby has been moving. She has not had an obstetrical ultrasound. On examination, this measures 36 cm by height of the uterus. The cervix is soft, 25% effaced, and 1 cm dilated. The fetus is vertex and appears to be approximately 6½ to 7 pounds in weight. The fetal heart rate is 142 and regular.

SELECT THE ONE BEST ANSWER TO THE FOLLOWING QUESTIONS

1. At this time, what would you do?
   a) tell her to come back in a week while you think about things
   b) arrange a biophysical profile and an obstetrical ultrasound examination; ask the ultrasonographer for estimated gestational age and weight
   c) book her for induction of labor
   d) book her for C-section just to be on the safe side
   e) do nothing now; make an appointment to see her in 1 week

2. A pregnancy is defined as being *postterm* if it exceeds how many days of gestation?
   a) 280 days
   b) 287 days
   c) 294 days
   d) 273 days
   e) 301 days

3. What is the approximate pseudoprevalence of post-term pregnancy?
   a) 25%-30%
   b) 15%-19%
   c) 10%-14%
   d) 5%-9%
   e) 2%-3%

4. What is the approximate true prevalence of postterm pregnancy?
   a) 25%-30%
   b) 15%-19%
   c) 10%-14%
   d) 5%-9%
   e) 2%-3%

5. Which of the following parameters is the most sensitive test for the prediction of fetal asphyxia and resultant perinatal mortality in post-term pregnancy?
   a) a nonstress test weekly
   b) a nonstress test biweekly
   c) lack of a 3-cm vertical pocket of amniotic fluid on ultrasound
   d) lack of a 1-cm vertical pocket of amniotic fluid on ultrasound
   e) a contraction stress test

6. What is the most common cause of a diagnosis of post-dates pregnancy?
   a) lack of an obstetrical ultrasound in pregnancy
   b) inaccurate or incorrect dates (based on the first day of the last normal menstrual period)
   c) the post-maturity syndrome
   d) intrauterine growth retardation
   e) none of the above

7. Which of the following statements regarding post-term pregnancy is(are) true?
   a) the perinatal mortality rate is increased in patients who have, in fact, gone past 42 completed weeks of gestation
   b) the incidence of meconium staining and meconium aspiration is increased in patients who have gone beyond 42 completed weeks of gestation
   c) the true post-term fetus may continue to gain weight in utero and present a problem at birth because of fetal size
   d) the intrauterine environment in a true post-term pregnancy may predispose to the development of a dysmature or dystrophic infant
   e) all of the above are true

8. To what does the term *post-mature* refer?
   a) all infants delivered by mothers diagnosed as post-term
   b) all infants delivered by mothers who are verified by objective criteria to be greater than 42 weeks gestation
   c) infants who display a specific subset of characteristics and who are delivered by mothers who are truly post-term
   d) no longer a useful description
   e) none of the above

9. A colleague of yours describes his approach to post-term gestation: "I deliver all my women at 42 weeks." Without inquiring about his perinatal morbidity and mortality statistics, which of the following is(are) reasons not to follow his example?

a) it is difficult to predict for certain which fetuses are likely to develop significant problems left in utero past 42 weeks
b) induction of labor is not always successful
c) delivery by C-section appreciably increases the risk of serious maternal morbidity
d) the great majority of fetuses who are truly more than 42 weeks fare well
e) all of the above are true

10. At this time, which of the following is(are) true regarding those women who have been established to be truly post-term greater than 42 weeks of gestation)?

a) there are two approaches to managing these pregnancies: one is conservative and the other is aggressive
b) there appears to be no difference in perinatal outcome between aggressive management and conservative management if conservative management includes an appropriate protocol for fetal surveillance
c) aggressive management appears to result in lower perinatal morbidity and mortality than conservative management
d) a and b
e) a and c

Short Answer Management Problem 44

You are a family physician doing obstetrics in your local hospital. You have been asked to develop a clinical practice guideline for the management of post-term pregnancy.
   Prepare this CPG based on your knowledge of the subject.

ANSWERS

1. B. Basically, you don't have a very good idea of what's going on here except for the following:
   A. This patient appears to be in the late part of the third trimester.
   B. She has had little prenatal care; she may be at high risk.
   C. The fetus shows no sign of fetal distress at this time, but your information is limited.
   D. The story of the sudden move is a bit strange and bears further investigation.
      The best things to do at this time would be the following:
      a) Ensure fetal well-being with a biophysical profile examination.
      b) Obtain an estimate of fetal gestation and fetal weight by ultrasonography.
      c) Book a follow-up appointment.
      d) Suggest that a public health nurse assess this patient in her home context.

2. C.

3. C.

4. E. A pregnancy is defined as post-term if it persists beyond 294 days (42 weeks) or more from the onset of the first day of the last normal menstrual period.
   The true prevalence of post-term pregnancy among all pregnant women is approximately 2%-3%. The pseudoprevalence of post-term pregnancy (the prevalence of the label of post-term pregnancy being applied or documented in the chart) is approximately

10%-14%. Thus, the conclusion is that the vast majority of pregnancies that are labeled as post-term are not post-term but really a case of mistaken dates.

5. C. The most sensitive test for the prediction of fetal asphyxia and resultant perinatal mortality in post-term pregnancy is the lack of a 3-cm amniotic fluid pocket on ultrasound. The 3-cm pocket is reassuring. A recent study has shown that the perinatal mortality using the lack of a 3-cm pocket as a test as a basis for intervention was associated with a lower perinatal mortality rate than using either nonstress testing or contraction stress testing. Thus the performance of a biophysical profile on a biweekly basis, with the demonstration of a 3-cm amniotic fluid pocket, is a reassuring sign that suggests that the fetus is in good condition.

6. B. The most common cause of a diagnosis of post-dated pregnancy is incorrect or inaccurate dates based on the first day of the last menstrual period. Although the lack of an obstetrical ultrasound in pregnancy will increase the probability of that diagnosis being made, it is not the true cause.

7. E. The perinatal mortality rate and the incidence of meconium staining and meconium aspiration are increased when the gestational age is 42 weeks or beyond. The true post-term pregnancy may even continue to gain weight in utero and thus be unusually large at birth. On the other hand, the intrauterine environment may predispose to loss of fetal weight, loss of subcutaneous fat and muscle, and a dystrophic or dysmature appearance. This is the more common and more sinister scenario.

8. C. The term *post-mature* as applied to infants delivered refers to a specific subset of infants delivered of mothers who are truly post-term and who display the following characteristics:
   A. Underweight due to loss of subcutaneous fat
   B. Long and thin in girth
   C. Skin with patchy areas of desquamation
   D. Skin sometimes covered with meconium
   E. Wrinkled hands and feet on the ventral surfaces
   F. Long nails stained with meconium

9. E.

10. D. At least five difficult problems persist that serve to discourage a policy of delivering all fetuses whose gestational age is merely suspected to be at least 42 weeks:
    A. Gestational age is not always known precisely, and thus the fetus may actually be less mature than believed.
    B. It is very difficult to identify with precision those fetuses who are likely to develop significant morbidity if left in utero.
    C. The great majority of these fetuses fare rather well.
    D. Induction of labor is not always successful.
    E. Delivery by C-section appreciably increases the risk of serious maternal morbidity not only in this pregnancy but also to a degree in subsequent ones.

    It becomes clear that there are two distinct approaches to the management of pregnancies determined to be 42 weeks or more. A randomized investigation comparing elective induction with antepartum surveillance (nonstress testing, amniotic fluid volume, fetal movement counting) was performed in Canada. Women were randomized to either induction of labor at 42 weeks or serial antenatal fetal testing.

    The results of this trial, the most comprehensive yet performed in the world, indicated the following:
    A. Induction of labor at 42 weeks resulted in a lower rate of C-section (21%) than in the antenatal surveillance group (25%).
    B. Infant outcomes were equivalent in the two study groups.

SOLUTION TO SHORT ANSWER MANAGEMENT PROBLEM 44

Following are the steps that probably should be in the guidelines you have prepared for the management of post-term pregnancy.

1. Review the entire prenatal history. Establish whether or not the last menstrual period and the last normal menstrual period are the same thing.
2. Review any and all obstetrical ultrasounds performed during the pregnancy.
3. Calculate the EDC from (1) and compare it to the EDC from (2). If more than one ultrasound was performed, use the date established by the ultrasound closest to 16-18 weeks' gestation.
4. Determine your best estimate of the EDC from all the information available.
5. At 41 weeks (from 4), perform a pelvic examination to determine cervical effacement and cervical dilatation.
6. Begin antenatal monitoring at 41 weeks:
   A. Nonstress tests twice/week
   B. Fetal movements charting daily
   C. Biophysical profile (especially amniotic fluid volume, looking for at least one 3-cm pocket of amniotic fluid)
7. Repeat the pelvic examination at 42 weeks and reevaluate cervical effacement and cervical dilatation.
8. Definitely obtain a consultation from an obstetrician at this time (if one has not already been done).
9. Continue antenatal monitoring at 42 weeks as at 41-42 weeks.
10. At 42 5/7 weeks (42 weeks/5 days) begin induction of labor. If cervix is not ripe, then ripening of the cervix with a prostaglandin gel is indicated prior to formal induction with oxytocin.
11. If induction not successful or if there is any sign of fetal distress during induction, proceed to C-section.

    The Canadian study suggests that this approach will lower the rate of C-section.

SUMMARY OF THE DIAGNOSIS AND MANAGEMENT OF POST-TERM PREGNANCY

A good summary of this chapter is provided by the clinical practice guideline given in the Solution to the Short Answer Management Problem.

SUGGESTED READINGS

Cunningham FG et al., eds. Preterm and postterm pregnancy and fetal growth retardation. In: Williams obstetrics. 19th Ed. Norwalk, CT: Appleton and Lange, 1993.

Hannah ME et al. Canadian multicenter post-term pregnancy trial group: Induction of labor as compared with serial antenatal monitoring in post-term pregnancy. N Engl J Med 1992; 326:1587.

PROBLEM 45   A 25-YEAR-OLD FEMALE, PARA 0 GRAVIDA 2, WITH VAGINAL BLEEDING

A 25-year-old female, para 0 gravida 2, presents to your office at 11 weeks' gestation with vaginal bleeding, mild lower abdominal cramping, and bilateral lower pelvic discomfort. She is crying and upset. Her previous pregnancy ended in miscarriage at 9 weeks.

On examination, a bright red flow is seen coming from the cervical os. Her cervix is closed. The uterus by palpation is 8-9 weeks' gestation.

Her blood pressure is 120/70 mm Hg and her pulse rate is 96. No other abnormalities are found.

SELECT THE ONE BEST ANSWER TO THE FOLLOWING QUESTIONS:

1. What is the most likely diagnosis of this patient's condition at this time?
   a) threatened abortion
   b) inevitable abortion
   c) incomplete abortion
   d) recurrent spontaneous abortion
   e) complete abortion

2. The vaginal blood flow in this patient increases slightly while in your office. She is now soaking through approximately 1 pad every 2 hours.
   What would you do at this time?
   a) observe carefully at home; order outpatient investigations
   b) admit the patient to hospital and investigate her condition further
   c) observe the patient at home; tell her not to worry about anything
   d) admit the patient to the hospital for observation only; no testing is indicated at this time
   e) it doesn't really matter

3. Taking into account your management, the patient goes on to abort the fetus 3 days later. On examination it appears that most of the placental tissue is present. What would you now recommend?
   a) no further treatment
   b) ergonovine maleate to contract the uterus
   c) prophylactic antibiotics to prevent infection
   d) dilatation and curettage
   e) b and c

4. What is the spontaneous abortion rate in North American women?
   a) 10%
   b) 20%
   c) 25%
   d) 50%
   e) 75%

5. Spontaneous abortion is defined as which of the following?

a) any miscarriage
b) termination of pregnancy before 20 weeks' gestation based on the last normal menses
c) delivery of a fetus-neonate under 250 g
d) delivery of a fetus-neonate under 500 g
e) none of the above

6. What is the most commonly recognized precipitating factor in spontaneous abortion?
   a) chromosomal abnormality
   b) advanced maternal age
   c) preexisting chronic maternal disease
   d) alcohol intake
   e) cigarette smoking

7. What is the most commonly recognized chromosomal anomaly associated with first-trimester spontaneous abortion?
   a) autosomal trisomy
   b) monosomy
   c) tetraploidy
   d) autosomal monosomy
   e) sex chromosome polysomy

8. Which of the following conditions is(are) associated with an increased incidence of abortion?
   a) hypothyroidism
   b) controlled diabetes mellitus
   c) uncontrolled diabetes mellitus
   d) all of the above
   e) none of the above

9. Which of the following statements regarding cigarette smoking and spontaneous abortion is(are) true?
   a) smoking has been associated with an increased risk of euploidic abortion
   b) in women who smoke >14 cigarettes/day, the risk of spontaneous abortion is twice that of women who do not smoke
   c) smoking increases the risk of abortion by a factor of 1.2 for each 10 cigarettes smoked/day
   d) all of the above are true
   e) none of the above are true

10. Which of the following statements regarding the risk of spontaneous abortion and alcohol intake is(are) true?
    a) the risk of spontaneous euploidic abortion is increased even when alcohol is consumed "in moderation" during pregnancy
    b) the spontaneous abortion rate is doubled in women who drink twice weekly
    c) the spontaneous abortion rate is tripled in women who consume alcohol daily
    d) all of the above are true
    e) none of the above are true

11. Which of the following antibodies is most clearly associated with spontaneous abortion?
    a) anticardiolipin antibody
    b) antithyroid antibody
    c) antinuclear antibody
    d) rheumatoid factor
    e) anti-smooth muscle antibody

Short Answer Management Problem 45

Describe the currently recommended classification of spontaneous abortion.

ANSWERS

1. A. The diagnosis is threatened abortion. Threatened abortion is defined as bloody vaginal discharge or vaginal bleeding that appears during the first 20 weeks of pregnancy. Mild abdominal cramping often accompanies the bleeding. The incidence of threatened abortion in pregnancy is 20-25%; of that number half go on to abort the fetus. Threatened abortion is associated with a higher risk of preterm labor, low birth weight, and perinatal mortality. There is, however, no increased risk of fetal malformations.

   Inevitable abortion is defined as vaginal bleeding during the first half of pregnancy accompanied by cervical dilatation and rupture of the gestational sac.

   Incomplete abortion is the incomplete evacuation of the products of conception during the abortion. It is often difficult, however, to be sure that all of the products of conception have been expelled without doing a dilatation and curettage.

   Recurrent spontaneous abortion refers to three or more consecutive abortions.

   Complete abortion refers to the complete evacuation of the products of conception from the uterus during the first half of pregnancy.

2. B. In any patient with more than slight bleeding, hospitalization is wise. With the associated cramping in this patient there is a high probability that she will go on to abort. Investigations in hospital should include a beta-HCG level and obstetric ultrasound to establish pregnancy and the viability of same.

3. D. Unless all of the fetus and placenta can be positively identified, dilation and curettage is indicated. It is often very difficult to be sure that an abortion is indeed complete. If the gestational age is less than 10 weeks, conservative management may be reasonable.

Ergonovine maleate and prophylactic antibiotics are most useful when excessive bleeding occurs in the postpartum period and is thought not to be due to retained products of conception.

4. C. The spontaneous abortion rate in North American women is approximately 25%. Several reports have indicated spontaneous abortion rates as high as 50%; this, however, has not been confirmed.

5. B. Spontaneous abortion is defined as the termination of pregnancy before 20 weeks' gestation based on the date of the last normal menstrual period.

6. A. The most commonly recognized precipitating factor in spontaneous abortion is chromosomal anomaly.

7. A. The most common recognized chromosomal abnormality associated with first-trimester spontaneous abortion is autosomal trisomy. It can be the result of an isolated nondisjunction, maternal or paternal balanced translocation, or balanced chromosomal inversion.

8. C. Uncontrolled diabetes mellitus has been associated with an increased incidence of spontaneous abortion. Well-controlled diabetes, however, is not. There is also no association between hypothyroidism and spontaneous abortion.

9. D. Cigarette smoking is associated with an increased risk of euploidic abortion. For women who smoke more than 14 cigarettes/day, the risk of spontaneous abortion is approximately twice that of nonsmokers. This is independent of either maternal age and alcohol ingestion. The risk of spontaneous abortion increases in a linear fashion by a factor of 1.2 for each 10 cigarettes smoked/day.

10. D. The incidence of spontaneous euploidic abortion is increased even when alcohol is consumed "in moderation." Recent studies have indicated that the abortion rate is doubled in women who consume alcohol twice weekly and is tripled in women who consume alcohol daily when compared to nondrinkers. Increased euploidic abortion is strong evidence that both tobacco and alcohol are embryotoxins.

11. A. Autoimmune mechanisms are those in which a cellular or humoral response is directed against a specific site within the host. Connective-tissue disorders such as SLE are associated with increased abortion and fetal death.

    Antiphospholipid antibodies, including the lupus anticoagulant and anticardiolipin antibodies, are examples of autoimmune disease states that are associated with recurrent abortion.

SOLUTION TO SHORT ANSWER MANAGEMENT PROBLEM 45

The classification of spontaneous abortion is as follows:

1. *Threatened abortion:* threatened abortion is defined as any bloody vaginal discharge or vaginal bleeding that occurs before 20 weeks of gestation (based on gestational age, not on embryologic age).
2. *Inevitable abortion:* inevitable abortion is defined as rupture of the membranes in the presence of cervical dilatation during the first 20 weeks of gestation.
3. *Missed abortion:* missed abortion is defined as retention of dead products of conception in utero for up to 4 weeks.
4. *Recurrent spontaneous abortion:* recurrent spontaneous abortion (previously known as habitual abortion) has been defined by various criteria of number and sequence. The most generally accepted definition refers to three or more consecutive spontaneous abortions.

SUMMARY OF THE DIAGNOSIS AND MANAGEMENT OF SPONTANEOUS ABORTION

1. **Classification:** see the Short Answer Management Problem in this chapter.
2. **Investigation of threatened abortion:**
   a) Serial beta-HCG levels
   b) Ultrasound (if questionable, repeat in 1-2 weeks)
3. **Management of threatened abortion:**
   a) Rest in hospital (unless there is only a small amount of blood in which case rest at home is reasonable)
   b) Observation
   c) Conservative management if bleeding slows down or stops (document live fetus by ultrasound)
   d) Dilatation and curettage if heavy bleeding continues and ultrasound reveals no evidence of a live fetus

SUGGESTED READING

Cunningham FG, MacDonald PC, Leveno KJ, Gant N, Gilstrap L. Williams obstetrics. 19th Ed. Norwalk, CT: Appleton and Lange,

PROBLEM 46   A 21-YEAR-OLD FEMALE WITH A VAGINAL DISCHARGE

A 21-year-old female presents to your office with a pruritic, thick, white, vaginal discharge. This is associated with vulvar erythema. There is no discharge present at the introitus. The consistency of the discharge is curdy, the viscosity is high, and the discharge is adherent to the vaginal walls. The pH is 4.0, and there is no amine odor.

SELECT THE ONE BEST ANSWER TO THE FOLLOWING QUESTIONS:

1. What is the most likely diagnosis in this patient?
   a) physiologic discharge
   b) bacterial vaginosis
   c) candidiasis
   d) trichomoniasis
   e) none of the above

2. What is the treatment of choice in this patient?
   a) metronidazole cream
   b) ampicillin
   c) miconazole (local)
   d) nystatin tablets
   e) none of the above

3. The patient does not respond to the treatment you prescribed. At this time, what should you do?
   a) repeat the treatment offered first
   b) repeat the treatment offered first and double the dose
   c) prescribe oral fluconazole in a single dose
   d) reculture the patient
   e) reconsider the diagnosis

4. Which of the following is(are) established risk factors for recurrent candidal vulvovaginitis?
   a) diabetes mellitus
   b) long-term antibiotic therapy
   c) HIV infection
   d) all of the above
   e) none of the above

5. A 25-year-old female presents to your office with a profuse, gray-green, malodorous discharge with irritation and pruritus. The discharge is present at the introitus. There is vulvar edema present. The discharge is adherent to the vaginal walls. The pH is 6.0. There is an amine odor present, and the microscopic examination shows 15 WBC/s/hpf.
   What is the most likely diagnosis in this patient?
   a) candidiasis
   b) trichomoniasis
   c) bacterial vaginosis
   d) physiologic discharge
   e) nonspecific vaginitis

6. What is the treatment of choice for the patient described in Question 5?
   a) intravaginal miconazole

   b) intravaginal clotrimazole
   c) metronidazole 250 mg tid
   d) ampicillin 500 mg tid
   e) a 2-g stat oral dose of metronidazole

7. A 29-year-old female presents with a 2-week history of profuse, malodorous discharge with irritation. On examination, the discharge is present at the introitus. It is gray in color. It is homogeneous and has a low viscosity. It is adherent to the vaginal walls. The pH is 6.5. An amine odor is present. On microscopic examination "clue cells" are present, but white blood cells are absent.
   What is the most likely diagnosis in this patient?
   a) a bacterial vaginal infection
   b) trichomoniasis
   c) candidiasis
   d) human immunodeficiency virus
   e) none of the above

8. What is the treatment of choice for the condition described?
   a) intravaginal miconazole (one tablet) for 7 days
   b) intravaginal clotrimazole (one tablet) for 7 days
   c) a 2-g stat dose of metronidazole
   d) oral metronidazole 250 mg-500 mg tid for 7 days
   e) oral erythromycin 500 mg tid

9. What is the most common type of bacteria associated with a vaginal bacterial infection?
   a) gram-positive aerobic cocci
   b) gram-negative aerobic rods
   c) gram-negative aerobic cocci
   d) anaerobic bacteria
   e) gram-positive rods

10. The "whiff test" or "amine odor" test is of use in diagnosing which of the following vaginal infections?
    a) trichomoniasis
    b) a bacterial vaginal infection
    c) candidiasis
    d) physiologic discharge
    e) all of the above

11. What is the most common form of vaginitis?
    a) vulvovaginal candidiasis
    b) trichomoniasis
    c) bacterial vaginal infection
    d) chlamydial vaginitis
    e) none of the above

Short Answer Management Problem 46

Describe the differentiation of a vaginal discharge based on the following:
a) pH
b) WBCs
c) Amine odor test
d) Consistency
e) Color
f) Presence of clue cells

ANSWERS

1. C. This patient has candidiasis. *Candida albicans* is a commensal organism in most women. When, however, *Corynebacterium sp.* and specific fungal inhibitory factors are suppressed, it can produce an infection.

   Pruritus is by far the most common symptom in vaginal candidiasis. Discharge may be normal or increased. It is usually described as a white and curdy cottage cheese. Burning, irritation, and soreness may be present. Dyspareunia and vulvar (external) dysuria are common. Erythema of the vulva is common.

   Predisposing factors for vaginal candidiasis include the premenstrual phase of the menstrual cycle, antibiotic use, and coitus. There is no direct relationship between vaginal candidiasis and the oral contraceptive pill.

   Physical examination often reveals vulvar erythema and edema. The discharge is often adherent to the vaginal walls. The vaginal pH is usually normal (<4.5). Amine odor is absent, and WBCs are not increased. Mycelia and/or spores may be seen on microscopy.

2. C. The treatment of choice in this patient is an imidazole cream/suppository, or clotrimazole cream/suppository. Many regimens utilizing imidazole or clotrimazole have shown high cure rates. The treatment regimens vary from 1 to 7 days. Because of the presence of both internal and external symptoms, the use of a preparation containing both vaginal miconazole ovules (one/night for 3 nights) plus external miconazole cream (to be applied to the vulvar area once or twice a day) can be recommended. Loose-fitting clothing and cotton underwear will decrease colonization rates.

   In recurrent candidiasis, 1% gentian violet or oral nystatin or ketoconazole can be used. In recurrent candidiasis the partner should be treated with an imidazole cream, locally applied to the foreskin and the glans.

3. C. A single dose of oral fluconazole is at least as effective as intravaginal treatment for vulvovaginal candidiasis, and many patients seem to prefer it. Gastrointestinal toxicity is fairly common with the oral drug, however. The recommended dose is a single 150-mg oral dose.

4. D. Risk factors for vaginal candidiasis include the following:
   a) Physical disruption of the integument
   b) Pregnancy
   c) Antibiotic therapy
   d) Diabetes mellitus
   e) Immunologic deficiencies (including HIV infection)
   f) Tight-fitting clothing
   g) Sexual behavior (including oral-genital and anal sex)

   The oral contraceptive pill does not seem to increase the incidence of symptomatic candidiasis, although it may increase the frequency of the carrier state.

5. B. This patient has trichomoniasis. The symptoms of trichomoniasis include a malodorous, copious, grayish-green vaginal discharge that adheres to the vaginal walls. Irritation, pruritus, and vulvar edema may be present. Erythema of the vaginal mucosa is common. The pH is usually greater than 5.0. Motile trichomonads and numerous white blood cells are often seen on light microscopy.

6. E. The treatment of choice for trichomoniasis is metronidazole. The recommended treatment protocol is a single oral dose of 2 g. Patients who fail to respond to a single oral dose of 2 g should be given extended therapy consisting of a dose of 500 mg of metronidazole for 7 days.

   Because trichomoniasis is a sexually transmitted disease, simultaneous treatment of the male partner(s) is essential. Reinfection is a major cause of recurrence.

7. A. This patient has a bacterial vaginal infection. Bacterial vaginal infections are the most common form of vaginitis. Bacterial vaginal infection has been known as nonspecific vaginitis, *Gardnerella* vaginitis, *Haemophilus* vaginitis, *Corynebacterium* vaginitis, mixed bacterial vaginitis, and anaerobic vaginitis. Bacterial vaginal infections are polymicrobial infections involving a synergistic interaction between Gardnerella vaginitis and anaerobic bacteria.

   Bacterial vaginal infections are frequently asymptomatic. Symptomatic patients usually present with a malodorous, profuse discharge. The discharge is present at the introitus, is gray in color, and is homogeneous. It has a low viscosity and is adherent to the vaginal walls. The pH is >5.0, and an amine odor is present on exposure to KOH. Clue cells (vaginal epithelial cells with an obscured border resulting from adherence of bacteria to the cell border) are often seen. WBCs are absent.

8. D. The treatment of choice for bacterial vaginal infections is oral metronidazole 250-500 mg tid for 7 days. It is generally recommended that the patient's partner also be treated.

9. D. The most common bacteria associated with bacterial vaginal infections are anaerobic bacteria. The anaerobic bacteria such as *peptostreptococci* interact with other bacteria including *Corynebacterium, Haemophilus,* and other species to produce the characteristic infection.

10. B. The whiff test or amine odor test is of use in the diagnosis of a bacterial vaginal infection. It reflects the production of amines by the anaerobic bacteria themselves.

11. C. The most common type of vaginitis is bacterial vaginal infection. Bacterial vaginal infection accounts for 35-50% of all cases of vaginitis. Candidiasis accounts for 20-40%, and trichomoniasis for 10-20%.

SOLUTION TO SHORT ANSWER MANAGEMENT PROBLEM 46

Vaginal discharge may be differentiated on the basis of several characteristics. These include pH, the presence or absence of WBCs, the amine odor test, the presence or absence of clue cells, consistency, and color.
The differentiation is as follows:
1. Normal vaginal discharge:
   a) Clear or white discharge
   b) Nonhomogeneous
   c) Scant to moderate
   d) pH < 4.5
   e) Amine odor negative
   f) Clue cells absent
   g) Trichomonads absent
   h) Mycelia absent
   i) The presence of normal epithelial cells and lactobacilli
2. Bacterial vaginal infection:
   a) Malodorous discharge
   b) White or gray; homogeneous
   c) Moderate in amount
   d) pH > 4.5
   e) Amine test positive
   f) Clue cells present
   g) Trichomonads absent
   h) Mycelia absent
   i) Predominance of coccobacilli
   j) Few to no leukocytes
3. Vulvovaginal candidiasis:
   a) Pruritus
   b) Thick, white discharge
   c) Homogeneous
   d) Thick clumps of curdy material
   e) Vulvar, introital, and vaginal edema and erythema
   f) pH < 4.5
   g) Amine test absent
   h) Clue cells absent
   i) Trichomonads absent
   j) Mycelia present
   k) Normal flora on microscopy
4. Trichomoniasis:
   a) Pruritus
   b) Fishy odor
   c) Gray or yellow-green
   d) Thin
   e) Homogeneous ± vulvar and vaginal erythema
   f) pH > 4.5
   g) Amine test absent
   h) Clue cells absent
   i) Trichomonads present
   j) Mycelia absent
   k) Many polymorphonuclear leukocytes, large amounts of cellular debris

SUMMARY OF THE DIAGNOSIS AND TREATMENT OF VULVOVAGINITIS

1. **Diagnosis:** See the differentiation given in the solution to the short answer management problem in this chapter.
2. **Treatment:**
   a) Normal vaginal discharge: no treatment necessary
   b) Bacterial vaginal infection: oral metronidazole 250-500 mg tid for 7 days
   c) Trichomoniasis: single stat oral dose of metronidazole—2 g
   d) Vulvovaginal candidiasis: imidazole cream or suppository; clotrimazole cream or suppository

SUGGESTED READINGS

Brooks L. Vulvovaginitis. In: Rakel R, ed. Conn's current therapy. Philadelphia: WB Saunders, 1994.
Oral fluconazole for vaginal candidiasis. The medical letter, volume 36(631), September 16, 1994, pp. 1-2.

PROBLEM 47   A 26-YEAR-OLD FEMALE WITH AN ABNORMAL PAP SMEAR

A 26-year-old female presents for her periodic health assessment. She is married, has two children, and has had no major medical illnesses. She has been a regular patient of yours for many years.

She is a current cigarette smoker (approximately 1 pack/day). She has been currently using the birth control pill as a means of contraception for 9 months.

She describes her adolescence as a period of turmoil. During her high school years she had approximately 10 sexual partners. She does not recall ever having contracted an STD.

Her blood pressure is 100/70 mm Hg, and her pulse is 72 and regular. On pelvic examination, her adnexa are normal and nontender. There is no cervical discharge, and her cervix looks normal.

Her pap smear comes back three days later and is graded as cervical intraepithelial neoplasia—grade 1 (CIN-1).

SELECT THE ONE BEST ANSWER TO THE FOLLOWING QUESTIONS

1. At this time, assuming that this patient is reliable in follow-up, what should you do?
   a) repeat the Pap smear in 1 year
   b) repeat the Pap smear in 4-6 months
   c) repeat the Pap smear in 1-3 months
   d) refer the patient for colposcopy
   e) refer the patient for a bone biopsy

2. A 26-year-old female presents for a routine periodic health assessment. A Pap smear is performed and the result comes back CIN-1 with Trichomonas vaginalis present.
   What would you do at this time?
   a) treat the infection and repeat the Pap smear at the next recommended screening interval
   b) treat the infection and repeat the Pap smear in 6 weeks
   c) treat the infection in the patient and her partner and repeat the Pap smear at the next recommended screening interval
   d) treat the infection in the patient and partner and repeat the Pap smear in 6 weeks
   e) refer the patient for colposcopy

3. Which of the following statements regarding carcinoma of the cervix and/or analysis of the Pap smear is false?
   a) carcinoma of the cervix can be regarded as an STD
   b) case-finding for carcinoma of the cervix can stop at age 65 providing the patient has been adequately screened before and has had no new sexual partners after that ime
   c) an Ayres spatula is a sufficient tool for obtaining a specimen of the endocervix for Pap smear analysis
   d) carcinoma of the cervix is a disease with a long lead time
   e) none of the above statements are false

4. Carcinoma of the cervix is usually associated with which of the following viruses?
   a) herpes simplex type I virus
   b) herpes simplex type II virus
   c) human papilloma virus
   d) human parvovirus
   e) adenovirus

5. Which of the following is not a documented direct risk factor for carcinoma of the cervix?
   a) a partner with multiple sexual partners
   b) an early age of first intercourse
   c) intercourse with more than three partners
   d) a clinical history of condyloma acuminata
   e) a herpes simplex type II viral infection

6. You are just beginning the transformation of your practice into an evidence-based practice, in which the recommendations of the United States Preventive Services Task Force on the Periodic Health Examination are followed. As you know, one of the most important recommendations made by that task force is regular screening of all women for cervical cancer.
   If this were to occur, and every female patient in your practice under the age of 65 years was screened at the recommended intervals for cervical cancer with the Pap smear, what percentage of cervical cancers could be prevented (actual effectiveness, not theoretical effectiveness)?
   a) 100%
   b) 92%
   c) 80%
   d) 64%
   e) 51%

7. The current recommendation for screening by Pap smear for carcinoma of the cervix includes which of the following classification structures or provisions?
   a) all women who are or who have been sexually active should have regular Pap smears
   b) all women who have reached the age of 18 years should have regular Pap smears
   c) after three normal Pap smears, the interval time between Pap smears can be increased in low-risk patients

d) Pap smear screening intervals are recommended on the basis of classification of women into three risk categories that include most women
e) all of the above are included in the current recommendation

8. Which of the following is the greatest concern when considering Pap smear interval screening?
a) the specificity of the Pap smear
b) the sensitivity of the Pap smear
c) the positive predictive value of the Pap smear
d) the method of performing the Pap smear
e) the decreased ability to interpret Pap smear slides because of air drying

9. A Pap smear report comes back on a patient of yours who had a smear performed 1 week ago. The report reads, "unsatisfactory for evaluation." At this time, what should you do?
a) phone the cytopathologist and tell him to get with it; you haven't time for his mistakes
b) repeat the Pap smear immediately

c) repeat the Pap smear; but repeat it no sooner than 6 weeks from the previous smear
d) repeat the Pap smear in 4-6 months if the patient is low risk
e) repeat the Pap smear only if it seems reasonable

10. What is the most cost-effective and least invasive mode of treating squamous intraepithelial lesions of the cervix?
a) laser therapy
b) 5-fluorouracil
c) cryotherapy
d) electrical cauterization
e) any of the above

11. At an anatomic level, carcinoma of the cervix and its precursor conditions are anatomically connected to which of the following?
a) the squamous epithelium
b) the columnar epithelium
c) the squamous-columnar epithelium
d) the exterior of the cervical os
e) the interior of the cervical os

Short Answer Management Problem 47

Discuss the new or Bethesda classification system for pap smear reporting. Compare it to the cervical intraepithelial classification system and correlate these results with cytopathologic findings on the Papanicolaou smear.

ANSWERS

1. B. The class system of Pap smear reporting has been significantly revised, and that aspect will be discussed in another question. With this change, the management of CIN-1 has become more conservative (and more controversial). Clinicians must make an educated guess until optimal management patterns are further defined by large epidemiological studies. Only 15%-20% of (CIN-1) lesions will progress to a higher-grade lesion. In light of this relatively slow temporal progression of CIN-1 lesions, expectant management of women with low-grade CIN on a single Pap smear is acceptable, assuming that they are good follow-up candidates. In this situation, Pap smears should be done every 4-6 months for three intervals, and if any subsequent Pap smear report over the next 12-18 months shows premalignant change, the woman must be referred for colposcopic evaluation. Conversely, if all Pap smears are reported as normal during this period of increased surveillance, the woman may return to a routine screening pattern afterward. Women who are not good follow-up risks should be advised to receive colposcopic evaluation of a single low-grade CIN Pap smear reading.

2. C. The recommended procedure in this case is to treat the Trichomonas vaginalis infection if it has not been treated in both the patient and her partner. As in the first case, the recommendations for follow-up have changed. Because the Pap smear is very specific for detecting Trichomonas, there is no need to perform "hanging drop" preparations or any other test to confirm Trichomoniasis. Repeat the Pap smear at the next routine screening interval, unless the narrative report mentions obscuring inflammation and indicates the need to repeat the Pap smear after treatment has been completed.

3. C. Carcinoma of the cervix is a sexually transmitted disease. Risk factors include early onset of intercourse, three or more sexual partners, a male sexual partner who has had other partners, a clinical history of condyloma acuminata, and cigarette smoking.

   Postmenopausal women may cease to have Pap smears after the age of 65 years provided they have no new sexual partners after that time. The other stipulation to this is that adequate screening has occurred previously.

   Carcinoma of the cervix is a disease with a long lead time. Lead time is the period of time between the detection of a medical condition by screening and the time when it ordinarily would have been diagnosed because an individual patient experienced symptoms and sought medical care. Diseases with long lead times usually lend themselves to effective screening programs.

The Pap smear should be obtained by using an Ayres or similar spatula for sampling the exocervix, and a brush sampling device to sample the endocervix. Both samples are put on the same slide and, in fact, one can be placed on top of the other.

The cervical sample should be obtained in the following manner:
A. Use a large cotton-tipped applicator in a gentle wiping motion to remove the excess cervical mucus.
B. The order of sampling is critical: first the exocervix, and then the endocervix.
C. Fix the sample immediately to avoid air drying.

4. C. Carcinoma of the cervix is usually associated with the human papilloma virus (HPV). The type of the human papilloma virus involved is very important in determining the malignant potential of the virus. Our knowledge to date indicates the following:
A. HPV types 6 and 11 frequently are isolated from cervical condylomata and low-grade lesions and are felt to be low risk low malignant potential.
B. HPV types 16, 18, 31, 33, and 35 are considered to be high-risk HPV types. Although they may be found in low-grade lesions, they are more commonly present in high-grade lesions in cervical squamous cell carcinoma and adenocarcinoma.

5. E. Human papilloma virus (HPV) alone is insufficient to initiate the development and proliferation of a premalignant lesion. Thus another factor, commonly referred to as a cofactor or a facilitating factor, is necessary to act in concert with HPV to initiate these premalignant changes. As an example, cigarette smoking has been identified as an extremely important cofactor—so important as to double a smoker's risk of cervical cancer in comparison with nonsmokers.

As well, epidemiologic data are consistent with the biological mechanism just cited. The primary epidemiological risk factors that have been estimated include the following:
A. Early onset of intercourse: this is defined as intercourse before the age of 20 years—metaplasia is most active during adolescence, making a young woman much more vulnerable to cervical cellular changes.
B. Three or more sexual partners: this refers to three or more sexual partners in one lifetime. The equation is simple: the greater the number of sexual partners, the greater the risk of acquiring a high-risk type of HPV.
C. Male sexual partner who has had other partners: this is especially true if a previous partner had cervical cancer.

D. Clinical history of condyloma acuminata

Herpes simplex virus type II is not considered an identifiable risk factor for carcinoma of the cervix. Indirectly, of course, as an STD, an episode of HPV type II tends to go hand in hand with the epidemiologic risk factors just listed.

6. B. A reproductive health care visit represents an ideal opportunity to offer cancer screening tests. The Pap smear, more than many other screening tests, has proven its cost-effectiveness over the years. If your office is equipped with an ideal information management system, and you were able to recall all of your female patients under the age of 65 at appropriate screening intervals, it is estimated that 92% of cervical cancers could be prevented. The other 8% would escape detection because of improper technique, imperfections in cytological technology, and the biological behavior of the malignant lesions.

The difference between theoretical effectiveness and actual effectiveness is the modus operandi in this case. This concept is extremely important in contraception and will be discussed in another chapter of this book.

7. E. In August 1987 a Pap smear consensus statement was issued by a number of medical organizations. It reads as follows: All women who are, or who have been sexually active, or who have reached 18 years of age (should) have an annual Pap test and pelvic examination. After a woman has three or more consecutive, satisfactory, normal annual exams, the Pap test may be performed less frequently at the discretion of the physician.

Pap smear screening intervals are determined by the risk status of the individual patient. The risk status is divided into three levels or categories of risk.
I. Extremely low-risk patients:
   1) Virginal patients
   2) Those patients with >5 benign Pap smears and a hysterectomy for benign disease
   3) Those patients with >10 benign Pap smears including one at age 60 or older, and who are presently over the age of 65 years
   Recommendation: Pap smear not necessary
II. Low-risk patients:
   1) Those patients with the onset of sexual activity at >20 years
   2) Those patients with <3 sexual partners (ever)
   3) Those patients who use barrier contraceptive methods
   4) Those patients who are nonsmokers
   5) Those patients with a previously normal Pap smear
   Recommendation: Pap smears yearly for 3 years, then every 2-3 years
III. High-risk patients:
   1) Onset of sexual activity at <20 years

2) Three or more sexual partners (ever)
3) History of HPV or STDs
4) Previously abnormal Pap smear
5) Cigarette smoker
Recommendation: Pap smear yearly

8. **B.** A central concern in determining the appropriate screening intervals for Pap smears is the risk of a false-negative Pap smear. A false-negative Pap smear will occur when a smear has been interpreted as normal when, in fact, it is not normal. The longer the sampling interval, the greater the risk that a falsely negative Pap smear will result in a delay of up to 6 years in lesion detection.

The currently quoted rate of false-negative Pap smear results is approximately 20%. The currently quoted specificity for the Pap smear is 70%. If two Pap smears are performed in a short interval, the rate of false negatives drop to 4%. If three smears are performed in a relatively short time interval, the false negative rate falls to 0.8%.

9. **C.** A Pap smear that comes back labeled "unsatisfactory for evaluation" may be due to inadequate sampling, air drying, excessive red or white blood cells, and other factors that make interpretation difficult or impossible. The recommended procedure in this case is as follows:
A. Repeat the Pap smear, preferably when the woman is at midcycle and has not had intercourse or used vaginal products for at least 24 hours.
B. Repeat the Pap smear in a time frame no less than 6 weeks after the previous smear.

The reason for this latter part of the recommendation is that repetitive sampling over short periods of time may actually increase the risk of falsely negative results due to decreased exfoliation of abnormal cells and a greater likelihood of reparative changes.

10. **C.** The most cost-effective and least invasive mode of treating squamous intraepithelial lesions of the cervix is cryotherapy. Lesions that have been identified by the application of acetic acid should be treated with cryotherpy rather than observed (as some authorities prefer).

11. **C.** At menarche, when estrogen levels rise and *Lactobacillus* sp. consequently colonize the vagina, the vaginal pH drops into an acidic range. This environment changes the exposed fragile columnar epithelial cells around the cervical os, leading to their replacement by squamous epithelium, a process referred to as squamous metaplasia. As this process proceeds over decades, the advancing edge of the squamous epithelium (referred to as the squamo-columnar junction, or SCI) migrates centrally toward the cervical os, and ultimately into the endocervical canal. Squamous metaplasia is most rapid during adolescence and accelerates further during pregnancy.

BETHESDA SYSTEM	CIN CLASSIFICATION	PAP SMEAR FINDINGS
1. Low-grade SIL*	A. HPV changes	A. Atypia, koilocytotic, warty, condylomatous,
	B. CIN-1	B. Mild dysplasia
2. High-grade SIL*	C. CIN-II	C. Moderate dysplasia
	D. CIN-III	D. Severe dysplasia; carcinoma-in-situ

*SIL = squamous intraepithelial lesion.

SUMMARY OF THE PAP SMEAR AND CERVICAL CANCER: FOCUS ON PREVENTION AND EARLY DETECTION

1. **Cost-effectiveness of the Pap smear:** the Pap smear has proven to be one of the most cost-effective preventive medicine tools for the primary care physician.
2. **Goal of screening and case-finding:** to ensure that every female patient between the ages of 18 years and 65 years of age is screened at appropriate intervals
3. **Specificity of Pap smear:** 70%. If two Pap smears are done 1 year apart the specificity for picking up cervical cancer increases to 96%.
4. **Interval of screening:** According to risk—very low risk, low risk, and high risk. See answer to Question 7.
5. **U.S. Preventive Task Force screening recommendation for low-risk women:** three normal Pap smears, one year apart, followed by screening every 2 or 3 years up to the age of 65
6. **New Bethesda reporting system for Pap smears:** old system includes HPV change; CIN-I, CIN-II, and CIN-III; new system is based on squamous intraepithelial lesion.

Bethesda system: low-grade SIL (corresponds to HPV change and CIN-I) and cellular changes including atypia and mild dysplasia

High-grade SIL: (corresponds to CIN-II and CIN-III) and cellular changes including moderate dysplasia, severe dysplasia, and carcinoma-in-situ
7. **Etiology of cervical cancer:** human papilloma virus types 16, 18, 31, 33, and 35 acting along with cofactors.

Cofactors include cigarette smoking and risk factors for cervical cancer, including early first intercourse, three or more partners, male partner with more partners, and a clinical history of condyloma acuminata.
8. **Abnormal descriptive diagnoses on Pap smear reporting:**
a) Infection:
1. Fungus consistent with *Candida* sp.
2. *Trichomonas vaginalis*
3. Predominance of coccobacilli consistent with shift in vaginal flora
4. Bacteria morphologically consistent with Actinomyces species (associated with IUD)

b) Reactive and reparative:
  1. Reactive cellular changes associated with inflammation
  2. Atrophy with inflammation
  3. Intrauterine contraceptive device
c) Squamous cell abnormalities:
  1. Atypical squamous cell of undetermined significance (ASCUS)
  2. Low-grade SIL
  3. High-grade SIL
  4. Atypical glandular cells of undetermined significance (AGCUS)

  5. Squamous cell carcinoma, endocervical adenocarcinoma
9. **Treatment of squamous intraepithelial lesions:**
  a) Cryotherapy is the treatment of choice for most lesions.
  b) Occasionally laser therapy is needed.

SUGGESTED READING

Hatcher R et al. Contraceptive technology. 16th Rev. Ed. New York: Irvington, 1994.

PROBLEM 48   A 35-YEAR-OLD FEMALE WITH MANY PREMENSTRUAL SYMPTOMS

A 35-year-old female presents with a 6-month history of fatigue, breast tenderness, abdominal bloating, fluid retention, anxiety, irritability, depression, difficulty concentrating, and insomnia. These symptoms occur on a regular basis during the 8 days before to the onset of her menstruation.

There is no significant lack of interest in life, no guilt, no hopelessness, no appetite disturbance, no psychomotor retardation or psychomotor agitation, and there are no other symptoms.

Her physical examination is normal. Her blood pressure is 110/75 mm Hg. Her pelvic examination reveals what appears to be a small cystic structure on the right ovary. The uterus is normal in size and feel.

SELECT THE ONE BEST ANSWER TO THE FOLLOWING QUESTIONS

1. What is the most likely diagnosis in this patient?
   a) generalized anxiety disorder
   b) masked depression
   c) major depressive illness
   d) premenstrual syndrome
   e) hypochondriasis

2. What is the prevalence of the disorder described among American women in the reproductive years?
   a) 1%
   b) 10%
   c) 25%
   d) 50%
   e) 75%

3. The most important element in establishing the diagnosis in a patient such as this is a good history. What is the most important information in the history?
   a) the severity of the symptoms
   b) the number of symptoms
   c) the timing of the symptoms in the menstrual cycle
   d) the presence and severity of the depression or anxiety
   e) all of the above are of equal importance

4. The symptoms described above are most common in what phase of the menstrual cycle?
   a) premenstrually for 1-14 days
   b) during menstruation
   c) after menstruation for 1-14 days
   d) premenstrually for 15-18 days
   e) after menstruation for 15-18 days

5. The etiology of the condition described is unknown. However, of the choices listed below, which is most compatible with the signs and symptoms of the syndrome?
   a) an estrogen-deficiency syndrome
   b) a progesterone-deficiency syndrome
   c) a progesterone-excess syndrome
   d) an estrogen-excess syndrome
   e) a combination estrogen-progesterone deficiency

6. What is the condition most commonly confused with this condition?
   a) generalized anxiety disorder
   b) panic disorder
   c) major depression
   d) schizoaffective disorder
   e) none of the above

7. What is the treatment of choice for patients manifesting mild symptoms of this disorder?
   a) intensive psychotherapy
   b) single-agent pharmacotherapy
   c) multiagent pharmacotherapy
   d) intensive psychotherapy and multiagent pharmacotherapy
   e) none of the above

8. Which of the following OTC medications may be helpful in the treatment of the condition described above?
   a) ibuprofen
   b) vitamin E
   c) vitamin C
   d) a and b
   e) all of the above

9. Regarding the use of hormone therapy in the disorder described, which of the following has(have) been shown to be effective?
   a) medroxyprogesterone acetate
   b) oral contraceptives
   c) natural progesterone suppositories
   d) a and b only
   e) all of the above

10. Regarding the use of pharmacologic therapy in the treatment of the disorder described, which of the following has/have been shown to reduce the severity of symptoms?

a) medroxyprogesterone acetate
b) nonsteroidal antiinflammatory drugs
c) fluoxetine

d) alprazolam
e) all of the above

Short Answer Management Problem 48

Discuss the prevalence, definition, and importance of the following terms and clearly distinguish between them. At the same time, discuss this statement: "Premenstrual syndrome is a psychiatric disorder."
1. Premenstrual symptoms
2. Premenstrual syndrome
3. Late luteal phase dysphoric disorder
4. Premenstrual dysphoric disorder

ANSWERS

1. D. This patient has premenstrual syndrome. Premenstrual syndrome is a syndrome of unknown etiology causing a recurrent profile of symptoms that are annoying for many women, but can debilitating for a small minority (especially in the decade before menopause).

   Symptoms include psychological symptoms and physical symptoms. Because of the multitude of symptoms, the diagnosis is often missed. The cyclic manifestation of these symptoms in rhythm with the menstrual cycle is pathognomonic for PMS.

   For the diagnosis of PMS to be established, the following criteria have to be met:
   1) Symptoms are present to some degree in each menstrual cycle and begin at or after ovulation.
   2) Symptoms resolve near menses.
   3) The patient is symptom free from the cessation of menses until the time of ovulation (at least 7 symptom-free days are present in each cycle).

   Symptoms of premenstrual syndrome include the following:
   Physical:
   Abdominal bloating
   Edema
   Weight gain
   Constipation
   Hot flashes
   Breast pain
   Headache
   Acne
   Rhinitis
   Palpitations
   Psychological:
   Anxiety
   Depression
   Irritability
   Wide mood swings
   Increased appetite
   Aggression
   Lethargy or fatigue
   Forgetfulness/reduced concentration
   Sleep disorders
   Phobias

2. B. Although premenstrual symptoms occur in up to 90% of women, severe symptoms that interfere with work or social activities occur in, at most, 10% of women in the reproductive years.

3. C. The timing of the symptoms to the rest of the menstrual cycle is the most important factor in establishing a diagnosis of premenstrual syndrome. The relationship of symptoms to the rest of the menstrual cycle is best established by a calendar that is kept for at least two consecutive menstrual cycles. Included in the calendar should be the first day of the cycle, a daily rating of the menstrual flow (slight, moderate, heavy, or heavy with clots), and the symptoms experienced (rated on a scale of 1 to 3).

4. A. The symptoms described occur in the premenstrual period. The symptoms last anywhere from 1 to 14 days.

5. B. Although the etiology of PMS is unknown, the most likely association is with progesterone deficiency.

   Other causes that have been speculated to contribute significantly include prostaglandin metabolism; relative endorphin lack; vitamin B_6 deficiency; and a biopsychosocial model where biologic, psychologic, and social factors interact in a complex manner.

6. C. The condition most closely associated with PMS is major depression. It is imperative that the physician rule out depression (including masked depression) before making a definitive diagnosis of PMS.

7. E. The treatment of choice for patients exhibiting mild PMS symptoms is basically lifestyle change and stress reduction.

There is some evidence that reactive hypoglycemia can exacerbate PMS symptoms. Frequent, low-fat, high-complex carbohydrate meals with adequate protein can decrease fatigue and improve weight control. Regular aerobic exercise decreases depression and stress-related symptoms. Generalized stress-reduction techniques can and often do have the same effect.

Increased consumption of caffeine is correlated with increased risk of PMS. Patients should decrease caffeine intake and limit the use of alcohol.

Several studies have shown that vitamin E can decrease PMS symptoms, especially breast tenderness. The recommended dosage is 400 IU/day.

8. D. Prostaglandin inhibitors such as mefenamic acid (Ponstel) and naproxen sodium (Anaprox) are effective therapies for dysmenorrhea and have also been shown in some studies to decrease the symptoms of PMS, including depression and irritability.

Vitamin C has not been shown to have any therapeutic advantage in the treatment of PMS. Vitamin E is discussed in the answer to question 7.

9. D. Medroxyprogesterone acetate (Depo-Provera) 100 mg-150 mg/month and oral contraceptives have been shown, in some studies, to have a beneficial effect on the symptoms of PMS. In many placebo-controlled studies, however, natural progesterone suppositories have not shown any significant advantage over placebo. Despite this, however, there are many physicians who continue to believe in natural progesterone suppositories and who treat patients with 800 mg to 1200 mg in three divided doses/day beginning at least 3 days before the anticipated symptoms.

10. E. In women with a main symptom of depression, fluoxetine has been shown to be effective. Due to a lengthy buildup of this drug to a therapeutic range, it should be used continuously. The average dose is 20 mg/day.

In women in whom the main symptom is anxiety, the two medications that have shown to be effective are alprazolam (Xanax) and buspirone (Buspar).

Medroxyprogesterone acetate and nonsteroidal anti-inflammatory drugs have already been discussed.

SOLUTION TO SHORT ANSWER MANAGEMENT PROBLEM 48

1. Prevalence:
   1. Premenstrual symptoms: 80% of all women in their reproductive years have premenstrual symptoms.
   2. Premenstrual syndrome: 10% to 20% of all women in their reproductive years have premenstrual syndrome.
   3. Late luteal phase dysphoric disorder and premenstrual dysphoric disorder: 2% to 3% of women in the reproductive years have late luteal phase dysphoric disorder/premenstrual dysphoric disorder.

2. Definition:
   1. Premenstrual symptoms: the presence of one or more of the many symptoms that have been discussed
   2. Premenstrual syndrome: the presence of a relatively large number of symptoms at the right time and with at least one symptom-free week following menstruation
   3. Late luteal phase dysphoric disorder (DSM-III-R) and premenstrual dysphoric disorder (DSM-IV) are two different names for the same disorder.

The critical difference between late luteal phase dysphoric disorder/premenstrual dysphoric disorder and premenstrual syndrome is that the symptoms are of sufficient severity and duration to interfere with social or occupational functioning, academic work, or productivity in whatever way that is defined.

The statement "Premenstrual syndrome is a psychiatric disorder" is false.

Only 2% to 3% of women have the symptoms and the syndrome to such a degree that it interferes with social functioning, occupational functioning, academic functioning, or productivity.

SUMMARY OF THE DIAGNOSIS AND MANAGEMENT OF PREMENSTRUAL SYNDROME

1. **Diagnosis:** multiple physical and psychologic symptoms occurring in the premenstrual period (See the list in the answer to Question 1.)
2. **Etiology:** unknown. Possibilities include relative progesterone deficiency in the luteal phase, prostaglandin excess, and endorphins.
3. **History:** history is most important. It must be confirmed by charting symptoms for at least 2 months.
4. **Treatment:**
   Nonpharmacologic:
   a) Low-fat, high-complex carbohydrate diet
   b) Aerobic exercise
   c) Avoid caffeine
   d) Avoid alcohol

e) Relaxation techniques

Pharmacologic:

a) Hormonal:
   1. Medroxyprogesterone acetate
   2. Oral contraceptive pill
   3. Danazol
b) Nonhormonal:
   1. Nonsteroidal antiinflammatories, such as mefenamic acid (Ponstel) and naproxen sodium (Anaprox)
   2. Fluoxetine (Prozac)
   3. Alprazolam (Xanax) and buspirone (Buspar)
c) Vitamin therapy:
   1. Vitamin E (400 IU/day)
   2. Vitamin B_6 (100 mg/day)

No evidence for effectiveness of spironolactone or natural progesterone suppositories.

SUGGESTED READING

Chihal HJ. Premenstrual syndrome. In: Rakel R, ed. Conn's current therapy. Philadelphia: WB Saunders, 1994.

PROBLEM 49   A 48-YEAR-OLD FEMALE WITH HOT FLASHES

A 48-year-old female presents to your office with a 1-year history of "feeling warm and sweaty." These feelings occur for short periods of time, frequently during the day. These symptoms began when her menstrual periods stopped. In addition to the feelings of being "warm and sweaty," she describes some night sweats, sleep disturbances, and anxiety.

SELECT THE ONE BEST ANSWER TO THE FOLLOWING QUESTIONS

1. What is the most likely diagnosis in this patient?
   a) pheochromocytoma
   b) hyperthyroidism
   c) menopausal hot flashes
   d) generalized anxiety disorder
   e) panic attacks

2. What is the treatment of choice for this patient?
   a) conjugated estrogen alone
   b) conjugated estrogen with oral progesterone
   c) oral progesterone only
   d) synthetic estrogen
   e) synthetic progesterone

3. What is the recommended dosage of the treatment regime of choice for this condition?
   a) 0.625 mg conjugated estrogen/day
   b) 0.625 mg conjugated estrogen/day plus 10 mg oral progesterone for first 13 days of calendar month
   c) 10 mg medroxyprogesterone acetate
   d) ethinyl estradiol 50 μg/day
   e) Depo-Provera 150 mg/month

4. What is the recommended dosage regime of the treatment above?
   a) continuous estrogen/cyclic progestin
   b) continuous estrogen/continuous progestin
   c) cyclic estrogen/cyclic progestin
   d) cyclic estrogen/continuous progestin
   e) it doesn't really matter

5. Calcium has been shown to be effective in the prevention and treatment of the condition described. At what time in the female life cycle should calcium be started?
   a) age 35-40
   b) age 50
   c) age 55
   d) at menopause (as soon as possible after it begins)
   e) within the first 2 years of menstrual cessation

6. Which of the following statements regarding estrogen in this condition is(are) true?
   a) estrogen used in treating the condition described significantly decreases the risk of coronary artery disease in women

b) estrogen used in treating this condition has no effect on coronary artery disease rates in women
   c) estrogen used in this condition increases the risk of coronary artery disease in women
   d) no firm relationship between estrogen use and coronary artery disease risk in women has been established
   e) the effect of estrogen on coronary artery disease risk in women is unknown

7. Hormone manipulation therapy is begun on a patient who presents with vasomotor menopausal symptoms. For this condition it is recommended that hormone therapy be given for how long?
   a) until the symptoms abate
   b) 1-2 years
   c) 3-5 years
   d) 10 years
   e) the ideal length of time for replacement is unknown at this time

8. The effect of estrogen replacement therapy on plasma lipids shows which of the following?
   a) estrogen increases serum LDL
   b) estrogen increases serum HDL
   c) estrogen decreases serum LDL
   d) estrogen decreases serum HDL
   e) estrogen increases serum HDL and decreases serum LDL

9. Which of the following is(are) risk factors for the most significant complication of this condition?
   a) cigarette smoking
   b) lean body mass
   c) sedentary lifestyle
   d) Caucasian race
   e) all of the above

10. Which of the following statements concerning this condition is(are) true?
   a) osteoporosis is the major complication
   b) exercise has been shown to decrease the incidence/prevalence of the complication
   c) hormone therapy appears not only to stabilize the complication but partially reverse it
   d) a and b only
   e) all of the above

11. Withdrawal bleeding following the initiation of estrogen replacement therapy may be difficult or embarrassing. The incidence of significant withdrawal bleeding in postmenopausal women who take exogenous estrogens is approximately 30%.

    Which of the following treatment regimes minimizes the occurrence of withdrawal bleeding?
    a) continuous estrogen/cyclic progestin
    b) continuous estrogen/continuous progestin
    c) cyclic estrogen/cyclic progestin
    d) cyclic estrogen/continuous progestin
    e) it doesn't really matter

12. Oral progestational agents have which of the following effects on plasma lipids?
    a) raise HDL/raise LDL
    b) lower HDL/lower LDL
    c) raise HDL/lower LDL
    d) lower HDL/raise LDL
    e) raise VLDL/lower LDL/lower HDL

Short Answer Management Problem 49

List four contraindications to the use of postmenopausal estrogens.

ANSWERS

1. C. The most likely diagnosis in this patient is menopausal hot flashes. The diagnosis is based on the right age of a female patient for menopause, the classical "hot flashes" coming on daily but coming on frequently, and the association of these symptoms with the cessation of menses.

   Hyperthyroidism would be a greater possibility in the absence of some of the other symptoms.

   Hot flashes may accompany generalized anxiety disorder and panic disorder. These disorders, however, have many other symptoms as well.

2. B. In this case, pheochromocytoma should receive brief (but only brief) consideration. The preferred treatment regime for hot flashes or other menopausal symptoms is a combination of conjugated estrogen (Premarin) and oral progesterone. The oral progesterone is added to protect the endometrium from hyperplasia and later endometrial carcinoma.

3. B.

4. A. At this time, the most commonly used treatment regimen of hormone replacement therapy in the United States for women with an intact uterus is conjugated estrogen 0.625 mg/day plus medroxyprogesterone acetate 10 mg/day for the first 13 days of each month.

5. E. The recommended time for beginning calcium therapy is during the 2 years following the cessation of menstruation. This maximizes the benefit of osteoporosis protection; however, better late than never. Considera-

tion of starting this type of regime (up to the age of 65 years) is reasonable.

6. A. One of the very positive side effects of estrogen replacement therapy in post-menopausal women is protection from coronary artery disease. Cardiovascular disease (CVD) is the leading cause of death among women in industrialized countries (an often forgotten fact), including a rate of greater than 50% of postmenopausal women. Estrogens have been thought to have a significant protective effect against atherosclerosis in postmenopausal women. As an example, the rate of cardiovascular mortality in premenopausal women is approximately 20% of age-matched men; following menopause, however, the risk among postmenopausal women quickly catches up to age-matched men unless the women are on estrogen replacement therapy.

   The relative risk of CVD among postmenopausal estrogen users compared to nonusers has been compared in several studies. All have shown reduced risk in estrogen users, although the decrease of risk reduction has been quite variable.

7. E. Some recent evidence has suggested that even if estrogens are started for hot flashes (if the patient is not a high risk candidate for osteoporosis), this may be reason enough to consider using estrogen indefinitely. At this point, it is fair to say that nobody really knows for sure. There are more opinions on this matter than there are schedules for combination estrogen/progestin replacement therapy.

8. E. Exogenous estrogens have a very favorable effect on the lipid profile: they raise HDL by 16-18% and they

lower atherogenic LDL by 15-19%. Both these changes significantly reduce cardiac risk.

9. E. The most significant risk of estrogen deficiency in postmenopausal women is osteoporosis. The risk factors for osteoporosis include the following:
   1) Female sex
   2) Postmenopausal status
   3) Caucasian race
   4) Northern European or Scandinavian ancestry
   5) Sedentary lifestyle
   6) Cigarette smoking
   7) Lean body mass
   8) Possibly family history of osteoporosis

10. E. Osteoporosis is the major complication of post-menopausal estrogen deficiency. Aerobic exercise has been shown to significantly decrease the probability of developing severe osteoporosis. Exogenous estrogen replacement therapy not only stabilizes osteoporosis but may partially reverse it.

11. B. The current recommendation to minimize withdrawal bleeding in postmenopausal women is as follows: conjugated estrogen 0.625 mg to 1.25 mg/day continuously plus progestin 2.5 mg/day continuously.

12. D. In contradistinction to estrogens, progestational agents have the opposite (and potentially deleterious) effect on plasma lipids. Progestational agents raise LDL and lower HDL. Having said that, however, the risk of cardiovascular morbidity and mortality in postmenopausal women who are on hormone replacement therapy is significantly lower than for women who are not on hormone replacement therapy. These results are based on combination therapy with estrogen and progesterone and thus are a measure of the overall benefit.

SOLUTION TO SHORT ANSWER MANAGEMENT PROBLEM 49

Four contraindications to the use of postmenopausal estrogen replacement therapy are as follows:
1. Known or suspected endometrial or breast cancer
2. Genital bleeding of uncertain origin
3. Active liver disease
4. Active thromboembolic disease or a history of estrogen-related thromboembolic disease

SUMMARY OF THE DIAGNOSIS AND TREATMENT OF POSTMENOPAUSAL SYMPTOMS AND THEIR SEQUELAE

1. **Classification of symptoms:**
   a) Vasomotor symptoms: hot flushes/hot flashes develop in 75% of postmenopausal women.
   b) Urogenital symptoms; dyspareunia, vaginal itching, vaginal dryness, burning, urgency and frequency of urination

2. **Investigations:** all patients being considered for hormonal replacement therapy should have a complete history and physical with special attention to blood pressure measurement, breast and pelvic examination, and Pap smear. Mammography should be performed initially to avoid estrogen administration in a patient with preexisting subclinical breast cancer; it should be repeated yearly after age 50. An endometrial biopsy should be performed if the patient is likely to have preexisting endometrial hyperplasia (risk factors are obesity and the presence of abnormal vaginal bleeding).

3. **Treatment:**
   a) Estrogen replacement therapy: Most commonly used regime: exogenous estrogen (Premarin) 0.625 mg/day throughout the cycle plus medroxyprogesterone acetate (Provera) 10 mg for the first 13 days of the cycle

   Most commonly used regime if withdrawal bleeding is a problem: exogenous estrogen (Premarin) 0.625 mg to 1.25 mg/day continually plus medroxyprogesterone acetate (Provera) 5 mg/day continually

   Alternative to oral estrogen: the Estroderm patch (50 μg) twice per week. The theoretical advantage of this regime is that it avoids first-pass metabolism through the liver.

   With this regime, the patient still has to take a pill (progesterone), but a combination estrogen/progesterone patch will soon be available.

   Length of time that estrogen should be given: unknown

   Best current advice: indefinitely

   Osteoporosis is a major cause of morbidity and mortality in elderly women and should be considered serious enough to use a prophylactic regime (as previously discussed), especially in high-risk women.
   b) Progesterone (Provera): progestins (Provera) relieve hot flashes in 70% of women who have a contraindication to estrogen. The usual dose of medroxyprogesterone acetate is 10 mg orally per day or 50 to 150 mg intramuscularly every 3 months.
   c) Alpha-adrenergic agonist (Clonidine): an alternative for the treatment of hot flashes (effective in 30% to 40% of cases) is Clonidine, a centrally acting alpha-adrenergic agonist. This drug, usually administered

in an initial dose of 0.1 mg twice/day has significant side effects (primarily orthostatic hypotension and typical anticholinergic effects).

d) Megestrol acetate: a recent report suggests that megestrol acetate may prevent and relieve hot flashes and hot flushes. This drug, an androgenic agent, given in a dosage of 20 mg/day, is well tolerated by menopausal women.

4. **Controversy:** should all postmenopausal women be treated with exogenous estrogen in the postmenopausal period to prevent osteoporosis?

Answer: probably not. Base your decision on risk factors.

SUGGESTED READINGS

Loprinzi C et al. Megestrol acetate for the prevention of hot flashes. N Engl J Med 1994; 331(6):347-352.

Walsh BW, Schiff I. Menopause. In: Rakel R, ed. Conn's current therapy. Philadelphia: WB Saunders, 1994.

PROBLEM 50   A 14-YEAR-OLD FEMALE WITH LOWER MIDABDOMINAL, COLICKY PAIN WITH HER MENSTRUAL CYCLE

A 14-year-old female presents to your office with a 6-month history of lower midabdominal pain. The pain is colicky in nature, radiates through to the back and upper thighs, begins within a few hours of the onset of menstruation, and lasts from 2 to 4 days. Menarche (initially irregular) began 18 months ago. The patient is not sexually active.

On physical examination the patient looks thin and is found to be on the fifth percentile of weight for height. No other abnormalities are detected.

SELECT THE ONE BEST ANSWER TO THE FOLLOWING QUESTIONS:

1. What is the most likely diagnosis in this patient?
   a) primary dysmenorrhea
   b) pelvic inflammatory disease
   c) secondary dysmenorrhea
   d) endometriosis
   e) psychogenic abdominal pain

2. Which of the following has(have) been shown to be consistently associated with the pain produced by the condition described?
   a) elevation of myometrial resting tone
   b) elevation of contractile myometrial pressure
   c) increased frequency of uterine contractions
   d) dysrhythmia of uterine contractions
   e) all of the above

3. The disorder described appears to be mediated by which of the following?
   a) increased levels of the enzyme prostaglandin synthetase
   b) decreased levels of the enzyme prostaglandin synthetase
   c) increased levels of cyclic AMP
   d) decreased levels of cyclic AMP
   e) none of the above

4. The pathophysiology of the disorder described involves which of the following?
   a) vasodilatation of the uterine arterial supply
   b) vasoconstriction of the uterine arterial supply
   c) venous vasodilatation of the uterine veins
   d) venous vasodilatation of the pelvic veins
   e) none of the above

5. The disorder described usually begins at what age?
   a) 30-40
   b) 15-25
   c) 40-45
   d) 20-30
   e) within 2 years of the onset of menstruation

6. Which of the following is not directly associated with the secondary form of the condition described?

   a) ectopic pregnancy
   b) endometriosis
   c) adenomyosis
   d) chronic PID
   e) placement of an IUD

7. What is the prevalence of the disorder described among American women of childbearing age?
   a) 5-10%
   b) 15-25%
   c) 30-40%
   d) 50-75%
   e) >90%

8. Which of the following drugs has(have) been demonstrated to be efficacious in the treatment of the disorder described?
   a) ibuprofen
   b) naproxen
   c) acetylsalicylic acid
   d) a and b
   e) all of the above

9. A patient with the condition described is being treated with a fenamate (Ponstel). She has received some benefit from this treatment (which was initiated 3 months ago), but it has only lowered the pain from a level of 7/10 to a level of 4/10. At this time, what would you do?
   a) continue the fenamate
   b) discontinue the fenamate and begin oxycodone
   c) switch to the oral contraceptive pill
   d) switch to danazol
   e) switch to a nonsteroidal anti-inflammatory of a different class

10. Endometriosis is associated with this condition. What is the pharmacologic treatment of choice for endometriosis?
    a) a progestational agent
    b) nonsteroidal anti-inflammatories
    c) danazol
    d) prednisone
    e) terbutaline

Short Answer Management Problem 50

Discuss the two most commonly recommended treatments for the primary form of the condition described and how you would decide on your treatment of choice.

ANSWERS

1. A. This young girl has primary dysmenorrhea. Primary dysmenorrhea is the most common gynecologic complaint experienced by young women. Fifty to seventy-five percent of menstruating women experience this symptom; in 10% it is severe.

   Primary dysmenorrhea usually begins within 6-12 months of menarche. The pain is lower abdominal and often colicky. The pain associated with each cycle usually begins within a few hours of the beginning of the onset of menstrual flow. Anovulatory cycles are usually not associated with dysmenorrhea. Symptoms associated with primary dysmenorrhea include nausea, vomiting, diarrhea, headache, breast tenderness, and fatigue.

   Secondary dysmenorrhea is dysmenorrhea due to underlying pelvic pathology. Pelvic inflammatory disease and endometriosis are the two primary causes of secondary dysmenorrhea.

   Psychogenic factors, although thought by some to be a cause of dysmenorrhea, are unlikely to be related to the disorder.

2. E. Primary dysmenorrhea is associated with the following:
   a) An elevation of myometrial resting tone to above 10 mm Hg
   b) An elevation of contractile myometrial pressure to above 120 mm Hg
   c) An increased frequency of uterine contractions
   d) Dysrhythmia of uterine contractions
   These physiologic changes increase production of prostaglandins. This causes uterine hypoxia.

3. A.

4. B. Primary dysmenorrhea is pathologically mediated by an increase in the level of the enzyme prostaglandin synthetase. Elevated levels of the enzyme produce vasoconstricting prostaglandins that are responsible for uterine hypoxia, or uterine angina, which produces the pain of dysmenorrhea. The vasoconstriction itself takes place in the branches of the uterine artery.

5. E. One of the most important distinguishing characteristics of primary dysmenorrhea is the age of onset. Primary dysmenorrhea almost always begins within 2 years of the onset of menstruation. If dysmenorrhea begins at a later time, secondary dysmenorrhea is much more likely.

6. A. Ectopic pregnancy is not directly associated with secondary dysmenorrhea. It is, however, indirectly related due to the secondary dysmenorrhea-PID link.

   Secondary dysmenorrhea is defined as dysmenorrhea due to a concurrent organic pelvic pathologic process; it can be caused by any one of the following:
   a) Endometriosis
   b) Myomas
   c) Adenomyosis
   d) Endometrial polyps
   e) Cervical stenosis
   f) Pelvic inflammatory disease
   g) The presence of an intrauterine device

7. D. Fifty to seventy-five percent of American women of childbearing age experience dysmenorrhea. The vast majority of these women (>90%) will have primary dysmenorrhea. As just discussed, however, there are numerous secondary causes. These secondary causes usually produce symptoms at a significantly later age.

8. E. Nonsteroidal anti-inflammatory agents are a mainstay of treatment for primary dysmenorrhea. This includes acetylsalicylic acid (aspirin). Nonsteroidal anti-inflammatory agents exert their effect by inhibiting the production of prostaglandins through inhibition of the enzyme prostaglandin synthetase.

9. E. Nonsteroidal anti-inflammatory drugs are an agent of choice for the treatment of primary dysmenorrhea. A reasonable length of time for a trial of one agent is 3 months. If, after that time, there has not been a significant change in the pain and discomfort, an agent of another class should be tried. Following are the classes of NSAIDs and examples of each:

GROUP	AGENT
1. Benzoic acid derivatives	Aspirin
2. Butyrophenone	Phenylbutazone
3. Indole acetic acid derivative	Indomethacin
4. Fenamates	Mefenamic acid (Ponstel)
5. Propionic acid derivatives	Ibuprofen (Motrin)
	Naproxen (Naproxen)
	Naproxen sodium (Anaprox)
6. Piroxacams	Feldene

   In general, the groups of choice include the fenamates and the propionic acid derivatives. In the patient described, a very reasonable choice would be to switch the patient to a propionic acid derivative such as naproxen sodium (Anaprox) for a 3-month period. If that was not effective, a switch to the oral contraceptive pill would be the next logical alternative.

10. A. The treatment of choice for endometriosis is a progestational agent. The progestational agents that have been used include medroxyprogesterone acetate (Depo-Provera) intramuscularly every 2 weeks for 4 doses and then monthly for 4 additional doses. Each dose contains 150 mg. Oral medroxyprogesterone acetate (Provera) in a dose of 30-50 mg for 4 to 6 months can also be used.

Other treatment options include the oral contraceptive pill, danazol, GnRH analogues, conservative surgery, and radical surgery.

SOLUTION TO SHORT ANSWER MANAGEMENT PROBLEM 50

The two recommended treatments for primary dysmenorrhea are the nonsteroidal anti-inflammatory drugs (discussed previously) and the oral contraceptive pill. Both of these treatments are highly effective in reducing the pain and symptoms associated with the condition. The manner in which you decide first and second choice depends on the additional need for contraceptive protection. If she is sexually active, then the OCP would be your first choice. If, on the other hand, she is not sexually active and does not intend to become sexually active, an NSAID may be preferable.

SUMMARY OF THE DIAGNOSIS AND TREATMENT OF DYSMENORRHEA

Diagnosis:

1. Primary dysmenorrhea: begins within 2 years of the onset of menarche. Presents with colicky, midabdominal pain, spasmodic in nature, starting with or a few hours after the onset of the menstrual flow and usually lasting for 2-4 days.

2. Secondary dysmenorrhea: usually begins later (in relation to menarche) and is often associated with irregular cycles and anovulatory bleeding. Causes include endometriosis, adenomyosis, endometrial polyps, myomas, cervical stenosis, pelvic inflammatory disease, and the IUD.

Treatment:

1. Primary dysmenorrhea:
   a) NSAIDs (in patients not needing contraceptive protection): most commonly used classes: fenamates and propionic acid derivatives. If a drug from one class is not effective after three cycles, try a drug from the other class. If this is not successful, proceed to the OCP.
   b) OCP is the treatment of choice in those young women requiring contraction.

2. Secondary dysmenorrhea: establish and treat the cause.

SUGGESTED READING

Barmat L, Schinfeld J. Dysmenorrhea. In: Rakel R, ed. Conn's current therapy. Philadelphia: WB Saunders, 1994.

PROBLEM 51   A 35-YEAR-OLD FEMALE WITH HEAVY MENSTRUAL PERIODS

A 35-year-old female presents to your office for her regular checkup. On functional inquiry you elicit that she is having extremely heavy, long, and irregular periods. She is not obese.

On physical examination, her blood pressure is 120/80 mm Hg. Examination of the head and neck, cardiovascular system, respiratory system, abdomen, musculoskeletal system and neurological systems are normal. Pelvic examination reveals a normal-sized uterus with ovaries that are barely palpable.

SELECT THE ONE BEST ANSWER TO THE FOLLOWING QUESTIONS

1. What would you do at this time?
   a) reassure the patient that the periods will eventually settle down
   b) prescribe estrogen replacement therapy with progesterone to take care of the problem
   c) provide a monthly injection of IM Depo-Provera to take care of the problem
   d) prescribe a sedative; the basic problem is rattled nerves due to heavy flow
   e) none of the above

2. Which of the following should be considered in the differential diagnosis of this patient's problem?
   a) uterine polyp
   b) submucous fibroid
   c) adenomatous hyperplasia
   d) adenomyosis
   e) all of the above

3. Providing that all of the conditions (and all or most of the secondary causes for the bleeding) are eliminated, what is the most likely diagnosis in this patient?
   a) menopause
   b) "nervous uterus"
   c) dysmenorrhea complicated by bleeding
   d) dysfunctional uterine bleeding
   e) none of the above

4. What is the most likely underlying cause of this patient's abnormal bleeding?
   a) anovulation
   b) multiple ovulation
   c) a coagulation defect
   d) uterine pathology
   e) none of the above

5. What is the average blood loss during menstruation?
   a) 10 cc
   b) 30 cc
   c) 50 cc
   d) 80 cc
   e) 100 cc

6. What is the most common physiologic correlate of dysfunctional uterine bleeding (DUB)?
   a) estrogen withdrawal
   b) estrogen breakthrough
   c) progesterone withdrawal
   d) progesterone breakthrough
   e) none of the above

7. What is the definition of DUB?
   a) irregular vaginal bleeding of endometrial origin that is either excessive (more than 80 ml), prolonged (more than 7 days), or unpatterned; an additional stimulation is the absence of a specific genital tract lesion
   b) painful, irregular bleeding secondary to systemic disease; no cause demonstrated
   c) abnormal vaginal bleeding of endometrial origin
   d) uterine bleeding at the extremes of life
   e) none of the above

8. Which of the following systemic diseases is(are) associated with abnormal vaginal bleeding?
   a) hypothyroidism
   b) hyperthyroidism
   c) cirrhosis
   d) renal failure
   e) all of the above

9. Which of the following laboratory investigations is (are) indicated in the evaluation of abnormal uterine bleeding?
   a) serum pregnancy test
   b) serum T4 and TSH
   c) basal body temperature charting
   d) pelvic ultrasound
   e) all of the above

10. Anovulatory DUB accounts for approximately what percentage of total DUB?
    a) 10%
    b) 25%
    c) 50%
    d) 75%
    e) 90%

11. The treatment(s) of choice for DUB include which of the following?
    a) reassurance and education
    b) oral contraceptives
    c) cyclic progesterone

d) all of the above
e) none of the above

12. A 24-year-old obese female with a history of irregular menstrual periods presents to the ER with a 10-day history of heavy uterine bleeding. She is soaking through 20 pads/day. Her hemoglobin, when last measured 6 months ago, was 14 grams%. Today it is 9.0 grams%.

You suspect significant blood loss caused by chronic anovulation. What is the treatment of choice at this time in this patient?
a) medroxyprogesterone acetate IM
b) Premarin IV
c) danazol IV
d) factor VIII cryoprecipitate
e) a high dose oral contraceptive pill

Short Answer Management Problem 51

Describe the origin of oligomenorrhea or amenorrhea in women athletes who exercise strenuously.

ANSWERS

1. E. All of the choices offered are inappropriate. The first and most important question you have to ask is this: is there a secondary cause for this heavy bleeding or is there not? If there is a secondary cause, then the cause should be identified and corrected if possible. Dysfunctional uterine bleeding refers to uterine bleeding for which no specific genital tract lesion or systemic cause is found.

2. E. This question asks you to identify the secondary causes of heavy menstrual periods, or menorrhagia. If the periods are heavy only, then the appropriate term is menorrhagia. If the periods are irregular only, then the appropriate term is metrorrhagia. If the periods are both heavy and irregular, then the appropriate term is menometrorrhagia.

   The secondary causes that should be considered in this case include the following:
   a) Uterine fibroids
   b) Submucous fibroids
   c) Endometriosis
   d) Adenomyosis
   e) Chronic pelvic inflammatory disease
   f) Endometrial polyps
   g) Coagulation defects
   h) Massive obesity
   i) Ovarian abnormalities
   j) Severe hypothyroidism
   k) Adenomatous hyperplasia
   l) Endometrial carcinoma

3. D. The most likely diagnosis in this patient is DUB.

4. A. The most common cause of DUB is anovulation. Ovulatory uterine bleeding may be associated with oligomenorrhea, menorrhagia, or menometrorrhagia.

DUB usually occurs during puberty and before menopause; it is less common in the reproductive years, although ovulatory dysfunctional uterine bleeding does occur during this time. Ovulatory dysfunctional uterine bleeding may be associated with midcycle spotting, premenstrual spotting, or postmenstrual spotting. Ovulatory DUB accounts for less than 10% of all DUB.

5. B. The usual duration of menstrual flow is 4-6 days and the average blood loss during that period of time is 30 cc. The duration of flow appears to be related to estrogen stimulation.

   In anovulatory DUB is the ability of the endometrium to synthesize prostaglandins is greatly increased. Thus, it is not surprising that NSAIDs (potent inhibitors of prostaglandin synthesis) may be extremely therapeutic in terms of blood flow reduction.

6. B. The most common physiologic correlate of anovulatory DUB is estrogen breakthrough. Anovulation results in a continuous endometrial estrogen stimulation; this eventually results in a buildup of the endometrial lining beyond the capacity of support.

7. A. This answer gives more detail regarding definition of DUB.

   Dysfunctional uterine bleeding can be defined as vaginal bleeding of endometrial origin that may be excessive (greater than 80 ml), prolonged (greater than 7 days), or unpatterned in which no specific genital tract lesion or systemic cause is found.

8. E. Dysfunctional uterine bleeding can be associated with hypothyroidism, hyperthyroidism, cirrhosis, renal failure, diabetes mellitus, hyperprolactinemia, polycystic ovarian syndrome, premature menopause, blood dyscrasia, emotional and physical stress, and nutritional disorders including morbid obesity and anorexia nervosa.

In the evaluation of abnormal uterine bleeding, it is often helpful to group causes according to age:

1. Menarche to age 20: greater than 95% of abnormal uterine bleeding is dysfunctional and anovulatory. A careful history and physical examination is usually all that is required in the evaluation. Oral contraceptive agents and NSAIDs are of particular therapeutic benefit.

2. Ages 20-40: anovulation is uncommon in this age group as a cause of dysfunctional uterine bleeding. A careful history and physical examination should precede any investigations. A hysteroscopy, endometrial sampling, and laparoscopy may, however, be eventually indicated in the evaluation.

3. Age greater than 40: anovulation is a major cause of abnormal uterine bleeding in this age group. Uterine fibroids, cervical polyps, and endometrial carcinoma, must, however, be excluded. Endometrial sampling is recommended.

9. E. Because of the numerous causes of abnormalities in uterine bleeding already discussed, serum T4, serum TSH, basal body temperature monitoring, serum pregnancy test, and pelvic ultrasound are all tests that may be indicated depending on the circumstances including history, physical examination, and age.

10. E. Anovulatory dysfunctional uterine bleeding accounts for greater than 90% of all dysfunctional uterine bleeding; ovulatory dysfunctional uterine bleeding accounts for the remaining 10%.

11. D. Treatments for dysfunctional uterine bleeding can be divided into pharmacologic and nonpharmacologic.

    The nonpharmacologic treatment that is both most common and most important includes reassurance about the benign nature of the disorder (once other causes have been excluded) and education about the self-limiting nature of the disorder with time.

    The other nonpharmacologic treatment is actually a dilatation and curettage of the uterus that can, in fact, be therapeutic as well as diagnostic.

    Pharmacologic treatments include the oral contraceptive pill, ethinyl estradiol, cyclic progestins, and nonsteroidal anti-inflammatory agents.

12. B. The treatment of choice for this type of heavy DUB is intravenous estrogen (Premarin 25 mg IV q4h for 3-4 doses). In this patient the endometrial lining that is remaining (the basal layer) will be less responsive to progestin therapy.

    As an alternative to IV Premarin the OCP can be given four times per day for 5-7 days. This, however, would likely be associated with significant nausea.

    For the long term in this patient you may wish to consider an NSAID.

SOLUTION TO SHORT ANSWER MANAGEMENT PROBLEM 51

Women who exercise excessively or very frequently commonly present not only with oligomenorrhea but often with amenorrhea itself that may have been going on for many months or even years. The origin of this oligomenorrhea or amenorrhea in nearly all cases is anovulation. Because of the potential danger of unopposed endometrial estrogen buildup without shedding, it is reasonable to try a uterine bleed with hormonal therapy (estrogen and/or progesterone depending on the circumstances of the individual case).

SUMMARY OF THE DIAGNOSIS AND TREATMENT OF DYSFUNCTIONAL UTERINE BLEEDING

1. **Definition:** abnormal uterine bleeding that cannot be attributed to any specific genital tract lesion or systemic disease

2. **Classification of dysfunctional uterine bleeding:**
   a) Anovulatory:
      Prevalence: 90%
        Oligomenorrhea
        Menorrhagia
        Menometrorrhagia
   b) Ovulatory:
      Prevalence: 10%
        Midcycle spotting
        Premenstrual spotting

3. **Considerations regarding patient age:** in patients over the age of 20 years, exclude pelvic pathology before making the diagnosis of DUB. Also consider the other etiologies that may be associated with DUB.

4. **Treatment:**
   a) Anovulatory dysfunctional uterine bleeding:
      1. Consider diagnostic and therapeutic D and C.
      2. NSAIDs
      3. OCP
      4. Cyclic progestins
      5. Endometrial ablation if none of these is effective
   b) Ovulatory dysfunctional uterine bleeding:
      1. Midcycle spotting: ethinyl estradiol or OCP
      2. Premenstrual spotting: cyclic progestins
      3. Postmenopausal spotting: NSAID or OCP
   c) Acute hemorrhage caused by DUB: Premarin IV, OCP 4 times/day for 5-7 days OCP or oral Provera to follow

SUGGESTED READING

Friedman C. Dysfunctional uterine bleeding. In: Rakel R, ed. Conn's current therapy. Philadelphia: WB Saunders, 1994.

PROBLEM 52   A 23-YEAR-OLD FEMALE WHO WISHES TO BEGIN TAKING THE ORAL CONTRACEPTIVE PILL

A 23-year-old female presents to your office for a complete physical assessment. She wishes to begin taking the pill. Before giving her a prescription, you establish whether or not she has any relative or absolute contraindications to the pill.

She has been previously healthy (according to her). She tells you that she has never had any major medical problems. You note that she is really quite obese.

She has no history of liver disease, no history of sexually transmitted diseases, no history of migraine headaches, no history of estrogen-dependent neoplasia, and she states that she is as healthy as a horse. (Horses, however, do not smoke 2½ packs of cigarettes/day, which this patient does.)

The patient has never been pregnant.

On examination, her blood pressure is 160/100 mm Hg (large cuff). Her weight is 220 lb, and she is 5 feet, 10 inches tall. She has an obese abdomen. Her Pap smear is performed (her cervix looks normal), and her pelvic examination is normal.

SELECT THE ONE BEST ANSWER TO THE FOLLOWING QUESTIONS

1. What would you do at this time?
   a) prescribe the OCP and be done with it
   b) prescribe an amphetamine to get things going with her weight reduction and see her in 1 month
   c) tell her to forget it; you are not interested in giving her the pill
   d) tell her that she is really far too fat to take the pill
   e) none of the above

2. What would your next step be?
   a) obtain a more detailed history today and retake her BP
   b) refer her to one of your partners who specializes in this area
   c) refer her to a rapid weight-loss center and tell her to come back when she has lost 100 lb and quit smoking
   d) just give her the pill; the whole thing is not worth the trouble
   e) none of the above

3. You see the same patient the next week and her blood pressure is 150/105 mm Hg (this is after 5 minutes of rest). What would you do at this time?
   a) give her the oral contraceptive pill
   b) give her a thiazide diuretic
   c) give her a stern lecture on the dangers of smoking
   d) start her on an 800-calorie diet
   e) none of the above

4. The patient returns in a week. Her blood pressure is 140/100 mm Hg. No other changes are found (in either history or physical examination). At this time, what would you do?
   a) start her on the oral contraceptive pill
   b) tell her to see your partner next week (another specialist who as yet doesn't know it)

   c) tell her to stop smoking
   d) put in an intrauterine device
   e) none of the above

5. Which of the following is(are) side effects of the oral contraceptive pill?
   a) headaches
   b) nausea and vomiting
   c) cervical ectopia
   d) hepatocellular adenomas
   e) all of the above

6. Which of the following cancers has the oral contraceptive pill definitely been associated with (either increasing the risk or decreasing the risk)?
   a) ovarian carcinoma
   b) breast carcinoma
   c) cervical carcinoma
   d) all of the above
   e) none of the above

7. Which of the following statements regarding the relationship between OCP and sexually transmitted diseases is(are) true?
   a) the OCP protects against gonococcal infections
   b) the OCP protects against chlamydial infections
   c) the OCP protects against both gonococcal and chlamydial infections
   d) the OCP protects against gonococcal infections but may promote chlamydial infections
   e) the OCP protects against chlamydial infections but may promote gonococcal infections

8. A 21-year-old female presents to your office for the pill. She is healthy, has had no major medical problems, and is a nonsmoker, a nondrinker, and an exercise enthusiast. She is not obese.

   On examination, her blood pressure is 110/70 mm Hg. Her pulse is 72 and regular. Examination of the rest of the body, including a Pap smear and a pelvic examination, is normal.

She states that she has a number of boyfriends and they are all sexual partners. What would you do at this time?

a) give her a prescription for the OCP and say good-bye

b) give her a prescription for the OCP and tell her to get rid of as many of her boyfriends as possible: the more boyfriends, the greater the risk

c) give her a prescription for the OCP but stress the importance of always using condoms as a protection against STDs

d) tell her to use condoms only: they will both protect against STDs and look after the contraceptive issue

e) none of the above

9. A 16-year-old female presents to the ER at 4 AM. She had sexual intercourse at 12 AM and is absolutely frantic because she is not on the OCP. You consider emergency contraception.

What is(are) the postcoital agent(s) of choice for this patient?

a) ethinyl estradiol 100 μg $\times$ 2 (12 hours apart)

b) 2.0 mg Norgestrel or 1.0 mg Levonorgestrel

c) trimethobenzamide (Tigan) 250 mg $\times$ 3 (8 hours apart)

d) a and b only

e) all of the above

10. Of the following oral contraceptive pills, which would be your first choice for a patient (all other things being equal)?

a) Loestrin 1/20 (20 μg ethinyl estradiol plus norethindrone)

b) Minovral (30 μg ethinyl estradiol plus levonorgestrel)

c) Ovral (50 μg ethinyl estradiol plus levonorgesterol)

d) any of the above

e) none of the above

11. A 17-year-old female presents to your office for a discussion. It is very difficult to get a commitment from her about what she wishes to discuss, but after time she tells you that she wants to talk about sex. She has a 16-year-old boyfriend who has been trying to get her to say yes, but she is confused. On the one hand, she is scared that if she says no that the word will get around the school that she is a square. On the other hand, if she says yes, she believes that she will be violating herself.

Based on this information, what would be the most prudent advice to her?

a) go for it; give the guy what he wants, but set limits: only three times/week

b) go for it; if she doesn't, she might as well change schools

c) go for it; just be careful

d) it is OK to say no; it is not an extremist position, especially in the age of STDs

e) it is OK to say no; you better think this through again; yes might be a better answer

12. Which of the following statements regarding condoms is(are) true?

a) condoms prevent both unintended pregnancy and sexually transmitted diseases

b) condoms are the most effective method for preventing HIV infection

c) except for coitus interruptus, condoms are the only readily reversible method of birth control for men

d) condoms rarely break during vaginal intercourse

e) a, b, and c

f) all of the above

13. Which of the following statements regarding vaginal spermicides is(are) true?

a) vaginal spermicides must be used with the cervical diaphragm, cervical cap, and the cervical sponge

b) vaginal spermicides reduce the risk of transmission of neisseria gonorrhea

c) vaginal spermicides reduce the risk of transmission of chlamydia trachomatis

d) vaginal spermicides reduce the risk of transmission of HIV infection

e) a and c

f) a, b, and c

g) all of the above

14. Which of the following are noncontraceptive health benefits?

a) decreased risk of benign breast changes

b) decreased rate of ectopic pregnancy

c) decreased incidence of iron-deficiency anemia

d) decreased incidence of endometrial carcinoma

e) all of the above

15. Which of the following statements concerning the use of the cervical diaphragm, cervical cap, and cervical sponge is(are) true?

It has been definitely established that:

a) DCS methods are simple and noninvasive

b) DCS methods reduce the risk of transmission of gonorrhea

c) DCS methods reduce the risk of transmission of chlamydia

d) DCS methods reduce the risk of transmission of human immunodeficiency virus

e) a, b, and c

f) all of the above

16. Which of the following statements concerning the use of the oral contraceptive pill during lactation is(are) true?

a) the very low dose combined oral contraceptive pill can be used in lactation

b) the small amount of estrogen in the low dose combined OCP does not decrease breast milk production

c) a small amount of estrogen in the low dose combined OCP does enter the breast milk
d) all of the above are true
e) none of the above are true

17. The long-acting intramuscular form of birth control that has finally been approved by the FDA in the United States (after having been proved successful in over 90 countries) is which of the following?
a) Danazol
b) Bromocriptine
c) Depo-Provera
d) Depo-Premarin
e) Norplant

18. The major indication for the use of the minipill is a woman who:
a) only wishes to expose her body to one hormone
b) wants to take the lowest possible dose of contraceptive
c) has no intention of staying on the pill for a long time

d) has relative or absolute contraindications to the estrogen component of the combined OCP
e) a patient in whom the combination OCP failed

19. A 22-year-old para 2 gravida 2 female with a history of thrombophlebitis during her last pregnancy and who is sure that she does not want to go through another pregnancy for at least 4 years (and perhaps never) is best placed on which of the following?
a) Depo-Provera
b) Norplant
c) a combined OCP
d) the minipill
e) a or b

20. Which of the following medications may interact with the combined oral contraceptive pill to decrease its efficacy?
a) phenytoin
b) rifampin
c) diazepam
d) amitriptyline
e) all of the above

Short Answer Management Problem 52

PART A: List the contraindications to the insertion of an intrauterine device.

PART B: Discuss the advantages and disadvantages of permanent female sterilization.

PART C: Discuss the advantages and disadvantages of permanent male sterilization.

ANSWERS

1. E. At this point, you need a lot more information than you have. For example, you have the following problems:
   1. Obesity (morbid)
   2. Elevated blood pressure reading (probably secondary to 1)
   3. Nicotine addiction (heavy)
   4. No stated reason for OCP use at this time
   5. No discussion about sexually transmitted diseases

2. A. At least you can get a better history before she leaves the office today and focus on some of these major questions:
   1. Is she sexually active at this time?
   2. If yes, one partner? Two partners? How many?
   3. Has she been sexually active in the past?
   4. Is she planning to use condoms as well as the OCP?
   5. Has she ever tried to stop smoking?
   6. Does she want to quit smoking?

7. Has she ever tried to lose weight?
8. Does she want to lose weight?
   At the same time, you can recheck her blood pressure under the following conditions:
   1. Left arm, supine after 5 minutes of rest
   2. Large BP cuff (or leg cuff)

3. E. This patient still cannot be labeled as hypertensive; she has only two readings that are elevated and separated by 1 week.
   It would seem reasonable today to begin discussing a stop-smoking regimen, begin discussing food intake, or begin discussing an exercise program. Certainly, it would not be appropriate to take on all three at the same time. In addition, the patient needs to have one more blood pressure reading taken at least 1 week from now.

4. E. This patient has one official relative contraindication to the oral contraceptive pill, but she also has three risk factors for thrombophlebitis, pulmonary emboli, and other cardiovascular diseases:

1. Smoker (heavy)
2. Obesity
3. Hypertension

On the basis of risk/benefit ratio in this patient, it would appear that another contraceptive alternative would be preferable if possible; if not, the oral contraceptive pill would have to be used with extreme caution and full written consent.

5. E. The disadvantages and cautions of the OCP are as follows:
   1. It must be taken every day.
   2. It is expensive.
   3. There may be unwanted menstrual cycle changes (missed periods, scanty bleeding, spotting, or breakthrough bleeding).
   4. Nausea and vomiting: nausea may occur in the first cycle or so of pill use; less commonly, it continues.
   5. Headaches may begin or worsen (tension, migraine, or tension-migraine).
   6. Decreased libido may be due to decreased free testosterone.
   7. Both cervical ectopia and chlamydia infection are more common on the OCP.
   8. Thrombophlebitis, pulmonary emboli, and other CV diseases in:
      a) Smokers
      b) Sedentary lifestyle
      c) Obese
      d) >50 years in age
      e) Hypertension
      f) Diabetes
      g) History of heart or vascular disease
   9. Glucose intolerance
   10. Gallbladder disease
   11. Hepatocellular adenomas

6. A. There is no evidence that the OCP leads to an increase in any type of cancer, including breast cancer and cervical cancer.

   There is, however, convincing evidence that the OCP leads to a decrease in the incidence of ovarian carcinoma and endometrial carcinoma.

7. D. The oral contraceptive pill protects against gonococcal infections but may actually promote chlamydial infections. Chlamydia cervicitis is more common in women on the OCP. The OCP can cause cervical ectopia, a condition in which part of the cervical surface near the opening of the canal becomes covered by a delicate mucus-secreting columnar cell that normally lines the cervical canal. With an ectropion, the cervix of the pill user is more vulnerable to *Chlamydia trachomatis* infection. No evidence exists, however, that this increased risk places women using oral contraceptive pills at a greater risk of pelvic inflammatory disease.

8. C. This is a very common scenario and one that is frequently mismanaged. What ends up happening in a lot of cases is that the patient is simply given a prescription for the OCP and allowed to leave the office without the benefit of a significant amount of both contraceptive counseling and STD counseling. Although you may argue that D would be a better choice, it would not. This patient has specifically requested the OCP and it is reasonable to give the OCP to her once you have done the following:
   1. Counseled her regarding the possible side effects of the OCP
   2. Counseled her regarding the risks and benefits of the OCP
   3. Counseled her about safe sexual practices
   4. Counseled her about the importance of always using condoms along with the OCP when she is in the present situation (that is, with a number of partners)

9. E. The postcoital treatment of choice is as follows:
   A. A combination OCP with a high dose of estrogen and progesterone (Ovral), 2 tabs × 12 hours apart, plus an antinauseant (such as Tigan), *or*
   B. Ethinyl estradiol 100 μg × 2 (12 hours apart) plus norgesterol 2.0 mg or levonorgesterol 1.0 mg plus an antinauseant (such as Tigan)

   Other options include Danazol treatment (two doses, 12 hours apart, totalling 800 mg or three doses, 12 hours apart, totalling 1200 mg), progestin-only pill (such as a pill containing 0.75 mg levonorgesterol with the first pill being taken no more than 8 hours after intercourse), or postcoital IUD insertion 5 to 7 days after ovulation in a cycle when unprotected intercourse has occurred.

10. A. The oral contraceptive pill with the lowest estrogen content would be the oral contraceptive of choice from those listed. There are so many OCPs on the market that it is a very good idea for a physician to become accustomed to using two or three and using them well. There are biphasic pills and triphasic pills; there are progestin-only pills and there are pills that vary in both the content of estrogen and progesterone and the particular progesterone.

    As general rules in prescribing the OCP you should ask yourself the following questions:

    Can this individual be prescribed an OCP with estrogen?

    If yes, then consider the following factors in your decision:
    1. The number of micrograms of ethinyl estradiol
    2. The availability of that particular OCP
    3. Ease of remaining on the schedule imposed by that particular OCP
    4. Price of pills to the clinic
    5. Price of pills to the patient
    6. Prior experience of this woman or the clinician caring for this woman with a special pill

If no, then consider the following:
1. A progestin-only pill
2. An IUD
3. Condoms
4. Diaphragm, cervical cap
5. Foam
6. Cervical sponge

11. D. In this particular case, it is obvious that the young girl is being hounded and almost forced into sex by her boyfriend. In a situation such as this, the most logical response is to say the following: "It is OK to say no: it is not an extremist position, especially in this age of viral STDs."

12. F. The following facts concerning condoms can be stated:
1. Unlike other, more effective nonbarrier contraceptives, condoms, if used consistently and correctly, prevent both unintended pregnancy and sexually transmitted infection.
2. When used consistently and correctly, condoms are the most effective method for preventing HIV infection.
3. Condoms can be used with other contraceptives when STDs are a concern. Other more effective contraceptives such as sterilization, oral contraceptives, Norplant implants, Depo-Provera, and intrauterine devices do not prevent HIV infection or other STDs.
4. Except for coitus interruptus, condoms are the only readily reversible method of birth control for men.
5. Condoms rarely break during vaginal intercourse. Further, not every broken condom results in pregnancy or infection.
6. The provision of condoms in large numbers at a low or no cost and the promotion of positive images of condoms need to become major public health priorities.

13. F. Vaginal spermicides have the following important qualities:
1. Vaginal spermicides are simple, free of systemic side effects, available without a prescription, and can be used intermittently, with little planning needed.
2. Vaginal spermicides are an integral component of vaginal barrier methods, including the cervical diaphragm, the cervical sponge, and the cervical cap.
3. Vaginal spermicides reduce the transmission of important sexually transmitted diseases including neisseria gonorrhea and chlamydia trachomatis.
4. Vaginal spermicides, however, have an unknown effect (positive, negative, or neutral) on the incidence of human immunodeficiency virus transmission.

14. E. The oral contraceptive pill is very effective in reducing the risk of the following:
1. Carcinoma of the endometrium (discussed earlier)
2. Carcinoma of the ovary (discussed earlier)
3. Benign fibrocystic breast changes
4. Iron-deficiency anemia (due to significantly decreased blood loss during menstruation)
5. Reduced incidence of *chlamydia trachomatis*-induced PID
6. Reduced incidence of ectopic pregnancy

15. E. The following are true of diaphragms, caps, and sponges (DCS):
1. They are simple to use and noninvasive.
2. Women who use a DCS method have reduced rates of gonorrhea, chlamydia, ectopic pregnancy, and the serious sequelae of pelvic inflammatory disease.
3. Regarding the impact of DCS methods on HIV risk of transmission, abstinence is the safest choice, and using latex condoms can reduce the risk.
4. Unlike male condoms or spermicide, a woman can use a vaginal barrier without the direct cooperation of her partner. Correct use does not require an interruption in lovemaking.
5. Consistent and correct use is essential for success with vaginal barrier methods; most failures occur because the method is not used.

16. D. It is recommended that a low dose combination OCP can be used in lactation. Even though a small amount of ethinyl estradiol is passed through the breast milk to the baby, this does not decrease breast milk production.

17. C. The form of progesterone that has finally been approved in the United States for IM use is Depo-Provera. A deep IM injection of 150 mg of Depo-Provera will act as an extremely effective contraceptive for at least 3 months. It should be repeated every three months. Depo-Provera works by inhibiting ovulation (FSH and LH suppression) and also by eliminating the LH surge.

Depo-Provera also produces a shallow and atropic endometrium and the development of a thick mucus that decreases sperm penetration.

18. D. This major indication for the Progestin-only pill, such as Norethindrone or Norgesterol, is for patients who have either an absolute or a relative contraindication to the estrogen component of the combined oral contraceptive pill.

19. E. If a patient provides information to you that she has no intention of getting pregnant for some time and has a contraindication to the combined oral contraceptive

pill (the estrogen component) then the two choices that make the most sense are Norplant (a long-acting contraceptive—up to 5 years) and Depo-Provera.

Although the minipill could be used, it is question of whether or not the patient wishes to take a pill every day for the next 5 years.

20. E. The medications that are known to interact with the oral contraceptive pill and decrease its efficacy can be divided into the following categories:
    1. The anticonvulsants: phenobarbital, carbamazepine, primidone, phenytoin, and ethosuximide.
    2. Lipid agents: some lipid-lowering drugs (especially Clofibrate)
    3. The antibiotics—rifampin, isoniazid, penicillin, ampicillin, metronidazole, tetracycline, neomycin, chloramphenicol, sulfonamides, and nitrofurantoin
    4. Sedatives, hypnotics, tricyclic antidepressants, and antipsychotics

SOLUTION TO SHORT ANSWER MANAGEMENT PROBLEM 52

PART A: The contraindications to the insertion of an intrauterine device are as follows:
A. Absolute contraindications:
   1. Active, recent, or recurrent PID
   2. Postpartum endometritis
   3. Postabortion infection
B. Relative contraindications:
   1. Risk factors for PID:
      a) Purulent cervicitis
      b) Recent positive test for gonorrhea or chlamydia
      c) Recurrent history of gonococcal or chlamydial cervicitis
   2. High risk for acquiring a sexually transmitted disease, including multiple sexual partners and a partner with multiple sexual partners
   3. Impaired response to infection: diabetes, steroid treatment, HIV disease
   4. Risk factors for HIV infection and/or HIV disease
   5. Undiagnosed, irregular, heavy, or abnormal vaginal bleeding
   6. Cervical or uterine malignancy (known or suspected)
   7. Unresolved Pap smear
   8. History of ectopic pregnancy. This is a particularly important consideration if future pregnancy is desired.
   9. Previous problems with the IUD including pregnancy, expulsion, perforation, pain, or heavy bleeding
   10. Past history of severe vasovagal reactivity or fainting
   11. Difficulty obtaining emergency follow-up care and treatment for pelvic infection
   12. Valvular heart disease such as aortic stenosis
   13. Anatomical abnormalities of the uterus:
       a) Leiomyomata
       b) Endometrial polyps
       c) Cervical stenosis
       d) Bicornate uterus
       e) Very small uterus
   14. Nulliparous women

PART B: The advantages and disadvantages of female sterilization are as follows:
A. Advantages and indications:
   1. Permanent
   2. Highly effective
   3. Cost-effective when cost is spread out over time
   4. Nothing to buy or remember
   5. No significant long-term side effects
   6. Partner compliance not required
   7. No interruption in lovemaking
   8. Very private/personal matter
B. Disadvantages and cautions:
   1. Permanent
   2. Reversibility difficult and expensive
   3. Sterilization procedures technically difficult
   4. Requires surgeon, operating room (aseptic conditions), trained assistants, medications, surgical equipment
   5. Expensive at the time performed
   6. Morbidity and mortality high when considered for 1 year
   7. If failure, then there is a high probability of ectopic pregnancy
   8. No protection from STDs, including HIV

PART C: The advantages and disadvantages of male sterilization are as follows:
A. Advantages and indications:
   1. Highly effective
   2. Relieves the female of the contraceptive burden
   3. Inexpensive in the long run
   4. Permanent
   5. Highly acceptable procedure to most clients
   6. Very safe
   7. Quickly performed
B. Disadvantages and cautions:
   1. Protection for the male (it is the female who is at risk for pregnancy)
   2. A surgical procedure requiring surgical training, aseptic conditions, medications, and technical assistance
   3. Expensive in the short term
   4. Permanent (although reversal is possible, it is expensive, requires a highly technical and major surgery, and its results cannot be guaranteed)
   5. Serious long-term effects suggested (although currently unproven)
   6. Regret in 5% to 10% of patients
   7. No protection against STDs including HIV

a) Sperm antibodies develop in 50% to 66% of all men who undergo a vasectomy. It has been suggested that there may be an association between sperm antibodies and atherosclerotic vascular disease.

Recent studies have found a weak positive association between vasectomy and prostate cancer.

SUMMARY OF THE MANAGEMENT OF CONTRACEPTION

1. **First things first:**
   a) History and physical examination
   b) Remember that contraception does not only equal contraception; it equals contraception plus prevention of sexually transmitted diseases. When a patient presents with requests for contraception, the physician must consider both contraception and protection against sexually transmitted diseases.
2. **Oral contraceptive pill:**
   a) For OCP users: use OCP plus a barrier method.
   b) Consider relative and absolute contraindications; also consider whether or not the risks outweigh the benefits.
   c) Use the lowest estrogen dose possible when using the oral contraceptive pill.
   d) Considerations that should be taken seriously:
      1. Smoking
      2. Obesity
      3. Hypertension
   e) Learn to use two or three OCPs well
   f) Lactation and combination OCP do not go together.
   g) The combination oral contraceptive pill is protective against ovarian cancer and endometrial cancer.
   h) The combination oral contraceptive pill is protective

against benign breast changes. It has no effect on the incidence of breast cancer.
3. **Barrier methods:**
   a) Condoms
   b) Cervical cap
   c) Cervical diaphragm
   d) Cervical sponge
4. **Abstinence:**
   a) Remember, when your young patients ask, tell them it is OK to say no!
5. **Intrauterine contraceptive device:**
   a) Efficacy: excellent
   b) Ninety-eight percent of IUD users say they are happy with this method, and 60% of women with IUDs are repeat users.
   c) The Cu T 380 A (ParaGuard) offers 8 years of very effective protection, with only about 2% of women becoming pregnant within the first year of use.
6. **Progesterone-containing contraceptives:**
   Main indication is a contraindication to the estrogen component of the combined oral contraceptive pill.
   a) The minipill
   b) Depo-Provera
   c) Norplant
7. **Permanent sterilization:**
   a) Female sterilization
   b) Male sterilization
      Consider long-term potential complications:
      1. Anti-sperm antibodies
      2. Prostate cancer

SUGGESTED READING

Hatcher R et al. Contraceptive technology. 16th Rev. Ed. New York: Irvington, 1994.

PROBLEM 53   A 28-YEAR-OLD FEMALE WITH PELVIC PAIN AND VAGINAL BLEEDING

A 28-year-old female presents to your office with a 2-week history of pelvic pain and scant vaginal bleeding. There has been no vaginal discharge. She is married, has no children, and has been trying to become pregnant for the past 18 months. Her menstrual periods have always been regular, but she is now 3 weeks past the date at which she would have expected her last period.

On examination, her uterus feels slightly enlarged and boggy. There is a small amount of blood, "dark brownish-red," in the vaginal pool. Her left adnexal is somewhat tender. Her right adnexa is normal.

SELECT THE ONE BEST ANSWER TO THE FOLLOWING QUESTIONS

1. At this time, what is the most important diagnosis to exclude?
   a) ruptured corpus luteum cyst
   b) acute pelvic inflammatory disease
   c) ectopic pregnancy
   d) threatened abortion
   e) incomplete abortion

2. In taking a complete history from this patient, which of the following questions would be of particular importance?
   a) a history of fever within the last 24 hours
   b) a history of dysmenorrhea
   c) a history of menorrhagia
   d) a history of any irregularity in the last menstrual period
   e) a history of previous miscarriages

3. What is the most important single laboratory/imaging test to be performed at this time in this patient?
   a) serum beta-HCG
   b) urine HCG
   c) culdocentesis
   d) pelvic ultrasound
   e) laparoscopy

4. Regarding the epidemiology of the condition described, which of the following statements is(are) true?
   a) there has been marked increase in the incidence of this condition in the United States over the past 20 years
   b) there has been marked increase in the prevalence of this condition among women in the childbearing years in the United States over the past 20 years
   c) the actual, absolute number of cases of this condition in the United States has increased out of proportion to population growth over the last 20 years
   d) all of the above statements are true
   e) none of the above statements are true

5. Regarding the risks of morbidity and mortality associated with this condition in the United States, which of the following statements is(are) true?
   a) this condition remains the second most common

cause of maternal death in the United States at this time
   b) the maternal death rate from this condition could be decreased by at least one-third with earlier diagnosis and management
   c) most maternal deaths from this condition occur as a result of intraabdominal hemorrhage
   d) all of the above are true
   e) none of the above are true

6. Anatomically speaking, the condition described is most commonly associated with which of the following structures?
   a) the ampulla of the fallopian tube
   b) the isthmus of the fallopian tube
   c) the interstitial portion of the fallopian tube
   d) the interstitial portion of the ovary
   e) the endometrial lining itself

7. The condition described often goes undiagnosed in a young woman for some time. Which of the following symptoms or signs is the earliest indication of this problem?
   a) tachycardia
   b) acute severe abdominal pain
   c) a vasovagal attack or a feeling of dizziness and light-headedness, especially on assuming the upright position
   d) severe vaginal hemorrhage
   e) severe swelling and bloating of the abdomen

8. The diagnosis you suspected in the patient described in the case history is confirmed. Which of the following is(are) common signs/symptoms in this condition?
   a) abdominal pain
   b) irregular vaginal bleeding
   c) abdominal tenderness
   d) amenorrhea
   e) all of the above

9. What is(are) the major complication(s) of the condition described?
   a) intraabdominal hemorrhage
   b) hypovolemia and shock
   c) fetal death
   d) a and b
   e) all of the above

10. Which of the following is(are) documented risk factors
    for ectopic pregnancy?
    a) endosalpingitis
    b) paratubal adhesions
    c) cigarette smoking
    d) a and b
    e) all of the above

11. Which of the following organisms is most closely asso-
    ciated with the condition described?
    a) *Bacteroides fragilis*
    b) *Klebsiella pneumoniae*

c) *Escherichia coli*
d) Group A beta-hemolytic *streptococcus*
e) all of the above

12. What is the medical treatment of choice for the condi-
    tion described?
    a) intravenous estrogen
    b) oral estrogen
    c) oral progesterone
    d) IM medroxyprogesterone acetate
    e) methotrexate

Short Answer Management Problem 53

Discuss the possible reason(s) for the marked increase in both the absolute number of ectopic pregnancies and the
incidence/prevalence of ectopic pregnancy in the United States for the past two decades.

ANSWERS

1. C. The most important diagnosis to exclude at this time
   in this patient is ectopic pregnancy. In a patient who is
   in the childbearing age group, any of the three A's should
   suggest the possibility of an ectopic pregnancy. The
   three A's are amenorrhea, abdominal pain, and abnormal vaginal bleeding.

   The differential diagnosis of ectopic pregnancy in-
   cludes the following:
   A. Ruptured corpus luteum cyst
   B. Pelvic inflammatory disease
   C. Threatened or incomplete abortion
   D. Dysfunctional uterine bleeding
   E. Torsion of the adnexa
   F. Degenerating fibroid
   G. Endometriosis
   H. Acute appendicitis

2. D. The most important question to ask at this time is to
   have the patient define for you the history of the last
   menstrual period. The patient, in fact, tells you that she
   missed her last menstrual period. In many women who
   end up with ectopic pregnancies, you obtain a history of
   menstruation occurring at the regular time, but the
   menstrual period itself being significantly different in
   quality, that is, being "lighter" in terms of amount of
   flow. This, in anatomic pathological terms, corresponds
   to the shedding of the uterine decidual tissue secondary
   to necrosis of the trophoblastic tissue.

3. A. Based on this patient's history and physical examination, the probability of an ectopic pregnancy is very
   high. Therefore, a serum beta HCG is the most important investigation to perform at this time. At the same

time as the serum beta HCG is ordered, it would certainly be reasonable to order an obstetrical ultrasound.
The presence of an intrauterine gestational sac virtually
excludes ectopic pregnancy. The absence of a gestational
sac *and* the presence of a high titer of beta HCG (>6500
mIU/ml) is strong evidence of ectopic gestation. When
the beta HCG level is <6000 mIU/ml, the situation is
less clear. Ectopic pregnancy should still be suspected,
and serial quantitative HCG levels should be performed
every 48 hours.

4. D. There has been a marked increase in incidence,
   prevalence, and absolute number and rate of ectopic
   pregnancies in the United States over the past two
   decades. The actual number has increased out of proportion to the growth in the population; in fact, it has
   quadrupled between 1970 and 1987.

5. D. The percentage of all maternal deaths due to ectopic
   pregnancy increased by 8% between 1970 and 1987 even
   though the maternal death rate as a reflection of total
   cases of ectopic pregnancy has decreased. The case-fa-
   tality rate itself decreased 95% from 35.5 per 10,000 ectopic pregnancies in 1970 to 3.4 per 10,000 pregnancies
   in 1987. This fall in death rate applies to both white and
   nonwhite women. When considered in the total picture,
   this death rate is really remarkable in view of the increasing incidence/prevalence of the condition that occurred in the United States during the same time period.

   The dramatic decrease in death rate from ectopic
   pregnancy is due to improved diagnosis and treatment.

6. A. The most frequent site of extrauterine implantation
   is the ampulla of the fallopian tube. The isthmus of the
   fallopian tube is the next most common site of implan-

tation. Interstitial tubal pregnancy is very uncommon; it represents only 3% of the total number.

7. C. The signs and symptoms of this condition will be discussed at length in a subsequent question. However, it is important to recognize the earlier signs and the earlier symptoms that will allow the diagnosis to be made before significant damage occurs or a major complication arises.

   An early response to moderate intraabdominal hemorrhage may range from no change in pulse, blood pressure, or syncope, to a slight rise in blood pressure, or a vasovagal response with bradycardia and hypotension. This can be manifested by any significant change in blood pressure that occurs upon assuming the upright position from a supine position. Thus either a vasovagal attack or significant difference in standing and supine blood pressures may indicate hypovolemia secondary to as-yet undetected bleeding into the abdominal cavity from an ectopic pregnancy that is, in fact, rupturing.

8. E. There are no absolutely pathognomonic signs or symptoms of an early ectopic pregnancy. The most common symptoms noted are *the three A's:* abdominal pain, abnormal vaginal bleeding, and amenorrhea. Between 96% and 100% of patients with ectopic gestation complain of pain, even before rupture. No specific type of pain is diagnostic. With tubal rupture, the pain becomes more severe.

   Amenorrhea or a history of abnormal menses is reported in 75% to 95% of patients with ectopic pregnancy. A careful history with respect to the character and timing of the last two or three menstrual cycles (amount of flow, days of flow) is extremely important. Initially patients will often state that they have not missed a period; however, when questioned carefully, they may describe the period as being different (lighter than usual or irregular in timing). This bleeding may, in fact, represent bleeding from an endometrial slough. Profuse bleeding is uncommon.

   Common symptoms of early pregnancy, such as nausea and breast tenderness, are present in only 10% to 25% of patients with ectopic pregnancies. Symptoms of dizziness and fainting (vasovagal symptoms as mentioned previously) are present in 20% to 35% of patients. A few patients will state that they, in fact, passed tissue (a decidual cast).

   Most patients are afebrile.

   Abdominal tenderness is present in most patients (80%-95%). Rebound tenderness may or may not be present.

   A mass is palpable in 50% of patients with ectopic pregnancy. If there is uterine enlargement, it is not to the degree that would be expected for the duration of amenorrhea.

9. D. The major complications of ectopic pregnancy are intraabdominal hemorrhage and hypovolemia and shock secondary to rupture. Rupture of the ectopic pregnancy is responsible for almost all maternal morbidity and mortality.

   Fetal death cannot be classified as a major complication because of its inevitability in ectopic pregnancy.

10. E. The following is a list of suggested risk factors. Beside each is indicated the level of evidence for or against the plausibility of the risk factor.
    A. Salpingitis, especially endosalpingitis: definite risk factor
    B. Paratubal adhesions (postabortal, puerperal infection, appendicitis, endometriosis): definite risk factor
    C. Developmental abnormalities of the tube (diverticuli, accessory ostia, hypoplasia); rare, but definite risk factor
    D. Previous ectopic pregnancy: definite risk factor; 7%-15% risk of recurrence
    E. Previous operations on the tube: definite risk factor
    F. Multiple previous induced abortions: definite risk factor
    G. External migration of the ovum: little evidence to support this as a risk factor
    H. Menstrual reflux: little evidence to support this as a risk factor
    I. Altered tubal mobility (progesterone-only contraceptives): some evidence to support this as a risk factor
    J. Cigarette smoking: unrecognized up to now but definite risk factor
    K. Oral contraceptive pill: this is a protective factor. Relative risk is decreased compared to nonusers.
    L. Intrauterine device: this is a protective factor. The relative risk of ectopic pregnancy in users of the IUD compared to nonusers is decreased.
    M. Traditional barrier methods of contraception: this is a protective factor.

11. A. *Bacteroides fragilis* and *Peptostreptococcus* are the anaerobic organisms that, in combination with a neisseria gonorrhea and/or chlamydiae trachomatis, are usually responsible for acute PID. Acute PID results in tubal adhesions and tubal scarring and occlusion that subsequently increase the risk of ectopic pregnancy.

12. E. The medical management of choice for ectopic pregnancy is methotrexate. Methotrexate should be considered only if the following conditions apply:
    A. Early gestation (preferably <8 weeks)
    B. Tubal mass <3.5 cm in diameter
    C. Fetus is not alive.
    D. Patient is hemodynamically stable
    E. Patient has normal hemoglobin, liver function, and renal function

    Methotrexate therapy fails in approximately 5% to 10% of patients.

SOLUTION TO SHORT ANSWER MANAGEMENT PROBLEM 53

The very significant increase in incidence, prevalence, and the absolute number of ectopic pregnancies in the United States during the last 20 years, plus the number of ectopic pregnancies out of proportion to the growth of the population, appears to be due to an increased risk of and increased rate of sexually transmitted disease, particularly acute PID and chronic PID. These STD increases are primarily due to infection with two organisms: neisseria gonorrhea and chlamydia trachomatis. Acute PID, however, is usually polymicrobial in origin and often involves a combination of gram-positive organisms, gram-negative organisms, and anaerobic organisms. The anaerobes implicated include *Bacteroides fragilis* and *Peptostreptococcus.*

SUMMARY OF THE DIAGNOSIS AND TREATMENT OF ECTOPIC PREGNANCY

1. **Prevalence:** females ages 15-44 years:
   1970: rate/10,000 females = 5.5
   1987: rate/10,000 females = 14.0
   Increasing prevalence appears to be due to increasing prevalence of sexually transmitted diseases, especially acute PID.
2. **Pathogenesis:** major risk factors include previous ectopic; acute or chronic PID with tubal scarring and tubal adhesions; and cigarette smoking.
3. **Signs and symptoms:**
   The three A's: Abdominal pain + Amenorrhea + Abnormal vaginal bleeding = Ectopic pregnancy until proven otherwise.

Vasovagal attacks and orthostatic hypotension are strong indicators of tubal rupture.
4. **Major complications:**
   Tubal rupture = intraabdominal hemorrhage/hypovolemia + shock
5. **Investigations:**
   a) If missed menstrual period or abnormal menstrual period then do serum beta-HCG
   b) Pelvic ultrasound should confirm.
6. **Treatment:**
   a) Medical management:
   1. Methotrexate: methotrexate should be used only in patients who are hemodynamically stable with a normal hemoglobin, normal liver function tests, and normal renal function.
   b) Surgical management:
   Laparotomy with:
   1. Salpingectomy
   2. Tubal sterilization
   3. Fallopian tube conservative surgery:
      i) Salpingostomy
      ii) Salpingectomy
      iii) Segmental resection and anastomosis
      iv) Fibrial evacuation

SUGGESTED READING

Cunningham FG et al., eds. Ectopic pregnancy. Williams obstetrics. 19th Ed. Norwalk, CT: Appleton and Lange, 1993.

PROBLEM 54   A COUPLE THAT HAS BEEN UNSUCCESSFUL IN CONCEIVING AFTER 18 MONTHS OF TRYING

A 28-year-old female and her 27-year-old husband have been trying to conceive for the past 18 months. They are extremely anxious, and during the interview the wife begins to cry.

You go through a short history on both members of the couple today in preparation for a more thorough investigation. You discover that the wife has a history of PID (one episode at age 18). The husband has been healthy and has had no major medical problems.

SELECT THE ONE BEST ANSWER TO THE FOLLOWING QUESTIONS

1. What is the next most appropriate step in the evaluation of this couple?
   a) tell the couple that the infertility is due to previous PID and refer them to an adoption agency
   b) refer the patient to a gynecologist to break the news of the infertility
   c) begin the wife on clomiphene citrate
   d) refer the couple to a psychiatrist
   e) none of the above

2. How is primary infertility defined?
   a) inability to ever achieve conception despite unprotected intercourse for 12 months
   b) inability to ever achieve conception despite unprotected intercourse for 18 months
   c) inability to ever achieve conception despite unprotected intercourse for 24 months
   d) inability to ever achieve conception despite unprotected intercourse for 6 months
   e) none of the above

3. How is secondary infertility defined?
   a) inability to achieve conception despite unprotected intercourse for 12 months following a previous conception
   b) inability to achieve conception despite unprotected intercourse for 18 months following a previous conception
   c) inability to achieve conception despite unprotected intercourse for 24 months following a previous conception
   d) inability to achieve conception despite unprotected intercourse for 6 months following a previous conception
   e) none of the above

4. In attempting to obtain a history from both husband and wife that will lead you to a diagnosis of infertility, which of the following is the most important question?
   a) the current medications that both partners (but especially the husband) are taking
   b) the frequency of intercourse
   c) the position(s) when intercourse takes place
   d) the amount of time that the female spends trying to maximize the tilt of the vagina after intercourse
   e) the age of the husband

5. What is the prevalence of primary infertility in American couples?
   a) <1%
   b) 4-6%
   c) 10-15%
   d) 20-25%
   e) 30-35%

6. In the United States, the male is principally responsible for what percentage of infertility in couples attempting to conceive?
   a) 10%
   b) 20%
   c) 30%
   d) 40%
   e) 50%

7. In the United States, the female is principally responsible for what percentage of infertility in couples attempting to conceive?
   a) 10%
   b) 20%
   c) 30%
   d) 40%
   e) 50%

8. Which of the following statements regarding the occurrence of ovulation is(are) true?
   a) the female partner should keep a basal body temperature chart for at least 6 months before ovulation can be precisely determined
   b) a woman who has a menstrual period every 6 months may still be ovulating on a monthly basis
   c) if a woman has regular menstrual cycles associated with cyclical premenstrual sensations or symptoms (molimina), she is almost certainly ovulating
   d) the only accurate method of determining ovulation is by endometrial biopsy
   e) if a woman has been anovulatory for a period of greater than 1 year, it is unlikely that she will ever ovulate again

9. Which of the following statements regarding the physiology of infertility is(are) false?
   a) normal quality and quantity of periovulatory cervical mucus is essential for fertilization to occur
   b) sufficient progesterone must be present in the luteal phase to properly prepare the endometrium for implantation
   c) the hypothalamic-pituitary-ovarian axis must be functioning properly in order to regulate normal folliculogenesis and ovulation
   d) sufficient progesterone levels must be present in the periovulatory phase in order to induce the luteinizing hormone (LH) surge
   e) none of the above are false

10. Which of the following statements concerning the investigation of infertility is(are) false?
    a) both male and female partners should be investigated simultaneously
    b) ovulation can be confirmed by the recording of the basal body temperature
    c) the adequacy of the luteal phase is well assessed by midluteal phase serum progesterone determinations
    d) the postcoital test is negative unless 25 sperm are seen per high power field (HPF)
    e) none of the above statements are false

11. The World Health Organization has issued parameters for the assessment of a normal sperm analysis. Which of the following is not part of the WHO's criteria for a normal sperm analysis?
    a) total count greater than 20 million sperm/ml
    b) sperm demonstrate greater than 50% motility
    c) sperm demonstrate greater than 50% normal morphology
    d) total semen volume is greater than 2.0 ml
    e) all of the above are part of WHO's definition

12. What is the most common identified female factor responsible for infertility?
    a) ovulatory/luteal phase dysfunction
    b) cervical mucus abnormality
    c) tubal adhesions and scarring

d) endometriosis
e) autoantibodies to sperm

13. What is the most common identified male factor responsible for infertility?
    a) previous mumps infection
    b) primary testicular failure
    c) idiopathic low motility
    d) testicular varicocele
    e) previous history of epididymitis

14. Which of the following is(are) true regarding varicoceles?
    a) varicoceles are due to incompetent valves in the testicular vein
    b) 90 percent of varicoceles occur on the left side
    c) treatment consists of operative ligation of the spermatic vein
    d) a and c
    e) all of the above are true

15. Which of the following statements most correctly describes the manner in which a family physician should conduct an infertility investigation?
    a) the partners should be assessed one at a time; if no cause is found in the wife, the husband should then be checked
    b) the family physician should assess one factor at time; the infertility investigation should be completed within approximately 9 months
    c) the family physician should recommend an immediate referral to a gynecologist for the woman; if no infertility factor is found, the physician should refer the husband to a urologist for a fertility workup
    d) the family physician should assess both husband and wife at the same time; preliminary investigations should be completed within 2 months
    e) none of the above are true

16. What is the drug of choice for induction of ovulation?
    a) clomiphene citrate
    b) danazol
    c) bromocriptine
    d) deprenyl
    e) none of the above

Short Answer Management Problem 54

Because of the significant impact of acute PID on future fertility, discuss how you would approach a young girl who asked you for a prescription for the oral contraceptive pill.

ANSWERS

1. E.

2. A.

3. A. The most appropriate first step is to perform a complete history and physical examination on both partners.

   Primary infertility is defined as the inability of a couple to achieve a pregnancy after at least 12 months of unprotected intercourse, with adequate frequency of intercourse a necessary prerequisite. Within 1 year, 95% of "normal" couples should achieve a pregnancy. Secondary infertility is defined as the inability to achieve conception despite unprotected intercourse for 12 months following a previous conception.

   If conception does not occur within that time, a complete evaluation of both partners is indicated. In the female, a complete history including the menstrual history, previous surgery, and previous pelvic infections should be documented. The physical examination of the woman should evaluate any signs of endocrine disorder, and a complete pelvic examination (including rectovaginal) should be performed. In the male, a history of mumps, current medications, and a history of epididymitis or other male genitourinary infection are important. The physical examination should include testicular size, location of the urethral meatus, and the presence or absence of a varicocele. The prostate should be examined.

4. B. There are many factors affecting reproductive performance. The most important of these factors include the following:
   A. The age of the female partner
   B. The age of the male partner
   C. The understanding (or lack of same) of reproductive biology
   D. Coital frequency
   E. Timing of intercourse
   F. Coital technique
   G. The use of lubricants
   H. The use of douching following intercourse
   I. A history of multiple sexual partners (in either partner, but especially in the female)
   J. A history of sexually transmitted diseases
   K. The history of previous pregnancies
   L. A history of sickle-cell disease
   M. Nutrition (especially in the female)
   N. Exposure to toxic agents
   O. A history of smoking and or alcohol use in either partner
   P. Medication use in either partner
   Q. A history of surgery involving reproductive structures in either partner

R. Exposure to radiation
S. Excessive physical exertion and heat
   Of the choices offered in the question, the most important factor listed is the frequency of intercourse. Often a couple who presents for assessment of infertility is found to have a problem with the frequency of intercourse (in that they are having intercourse only one or two times per month). This will greatly increase the time required to achieve a successful pregnancy.

5. C. The prevalence of infertility in American couples is approximately 10%-15%. This represents the number of couples who are not able to conceive within 12 months if they are using no contraception and attempting to achieve a pregnancy. It must be recognized that this merely represents an aggregate summary statistic and usually is of little value when counseling an individual or couple regarding the chance of conception. The factors listed in the answer to Question 3 all influence this infertility prevalence.

6. D.

7. D. In the United States the male and the female are principally responsible for 40% of infertility each. In 20% the cause is unknown or problems exist with both partners.

8. C. If a woman has regular menstrual cycles associated with cyclical premenstrual sensations or symptoms (molimina), then she is almost certainly ovulating. A woman who is menstruating regularly does not have to keep taking her basal body temperature for 6 months; to do so is both unnecessary and anxiety provoking. On the other hand, a woman who has a menstrual period only every 6 months is almost certainly not ovulating.

   Ovulation is most easily assessed by a history of regular cyclical menses; endometrial biopsy is rarely necessary. Many women who are anovulatory for long periods of time can have ovulation induced with clomiphene; therefore a 1-year history of anovulation is not at all hopeless.

9. D. A successful pregnancy is dependent on the following male and female factors:
   A. 1. Successful vaginal intercourse with the deposition of motile spermatozoa in the upper vagina before ovulation
      2. A normal female hypothalamic-pituitary-ovarian axis that is capable of producing a luteinizing hormone (LH) surge
      3. Stimulation of the production of normal cervical mucus
      4. Production of sufficient progesterone during the luteal phase to maintain the corpus luteum and prepare the endometrium for implantation

B. A normal quality and quantity of periovulatory cervical mucus and normal sperm-mucus interaction
C. Normal, patent, fallopian tubes that allow ovum pickup, transport, and fertilization
D. A normally hormonally stimulated uterus that is capable of supporting and maintaining implantation

The luteinizing hormone surge does not occur in the periovulatory phase.

10. D. Both male and female partners should be investigated simultaneously.

A semen analysis should be performed.

In the male, a semen analysis should be obtained, preferably by masturbation. The World Health Organization's normal parameters of sperm count are >20 million sperm/ml, >50% motility, and >50% normal morphology. An abnormal semen analysis should be repeated at least twice.

In the female, ovulation should be assessed by basal body temperature (BBT) charting. Normally an increase in BBT of 0.5-1.0° F follows ovulation. Prolonged use of BBT records can become a significant source of anxiety and should be avoided. A 2- or 3-month period of charting is recommended. Ovulation can be predicted prospectively with one of several rapid monoclonal antibody assay kits for the detection of urinary LH. These kits, however, are expensive.

Luteal phase function can be assessed by the measurement of midluteal phase progesterone. A midluteal serum progesterone level above 10-15 ng/ml is considered evidence of an adequate luteal phase. Endometrial biopsy can also be used to diagnose a luteal phase defect.

The postcoital test measures the cervical factor in infertility. During the periovulatory period the cervical mucus should be thin, clear, acellular and exhibit ferning and spinnbarkeit. The sperm-mucus interaction is assessed by counting the number of motile sperm per high-power field. If at least one motile sperm/HPF is found, the postcoital test is positive.

Tubal patency is assessed by laparoscopy plus intraoperative dye hydrotubation.

The uterine factor is best assessed by hysteroscopy.

Immune factors that may be involved in unexplained infertility can be assessed by measuring antisperm antibodies.

11. D. The World Health Organization's definition of a normal sperm analysis is as follows:
A. Number: >20 million (15-20 million is suboptimal but still capable of producing a pregnancy.)
B. Percentage of sperm that demonstrate forward motility: >50% of total number
C. Percentage of sperm that exhibit what is considered to be a "normal morphology": >50%

The World Health Organization does not comment on semen volume in its "normal" parameters.

12. C. The most common identified female cause of infertility is associated with tubal factors, particularly tubal adhesions and scarring from previous pelvic inflammatory disease. Other factors are ovulatory/luteal phase defects (10-15%), cervical factors (10%), and male factors (40%).

13. D. The most commonly identified male factor associated with infertility is a testicular varicocele. Second on the list is primary testicular failure followed by epididymitis as the third most common factor.

14. E. Varicocele is the most common identifiable cause of male infertility. Varicocele is due to incompetent valves in the testicular vein, permitting the transmission of hydrostatic venous pressure; distention and tortuosity of the pampiniform plexus results. Varicoceles are present on the left side in 90% of cases, presumably due to venous drainage of the left testes to the left renal vein, causing increased retrograde venous pressure.

Surgical treatment of varicoceles should take place only if the varicocele appears to be a cause of infertility *or* the varicocele is symptomatic (a dragging scrotal sensation is a problem).

15. D. Infertility investigations should be conducted quickly, and both husband and wife should be evaluated at the same time. The emotional impact of infertility can be very traumatic to a young couple. The longer the time taken to complete the investigations, the greater is the emotional trauma. The family physician can perform baseline complete histories and baseline physical examinations on both members of the couple, semen analysis on the husband (repeated), basal body temperature charting on the female, postcoital testing, and serum LH and FSH determinations along with midluteal serum progesterone determination on the female partner. These investigations can be completed in a short period of time. If no cause is found (and this would suggest a tubal or peritoneal factor), a referral to a gynecologist should be made as quickly as possible.

16. A. If the female partner is not ovulating or has very irregular cycles, the drug of choice for induction of ovulation is clomiphene citrate. Although a number of regimens are available, a common regime is to give clomiphene for the first 5 days of the cycle. Multiple pregnancy is a risk.

SOLUTION TO SHORT ANSWER MANAGEMENT PROBLEM 54

The advice you would give your young client should include the following:

1. Because of the risk of STDs (including AIDS) and subsequent PID, you would recommend the use of a barrier

method of contraception (such as condoms) along with the OCP.

2. You should make the patient aware that although the OCP may protect against one type of PID (gonococcal PID), it does not protect against, and may even promote, chlamydial PID.

3. Reinforce the importance of limiting sexual partners (to one) if possible.

4. Reinforce the importance of telling your young client that she should *not* have sex if her partner refuses to wear a condom.

5. Ask her to return regularly for counseling and support.

SUMMARY OF THE DIAGNOSIS AND MANAGEMENT OF INFERTILITY

1. **Definition** (primary): failure to achieve a pregnancy after at least 12 months of unprotected intercourse

2. **Prevalence:** the prevalence of infertility in the American population is 10%-15%.

3. **Most common causes:**
   Female:
   a) Tubal adhesions and scarring from PID
   b) Anovulatory cycles
   c) Other abnormalities in tubes and uterus
   d) Amenorrhea due to anorexia nervosa or continuing vigorous exercise (long-term)
   e) Hyperprolactinemia
   Male:
   a) Varicocele
   b) Primary testicular failure
   c) Previous epididymitis or mumps orchitis

4. **Investigations:**
   a) Complete histories (both partners)
   b) Complete physical examinations (both partners)
   c) Semen analysis (repeated twice): male factor
   d) Basal body temperature monitoring and/or assessment of regular menstrual cycles: ovulatory factor
   e) Postcoital test: cervical factor
   f) Midluteal progesterone: luteal phase factor

5. **Referrals:**
   a) Referral to a gynecologist for assessment of tubal and peritoneal factors
   b) Referral to a urologist if a varicocele is detected

6. **Treatment options:**
   a) Male infertility:
      1. Artificial donor insemination (ADI): particular attention must be paid to ensuring that the donor is free from sexually transmitted diseases (especially AIDS). The current recommendation is for the sperm to be stored for 6 months and if the donor is still HIV negative to inseminate at that time.
   b) Female infertility:
      1. Cervical mucus problems: cervical mucus problems impairing conception may be treated with insemination or uterine instillation of a small amount of specially prepared sperm.
      2. Cervical incompetence: if cervical incompetence is interfering with continuing pregnancy, the treatment of choice is cervical cerclage, bed rest, or both.
      3. Ovarian disorders: ovulation disorders can be treated with drugs to induce ovulation. Clomiphene citrate suppresses estrogen's ovulation-suppressive effect. In women whose ovulation is suppressed by hyperprolactinemia (high blood levels of the pituitary hormone prolactin), ovulation may be induced with prolactin-suppressing drugs such as bromocriptine.
      4. Uterine/tubal abnormalities:
         i) Specific corrective surgical procedures (for PID adhesions and scarring and for endometriosis)
         ii) Gamete intrafallopian tube transfer (GIFT)
         iii) In vitro fertilization
      5. Adoption: adoption may be the only vehicle left to some couples. To maximize the ability to cope, it is recommended that this subject be raised early rather than later.

SUGGESTED READING

Hatcher RA et al., eds. Infertility. In: Contraceptive technology. 16th Rev. Ed. New York: Irvington, 1994.

Psychiatry/Behavioral Science and Communication

PROBLEM 55   A 34-YEAR-OLD FEMALE WHO IS TEARFUL AND SAD

A 34-year-old female presents to your office in a state of depression. She tells you that she has been "way down" for the past 4 months and has not felt much like doing anything. She had a previous "nervous breakdown" when she was 22 years old. She worked as a business executive until 4 months ago but has found it impossible not only to work but to do anything else. She had worked at her present position for approximately 18 months but was finding work an increasing stress; she was working approximately 75 hours/week and having to deal with daily difficulties and conflicts. She is currently on long-term sick leave.

She expresses her current situation best by saying, "I have no joy left in life; I don't enjoy doing anything, nor do I have any interest in any of my previous activities." Her other symptoms include sleeping approximately 14 hours/day, almost continual feelings of guilt and hopelessness, a state of having almost no energy "all of the time," decreased concentrating ability, no appetite plus a 24-lb weight loss, and being unable to "move around" or get anything done.

She is married and has three children. Her past health has been excellent apart from the previously mentioned "nervous breakdown."

Her marriage is described as "excellent;" her husband is very supportive. She does admit, however, to a significant decrease in sexual interest and activity.

Her family history is significant for alcoholism in both her mother and father.

She is on no drugs and has no allergies.

Her physical examination is completely normal in all systems.

SELECT THE ONE BEST ANSWER TO THE FOLLOWING QUESTIONS

1. What is the most likely diagnosis in this patient?
   a) adjustment disorder secondary to work stress
   b) generalized anxiety disorder
   c) major depressive disorder
   d) organic affective disorder
   e) dysthymia

2. Which of the following types of psychotherapy is most commonly used in the illness above?
   a) psychoanalytic psychotherapy
   b) behavioral psychotherapy
   c) psychodynamic psychotherapy
   d) cognitive psychotherapy
   e) supportive psychotherapy

3. The aims or goals of the psychotherapy for this condition include which of the following?
   a) providing a therapeutic rationale or explanation for the patient's symptoms
   b) providing ongoing education regarding the illness, prognosis, and treatment
   c) guiding the patient with respect to interpersonal relationships, work, and major life adjustments
   d) helping to bolster the patient's morale
   e) all of the above

4. What is the pharmacologic agent of choice in the disorder described?
   a) a selective serotonin reuptake inhibitor (SSRI)
   b) a tricyclic antidepressant
   c) a nonselective MAO inhibitor
   d) a selective MAO inhibitor
   e) lithium carbonate

5. A 41-year-old male presents with a 3-year history of a "depressed mood." He states that he feels "depressed most of the time," although there are periods when he feels better than others. He feels chronically tired, has some difficulty concentrating at work, and has found it difficult to remain productive and efficient as CEO of a major company. He has had no other symptoms. His health is otherwise good. He is on no medications.
   What is the most likely diagnosis?
   a) adjustment disorder
   b) dysthymic disorder
   c) major depressive disorder
   d) organic affective disorder
   e) none of the above

6. What is the treatment of choice for the patient described in Question 5?
   a) a tricyclic antidepressant
   b) a serotonin reuptake inhibitor
   c) supportive and/or cognitive psychotherapy

d) a and c
e) b and c

7. A 35-year-old female presents to your office with a 3-month history of depressed mood. She feels "extremely distressed at work" and tells you that she is "burned out." You discover that she moved into a managerial position at work 4 months ago and is having a great deal of difficulty (interpersonal conflict) with two of her employees.

   The patient has no history of psychiatric illness. She has no other symptoms. She is on no medications.

   What is the most likely diagnosis in this patient?
   a) adjustment disorder with depressed mood
   b) dysthymic disorder
   c) major depressive disorder
   d) organic affective disorder
   e) burnout

8. What is the treatment of choice for the patient described in Question 7?
   a) a tricyclic antidepressant
   b) a selective serotonin reuptake inhibitor (SSRI)
   c) supportive psychotherapy
   d) a and c
   e) b and c

9. A complete psychiatric history is most important in evaluating depressed patients. In taking a history from a patient with depression, which of the following questions is the most important question to ask?
   a) inquiry into the family history of psychiatric disorders
   b) inquiry into the personal history of previous episodes of depression
   c) inquiry into suicidal ideation
   d) inquiry into the presence or absence of hallucinations
   e) inquiry into the presence or absence of delusions

10. A 45-year-old male, a "hard-driving executive," presents with a 4-month history of feelings of sadness, irritability, loss of appetite, inability to concentrate, and a significantly decreased ability to function in his role as the manager of a major corporation subsector. He tells you that he is "completely burned out."

    When you question him he tells you that "he has been using anything and everything possible to try and relax." He has missed a number of days of work recently because he "just hasn't felt up to it." He also complains of increasing stomach pains and headaches over the last 2 months.

    From the history given, what is the most likely diagnosis?
    a) major depressive disorder
    b) dysthymic disorder
    c) mood disorder due to a general medical condition
    d) substance-induced mood disorder
    e) adjustment disorder with depressed mood

11. What is the treatment of choice for the patient described in Question 10?
    a) a selective serotonin reuptake inhibitor (SSRI)
    b) a tricyclic antidepressant
    c) an MAO inhibitor
    d) lithium carbonate
    e) none of the above

12. A 61-year-old male, a patient whom who you have known for 20 years, presents with a 4-month history of depression. He has no previous history of psychiatric illness, nor is there any evidence of psychiatric illness in his family. He has also been feeling extremely fatigued, has lost his appetite, has lost 20 lb in weight, and has begun to experience "stomach pains" diagnosed by an ER doctor as "irritable bowel syndrome."

    The other significant factor is that this patient retired from his position as an administrative assistant with the Internal Revenue Service 6 months ago. His symptoms began 2 months after that event.

    On examination, the patient fits the criteria for major depressive disorder. However, he also has other findings that concern you. He is having many more episodes of the "irritable bowel syndrome" pain than he previously did. He is also experiencing more "constipation." There is a definite difference in the periumbilical region on percussion: tympany changes to dullness over a 6-cm area.

    On the basis of the information given, which of the following conditions is the most likely possibility in this patient?
    a) major depressive disorder
    b) late-onset depressive disorder: DSM-IV "brief depressive disorder"
    c) adjustment disorder with depressed mood
    d) mood disorder due to a general medical condition
    e) dysthymia

13. What is the primary treatment for the patient described in Question 12?
    a) a selective serotonin reuptake inhibitor (SSRI)
    b) a tricyclic antidepressant
    c) an MAO-B inhibitor
    d) lithium carbonate
    e) none of the above

14. What is the single most likely diagnosis based on the signs and symptoms reported in Question 12?
    a) carcinoma of the stomach
    b) carcinoma of the pancreas
    c) early delirium
    d) early Alzheimer's disease
    e) dysthymic disorder

15. As physicians, we need to convince our patients that depression is a disease like any other; it originates from dis-

ordered body chemistry, just as diseases such as hypothyroidism, hyperthyroidism, and diabetes mellitus do.

Which of the following hypotheses supports this argument?

a) loss of the normal feedback mechanism inhibiting adrenocorticotropic hormone
b) The lack of normal suppression of blood cortisol following the administration of dexamethasone
c) The generalized decrease in noradrenergic function in depressed patients

d) a and b
e) all of the above

16. Which of the following neurotransmitters appears to be the most important mediator of depressive illness in humans?

a) norepinephrine
b) acetylcholine
c) dopamine
d) serotonin
e) tryptophan

Short Answer Management Problem 55

Discuss a strategy for the pharmacologic management of major depressive disorder.

ANSWERS

1. C. The diagnosis in this patient is major depressive disorder. The criteria for major depressive disorder according to the *Diagnostic and Statistical Manual of Mental Disorders—Fourth Edition (DSM-IV)* follow:

A. Five or more of the following symptoms present during the same 2-week period and representing a change from previous functioning. At least one of those two symptoms must be either (1) or (2):
   1. Depressed mood most of the day, nearly every day, as indicated by either subjective report (such as feeling sad or empty) or observation made by others (for example, appears tearful)
   2. Markedly diminished interest or pleasure in all, or almost all, activities most of the day, nearly every day (as indicated by either subjective account or observation made by others)
   3. Significant weight loss when not dieting or weight gain (for example, a change of more than 5% of body weight in a month), or decrease or increase in appetite nearly every day
   4. Insomnia or hypersomnia nearly every day
   5. Psychomotor agitation or retardation nearly every day (observable by others, not merely subjective feelings of restlessness or being slowed down)
   6. Fatigue or loss of energy nearly every day
   7. Feelings of worthlessness or excessive or inappropriate guilt (which may be delusional) nearly every day (not merely self-reproach or guilt about being sick)
   8. Diminished ability to think or concentrate, or indecisiveness, nearly every day (either by subjective account or observed by others)
   9. Recurrent thoughts of death (not just fear of dying), recurrent suicidal ideation without a specific plan, or a suicide attempt, or a specific plan for committing suicide

B. The symptoms do not meet the criteria for a mixed episode (manic-depression).
C. The symptoms cause clinically significant distress or impairment in social, occupational, or other important areas of functioning.
D. The symptoms are not due to the direct physiological effects (such as drug abuse or a medication) or a general medical condition (hypothyroidism).
E. The symptoms are not accounted for by bereavement (after the loss of a loved one); the symptoms persist for longer than 2 months or are characterized by a marked functional impairment, morbid preoccupation with worthlessness, suicidal ideation, psychotic symptoms, or psychomotor retardation.

A mnemonic for major depressive disorder is as follows: SIG: EM CAPS (5 out of 9, including 4 or 5).
   1. S = sleep (hypersomnia or insomnia)
   2. I = interest (lack of interest in life in general)
   3. G = guilt or hopelessness
   4. E = energy or fatigue
   5. M = mood (depressed, sadness)
   6. C = concentration (lack of)
   7. A = appetite (increased or decreased; weight loss or gain)
   8. P = psychomotor (retardation or agitation)
   9. S = suicidal ideation

The other choices in this question are discussed in various other chapters of this book.

2. E.

3. E. There are a wide range of psychotherapeutic interventions that may be useful in the treatment of mood disorders, particularly depressive mood disorders. The

establishment of a supportive therapeutic relationship is often crucial in the treatment of the depressed patient. Supportive psychotherapy generally consists of the following:

1. Providing a therapeutic rationale or explanation for the patient's symptoms
2. Providing ongoing education and feedback about the patient's illness, prognosis, and treatment
3. Guiding the patient with respect to interpersonal relationships, work, and major life adjustments
4. Helping to bolster the patient's morale
5. Setting realistic goals
6. Being available in time of crisis

Supportive psychotherapy in this patient's case would focus on this patient's work environment and the stress associated with it.

Cognitive psychotherapy, the other major psychotherapy used in major depression, is a method of brief psychotherapy developed over the last two decades by Aaron T. Beck. It is primarily used for the treatment of mild to moderate depression and for patients with low self-esteem. It is similar to behavioral therapy in that it aims at the direct removal of symptoms rather than the resolution of underlying conflicts, such as is attempted in psychodynamic psychotherapies. Cognitive therapists view the patient's conscious thoughts as central to production. Both the content of thoughts and thought processes are seen as disordered in people with such symptoms. Therapy is directed at identifying and altering these cognitive distortions.

4. A. The pharmacologic treatment of choice in patients with major depressive disorder is now a member of the class of drugs known as selective serotonin reuptake inhibitors (SSRIs). The agents in this new class include fluoxetine (Prozac), sertraline (Zoloft), and paroxetine (Paxil). These agents have significantly fewer side effects than the tricyclic antidepressants. The major side effects include gastrointestinal distress, tremor, insomnia, somnolence, and dry mouth. The SSRIs have replaced the tricyclic antidepressants as the drugs of first choice for major depressive disorder in adults. The SSRIs act exactly as they are named: they block the reuptake of serotonin in the brain.

The tricyclic antidepressants are now the drugs of second choice. A tricyclic antidepressant should be tailored to the individual patient's needs. If the patient's symptoms include fatigue, hypersomnia, lethargy, an inability to concentrate, then a drive-enhancing tricyclic such as desipramine or nortriptyline should be used. If, on the other hand, the patient's symptoms include anxiety, insomnia, and irritability, an anxiety-reducing tricyclic such as amitriptyline or doxepin would be more appropriate. If the patient has symptoms that require both drive enhancement and anxiety reduction, an agent such as imipramine or maprotiline would be most appropriate.

The tricyclic antidepressants exert multiple effects on central and autonomic nervous system pathways, at least partially by presynaptic blockade of norepinephrine or serotonin reuptake.

In selecting a TCA the physician must consider the presenting symptoms, the side effect profile (especially the anticholinergic side effects), and the cost when deciding on therapy. A drug with low anticholinergic side effects is nortriptyline. A drug with a higher anticholinergic side effect profile is amitriptyline. The major anticholinergic side effects exhibited by TCAs include dry mouth, urinary retention, constipation, and blurred vision. Other serious significant side effects include orthostatic hypotension (an alpha-blockade side effect), cardiac conduction abnormalities (an increased risk for patients with second-degree and third-degree heart block, or right or left bundle branch block due to a quinidine-like action), and excessive sedation due to an antihistamine-like action.

Monamine oxidase inhibitors (such as phenelzine or tranylcypromine) may be effective in cases of resistant major depressive disorder. MAO inhibitors are effective antidepressants whose mode of action is to block irreversibly postsynaptic inactivation of epinephrine, norepinephrine, dopamine, and serotonin.

MAO inhibitors do not exhibit the anticholinergic side effects seen with tricyclics. The most common side effects of these drugs are dizziness, orthostatic hypotension, sexual dysfunction, insomnia, and daytime sleepiness. The greatest risk with MAO inhibitors is the occurrence of hypertensive crises; hypertensive crises can be caused by the consumption of large amounts of certain foods (aged cheese, red wine) or drugs containing sympathetic stimulant activity.

If the antidepressant drugs just described fail as single agents, the next step is augmentation with low-dose lithium for 1 to 2 weeks.

Pharmacologic treatment of major depressive disorder is effective in approximately 70%-75% of cases.

5. B. This patient has a dysthymic disorder. Dysthymic disorder is defined as a depressive syndrome in which the patient is bothered all or most of the time by depressive symptoms; these symptoms are not of sufficient severity to warrant a diagnosis of major depressive episode.

6. E. Because of the long history, this patient should probably be treated with a combination of psychotherapy and pharmacotherapy.

The pharmacologic agent class of choice at this time is the serotonin reuptake inhibitors (SSRIs). Agents such as fluoxetine (Prozac) 20-40 mg/day, sertraline (Zoloft) 50-200 mg/day, or paroxetine (Paxil) 20-50 mg/day.

Psychotherapy (either supportive psychotherapy or cognitive psychotherapy as described earlier) is an important component of the treatment of this condition.

7. A. This patient has an adjustment disorder with depressed mood. Adjustment disorder with depressed mood is defined as a reaction to an identifiable psychosocial stressor(s) that occurs within 3 months of the onset of the stressor. The major characteristic of the disorder is an impairment in occupational or social functioning.

The term *burnout* is being used more and more in this era of cutbacks, job losses, and flattening of organizational structure. The end result is that individuals are being asked to do more and more with less and less. Thus individuals get to a point where they can no longer cope, and psychologic illness sets in. Inappropriate coping mechanisms such as the use of alcohol and/or drugs are becoming more and more common in this situation. It is important to rule out a major depressive disorder in a patient like this and to do what is possible to help the patient remove or modify the stressor(s). Burnout, however, is not a diagnosis.

8. C. The treatment of choice for adjustment disorder is supportive psychotherapy. If possible, the stressor should be removed. If not possible, ways of managing the stressor (relaxation therapy, biofeedback, aerobic exercise) should be employed. The physician should discuss these specific coping strategies with specific goals and objectives negotiated with the patient.

9. C. The single most important question to ask in a patient who presents with signs and symptoms of depression is whether or not they have contemplated suicide. The questioning and the rationale should proceed as follows:
   1. Have you ever considered that "life really isn't worth it" and that "you should end it all"?
   2. If you have, have you thought of the means by which you would do it?
   3. Have you considered a specific plan for ending your life?
   4. Would you consider a contract with me, a promise that if life got too unbearable you would call me?

10. D.

11. E. This patient most likely has a substance-induced mood disorder. The "tipoffs" to this diagnosis in this patient are as follows:
    1. Symptoms and signs of depression
    2. A self-described "burnout syndrome"
    3. The missing of a number of days of work recently
    4. The clue of "I am using anything and everything to try and relax."

    The sequence of events that likely took place in this patient are as follows. The drive to keep going faster and faster to "stay on the treadmill" eventually lead to a depressive disorder and occupational burnout. This was followed by inappropriate "coping mechanisms"

including the use of alcohol and/or drugs to keep going. Eventually he reached a point where he was unable to function because of (1), (2), and (3) above, and his occupational functioning was impaired.

The steps that should be pursued in this patient's case are as follows:
A. Ask the patient about alcohol: specific amounts, specific times, total intake.
B. Administer an alcohol abuse questionnaire if possible.
C. Interview the patient's wife.
D. Speak to the patient's colleagues if possible.
E. Confirm or refute the hypothesis of depressive disorder due to substance-induced mood disorder.
F. If confirmed, begin aggressive intervention.
G. Aggressive intervention should include an intensive inpatient rehabilitation program. This should include a detoxification program if necessary.
H. G should include individual counseling, group psychotherapy, and family psychotherapy.

12. D.

13. E.

14. B. This patient most likely has a mood disorder due to a general medical condition. The single most likely diagnosis is carcinoma of the pancreas. This is especially suspicious based on the change in the percussion note from tympany to dullness and the associated symptoms including weight loss and stomach pains.

The major differential diagnosis in this patient would be adjustment disorder with depressed mood associated with his retirement. The physical signs, however, point away from this.

The "primary treatment" in this case is to confirm "mood disorder secondary to general medical condition. An antidepressant agent, particularly an SSRI with few side effects, would not be inappropriate in this patient at this time. This is, however, a secondary treatment.

15. E.

16. D. One of the most difficult challenges that we face as physicians is trying to impress on our patients the "biological basis" for major depressive illness, in other words, trying to convince our patients that depression is a biological illness, just as any other illness, and has physiologic markers or characteristics to accompany it.

In the case of major depressive disorder, we are aware of the following physiologic abnormalities.
    1. There is a "neurotransmitter imbalance" that appears to be due to a relative deficiency of the neurotransmitter serotonin. The new SSRIs add confirmatory evidence to this hypothesis.

2. We know that patients with major depressive disorder have hyperactivity of the hypothalamic-pituitary-adrenal (HPA) axis. This results in elevated plasma cortisol levels and nonsuppression of cortisol following dexamethasone (DST).

3. There is blunting of the normally expected increase in plasma growth hormone induced by alpha-2-adrenergic receptor agonists.

4. There is blunting of serotonin-mediated increases in plasma prolactin.

SOLUTION TO SHORT ANSWER MANAGEMENT PROBLEM 55

A strategy for the pharmacologic management of major depressive disorder is as follows:

Step 1: identify and treat causes unrelated to major depressive disorder (such as hypothyroidism).

Step 2: use single-agent pharmacotherapy as first step. (Unless contraindicated the use of a selective serotonin reuptake inhibitor is now the drug of first choice.) This class includes the following:
- Sertraline (Zoloft)
- Paroxetine (Paxil)
- Fluoxetine (Prozac)

Step 3: Augment first agent with:
A) Lithium carbonate
B) Folic acid
C) T-3 or T-4
D) L-tryptophan

Step 4: alternative drug selection: if a combination of 2 and 3 is ineffective, consider the addition of another agent in the Step 3 class or a tricyclic antidepressant. If you decide to use a tricyclic antidepressant, then choose nortriptyline if the patient requires sedation, and choose desipramine if the patient requires activation.

Step 5: if step 4 is ineffective, consider substituting either bupropion (a unique antidepressant) or an MAO inhibitor.

Each one of these therapies should be used for at least 8 weeks before they are considered a therapeutic failure.

Step 6: Electroconvulsive therapy: ECT should be used only after at least three primary agents and two augmented drugs have been used; (for example, primary agents: sertraline, nortriptyline, and bupropion; plus augmented drugs: lithium carbonate or L-tryptophan).

SUMMARY OF THE DIAGNOSIS AND MANAGEMENT OF MAJOR DEPRESSIVE DISORDER

1. **Prevalence:**
   a) Major depressive disorder:
      1. Lifetime prevalence: 3.5% to 5.8% of the population
      2. Gender difference: higher in women than in men
   b) Dysthymia:
      1. Lifetime prevalence: 2.1% to 4.7%
      2. Gender difference: higher in women than in men
   c) Prevalence in general medical settings: in general medical settings, which select for patients with emotional distress and physical illness, the prevalence rates for depression has been reported to be as high as 15%.

2. **Differential diagnosis of major depressive disorder:**
   DSM-IV criteria: American Psychiatric Association, 1994
   a) Major depressive disorder
   b) Dysthymia
   c) Depression due to a general medical condition
   d) Adjustment disorder with depressed mood
   e) Substance-induced mood disorder
   f) Manic episodes with irritable mood
   g) Mixed episodes (depression/hypomania)

3. **Major depressive disorder (MDD) versus dysthymia:**
   a) MDD: Follow the mnemonic (p. 259) SIG: EM CAPS (5/9 with one being either E or M).
   b) Dysthymia: perhaps best described as "chronic ongoing depression"—lasts years rather than weeks or months.

4. **Subclassifications of major depressive disorder:**
   Once a diagnosis of depression has been made, the clinician should further characterize the syndrome if possible into the following categories:
   a) Unipolar versus bipolar
   b) Melancholic versus nonmelancholic
   c) Psychotic versus nonpsychotic
   d) Atypical depression
   e) Masked depression
   A. Unipolar depression versus bipolar depression:
   Best characterized as:
      1. Major depressive disorder (unipolar)
      2. Bipolar affective disorder
   B. Melancholic versus nonmelancholic
   Best characterized as melancholic: 40% to 60% of all hospitalizations for depression. Symptoms include anhedonia, excessive or inappropriate guilt, early morning waking, anorexia, psychomotor disturbance, and diurnal variation in mood. The depressed melancholic patient may appear frantic, fearful, agitated, or withdrawn.
   C. Psychotic versus nonpsychotic: psychotic depressions are not rare. Studies suggest that approximately 10%-25% of patients hospitalized for major depression have a psychotic depression.
   D. Atypical depression: atypical depression denotes neurovegetative symptoms that are generally the opposite of what is seen in melancholia. This includes hypersomnia instead of insomnia, hyperphagia (sometimes as a carbohydrate craving) rather than anorexia, and reactivity (mood changes with en-

vironmental circumstances) as well as a long-standing pattern of interpersonal rejection sensitivity. Patients with atypical depression are frequently reported to have an anxious or irritable mood rather than dysphoria.

E. Masked depression: Masked depression is similar to atypical depression. Instead of overt depression, the depression is expressed as many psychosomatic signs and symptoms.

5. **Treatment:**
   a) Follow guidelines written in the Short Answer Management Problem.
   b) Consider the SSRIs as the drugs of first choice at this time except in the very young and the very old.
   c) Treat for at least 8 weeks before you consider the therapy you are using a therapeutic failure.
   d) Remember that major depressive disorder is a recurrent disease: at 1 year following the start of therapy, 33% will be free of the disease, 33% will have had a relapse, and 33% will still be depressed
   e) Remember that major depressive disorder should be treated with a combination of pharmacotherapy and psychotherapy (psychotherapy to be discussed in another chapter in this book).

6. **Three-phase approach to the treatment of depression:**
   a) Acute treatment phase, phase 1: time = 6 weeks to time = 12 weeks
      Goal: the goal of this phase is the remission of symptoms of depression.
   b) Continuation treatment, phase 2: time = 4 months to time = 9 months
      Goal: the goal of this phase is to prevent a relapse of the depressive symptoms.
   c) Maintenance treatment, phase 3: time = 1 year to ??
      Goal: The goal of this phase of therapy is to treat patients who have had three or more episodes of depression. Prevention of recurrence is the treatment end point.

   There is broad consensus among consultants that the continuation treatment phase is the most critical in determining a successful clinical outcome. The panel recommends that through the continuation treatment phase that medication is indicated at full dose.

The danger that needs to be avoided is as follows:

"Too often medication is tapered or discontinued shortly after symptoms have been brought under control; this greatly increases the patient's risk of relapse. There is no justification for lowering the effective dose of an antidepressant drug during maintenance treatment." (from: American Psychiatric Association. Diagnostic and statistical manual of mental disorders [DSM-IV]. Washington, DC: American Psychiatric Association Press, 1994.) During this phase you should see the patient once per week for the first 6-8 weeks, depending on the individual. Once stable, you should see the patient every other week for 4 weeks; following that, once a month. If the patient is on one of the tricyclics and there is a partial or inadequate response, plasma concentrations of the drug should be obtained.

Once the patient is asymptomatic for at least six months following a depressive episode, recovery from the episode is declared.

The termination of therapy must be accompanied by patient education. The key concern here is the likelihood of a recurrent episode. If this is the patient's first bout of depression that needed to be treated, the recurrence rate is approximately 50%. If there have been previous episodes of depression and/or a family history of depression, the probability of a recurrence is increased significantly. The patient must be made aware of the symptoms that indicate when another episode is likely. You need to remember that if therapy is initiated early in the disease course, it is more likely to be effective faster. You need to tell the patient that subsequent attacks can be treated effectively.

SUGGESTED READINGS

American Psychiatric Association. Diagnostic and statistical manual of mental disorders (DSM-IV). Washington, DC: American Psychiatric Association Press, 1994.

Bell I, Gelenberg A. Mood disorders. In: Rakel R, ed. Conn's current therapy. Philadelphia: WB Saunders, 1994.

Risby E, Risch SC, Stoudemire A. Mood disorders. In: Stoudemire A, ed. Clinical psychiatry for medical students. 2nd Ed. Philadelphia: JB Lippincott, 1990.

PROBLEM 56 A 42-YEAR-OLD COMPUTER SCIENCE PROFESSOR WHO HAS JUST BEEN ANOINTED BY GOD AS THE NEW HEAD OF THE COMPUTER AGE

A 42-year-old computer science professor is brought to the ER by his wife, who complains that for the last 4 weeks her husband has become increasingly irritable, angry, and suspicious. She states that "his personality has completely changed." He has not slept for six nights and has been found by the local police every night working on his computer programs on a major street, with the computer plugged in by a long extension cord to the nearest house.

He has become preoccupied with the belief that God has anointed him as the "new leader of the computer age." Fearing that his ideas will be stolen by INTERPOL, the KGB, the State Police, and, for some reason, the "Red Coated Mounties" from Canada, he has constructed an elaborate mathematical code that allows only him and his appointed (and for that matter, anointed) prophets to understand the programs. He quite proudly states that "Albert Einstein wouldn't have a chance at this; it's even too clever for him!" Fearing that all of these various police forces of the world will want to steal the programs, he has bought a very smart disguise (a Royal Canadian Mounted Police Colored trench coat) along with a Mountie hat and dark sunglasses. He tells you that "they will now see me as one of their own—what a brilliant disguise."

During the interview he is extremely agitated and paces the floor. He makes a number of sexual advances toward the nurse who is observing him.

The patient's wife states that the patient has been depressed on and off throughout his life and has been on "all kinds of crap" for the depression, none of which helped at any time. She describes her husband's family as "a whole bunch of nuts."

The patient's wife goes on to tell you that his mother calls him at 3 AM each morning (just as he is getting his equipment and extension cords set up outside, rooting through the garage, knocking everything over, and waking up the entire neighborhood). He has devised the "world's longest telephone cord" (he takes the calls from his mother in the middle of the street). His father has been admitted to a psychiatric hospital on a number of occasions, sometimes for alcoholism and sometimes for "weird behavior." He has been treated with shock treatments. One of his sisters is a drug addict; another sister is a "friend of the earth" and lives in a commune.

According to the patient's wife, the patient has never had a substance abuse problem of any kind.

SELECT THE ONE BEST ANSWER TO THE FOLLOWING QUESTIONS

1. Based on the history given, what is the best term to describe the behavior exhibited in this patient?
   a) acute hypomania
   b) acute mania
   c) acute organic psychosis
   d) acute confusional state
   e) delirium

2. Based on the patient's personal history, the descriptive term applied in Question 1, and the family history described, this is most likely a part of a condition known as which of the following?
   a) bipolar affective disorder
   b) unipolar affective disorder
   c) major depressive disorder
   d) schizoid personality disorder
   e) schizophrenia

3. The DSM-IV would further subclassify this into which of the following?
   a) schizophrenia: catatonic type
   b) schizophrenia: paranoid type
   c) BAD (bipolar affective disorder): subtype I
   d) BAD (bipolar affective disorder): subtype II
   e) this is all irrelevant; we all know that this gentleman is "just plain nuts"

4. At this time, what would you do?
   a) prescribe diazepam and tell his wife that you will review the situation tomorrow (if you have time)
   b) prescribe lithium carbonate on an outpatient basis and see the patient in 3 months
   c) prescribe fluphenazine on an outpatient basis and see the patient in 1 week
   d) prescribe a tricyclic antidepressant on an outpatient basis and see the patient in 1 week
   e) none of the above

5. Your mother has just been told that she has the illness that has just been described. You begin to wonder about the heritability of such a disorder. What is your relative risk of developing the disorder described compared to someone without a first-degree relative with the disease?
   a) relative risk: 0.5
   b) relative risk: 1.0
   c) relative risk: 24.0
   d) relative risk: 2.0
   e) relative risk: 3.5

6. Which of the following statements regarding lithium carbonate in the treatment of the disorder described is(are) true?
   a) lithium carbonate is the drug of choice in the treatment of this disorder
   b) lithium prevents relapses as effectively in unipolar affective disorder as in bipolar affective disorder

c) lithium is not metabolized and therefore problems related to active metabolites or inactive metabolites do not exist

d) the average daily dose of lithium required to treat bipolar affective disorder is 900 mg

e) all of the above

7. Patients with this disorder who are refractory to lithium carbonate should be treated with which of the following?
   a) carbamazepine
   b) L-tryptophan
   c) valproic acid
   d) a and c only
   e) all of the above

8. Which of the following neurotransmitters is(are) involved in the etiology of the acute manic or acute hypomanic episodes in bipolar affective disorder?
   a) norepinephrine
   b) dopamine
   c) serotonin

d) a and b
e) all of the above

9. Which of the following best conceptualizes the definition of the disorder *cyclothymia*?
   a) cyclothymia is best described as a less severe form of bipolar affective disorder
   b) cyclothymia and dysthymia are virtually identical
   c) cyclothymia is a more severe, more chronic form of bipolar affective disorder
   d) cyclothymia, by definition, has none of the elements of positive family history that characterize bipolar affective disorder
   e) none of the above are true

10. Which is the treatment of choice for cyclothymia?
    a) an SSRI
    b) a tricyclic antidepressant
    c) an MAO inhibitor
    d) valproic acid
    e) lithium carbonate

Short Answer Management Problem 56

Describe the basic diagnostic features of bipolar disorder: manic episode and bipolar disorder: hypomanic episode.

ANSWERS

1. B.

2. A.

3. C.

4. E.

5. C.

6. E.

7. D. The most likely diagnosis in this patient at this time is *acute mania*. Mania is defined as a distinct period of abnormally and persistently elevated, expansive, or irritable mood. It may include inflated self-esteem or grandiosity, decreased need for sleep, loquaciousness, flight of ideas, distractibility, increase in goal-directed activity, activities such as unrestrained buying sprees, sexual indiscretions, and foolish business investments. These symptoms cause a marked impairment in occupational functioning.

The basic difference between mania and hypomania is as follows: in mania there are psychotic symptoms and a marked impairment in normal functioning (social, occupational, and so on). In addition, the mood disturbance is more severe.

With no history of drug dependency problems, an organic mood disorder (an acute confusional state, delirium) is less likely.

Schizophrenia is less likely because of the good premorbid functioning and the family history of affective disorder. Schizoaffective disorder is unlikely because the patient's delusions are associated in time with his affective symptoms only.

This episode of acute mania is part of a bipolar affective disorder. To make the diagnosis of bipolar affective disorder you need at least one episode of mania or hypomania. This patient has a past history that is very suggestive of major depression, and this provides the link to bipolar affective disorder.

He almost certainly has a mother with bipolar affective disorder, indicated by her 3 AM phone calls. Also, his father obviously had a major depressive disorder treated with ECT.

The American Psychiatric Association has subdivided bipolar affective disorder into two types: bipolar I and bipolar II. Bipolar I disorder identifies a patient who has had at least one true manic episode. A history of depression or hypomania may also be present in the bipolar I patient, but neither of these conditions is essential for the diagnosis. In bipolar II patients, there is a history of hypomania and major depressive episodes but no history of mania.

The treatment of choice at this time is admission to a hospital and treatment with an antipsychotic agent such as haloperidol (IM) until the psychotic symptoms subside. He should be placed on lithium carbonate at the same time. Lithium carbonate is the drug of choice for the treatment of BAD. The usual dosage is 900 mg-1200 mg (with blood level monitoring).

Lithium carbonate also prevents relapses in unipolar affective disorder. In the treatment of acute mania, it may be 10 to 14 days before the full therapeutic effect of lithium is felt. Lithium is not metabolized and therefore does not accumulate metabolism.

There is good evidence that patients with bipolar affective disorder who do not respond to lithium carbonate should be treated with either one of two anticonvulsants medications: carbamazepine or valproic acid. These agents have proven to be just as effective as lithium carbonate in the treatment of BAD. It is generally recognized that 10% to 20% of BAD patients will not respond to lithium and will have to be treated with other agents.

Outpatient therapy is not indicated in patients with acute mania. Diazepam or a tricyclic antidepressant are not the recommended agents for the treatment of acute mania.

The genetic evidence is very strong for bipolar affective disorder. First-degree relatives of patients with bipolar illness are reported to be at least 24 times more likely to develop bipolar illness than relatives of control subjects. The incidence of bipolar illness and unipolar depression is much higher in first-degree relatives of patients with bipolar illness than in the general population. On the other hand, first-degree relatives of patients with unipolar illness have an increase in the incidence of unipolar depression only.

8. D. The most striking pharmacologic data relating to theories of acute mania and acute hypomania is the consistent finding that direct or indirect norepinephrine and dopamine agonists (those drugs that stimulate the noradrenergic and dopaminergic receptors or increase concentrations of these neurotransmitters in the brain) can precipitate mania or hypomania in patients with underlying bipolar illness. Stimulants such as amphetamines and cocaine can induce manic-like syndromes in patients who do not appear to have an underlying vulnerability to develop a bipolar disorder. Thus the association of mania or hypomania with hyperadrenergic and/or hyperdopaminergic states is firmly established.

9. A.

10. E. Cyclothymia is best conceptualized as a relatively less severe form of bipolar illness. The data indicate that approximately 30% of cyclothymics have a positive family history for bipolar illness. By definition, cyclothymia is a chronic mood disturbance of at least 2 years' duration and involving numerous hypomanic and mild depressive episodes (that do not meet the diagnostic criteria for mania or major depression), with no periods of euthymia greater than 2 months.

As with bipolar affective disorder, the treatment of choice is lithium carbonate.

SOLUTION TO SHORT ANSWER MANAGEMENT PROBLEM 56

I. Key features of bipolar disorder: manic episode:
1. A distinct period of abnormality and persistently elevated, expansive, or irritable mood, lasting at least 1 week, and of sufficient severity to cause marked impairment in social or occupational functioning
2. During this period of time, at least three of the following symptoms are also present:
   A. Grandiosity
   B. Decreased need for sleep
   C. Hyperverbal or pressured speech
   D. Flight of ideas or racing thoughts
   E. Distractibility
   F. Increase in goal-directed activity or psychomotor agitation
   G. Excessive involvement in pleasurable activities that have a high potential for painful consequences
3. There is no evidence of a physical or substance-induced etiology or the presence of another major mental disorder to account for the patient's symptoms.

II. Key features of hypomanic episodes:
1. A distinct mood of sustained elevated, expansive, or irritable mood, lasting for at least 4 days, that is clearly different from the individual's nondepressed mood yet does not cause marked impairment in social or occupational functioning such as in acute mania
2. During the mood disturbance, at least three of the following symptoms are also present to a significant degree:
   A. Inflated self-esteem or grandiosity
   B. Decreased need for sleep
   C. More talkative than usual
   D. Flight of ideas or racing thoughts
   E. Distractibility
   F. Increase in goal-directed activity or psychomotor agitation

G. Excessive involvement in pleasurable activities that have a high potential for painful consequences

3. The episode is not due to a physical or substance-induced etiology.

SUMMARY OF THE DIAGNOSIS AND TREATMENT OF BIPOLAR AFFECTIVE DISORDER

1. **Prevalence:**
   a) The prevalence of bipolar disorders varies from 0.7% to 1.6% (lifetime).
   b) The prevalence is greater in women than in men.
   c) In general medical settings (settings that select for patients with emotional distress and physical illness), the prevalence rate is probably between 5% and 10% (lifetime).

2. **Classification of bipolar affective disorders:**
   a) Bipolar affective disorder I: a patient with BAD who has had at least one episode of true mania
   b) Bipolar affective disorder II: a patient with BAD who has not had at least one episode of true mania
   c) Cyclothymia: a less severe form of bipolar affective disorder

3. **Heritability of bipolar affective disorder:**
   a) First-degree relatives of patients with bipolar affective disorder are at least 24 times more likely to develop bipolar illness than relatives of control subjects.
   b) The incidence of both bipolar illness and unipolar illness is much higher in first-degree relatives of patients with bipolar illness than in the general population.

4. **Diagnostic criteria:**
   a) See diagnostic criteria for acute mania and acute hypomania in Short Answer Management Problem 56.
   b) The other half of bipolar disorder is, of course, depression, which is discussed in Chapter 55.

5. **Cyclothymia:**
   a) Cyclothymia is defined as a more chronic, less severe form of bipolar affective disorder. By definition, it is a chronic mood disturbance of at least 2 years' duration and involves numerous hypomanic and mild depressive episodes. These episodes do not meet the diagnostic criteria for bipolar affective disorder or major depression.
   b) In cyclothymia there are no periods of euthymia greater than 2 months in duration.

6. **Treatment:**
   a) Acute treatment:
      1. Hospitalization for acute mania
      2. Neuroleptic agents (haloperidol, thioridazine)
   b) Maintenance and prevention of relapse:
      1. Lithium carbonate is the agent of first choice (usual dosage is 900 mg-1200 mg/day).
      2. Anticonvulsants: carbamazepine and valproic acid are agents of second choice.

SUGGESTED READINGS

American Psychiatric Association. Diagnostic and statistical manual of mental disorders. 4th Ed. Washington, DC: American Psychiatric Association Press, 1994.

Stoudemire A. Clinical psychiatry for medical students. 2nd Ed. Philadelphia: JB Lippincott, 1994.

PROBLEM 57   AN INTRODUCTION TO "THE GOD OF THE MILKY WAY"

A 22-year-old male is brought to the ER by the paramedics accompanied by his parents. He had begun to cut himself with a sharp knife at home and his father had called 911.

The father tells you that this was the last straw. He tells you that his son has been acting very strangely for the past 15 months.

The patient himself stares straight ahead and refuses to answer any questions. He does, however, ask the nurse if she wants to kneel and kiss his hand. When she says, "No, sir, I do not," the patient replies by saying, "You are the first woman who has refused the invitation to kiss the god of the Milky Way's hand." He points to the door entrance and remarks to the nurse, "You know, I could have you killed by my space-soldiers; all it would take is one zap with the green ray gun from one of them."

The patient's father tells you that his son has essentially locked himself in his room for the past year. He eats all his meals there. He has some carpentry skills, and he built a large "dinner decontamination center" by knocking out three of the major upstairs walls. This occurred while his father and mother were on holiday.

When they do see him, he seems very sad and depressed, and his voice can sometimes barely be heard.

The patient had a job at a fast-food restaurant but was fired 9 months ago when he started to "inject all the hamburgers with a decontamination substance," which turned out to be a thick mixture of pulverized leeches. It was at that point that he locked himself in his room for good.

He has had no other medical conditions in the past 7 years. Prior to that he had suffered from episodes of major depression. He dropped out of school halfway through grade 8. His other significant history includes enuresis, encopresis, and separation anxiety as a child.

His father is confident that his son is on no drugs, prescription or otherwise.

When you ask about family history of psychiatric disorders, alcoholism, or drug use, the father replies that "some quack of a psychiatrist labeled me as an alcoholic, which of course I am not." When you ask the patient's father what he drinks, he replies, whiskey. You deliberately overestimate the amount: "Sir, would you drink two bottles per day?" He replies, "No, of course not; one 26-oz would be tops."

You realize that you need more information about the patient's appointment as the god of the Milky Way. He tells you that this title was first bestowed upon him 14 months ago when the spaceship first landed in the back yard and he was invited in to speak to the Grand Poobah of Intergalactic Space Travelers. After an elaborate two-hour ceremony at which the Grand Poobah announced that the IGSTO (Intergalactic Space Traveler's Organization) had been searching for him for 400 years, he was officially crowned.

The mental status examination on this patient is next to impossible. The patient's blood pressure is normal, as is the rest of the physical examination.

SELECT THE ONE BEST ANSWER TO THE FOLLOWING QUESTIONS

1. What is the most likely diagnosis in this patient at this time?
   a) schizoaffective disorder
   b) schizophrenia
   c) schizophreniform disorder
   d) bipolar affective disorder
   e) delusional disorder

2. Of the following features, which one is most classical of the diagnosis?
   a) disorganized speech
   b) delusions
   c) hallucinations
   d) the presence of both positive and negative symptoms
   e) disorganized or catatonic behavior

3. How is the term delusion defined?
   a) a false belief that is fixed and not explainable based on the cultural background of the individual
   b) a disorder of the form of thought

   c) a convincing feeling that one is being persecuted
   d) a convincing feeling that one is being controlled by a supernatural force
   e) the experiencing of stimuli in any of the senses in the absence of external stimulation

4. The differential diagnosis of this disorder described includes which of the following?
   a) bipolar affective disorder
   b) schizoaffective disorder
   c) delusional disorder
   d) brief psychotic disorder
   e) all of the above

5. How is the term psychosis best defined?
   a) behavior marked by a break from reality
   b) behavior marked by a fixed false belief not in keeping with current life situation or circumstance
   c) behavior not in keeping with the current environment in which the individual finds himself or herself
   d) behavior marked by the sight of objects that are not present
   e) behavior marked by the hearing of sounds that are not present

6. A patient presents to the ER with almost identical symptoms to the patient described in Question 1. However, the time from the beginning of the illness (the onset of the first symptom) to the termination of all symptoms is only 4 months. What is the most likely diagnosis in this patient?
   a) schizophrenia
   b) schizoaffective disorder
   c) schizophreniform disorder
   d) bipolar affective disorder
   e) brief psychotic disorder

7. A patient who develops acute psychiatric symptoms much like those described in Question 1, but in whom the symptoms of depression and/or mania are more prominent than the psychotic symptoms, would most likely have developed which of the following conditions?
   a) schizophrenia
   b) schizoaffective disorder
   c) schizophreniform disorder
   d) bipolar affective disorder
   e) brief psychotic disorder

8. The condition described in Question 1 is associated with a certain neurotransmitter imbalance. This imbalance is primarily characterized by which of the following?
   a) a relative deficiency of dopamine receptors
   b) a relative deficiency of serotonin receptors
   c) a relative excess of dopamine receptors
   d) a relative excess of serotonin receptors
   e) a relative deficiency of acetylcholine receptors

9. What is the drug of first choice for the patient presented in the case history?
   a) risperidone
   b) clozapine
   c) haloperidol
   d) lithium carbonate
   e) fluoxetine

10. Which of the statements regarding the condition described in Question 1 is(are) true?
   a) there is a documented genetic component in the etiology of the condition described above
   b) the gene that is involved in the transmission of this condition is located on the fifth chromosome
   c) lateral ventricular enlargement is common in this condition
   d) increased width of the third ventricle is common in this condition
   e) all of the above statements are true

Short Answer Management Problem 57

Describe the differential diagnosis of psychosis.

ANSWERS

1. B.

2. D. The most likely diagnosis in this patient is schizophrenia. Schizophrenia is characterized by the following features:
   1. Psychotic symptoms, at least two, present for at least 1 month.
      A. Hallucinations
      B. Delusions
      C. Disorganized speech (incoherence, evidence of a thought disorder)
      D. Disorganized or catatonic behavior
   2. Negative symptoms (flattening of affect, lack of motivation)
   3. Impairment in social or occupational functioning
   4. Duration of the illness for at least 6 months
   5. Symptoms are not primarily due to a mood disorder or schizoaffective disorder
   6. Symptoms are not due to a medical, neurologic, or substance-induced disorder.

The most classical symptom of schizophrenia is the presence of both positive and negative symptoms.

Positive symptoms include the psychotic symptoms just described. Negative symptoms include the flattening of affect and the lack of motivation.

In greater detail, the most reliably recognized symptoms of the illness are its more dramatic ones such as hallucinations, delusions, and bizarre behavior. These are called positive symptoms because they are symptoms that are added to the premorbid state. However, there is a long tradition in not considering these the central elements of schizophrenia. Negative symptoms such as emotional blunting, apathy, and lack of motivation are symptoms marked by the absence of the ability to function in some ways. These negative symptoms are less dramatic in presentation. Some authorities believe the negative symptoms to be the core symptoms of schizophrenia. Thus an illness defined purely by its more dramatic presentations could correctly label one group of patients who suffer predominantly from the core negative expressions that result from the pathophysiology of the illness, but without its more dramatic manifestations.

3. A. A delusion is defined as a fixed false belief that cannot be explained on the basis of the cultural background of the individual.

4. E. The differential diagnosis of schizophrenia includes the following:
   1. Delusional disorder: a delusional disorder is a condition in which the patient has a delusion lasting for at least one month in the absence of prominent hallucinations or bizarre behavior.
   2. Brief psychotic disorder: a brief psychotic disorder is a disorder characterized by a relatively sudden onset of psychosis that lasts for a few hours to a month with a return to normal premorbid functioning at that time.
   3. Schizophreniform disorder: a schizophreniform disorder is a disorder displaying the signs and symptoms of schizophrenia but in which the patient completely recovers within a 6-month period.
   4. Schizoaffective disorder: a schizoaffective disorder is a psychotic disorder that is differentiated from schizophrenia by either depressive symptoms or manic symptoms which are prominent and consistent features of a patient's long-term psychotic illness.
   5. Bipolar affective disorder (manic phase): a bipolar affective disorder (manic phase) is differentiated from Schizophrenia by a relatively shorter course (significantly less than 6 months), the bipolar recurring nature of the symptoms with significant time intervals in between, and the separation of positive symptoms and negative symptoms.
   6. Psychotic disorder due to a general medical condition
   7. A substance-induced psychotic disorder: this latter category applies primarily to drugs such as amphetamine-like substances.

5. A. *Psychosis* is a generic descriptive term applied to behavior marked by a break or loss of contact with reality. This often presents as disorganization of mental processes, emotional aberrations, difficulty in interpersonal relationships, and a decrease in functional capacity. In a patient with psychosis, mundane daily responsibilities may become burdensome or impossible to manage.

6. C. A patient who presents with schizophrenia-like symptoms that last for a period of time shorter than 6 months is classified as having schizophreniform disorder.

   Patients with schizophreniform disorder can be classified into those with or without good prognostic features. Good prognostic features include an acute onset, good premorbid functioning, and the absence of a flat affect. In patients who meet the criteria for schizophreniform disorder but have not recovered, the diagnosis must be provisional.

7. B. This patient has a schizoaffective disorder. A schizoaffective disorder is usually diagnosed when depressive or manic symptoms are a prominent and consistent feature of a patient's long-term psychotic illness. The diagnosis can be substantiated if the longitudinal course is consistent with schizophrenia and if residual schizophrenic-like symptoms persist when the patient is not depressed or manic. If, on the other hand, the psychotic symptoms are present only when the patient is depressed or manic and the patient has a relatively good interim functioning between episodes, then the patient should be considered to have a primary mood disorder (either a major depressive disorder (with psychotic features) or a bipolar affective disorder.

8. C. The neurochemical basis of schizophrenia is shown to be a relative increase in the number of type 2 dopamine (D_2) receptors. The drugs that stimulate dopamine receptors (such as amphetamines) can produce schizophrenic-like symptoms.

9. A. An exciting advance has been made in the therapy of schizophrenia with the introduction of the drug Risperidone. Risperidone is unique in that it treats both the negative symptoms and the positive symptoms of schizophrenia.

   The previously available agents used to treat schizophrenia such as haloperidol and clozapine are effective in treating only the positive symptoms.

   The mechanism of antipsychotic action of risperidone is unknown. The drug has affinity, like clozapine, for serotonin type 2 receptors and, like haloperidol, for dopamine type 2 receptors. Risperidone also binds to alpha-adrenergic and histamine H-1 receptors.

   Clozapine has been found to have significantly fewer extrapyramidal effects than haloperidol.

10. E. First, there is considerable evidence that schizophrenia is an illness that runs in some families, although the majority of patients do not have a first-degree relative. The morbid risk of a first-degree relative of a schizophrenic developing schizophrenia is approximately 4% to 9%.

    Second, advances in molecular biology have allowed the gene that transmits schizophrenia to be isolated. It is in close proximity to a known DNA marker on the fifth chromosome.

    Third, CT and MRI studies have demonstrated that in schizophrenic patients there is enlargement of the lateral ventricles, there is increased width of the third ventricle, and there is sulcal enlargement suggestive of cortical atrophy.

SOLUTION TO SHORT ANSWER MANAGEMENT PROBLEM 57

A differential diagnosis of psychosis is as follows:
1. Schizophrenia
2. Schizophreniform disorder

3. Schizoaffective disorder
4. Bipolar affective disorder (manic phase)
5. Delusional disorder
6. Brief psychotic disorder
7. Psychotic disorder due to a general medical condition
8. Substance-induced psychotic disorder

SUMMARY OF THE DIAGNOSIS AND TREATMENT OF SCHIZOPHRENIA

1. **Prevalence:** the lifetime prevalence of schizophrenia is 1% to 2%.

2. **Characteristics of psychotic symptoms:**
   a) Psychotic symptoms are nonspecific and occur in a variety of medical, psychiatric, neurological, and substance-induced disorders.
   b) First-onset psychosis after the age of 45 generally indicates a neurologic, a medical, substance-induced disorder, or a psychotic depression. The onset of schizophrenia after the age of 45 is rare.

3. **Main diagnostic clues to the diagnosis of schizophrenia:**
   a) Positive symptoms plus negative symptoms: Positive symptoms include hallucinations, delusions, and bizarre behavior. Negative symptoms include emotional blunting, apathy, or avolition.

4. **Differential diagnosis of schizophrenia and clues to each one:**
   a) Delusion disorder: a disorder in which a delusion lasts at least one month. No other positive symptoms or negative symptoms of schizophrenia are present.
   b) Brief psychotic disorder: a disorder that is characterized by a relatively sudden onset of psychosis that lasts for a few hours to a month with a return to premorbid functioning thereafter. No other positive or negative symptoms are present.
   c) Bipolar affective disorder: subtype I: a disorder in which the psychotic symptoms are present only when the patient is depressed or manic and the patient has relatively good interim functioning between episodes.
   d) Schizophreniform disorder: both the positive and the negative symptoms of schizophrenia are present, but the patient recovers without residual symptoms within a 6-month period.
   e) Schizoaffective disorder: if a patient has symptoms of depression or mania with psychosis, and the depressive or manic symptoms are a prominent and consistent feature of the patient's long-term psychotic illness, schizoaffective disorder is the most likely diagnosis.
   f) Psychotic disorder due to a general medical condition: disorders that may produce psychotic symptoms include cerebral neoplasms, cerebrovascular disease, epilepsy, thyroid disorders, parathyroid disorders, hypoxia, hypoglycemia, hepatic disorders, renal disorders, and autoimmune disorders.

   g) Substance-induced psychotic disorder: this most commonly occurs with the amphetamines.

5. **Symptoms and signs of schizophrenia:**
   a) Psychotic symptoms are present for at least 1 month including two of hallucinations, delusions, disorganized speech (incoherence, evidence of a thought disorder), and disorganized or catatonic behavior.
   b) Negative symptoms are present (affective flattening, lack of motivation).
   c) Impairment in social or occupational functioning
   d) Duration of the illness for at least 6 months.
   e) Symptoms are not due to a mood disorder or schizoaffective disorder.
   f) Symptoms are not due to a medical, neurologic, or substance-induced disorder.

6. **Subtypes of schizophrenia:**
   a) Catatonic: dominated by motoric abnormalities such as rigidity and posturing
   b) Disorganized: marked by flat affect and disorganized speech and behavior
   c) Paranoid: paranoid symptoms in the absence of catatonic and disorganized features
   d) Undifferentiated
   e) Residual

7. **Causation:**
   a) Schizophrenia is believed to have a pathogenesis that consists of an interaction between genetic influences and environmental variables.
   b) There is an increase in the number of dopamine receptors in certain areas of the brains of schizophrenics.

8. **Treatment:**
   a) Acute phase:
      1. Hospitalization
      2. Neuroleptics
      3. Risoperidone is the drug of choice (only drug to treat the positive and negative symptoms)
   b) Chronic phase:
      1. Risperidone
      2. Psychosocial treatment: underlying goals are treatment of symptoms, reduction of stress, mobilization of social supports, assistance with deficits in daily living skills caused by the illness, and gradual rehabilitation to the most autonomous level of functioning possible for the individualized patient.

SUGGESTED READINGS

American Psychiatric Association. Diagnostic and statistical manual of mental disorders. 4th Ed. Washington, DC: American Psychiatric Association Press, 1994.

Ninan P, Mance R. Schizophrenia and other psychotic disorders. In: Stoudemire A, ed. Clinical psychiatry for medical students. 2nd Ed. Philadelphia: JB Lippincott, 1994.

PROBLEM 58   A 45-YEAR-OLD MALE WITH AN ENLARGED LIVER

A 45-year-old executive comes to your office for his periodic health assessment. He tells you that he has been feeling "tired, and just not myself lately." He also tells you that he has been so tired that he "has had to stay home from work for many days at a time." He is beginning to question his ability to provide the leadership role that he needs to provide as the CEO of a major transportation company.

When you inquire about other symptoms, he tells you that he has also suffered from "profound headaches" and that his sex life with his wife is "the *pits.*" On direct questioning he tells you that the headaches "have been a problem for the past 6 months" and his "lack of interest in sex" for about the same amount of time.

He has had no serious medical, surgical, or psychiatric illnesses to date. He tells you that he is taking no OTC drugs or prescription drugs.

The patient describes himself as a "social drinker," and his use of alcohol as "strictly to relax." He then states, "I certainly hope you do not think I am an alcoholic, Doc!" There is no evidence of acute intoxication at this time.

He does state, on more persistent questioning, "Well, maybe I am using more alcohol than I did a few years ago;" "Well, I do get a few shakes the next day if I have had too many drinks;" and "Well, I have spent some time trying to hide it around the house, Doc." His last statement, however, is "but Doc, I am not an alcoholic, you know."

His father died of complications of "yellow jaundice" at age 61. His mother died of complications of "heart failure" at age 69. He has three brothers and two sisters; all are well.

On P/E his blood pressure is 160/104 mm Hg. His pulse is 96 and regular. Examination of the head and neck, respiratory system, and musculoskeletal system are normal.

Examination of the cardiovascular system reveals a PMI (point of maximum impulse) in the fifth intercostal space in the anterior axillary line). He subsequently describes recent episodes of "waking up at night short of breath" as well as "shortness of breath on exertion."

Examination of the gastrointestinal system reveals no tenderness or rebound tenderness. The liver edge is palpated approximately 8 cm below the right costal margin.

Examination of the neurological system reveals a fine tremor on extension of both hands. He cannot perform serial 7's and has difficulty with recall of information on the mental status examination.

SELECT THE ONE BEST ANSWER TO THE FOLLOWING QUESTIONS

1. With the history given, what is the best description of the most likely diagnosis in this patient?
   a) masked depression
   b) the old "burnout syndrome"
   c) major depressive disorder
   d) alcohol dependence
   e) abuse

2. Which of the following signs and/or symptoms further substantiate your diagnosis in this patient?
   a) the location of the PMI (point of maximum impulse)
   b) the patient's elevated blood pressure
   c) the abdominal signs on physical examination
   d) none of the above; these are related to another problem
   e) all of the above

3. The disorder diagnosed in Question 1 cost the American economy how many dollars in the year 1988?
   a) What is this, a class in economics? How should I know?
   b) I know but I prefer not to say
   c) $8,500,800 (according to my calculations)

   d) $8,500,800 (according to someone else's calculations)
   e) $85,800,000,000

4. What is the most likely cause of the patient's liver edge palpated at 8 cm below the right costal margin?
   a) tricornute liver (congenital malformation)
   b) alcoholic hepatitis
   c) alcoholic (Laennec's) cirrhosis
   d) "the deep diaphragm pushing the liver down" syndrome
   e) hepatorenal syndrome

5. There is a high correlation between the disorder diagnosed in Question 1 and which of the following syndromes?
   a) generalized anxiety disorder
   b) major depressive disorder
   c) schizophrenia
   d) opioid abuse
   e) all of the above
   f) b and d only

6. The patient's inability to perform serial 7's and information recall is most likely due to which of the following?
   a) benign senile forgetfulness syndrome

b) alcoholic dementia
c) alcoholic amnestic syndrome
d) all of the above are equally likely
e) b or c

7. Which of the following neurotransmitters has been implicated in the disease process established by the diagnosis made in Question 1?
   a) dopamine
   b) angiotensin
   c) serotonin
   d) aldosterone
   e) acetylcholine

8. Regarding risk factors for the condition diagnosed in Question 1, which of the following statements most accurately reflects risk factor status and identification?
   a) there are no risk factors for this disease; it just happens
   b) there is no single factor that accounts for increased relative and absolute risk in first-degree relatives of patients with this disorder
   c) genetic, familial, environmental, occupational, socioeconomic, cultural, personality, life stress, psychiatric comobidity, biologic, social learning, and behavioral conditioning are all risk factors or risk environments for this disorder
   d) there is a clear risk factor stratification for this disorder
   e) b and c

9. What are the concordance rates for this disorder among identical twins and fraternal twins, respectively?
   a) 35% and 70%
   b) 3% and 3%
   c) 70% and 35%
   d) 50% and 50%
   e) 25% and 75%

10. How is *alcohol dependence syndrome* best defined?
    a) a state in which a syndrome of drug-specific withdrawal signs and symptoms follows reduction or cessation of drug use
    b) a state in which the physiologic or behavioral effects of a constant dose of a psychoactive substance decreases over time
    c) a physiologic state that follows cessation or reduction in the amount of drug used
    d) a and b
    e) all of the above

11. How is *alcohol withdrawal syndrome* best defined?
    a) a state in which a syndrome of drug-specific withdrawal signs and symptoms follows the reduction or cessation of drug use
    b) a state in which the physiologic or behavioral effects of a constant dose of a psychoactive substance decreases over time

c) a pathological state that follows cessation or reduction in the amount of drug used
d) a and b
e) all of the above

12. How is *alcohol abuse syndrome* best defined?
    a) a maladaptive state leading to clinically significant impairment
    b) a maladaptive state leading to clinically significant distress
    c) a maladaptive state leading to laboratory significant impairment
    d) either a or c
    e) either a or b

13. Considering the patient described, which of the following diagnostic imaging procedures are definitely indicated?
    a) chest X-ray
    b) cardiac echocardiogram
    c) CT scan of the head
    d) a and b only
    e) all of the above

14. Which of the following explanations is the most likely explanation for the tremors observed on physical examination?
    a) delirium tremens (early)
    b) alcohol withdrawal syndrome
    c) thiamine deficiency
    d) alcoholic encephalopathy (early)
    e) Korsakoff's psychosis

15. A 26-year-old male presents to your office for a periodic health examination prior to marriage. When you question him about lifestyle and ask him about his alcohol intake, he replies that he is a "social drinker."
    Once that is established what should you do?
    a) congratulate him; tell him that you are a "social drinker also" and that it's good that at least some people can avoid getting into problems with alcohol
    b) accept "social drinking" at face value and move onto the next question
    c) ask him the following question: "How social is social in the strictly social sense?"
    d) ask him to very specifically define social drinking
    e) first establish what he drinks; following that, overestimate the daily consumption and then come down from there

16. A patient whom you suspect of alcohol dependence demonstrates significant short-term memory deficits. He then tries to cover up those deficits by, in your opinion, making up answers to questions. This is known as which of the following?
    a) Wernicke's alcoholic encephalopathy

b) Korsakoff's psychosis
c) Alcohol amnestic disorder
d) Alcoholic dementia
e) Alcoholic hallucinosis

17. The feature described as "making up answers to questions" is known as which of the following?
a) confabulation
b) alcoholic lying
c) alcoholic delirium
d) alcoholic paranoia
e) memory loss encephalopathy

18. What is the cause of the disorder described in Question 16?
a) riboflavin deficiency
b) thiamine deficiency
c) zinc deficiency
d) cerebral atrophy due to alcohol abuse
e) cerebellar atrophy due to alcohol abuse

19. The word *alcoholism* means different things to different people. Of the following, which is the best definition of alcoholism?
a) alcohol abuse and alcohol dependency
b) alcohol abuse but not alcohol dependency
c) alcohol abuse or alcohol dependency
d) alcohol abuse and/or alcohol dependency
e) none of the above represent an adequate definition of alcoholism

20. What is the percentage of the American population who use at least some alcohol (or have used some alcohol)?
a) 50%
b) 60%
c) 70%
d) 90%
e) 94%

Short Answer Management Problem 58

PART A: Provide a screening test for alcohol abuse that can be easily administered in the office setting.

PART B: List five objectives for short-term treatment of the patient and the patient's family in a case of alcohol dependence.

ANSWERS

1. D.

2. E. This patient has *alcohol dependence,* which is defined as follows: at least three of the following occurring over a 12-month period of time:
   1. Tolerance: the need for increased amounts of a substance in order to achieve intoxication or another desired effect; or markedly diminished effect with use of the same amount of the substance.
   2. Characteristic withdrawal symptoms or the use of the alcohol (or a closely related substitute) to relieve or avoid withdrawal
   3. Substance often taken in larger amounts over a longer period of time than the person intended
   4. Persistent desire or one or more unsuccessful attempts to cut down or quit drinking
   5. A great deal of time spent in getting the alcohol, drinking it, or recovering from its effects
   6. Important social, occupational, or recreational activities are given up or reduced because of the alcohol
   7. Continued alcohol use despite the knowledge of having a persistent or recurrent social, psychological, or physical problem that is caused by, or exacerbated by, use of alcohol

The physical signs and symptoms actually substantiate the diagnosis of alcohol dependence, not alcohol abuse. Alcohol dependence is defined as a maladaptive pattern of alcohol use with adverse clinical consequences. These include the following:
1. The PMI (point of maximum impulse): the location of the PMI in the fifth intercostal space suggests cardiomegaly. This could be on the basis of either alcoholic cardiomyopathy or hypertension (most likely also related to alcohol intake).
2. The obvious hepatomegaly suggests either alcoholic hepatitis or cirrhosis of the liver.
3. The fine tremor suggests early alcoholic encephalopathy. This is substantiated by the cognitive dysfunction (lack of ability to perform serial 7's).
4. The patient's hypertension suggests alcohol as a potential cause.

3. E. In 1988 alcohol abuse cost the United States health care system $85,800,000,000 (over $85 billion). This cost measures only the direct costs to the system. Indirect costs such as marital breakup and family dysfunction are not considered.

4. C. The most likely cause of the hepatomegaly is alcoholic (Laenec's) cirrhosis. Although in many patients this

could represent alcoholic hepatitis, the presence of other CNS symptoms and signs suggests alcoholic cirrhosis.

5. E. The National Institute of Mental Health Epidemiologic Catchment Area Program found a very high correlation rate between alcoholism and the following:
   A. Suicide
   B. Homicide
   C. Accidents
   D. Anxiety disorders
   E. Major depressive disorder
   F. Schizophrenia
   G. Narcotic drug abuse
   H. Cocaine abuse

6. E. Chronic alcohol use is associated with the cognitive and memory deficits of *alcoholic dementia* (alcohol-persisting dementia) and the more restrictive memory deficits of *alcohol amnestic disorder*. Patients with alcohol-related amnestic syndrome have the most difficulty with short-term memory (remembering recent events). However, deficits may be noted in long-term memory as well.

7. C. Ethyl alcohol (ethanol) has been demonstrated to have significant effects on several brain neurotransmitter systems. Acute exposure to alcohol appears to inhibit excitatory NMDA receptors, whereas chronic alcohol exposure causes a sensitization of these receptors. Alcohol also affects the activity of the beta-adrenergic receptors and the adenosine neurotransmitter receptors linked to adenylate cyclase. Alcohol causes the release of serotonin from neurons, and chronic use may lead to depletion of brain serotonin. Alcohol has been shown to modify the binding of GABA (gamma-amino-butyric acid) to its receptors and augments the electrophysiologic and behavioral effects of GABA in animals.

8. E. Factors that determine an individual's susceptibility to a substance-use disorder are not well understood. Studies of populations at risk for developing substance abuse have identified many factors that foster the development and continuance of substance use, including genetic, familial, environmental, occupational, socio-economic, cultural, personality, life stress, psychiatric comorbidity, biologic, social learning, and behavioral conditioning.

9. C. The concordance rate for alcoholism among identical twin pairs is twice that of fraternal twin pairs. The rates are 70% and 35%, respectively.

10. D. See the answer to Question 1.

11. A. Alcohol withdrawal syndrome is a substance-specific syndrome that develops following cessation of, or reduction in dosage of, alcohol.

12. A. Alcohol abuse is a "residual category" that describes patterns of alcohol use that do not meet the criteria for alcohol dependence. *Alcohol abuse* is defined as a maladaptive pattern of substance use that causes clinically significant impairment. This may include impairments in social, family, or occupational functioning; the presence of psychological or physical problems; or the use of alcohol while or before driving a motor vehicle.

13. D. The imaging studies that are definitely indicated in this patient include chest X-ray and echocardiogram. An echocardiogram should be done to define the thickness of the left ventricular wall (to determine whether or not left ventricular hypertrophy is, in fact, present, as is indicated by the position of the point of maximum impulse).

    A chest X-ray can be justified on the basis of probable cardiac enlargement, that is, to measure the cardiac-thoracic ratio.

14. D. The tremor that is demonstrated on physical examination suggests the early diagnosis of Wernicke's or alcoholic encephalopathy. The fine tremor of his hands on extension is what is called "liver flap" and confirms the nature of the disorder.

15. E. Remember, social drinking is very unlikely to be social drinking.

    The first step is to determine whether or not a patient drinks.

    The second step is to determine how much a patient drinks. This is done by greatly overestimating what you believe to be the worst case scenario and coming down. For example, you might say, "Well, if its beer you drink, do you drink one case (24 cans) per day?"

    It will surprise you how often the response comes back: "Oh no, Doctor, it wouldn't be any more than one-half that much."

    The most sensitive and most specific instrument for screening for alcoholism in the primary care office setting is the CAGE questionnaire. The CAGE questionnaire includes four questions:
    1. Have you ever felt the need to cut down on your drinking?
    2. Have you ever felt annoyed by criticisms of your drinking?
    3. Have you ever had guilty feelings about drinking?
    4. Have you ever taken a morning eye-opener?
    With the CAGE questionnaire, any more than one correct answer may suggest alcohol abuse.

    Another reliable screening tool for heavy alcohol use is the Michigan Alcohol Screening Test (MAST). This 25-item scale identifies abnormal drinking through its social and behavioral consequences with a sensitivity of 90% to 98%. The Brief MAST, a shortened 10-item test, has been shown to have similar efficacy.

16. B.

17. A.

18. B. This patient has *Korsakoff's psychosis*. Patients with alcohol-related amnestic disorder have the most difficulty with short-term memory (remembering recent events), although deficits in long-term memory may be noted as well. Patients who try to conceal or compensate for their memory loss by *confabulation* (making up answers or talking around questions that require them to use their memory) have definite evidence of a chronic (probably terminal) alcohol problem. The cause of this particular disorder is a deficiency in the vitamin thiamine. For that reason, whenever a patient presents in an unconscious state that may be related to alcohol abuse, intravenous thiamine should be administered.

19. E.

20. D. The definition of *alcoholism* is as follows: alcoholism is a repetitive but inconsistent and sometimes unpredictable loss of control of drinking that produces symptoms of serious dysfunction or disability. It is estimated that 90% of the American population uses at least some alcohol.

SOLUTION TO SHORT ANSWER MANAGEMENT PROBLEM 58

PART A: A good primary care screening test for alcoholism is the CAGE questionnaire. The CAGE questionnaire has been described. Alternatives are the Michigan Alcohol Screening Test (25 items) and the Brief Michigan Alcohol Screening Test (10 items).

PART B: Five objectives for the short-term treatment of alcohol dependence in the patient and the patient's family include the following:

A. Relieving subjective symptoms of distress and discomfort due to intoxication or withdrawal
B. Preventing and/or treating serious complications of intoxication, withdrawal, or dependence
C. Establishing an alcohol-free state
D. Preparing for and referral to longer-term treatment or rehabilitation
E. Engaging the family in the treatment process

SUMMARY OF THE DIAGNOSIS AND TREATMENT OF ALCOHOL DEPENDENCE AND ALCOHOL ABUSE

1. **Prevalence:** an estimated 5% to 7% of Americans have alcoholism in any given year and 13% will have it sometime during their lifetime.
2. **Economic costs:** the *direct* economic costs of alcoholism in the United States are staggering. In 1988 total economic losses in the United States were $85.8 billion. This does not include indirect economic costs and noneconomic costs and losses.
3. **Definitions:**
   a) *Alcoholism:* alcoholism is defined as a repetitive but inconsistent and sometimes unpredictable loss of control of drinking that produces symptoms of serious dysfunction or disability.
   b) *Alcohol dependence:* a maladaptive pattern of alcohol use that includes three of the following:
      1. Tolerance
      2. Withdrawal
      3. Increasing amounts of consumption
      4. Desire or attempts to cut down or quit
      5. Substantial time spent in "hiding habit"
      6. Important social, occupational, or recreational malcoping
      7. Continued use of alcohol despite knowledge of having a persistent or recurrent social, psychological, or physical problem
   c) *Alcohol abuse:* a residual category that describes patterns of alcohol use that do not meet the criteria for alcohol dependence
   d) *Alcohol intoxication:* reversible, alcohol-specific physiological and behavioral changes due to recent exposure to alcohol
   e) *Alcohol withdrawal:* an alcohol-specific syndrome that develops following cessation of, or reduction in amount of, alcohol.
   f) *Alcohol-persisting disorder:* an alcohol-specific syndrome that persists long after acute intoxication or withdrawal abates (such as memory impairments or dementia)
4. **Systemic disease association:** the following disease states are directly linked to the toxic effects of alcohol:
   a) Alcoholic cardiomyopathy
   b) Systemic hypertension
   c) Alcoholic hepatitis
   d) Laennec's (alcoholic) cirrhosis
   e) Esophageal varices, gastritis, ascites, edema
   f) Peripheral neuropathy
   g) Alcoholic encephalopathy
5. **Neurological syndromes:**
   a) Alcoholic dementia
   b) Alcoholic amnestic disorder
   c) Korsakoff's psychosis
   d) Wernicke's encephalopathy
   e) Alcoholic hallucinosis
   f) Alcoholic paranoia
   g) Alcohol delirium
6. **Screening:**
   a) The CAGE questionnaire
   b) The MAST questionnaire
   c) The Brief MAST questionnaire
7. **Laboratory testing:** there are no diagnostic tests that are specific for alcohol dependence, but MCV (mean corpuscular volume), liver transaminases (SGOT, SGPT), and gamma-glutamyl transferase are the three

most common tests. The accuracy of a diagnosis of alcoholism increases when all three tests are used together.

8. **Treatment:**
   a) General considerations: see Short Answer Management Problems.
   b) Long-term treatment must have the following characteristics to maximize its potential:
      1. Inpatient treatment program
      2. All-inclusive and usually prolonged (4-6 weeks)
      3. Must be targeted for patient and family
   c) Goals of long-term treatment:
      1. Maintain alcohol-free state
      2. Make significant changes in lifestyle, work, and friendships
      3. Treat underlying psychiatric illness (dual diagnosis)
      4. Alcoholics Anonymous for long-term counseling

SUGGESTED READINGS

American Psychiatric Association. Diagnostic and statistical Manual. 4th Ed. Washington, DC: American Psychiatric Association Press, 1994.

Swift R. Alcoholism and substance abuse. In: Stoudemire A, ed. Clinical psychiatry for medical students. 2nd Ed. Philadelphia: JB Lippincott, 1994.

PROBLEM 59   A 32-YEAR-OLD CHIEF EXECUTIVE OFFICER WITH "RAPIDLY SWINGING MOODS"

A 32-year-old man is brought into the ER by his wife one evening. She tells you that "something is desperately wrong with my husband." She states he used to be kind, even-keeled, and fun to be with, but during the last year, she says, he has "changed drastically."

He now exhibits behavior that can best be described as "very erratic." He will go from periods of extreme depression to short intervals of "being on top of the world," "extremely elated," with "extremely fast speech and restlessness." After a few hours, he goes back into a state of depression. His wife brought him into the ER tonight because he was in a period of elation and euphoria.

She also tells you that her husband has not been performing well at work lately, and that "some of his colleagues have noticed some strange behavior." In addition, his wife tells you that "money seems to be disappearing from our bank account at a rate far faster than I can explain."

On examination, the patient is obviously euphoric and elated. When you ask him why he agreed to come tonight, he tells you that he feels so good, he would do anything to please his wife. His speech appears extremely pressured.

On physical examination his blood pressure is 190/110 mm Hg. His pulse is 128 and regular. His pupils are widely dilated, and he is sweating profusely.

SELECT THE ONE BEST ANSWER TO THE FOLLOWING QUESTIONS:

1. With this history and physical examination, what is the most likely diagnosis?
   a) rapid-swing bipolar affective disorder—subtype I
   b) rapid-swing bipolar affective disorder—subtype II
   c) amphetamine intoxication
   d) cocaine intoxication
   e) schizophrenia: catatonic subtype

2. At this time, what would be the most appropriate course of action?
   a) arrange for a psychiatric consultation on an elective basis; leave the room and hurry on to the next patient
   b) arrange for a social worker to see the patient and his wife now
   c) arrange for a stat psychiatric consult
   d) call the appropriate consultant and relate the history, your findings and diagnosis, and appropriate acute intervention
   e) reach for the diazepam in an effort to "calm everybody down"

3. The term *dual diagnosis* in psychiatry refers to which of the following?
   a) any two closely related psychiatric disorders in the same patient
   b) any two relatively unrelated psychiatric disorders in the same patient
   c) the upper phase (the high) and the lower phase (the low) of a bipolar affective disorder
   d) the existence of both a psychiatric disorder and a substance abuse disorder in the same patient
   e) the existence of both a chronic medical disorder and a psychiatric disorder in the same patient

4. In obtaining information regarding this disorder from the patient, which of the following is the most effective interview strategy considering the history?
   a) to focus on the precise details of the euphoria and the elation the patient is experiencing
   b) to focus on the precise details of the longer periods of the depression the patient is experiencing
   c) to focus on the precise details of the negative consequences that have resulted from the patient's symptoms
   d) to focus on the relationship between the patient's symptoms and the possible use or abuse of alcohol
   e) focusing on the relationship between the patient's symptoms and the relationship with his wife

5. Of the substances listed below, which has undergone the most dramatic epidemic increase in the last decade in the United States?
   a) anabolic steroids
   b) crack cocaine
   c) hallucinogens
   d) cannabis
   e) volatile organic inhalants

6. Following informed consent, which of the following laboratory tests will yield the most significant information concerning the confirmation of the diagnosis made in this patient?
   a) serum cotinine level
   b) urine benzoylecognine level
   c) urine opioid and serum opioid metabolite levels
   d) serum gamma glutamyl transferase
   e) serum barbiturate level

7. Which of the following is(are) complications of the disorder diagnosed in the patient described?
   a) sudden cardiac death

b) cerebral hemorrhage
c) respiratory arrest
d) convulsions
e) all of the above

8. Which of the following statements regarding opioid abuse in the United States is(are) true?
   a) IV drug abusers are now the largest growing group of persons with new cases of AIDS in the U.S.
   b) opioid overdose should be suspected in any patient who presents with coma and respiratory depression
   c) nausea, vomiting, cramps, and diarrhea are symptoms of opioid withdrawal
   d) b and c
   e) all of the above are true

9. Which of the following substances is classified as the most lethal substance in our society?
   a) nicotine
   b) alcohol
   c) cocaine
   d) heroin
   e) cannabis

10. Which of the following drugs has been shown to suppress the signs and symptoms of opioid withdrawal?
    a) naloxone
    b) naltrexone
    c) clonidine
    d) disulfiram
    e) methadone

11. Which of the following is a specific benzodiazepine antagonist recently approved by the FDA?
    a) flumazenil
    b) naltrexone
    c) clonidine
    d) methadone
    e) sertraline

12. Which of the following drugs has been shown to be effective for sedative detoxification?
    a) flumazenil
    b) naltrexone
    c) carbamazepine
    d) sertraline
    e) clonidine

Short Answer Management Problem 59

Describe the general principles of interviewing a patient you suspect of having a substance-abuse problem but who denies the problem.

ANSWERS

1. D. This patient has cocaine intoxication. Cocaine intoxication is characterized by elation, euphoria, excitement, pressured speech, restlessness, stereotyped movements, and bruxism. Sympathetic stimulation occurs, including tachycardia, hypertension, mydriasis, and sweating. Paranoia, suspiciousness, and psychosis may occur with prolonged use. Overdosage produces hyperpyrexia, hyperreflexia, seizures, coma, and respiratory arrest.

2. D. The treatment of choice is detoxification and rehabilitation in an inpatient treatment center. The therapy must be include individual psychotherapy and group (family) psychotherapy.

3. D. The term *dual diagnosis* means the coexistence of substance abuse and another psychiatric illness.

4. C. The most effective strategy in the treatment of cocaine intoxication is to focus on fallout from the negative consequences resulting from drug abuse. This will produce the greatest likelihood of convincing the patient that he or she has a problem.

5. B. The drug having undergone the most substantial increase in use over the last few years is cocaine (especially crack cocaine).

6. B. The metabolite of cocaine that can be detected in the urine is benzoylecognine. It should be tested for as soon as possible.

7. E. The complications of cocaine intoxication include the following:
   1. Sudden cardiac arrhythmias
   2. Convulsions
   3. Respiratory arrest
   4. Cerebral hemorrhage
   5. Sudden cardiac death

8. E. IV drug abusers are now the largest growing group of persons with new cases of AIDS in the U.S.
   Opioid overdose should be suspected in any patient

who presents to the ER with coma, convulsions, and respiratory depression.

Nausea, vomiting, cramps, and diarrhea are signs and symptoms of opioid withdrawal.

9. A. Nicotine addiction and tobacco use are legally sanctioned forms of substance abuse. Tobacco is clearly the most lethal substance in our society, accounting for over 350,000 premature deaths per year in the United States.

10. C. The alpha$_2$-adrenergic agonist clonidine hydrochloride may be used to suppress many of the signs and symptoms of opioid withdrawal. Clonidine acts at presynaptic noradrenergic-nerve endings in the locus ceruleus of the brain and blocks the adrenergic discharge produced by opioid withdrawal. In most studies clonidine has been shown to suppress approximately 75% of opioid withdrawal signs and symptoms, especially autonomic hyperactivity and gastrointestinal symptoms. Withdrawal symptoms that are not significantly ameliorated by clonidine include drug craving, insomnia, arthralgias, and myalgias.

11. A. Flumazenil (Mazicon) is the first benzodiazepine *antagonist* to be approved by the FDA in the United States. Flumazenil binds competitively and reversibly to the GABA-benzodiazepine receptor complex and inhibits the effects of the benzodiazepines. The drug is approved for the treatment of benzodiazepine overdose and/or the reversal of benzodiazepine oversedation.

12. A. Two recent double-blind controlled trials have clearly demonstrated that a new benzodiazepine antagonist (flumazenil) is effective for sedative detoxification.

SOLUTION TO SHORT ANSWER MANAGEMENT PROBLEM 59

The general principles of interviewing a drug-abusing patient who initially denies drug abuse (and that includes most patients) includes the following:

A. Attempt to obtain as detailed a history of any substance use (start with nicotine and alcohol).
B. Inquire about physical and/or behavioral problems.
C. Provide empathy and concern in an effort to instill trust on the part of the patient.
D. Avoid judgmental attitudes and pejorative statements.
E. The most effective interview strategy is to focus on whether or not the patient has experienced negative consequences due to his or her use of psychoactive substances, has poor control of use, or has been criticized by others concerning his or her pattern of behavior or use of the substance.

F. Confront the patient if you have absolute evidence.
G. Always include at least one close family member.

SUMMARY OF THE DIAGNOSIS AND TREATMENT OF DRUG ABUSE

Many definitions that concern drug abuse have been completely covered in the chapter on alcoholism.
1. **Cycle of progression:** drug seekers often have a very established pattern of abuse: alcohol to marijuana to cocaine (or another highly addictive substance).
2. **Substance that is overall the most lethal in the world:** nicotine, via cigarette smoking
3. **Drug epidemic:** crack cocaine use is epidemic in the United States and is quickly escalating.
4. **Opioid abuse:** IV opioid users are now the second largest group of patients with AIDS in the United States.
5. **Specific drugs:**
   a) Cocaine: cocaine is a sympathetic stimulator and increases the sympathetic stimulation of the central nervous system while producing euphoria as well as a high.
      Cocaine (crack) is highly lethal, highly potent, and significantly less expensive than many other drugs.
   b) Caffeine: caffeine and related methylxanthines are ubiquitous drugs in our society. These drugs produce sympathetic stimulation, diuresis, bronchodilatation, and central CNS stimulation.
   c) Cannabis: marijuana, although illegal, has been used at one time or another by 64.8% of adult Americans. Cannabis intoxication is characterized by tachycardia, muscle relaxation, euphoria, and a sense of well-being. Tachycardia, time sense alteration, and emotional lability alteration are common.
   d) Anabolic steroids: a recent study has determined that 6.5% of adolescent American boys and 1.9% of adolescent American girls report anabolic steroid use.
      The medical complications of these drugs include myocardial infarction, stroke, and hepatic disease. Psychiatric symptoms associated with anabolic steroid use include severe depression, psychotic (paranoid) symptoms, aggressive behavior, homicidal impulses, euphoria, irritability, anxiety, racing thoughts, and hyperactivity. (All of these symptoms will decline or be eliminated on discontinuation of the drug.)
   e) Hallucinogens: the hallucinogens include lysergic acid diethylamide (LSD), mescaline, psilocybin, dimethyltryptamine (DMT), hallucinogenic amphetamines, and methylenedioxyamphetamine. The mechanism of action of these substances include stimulation of CNS dopamine or serotonin.
   f) Inhalants: inhalants are volatile compounds that are inhaled for their psychotropic effects. Substances in this class include organic solvents (such as gasoline, toluene, and ethyl ether). Inhalants are ubiquitous and readily available in most households.

These are drugs of choice for many very poor people, especially those crowded in deplorable housing conditions such as Indian reservations.

g) Nicotine: more than 50 million Americans smoke cigarettes daily, and another 10 million use another form of tobacco. Nicotine addiction and tobacco use are legally sanctioned forms of substance abuse. Tobacco is clearly the most lethal substance in our society, accounting for over 350,000 premature deaths per year, primarily due to cardiovascular disease and cancer.

h) Opioids: opioid dependence and abuse remain very significant sociologic and medical problems in the United States, with an estimated 500,000 opioid addicts. The patients are frequent users of medical use and surgical services due to multiple medical sequelae of IV drug use and associated lifestyle.

6. Treatment:

a) The general characteristics of drug abuse treatment have already been outlined. Most important principles include the following:

1. Detoxification and elimination of withdrawal symptoms

2. Initial admittance of a problem and alignment of social support systems (the family)

3. Long-term intensive individual and group therapy

4. Inclusion of the family members in item 3

b) Special treatments:

1. Methadone: for opioid withdrawal

2. Naltrexone (a long-acting orally active opioid antagonist), which when taken regularly entirely blocks mu-opioid receptors, thus blocking the opioid euphoric, analgesic, and sedative properties

3. Clonidine: blocks many symptoms of opioid withdrawal

4. Flumazenil (Mazicon) is the first benzodiazepine antagonist to be approved by the FDA.

5. Tegretol: carbamazepine has been shown to be effective for ethanol and sedative detoxification.

SUGGESTED READINGS

American Psychiatric Association. Diagnostic and statistical manual for psychiatric disorders. 4th Ed. Washington, DC: American Psychiatric Association Press, 1994.

Swift R. Alcoholism and substance abuse. In: Stoudemire A, ed. Clinical psychiatry for medical students. 2nd Ed. Philadelphia: JB Lippincott, 1994.

PROBLEM 60   A 19-YEAR-OLD FEMALE WITH RAPID WEIGHT LOSS, AN INTENSE FEAR OF GAINING WEIGHT, AND AMENORRHEA

A 19-year-old female presents to your office with a 30-lb weight loss during the last 6 months. She states that she has an intense fear of gaining weight. She also admits to amenorrhea of 4 months' duration. When questioned about her perception of her weight, she states she "still feels fat."

She denies episodes of binge eating and purging. She also denies the use of laxatives or diuretics.

On examination, the patient is approximately 25% below expected body weight. There is evidence of significant muscle wasting. Her blood pressure is 90/70 mm Hg and her heart rate is 52 and regular. There appears to be a significant fine hair growth over her entire body.

SELECT THE ONE BEST ANSWER TO THE FOLLOWING QUESTIONS

1. What is the most likely diagnosis in this patient?
   a) borderline personality disorder
   b) bulimia nervosa
   c) anorexia nervosa
   d) generalized anxiety disorder
   e) masked depression

2. This disorder requires the maintenance of body weight at what percentage below ideal body weight?
   a) 5%
   b) 10%
   c) 15%
   d) 20%
   e) 25%

3. What percentage of individuals with the disorder described have an accompanying major depressive disorder or a coexisting anxiety disorder?
   a) 10%
   b) 20%
   c) 30%
   d) 50%
   e) 75%

4. What is the lifetime prevalence of obsessive-compulsive disorder in patients with this disorder?
   a) 5%
   b) 15%
   c) 25%
   d) 50%
   e) 75%

5. What is the most serious complication of the disorder described?
   a) muscle wasting
   b) generalized fatigue and weakness
   c) hypokalemia
   d) bradycardia
   e) hypotension

6. Which of the following is(are) true regarding the DSM-IV classification of eating disorders?
   a) there are two types of anorexia nervosa specified in DSM-IV: the restricting type and the binge eating/purging type
   b) there are two types of bulimia nervosa specified in DSM-IV: the purging type and the nonpurging type
   c) the two disorders *anorexia nervosa* and *bulimia nervosa* are mutually exclusive
   d) a and b
   e) all of the above are true

7. A 26-year-old patient presents with recurrent episodes of binge eating (approximately 4 times/week) after which she vomits to prevent weight gain. She says that "she has no control" over these episodes and becomes depressed because of being unable to control herself. These episodes have been occurring for the past 2 years.

   She admits to using self-induced vomiting, laxatives, and diuretics to lose weight.

   On examination, the patient's blood pressure is 110/70 mm Hg and her pulse is 72 and regular. Examination also shows that the cardiovascular system, the respiratory system, the abdomen, the musculoskeletal system, and the neurological systems are all normal.

   What is the most likely diagnosis in this patient?
   a) borderline personality disorder
   b) anorexia nervosa
   c) bulimia nervosa
   d) masked depression
   e) generalized anxiety disorder

8. Examination of which of the following is most likely to be abnormal in patients with the disorder described in Question 7?
   a) the mouth
   b) the cervical and axillary lymph nodes
   c) the right upper quadrant of the abdomen
   d) the sensory component of the neurological system
   e) the motor component of the neurological system

9. Regarding the prevalence of the disorders described in Question 1 and 7, which of the following statements is(are) true?
   a) the prevalence of the disorder in Question 1 is increasing, whereas the prevalence of the disorder described in Question 7 is decreasing
   b) the prevalence of the disorder described in Question 1 is decreasing, whereas the prevalence of the disorder described in Question 7 is increasing
   c) the prevalence of both disorders is increasing
   d) the prevalence of both disorders is decreasing
   e) the prevalence of both disorders has remained unchanged over the past decade

10. The patient described in Question 1 should be treated in which manner?
   a) as an outpatient: treatment focused on pharmacotherapy, psychotherapy, and behavior modification
   b) as an inpatient: treatment focused on pharmacotherapy, psychotherapy, and behavior modification
   c) as an inpatient: treatment focused on psychotherapy and behavior modification
   d) as an outpatient: treatment focused on psychotherapy and behavior modification
   e) as an outpatient: treatment focused on pharmacotherapy

11. Which of the following drugs have been shown to be of benefit in the treatment of the disorder described in Question 7?
   a) MAO inhibitors
   b) tricyclic antidepressants
   c) selective serotonin reuptake inhibitors (SSRIs)
   d) b and c
   e) all of the above

12. Which of the following psychotherapies has been shown to be superior in the treatment of the disorder described in Question 7?
   a) supportive psychotherapy
   b) psychodynamic psychotherapy
   c) psychoanalytic psychotherapy
   d) cognitive-behavioral psychotherapy
   e) a, b, or d

Short Answer Management Problem 60

List the psychiatric disorders and associated conditions that have been shown to be related to the conditions described in this chapter.

ANSWERS

1. C.

2. C.

3. E.

4. C.

5. C. This patient has anorexia nervosa. Anorexia nervosa is characterized by:
   a) A patient who refuses to maintain her minimal normal body weight for age and height leading to maintenance of body weight 15% below expected; or failure to gain weight as expected during growth, leading to body weight 15% below expected
   b) Even though underweight, intense fear of gaining weight or becoming fat
   c) The patient experiences her body weight, size, or shape in a disturbed fashion, such as claiming to feel fat even when she is clearly underweight.
   d) In female patients, at least three menstrual periods that should otherwise have been expected to occur have not occurred.
   e) Two subtypes are recognized:
      A. The restricting type: restrictors don't usually engage in binge eating, self-induced vomiting, or misuse of diuretics or laxatives.
      B. The binge eating/purging type: these patients, regularly engage in binge eating and/or self-induced vomiting, and misuse of laxatives or diuretics.

      The medical complications of anorexia nervosa include muscle wasting, fatigue, depression of cardiovascular function leading to bradycardia and hypotension, and depression of body temperature mechanisms leading to hypothermia. The most serious abnormality, however, is hypokalemia, with resultant cardiac dysrhythmias and possibly sudden death.

      Up to 75% of anorexia nervosa patients have a coexisting major depressive disorder or anxiety disorder, and up to 25% of anorexia nervosa patients will develop an obsessive-compulsive disorder in their lifetimes.

6. D. There are two types of anorexia nervosa and two types of bulimia nervosa. The two types of anorexia nervosa are the restricting type and the binge eating/purging type. The two types of bulimia nervosa are the purging type and the nonpurging type. Anorexia nervosa and bulimia nervosa are not mutually exclusive; there appears to be a continuum among patients of the two symptom complexes of self-starvation and binge-purge cycles: about 50% of patients with anorexia nervosa will also have bulimia nervosa, and many patients with bulimia nervosa may previously have had at least a subclinical form of anorexia nervosa.

7. C.

8. A. This patient has bulimia nervosa. Bulimia nervosa is characterized by the following:
   A. Repeated episodes of binge-eating large amounts of food in brief periods of time
   B. The patient regularly engages in severe compensatory behaviors to prevent weight gain, such as self-induced vomiting, misuse of large amounts of laxatives or diuretics, diet pills, fasts, very strict diets, and/or very vigorous exercise.
   C. At least two binge eating and purging/severe compensatory behaviors/week for a minimum of 3 months
   D. Unrelenting overconcern regarding weight and body shape
   E. Two subtypes are recognized:
      1. Purging type: these patients regularly engage in self-induced vomiting and/or misuse of laxatives or diuretics.
      2. Nonpurging type: these patients don't usually self-induce vomiting or misuse laxatives or diuretics to lose weight. Instead, they engage in other severe compensatory behaviors such as fasting or excessive exercise.

   The most frequently observed abnormality in bulimia nervosa is an abnormality in the examination of the head and neck (specifically the mouth). Examination of the mouth reveals the evidence of dental caries and peridontal disease that occur because of the effects of repeated vomiting.

9. C. Studies suggest that among adolescent and young adult women in certain high school and college settings, the prevalence of clinically significant eating disorders is approximately 4% and for more broadly defined syndromes may be as high as 8%. The prevalence of these disorders seems to have increased dramatically over the past several decades. The prevalence of eating disorders in many ways appears to parallel the society's attitudes regarding beauty and fashion.

10. C. First, it is important to establish how ill this patient really is. Based on what is known (a 30-lb weight loss in 6 months), this patient is very ill. Most authorities in this circumstance would suggest inpatient therapy with a focus on reestablishing a reasonable weight, individual psychotherapy, and behavior modification. The only justifiable pharmacotherapy would be antidepressant medication for the depression that persists following weight gain and for depression in the still-underweight patient. The drug class of choice is one of the SSRIs (selective serotonin reuptake inhibitor agents).

11. E. Controlled studies indicate that tricyclic antidepressants (particularly imipramine and desipramine), MAO inhibitors such as phenelzine, along with SSRI agents such as fluoxetine or sertraline have been shown to be successful in reducing binge eating and purging episodes.

12. E. Psychotherapies that have been shown to be successful in the treatment of bulimia nervosa include supportive psychotherapy, psychodynamic psychotherapy, and cognitive-behavioral psychotherapy.

    The major success appears to come with cognitive-behavioral psychotherapy. This includes several stages, each consisting of several weeks or biweekly individual and/or group sessions. The first stage emphasizes the establishment of control over eating; this utilizes behavioral techniques such as self-monitoring. The second stage focuses on attempts to restructure the patient's unrealistic cognitions and instill more effective modes of problem solving. The third stage emphasizes maintaining the gains and preventing relapse, and often provides 6 months to a year of weekly sessions to provide close follow-up during times when relapse is common.

SOLUTION TO SHORT ANSWER MANAGEMENT PROBLEM 60

The psychiatric disorders that are related to the eating disorders described include the following:

1. Major depressive disorder
2. An anxiety disorder
   (75% of patients with an eating disorder have either item 1 or item 2 at the same time.)
3. Chemical dependency and substance abuse
4. Personality disorders

SUMMARY OF THE DIAGNOSIS AND TREATMENT OF EATING DISORDERS

1. **Prevalence:**
   a) The prevalence of eating disorders is 4%.
   b) The prevalence of broadly defined syndromes may be as high as 8%.
   c) The prevalence of these disorders has increased significantly over the past several decades.
2. **Symptoms:** the symptoms of both anorexia nervosa and bulimia nervosa have been described previously.
   a) Diagnostic clues:
      Anorexia nervosa: a 15% weight loss, a distorted body image (feeling fat in spite of being grossly underweight), and an intense fear of gaining weight
   b) Diagnostic clues:
      Bulimia nervosa: repeated episodes of rapid binge eating, severe compensatory behaviors to lose weight, and unrelenting overconcern with weight and body image
3. **Relationships between the two disorders:** there appears to be a continuum between the two disorders: 50% of patients with anorexia nervosa also have bulimia nervosa.
4. **Complications:**
   a) Anorexia nervosa: the physical complications of starvation:
      1. Depletion of fat
      2. Muscle wasting (including cardiac muscle in severe wasting)
      3. Bradycardia
      4. Cardiac arrhythmias (sudden death may follow)
      5. Leukopenia, hypercortisolemia, osteoporosis
      6. Cachexia
      7. Lanugo (fine baby hair)
   b) Bulimia nervosa:
      1. Dental caries and dental disease
      2. Metabolic abnormalities (hypokalemia secondary to vomiting)
      3. Melanosis coli from laxative abuse
5. **Treatment:**
   a) Anorexia nervosa:
      1. Hospitalization to reestablish weight and correct metabolic abnormalities
      2. Individual psychotherapy and insight-oriented behavior modification
      3. Pharmacologic agents limited to treatment of co-existing depression
   b) Bulimia nervosa:
      1. Supportive psychotherapy, psychodynamic psychotherapy, and cognitive-behavior psychotherapy
      2. Tricyclics, MAOs, and SSRIs are used to treat the binge eating component.

SUGGESTED READINGS

American Psychiatric Association. Diagnostic and Statistical Manual. 4th Ed. Washington, DC: American Psychiatric Association Press, 1994.

Yager U. Eating disorders. In: Stoudemire A, ed. Clinical psychiatry for medical students. 2nd Ed. Philadelphia: JB Lippincott, 1994.

PROBLEM 61   A 36-YEAR-OLD FEMALE WITH SHORTNESS OF BREATH AND PALPITATIONS

A 36-year-old female presents to your office with an 8-month history of shortness of breath, palpitations, dizziness, trouble swallowing, restlessness, fatigue, and anxiety regarding her job and the health of her two children. She tells you that she constantly worries about what could happen to her children when they are playing with other children in their homes (where she cannot be constantly supervising their play activities). She also worries about them dying in a car crash. She tells you: "Well, I'm very concerned about them not only being in an automobile accident but also about the possibility of the seat belts coming loose."

When you directly question her about some of these worries she readily admits to you that "I know I'm worrying too much, Doctor, but I just can't help it."

She also admits to muscle tension, easy fatigability, difficulty concentrating, having trouble falling and staying asleep, and irritability.

At this point in the interview she becomes very tense and tells you, "You know, Doctor, this is really getting out of control; it's getting so bad that it is interfering with my everyday life."

On P/E, the patient's thyroid gland is slightly larger than normal, but still within normal limits. Her blood pressure is 160/60 mm Hg and her pulse is 108 and regular. Examination of the abdomen is completely normal. All other systems are completely normal.

SELECT THE ONE BEST ANSWER TO THE FOLLOWING QUESTIONS

1. What is the most likely diagnosis in this patient?
   a) panic disorder
   b) major depressive disorder
   c) generalized anxiety disorder
   d) hypothyroidism
   e) hypochondriasis

2. Of patients with the disorder described, what percentage have at least one other anxiety disorder at some time in their life?
   a) 10%
   b) 30%
   c) 50%
   d) 80%
   e) nobody really knows for sure; everything in medicine is basically speculation

3. What is the most common error made in the diagnosis of the disorder described?
   a) misdiagnosing this disorder as a related anxiety disorder instead of generalized anxiety disorder
   b) misdiagnosing this disorder as depression
   c) misdiagnosing this disorder as hyperthyroidism
   d) misdiagnosing this disorder as pheochromocytoma
   e) misdiagnosing this disorder as a multiple endocrine neoplasia syndrome

4. Which of the following symptoms is(are) generally not characteristic of the disorder described?
   a) awakening with apprehension and unrealistic concern regarding future misfortune
   b) worry out of proportion to the likelihood or impact of feared events

   c) a 6-month or longer course of anxiety and associated symptoms
   d) association of the anxiety described with depression
   e) anxiety regarding health concerns

5. Which of the following statements regarding the disorder described above is(are) true?
   a) this disorder may develop between attacks in panic disorder
   b) the symptoms of this disorder are often present in episodes of depression
   c) medical conditions that produce the major symptom associated with this disorder must be excluded
   d) the disorder is accompanied by symptoms of motor tension, autonomic hyperactivity, vigilance, and scanning
   e) all of the above are true

6. What is the psychotherapy or therapy of choice in the disorder?
   a) biofeedback
   b) progressive muscle relaxation
   c) cognitive therapy
   d) psychoanalytic psychotherapy
   e) supportive psychotherapy

7. What is the pharmacologic agent of choice in this disorder?
   a) alprazolam
   b) buspirone
   c) amitriptyline
   d) fluoxetine
   e) lorazepam

8. Which of the following pharmacologic agents is not recommended in the treatment of this disorder?
   a) flurazepam

b) clorazepate

c) temazepam

d) clozapine

e) clonazepam

9. This disorder is more common in which of the following?

a) young to middle-aged females

b) nonwhites

c) those currently not married

d) those of lower socioeconomic class

e) all of the above

10. Which of the following statements is(are) true regarding the disorder?

a) this disorder displays definitive genetic transmission

b) the major symptom of this disorder may be a conditioned response to a stimulus that the individual has come to associate with danger

c) there is little relationship between the onset of this disorder and the cumulative effects of stressful life events

d) b and c

e) all of the above

Short Answer Management Problem 61

PART A: List three substances that may precipitate the major symptom associated with this condition.

PART B: List two contraindications to using benzodiazepines to treat this disorder.

ANSWERS

1. C.

2. D. This patient has generalized anxiety disorder (GAD). *Generalized anxiety disorder* is defined as unrealistic or excessive worry about several life events or activities, for a period of at least 6 months, during which the person has been bothered more days than not by these concerns. In addition, the following six symptoms are present: muscle tension, restlessness or feeling keyed up or on edge, easy fatigability, difficulty concentrating or a sensation of the "mind going blank" because of anxiety, trouble falling or staying asleep, and irritability. Finally, the anxiety, worry, or physical symptoms significantly interfere with the person's normal routine or usual activities, or caused marked distress.

    Of patients with GAD, at least 80% of patients have had at least one other anxiety disorder in their lifetime.

3. A. The most common diagnostic error made in diagnosis related to GAD is misdiagnosing GAD when another anxiety disorder is the actual cause. This leads to inappropriate and ineffective treatment decisions. The symptom of anxiety is prominent in a number of conditions, including the following:
    A. Depressive disorders
    B. Psychotic disorders
    C. Substance abuse disorders
    D. Somatoform disorders
    E. Other medical conditions (especially those associated with dyspnea)
    F. Medication side effects (sympathomimetic agents)

4. E. Generalized anxiety disorder is characterized by awakening with apprehension and concern regarding future misfortune, worry out of proportion to the likelihood or impact of feared events, a duration of 6 months or more of anxiety or associated symptoms, and an association of the described anxiety with depression.

    Generalized anxiety disorder is usually not associated with health concerns. When health concerns become the focus of worry, the diagnosis shifts to a diagnosis in favor of a somatoform disorder.

5. E. Generalized persistent anxiety may develop between attacks in panic disorder. GAD symptoms are often present during episodes of depression. As with panic disorder, medical conditions that may produce anxiety symptoms such as hyperthyroidism or caffeinism must be excluded.

    GAD is characterized by chronic anxiety about life circumstances accompanied by symptoms of motor tension, autonomic hyperactivity, vigilance, and scanning.

6. B. Preliminary studies of behavioral treatment of GAD suggest positive results with progressive muscle relaxation and anxiety management.

    Biofeedback does not appear to have a specific value. Cognitive therapy, especially when combined with systematic desensitization in imagination or relaxation, improves GAD symptoms; however, cognitive therapy alone is not effective.

7. B. Buspirone, a nonbenzodiazepine anxiolytic, has become the pharmacologic treatment of choice for GAD. The mechanism of action is not established, but phar-

macologic activity includes a decrease in serotonin and an increase in dopamine and norepinephrine cell firing. Buspirone does not produce drowsiness or impair driving skill and thus lacks abuse potential or withdrawal symptoms with abrupt discontinuation.

8. D. Commonly used benzodiazepines include the following: diazepam (Valium), flurazepam (Dalmane), halazepam (Prazepam), chlordiazepoxide (Librium), alprazolam (Xanax), triazolam (Halcion), clorazepate (Tranxene), prazepam (Centrax, Vestran), midazolam (Versad), lorazepam (Ativan), temazepam (Restoril), oxazepam (Serax), and clonazepam (Klonopin).

Clozapine is an atypical antipsychotic agent that has shown superior efficacy over other typical neuroleptics in the treatment of refractory schizophrenic patients.

9. E. GAD is slightly more common in young to middle-aged females, nonwhites, those not currently married, and those of lower socioeconomic class status.

10. B. There is no convincing evidence of genetic transmission of GAD. Behavioral theories consider anxiety, like panic disorder, a conditioned response to a stimulus that the individual has come to associate with danger. There is also some suggestion that the onset of GAD may be related to the cumulative effects of several stressful life events.

SOLUTION TO SHORT ANSWER MANAGEMENT PROBLEM 61

PART A: Five substances that can produce significant anxiety include the following:
A. Caffeine
B. Cocaine
C. Amphetamines (methylphenidate, dextroamphetamine)
D. Lysergic acid diethylamide (LSD), mescaline, psilocybin, dimethyltryptamine
E. Alcohol

PART B: Two substances that contraindicate benzodiazepine use include the following:
A. A history of alcohol abuse
B. A history of substance (other than alcohol) abuse

Note: Buspirone is not contraindicated with a history of alcohol or drug abuse.

SUMMARY OF THE DIAGNOSIS AND TREATMENT OF GENERALIZED ANXIETY DISORDER

1. **Epidemiology:** a 1-month prevalence rate of 2.5% for GAD using research diagnostic has been demonstrated.
2. **Differential diagnosis:**
   a) Panic disorder
   b) Somatoform disorder
   c) Hypochondriasis
   d) Psychoactive substance use
   e) Depression (with secondary anxiety)
   f) Hyperthyroidism
   g) Caffeinism
3. **Symptoms:**
   a) GAD is characterized by chronic excessive activity concerning life circumstances accompanied by symptoms of motor tension, autonomic hyperactivity, vigilance, and scanning.
   b) The symptoms of anxiety, worry, or physical symptoms significantly interfere with the person's normal routine of usual activities and caused marked distress.
4. **Treatment:**
   a) Nonpharmacologic treatment:
      1. Progressive muscle relaxation and anxiety treatment
      2. Cognitive therapy with systemic desensitization in imagination or relaxation
   b) Pharmacologic treatment:
      1. Buspirone, a nonbenzodiazepine anxiolytic, is the treatment of choice for GAD.
      2. Use antidepressants if anxiety is secondary to depression.

SUGGESTED READINGS

American Psychiatric Association. Diagnostic and Statistical Manual. 4th Ed. Washington, DC: American Psychiatric Association Press, 1994.

Nagy L, Krystal J, Charney D. Anxiety disorders. In: Stoudemire A, ed. Clinical psychiatry for medical students. 2nd Ed. Philadelphia: JB Lippincott, 1994.

PROBLEM 62   A 48-YEAR-OLD MALE WITH A 6-MONTH HISTORY OF SNORING, NOCTURNAL BREATH CESSATIONS, AND EXCESSIVE DAYTIME SLEEPINESS

A 48-year-old male presents to your office with his wife. His wife complains to you that "he is constantly snoring" and she has put up with all she can. This has been going on for a number of years, but it has been getting worse lately. His wife also tells you that "sometimes he even stops breathing during the night."

When you ask the patient directly, he says, "Well, I may snore a bit, but I think my wife is exaggerating." You somehow doubt the latter statement.

On examination, the patient weighs 310 pounds. His blood pressure is 200/105 mm Hg (measured with a large cuff). There is a grade III/VI systolic murmur present along the left sternal edge. You believe that there is elevated jugular venous pressure when he lies at a 45-degree angle.

SELECT THE ONE BEST ANSWER TO THE FOLLOWING QUESTIONS

1. What is the most likely diagnosis in this patient?
   a) narcolepsy
   b) obstructive sleep apnea syndrome
   c) generalized poor physical condition
   d) central sleep apnea syndrome
   e) adult onset adenoid hypertrophy

2. To what is the pathophysiology of this condition related?
   a) collapse of the pharyngeal walls repetitively during sleep
   b) failure of the genioglossus and other upper airway dilator muscles
   c) sleep-related upper airway obstruction and cessation in ventilation (apneas)
   d) a and c
   e) all of the above

3. This condition is accompanied by which of the following?
   a) hypoxemia
   b) hypercarbia
   c) metabolic acidosis
   d) respiratory acidosis
   e) a, b, and d
   f) all of the above

4. What is(are) the major symptom(s) of this disorder?
   a) loud snoring
   b) daytime hypersomnolence
   c) disturbed nonrefreshing sleep
   d) weight gain
   e) a, b, and c
   f) all of the above

5. What is(are) the clinical feature(s) associated with the condition described?
   a) systemic hypertension
   b) inhibited sexual desire
   c) depression

   d) a and b
   e) all of the above

6. What is(are) the factor(s) that predispose to this condition?
   a) alcohol intake
   b) benzodiazepines
   c) hyperthyroidism
   d) a and b
   e) all of the above

7. What is the treatment of first choice for this disorder?
   a) uvulopalatopharyngoplasty surgery (UPP)
   b) tracheostomy
   c) continuous positive airway pressure (CPAP)
   d) nortriptyline
   e) alprazolam

8. Which of the following drugs is contraindicated in the treatment of the disturbed, nonrefreshing sleep that is associated with the condition described?
   a) fluoxetine
   b) sertraline
   c) alprazolam
   d) phenelzine
   e) paroxetine

9. A 35-year-old male presents to your office with a chief complaint of "weak muscles," especially after laughing. On further questioning you discover that the patient has excessive daytime sleepiness and "weird imaginings" just before going to sleep at night. The patient appears anxious and tense. What is your tentative diagnosis?
   a) narcolepsy
   b) hysterical conversion reaction
   c) psychosomatic symptoms secondary to chronic anxiety
   d) hypochondriasis
   e) obstructive sleep apnea

10. Which of the following is not a symptom of the disorder described?
    a) catalepsy

b) hypnagogic hallucinations
c) sleep paralysis
d) restless and disturbed sleep
e) persistent daytime sleepiness

11. The "daytime symptoms" of the disorder described is(are) treated well with which of the following medications?
    a) methylphenidate
    b) dextroamphetamine
    c) mazindol
    d) a and b only
    e) all of the above

12. The "nighttime symptoms" of the disorder described is(are) best treated by which of the following?
    a) alprazolam
    b) nortriptyline
    c) protriptyline
    d) b or c
    e) all of the above

13. The diagnosis described in Question 9 is best established by which of the following?
    a) nocturnal polysomnogram (NPSG)
    b) multiple sleep latency test (MSLT)
    c) either a or b
    d) a and b together
    e) neither a nor b

14. What percentage of adult Americans experience significant sleep difficulties in any given year?
    a) 5%
    b) 10%
    c) 15%
    d) 25%
    e) 50%

15. Insomniacs often compensate for lost sleep by delaying their morning awakening time or by napping, which actually may have the effect of further fragmenting their nocturnal sleep. What is this disorder known as?
    a) mixed-up insomniac syndrome
    b) insufficient sleep syndrome
    c) inadequate sleep hygiene
    d) adjustment sleep disorder
    e) psychophysiologic insomnia

16. Insomniacs who voluntarily curtail their time in bed, usually in response to social and/or occupational demands, is best diagnosed as which of the following?
    a) workaholic sleep loss syndrome

b) inadequate sleep hygiene
c) insufficient sleep syndrome
d) adjustment sleep disorder
e) psychophysiologic insomnia

17. Insomniacs who develop anticipatory anxiety over the prospect of another night of sleeplessness followed by another day of fatigue in response to a previously resolved stressor is known as which of the following?
    a) adjustment sleep disorder
    b) psychophysiologic insomnia
    c) inadequate sleep hygiene
    d) insufficient sleep syndrome
    e) generalized anxiety disorder insomnia

18. A 73-year-old male is admitted to the hospital for a TURP procedure. The procedure is postponed because of some abnormal test results. The patient tells you that he has had extreme difficulty in sleeping since coming into the hospital. What is the most likely diagnosis in this patient?
    a) adjustment sleep disorder
    b) psychophysiologic insomnia
    c) inadequate sleep hygiene
    d) insufficient sleep syndrome
    e) sudden-onset central sleep apnea

19. What is the major difference between idiopathic hypersomnolence and narcolepsy?
    a) daytime somnolence
    b) frequent daytime naps
    c) awakening unrefreshed versus awakening refreshed from these frequent daytime naps
    d) significant differences in treatment
    e) none of the above

20. What is the difference between periodic limb movement disorder (nocturnal myoclonus) and restless legs syndrome?
    a) kicking of the lower extremities in nocturnal myoclonus versus sensory loss in restless legs syndrome
    b) patient awareness with nocturnal myoclonus versus patient unawareness with restless legs syndrome
    c) kicking of the lower extremities in restless legs syndrome versus sensory loss in nocturnal myoclonus
    d) patient awareness with restless legs syndrome versus patient unawareness in nocturnal myoclonus
    e) none of the above

Short Answer Management Problem 62

Discuss the principles of the use of hypnotic agents in the management of sleep disorders.

ANSWERS

1. B. This patient has obstructive sleep apnea. The major symptoms of obstructive sleep apnea syndrome are as follows:
   A. Loud snoring
   B. Reports of prolonged pauses in respiration during sleep
   C. Daytime hypersomnolence
   D. Disturbed nonrefreshing sleep
   E. Weight gain

2. E. The pathophysiology of obstructive sleep apnea syndrome (OSA) includes the following:
   A. The pharyngeal walls collapse repetitively during sleep, causing intermittent sleep-related upper airway obstruction and cessation in ventilation (apneas).
   B. The cessation of ventilation is related to a concomitant loss of inspiratory effort.
   C. Upper airway closure in OSA occurs due to a failure of the genioglossus and other upper airway dilator muscles. Apnea results.

3. E. Obstructive sleep apnea produces the following acid-base balance situation:
   A. Apnea causes hypercarbia, hypoxemia, and a resulting respiratory acidosis.
   B. Only if there is another preexisting condition associated with OSA will metabolic acidosis be produced.

4. F. See the answer to Question 1.

5. E. Associated clinical features of OSA include systemic hypertension; inhibited sexual desire; impotence; ejaculatory impairment; depression; deficits in attention, motor efficiency, and graphomotor ability; deterioration in interpersonal relationships; marital discord; and occupational impairment.

6. D. Factors that predispose to OSA include sedating pharmacologic agents including alcohol and benzodiazepines (all are contraindicated in OSA); nasal obstruction; large uvula; low-lying soft palate; retrognathia, micrognathia, and other craniofacial abnormalities; pharyngeal masses such as tumors or cysts; macroglossia; tonsillar hypertrophy; vocal cord paralysis; obesity; hypothyroidism; and acromegaly.

7. C.

8. C. The most established management options, in order of most preferred option first, are as follows:
   1. Continuous positive airway pressure (CPAP)
   2. Uvulopalatopharyngoplasty (UPP)
   3. Tracheostomy
   Additional measures:
   1. Weight loss should be encouraged.
   2. Antidepressants that are stimulating, such as protriptyline, fluoxetine, sertraline, and paroxetine, are best suited to manage coexistent depression.
   Chronic anxiety, which may complicate the OSA picture should not be managed with benzodiazepines. Instead, the nonbenzodiazepine *buspirone*, which does not appear to aggravate OSA, should be used, along with behavioral treatments. Thus alprazolam is contraindicated.

9. A.

10. A. This patient has narcolepsy. The major symptoms of narcolepsy are as follows:
    A. Persistent daytime sleepiness
    B. Cataplexy (*not* catalepsy)
    C. Hypnagogic or hypnopompic hallucinations
    D. Sleep paralysis
    E. Restless and disturbed sleep
    Definitions:
    1. *Cataplexy:* cataplexy is defined as an abrupt paralysis or paresis of skeletal muscles that usually follows emotional experiences such as anger, surprise, laughter, or physical exercise.
    2. *Hypnagogic (or hypnopompic) hallucinations:* these are hallucinations that are vivid and often frightening dreams occurring after falling asleep (or upon awakening).
    3. *Sleep paralysis:* sleep paralysis is a global paralysis of voluntary muscles that usually occurs shortly after falling asleep and lasts a few seconds or minutes.
    Cataplexy, hypnagogic hallucinations, and sleep paralysis are thought to be manifestations of an underlying aberration in the control of the timing of REM sleep that in turn results in "attacks" of REM sleep during wakefulness.

11. E. Commonly used medications used to control excessive daytime sleepiness include pemoline 18.75 mg to

112.5 mg/day, methylphenidate 5 to 60 mg/day, and dextroamphetamine 5 to 60 mg/day. In refractory cases, mazindol 3 to 6 mg/day, a tricyclic compound with anorexic properties, may be utilized. Tolerance may be minimized by prescribing the lowest effective dose and asking patients to take regular drug holidays on days when their need for alertness is lowest.

12. D. The REM-related symptoms of cataplexy—hypnagogic hallucinations and sleep paralysis—can be controlled with REM-suppressant medications such as the tricyclic antidepressants protriptyline 5 to 30 mg/day, imipramine 50 to 200 mg/day, or nortriptyline 50 to 100 mg/day. Many narcoleptics also require emotional support.

13. D. Other than the obvious behavioral manifestations of excessive daytime sleepiness (yawning, drooping eyelids, psychomotor retardation), physical examination is typically unrevealing in narcolepsy. If the diagnosis is suspected, it must be confirmed by nocturnal polysomnogram (NPSG) and multiple sleep latency test (MSLT).

14. D. Approximately 25% of all American adults express sleep-related complaints over the course of a 1-year period.

15. C. Many individuals unknowingly engage in habitual behaviors that harm sleep. Insomniacs, for example, often compensate for lost sleep by delaying their morning awakening time or by napping. These behaviors actually have the effect of further fragmenting nocturnal sleep. Instead, insomniacs should be advised to adhere to a regular awakening time regardless of the amount of sleep that they have gotten and to avoid naps.

16. C. Individuals who voluntarily curtail this time in bed, usually in response to social and occupational demands have what is best termed *insufficient sleep syndrome*. Although sleep reduction may be as little as 1 hour per night, over long periods of time such a pattern may lead to daytime hypersomnolence and result in impairment.

17. B. Patients who develop anticipatory anxiety over the prospect of another night of sleeplessness followed by another day of fatigue have what is known as psychophysiologic insomnia. Anxiety typically increases as bedtime approaches and reaches maximum intensity following retirement. Sufferers often spend hours in bed awake focused on and brooding over their sleeplessness, which in turn aggravates their insomnia even further. Persistent psychophysiologic insomnia often complicates other insomnia disorders.

18. A. This patient has adjustment sleep disorder. This common disorder is caused by acute emotional stressors such as job loss or hospitalization. The result is insomnia, typically a difficulty in falling asleep, mediated through tension and anxiety. Symptoms usually remit shortly after abatement of the stressors. Treatment is warranted if daytime sleepiness and fatigue interfere with functioning or if the disorder lasts for more than a few weeks.

19. C. Idiopathic hypersomnolence is a lifelong and incurable disorder that has a variable age of onset. The most prominent symptom of this disorder is unrelenting daytime somnolence. Patients spend lengthy period of time sleeping at night only to awaken feeling more sleepy. They take frequent and lengthy daytime naps. However, unlike patients with narcolepsy, they awaken from these naps feeling unrefreshed.

20. D. Periodic limb movement disorder (nocturnal myoclonus) is characterized by the repetitive (usually every 20 to 40 seconds) twitching or kicking of the lower extremities during sleep. Patients usually present with the complaint of unrelenting insomnia, most often characterized by repeated awakenings following sleep onset.

Restless legs syndrome is a creeping, crawling sensation in the lower extremities manifested by irresistible leg kicks that affect patients upon reclining prior to falling asleep. Unlike periodic limb movement disorder, however, the patient is very aware of this phenomenon and resorts to moving the affected extremity by stretching, kicking, or walking to relieve symptoms. Many patients are depressed, irritable, and angry. Psychosocial impairment such as job loss and relationship difficulties are quite common.

SOLUTION TO SHORT ANSWER MANAGEMENT PROBLEM 62

The use of hypnotic agents in sleep disorders is a subject of great controversy (mainly because of their very wide and sometimes very inappropriate use). There are many factors that influence the decision of whether to prescribe a hypnotic agent and which hypnotic agent to prescribe.

The disadvantages of prescribing a hypnotic agent are as follows:

1. There is a propensity for daytime somnolence with the use of an agent that has either a medium half-life or a long half-life.

2. A second factor is the propensity for the development of drug tolerance. Larger and larger quantities of the drug are needed to produce the same effect.

3. A third factor is the ability of hypnotics to produce rebound anxiety the following day. This is especially true of those agents that have a short half-life.

4. Hypnotics may produce symptoms of autonomic hyperactivity and irritability the following day. This is a particular problem with those hypnotics that have a very short half-life. Next-day tremor and nervousness is a very good example of this phenomenon.

5. In the vast majority of cases, although hypnotics are specifically indicated for only short periods of time, they are used for longer and longer periods of time. The result of this is that after a period of approximately 3 weeks, the hypnotic agents begin working in the opposite manner to which they were intended: instead of helping sleep, they actually hinder sleep.

SUMMARY OF THE DIAGNOSIS AND TREATMENT OF SLEEP DISORDERS

1. **Prevalence:** the overall prevalence of sleep disorders and sleep difficulties in the American population is estimated to be approximately 25% in any given year. This includes, of course, all forms of sleep disturbance, both long and short.

2. **Sleep phases and laboratory investigation:**
   a) Human sleep: human sleep is made up of basically two types of sleep patterns: non-REM sleep and REM sleep (REM = rapid eye movement). Non-REM sleep has four stages and accounts for approximately 75% of total sleep. REM sleep occupies approximately 25% of total sleep.
   b) Sleep investigations: all sleep investigations should be performed in a proper, accredited sleep laboratory. The two basic tests indicated in sleep disorders are the nocturnal polysomnogram (NPSG) and the multiple sleep latency test (MSLT).

3. **Specific sleep disorders:**
   a) Obstructive sleep apnea: obstructive sleep apnea consists of loud snoring; prolonged pauses in breathing during sleep; daytime hypersomnolence; disturbed, nonrefreshing sleep; and weight gain.
      Pathophysiologic abnormalities produce apnea.
      Associated conditions include obesity, systemic hypertension, sexual dysfunction, depression, and anxiety.
      Treatment of choice for OSA is continuous positive airway pressure (CPAP). Second and third management choices include UPP surgery and tracheostomy.
      Weight loss should be encouraged; alcohol should be discouraged; benzodiazepines should be prohibited; and systemic hypertension should be treated.

Depression should be treated with a nonsedating antidepressant (SSRIs or protriptyline).
   b) Central sleep apnea: this is a rare syndrome on its own and is characterized by cessation of ventilation related to a concomitant loss of inspiratory effort.
   c) Narcolepsy: this disorder produces the following classical symptoms: cataplexy, hypnagogic or hypnopompic hallucinations, and sleep paralysis. There is associated persistent daytime sleepiness and restless and disturbed sleep.
      Medications used to combat excessive sleepiness include pemoline, methylphenidate, and dextroamphetamine. Mazindol is used in resistant cases. The REM-related symptoms of cataplexy and hypnagogic hallucinations are best treated with a stimulating tricyclic antidepressant such as nortriptyline or protriptyline.
   d) Idiopathic hypersomnolence: this is a lifelong and incurable disorder that has, as its most prominent feature, unrelenting daytime somnolence. Patients spend lengthy periods of time sleeping at night only to awaken feeling more sleepy. Unlike the narcoleptic, they awaken from their frequent daytime naps feeling unrefreshed.
   e) Periodic limb movement disorder (nocturnal myoclonus): this disorder is characterized by repetitive (usually every 20 to 40 seconds) twitching or kicking of the lower extremities during sleep. Patients usually present with the complaint of unrelenting insomnia, most often characterized by repeated awakenings following sleep onset.
      Baclofen, clonazepam, and carbidopa-levodopa may relieve these symptoms
   f) Restless legs syndrome: the hallmark of this disorder is a "creeping sensation" in the lower extremities and irresistible leg kicks that affect patients upon reclining prior to falling asleep. Unlike periodic limb movement disorder, the patients are very well aware of these symptoms and resort to moving the affected extremity by stretching, kicking, or walking to relieve the symptoms.

4. **Hypnotic agents:** in most primary care practices, the distinct disadvantages just described outweigh any possible benefit, especially on a long-term basis.

SUGGESTED READINGS

American Psychiatric Association. Diagnostic and Statistical Manual. 4th Ed. Washington, DC: American Psychiatric Association Press, 1994.

Doghramji K. The evaluation and management of sleep disorders. In: Stoudemire A, ed. Clinical psychiatry for medical students. 2nd Ed. Philadelphia: JB Lippincott, 1994.

PROBLEM 63   A 26-YEAR-OLD FEMALE WITH AN "ABDOMEN FULL OF SCARS"

A 26-year-old female presents to the ER with a 6-month history of "severe abdominal pain" that is relieved only by Demerol. The patient self-reports "many, many, operations" on her stomach, gallbladder, common bile duct, pancreas, large bowel, small bowel, spleen, and others that she can't remember.

She tells you when you introduce yourself that "she has heard all about you" and is certainly glad that "you are here to solve her problems." She further tells you that she "was on the brink" until she called the emergency department and found out that you were the ER doctor in charge of care today.

When you try and obtain more of a complete history regarding all of her abdominal problems, she tells you that she has been in 57 different hospitals in the last 37 months. She goes back to her original line about her delight with you being on duty today.

On examination, the patient's blood pressure is 120/79 mm Hg. Her pulse is 72 and regular. Examination of the head and neck reveals "multiple scars" on her face from "gland surgery." Her abdomen has 9 different scars in different locations. When you press gently on her abdomen she screams very loudly. It is 3 AM and anyone in the 36-room ER who did happen to be asleep is no longer in that state.

SELECT THE ONE BEST ANSWER TO THE FOLLOWING QUESTIONS

1. On the basis of the history and physical examination, what is the most likely diagnosis in this patient?
   a) borderline personality disorder
   b) antisocial personality disorder
   c) somatoform disorder
   d) factitious disorder with predominant physical signs and symptoms (Munchausen syndrome)
   e) malingering

2. Which of the following descriptions best fits patients with this disorder?
   a) "scarface personality"
   b) "gridiron abdomen"
   c) "lostlove syndrome"
   d) "deceptive fever syndrome"
   e) multiple personality disorder

3. In which of the following demographic groups does this disorder occur more commonly?
   a) males
   b) females
   c) health care workers
   d) b and c
   e) a and c

4. The prevalence of factitious disorders among patients admitted to general hospitals (primary and secondary care) in the United States is approximately which of the following?
   a) 0.05% of all admissions
   b) 0.1% of all admissions
   c) 0.5% of all admissions
   d) 1.0% of all admissions
   e) 5.0% of all admissions

5. Which of the following criteria is(are) important in establishing the diagnosis?
   a) intentional production or feigning of physical symptoms
   b) intentional production or feigning of psychological symptoms
   c) motivation to assume the sick role
   d) a and b only
   e) all of the above

6. Which of the following signs or symptoms is most predictive of this disorder?
   a) signs and symptoms of a major depressive disorder or a brief depressive disorder
   b) an obvious, recognizable goal in producing the signs and symptoms
   c) pathological lying; lack of close relationships with others; hostile and manipulative manner; associated substance and criminal behavior
   d) multiple admissions to different hospitals, multiple referrals to different physicians, and multiple surgical procedures
   e) the involuntary production as opposed to the voluntary production of multiple symptoms

7. When physical symptoms predominate in this disorder, what is the diagnosis?
   a) Briquet's syndrome
   b) Ganser's syndrome
   c) Munchausen syndrome
   d) doctor abuse syndrome
   e) none of the above

8. A patient who presents to your local ER with these signs and symptoms is likely to produce which of the following behaviors?
   a) self-injection of insulin when not a diabetic

b) self-bloodletting and putting of same into urine to imitate hematuria

c) allowing the thermometer used to take temperature to be immersed in hot water

d) when producing a urine sample contaminating it with feces

e) all of the above

9. Which of the following disorders is(are) part of the differential diagnosis of the condition described?
a) somatoform disorder
b) antisocial personality disorder
c) malingering
d) Ganser's syndrome
e) all of the above

10. Which of the following disorders is likely to have occurred previously in a patient who has the disorder described?
a) major depressive disorder
b) generalized anxiety disorder

c) childhood abuse or deprivation
d) childhood depression
e) infantile autism

11. Which of the following traits are often present in patients who present with this disorder?
a) decreased self-worth and self-esteem
b) poor identity formation
c) masochistic personality traits
d) all of the above
e) a and b only

12. What is the single most important factor in treating this disorder?
a) early recognition by the physician
b) long, drawn-out, protracted, weekly, repetitive psychoanalysis by a Freudian-type psychoanalyst
c) cognitive psychotherapy
d) behavioral-oriented psychotherapy
e) helping the patient understand how bizarre this really is

Short Answer Management Problem 63

Discuss the manner in which the condition described begins.

ANSWERS

1. D.

2. B. This patient has a factitious disorder of the predominantly physical subtype. This is known as *Munchausen syndrome*.

The essential feature of patients with this disorder is their ability to present physical symptoms so well that they are able to gain admission to a hospital. To support their history, the patients may feign symptoms suggestive of a disorder involving any organ system. They are familiar with most diagnoses in *Harrison's Principles of Internal Medicine*. They give excellent histories capable of deceiving even the most experienced physician.

The presentations that these patients manifest are myriad and include the following: hematoma, hemoptysis, abdominal pain, fever, hypoglycemia, lupus-like syndrome, nausea, vomiting, dizziness, and seizures. As well, the urine of these patients is often contaminated with blood or feces; anticoagulants are taken to simulate bleeding disorders; insulin is used to produce hypoglycemia. (These are just a few of the symptoms produced in this disorder and the lengths gone to produce disease.)

One of the most common acts in factitious disorder patients is the "heat the thermometer" syndrome. In this case, a patient who does not appear to be ill presents with a temperature of $\geq 104°F$. This is often produced by hot water or a hot lamp.

The patients may acquire what is classically referred to as a "gridiron abdomen" from the multiple procedures. Complaints of pain, especially that simulating renal colic, are common. The classical description of this patient includes someone who comes in seeking Demerol. In one of the typical scenarios, once the patient is in hospital he or she will continue to be demanding and difficult. As each test is returned and the result is negative, the patient may actually acuse the doctor of incompetence, threaten litigation, and become abusive. Some patients may discharge themselves abruptly; especially when and if they begin to suspect that the staff is catching on or when the staff begins to confront the patient.

From there the patient moves on to another hospital in the same or another city and the cycle begins again.

Some of the risk factors for this behavior and this disorder include the following:
1. Specific predisposing factors and true physical disorders during childhood leading to extensive medical treatment

2. A "grudge" against the medical profession
3. Employment as a medical professional or medical paraprofessional
4. Any type of important relationship with a physician in the past

3. E. Factitious disorder is more common in the following:
   A. Males
   B. Health care workers
   C. Health care professionals
   D. Individuals with a history of abuse in their family

4. E. The prevalence of factitious disorders in admissions to primary and secondary general hospitals in the United States is thought to be about 5%. This may seem high, but this disorder, like other serious disorders with grave psychological implications (such as spousal abuse), continue to be underestimated by health professionals.

5. E. The *Diagnostic and Statistical Manual of Mental Disorders—Fourth Edition* (DSM-IV) has established the following diagnostic criteria for factitious disorder:
   1. Intentional production or feigning of physical or psychological signs or symptoms
   2. The motivation for the patient is to assume the "sick role."
   3. External incentives for the behavior (such as economic gain, avoiding legal responsibility, or improving physical well-being) are absent.
   The subtypes of factitious disorder are as follows:
   A. Factitious disorder with predominantly psychological signs and symptoms (if psychological signs and symptoms predominate in the clinical presentation)
   B. Factitious disorder with predominantly physical signs and symptoms (if physical signs and symptoms predominate in the clinical presentation)
   C. Factitious disorder with combined psychological and physical signs (the classification when combined psychological and physical signs and symptoms are present, but neither predominate.

6. D. The most characteristic finding in factitious disorder is the multiple doctors, multiple referrals, multiple hospitals, and multiple surgical procedures. Although C is also correct (lying, failure to form close relationships, hostile manners, and so on), this is often seen in antisocial personality disorder. The symptoms produced by factitious disorder patients are voluntary, not involuntary.

7. C. Factitious disorder with predominantly physical signs and symptoms has been designated as *Munchausen syndrome.* This syndrome is named after an 18th-century German baron named Baron von Munchausen. Other names for the condition are hospital addiction, polysurgery addiction, and professional patient syndrome.

8. E. A patient who presents to your local ER with signs and/or symptoms of a factitious disorder may well self-inject insulin when not a diabetic, produce by bloodletting enough blood to simulate macroscopic or microscopic hematuria after mixed with urine, heat a thermometer either with hot water or under a lamp to produce a grossly elevated temperature reading, or mix feces with urine to simulate the possible diagnosis of an abdominal or pelvic fistula.

   All of these behaviors are designed by the patient to generate among his or her physicians and other health care workers an appearance of serious organic illnesses.

9. E. Any disorder in which the physical signs and symptoms are prominent should be considered in the differential diagnosis of factitious disorder. The possibility of many organic diseases that may mimic factitious disorder or are part of the total disease picture must be considered. The major differential diagnosis lies between factitious disorder and the following:
   A. Somatoform disorders: The somatoform disorders consist of the following:
      1. Somatization disorder: A factitious disorder is differentiated from somatization disorder (Briquet's syndrome) by the voluntary production of factitious symptoms, the extreme course of multiple hospitalizations, and the patient's seeming willingness to undergo an extraordinary number of mutilating procedures.
      2. Conversion disorder: A factitious disorder is differentiated from conversion disorder by the following: conversion patients are not usually conversant with medical terminology and hospital routines, and conversion patients have symptoms that bear a direct temporal relation or symbolic reference to specific emotional conflicts.
      3. Hypochondriasis: A factitious disorder is differentiated from hypochondriasis in that hypochondriac patients do not usually voluntarily initiate the production of symptoms, and hypochondriac patients typically have a later age of onset.
   B. Personality disorders: Antisocial personality disorder has been discussed. Histrionic personality disorder is associated with a "dramatic flair"; this, however, is not found in all factitious disorder patients. Borderline personality disorders and schizotypal personality disorders need to also be considered.
   C. Malingering: factitious disorders must be distinguished from malingering. Malingerers have an obvious recognizable, environmental goal in producing the signs and symptoms that they exhibit (for example, they don't want to return to work). Reasons for not wanting to return to work include financial renumeration or compensation (by far the

most common), evading the police, avoiding having to go back to a job that they detest, or simply wanting a free bed and room for the night.

D. Substance abuse: if a patient who has a documented factitious disorder also has a substance abuse problem, it is very important that the diseases be evaluated separately, diagnosed separately, investigated separately, and treated separately.

E. Ganser's syndrome: Ganser's syndrome is a controversial condition almost always found in inmates in penitentiaries. It is characterized by the subject's using an approximate answer. For example, patients with the disorder may respond to a simple question with astonishingly incorrect answers. For example, an inmate is asked the color of a blue sweater; he says, "red."

10. C. The most common quoted series of events associated with the etiology of factitious disorders is the following:
1. The patient's family of origin usually contained either a rejecting mother or an absent father.
2. There is a very high prevalence of child abuse and child deprivation with the patient in the family of origin.
3. The patient perceives one or both parents as rejecting figures who are unable to form close relationships.
4. The facsimile of genuine illness, therefore, is used to recreate the desired positive parent-child bond.
5. The disorder forms a repetition compulsion—repeating the basic conflict of needing and seeking acceptance and love while expecting that they will not be forthcoming. Therefore, the patient transforms the physician and staff members into rejecting parents.

11. D. Factitious disorder is associated with:
1) Decreased self-worth and self-esteem
2) Inadequate identity formation
3) Masochistic personality traits
4) Learned helplessness as a child if abuse was present
5) Tendency to seek approval from anyone and everyone

12. A. Treatment is best focused on management rather than on cure. The single most important factor in successful management of this condition is a physician's early recognition of the disorder before iatrogenic disease has precluded a condition beyond repair. Again, as with spousal abuse, for example, you will not make the diagnosis unless you think about the diagnosis!

SOLUTION TO SHORT ANSWER MANAGEMENT PROBLEM 63

Factitious disorders usually begin in early adult life. They occasionally begin in childhood or in adolescence. Characteristically, the following series of events begins the chain reac-

tion of doctors, referral to more doctors, admission to hospital, admission to more hospitals, voluntary discharge from hospital if the situation becomes uncomfortable, and quickly checking into a new hospital.

1. The onset of the disorder or of discrete episodes of treatment seeking may follow a real illness, a loss (and subsequent adjustment reaction), or an abandonment (and subsequent adjustment reaction).
2. Usually the patient or a close relative of the patient had a hospitalization in childhood or early adolescence for a genuine physical illness. Thereafter a long pattern of successive hospitalizations unfolds, beginning insidiously, and progressing in a spiral that is difficult to stop.

A SUMMARY OF THE DIAGNOSIS AND MANAGEMENT OF FACTITIOUS DISORDER

1. **Prevalence:** approximately 5% of admissions to primary and secondary care hospitals
2. **Etiology:** etiology is associated with child abuse in the family of origin, child deprivation in the family of origin, a mother who rejected the child, and a family who was absent a great percentage of the time, that is, a very traumatic childhood.
3. **The cycle begins:** the cycle begins in early adult life usually following discrete episodes of treatment seeking following a real illness. Thus, in factitious patients, usually either the patient or a close relative of the patient had a hospitalization in childhood or early adolescence for a genuine physical illness. Thereafter a long pattern of successive hospitalizations unfolds, beginning insidiously.
4. **Demographic characteristics:** factitious disorder is more common in males, hospital workers, and health care workers.
5. **DSM-IV criteria for factitious disorder:**
   a. Intentional production or feigning of physical or psychological signs or symptoms
   b. The motivation for the behavior is to assume the sick role.
   c. External activities for the behavior (such as economic gain, avoiding legal responsibility, or improving physical well-being (as in malingering) are absent.
   DSM-IV subtypes:
   1. Predominantly psychological signs and symptoms
   2. Predominantly physical signs and symptoms (Munchausen syndrome)
   3. Combined psychological and physical signs and symptoms
6. **Differential diagnosis of factitious disorder:**
   a) Somatoform disorders:
   1. Somatization disorder
   2. Conversion disorder
   3. Hypochondriasis
   b) Personality disorders:
   1. Antisocial personality disorder
   2. Histrionic personality disorder

c) Malingering: most important distinguishing feature of factitious disorder from malingering is that in malingering there is an obvious, recognizable, environmental goal in producing signs and symptoms.

d) Substance abuse syndrome

e) Ganser's syndrome: usually confined to the prison population. Patients intentionally give the wrong answers to questions.

7. **Course and prognosis:**

a) Begins in early adult life.

b) Usual history is one of severe, incapacitating trauma or untoward reactions.

c) Overall prognosis for establishing a normal life is very poor.

8. **Treatment:** most important factor in any kind of successful management is to get to the patient and make the diagnosis before the abdomen looks like a football field. If you don't think of the diagnosis, then you won't make the diagnosis!

SUGGESTED READINGS

American Psychiatric Association. Diagnostic and statistical manual. 4th Ed. Washington, DC: American Psychiatric Association Press, 1994.

Kaplan HI, Sadock BJ, Grebb JA. Synopsis of psychiatry/behavioral sciences/clinical psychiatry. 7th Ed. Baltimore: Williams and Wilkins, 1994.

PROBLEM 64   A 27-YEAR-OLD FEMALE WITH 22 DIFFERENT SYMPTOMS

A 27-year-old female presents to your office for an initial consultation. She has heard from her best friend that "you are the best in town."

The symptoms described include the following: chest pain, palpitations, "beating thyroid gland," nausea, periodic vomiting, abdominal pain, diarrhea, dizziness, gait disturbance, double vision, blurred vision, "seizures" (she falls down in the middle of crowds of people), pain on urination, pain in the back, pain in the abdomen, pain in the neck, headaches, feelings of a "frozen vagina," intolerance to fatty foods, intolerance to high-fiber foods, heartburn, and "constant gas."

She tells you in a very dramatic, effective, and authoritive manner, "I just can't take it any more, Doctor, and I guess that is why I have come to you. I hear you are so good!"

Although you know that you should pursue more of a past history, you (for some reason) don't feel like it and decide to take an educated guess as to the diagnosis.

SELECT THE ONE BEST ANSWER TO THE FOLLOWING QUESTIONS

1. What is your educated guess?
   a) somatization disorder
   b) conversion disorder
   c) somatoform disorder
   d) hypochondriasis
   e) masked depression

2. At this time, what would you do?
   a) step out of the room and ask your secretary to call you on your cellular phone, which is in your pocket
   b) interrogate the patient until you have the friend's name
   c) prescribe a benzodiazepine (alprazolam)
   d) make another appointment for the patient to go into the patient's past history and family history
   e) tell the patient that you have to deliver a baby and that you are planning on closing your practice next week

3. What is the treatment of choice for the disorder described?
   a) a benzodiazepine
   b) a tricyclic antidepressant
   c) an SSRI (selective serotonin reuptake inhibitor)
   d) an MAO inhibitor
   e) none of the above

4. A 23-year-old female presents to your office with a chief complaint of having "the most prominent jaw in the world." She tells you that she has seen a number of plastic surgeons about this problem, but every one has "refused to do anything."

   On examination, her jaw appears to you to be completely normal. There is no protrusion that you can see, and it appears to you that she has not only has a completely normal jaw but also a completely normal face.

   Her mental status examination and her *Beck Depression Inventory* suggest some degree of underlying depression.

   The rest of her physical examination is completely normal.

   What is the most likely diagnosis in this patient?
   a) dysthymia
   b) major depressive disorder—subtype: masked depression
   c) somatization disorder
   d) body dysmorphic disorder
   e) hypochondriasis

5. Therapies that have produced successful results in this disorder include which of the following?
   a) the antipsychotic drug *pimozide*
   b) an SSRI
   c) a tricyclic antidepressant
   d) individual or group psychotherapy
   e) all of the above

6. A 29-year-old female patient (and a mother of five) presents to your office with a "constant headache."

   After performing a complete history, a complete physical examination, and a complete laboratory and radiologic workup, you make the diagnosis of tension headache. She then tells you that she has seen a number of other physicians about the same problem and that they have come to the same conclusion (which she believes is totally incorrect). You ask her to return for a further discussion about this problem next week, shake hands, and are about to leave.

   Before you can leave, however, she says, "Oh, by the way, Doctor, I want to talk to you about my neck pain, my abdominal pain, my pelvic pain, and my rib pain." She goes on to say that she has been diagnosed as having fibromyalgia, but she also believes that this is completely incorrect as well.

   She very dramatically illustrates to you by walking with her four canes (she has two canes in each hand; each of the two canes serves a different purpose) that these multiple pain symptoms are producing profound difficulty in her occupational and social functioning.

You tell her that you will continue discussion of these problems with her when you see her next week. You again attempt to leave the office.

What is the most likely diagnosis in this patient?
a) fibromyalgia
b) somatoform pain disorder
c) pain disorder associated with psychological factors
d) somatization disorder
e) none of the above

7. What is the preferred treatment for this patient?
a) repeated weekly (daily if needed) visits with you
b) group psychotherapy
c) individual cognitive psychotherapy
d) individual behavior modification therapy
e) treatment in a multidisciplinary pain clinic

8. A 27-year-old patient presents to the ER with a complaint of "having suddenly gone blind." Apparently, she was walking down the street on her way to work and suddenly, she could not see.

The visual impairment that she describes is bilateral, complete (no vision), and associated with "complete numbness and tingling" in both lower extremities.

Her husband accompanies her to the ER and gruffly tells you, "Whatever it is, Doc, fix it and fix it fast."

The P/E of the patient suggests a significant difference between the subjective symptoms and the objective complaints. Specifically, both the knee jerks and the ankle jerks are present and brisk; there is, however, no motor power in either lower extremity.

Based on the information provided, what is the most likely diagnosis?
a) somatization disorder
b) conversion disorder
c) bilateral: ophthalmic artery occlusion and spinal artery occlusion
d) hysteria
e) none of the above

9. What is the most appropriate step at this time?
a) call ophthalmology stat
b) call neurology stat
c) call psychiatry stat
d) call social work stat
e) don't call anybody stat; there is a better solution

10. A 41-year-old male presents to you for his first visit. He was (as many of your patients seem to be) referred by a friend because he was told you were the best of the best.

He has come to you for a "complete cancer checkup."

This patient, you come to understand, has had eight complete cancer checkups already this year. He has had four of the eight done at "executive check-up cen-

ters." He is the CEO of one of the largest oil field repair companies in the United States and thus has the opportunity to take advantage of some "health perks." He kindly provides a list of the tests he wishes to have done:

They include a complete history, a complete physical examination, a complete lab profile (this includes 157 different tests), a colonoscopy, a gastroscopy, a skeletal survey, X-rays of all body parts, "head-to-toe" CT, and "head-to-toe" MRI.

You learn that this patient is very afraid that he has cancer, especially afraid that he has cancer of the colon. His third aunt three times removed had a colon cancer resected 2 years ago and advised him to "get checked as often as possible."

You are amazed that he actually has time to function as the CEO of his company. The truth is, however, that he doesn't. He admits that this fear is very greatly interfering with his work and social life.

What is the most likely diagnosis in this patient?
a) somatization disorder
b) hypochondriasis
c) Munchausen syndrome
d) single obsessive disorder
e) masked depression

11. What is the treatment of choice for the patient described?
a) weekly reassurance that he does not have cancer after performing all the tests he has requested
b) weekly assurance that he does not have cancer without performing all the tests he has requested
c) weekly assurance that he does not have cancer after refusing to perform all the tests he has requested
d) collaboration between yourself (the primary care physician) and a psychiatrist, the goal of which is the development of a plan for regularly assessing this patient's ongoing psychosocial history and its manifestations, educating the patient, and providing appropriate supportive, behavioral, and/or cognitive psychotherapy
e) all of d plus lithium carbonate prophylactically and an SSRI agent

12. The term *somatothymia:*
a) does not exist; it is a "red herring"
b) exists but is virtually useless from a practical standpoint
c) communicates the inability to express physical distress in psychological language
d) communicates the inability to express psychological distress in psychological-based verbal language
e) has nothing to do with existence, herrings, or language

Short Answer Management Problem 64

Describe the difference in classification (DSM-II-R versus DSM-IV) with respect to pain as a presenting feature in the group of disorders labeled *somatoform disorders*.

ANSWERS

1. A.

2. D.

3. E. This patient has somatization disorder. Somatization disorder is characterized by the following symptoms:

   A. Multiple physical complaints of long-standing occurrence
   B. These have usually resulted in significant medical diagnostic testing, medical intervention, and other iatrogenic problems.
   C. The symptoms have resulted in significant occupational or social malfunction.
   D. The symptoms that have occurred include symptoms that are not fully explained by a known medical condition or by clinical findings.
   E. The symptoms include pain symptoms in at least four different sites, including headache or related pain, abdominal pain, back pain, joint pain, extremity pain, chest pain, rectal pain, dyspareunia.
   F. The symptoms include two or more of the following gastrointestinal symptoms: nausea, diarrhea, bloating, vomiting, and food intolerance.
   G. The symptoms include one or more of the following sexual dysfunction symptoms: erectile or ejaculatory dysfunction, irregular or excessive bleeding, or decreased libido or indifference.
   H. The symptoms include one or more pseudoneurologic symptoms, including a conversion symptom or a dissociative symptom.

   In this patient another visit is reasonable to try and establish some reasonable baseline history and physical examination.

   Somatization disorder must be considered under the following principles:

   1. The presentation must be considered in terms of the psychosocial nature of the symptoms, both current and past.
   2. The diagnostic procedures and therapeutic interventions must be based on objective, rather than subjective, findings.
   3. The physician must form a good "therapeutic alliance" with the patient.
   4. The patient's social network and social support system must be both extensively reviewed and utilized to maximum potential.
   5. A regular appointment schedule must be established for the patient with the physician.
   6. The dialogue that occurs between doctor and patient must address symptoms and signs from a somatic viewpoint.
   7. The need for referral should be recognized early, especially in chronic cases where "many physicians have been involved and done many things."
   8. The physician should assume that a coexisting or underlying psychiatric disorder exists until proven otherwise.
   9. The significance of personality features, addictive potential, and self-destructive behavior must be determined and addressed.
   10. The therapeutic alliance between physician and patient must be refocused to address the problem from the perspective of management rather than cure.

4. D.

5. E. This patient has body dysmorphic disorder.

   Body dysmorphic disorder is a condition characterized by the following:

   A. A preoccupation with an imagined or grossly exaggerated bodily defect.
   B. Clinically apparent distress associated with social, occupational, or functional impairment.
   C. Anorexia nervosa, psychotic, or other psychiatric disorder cannot account for the preoccupation and the impairment.

   The differential diagnosis of body dysmorphic disorder includes the following:

   A. Anxiety disorder
   B. Major depressive disorder
   C. Hypochondriasis
   D. Other somatoform disorders
   E. Factitious disorders
   F. Malingering

   Associated features of body dysmorphic disorder include the following: "doctor shopping," medication problems, conflicting opinions from multiple physicians, and iatrogenic disease.

Therapies that have been found to be most helpful are pharmacologic in nature. They include the SSRI inhibitors, the tricyclic antidepressants, the MAO inhibitors, and the antipsychotic drug-pimozide. Ideally, one or more of these pharmacologic therapies should be combined with the general principles discussed for somatization disorders discussed in the previous question, and either individual or group psychotherapy.

6. C.

7. E. The diagnosis in this patient is *pain disorder associated with psychological factors*. The treatment of choice for this patient is treatment is a multidisciplinary pain clinic. In DSM-II-R the disorder was identified as somatoform pain disorder but was changed to pain disorder associated with psychological factors in DSM-IV.

The criteria for pain disorder associated with psychological factors are as follows:
1. Pain is the prominent clinical presentation and is of sufficient severity to require assessment.
2. The pain results in social, occupational, or functional impairment or clinically significant distress.
3. Psychologic factors precipitate, exacerbate, or maintain the pain, or contribute to the severity of the pain.
4. The pain is not a component of somatization disorder or other psychiatric disorders including sexual dysfunction.

In many situations, however, the patient may have a bona fide physical illness (such as lumbar disk disease), but psychological factors appear to predominate. If the medical disorder appears to be present and be making a significant contribution to the patient's pain complaints, then the patient may be diagnosed with pain disorder associated with both psychological factors and a general medical condition.

As many as 40% of pain patients exhibit pain that is psychogenic in origin. Pain that is associated with prominent psychological features is diagnosed in women twice as frequently as in men. Evidence exists to suggest a familial pattern, with first-degree biological relatives being at higher risk for developing the disorder. A known familial pattern that includes a history of anxiety, depression, or alcohol dependence occurs at greater frequency than would be expected in the general population.

The differential diagnosis of pain must take into consideration other psychiatric syndromes such as somatization disorder, depressive disorder, malingering, and psychophysiologic disorders, hypochondriasis, or primary anxiety disorder.

Full appreciation of the etiologic factors involved in any form of pain that appears to be exacerbated by psychological factors is complicated because the clinician must account for secondary gain or reinforcement.

Psychological tests, most commonly the Minnesota Multiphasic Personality Inventory (MMPI) are used routinely to identify psychological factors.

In treating patients with pain disorder associated with psychological factors the initial strategy is to minimize doctor shopping and other interpersonal games while establishing a strong therapeutic alliance. A major task is to convince patients that they must work to modify their therapeutic expectations and attempt to manage or live with their pain.

A number of nonpharmacologic treatments are useful in chronic pain syndromes, including transcutaneous nerve stimulation, biofeedback, and other forms of behavioral psychotherapy. The tricyclic antidepressants often afford pain relief, especially desipramine, amitriptyline, and nortriptyline. However, the overall best management for a patient with a chronic pain syndrome that fulfills the criteria of DSM-IV is treatment at a multidisciplinary pain clinic. This treatment may take several weeks or longer; the overall success of this approach, however, appears much better than any other approach.

8. B.

9. E. This patient has a conversion disorder. Conversion disorders represent a type of somatoform disorder in which there is a loss or alteration in physical functioning that suggests a physical disorder but that cannot be explained on the basis of known physiologic mechanisms. Conversion disorders are usually seen in ambulatory care settings or emergency departments. Conversion symptoms are exceedingly common; estimates of 20% to 25% prevalence are given for patients admitted to a general medical setting. General hospital patients have consistently shown conversion symptoms in 5% to 14% of all psychiatric consultations.

Conversion symptoms result from stressful environmental events acting on the affective part of the brain in predisposed individuals. The DSM-IV criteria for conversion disorder are as follows:
1. The symptom(s) or deficit(s) are under voluntary control, affecting motor or sensory function. This suggests a medical condition.
2. The initiation or exacerbation of the symptom(s) or deficit(s) is preceded by conflicts or stressors, psychologic factors are prominent.
3. The symptom(s) or deficit(s) are not consciously or intentionally produced.
4. The symptom(s) or deficit(s) are not fully explained after clinical assessment as a medical condition or culturally sanctioned phenomenon.
5. The symptom(s) or deficit(s) impair social or occupational functioning, create significant distress, or require medical intervention.

6. The symptom(s) or deficit(s) are not limited to pain or sexual dysfunction or are not a component of somatization disorder or other psychiatric syndrome.

Common examples of conversion symptoms include paralysis, abnormal movements, aphonia, blindness, deafness, or pseudoseizures.

In this patient, the first consideration would be some type of domestic violence, particularly spousal abuse, as a cause of the conversion disorder symptoms. This would certainly fit in with the demands of the individual accompanying her. If this is true, therapy should be directed at treating the abuse first and foremost. If it is not the reason for the conversion disorder, it should nonetheless be asked about.

A wide variety of treatment techniques have been successfully used for the treatment of conversion disorder. Brief psychotherapy focusing on stress and coping and suggestive therapy and sometimes hypnosis may be extremely effective. A short hospitalization may also be helpful, particularly when symptoms are disabling or alarming. Hospitalization may serve to remove the patient from the stressful situation, demonstrating the importance of psychological factors. This would be a prime consideration in this patient.

10. B.

11. D. This patient has the disorder known as hypochondriasis. Hypochondriasis is defined as a concern with health or disease in one's self that is present for the major portion of time. The preoccupation must be unjustified by the amount of physical pathology and must not respond more than temporarily to clear reassurance given after a thorough examination. The core features of hypochondriasis consist of a complex of attitudes: disease fear, disease conviction, and bodily preoccupation with multiple somatic complaints. On presentation, the medical history is often related in great detail in the context of doctor-shopping, deteriorating doctor-patient relationships, and associated feelings of frustration and anger. The clinical course is chronic, with waxing and waning of symptoms.

The DSM-IV diagnostic criteria for hypochondriasis include the following:

1. A preoccupation or fear of serious disease with misinterpretation of bodily symptoms for 6 months or longer
2. Medical evaluation and reassurance are ultimately not therapeutic.
3. The preoccupation is not delusional or is not consistent with body dysmorphic disorder or not a component of another psychiatric disorder.
4. Significant social, occupational, or functional impairment occurs together with clinically significant distress.

The differential diagnosis of hypochondriasis includes other anxiety disorders, major depressive disorder, factitious disorders (including Munchausen syndrome), malingering, and psychotic disorders manifesting hypochondriacal delusions.

Munchausen syndrome would be the number one differential diagnosis. It is less likely because there is no evidence of pathologic lying or recurrent, feigned, or simulated illness.

The most crucial management technique in caring for the hypochondriacal patient is the inclusion of a legible psychosocial history in a prominent place in the patient's record. The general principles in caring for patients with somatization disorders should be followed.

Generally, the most effective treatment takes place in the context of collaboration with a family physician, a psychiatrist, and other health care workers such as a psychologist and social workers. Regular visits are essential to monitor symptoms, monitor anxiety and/or depression associated with the hypochondriacal symptoms, and help the patient come to terms with the condition.

12. D. The term *somatothymia* conveys the inability or the limited capacity of some individuals to articulate their feelings and intrapsychic conflicts in psychologically based verbal language.

SOLUTION TO SHORT ANSWER MANAGEMENT PROBLEM 64

The fundamental difference between DSM-III-R and DSM-IV regarding the symptom of pain is found in the change in terminology regarding from "somatoform pain disorder" to "pain disorder associated with psychological factors."

Pain is a prominent symptom in somatoform disorders and must be completely evaluated. As well, the symptom of pain must be considered in both a medical-based context and a psychological-based context. The symptom of pain cannot and should not be dismissed; neither must it be misinterpreted as something it is not. The most fundamental question requiring an answer is this: is this symptom of pain expressed primarily a symptom of a physical disorder or is it a symptom of a psychological disorder?

SUMMARY OF THE DIAGNOSIS AND TREATMENT OF SOMATOFORM DISORDERS

This chapter has produced extensive discussion of somatoform disorders. The summary, therefore, will be concise and short.

1. **Somatization disorder:**
   Diagnostic clues: multiple physical complaints with onset before the age of 30. Tendency of these complaints is to be both chronic and long-standing. The complaints involve each of the following: pain symptoms, GI symp-

toms, sexual dysfunction symptoms, and pseudoneurologic symptoms. There is impairment of social or occupational functioning associated with these symptoms.

2. **Conversion disorder:**
   Diagnostic clues: physical symptoms primarily involving neurologic symptoms are produced because of psychologic conflicts or stressors. They cannot be fully explained on an anatomical basis and result in impairment in social or occupational functioning. Conversion disorder often involves patients in the lower socioeconomic classes; it may also be a manifestation of a disturbed family or marital situation.

3. **Pain disorder associated with psychological factors:**
   Diagnostic clues: Pain is the prominent clinical presentation, and it results in social, occupational, or functional impairment. This diagnosis is made when psychological factors are believed by the physician to have a very significant role in the outset, severity, exacerbation, or perpetuation of the pain syndrome. Major depression and/or anxiety are often present and may be a component of the pain syndrome. The best therapeutic strategy is to limit doctor-shopping and modify the patient's therapeutic expectations from cure to management of the pain while attempting to appreciate the role of psychosocial or psychological factors, as well as stress. A multidisciplinary pain clinic is, in many or most of the patients, the treatment of choice.

4. **Hypochondriasis:**
   Diagnostic clues: hypochondriasis is characterized by a concern or preoccupation with health or disease in oneself that is present most of the time and is not justified by physical pathology. The core features of the disease include disease fear, disease conviction, and bodily preoccupation associated with multiple amplified somatic complaints. As with pain, the possibility of an underlying or secondary anxiety or depression should be strongly considered, and physical disease should be excluded. Treatment is most effective when there is collaboration between a primary care physician who continues regular appointments and a consulting psychiatrist. Again, the diagnosis requires significant social, occupational, or functional impairment.

5. **Body dysmorphic disorder:**
   Diagnostic clues: the fundamental diagnostic feature is a pervasive feeling of ugliness or physical defect that the patient believes is readily apparent to others. Patients frequently consult multiple primary care physicians, derma-

tologists, and plastic surgeons. Depressive symptoms, anxiety symptoms, obsessive personality traits, and psychosocial distress frequently coexist. Intervention focuses on psychosocial distress and group or family therapy as appropriate.

6. **Malingering:**
   Diagnostic clues: the essential feature of malingering is the intentional production of illness consciously motivated by external incentives such as avoiding military duty, obtaining financial compensation through litigation or disability, evading criminal prosecution, obtaining drugs, or securing better living conditions. Malingering should be suspected when medical/legal context overshadows the presentation, marked discrepancy exists between the clinical presentation and objective findings, and a lack of cooperation is experienced with the patient. Confrontation in a confidential and empathic but firm manner that allows an opportunity for constructive dialogue and appreciation of any psychological or psychosocial problems is imperative.

7. **Somatoform disorders as a public health problem:**
   a) 60%-80% of Americans have at least one somatization symptom/week.
   b) The economic costs of somatization are enormous: one study performed over 10 years ago established the cost for physicians seeing people with somatization symptoms at $20 billion (10% of the nation's total annual health care budget). We can assume that this figure has increased in proportion to the nation's rising health care costs since that time.
   c) Predictions suggest that this public health problem is going to increase as an increasingly stress-filled world predominates in a backdrop of family disruption, rapid cultural change, and attention to and care of the body.

SUGGESTED READINGS

American Psychiatric Association. Diagnostic and statistical manual. 4th Ed. Washington, DC: American Psychiatric Association, 1994.

Folks D, Ford CV, Houck CA. Somatoform disorders, factitious disorders, and malingering. In: Stoudemire A, ed. Clinical psychiatry for medical students. 2nd Ed. Philadelphia: JB Lippincott, 1994.

Goodman B. When the body speaks, who listens? Psychology Today 1995; 28(1):26-28.

PROBLEM 65   A 29-YEAR-OLD FEMALE WITH A POUNDING HEART, SHORTNESS OF BREATH, CHEST PAIN, DIZZINESS, AND FEELINGS THAT SHE IS "LOSING HER MIND"

A 29-year-old female teacher presents to your office with recurrent attacks of anxiety associated with a "pounding heart," "shortness of breath," "chest pain," dizziness, and "feelings that she is losing her mind."

These attacks have been ongoing for at least 8 months and only seem to occur during school days. She tells you that these symptoms begin when she gets up in front of the class in the morning.

When you question her carefully, you learn that she also develops what she describes as "fear" when she gets into crowded stores or shopping malls.

Her past history includes what a child psychiatrist labeled as *separation anxiety*. She states that her mother ran away with another man when she was 5 years old, and she was raised by her father.

Her physical examination is essentially unremarkable. Her blood pressure is 130/70 mm Hg and the examination of the CV system and the respiratory system is normal, as is the rest of the examination.

SELECT THE ONE BEST ANSWER TO THE FOLLOWING QUESTIONS

1. What is the most likely diagnosis in this patient?
   a) pheochromocytoma
   b) hyperthyroidism
   c) panic disorder
   d) paroxysmal atrial fibrillation
   e) generalized anxiety disorder

2. The symptom that this patient displays in relationship to her "fear of crowded stores or shopping malls" is known as the following:
   a) social phobia
   b) specific phobia
   c) claustrophobia
   d) agoraphobia
   e) generalized phobia

3. Which of the following is(are) characteristic of this disorder?
   a) smothering sensations
   b) fear of going crazy
   c) fear of not being able to control a particular situation
   d) fear of dying
   e) all of the above

4. The "phobia" that is described in the case and that is specified in Question 2 is characterized by which of the following?
   a) an intense fear of being in public places
   b) acute bursts of terrifying levels of anxiety
   c) avoidance of places where help may be unavailable or escape is difficult
   d) a loss of contact with reality, including hallucinations and delusions
   e) a, b, and c
   f) all of the above

5. Which of the following is(are) true of the disorder described in the case history?
   a) it is more common in males
   b) it usually begins in middle age
   c) it is rarely confused with coronary artery disease
   d) none of the above
   e) all of the above

6. Which of the following statements regarding the pharmacologic treatment of the disorder described in this case is(are) true?
   a) pharmacologic therapy is effective in blocking the symptoms of the disorder described
   b) pharmacologic therapy is effective in treating the "avoidance" of the specific situation
   c) a combination of pharmacologic therapy, psychoeducation, and biofeedback may be very helpful in the treatment of this disorder
   d) all of the above
   e) a and c only

7. What is the "gold standard" against which all other pharmacologic treatments must be measured?
   a) alprazolam
   b) phenelzine
   c) clomipramine
   d) desipramine
   e) amitriptyline

8. Which of the following drugs has recently been shown to be very effective in the treatment of this condition?
   a) imipramine
   b) phenelzine
   c) paroxetine
   d) atenolol
   e) alprazolam

9. A 29-year-old musician consults you regarding what he describes as "an intense fear" before he begins his

nightly performance with a world-famous orchestra. He tells you that it is only a question of time before he "really makes a major mistake."

What is the most likely diagnosis in this patient?
a) a specific phobia
b) a social phobia
c) a mixed phobia
d) panic disorder without agoraphobia
e) panic disorder with agoraphobia

10. What is the treatment of choice for the patient described in Question 9?
a) alprazolam prior to his nightly music performance
b) phenelzine prior to his nightly performance
c) atenolol prior to his nightly performance
d) clomipramine prior to his nightly performance
e) paroxetine prior to his nightly performance

Short Answer Management Problem 65

List four psychiatric disorders with which the condition described in the case presentation at the beginning of this chapter is associated?

ANSWERS

1. C. The most likely diagnosis in this patient is panic disorder. Panic disorder is defined as recurrent episodes of panic attacks (discrete periods of intense fear or discomfort) associated with other symptoms including dyspnea, dizziness, trembling, palpitations, choking sensations, nausea, feelings of depersonalization, numbness, hot flushes, chest pain, a fear of dying, a fear of going crazy, or a fear of not being able to control a situation to which you may be exposed.

   Although organic disease must be considered (especially thyroid dysfunction), the constellation of symptoms is almost diagnostic of panic disorder.

2. D. Agoraphobia is characterized by the following clinical features: an intense fear of being alone or in a public place; acute bursts of terrifying levels of anxiety (panic attacks); fear of panic attacks or other calamities leading to chronic anxiety and restriction of activities, often to the point of becoming housebound; and avoidance of supermarkets, shopping malls, church services, meetings, parties, elevators, tunnels, bridges, buses, subways, and other places where help is unavailable or escape is difficult.

3. E. Symptoms of a panic attack include the following:
   A. A discrete period of intense fear or discomfort, in which at least four of the following symptoms develop abruptly and reach a peak within 10 minutes:
   i) Palpitations, pounding heart, or accelerated heart rate
   ii) Sweating
   iii) Trembling or shaking
   iv) Sensations of shortness of breath or smothering
   v) A feeling of "choking"
   vi) Chest pain or discomfort
   vii) Nausea or abdominal distress
   viii) Feeling dizzy, unsteady, lightheaded, or faint
   ix) Derealization (feelings of unreality) or depersonalization (becoming detached from oneself)
   x) Fear of losing control or going crazy
   xi) Fear of dying
   xii) Paresthesia (numbness or tingling sensations)
   xiii) Chills or hot flushes

4. E. As discussed in the answer to Question 2, agoraphobia has the characteristics that are listed in choices a, b, and c.

   Agoraphobia is not, however, characterized by a loss of contact with reality, although patients may complain of "being in a daze" or "being in a fog" (feelings of derealization or depersonalization).

5. D. Panic disorder is a common medical illness. It usually begins in the twenties or thirties, although children and elders may develop the disorder. It is twice as common in women as it is in men.

   Genetic and epidemiologic studies have consistently demonstrated increased rates of panic disorder among first- and second-degree relatives of panic disorder patients. This could be a result of genetic factors, nongenetic biological factors, and/or cultural factors shared by family members. Between 15% and 18% of first-degree relatives of patients with panic disorder develop the condition.

   Chest pain is a common presenting complaint among patients with panic disorder. Many patients with chest pain have even been referred for coronary angiography. Other than cardiovascular symptoms, the two most common classes of symptoms are neurologic symptoms and gastrointestinal symptoms.

6. E. Pharmacologic treatments for panic disorder up to now have centered on treating the symptoms produced by the disorder itself. Pharmacologic agents have not really been effective in treating the "avoidance" of the actual panic-inducing situation itself. This may change in the future with the development of newer drugs (discussed later) that have been shown to be effective in the treatment of the panic disorder itself.

At this time, the best therapy for panic disorder is as follows:

A. Pharmacologic treatment (discussed below)
B. Behavioral treatment including the following:
   i) Graduated exposure to the phobic situation
   ii) Cognitive therapy (reduces irrational beliefs)
   iii) Relaxation training and biofeedback
   iv) Panic control treatment (PCT): comprised of breathing retraining, cognitive restructuring, and exposure to somatic cues
   v) Assertiveness training (can help with dependency, passivity, and suppressed anger)
   vi) Psychoeducation (a presentation of knowledge to the patient that includes symptoms, theories of causation, reassurance that what they believe will happen will actually not happen, and treatment strategies
   vii) Group therapy (which helps confirm to individuals with panic disorder that they are not alone)

7. C. The "gold standard" of pharmacologic therapy for panic disorder (and the agent against which all others must be measured) is the tricyclic antidepressant clomimipramine.

The "groups" of agents that have been tried and that have proven effective in patients up to this time include the following:

A. The tricyclic antidepressants: clomipramine is the "gold standard." Very close to clomipramine is imipramine.
B. The monoamine oxidase inhibitors: monoamine oxidase inhibitors such as phenelzine and tranylcypromine are effective at reducing the anxiety associated with panic disorder. The concern regarding a low tyramine diet is an issue that can be looked on as giving panic disorder patients "one more thing to worry about."
C. The benzodiazepines: the benzodiazepine of choice is alprazolam. This group of drugs should probably be tried, however, only after other drugs have failed due to concerns regarding discontinuation. Other commonly used agents in this class include lorazepam, clonazepam, and diazepam.

   Although the nonbenzodiazepine anxiolytic agent buspirone is effective in treating generalized anxiety disorder, it is probably ineffective in treating panic disorder.

D. The beta-blockers: although the beta blockers may block symptoms such as palpitations and tremor they are generally not as effective in treating panic attacks as either the tricyclic antidepressants, the MAO inhibitors, or the benzodiazepines.

The new pharmacologic approach to treatment of panic disorder will be discussed in the following question.

8. C. The drug that has recently been demonstrated to be extremely effective in treating panic disorder is *paroxetine,* a selective serotonin reuptake inhibitor. The starting dose is 20 mg/day.

It may well be the case that the other SSRI agents such as fluoxetine, sertraline, and fluvoxamine are just as effective. Paroxetine *(Paxil)* has, however, been studied in more patients up to this time.

9. B.

10. C. This patient has what is referred to as *performance anxiety* and is classified as a social phobia. This social phobia is really quite special, though, and is not at all uncommon. More often than not it is only in the situation of performance of the particular activity in question that symptoms develop.

The treatment of choice in this patient is a beta-adrenergic blocking agent. The most commonly used agents at this time include atenolol, oxprenolol, and metoprolol. Although propranolol is considered "the gold standard," a more selective beta blocker (selective in not crossing the blood-brain barrier) will not produce the side effects of lightheadedness or dizziness.

SOLUTION TO SHORT ANSWER MANAGEMENT PROBLEM 65

Attempts to "decrease the anxiety" associated with panic attacks and panic disorder may in fact cause individuals to self-medicate. This leads to a possible association between panic attacks, alcoholism or substance abuse.

Because of the nature of the symptoms, individuals with panic attacks and panic disorder more commonly develop other associated psychiatric conditions. These include generalized anxiety disorder and major depressive disorder.

SUMMARY OF THE DIAGNOSIS AND TREATMENT OF PANIC DISORDER

1. **Prevalence:**
   a) Lifetime prevalence: 1.4% to 1.5%
   b) Lifetime prevalence: 2.4-4.3 times greater for females than males
2. **Genetics:** risk of panic disorder in first-degree relatives of patients is 15% to 18%.

3. **Biochemistry:**
   a) Yohimbine, an alpha-2 adrenergic receptor antagonist, produces greater increases in the plasma levels of norepinephrine metabolite MHPG in panic disorder than in healthy subjects. This responsiveness appears to be specific for panic disorder.
   b) Preclinical studies have suggested possible serotonergic involvement in anxiety (this is compatible with newer pharmacologic therapies).

4. **Symptoms:**
   a) A panic attack is diagnosed when there is intense fear or discomfort associated with 4/10 of (1) palpitations/pounding heart/tachycardia, (2) sweating, (3) trembling or shaking, (4) shortness of breath/smothering, (5) choking, (6) chest pain/discomfort, (7) nausea/abdominal distress, (8) derealization/depersonalization, (9) fear of dying, (10) fear of losing control/going crazy, (11) paresthesiaes, (12) dizzy/unsteady/lightheaded, (13) chills/hot flushes
   b) Recurrent attacks of (a) above = panic disorder
   c) Panic disorder is subclassified according to whether or not it is accompanied by agoraphobia. Agoraphobia is defined as anxiety about being in places or situations in which escape might be difficult (or embarrassing) or in which help may or may not be available in the event of having an unexpected or situationally predisposed panic attack.

      Agoraphobia may involve travel, driving, proximity of safety, public places, or other situations such as sitting in a meeting or waiting in line.

5. **Concurrent psychiatric conditions:** panic disorder is associated with the following:
   a) Alcoholism
   b) Substance abuse
   c) Generalized anxiety disorder
   d) Major depressive disorder

6. **Treatment:**
   a) Nonpharmacologic:
      1. Behavioral treatment: gradually increasing exposure
      2. Cognitive therapy (reduces irrational beliefs, especially "I am going crazy," and so on)
      3. Biofeedback/relaxation therapy
      4. PCT = panic control treatment: this helps the patient to focus on breathing retraining, cognitive restructuring, and exposure to somatic cues (may be effective in desensitization).
      5. Assertiveness training: deals with dependency issues from childhood (high correlation of panic disorder with previous separation anxiety as a child); passivity; suppressed anger
      6. Psychoeducation: education about all aspects of the condition, especially the fact that it is common
      7. Group therapy: sharing of experiences reinforces item 6.
   b) Pharmacologic:
      1. Gold standard: clomipramine (a TCA) (close second: imipramine)
      2. MAO inhibitors
      3. Benzodiazepines: especially alprazolam
      4. Beta blockers (especially for social phobia: performance anxiety)
      5. SSRIs (especially paroxetine = Paxil) may become the drug of first choice very quickly.

SUGGESTED READINGS

American Psychiatric Association. Diagnostic and statistical manual. 4th Ed. Washington, DC: American Psychiatric Association Press, 1994.

Nagy L, Krystal JH, Charney DS. Anxiety disorders. In: Stoudemire A, ed. Clinical psychiatry for medical students. 2nd Ed. Philadelphia: JB Lippincott, 1994.

PROBLEM 66   A 22-YEAR-OLD LAW STUDENT WHO IS UNABLE TO ANSWER QUESTIONS IN CLASS

A 22-year-old law student presents to your office in a state of anxiety. He is currently taking a law class in which 50% of the class mark is based on class participation. Although he knows the material well, he is unable to answer the questions when posed to him by the professor. He has now gone through 2 months of the 6-month class and has not been able to answer one of the 14 questions that the professor has asked him in class.

The professor asked him to make an appointment for a "little chat" the other day. At that time, he was told that he would (in the professor's words) fail the class unless he began to participate.

The student describes himself as a loner. He tells you that he has always been shy, but this is the first time the shyness has really threatened to have a major impact on him.

His family history is significant for what he terms "this shyness."

His mother has the same characteristics, but for her it doesn't seem to be causing the kind of "life difficulties" it is causing for him.

His mental status examination is essentially normal.

SELECT THE ONE BEST ANSWER TO THE FOLLOWING QUESTIONS

1. What is the most likely diagnosis in this patient?
   a) panic disorder with agoraphobia
   b) panic disorder without agoraphobia
   c) panic disorder with social phobia
   d) social phobia
   e) specific phobia

2. Which of the following IS NOT a characteristic of the disorder described?
   a) persistent fear of humiliation
   b) exaggerated fear of humiliation
   c) embarrassment in social situations
   d) high levels of distress in particular situations
   e) fear of crowds or fear of closed in spaces

3. Which of the following physiologic symptoms is not characteristic of the disorder described?
   a) blushing
   b) trembling
   c) bradycardia
   d) sweating
   e) elevated blood pressure

4. The neurochemical basis of the disorder described is most closely associated with which of the following neurotransmitters or neurohormones?
   a) epinephrine
   b) norepinephrine
   c) serotonin
   d) a and b only
   e) all of the above

5. Pharmacologic intervention is one component of the treatment of this disorder. Which of the following pharmacologic agents has, until recently, been the drug of choice for this disorder?
   a) clonazepam
   b) alprazolam
   c) phenelzine
   d) a and b only
   e) all of the above

6. With respect to this disorder, which of the following drugs has(have) recently been shown to be of marked benefit in its treatment?
   a) fluoxetine
   b) sertraline
   c) risperidone
   d) a and b only
   e) all of the above

7. A change in nomenclature has recently occurred in relationship to certain phobias. This change has been to do which of the following?
   a) group all phobias under the general term *panic disorder*
   b) group all phobias under the general term *specific phobias*
   c) change the disorder name *simple phobia* to *specific phobia*
   d) change the disorder name *specific phobia* to *simple phobia*
   e) eliminate the classification of *with or without agoraphobia* that previously applied to panic disorder

8. A 73-year-old male is brought to your office by his wife. His wife states that for the "past 20 years this man has really never slept; he usually manages to keep me awake as well, and I am tired of it." She goes on to tell you that she thinks that he has had "Alzheimer's disease" for the past 10 years but will not admit it. She has heard that "shock

treatments once a day for a year will often work in these cases," and she asks you to "book him in."

Before you do any "booking," you decide that it may be in your best interest to obtain more detailed information.

In private, the patient tells you that "the old bird is exaggerating." He admits to having difficulty with sleep, but it didn't seem to be a problem for anyone until he lost his job as a customer service attendant at a 24-hour convenience store 1 year ago. Prior to that, he would work 6 nights/week at the convenience store and run his contracting business during the day (usually working all 7 days "to keep out of the old bird's hair").

You begin to get the impression that there is more here than meets the eye. On careful questioning you find out that he was a veteran of the Korean War and was "decorated for bravery with several medals." You further learn that it was during this time that his sleep habits became irregular for the first time. After the war, everything settled down for about 10 years, but after that he became (as he describes) "just unable to sleep."

What is the most likely diagnosis in this patient?
a) insomnia
b) obstructive sleep apnea
c) cataplexy
d) masked depression and anxiety
e) none of the above

9. Characteristics of this disorder include which of the following?
a) recurrent and intrusive recollections of some memories
b) efforts to avoid thinking about what has happened in the past
c) irritability or outbursts of anger
d) a and b only
e) all of the above

10. Regarding the treatment of the disorder described, which of the following statements is(are) true?
a) treatment relies on a combination of nonpharmacologic and pharmacologic treatments
b) nonpharmacologic treatment centers on the learning of behaviors to avoid anxiety from the conditioned stimulus
c) tricyclic antidepressants have been used with some success in the treatment of this disorder
d) monamine oxidase inhibitors have been used with some success in the treatment of this disorder
e) all of the above statements are true

11. Which of the following drugs is contraindicated in the treatment of this disorder?
a) lithium carbonate
b) phenelzine
c) fluoxetine
d) alprazolam
e) desipramine

12. At this time (although further studies are needed to confirm this), which of the following drugs is tentatively considered the best drug to treat all symptom clusters in this disorder?
a) lithium carbonate
b) phenelzine
c) fluoxetine
d) alprazolam
e) desipramine

13. A 26-year-old male, recently married, presents to your office with his new wife. They have been married for 3 months, and she tells you that she is very concerned about "some of his behaviors." Apparently, when they go out the door in the morning and close the garage door, he goes around the block "at least eight times to make sure it is closed." Also, when he washes his hands before a meal, he will often go back and wash them at least three or four times during the meal itself "just to make sure they are clean."

The husband sits there and doesn't really have anything to say. He lived with his parents until he was married and his wife tells you that apparently he "was always very well-protected" by his mother.

When the patient finally begins to talk he admits that everything his wife has just told you is true; he goes on to add, however, that his behaviors are simply "a way of protecting her."

His past history is fairly unremarkable except for his "being a loner." Both his family and his mother have a history compatible with depression.

What is the most likely diagnosis in this patient?
a) atypical depression
b) schizophreniform disorder
c) obsessive-compulsive disorder
d) SPP (spousal protective phobia)
e) specific phobia

14. Until very recently, the drug of choice for the treatment of this disorder has been which of the following?
a) clomipramine
b) phenelzine
c) lithium carbonate
d) buspirone
e) pimozide

15. A new agent that appears (initially, and up to this point) to be the "new" drug of choice is which of the following?
a) fluvoxamine
b) fluoxetine
c) buspirone
d) trazodone
e) sertraline

Short Answer Management Problem 66

List five common obsessions and five common compulsions associated with obsessive-compulsive disorder.

ANSWERS

1. D. This patient has a social phobia.

   Social phobias are characterized by a marked and persistent fear of one or more social or performance situations in which the person is exposed to unfamiliar people or to possible scrutiny by others. They fear that they may act in a manner that will be humiliating or embarrassing. Examples include (as in this patient) not being able to talk when asked to speak in public, choking on food when eating in front of others, being unable to urinate in a public lavatory, hand-trembling when writing in the presence of others, and saying foolish things or not being able to answer questions (as in this patient) in social situations.

   In addition to these, exposure to the feared social situation almost invariably provokes anxiety; the individual realizes that his or her behavior is abnormal and unreasonable; the feared social or performance situation is either avoided or endured with intense anxiety; and the avoidance, anxious participation, or distress in the feared social or performance situation interfere significantly with the person's normal routine, occupational (or, in this case, academic) functioning, or social activities and relationships with others.

2. E. Fear of crowds (in which escape may not be possible) is known as *agoraphobia*. Fear of closed spaces is known as *claustrophobia*. The other characteristics of social phobia are discussed in the answer to Question 1.

3. C. The fear of speaking, meeting people, eating, or writing in public is related to the fear of "appearing nervous or foolish," making mistakes, being criticized, or being laughed at. Physical symptoms include blushing, trembling, sweating, elevated blood pressure, and tachycardia (not bradycardia).

4. E. Symptoms reported by social phobia patients in phobic situations suggest heightened autonomic arousal. When placed in a phobic situation, social phobics experience significant increases in heart rate that are highly correlated with self-perceived physiologic arousal (in contrast to claustrophobics, who experience less heart rate increase and negative correlations between perceived and actual physiologic arousal). Stressful public speaking situations result in two- or threefold increases in plasma epinephrine levels. Norepinephrine increases are also seen.

   Until recently, the answer to this question would be d: epinephrine and norepinephrine only. However, now that the new SSRI agents have been shown to be effective in social phobic situations, serotonin is also involved. In this case, it would seem that social phobics would demonstrate a relative deficiency of serotonin rather than an excess as seen with epinephrine and norepinephrine. Thus the answer is e: all of the above.

5. C. Up until this time, the drugs of first choice for the treatment of social phobias have been the monamine oxidase inhibitors, specifically phenelzine (45-90 mg/day).

   In addition to the MAOs, the other drug groups that have been shown to be effective in social phobias have been the beta blockers (such as atenolol 50-100 mg/day) and the benzodiazepines (especially alprazolam 0.75 mg-1.5 mg bid).

6. D. Recently the selective serotonin reuptake inhibitors have been shown to be of marked benefit in the treatment of social phobias. This would suggest, as has been discussed previously, that in addition to the neurochemical basis of epinephrine/norepinephrine, social phobics also have a relative serotonin deficiency. The two SSRIs that in clinical trials have proven effective have been fluoxetine (Prozac) and sertraline (Zoloft).

7. C. The DSM-III name for the disorder *simple phobia* has been changed to *specific phobia* in the DSM-IV and differentiated from other anxiety disorders, including obsessive compulsive disorder, post-traumatic stress disorder, panic disorder with agoraphobia, agoraphobia without history of panic disorder, and social phobia.

8. E. The most likely diagnosis in this patient is post-traumatic stress disorder. The "clue" to the diagnosis is his involvement in the Korean War and the temporal association between the insomnia and that particular time in his life. Further discussion follows.

9. E. There are five major categories of criteria for the diagnosis of post-traumatic stress disorder listed in the DSM-IV:

   I. The person has experienced or witnessed an event that involves death, threat to life, or serious injury to himself or others that was experienced with intense fear, helplessness, or horror.

   II. The traumatic event is persistently reexperienced in ways such as recurrent and intrusive distressing recollections, dreams, feelings of thoughts that the event is recurring, psychological distress at exposure to symbolic events of that time, and physiologic reactivity upon exposure to cues of that event.

III. Persistent avoidance of stimuli associated with the trauma or numbing of general responsiveness, including efforts to avoid thoughts or feelings of the event; efforts to avoid activities, situations, or people associated with the event; inability to recall some aspect of the event (psychologic amnesia); feelings of detachment or distance from others; diminished ability to have "affective feelings"; and a sense of a foreshortened future

IV. Persistent symptoms of *increased arousal* (this is very common in war veterans) indicated by difficulty falling or staying asleep, irritability or outbursts of anger, difficulty concentrating, hypervigilance, and exaggerated startle response

V. Duration of symptoms must be at least 1 month.

VI. The disturbance causes marked distress or significant impairment in social or occupational functioning.

10. E.

11. D.

12. C. As with other anxiety disorders, treatment for posttraumatic stress disorder often is best accomplished with a combination of pharmacologic and nonpharmacologic therapies. It has been suggested that pharmacologic treatment may be required to control the physiological symptoms enabling the patient to tolerate working through the highly emotional material in psychotherapy.

The treatment of PTSD is often complicated by comorbid disorders. The most common of these disorders are alcoholism and other substance abuse.

In terms of psychotherapies the following is known:

A. Behavioral therapies including systematic desensitization and flooding produce a decrease in reexperiencing and hyperarousal, but not in avoidant/numbing symptoms.

B. Cognitive therapy has been found to be effective through stress inoculation training (relaxation, thought sleeping, breathing control, communications skills, and cognitive restructuring) to reduce PTSD symptoms early in treatment; long-term results appear improved when combined with prolonged exposure.

C. Hypnotherapy has produced results similar to desensitization, with more improvement in reexperiencing symptoms and less improvement in avoidance.

D. Psychodynamic therapy, on the other hand, had a greater effect on avoidance and less effect on reexperiencing.

There are few controlled trials to make a very informed decision regarding the superiority of one class of drugs over another in the treatment of this disorder. Both phenelzine (an MAO) and imipramine (a TCA) have been shown to reduce intrusion (reexperiencing symptoms) but not to affect avoidance terms.

Alprazolam (a benzodiazepine used in some phobic situations) is relatively contraindicated in this patient due to the sleep disorder that this patient has experienced.

Again, as with many other phobias, the SSRIs are appearing to come out on top in initial studies; fluoxetine, for example, was effective in treating all three symptom clusters. Confirmatory evidence is awaited with interest.

Other drugs that have shown some efficacy include clonidine, propranolol (both of which relieved startle, explosiveness, nightmares, and intrusive reexperiencing), lithium (which decreased autonomic arousal and reexperiencing of symptoms), and buspirone.

13. C.

14. A.

15. A. This patient has obsessive-compulsive disorder. Obsessive-compulsive disorder consists of either recurrent obsessions or recurrent compulsions.

The recurrent obsessions include persistent thoughts, impulses, or images that the patient attempts to ignore but that cannot be ignored. Additionally, the obsessions are not just excessive worries about real-life problems; the patient also recognizes that these obsessions are, in fact, the product of his or her own mind.

Common obsessions include obsessions regarding contamination or illness; violent images; fear of harming others or harming oneself; perverse/forbidden sexual thoughts, images, or impulses; symmetry or exactness; somatic situations; or religious thoughts.

Compulsions are repetitive behaviors or mental acts that the individual feels driven to perform in response to an obsession or according to rigid rules. The behavior or mental act is aimed at preventing or reducing distress or preventing a dreaded event or situation. These behaviors, however, are not connected in a realistic manner with what they are designed to neutralize or prevent and are clearly excessive.

The individual realizes that the compulsions are excessive and unreasonable. They caused marked distress in the person's life or significantly interfere with the person's normal routine, occupation, or social activities.

Common compulsions include checking things (door locks, water taps, and so on), cleaning and/or washing articles or parts of the body, counting objects or things, hoarding or collecting articles or things, ordering or arranging articles or things, or repeating things.

Until very recently, the "gold standard" of pharmacologic therapy for obsessive-compulsive disorder has been clomipramine. At this time, however, the SSRIs (selective serotonin reuptake inhibitors) have become the drugs of choice. Of the SSRIs, the single best agent in trials to date appears to be fluvoxamine. Other SSRIs found to be effective include fluoxetine and sertraline.

SOLUTION TO SHORT ANSWER MANAGEMENT PROBLEM 66

Here are some common obsessions:
1. Obsessions re: contamination and illness
2. Obsessions re: fear of harming others or self
3. Obsessions re: perverse/forbidden sexual thoughts, images, or impulses
4. Obsessions re: violent images
5. Obsessions re: symmetry/exactness
6. Obsessions re: somatic complaints/conditions
7. Obsessions re: religious thoughts

Here are some common compulsions:
1. Compulsions re: "checking" (doors, locks, and so on)
2. Compulsions re: cleaning or washing
3. Compulsions re: counting objects of various types
4. Compulsions re: hoarding or collecting objects of various types
5. Compulsions re: ordering/arranging articles of various types
6. Compulsions re: repeating things, speech, and so on

SUMMARY OF THE DIAGNOSIS AND TREATMENT OF SOCIAL PHOBIA, POST-TRAUMATIC STRESS DISORDER, AND OBSESSIVE-COMPULSIVE NEUROSIS

1. **Social phobia:**
   a) Epidemiology: estimated 6-month prevalence rate of social phobia is 1.2% to 2.2%.
   b) Definition: social phobia can be regarded as persistent and overwhelming fear of one or more social or performance situations in which the individual is exposed to unfamiliar people or to possible scrutiny by others. Fear of speaking in public, hand-trembling, and answering questions are particular examples. The fear is one of not being able to perform the particular activity and of being humiliated in public because of this. It produces both embarrassment and high levels of distress.

   The individual either avoids the situation or endures it with intense anxiety. The individual also realizes that the fear is unreasonable but is powerless to do anything about it. As well, the individual ex-periences occupational, social, or academic interference with normal life schedule and/or goals because of it.
   c) Symptoms: not only is intense anxiety and fear produced but also symptoms of autonomic hyperactivity, such as blushing, trembling, tachycardia, and elevated blood pressure.
   d) Neurochemistry: probable excess of norepinephrine and epinephrine; probable deficiency of serotonin
   e) Treatment:
      1. Nonpharmacologic:
         i) Behavioral techniques and cognitive restructuring
      2. Pharmacologic:
         i) Drug class of choice at this time: the SSRI inhibitors: fluoxetine and sertraline
         ii) Other drug classes of benefit:
            i) MAO inhibitors, particularly phenelzine
            ii) Beta blockers: atenolol, oxprenolol, propranolol
   f) Concomitant disorders: one-third of patients with social phobia report a history of major depressive disorder.

2. **Post-traumatic stress disorder:**
   a) Epidemiology: particularly important and common in war veterans. Lifetime prevalence rates as high as 30% have been reported.
   b) Definition: Post-traumatic stress disorder can be defined as an immediate or a delayed response to a catastrophic life event. The symptoms include recurrent or intrusive distressing recollections of the event, recurring distressing dreams of the event, fear and feelings of recurrence of the event, psychologic distress at exposure to events that symbolize or resemble the event, and physiologic reactivity upon exposure to internal or external cues. As well, there is persistent avoidance of stimuli associated with the trauma or numbing of the general responsiveness and persistent symptoms of increased arousal (such as being unable to fall or stay asleep).
   c) Examples of typical traumatic events that can generate post-traumatic stress disorder:
      1. Combat or war experiences
      2. Serious accidents (automobile, bus, plane, or train crashes)
      3. Natural disasters (tornado, hurricane, flood, or earthquake)
      4. Physical assault (rape, physical or sexual abuse, mugging, or torture)
      5. Other serious danger of death or severe injury to oneself
      6. Witnessing the mutilation, serious injury, or violent death of another person
   d) Treatment:
      1. Nonpharmacologic therapy:
         i) Behavioral therapy
         ii) Psychodynamic therapy

iii) Hypnotherapy
iv) Cognitive therapy
2. Pharmacologic therapy:
Drug classes that have been shown to be effective for various symptom complexes include the following:
   i) The SSRIs (may become the drugs of choice); initially appear to be drug class of choice to treat all symptom clusters
   ii) The MAO inhibitors
   iii) The tricyclic antidepressants
   iv) The beta blockers
   v) Central alpha-antagonists (clonidine)
   vi) Anti-manic agents: lithium
   vii) Nonbenzodiazepine anxiolytics: buspirone
e) Risk factors for development of PTSD: the risk factors for development of PTSD include separation from parents during childhood, family history of anxiety, preexisting anxiety or depression, family history of antisocial behavior, female sex, and neuroticism.

3. **Obsessive-compulsive disorder:**
a) Epidemiology: The measured 6 month prevalence rate has been estimated at 2% to 3%.
b) Definition: Obsessive-compulsive disorder is a mental disorder in which either *obsessions* (recurrent distressing thoughts, ideas, or impulses) are experienced as both unwanted and senseless but at the same time irresistible. *Compulsions* are repetitive, purposeful, intentional behaviors, usually performed in response to an obsession, which are recognized as unrealistic and unreasonable but are again irresistible.
c) Common obsessions and compulsions: See the solution to Short Answer Management Problem 66.

d) Treatment:
   1. Nonpharmacologic:
      i) Prolonged exposure to ritual-eliciting stimuli together with prevention of the compulsive response.
   2. Pharmacologic:
      i) Gold standard: clomipramine
      ii) Clomipramine is quickly being replaced by the SSRI inhibitors, especially fluvoxamine, but including fluoxetine and sertraline.
      iii) MAO inhibitors
      iv) Lithium carbonate
      v) Benzodiazepines
      vi) Trazodone
e) Coexisting disorders:
   1) Other anxiety disorders
   2) Eating disorders
   3) Gilles de la Tourette's syndrome
   4) Schizophrenia
   5) Separation anxiety in childhood

SUGGESTED READINGS

American Psychiatric Association. Diagnostic and statistical manual. 4th Ed. Washington, DC: American Psychiatric Association Press, 1994.

Nagy L, Krystal J, Charney DS. Anxiety disorders. In: Soudemire A, ed. Clinical psychiatry for medical students. 2nd Ed. Philadelphia: JB Lippincott, 1994.

PROBLEM 67   A 65-YEAR-OLD HYPERTENSIVE MALE WITH IMPOTENCE

A 65-year-old male with hypertension, congestive cardiac failure, and peptic ulcer disease presents to your office for his regular blood pressure check. You have managed to effectively control his blood pressure. Although his blood pressure is now under control, he complains of an inability to maintain an erection. He is currently taking the following medications: alpha-methyldopa, propranolol, verapamil, hydrochlorothiazide, and cimetidine.

On examination, his blood pressure is 140/70 mm Hg. His pulse is 56 and regular. The rest of the cardiovascular examination and the rest of the physical examination are normal.

SELECT THE ONE BEST ANSWER TO THE FOLLOWING QUESTIONS

1. Which of the medications listed is the least likely to be the cause of this man's sexual dysfunction?
   a) alpha-methyldopa
   b) propranolol
   c) verapamil
   d) hydrochlorothiazide
   e) cimetidine

2. Which of the following is the most common cause of sexual dysfunction in both males and females?
   a) pharmacologic agents
   b) panic disorder
   c) generalized anxiety disorder
   d) major depressive disorder
   e) dysthymia

3. Which of the following agents, previously thought not to be a cause of sexual dysfunction, has recently been shown to affect sexual dysfunction?
   a) captopril
   b) labetalol
   c) hydromorphone
   d) hydralazine
   e) methadone

4. Which of the following is the most common sexual dysfunction in males?
   a) hypoactive desire disorder
   b) erectile disorder
   c) orgasmic disorder
   d) premature ejaculation
   e) none of the above

5. Which of the following is the least likely sexual dysfunction in males?
   a) hypoactive desire disorder
   b) erectile disorder
   c) orgasmic disorder
   d) premature ejaculation
   e) none of the above

6. Which of the following statements regarding the etiology of male sexual dysfunction is most accurate?
   a) male sexual dysfunction is almost always psychologic in origin
   b) male sexual dysfunction is almost always organic in origin
   c) psychologic factors seem to predominate in male sexual dysfunction, both in primary and secondary forms
   d) male sexual dysfunction in a younger patient has a greater probability of being organic in origin
   e) male sexual dysfunction in an older patient has a greater probability of being psychologic in origin

7. Which of the following organic disorders is the most common cause of organic male sexual dysfunction?
   a) benign prostatic hypertrophy
   b) hyperthyroidism
   c) Parkinson's disease
   d) diabetes mellitus
   e) atherosclerosis of the abdominal aorta

8. What is the single most important aspect of the evaluation of male sexual dysfunction?
   a) the history
   b) the physical examination
   c) nocturnal penile tumescence measurement
   d) ratio of penile/brachial blood pressure
   e) serum testosterone measurement

9. Which of the following investigations is(are) indicated in a male patient with sexual dysfunction?
   a) CBC
   b) BUN, serum creatinine
   c) thyroid function studies
   d) serum testosterone level
   e) all of the above

10. Which of the following is(are) important in the treatment of male sexual dysfunction?
    a) reducing performance anxiety by prohibiting intercourse
    b) anxiety reductions by identification and verbalization

c) introduction of the process of "sensate focus"
d) instruction in interpersonal communication skills
e) all of the above

11. Which of the following is specifically indicated as a treatment for premature ejaculation?
a) the penile squeeze technique
b) the injection of testosterone
c) structured behavior modification programs
d) the intermittent injection of medroxyprogesterone
e) interarterial penile injection of local vasoconstrictors

12. A 24-year-old female who has been married for 6 months presents to your office in tears. She and her husband have been unable to have sexual intercourse. She says that when he tries to penetrate her she "tenses up" and is "unable to go any further."

Her past significant history includes being raped at the age of 12. The patient has vivid memories of this event.

Her general physical examination is normal. You do not attempt a vaginal examination.

Which of the following statements regarding vaginismus is false?
a) most women with vaginismus also have difficulty with sexual arousal
b) there is a strong association between vaginismus and an intense childhood and adolescent exposure to religious orthodoxy
c) there is a strong association between vaginismus and a traumatic sexual experience
d) vaginismus is a condition of involuntary spasm or constriction of the musculature surrounding the vaginal outlet
e) vaginismus may begin with a poorly healed episiotomy following childbirth

13. Regarding the diagnosis and treatment of vaginismus, which of the following statements is false?
a) throughout the diagnostic examination the woman must feel that she is in control and may terminate the examination at any time
b) the diagnosis of vaginismus can often be made without inserting a speculum
c) the sexual partner should be involved in all aspects of the treatment process
d) the insertion of vaginal dilators is not a recognized part of the treatment protocol
e) "sensate focus techniques" are an important part of the treatment protocol

14. Which of the following is the most common female sexual dysfunction disorder?
a) orgasmic disorder: anorgasmy
b) orgasmic disorder: delayed orgasm

c) hypoactive sexual desire disorder
d) sexual aversion disorder
e) none of the above

15. Which of the following statements regarding female sexual arousal disorder is false?
a) sexual arousal disorder is more common in women than in men
b) the diagnosis takes into account the focus, intensity, and duration of the sexual activity
c) if sexual stimulation is inadequate in focus, intensity, or duration, the diagnosis cannot be made
d) sexual arousal disorder in women is not associated with inadequate vaginal lubrication
e) female sexual arousal disorder is often associated with inhibited female orgasm

16. Of the following listed causes, which is the most common cause of hypoactive sexual desire disorder in women?
a) major psychiatric illness
b) major psychiatric illness in the woman's partner
c) dual-career families, with increased responsibilities on the woman both at work and in the home
d) major physical illness in the woman
e) alcoholism in the woman's partner

17. Which of the following statements regarding the orgasmic disorder "inhibited female orgasm" is false?
a) inhibited female orgasm is the most common female sexual dysfunction
b) primary anorgasmia is more common among unmarried women than among married women
c) women over the age of 35 years have increased orgasm potential
d) women may have more than one orgasm without a refractory period
e) fear of impregnation is a common cause of inhibited female orgasm

18. Which of the following statements regarding dyspareunia is(are) true?
a) it may be caused by endometriosis
b) it may be caused by vaginitis or cervicitis
c) it may be caused by an episiotomy scar
d) all of the above
e) none of the above

19. Which of the following methods is(are) useful in the treatment of female sexual dysfunction?
a) sexual anatomy and physiology education
b) sensate focus exercises
c) treatment of underlying anxiety and depression
d) none of the above
e) all of the above

20. Which of the following major psychiatric conditions is most closely linked to sexual dysfunction?
    a) panic attacks/panic disorder
    b) generalized anxiety disorder
    c) major depressive disorder
    d) schizoaffective disorder
    e) schizophrenia

Short Answer Management Problem 67

Describe the goal, selection, types, and duration of sexual dysfunction psychotherapies most commonly practiced today.

ANSWERS

1. C.

2. A.

3. A. Drugs are definitely the most common cause of sexual dysfunction. Although drugs are more of a problem in males than in females, they have certainly been shown to have a major effect in women as well as men. Many different classes of drugs have been implicated in sexual dysfunction, with the main offenders being the antihypertensive drugs; the tricyclic antidepressants; the major tranquilizers; and other miscellaneous drugs including lithium, digoxin, indomethacin, antiparkinsonian drugs, and cimetidine.

    Here is a safe rule to follow: "assume that the dysfunction is due to drugs until proven otherwise."

    In the patient described in Question 1, the only antihypertensive agent that has not been associated with sexual dysfunction is verapamil (a calcium-channel blocker).

    Recently ACE inhibitors (particularly captopril) have been associated with sexual dysfunction. One recent study has confirmed that 19% of males taking captopril have worsening of their sexual function.

4. D.

5. B. The estimated prevalence of male sexual dysfunction among the general population is as follows:
    1. Premature ejaculation: 37%
    2. Hypoactive sexual desire disorder: 16%
    3. Orgasmic disorder: 7%
    4. Erectile disorder: 6%

6. C. The etiology of male sexual dysfunction may be psychologic, organic, or a combination of both. Psychologic dysfunction predominates, even when a significant organic factor is present. As well, male organic sexual dysfunction is complicated by the relationship of the male with his partner. In young men, most cases of male sexual dysfunction will be psychologic in origin. In older men, as the incidence of concurrent disease rises, so does the prevalence of organic sexual dysfunction.

7. D. Diabetes mellitus is the most common organic cause of male sexual dysfunction. The pathophysiology of diabetes-induced male sexual dysfunction is diabetic neuropathy.

    Other common causes of organic male sexual dysfunction include the following:
    A. Atherosclerotic vascular disease
    B. Congestive heart failure
    C. Renal failure
    D. Hepatic failure
    E. Respiratory failure
    F. Genetic causes (Klinefelter's syndrome)
    G. Hypothyroidism
    H. Hyperthyroidism
    I. Multiple sclerosis
    J. Parkinson's disease
    K. Surgical procedures:
        1. Radical prostatectomy
        2. Orchidectomy
        3. Abdominal-perineal colon resection
        4. Radiation therapy

8. A. The single most important aspect in the evaluation of male (and female) sexual dysfunction is the history. For example, in a patient with an erectile disorder, if erections are achieved under certain conditions but not others, the likelihood is high that the dysfunction is psychogenic. Normal erectile function during masturbation, extramarital sex, and in response to erotic material suggests a psychologic cause. Similarly, if a normal erection is lost during vaginal insertion, a psychologic cause is suspected. A complete drug history is essential.

    The history should include present and previous birth control, a complete past psychiatric history, a complete family history; a history of surgical procedures, a history of the marital relationship, and a history of present job satisfaction and hours of work. The recurrence or persistence of the presenting sexual problem should be sought.

A complete physical examination should be performed. The physical examination will determine whether there is any evidence of organic pathology associated with the sexual dysfunction.

Measurement of nocturnal penile tumescence (most simply done using a strain gauge), the ratio of penile/brachial blood pressure, and the serum testosterone are investigations that have an important role to play in the overall evaluation of impotence, but they do not take the place of a good history.

9. E. Based on the organic etiologies discussed in the answer to Question 7, baseline screening bloodwork is indicated. This should include a CBC, BUN and serum creatinine, fasting blood sugar, fasting cholesterol, thyroid function studies, liver function tests, and a serum testosterone level.

10. E. Most cases of sexual dysfunction have, as discussed previously, a very significant psychological component. After a complete history, a complete physical examination, screening bloodwork, and discontinuation of offending medications, the treatment of male sexual dysfunction (and female sexual dysfunction) has several important steps:
    A. Reduction or, hopefully, elimination of performance anxiety by prohibiting intercourse
    B. Anxiety reduction by identification and verbalization of the problem
    C. Introduction of the process of sensate focus (semistructured touching that will permit focus on sensory awareness without any need to perform sexually)
    D. Instruction to interpersonal communication skills

11. A. The initial treatment of premature ejaculation is the same as other therapies described here. In addition, an exercise known as the "penile squeeze technique" is used to raise the threshold of penile excitability. The penis is stimulated until impending ejaculation is perceived. At this time, the woman squeezes the coronal ridge of the glans penis, resulting in diminished erection and inhibited ejaculation. Eventually, with repeated practice, the threshold for ejaculatory inevitability is raised.

12. A. *Vaginismus* is defined as recurrent or persistent involuntary spasm of the musculature of the outer third of the vagina that interferes with coitus.

There is a strong association between vaginismus and an intense childhood and adolescent exposure to religious orthodoxy. Vaginismus may occur when an episiotomy fails to properly heal following childbirth. Most women with vaginismus have normal sexual arousal.

In this patient, the etiology of vaginismus is most likely from the traumatic sexual experience that took place during her childhood.

13. D. The evaluation and treatment of vaginismus begins with a carefully performed physical examination in which the patient is always in full control. She may terminate the examination at any time.

On inspection of the external genitalia, spasm and rigidity of the perineal muscles are often felt. In this case, the diagnosis can be made even without inserting a speculum. From inspection, the examination may proceed to the insertion of one or more of the examiner's fingers.

The use of vaginal dilators in gradually increasing sizes has proved helpful in the treatment of vaginismus. Beginning with the smallest size, the woman inserts these herself until she becomes both comfortable and relaxed with their insertion. When the largest plastic dilator can be inserted, the couple can proceed to intercourse.

The partner must be involved in all aspects of assessment and treatment. Ideally, he should be present to observe the entire evaluation and treatment. Together with anatomy and physiology education, the couple learns the concept of sensate focus exercises, which play a major part in the therapy of any sexual dysfunction.

14. C. The most common female sexual dysfunction disorder is hypoactive sexual desire disorder. It is present in 34% of women according to one study. Orgasmic disorder, on the other hand, is present in 4% to 9% in the same study. The prevalence of female arousal disorder, dyspareunia, and vaginismus are less clear.

15. D. *Female sexual arousal disorder* is defined as persistent or recurrent partial or complete failure to attain or maintain the lubrication-swelling response of sexual excitement until completion of the sexual activity. The diagnosis includes the subjective sense of sexual excitement and pleasure and requires the focus, the intensity, and the duration of stimulation to be adequate.

Sexual arousal disorder is often associated with inhibited female orgasm.

16. C. *Hypoactive sexual desire disorder* is defined as persistent or recurrent deficient or absent desire for sexual activity. The definition includes a lack of sexual fantasies. The major reasons for hypoactive sexual desire disorder are major marital dysfunction, in which the lack of desire to have sexual intercourse is a symptom of the dysfunction, and a change in the family structure from single-career families to dual-career families. The woman now, as well as having major work responsibilities, is still often left with the majority of the child care and home care in the evenings. By the time she gets everything done, she is "just too tired for sex."

17. A. *Inhibited female orgasm* is defined as persistent or recurrent delay in, or absence of, orgasm in a female following a normal sexual excitement phase during sexual activity. The definition takes into account the adequacy of focus, intensity, and duration of the sexual activity.

   Inhibited female orgasm (as one of the orgasmic disorders) is not the most common disorder of female sexual dysfunction (4%-9%). It is surpassed by hypoactive sexual desire disorder (34%).

   Primary anorgasmia (never having had an orgasm) is more common in unmarried women than in married women. Women over the age of 35 appear to have an increased orgasmic potential.

   Women may have more than one orgasm without a refractory period.

   Causes for inhibited female orgasm include fear of impregnation, rejection by the woman's sexual partner, hostility toward men, and feelings of guilt regarding sexual impulses.

18. D. *Dyspareunia* is defined as recurrent or persistent genital pain before, during, or after sexual intercourse. This dyspareunia cannot be caused exclusively by lack of lubrication or by vaginismus.

   In many cases, however, vaginismus and dyspareunia are closely associated. Other causes of dyspareunia include episiotomy scars, vaginitis, cervicitis, endometriosis, postmenopausal vaginal atrophy, and anxiety regarding the sexual act itself.

19. E.

20. C. One approach often used in the therapy of sexual dysfunction in couples is called *the LEDO approach.* The LEDO approach centers on the following:
   1. Lowering stress, tension, and anxiety levels through discussion, examination, and observation
   2. Ensuring that both parties understand each other's desires, pleasures, and difficulties
   3. Determining the partner's genuine awareness and knowledge of their own and each other's sexual autonomy and the process of intercourse
   4. Outlining, drawing, and explaining alternative approaches to arousal and excitation and intercourse techniques

   In the absence of other psychiatric pathology (remembering that the most common psychiatric condition associated with sexual dysfunction is major depressive illness in one or both mates), dual sex therapy is the most accepted approach to the treatment of sexual dysfunction.

   The sexual problem often reflects other areas of marital disharmony or marital misunderstanding. The marital relationship as a whole is treated, with emphasis on sexual functioning as a part of that relationship. Both a female and a male therapist should be involved in the treatment of the couple's sexual problem. The therapy is short-term and behaviorally oriented. The goal is to reestablish communication within the marital unit. Information regarding anatomy and physiology are given. Specific sensate focus exercises are prescribed. The couple proceeds from nongenital touching and sensory awareness to genital touching to sensory awareness to genital touching and finally to intercourse. The couple learns to communicate with each other through these graded exercises.

   If underlying major depressive disorder, dysthymia, generalized anxiety disorder, or other anxiety disorders are present, they must be treated separately.

SOLUTION TO SHORT ANSWER MANAGEMENT PROBLEM 67

The answer to this question is really a refinement of, reinforcement of, and expansion of the Ledo approach to sexual dysfunction psychotherapies.

I. Goal: resolution of specific sexual dysfunctions
II. Selection:
   1. Couples: all sexual dysfunction psychotherapy should ideally be performed with both partners.
   2. Sexual dysfunction most suited for psychotherapy:
      a) Impotence
      b) Premature ejaculation
      c) Vaginismus
      d) Orgasmic dysfunction
   3. Make sure all medical causes are ruled out.
III. Types of psychotherapies employed:
   1. Behavior modification techniques (including systemic desensitization), homework, and education
   2. Psychodynamic approaches
   3. Hypnotherapy
   4. Group therapy
   5. Couples therapy as needed to deal with system dynamics
IV. Duration: weeks to months

SUMMARY OF THE DIAGNOSIS AND TREATMENT OF SEXUAL DYSFUNCTION DISORDERS

1. **Prevalence:** it is extremely difficult to estimate the prevalence of sexual dysfunction disorders. However, estimates have stated that 40% of American couples at one time or another have sexual dysfunction of some type.
   b) Prevalence of certain disorders:
      1. Males:
         i) Premature ejaculation: 37% (most common)
         ii) Hypoactive sexual desire: 16%
         iii) Orgasmic disorder: 6%
         iv) Erectile disorder: 7%

   2. Females:
      i) Hypoactive sexual desire: 34% (most common)
      ii) Dyspareunia/vaginismus: n/a
      iii) Orgasmic disorder: 7%

2. **Most common causes:**
  a) Pharmaceutical agents appear to be the most common cause of sexual dysfunction—antihypertensives and mood-modifying drugs are especially important.
  b) Diabetes mellitus is the single most common organic disorder responsible for sexual dysfunction. (See the complete list in the answer to Question 7.)
  c) Remember that psychological causes are the predominant cause of most sexual dysfunction disorders.

3. **Approach to sexual dysfunction:**
  a) Always begin by treating this relationship in reference to the couple.
  b) Complete histories from both partners
  c) Complete physical examinations
  d) Laboratory testing must include CBC, renal function, liver function, thyroid function, blood glucose, serum cholesterol, and hormone levels (testosterone, FSH, LH, estrogen, and progesterone).
  e) Remember association between dyspareunia/vaginismus and previous sexual abuse.
  f) Remember the possibility of family violence in the present (such as wife abuse leading to rape).
  g) Use the LEDO general approach.
  h) Utilize the guidelines described in the solution to the Short Answer Management Problem.

SUGGESTED READINGS

American Psychiatric Association. Diagnostic and statistical manual. 4th Ed. Washington, DC: American Psychiatric Association Press, 1994.

Fagan PJ, Schmidt CW. Psychosexual disorders. In: Stoudemire A, ed. Clinical psychiatry for medical students. 2nd Ed. Philadelphia: J.B. Lippincott, 1994.

PROBLEM 68   A 29-YEAR-OLD WORKING MOTHER WITH THREE CHILDREN WHO IS UNABLE TO COPE

A 29-year-old mother who holds a full-time out-of-the-home job has just gone back to work after the birth of her third child. The child is currently 6 weeks old. She works as a registered accountant for a major American oil company. Her company is currently going through downsizing. Her husband has just lost his job as an assembly line worker at one of the major automobile corporations.

When she returned to work, she was immediately made to feel guilty by the upper management for "taking so much time off to have a baby" when they (all men) were loaded down with work. She is staying up to 3 AM and 4 AM to get her work done every evening. At this time, she has virtually no time to spend with her children. She is crying, fatigued, and absolutely exhausted after 10 days back on the job. She tells you, "I just can't take it any longer. I have to work to pay the mortgage and put food on the table. There are no other jobs available. What am I going to do? I just can't go on this way."

She finds herself becoming "very sleepy every day at work," and the management has commented on that as well.

She has no history of previous psychiatric problems, previous sleep disorders, family history of psychiatric disorder, or personal or family history of drug or alcohol use. She is not taking any drugs at present.

SELECT THE ONE BEST ANSWER TO THE FOLLOWING QUESTIONS

1. What is the major diagnosis in this patient at this time?
   a) major depressive disorder
   b) generalized anxiety disorder
   c) adjustment disorder
   d) dysthymia
   e) panic disorder

2. How is the "sleep disorder" that this patient exhibits most properly labeled?
   a) psychophysiologic insomnia
   b) adjustment sleep disorder
   c) inadequate sleep hygiene
   d) insufficient sleep syndrome
   e) idiopathic hypersomnolence

3. You decide to initiate psychotherapy. At this time, in this patient, and given this diagnosis, what is the single best psychotherapy to use?
   a) cognitive psychotherapy
   b) brief psychodynamic psychotherapy
   c) behavioral psychotherapy (behavior modification)
   d) supportive psychotherapy
   e) intensive psychoanalytically oriented psychotherapy

4. What is the major goal of the psychotherapy in this patient's situation?
   a) identify and alter cognitive distortions
   b) understand conflict area and particular defense mechanisms used
   c) maintain or reestablish the best level of functioning
   d) eliminate involuntary disruptive behavior patterns and substitute appropriate behaviors
   e) resolve symptoms and rework major personality structures related to childhood conflicts

5. What is the first priority at this time?
   a) foster a good working relationship with the patient
   b) approach the patient as a "blank screen"
   c) develop a "therapeutic alliance" with the patient
   d) begin the assignment of tasks for the patient to complete
   e) develop "free association" with the patient

6. What is the second priority at this time?
   a) reinforce and agree with her concerns; reinforce the fact that, given the circumstances, her feelings are prefectly normal
   b) act as a guide or mentor to help the patient extricate herself from her current working environment
   c) prescribe a hypnotic to "get things under control"
   d) have the patient "intellectualize" her concerns
   e) have her "lie down on the old couch" and act like "good old Dr. Freud"

7. Which of the following is(are) technique(s) of supportive psychotherapy?
   a) supporting intellectualization
   b) develop a short-term "mentoring" relationship
   c) develop a short-term "guiding" relationship
   d) suggest, reinforce, advise, and reality test
   e) all of the above

8. Which of the following psychotherapies has been shown to be most efficacious in the treatment of psychiatric conditions encountered in primary health care settings?
   a) intensive analytically oriented psychotherapy
   b) psychoanalysis
   c) cognitive psychotherapy
   d) brief psychodynamic psychotherapy
   e) behavioral psychotherapy

9. A 39-year-old female presents to your office with a 4-month history of depression. She meets the DSM-IV criteria for major depressive illness. She was started on sertraline 6 weeks ago and it appears to be helping significantly. Which of the following statements is(are) true regarding the therapeutic approach to this patient?
   a) most primary care physicians treat major depressive illness only with antidepressant medication
   b) supportive psychotherapy is the ideal psychotherapy for this patient
   c) there is little evidence to support a combination of medication plus psychotherapy in preference to psychotherapy alone
   d) brief psychodynamic psychotherapy has been shown to be the most effective psychotherapy when used with an SSRI (selective serotonin reuptake inhibitor)
   e) none of the above statements are true

10. Which of the following statements regarding cognitive psychotherapy is(are) true?
    a) the cognitive psychotherapist sees the interpretations that depressed patients make about life as different than those of nondepressed patients
    b) cognitive psychotherapy is best suited to patients who have unipolar, nonpsychotic illness

   c) cognitive psychotherapy is generally conducted over a period of 15 to 25 weeks in once-weekly sessions
   d) cognitive psychotherapy may be useful in patients who refuse to take, fail to respond to, or are unable to tolerate antidepressant medications
   e) all of the above statements are true

11. What is the major goal of cognitive psychotherapy?
    a) to help patients "pick themselves up by the bootstraps" and change their lives
    b) to reestablish their previous best level of functioning
    c) to understand the major conflict area and the particular defense mechanisms they are currently using
    d) to identify and alter cognitive distortions
    e) to clarify and resolve the focal area of conflict that interferes with current functioning

12. At this time, what is the ideal therapy for a patient with major depressive illness (unipolar)?
    a) cognitive psychotherapy plus a tricyclic antidepressant
    b) cognitive psychotherapy plus an SSRI
    c) supportive psychotherapy plus a tricyclic antidepressant
    d) supportive psychotherapy plus an SSRI
    e) brief dynamic psychotherapy alone

Short Answer Management Problem 68

Describe your philosophy regarding different types of psychotherapy to treat different primary care conditions.

ANSWERS

1. C.

2. D.

3. D. This patient has an adjustment disorder. Although this is detailed in another chapter of the book, the basic characteristics of adjustment disorder are as follows:
   1. The development of a psychological reaction to identifiable stressors or events
   2. The reaction reflects a change in the individual's normal personality and is different from the person's usual style of functioning.
   3. The psychological reaction is either "maladaptive," in that normal functioning (including social and occupational functioning) is markedly impaired, or the reaction is greater than normally expected of others in similar circumstances.
   4. The psychological reaction does not represent an exacerbation of another psychiatric disorder.

The sleep disorder that this patient has developed secondary to the "work demands" is known as insufficient sleep syndrome. Persons affected with this disorder voluntarily curtail their time in bed, usually in response to social and occupational demands. This results in daytime hypersomnolence and in impairment.

The type of psychotherapy that best fits treatment of this patient's life situation at this time is supportive psychotherapy. Supportive psychotherapy is discussed in detail in a subsequent question.

4. C. The major goal of supportive psychotherapy is to reestablish the best possible level of functioning given the limitations of the illness, personality, native ability, and life circumstances. In general, this distinguishes supportive psychotherapy from the change-oriented psychotherapies that aim to either reverse primary disease processes and symptoms or restructure personality.

There is unanimous agreement among authorities that the first priority of supportive psychotherapy is to foster a good working relationship with the patient.

5. A.

6. B. The next priority once the "working relationship" is established between patient and therapist is to act as a guide or a mentor in an effort to help her extricate herself from her current working environment. The best way to accomplish this is likely to be short-term disability or sick leave. During that time, the patient's goals will be to refocus her life and negotiate a "reasonable working relationship" with her employers. In the event this goal cannot be or is not reached, then long-term disability is an ethical, reasonable, and referable option. Ultimately, it would seem that a change in jobs would be the best solution; however, that is easier said than done.

    The prescription of a hypnotic is contraindicated because of her already-established sleep disorder. Adding a hypnotic would quite simply make one problem into two.

7. E. Some of the specific techniques employed in supportive psychotherapy include the following:
    A. Regular, weekly sessions where therapy for the patient is consistently available
    B. The support by the therapist of intellectualization in the patient
    C. Guiding and/or mentoring on the part of the therapist
    D. The concomitant use of medication (especially antidepressant medication)
    E. The specific techniques of suggestion, reinforcement, advice, teaching, reality testing, cognitive restructuring, reassurance, an active stance on the part of the therapist, the discussion of alternative behaviors, and the discussion of social/interpersonal skills.

8. C. In contrast to other psychotherapies, there is a growing amount of literature that supports the efficacy of cognitive psychotherapy. Although the number of studies is still small, the studies examining the outcome of cognitive psychotherapy have found it to be an effective treatment in ambulatory outpatients with mild to moderate degrees of depression. Cognitive psychotherapy is certainly more effective than no psychotherapy in treating both depressed volunteers and psychiatric patients who have a DSM-IV unipolar depression.

9. A. The only true statement in the series of choices offered is that most primary care physicians treat major depressive illness with antidepressive medicine. If psychotherapy is used at all, it is most commonly what is best described as a very brief supportive psychotherapy that is used to explain "the method by which the antidepressant medications work."

    The other important statements that need to be emphasized here are as follows:
    A. A combination of psychotherapy and pharma-

cotherapy is more effective than either method alone in major nonpsychotic unipolar depression.
    B. The psychotherapy of choice in the treatment of major depressive illness is cognitive psychotherapy, not supportive psychotherapy.

Studies suggest that there is about a 70%-75% success rate with each modality; if these are combined the success rate is increased to somewhere between 85% and 90%.

10. E.

11. D. Cognitive psychotherapy is a method of brief psychotherapy developed over the last two decades primarily for the treatment of mild to moderate depression and for patients with low self-esteem.

    Cognitive psychotherapists see the conclusions about life that nondepressed patients reach as different from those of depressed patients. Depressed persons tend to have very negative interpretations of the world, themselves, and the future. As well, depressed patients interpret events as reflecting defeat, deprivation, or disparagement and see their lives as being filled with obstacles and burdens. They also view themselves as unworthy, deficient, undesirable, or worthless and see the future as bringing a continuation of the miseries of the past.

    Cognitive therapy is best suited to patients with unipolar, nonpsychotic illness and is best conducted over 15 to 25 once-weekly sessions.

    Cognitive therapy can also be used in patients who refuse to take antidepressant medication, fail to respond to antidepressant medication, or are unable to tolerate antidepressant medications.

    The major goal of cognitive psychotherapy is to identify and alter cognitive distortions and thoughts. The techniques that are used include behavioral assignments, reading materials, and teaching that helps these patients recognize the difference between positively and negatively biased automatic thoughts. It may seem, at first glance, completely straightforward, but it is sometimes very difficult for the patient to tell the difference between the two. Also, it helps patients to identify negative schemes, beliefs, and attitudes.

12. B. At this time, the best combination of therapies for unipolar depressive illness is a combination of a selective serotonin reuptake inhibitor and cognitive psychotherapy plus an SSRI.

SOLUTION TO SHORT ANSWER MANAGEMENT PROBLEM 68

Primary care presents an opportunity to provide significant relief to patients through psychotherapy. There are many different forms of psychotherapy:

1. Psychoanalysis
2. Intensive (long-term) psychoanalytically oriented psychotherapy
3. Brief psychodynamic psychotherapy
4. Cognitive psychotherapy
5. Supportive psychotherapy
6. Behavioral psychotherapy

The goals of the various psychotherapies are as follows:

1. Psychoanalysis: the goal of psychoanalysis is to resolve symptoms and perform major reworking of personality structures related to childhood conflicts.
2. Psychoanalytically oriented psychotherapy: the goal of psychoanalytically oriented psychotherapy is to understand a conflict area and the particular defense mechanisms used to defend it.
3. Brief psychodynamic psychotherapy: the goal of brief psychodynamic psychotherapy is to clarify and resolve focal areas of conflict that interfere with current functioning.
4. Cognitive psychotherapy: the goal of cognitive psychotherapy is to identify and alter cognitive distortions.
5. Supportive psychotherapy: the goal of supportive psychotherapy is to reestablish the most optimal level of functioning possible in the patient.
6. Behavioral therapy (behavioral modification): the goal of behavioral therapy is to eliminate involuntary disruptive behavior patterns and substitute appropriate behaviors.

The two most important types of psychotherapy in primary care are cognitive psychotherapy and supportive psychotherapy.

Cognitive psychotherapy in primary care is useful mainly in the treatment of depression (unipolar, nonpsychotic).

Supportive psychotherapy in primary care has a much broader scope, and its use is indicated in the following: generalized anxiety disorders and other anxiety disorders, family dysfunction, marital therapy, and any condition to which importance is attached by the patient.

In addition, group psychotherapy provides significant support to groups of primary care patients in certain situations such as smoking cessation, stress reduction, and specific phobias including panic disorder.

SUMMARY OF THE DIAGNOSIS AND TREATMENT OF PRIMARY CARE PATIENTS WITH PSYCHOTHERAPIES

The "do's" and the "don'ts" of psychotherapy in family medicine:

1. *Do* consider the use of supportive psychotherapy in any condition built around the biopsychosocial model of illness.
2. *Do* consider the increased efficacy of treating unipolar depression with a combination of selective serotonin reuptake inhibitors and cognitive psychotherapy.
3. *Do* realize that good results with psychotherapy require time: cognitive psychotherapy, 15-25 weekly sessions, and supportive psychotherapy, weekly sessions for various lengths of time.
4. *Do* realize that some studies point to significant cost-effectiveness of psychotherapy in relationship to other interventions.
5. *Do* realize that to properly perform any type of psychotherapy other than brief supportive psychotherapy you will require extra training.
6. *Do not* underestimate the effect of both transference and countertransference on both patient and therapist.
7. *Do not* underestimate the potential of patient manipulation. Recognize the prevalence of somatoform disorders in family medicine and the relative difficulty of treating them successfully.
8. *Do not* prescribe narcotic analgesics for patients that are undergoing significant psychotherapy in your clinic. If you do, the drugs you prescribe will become the focus of the therapy rather than the condition itself.
9. *Do not* be afraid to refer a patient to a psychologist or a psychiatrist after five sessions of psychotherapy in which it is apparent that no progress in being made.
10. *Do* be extremely careful in deciding what conditions you treat with psychotherapy. The more complicated the condition, the longer the duration of the condition, and the larger the number of coexisting factors, the more difficult the task you face and the more training you need.

SUGGESTED READINGS

American Psychiatric Association. Diagnostic and statistical manual. 4th Ed. Washington, DC: American Psychiatric Association Press, 1994.

Ursano R, Siberman E, Diaz A. The psychotherapies: Basic theoretical principles and techniques. In: Stoudemire A, ed. Clinical psychiatry for medical students. 2nd Ed. Philadelphia: JB Lippincott, 1994.

PROBLEM 69   A 6-YEAR-OLD CHILD WHO IS "ALWAYS ON THE GO," "INTO EVERYTHING," AND "EASILY DISTRACTABLE"

A mother brings her 6-year-old boy to the office for a complete assessment. She states that "there is something very wrong with him." He just sprinkled baby powder all over the house, and last night he opened a bottle of ink and threw it on the floor. He is unable to sit still at school, is easily distracted, has difficulty waiting his turn in games, has difficulty in sustaining attention in play situations, talks all the time, always interrupts others, does not listen when talked to, and is constantly shifting from one activity to another.

As you enter the examining room, the child is in the process of destroying it.

On examination (what examination you can manage), you discover that there are no physical abnormalities demonstrated.

SELECT THE ONE BEST ANSWER TO THE FOLLOWING QUESTIONS

1. What is the most likely diagnosis in this patient?
   a) mental retardation
   b) childhood depression
   c) attention-deficit hyperactivity disorder
   d) maternal deprivation
   e) childhood schizophrenia

2. Which of the following is(are) associated with the disorder described?
   a) feelings of low self-esteem
   b) feelings of depression
   c) feelings of demoralization
   d) none of the above
   e) all of the above

3. Who is the person who usually makes this diagnosis?
   a) the child psychiatrist
   b) the family physician
   c) the mother or father
   d) the schoolteacher
   e) the grandparents

4. The differential diagnosis of this disorder includes which of the following?
   a) adjustment disorder
   b) bipolar disorder
   c) anxiety disorder
   d) childhood schizophrenia
   e) a, b, and c
   f) all of the above

5. What is the approximate prevalence of the disorder described among preschool and kindergarten boys?
   a) 1%-3%
   b) 5%-10%
   c) 11%-13%
   d) 14%-20%
   e) 21%-25%

6. This disorder is most closely linked to which of the following disorders?
   a) childhood depression
   b) childhood anxiety
   c) conduct disorder
   d) oppositional defiant disorder
   e) c and d

7. The diagnosis of conduct disorder is made when which of the following criteria is(are) fulfilled?
   a) repetitive and persistent patterns of behavior that violate the rights of others
   b) stealing
   c) lying
   d) vandalism
   e) any of two b, c, and d
   f) all of the above

8. What is the best definition of the term *oppositional defiant disorder*?
   a) chronic behavior patterns in children and adolescents that are more severe than those in conduct disorder
   b) chronic behavior patterns in children and adolescents that result in serious violation of the law and incarceration
   c) chronic behavior patterns in children and adolescents that are less severe than those seen in conduct disorder
   d) a and b
   e) none of the above

9. Which of the following disorders often appear together in the same individual at various life stages?
   a) mental retardation—ADHD—learning disability
   b) childhood depression—ADHD—early-onset adult schizophrenia
   c) ADHD—conduct disorder—antisocial personality disorder
   d) adjustment disorder—ADHD—major depression
   e) ADHD—bipolar disorder—conduct disorder

10. Conduct disorder appears to result from an interaction of which of the following factors?
    a) temperament
    b) attention to problem behavior and ignoring good behavior

c) association with a delinquent peer group
d) a and c only
e) all of the above

11. What is the pharmacologic treatment of choice for ADHD?
a) methylphenidate
b) dextroamphetamine
c) magnesium pemoline
d) all of the above
e) a or b only

12. What is the pharmacologic treatment of choice for ADHD in patients who do not respond to stimulants?
a) desipramine
b) fluoxetine
c) phenelzine
d) clonidine
e) amitriptyline

13. Regarding the comparison between the effects of stimulants on children, adolescents, and adults, which of the following statements is(are) correct?
a) in children and adolescents the use of stimulants has a paradoxical effect: they are "slowed down," as opposed to adults, in whom stimulants increase activity and awareness
b) normal and hyperactive children, adolescents, and adults have similar cognitive responses to comparable doses of stimulants
c) normal and hyperactive children, adolescents, and adults have similar behavioral responses to comparable doses of stimulants
d) b and c

e) nobody really knows for sure; it depends on the patient

14. A given child who is being treated with methylphenidate does not respond well to the medication; there is essentially no change in this behavior after 3 months of therapy.

At this time, what would you do?
a) continue methylphenidate at one and one-half times the dose (for another 3 months)
b) switch the child to dextroamphetamine
c) switch the child to magnesium pemoline
d) discontinue stimulants altogether and prescribe to desipramine
e) b or c

15. What is the most appropriate time to give methylphenidate to a child with ADHD?
a) twice per day: early morning and noon
b) three times per day: early morning, noon, and evening
c) once per day: early morning
d) four times per day: every 6 hours
e) it does not matter

16. What is the most common reason for referral to either a child psychiatry service or an adolescent psychiatry service?
a) conduct disorder
b) attention-deficit hyperactivity disorder
c) oppositional defiant disorder
d) childhood-adolescent depression
e) childhood-adolescent schizophrenia

Short Answer Management Problem 69

PART A: List four psychiatric disorders that are associated with attention-deficit hyperactivity disorder.

PART B: List five parental behaviors/disorders/situations that may be associated with attention-deficit hyperactivity disorder.

PART C: Comment on the association between attention-deficit hyperactivity disorder and schoolteachers.

ANSWERS

1. C. This child has attention-deficit hyperactivity disorder (ADHD). Diagnostic criteria for ADHD require a pattern of behavior that appears no later than the age of 7 years, has been present for at least 6 months, and is excessive for age and intelligence. The symptoms of the disorder are divided into inattention and hyperactivity/impulsivity; they must be present often, although not necessarily all of the time or in every situation. Possible symptoms are listed here, but all are not required in a specific child:
   1) Fidgety or restless
   2) Difficulty staying seated
   3) Easily distracted
   4) Difficulty waiting in lines or awaiting his or her turn

5) Impulsive speech
6) Difficulty following instructions
7) Short attention span at work and at play
8) Difficulty playing quietly
9) Doesn't seem to listen
10) Loses things
11) Makes careless mistakes
12) Difficulty organizing
13) Avoids engaging in effortful mental activities, particularly when not interested
14) Forgetful
15) Runs about or climbs excessively in situations where these activities are inappropriate

Hyperactive behavior per se is no longer considered the key or even a necessary feature of this disorder, although the term is often used as shorthand for ADHD. Others interpretations of primary deficits follow:

A. Lack of investment, organization, and maintenance of attention and effort in completing tasks
B. Inability to inhibit impulsive action
C. Lack of modulation of arousal levels to meet the demands of the situation
D. Unusually strong inclination to seek immediate reinforcement

2. E. Commonly associated features of ADHD are low self-esteem, feelings of depression, feelings of demoralization, and lack of ability to take responsibility for one's actions. In social situations these young children are immature, bossy, instrusive, loud, uncooperative, out of synchrony with situational expectations, and irritating to both adults and peers.

3. D. The most common person to make the diagnosis of ADHD is the schoolteacher. There is considerable controversy concerning the fact that many hyperactive children are "on Ritalin" because of "the remarks or diagnosis of the schoolteacher." There certainly is some truth to this statement. Inexperienced or overly critical teachers may in fact confuse normal age-appropriate overactivity with ADHD.

4. E. The differential diagnosis of ADHD includes the following:
   1. Adjustment disorder (an identifiable stressor is identified at home and the duration of symptoms is less than 6 months)
   2. An anxiety disorder (instead of or in addition to the diagnosis of ADHD)
   3. Bipolar disorder (bipolar disorder in children may manifest as a chronic mixed affective state marked by irritability, overactivity, and difficulty concentrating)
   4. Mental retardation
   5. A specific developmental disorder
   6. Drugs (phenobarbital in children is prescribed as an anticonvulsant, and Theophylline is prescribed for asthma)
   7. Systemic disorders (hyperthyroidism)

5. D. Between 14% and 20% of preschool and kindergarten boys and approximately a third as many girls have ADHD. In elementary schools, 3% to 10% of students have ADHD symptoms.

6. E. In clinical settings, at least two-thirds of patients with ADHD also have either oppositional defiant disorder or conduct disorder. The characteristics of these two disorders will be discussed in subsequent questions.

7. F. The diagnosis of conduct disorder requires a repetitive and persistent pattern of behavior that violates the basic rights of others or age-appropriate rules of society, manifested by at least three of the following behaviors:
   A. Stealing
   B. Running away from home
   C. Staying out after dark without permission
   D. Lying in order to "con" people
   E. Deliberate fire-setting
   F. Repeated truancy (beginning before the age of 13)
   G. Vandalism
   H. Cruelty to animals
   I. Bullying
   J. Physical aggression
   K. Forcing someone else into sexual activity

   Conduct disorder is a purely descriptive label for a heterogenous group of children and adolescents. Many of these individuals also lack appropriate feelings of guilt or remorse, lack empathy for others, and lack a feeling of responsibility for their own behavior.

8. C. Oppositional defiant disorder is best described as a milder form of conduct disorder. Children who are diagnosed as having oppositional defiant disorder are certainly at risk for developing conduct disorder.

9. C. ADHD commonly leads to conduct disorder. Adolescents who develop conduct disorder are predisposed to develop antisocial personality disorder and/or alcoholism as adults.

10. E. Conduct disorder appears to result from an interaction among the following factors:
    A. Temperament
    B. Parents who provide attention to problem behavior and ignore good behavior
    C. Association with a delinquent peer group
    D. A parent "role model" of impulsivity and rule-breaking behavior
    E. Genetic predisposition
    F. Marital disharmony in the family

G. Placement outside of the home as an infant or toddler

H. Poverty

I. Low IQ or brain damage

11. D. The pharmacological agents of choice for the management of ADHD are the following stimulant medications:

A. Methylphenidate

B. Dextroamphetamine

C. Magnesium pemoline

Up to 96% of children with ADHD have at least some positive behavioral response to methylphenidate and/or dextroamphetamine, although side effects may limit efficacy or require discontinuation of medication in some children. Both preschool children and adolescents may require lower weight-adjusted doses than school-aged children and manifest a greater likelihood of side effects and somewhat lower therapeutic efficacy.

12. A. Desipramine is the drug of choice in patients who do not respond to stimulants, who develop significant depression on stimulants, who have a personal or family history of tics, or who develop tics when on a stimulant.

The other choice that is partially correct is clonidine. The alpha-adrenergic agent clonidine, when given either in pill form or transdermal form, is useful for a subgroup of children with ADHD, including those with tics or a family history of Tourette's syndrome or those in whom a stimulant is only partially effective.

13. D. Contrary to previous belief, normal and hyperactive children, adolescents, and adults have similar cognitive and behavioral responses to comparable doses of stimulants. Stimulants do not have a paradoxical sedative action; they do not lead to drug abuse or addiction, and many adolescents with ADHD continue to require and benefit from their use.

14. E. Up to 25% of children who respond poorly to one stimulant have a positive response to another stimulant. Stimulants reliably decrease physical activity, especially during times when children are expected to be less active (such as during school but not during free time). They also decrease vocalization, noise, and disruption in the classroom to the level of normal peers and improve handwriting. Stimulants consistently improve compliance to adult commands.

Stimulants also produce improvement on cognitive laboratory tasks measuring sustained attention, distractibility, impulsivity, and short-term memory. Stimulants increase productivity and decrease errors in tests of arithmetic, reading comprehension, sight vocabulary, and spelling, and increase the percentage of assigned work completed.

Because of these benefits, it is strongly suggested that if one of the stimulants is not effective, try another one before switching to a drug of another class.

15. A. The best dosing schedule for stimulant medications used to treat ADHD is twice per day: early morning and noon. By giving the stimulants at this time, the maximal effectiveness will be during school hours when needed most. A "drug holiday" should be considered on the weekends.

16. A. The single most common reason for referral to a child or adolescent psychiatry clinic or hospital is conduct disorder.

SOLUTION TO SHORT ANSWER MANAGEMENT PROBLEM 69

PART A: Four psychiatric disorders that are associated with attention-deficit hyperactivity disorder include the following:

A. Childhood depression

B. Conduct disorder

C. Oppositional defiant disorder

D. Alcoholism

PART B: Five parental behaviors/disorders/situations that may be associated with attention-deficit hyperactivity disorder include the following:

A. Providing attention to problem behavior and ignoring good behavior

B. Parental modeling (impulsivity and rule-breaking)

C. Parental marital conflict

D. Family poverty

E. Inheritance (genetic-predisposition)

These factors are more often associated with oppositional defiant disorder than true attention-deficit hyperactivity disorder. However, as just mentioned, ADHD is related to ODD.

PART C: The relationship between attention-deficit hyperactivity disorder and schoolteacher input is as follows: in many cases, the diagnosis of ADHD is made by the teacher, not by the physician. Instead of carefully considering the diagnostic criteria elaborated by the DSM-IV, the physician may simply accept the word of the schoolteacher and begin treatment with stimulant medication. The basic problem is the inability, in some cases on the part of the schoolteacher and ultimately on the part of the physician, to distinguish between attention-deficit hyperactivity disorder and normal appropriate-for-age overactivity.

SUMMARY OF THE DIAGNOSIS AND TREATMENT OF ADHD, CONDUCT DISORDER, AND OPPOSITIONAL DEFIANT DISORDER

1. **Attention-deficit hyperactivity disorder:**
   a) Prevalence: prevalence (preschool and kindergarten): 14%-20% male, 3% to 10% female

b) Signs and symptoms: see the diagnostic criteria just described.

c) Treatment:

1. Nonpharmacologic: behavior modification can improve both academic achievement and behavioral compliance if they are specifically targeted.

2. Pharmacologic:

First choice:

i) Methylphenidate

ii) Dextroamphetamine

iii) Magnesium pemoline

Second choice:

i) Desipramine is the drug of choice in cases of stimulant failure.

ii) Clonidine may also be considered.

Stepwise therapy:

i) Begin stimulant 1 (usually methylphenidate)

ii) Increase dose gradually

iii) End of dose failure: consider another one of the two recommended stimulants.

iv) Failure: go to desipramine.

Length of time/dosing:

i) Consider early morning and noon dosing.

ii) Consider drug holidays on the weekend.

iii) Use for as long as is needed.

2. **Conduct disorder:**

a) Prevalence: the prevalence of conduct disorder has been estimated at 3% to 7%; males predominate.

b) Signs and symptoms: see the criteria listed earlier. Conduct disorder is the most common reason for referral to a child or adolescent psychiatry service.

c) Treatment:

1. Nonpharmacologic: cognitive-behavior modification (when used together) is single most effective nonpharmacologic therapy.

2. Pharmacologic:

i) Lithium: for severe impulse aggression

ii) Carbamazepine: for severe impulse aggression accompanied by emotional lability and irritability

iii) Propranolol: for uncontrollable rage reactions, especially when associated with impulse aggression

iv) Neuroleptics (such as haloperidol) may reduce aggression, hostility, negativism, and explosiveness in severely aggressive children.

v) Antidepressants: if the conduct disorder is secondary to major depression, successful treatment with antidepressants is indicated.

3. **Oppositional defiant disorder:**

a) Prevalence: the prevalence of this disorder is 6% to 10%; males predominate.

b) Differential diagnosis: "stubbornness."

c) Signs/symptoms: this disorder is best described simply as a less severe form of conduct disorder.

d) Treatment:

1. Nonpharmacologic: an operant approach using environmental positive and negative contingencies to increase or decrease the frequency of behaviors is most useful.

2. Pharmacologic: if ADHD and ODD coexist, treat with stimulant medication.

4. **Order of progression:** ADHD to conduct disorder or oppositional defiant disorder to antisocial personality disorder to alcoholism

5. **Major differential diagnosis of disruptive behavior disorders:**

a) Major depressive illness

b) Bipolar affective disorder

c) Anxiety disorder (one of)

d) Mental retardation

e) Specific developmental disorder

f) Adjustment disorder

g) Pharmacotherapy (phenobarbital, theophylline)

h) Systemic disorders (hyperthyroidism)

SUGGESTED READINGS

American Psychiatric Association. Diagnostic and statistical manual of mental disorders. 4th Ed. Washington, DC: American Psychiatric Association Press, 1994.

Dulcan MK. Psychiatric disorders of childhood and adolescence. In: Stoudemire A, ed. Clinical psychiatry for medical students. 2nd Ed. Philadelphia: J.B. Lippincott, 1994.

PROBLEM 70   A 35-YEAR-OLD FEMALE WITH METASTATIC CANCER OF THE CERVIX

A 35-year-old female, a new patient to your practice, presents to your office to seek help in obtaining a referral to the Mexican Cancer Cure Center in a small town near Mexico City. She has metastatic carcinoma of the cervix, which has been treated with chemotherapy and radiation therapy but has now spread to her entire axial skeleton. The patient excitedly shows you the brochure that describes the brand-new facility. She tells you that she has contacted the facility and has been accepted for treatment even though there is an extremely long waiting list and it is very difficult to get in. You need to formally refer her, she tells you, to the chief of staff in the center.

SELECT THE ONE BEST ANSWER TO THE FOLLOWING QUESTIONS

1. At this time what should you do?
   a) phone the chief of staff at the center and make the necessary arrangements
   b) ask the patient to provide you with more information so that you can study it and make an informed decision on her behalf
   c) tell the patient that there is no way that you will have anything to do with "quack" medicine; if she wants a referral she will have to see another physician
   d) ask the patient to reconsider her request and come back to see you in 6 weeks; by that time you will have had time to discuss her case with the oncologists and will have been able to determine more reasonable therapy for her
   e) none of the above

2. Regarding alternative therapy for the treatment of cancer and other serious diseases, which one of the following statements is true?
   a) alternative therapy and alternative therapy clinics are on the decline in North America
   b) alternative therapy is unlikely to produce any significant adverse effects
   c) alternative therapy clinics usually provide their services at nominal cost to patients and their families
   d) alternative therapy clinics are often run by American-trained MDs; foreign-trained MDs are a less frequent occurrence in today's modern alternative therapy clinics
   e) alternative therapy has been shown to be beneficial in some patients

3. Regarding patients who attend alternative therapy clinics, which of the following is not a common characteristic?
   a) high education level
   b) higher income level
   c) common coexistent psychiatric disorder
   d) previous or current conventional therapy
   e) Caucasian race

4. Regarding the total cost to patients and their families of alternative therapy centers is North America, which

of the following statements is true?
   a) the national (American) cost may be as high as $10 billion annually
   b) the cost is likely to reflect only the cost of the products involved in making the alternative preparations; most alternative practitioners are very altruistic in their treatments and beliefs and consequently little money changes hands between doctor and patient
   c) alternative therapy costs are generally funded by the major health care plans in the United States and Canada
   d) alternative therapy costs may be difficult to quantify due to the lack of even the most primitive facilities for keeping track of the books, accounts, and records.
   e) alternative therapies, in contradistinction to conventional therapies, are less likely to continue for long periods of time

5. Regarding alternative therapies, which of the following statements is true?
   a) a major advantage of alternative cancer therapies over conventional cancer therapies is their lack of side effects
   b) alternative therapies have been shown, in randomized controlled trials, to increase longevity in some cancer patients
   c) the U.S. Congress has decided not to fund any research trials involving alternative therapies or other unconventional medical practices
   d) the use of alternative therapies and conventional therapies at the same time is extremely uncommon
   e) none of the above are true

6. Physicians who are trained in the diagnosis and treatment of disease using conventional and scientifically proven techniques are often asked by patients about their "views on alternative forms of therapy." The patients who ask these questions are by and large patients who are ill with cancer or other serious conditions. Regarding opinions physicians hold about alternative therapies and involvement physicians have with alternative therapies, which of the following statements is most accurate?
   a) most young practitioners hold views that can be classified as at least neutral toward, and perhaps even supportive of, at least some types of alternative therapy

b) most unorthodox practitioners are MDs

c) most practitioners go out of their way to discourage patients from pursuing alternative therapies

d) most physicians who have examined the most common types of alternative therapies (discussed later) disregard them all as useless and/or harmful

e) patients who seek alternative therapies usually do not cause their physician any amount of anxiety or concern about that decision

7. Regarding the proportion of patients with cancer who seek alternative therapy(ies), which estimate is most widely accepted?
a) 10%
b) 25%
c) 50%
d) 70%
e) 85%

8. Which of the following statements regarding alternative cancer therapy and conventional cancer therapy is true?
a) most patients who seek treatment with alternative cancer therapies abandon conventional cancer therapies when alternative therapy begins
b) most patients who seek treatment with alternative cancer therapies continue conventional cancer therapies
c) most patients who seek treatment with alternative cancer therapies never return to the cancer clinic or to their former personal physician
d) most patients who seek treatment with alternative cancer therapy(ies) believe that conventional cancer therapy(ies) have irreversibly poisoned their organ systems
e) most patients who seek treatment with alternative cancer therapies have developed a confusional state

9. What is the single most important difference between alternative cancer therapies and conventional cancer therapies from the point of view of the patient?
a) alternative cancer therapies are directed at the target of the cancer, whereas conventional cancer therapies are not
b) alternative cancer therapies are much more likely to be successful in actual cure than conventional cancer therapies
c) alternative cancer therapies are less likely to produce fatigue than conventional cancer therapies
d) alternative cancer therapies are usually accompanied by a significant decision-making role on the part of the patient; such a decision-making role is much less common in conventional cancer therapies
e) alternative cancer therapies are more carefully administered than conventional cancer therapies

10. Regarding the relationship between the quality of the cancer patient's experience with conventional cancer therapy and his or her use of alternative cancer therapy, which of the following statements is the best description between quality of time, quantity of time, conventional cancer therapies and alternative cancer therapies?
a) there is a highly significant directly proportional relationship between the quantity of the patient's experiences with conventional cancer medicine and the patient's use of alternative medicine—the more often the patient is seen in the cancer clinic, the more likely he or she is to seek alternative therapies
b) there is a highly significant inversely proportional relationship between the quality of the patient's experiences with conventional cancer medicine and the patient's use of alternative therapies
c) there is no relationship between the quantity of the patient's experiences with conventional cancer medicine and use of alternative therapies
d) there is no relationship between the quality of patients' experiences with conventional cancer medicine and the patients' use of alternative therapies
e) there is no relationship among any of the items described

11. Which of the following statements regarding patients seeking treatment with alternative treatments is true?
a) it is difficult if not impossible to prevent a patient who wishes to use alternative therapies from doing so
b) the probability of a patient's using alternative therapies bears no relationship to either the personality or the belief system of his or her primary care physician
c) alternative therapies appear attractive to patients due to a patient sense of "naturality" and "non-toxicity"
d) physicians who provide patients with a sense that when physical deterioration approaches abandonment will not occur, and who concentrate on maximizing the patient's quality of life, are less likely to have their patients seeking alternative therapies
e) alternative therapies concentrate on the concept of treating the cancer itself, not on treating the body as a whole

12. Of the following alternative therapies, which, at present, is the most commonly used?
a) metabolic therapy
b) diet therapy
c) megavitamin therapy
d) imagery therapy
e) immune therapy

13. Consider the following characteristics of a certain alternative therapy:
1) It is based on the principle that toxins and waste material in the body interfere with metabolism and healing, and that therefore cells lack the nutrients essential to health.

2) It considers cancer and chronic illnesses based on degeneration of the pancreas, as well as on the immune system and the "oxidation system"

3) It directs treatment to "detoxification," typically through chronic cleansing with coffee grounds enemas, special diets, vitamins and minerals, enzymes, and laetrile.

This set of characteristics best describes which of the following alternative therapies?
a) metabolic therapy
b) diet therapy
c) megavitamin therapy
d) imagery therapy
e) immune therapy

14. Consider the following characteristics of a certain alternative therapy:

1) It is limited to treatment with specialized food products.

2) It is based on the principle, "You are what you eat."

3) It includes very specific instructions for food preparation and consumption.

This set of characteristics best describes which of the following alternative therapies?
a) metabolic therapy
b) specialized *yin-yang* diet therapy
c) megafood diet therapy
d) imagery diet therapy
e) none of the above

15. Consider the following characteristics of a certain alternative therapy:

1) It is based on Eastern *yin-yang* philosophical principles.

2) It is a fully formulated alternative concept of physiology and disease.

3) It is based on the principle of a "mother red blood cell" housed in the intestine as the progenitor of all body cells, tissues, and organs.

4) It specifies that food intake must be carefully balanced to counteract bodily dysfunction.

5) Further to the notion of balance, *yin* foods are prescribed for *yang* cancers and *yang* foods are prescribed for *yin* cancers

This set of characteristics best describes which of the following alternative therapies?
a) metabolic therapy
b) diet therapy
c) megavitamin therapy
d) macrobiotic diet therapy
e) immune physiology therapy

16. Consider the following characteristics of a certain alternative therapy:

1) It prescribes one or several vitamins daily in varying but always high dosages.

2) It is based on the belief that high-dose vitamins strengthen the body's capacity to destroy malignant cells.

This set of characteristics best describes which of the following alternative therapies?
a) megavitamin therapy
b) toxin-killing vitamin therapy
c) high-dose immune target diet therapy
d) macrobiotic diet therapy
e) none of the above

17. Regarding imagery therapy as a form of alternative therapy, which of the following statements is(are) true?
a) imagery therapy is a commonly practiced alternative therapy
b) imagery therapy requires the patient to visualize or imagine the destruction of malignant cells in the body
c) imagery therapy suggests that the reversal of the malignant process is based on the result of psychological influences on the body's capacity to counteract the malignant process
d) imagery therapy is unlikely to produce any toxic side effects
e) all of the above are true

18. Regarding spiritual therapy as a form of alternative therapy, which of the following statements is(are) true?
a) spiritual therapy involves the use of intense prayer
b) spiritual therapy often includes the laying on of hands
c) spiritual therapy is based on divine intervention
d) spiritual therapy is based on exorcism of the evil represented by the disease
e) all of the above are true

19. Regarding immune therapy as a form of alternative therapy, which of the following statements is(are) true?
a) immune therapy refers to injections of interferon, autogenous vaccines, fetal tissue, and other "immune supportive agents"
b) proponents of immune therapy believe that cancer develops and thrives due to the production of immune toxins
c) immune therapy is more commonly used as an alternative therapy than metabolic therapy
d) the use of some of the agents used for injection in immune therapy have no place in conventional cancer treatment
e) all of the above are true

20. Regarding the frequency of use of alternative therapies, which of the following lists most closely represents the order of alternative therapies, from most common to least common?
a) metabolic therapy, diet therapy, megavitamin therapy, imagery therapy, spiritual therapy, immune therapy

b) metabolic therapy, macrobiotic diet therapy, diet therapy, megavitamin therapy, spiritual therapy, immune therapy

c) metabolic therapy, immune therapy, spiritual therapy, diet therapy, megavitamin therapy, imagery therapy

d) metabolic therapy, macrobiotic diet therapy, microbiotic diet therapy, diet therapy, megavitamin therapy, imagery therapy, spiritual therapy, immune therapy

e) metabolic therapy, spiritual therapy, megavitamin therapy, immune therapy, diet therapy, imagery therapy

Short Answer Management Problem 70

PART A: A 56-year-old male diagnosed with carcinoma of the pancreas presents to your office for review of his narcotic pain medications. There is no doubt that this patient is palliative. He tells you that he has begun to take "shark's cartilage" as a chemotherapeutic agent. He explains to you that "sharks don't get cancer and it seems that shark's cartilage works by zeroing in on the cancer cells in the pancreas." Describe how you would respond to the news that this patient (your patient) is taking shark's cartilage.

PART B: A 36-year-old male with carcinoma of the colon and liver metastases presents to your office for his regular narcotic medication review. There is no doubt that this patient is palliative. He tells you that he has booked a flight to the Bahamas to be treated at "the Jones Center for Cancer Eradication and Research." He asks you to sign a form that will allow him to be partially reimbursed for the medications that he will be using while in the Jones Center. He further explains to you that the has received extensive information from the Jones Center and has been advised that the 2-week course of therapy should produce a cure within 4 months and will cost around $125,000 (everything is included in this price). Describe how you would counsel this patient and respond to his request.

ANSWERS

1. E. You, as the patient's family physician, should carefully discuss with the patient the following:
   a) Her previous therapy and her feelings about its benefit and its effect on her quality of life
   b) Her relationship and feeling regarding the other physicians involved in her care
   c) Her current condition including pain control, symptom control, fears, and feelings about the future
   d) Her reason for wanting to go to Mexico, her hopes and thoughts for what can be accomplished, and want she thinks will be the result of her visit
   e) Her thoughts and wishes regarding further conventional therapy
   f) The need for someone to "coordinate her care" and act as her "advocate" from this point on, no matter what
   It would be preferable to indicate to the patient that you, as her new family physician, are willing to do this. You are willing to discuss any and all options and to direct her in way that you feel are in her best interest. By doing this you have the best chance of gaining the confidence of the patient and being able to influence her in a manner that may have her reconsider her decision.

2. D. It may be surprising to some to learn that most of the alternative therapy clinics in North America are run by American-trained MDs, many of whom are Board certified in various specialties (excluding oncology).

3. C. Patients who seek alternative therapies are generally well-educated patients with a relatively high income. They most commonly have been in or are currently in conventional therapy. Most are Caucasian and do *not* have any serious psychiatric disorder.

4. A. We do not know precisely the total cost of alternative therapies in the United States. The most recent estimates, however, have put the cost at between $4 billion and $10 billion annually. Physicians in charge of such clinics or working in such clinics appear to demonstrate the complete antithesis of altruism. A recent patient of mine, who just returned from such a clinic suggested that money changed hands more quickly in that clinic than in a bank. Although some health plans may provide limited coverage for certain alternative therapies, this is the exception rather than the rule. Also, accounts and records are not difficult to keep in the usual brand-new and plush facilities that are home to many alternative therapy clinics. The same patient who compared the alternative therapy clinic to a bank pointed out that this was the first clinic that she had been in that needed a supercomputer to track all present patient financial information.

5. E. Contrary to public opinion, alternative therapies are not free of side effects. This will be detailed in another question. There is debate over whether scien-

tific evidence exists that alternative therapies increase longevity in some patients with certain cancers.

The U.S. Congress in January 1992 appropriated $2 million toward the creation of the Office for the Study of Unconventional Medical Practices. As mentioned previously, many patients are undergoing conventional cancer therapy and alternative cancer therapies at the same time.

6. A. In one study of medical graduates who had been practicing medicine for a short time in the United Kingdom (5 years or less), 86% held favorable views toward alternative medicine and 43% had referred patients for such treatment. Although such data are not available for the United States, this is rather sobering. It certainly implies the need for continuing education of all physicians regarding the growth of this "movement."

The majority of practitioners of alternative medicine are medical practitioners. In addition, the majority of North American physicians are at least neutral, and more commonly somewhat supportive, of patients beginning alternative therapies. It seems that many (perhaps even the majority) have adopted a "wait-and-see attitude" about these therapies. Having said all that, however, it seems that physicians, when faced with a real-life situation, do become a little concerned, especially when the patient is leaving their care for something that is totally unknown.

7. C. Although there is considerable debate about the figure, the most widely accepted figure suggests that 50% of patients with cancer (excluding nonmelanotic skin cancer) seek treatment with one or more forms of alternative therapy at one point or another in their treatment program.

8. B. Most cancer patients who seek treatment with alternative cancer therapies continue to receive either chemotherapy or radiotherapy following their return from the alternative therapy clinic.

9. D. The single most important difference between alternative cancer therapies and conventional cancer therapy has nothing to do with the therapies themselves. Rather, it has much more to do with the control and input into decision making that patients feel when going through their alternative therapies. In contrast, many patients undergoing conventional cancer therapies feel that their involvement in their own care is minimal; some feel that the major interest of their physician is their "possible recruitment" for another trial.

10. B. There is a highly significant inverse relationship between the quality of patients' experience with conventional medicine and their use of unproven methods of treatment or alternative medicine.

11. D. Physicians who provide patients with a sense that when deterioration begins abandonment will not occur, and who clearly indicate to the patient their primary interest in enhancing the quality of life remaining, are much less likely to have patients seeking alternative therapies.

Alternative therapies concentrate on treating the whole person and all body systems. That is, their efforts center on improving "general health" and providing the body an opportunity to fight the cancer more effectively itself. Alternative therapies do not, on the other hand, concentrate so much on treating the cancer in isolation.

Alternative therapies appear attractive to patients at least in part because of the misperception that they are natural and nontoxic. Many of these therapies are, in fact, extremely toxic and cause multiple complications.

12. A. The most common alternative therapy used today is metabolic therapy. The characteristics of all of the major alternative therapies will be discussed in subsequent questions.

13. A.

14. E.

15. D.

16. A.

17. E.

18. E.

19. A.

20. A. Questions 13 through 20 deal with the characteristics of all commonly practiced alternative therapies and the frequency of each.

The characteristics listed in the question carefully outline the principles of each of the alternative therapies, so they will not be repeated in the answers presented here. Several critical points, however, will be highlighted.

First, metabolic therapy, the most commonly used alternative therapy, has numerous complications. These complications are almost always the result of the medical toxicity produced by colonic irrigation (most commonly with coffee). These complications include electrolyte imbalance, bowel necrosis and perforation, toxic colitis, amebiasis, hypokalemia, and sepsis.

Second, macrobiotic diet therapy (as the most commonly used form of diet therapy) is usually associated with "iridology," cancer diagnosis based on determining which pie-shaped segment of the iris is abnormal. In addition, many of the macrobiotic diets recommended include such regimes as daily multiple milkshakes of liver extract and other rather unpalatable concoctions.

Third, megavitamin therapy may be very toxic. A prime example of megavitamin toxicity is the peripheral neuropathy produced by the excessive intake of vitamin B_6.

Fourth, immune therapy is not necessarily always an "alternative therapy." Alpha-interferon, for example, is well-established as a therapy for certain cancers including non-Hodgkin's lymphoma, hairy cell leukemia, and Kaposi's sarcoma.

Fifth, imagery therapy and spiritual therapy do not seem to produce many (if any) significant adverse effects. In addition, with spiritual therapy it is difficult to draw the line between normal spirituality (which could certainly be regarded as a necessary component of health) and the belief in exorcism and daily miracles.

Finally, with respect to frequency of use of alternative therapies, the order most frequently quoted is as follows:

1) metabolic therapy
2) diet therapy (including macrobiotic diets as the most common form of diet)
3) megavitamin therapy
4) imagery therapy
5) spiritual therapy
6) immune therapy

SOLUTION TO SHORT ANSWER MANAGEMENT PROBLEM 70

PART A: As previously discussed, approximately 50% of patients with cancer or other life-threatening illnesses will decide, at one point or another to try an alternative therapy. You, as the attending physician, have two basic responsibilities in this situation:

1) Reassure the patient that in spite of the decision to try alternative therapy, you will continue support for both her and her family throughout.
2) Clearly indicate to the patient and family what your opinions are regarding the alternative therapy that has been decided on. This should be done in a nonjudgmental but informative manner.

The literature suggests that a majority of physicians will either support the patient's decision to seek alternative therapy or actively recommend it. This is not surprising considering the desire of the physician (as well as the patient) to try anything that might possibly work. The literature suggests that a majority of patients who have tried one or more alternative therapies feel that it has, to some extent, helped their condition. In addition, it is extremely important that the patient's family physician facilitate hope, not unrealistic hope or hope for a cure, but rather hope for minimization or elimination of pain and symptoms leading to an improved quality of life however short.

In this particular instance, it appears that "shark's cartilage" is unlikely to produce any significant toxic side effects.

A reasonable response on the part of the physician to this patient's admission of "shark cartilage therapy" may be something like this:

> I understand that this period of time is extremely difficult for you and your family. I realize that we, as physicians, have not been able to offer you anything to slow down the growth of the cancer. That must be very frustrating for you, and it certainly is frustrating for us.
>
> My understanding of "shark's cartilage" and cancer in sharks is that, contrary to some people's opinion, sharks do, in fact, get cancer. Nevertheless, it appears that shark's cartilage is relatively harmless (I would check this out carefully!) and if you feel that this therapy is making you feel better and your quality of life is improved then I certainly am not going to try to dissuade you. I think, however, that you realize that the most important issue from my point of view is that you have both excellent pain and symptom control, and this is best accomplished with the drugs that we are giving you. I want your quality of life to be as good as it possibly can be; I am here to help you realize that, and I will continue to support you, treat you, and help you and your family in any way that I can.

PART B: Most of the general comments that were made about the first patient apply to the second patient as well. There is, however, a significant difference between the two patients and the two alternative therapies.

There is a high probability that The Jones Center for Cancer Eradication and Research does not operate altruistically. One may speculate, in fact, that the major purpose of the clinic is to make as much money as possible from people who are most vulnerable and at the most traumatic and difficult time in their lives. It is difficult to be sure what therapies are being used at the Jones Center, but the most likely would be corticosteroid therapy. Because of the significant risk to the patient from toxic side effects, the incredible prices charged, and the promise of something that cannot be delivered, I would phrase my remarks to this patient in the following way:

> I am your family physician and wish to remain your family physician. I will do anything I can to help you cope with the illness that you have. My main concerns are that you are able to be as pain free and symptom free as possible, and that your quality of life be maximized. I must tell you that, in my opinion, the therapy that you are about to embark on at the Jones Clinic will not improve your condition in any way; I am also concerned that you may develop some significant side effects as a result of this therapy.
>
> As your family physician I am also your advocate; as your advocate I must help you obtain whatever funding and other benefits that you can. Although I will sign the form, you must realize that if I am asked my opinion concerning the therapy you are about to undergo, I will tell the truth and indicate I have recommended against it.
>
> I realize that we are not able to offer you any other active, possibly curative therapy and for that I am truly sorry. I believe I understand how you have come to make this decision about going to the Jones Clinic. If and when you go, I would

ask you to contact me at least once per week while there and to let me know how you are feeling. When you return I want to see you as soon as possible. Remember, above anything else, that I am your doctor.

SUMMARY OF ALTERNATIVE THERAPIES IN PATIENTS WITH CANCER AND OTHER LIFE-THREATENING DISEASES

1. Approximately 50% of cancer patients will avail themselves of one or more kinds of alternative therapy at some time.
2. Alternative therapies vary from those that have the potential to produce very significant side effects to those that are unlikely to produce any harm.
3. Major alternative therapies in order of frequency of use:
   a) metabolic therapy
   b) diet (including macrobiotic diets)
   c) megavitamin therapy
   d) imagery therapy
   e) spiritual therapy
   f) immune therapy
4. Discuss honestly and openly your feeling about alternative therapy and the types of alternative therapies that your patient is considering with the patient and family.
5. Indicate your concern about unfounded claims, false promises, toxic side effects, and the incredible costs of some alternative therapies.
6. Remind the patient that no matter what, you will remain the patient's advocate and physician.
7. Encourage the patient to keep in regular contact if he or she decides to pursue an alternative therapy in a distant location.
8. Alternative therapy in the United States is a multi-billion-dollar industry. There is every reason to believe that it will increase, not decrease.
9. Decide what you, as a family physician, can ethically accept regarding the various alternative therapies. Communicate this to your patients.
10. Remind your patients that your primary concern is their quality of life and the pain and symptom control that increases it.
11. Never leave the patient without hope!

SUGGESTED READINGS

American Psychiatric Association. Diagnostic and statistical manual. 4th Ed. Washington, DC: American Psychiatric Association Press, 1994.

Cassileth B, Brown H. Unorthodox cancer medicine. Ca-A Journal for Clinicians 1988;38(3):176-186.

Cassileth B et al. Contemporary unorthodox treatments in cancer medicine. Annals of Internal Medicine 1984; 101:105-112.

Hauser S. Unproven methods in cancer treatment. Current Opinion in Oncology 1993;5:646-654.

McGinnis L. Alternative therapies, 1990. Cancer 1992; 67:1788-1792.

PROBLEM 71   A 24-YEAR-OLD MEDICAL STUDENT WHO DOUBTS THE VALUE OF FAMILY MEDICINE

A 24-year-old medical student presents to you, his faculty advisor, to discuss the specialty of family medicine. He has been told by his classmates that family medicine is the specialty that you enter if you aren't able to do anything else. You are, in addition to being his faculty advisor, also a family physician. You attempt to educate him about your specialty and also encourage him to consider a career in family medicine. In describing your specialty, you illustrate many of the key features of the specialty.

SELECT THE ONE BEST ANSWER TO THE FOLLOWING QUESTIONS

1. Which of the following statements concerning family physicians and specialists is(are) true?
   a) the family physician has to cover the whole field of medical knowledge
   b) in any given field of medicine, the specialist always knows more than the family physician
   c) by specializing in medicine, one can eliminate uncertainty
   d) only by specializing can one attain depth of knowledge
   e) none of the above are true

2. Which of the following statements concerning family physicians is(are) true?
   a) although all family physicians are generalists, not all family physicians must have identical knowledge and skills
   b) family physicians may be differentiated, but this should not lead to fragmentation of the specialty
   c) the family physician acts not only across clinical boundaries but across the difficult boundary between medical, psychologic/emotional, and social problems
   d) family physicians must coordinate and manage the input of specialists and other health care professionals
   e) all of the above are true

3. Which of the following is not a characteristic of the biomedical model of illness?
   a) patients suffer from diseases that can be categorized in the same way as other natural phenomena
   b) a disease can be viewed independently from the person who is suffering from it and from his or her social context
   c) each disease has a specific causal agent, and it is a major objective of research to discover these agents
   d) the biomedical model considers the context of the disease in the patient's life and the meaning of the disease in that context
   e) mental and physical diseases can be considered separately, with provision for a group of psychosomatic diseases in which the mind appears to act on the body

4. Which of the following statements regarding illness, disease, and suffering is true?
   a) illness and disease are basically identical; to consider them as different is to split hairs
   b) illness and disease, although different, should not be considered as separate
   c) illness and suffering are intensely personal experiences, experiences that are significantly different from disease
   d) physicians rarely equate suffering with pain and disease
   e) trying to establish differences among these terms is likely to turn out to be a waste of time for everyone

5. Which of the following best describes the biopsychosocial model of illness?
   a) the illness/disease anomaly
   b) the specific etiology anomaly
   c) the interaction of the illness with the patient's being and the patient's world
   d) the mind/body anomaly
   e) the biological/psychological anomaly

6. Which clinical method best describes the role of the family physician in patient care?
   a) the patient-centered clinical method
   b) the problem-oriented clinical method
   c) the illness-oriented clinical method
   d) the disease-oriented clinical method
   e) the doctor-centered clinical method

7. In viewing the prevalence of illness and the utilization of medical services among adults, how many adults will be referred to a university medical center per month from a population of 1000 adults at risk?
   a) 250
   b) 125
   c) 50
   d) 25
   e) 1

8. Which of the following best describes the difference between family medicine and general practice?
   a) there is no real difference; these are simply two names for the same thing
   b) family medicine as a specialty is the summation of all other specialties

c) general practice is concerned with all medical illnesses; family medicine is somewhat more specialized
d) family medicine treats illness in the context of the individual and his or her family; general practice does not have that same family-based orientation
e) family medicine is more psychologically oriented than general practice

9. Which of the following is not among the 25 most common reasons for visits to family physicians?
a) sore throat
b) cough
c) head cold
d) chest pain
e) angina pectoris

10. Which of the following methods of problem solving is most commonly used by family physicians in day to day practice?
a) intuition
b) the hypothetical-deductive reasoning method
c) the pattern recognition method
d) the clinical practice guidelines method
e) nobody really knows for sure

Short Answer Management Problem 71

A 37-year-old mother of five presents to your office with her sixth migraine headache in the past 2 weeks. You have known this patient and her family for many years. In the past she has had occasional migraine headaches (once or twice a year) but never a frequency approaching anything like this. She appears to you to be tired and withdrawn. You are about to reach for your prescription pad when something in the back of your mind stops you. List the five most important questions you would ask this patient at this time.

ANSWERS

1. E. Much of the apprehension about becoming a family physician is based on six myths about the respective roles of family physicians and specialists.

Myth 1: the family physician has to cover the whole field of medical knowledge. The family physician's knowledge is just as selective as the specialist's. Although different, the family physician must select that body of knowledge that best meets the needs of his individual patients, needs that allow prevention, early diagnosis, early treatment, and, if necessary, early referral.

Myth 2: in any given field of medicine, the specialist always knows more than the family physician. Family physicians become knowledgeable about common conditions that rarely reach specialists. Sometimes this comes as a surprise to family physicians themselves. The most common example of that would be the one of the patient who pressures the family physician to refer him to a specialist, even though the family physician feels in full command of the situation. Here family physicians often find to their surprise that the specialist is out of his or her depth, because common variants of the disease are, for the specialist, often as difficult as uncommon variants of the disease for family physicians.

Myth 3: by specializing, one can eliminate uncertainty. It has been suggested that the only way to eliminate uncertainty is to reduce problems to their simplest elements and isolate them from their surroundings. This would quickly spell the end of the specialty in question.

Myth 4: only by specializing can one attain depth of knowledge. This myth confuses the concept of depth with the concept of detail. The depth of a person's knowledge depends on the quality of his or her mind, not on information content.

Myth 5: as science advances, the load of information increases. Actually, the contrary is true. Authorities have established that it is the immature branches of science that have the greatest load of information. As eloquently put by Sir Peter Medawar:[1]

> As science advances, particular facts are comprehended within, and therefore, in a sense annihilated by, general statements of increasing power and compass— whereupon the facts need no longer be known explicitly—that is, spelled out and kept in mind.

Myth 6: error in medicine is usually caused by lack of information. Actually, very little medical error is caused by physicians' being ill-informed. Much more is caused by carelessness, insensitivity, failure to listen, administrative inefficiency, failure of communication, and many other factors that have significantly more to do with **attitudes** and **skills** of the physician than lack of factual knowledge.

2. E. The fact that family physicians are by definition generalists does not mean that they all have identical knowledge and skills. All family physicians should share the same commitment to patient care. However, by virtue of special interest or training, a family physician

may have knowledge that is not shared by his or her colleagues. In a group of family physicians this will often serve as a source of enrichment. The danger, however, in this is the possible fragmentation of the specialty. Family physicians may be differentiated, but family medicine should not fragment.

The family physician is distinguished not by being the only person responsible for performing the generalist function, but by the personal ability for acting across clinical and multidimensional boundaries. The latter boundary is best exemplified by what we term the *biopsychosocial model of illness.* This is currently expanding to include multiple primary health professionals as well as health care resource management.

3. D. The biomedical model of illness, a model that has dominated medicine for decades, is finally beginning its decline. For some of us, the decline cannot come soon enough. The biomedical model, also referred to by some as the "old paradigm" of medicine, can be described in the following manner:

Patients suffer from diseases that can be categorized in the same manner as all other natural processes. Disease can be and is viewed separately from the person who is suffering from it, and separately from the person's social context. Mental and physical diseases are considered separately, and there is special provision in the biomedical model for psychosomatic diseases in which the mind appears to influence and act on the body. For every disease there is a cause, and a major research agenda item is to discover those causes.

The biomedical model does not consider the context of the disease in the patient's life and the meaning of the disease in that context. The latter is the essential feature of the biopsychosocial model.

4. C. A very significant gap exists between the way we, as physicians, view disease and the way patients experience illness. Disease can best be described as a specific, definable, physiologic or psychologic entity that has a negative effect on bodily functioning. Although physicians often see illness in this context, patients see illness as a disruption of their "being in the world." Furthermore, illness is an intensely personal experience, one that can only be understood by the patient in terms of not only their world but of everything that is in it. Suffering, which is really an extension of illness, is the manner in which illness affects the individual in a negative way. As family physicians, it is extremely important that we are sensitive to suffering, listen to our patients' accounts of their suffering, be with our patients during that time, and offer support to them and their families, especially in the terminal stages of life.

5. C. The biopsychosocial model of illness describes the patient's reaction to what we call disease and, as previously discussed, what is better called illness. How the illness affects the patient, the patient's being, and the patient's interaction with his or her world in the biological, psychological, sociological, and spiritual sense is the best description of this model.

The illness/disease theory, the specific etiology theory, the mind/body theory, and the biological/psychological theory are all examples of what was previously referred to as the medical model.

6. A. The clinical model that best describes the role of the family physician in patient care is called the patient-centered clinical method. The patient-centered clinical method is the only model that allows the physician to explore with the patient the origin of illness in the true biopsychosocial sense.

7. E. The prevalence of illness and utilization of medical resources among 1000 adults in the United States has been extensively studied. For every 1000 members of the adult population, 750 will report one or more illnesses or injuries per month. Of those 750 adults, 250 will consult a physician one or more times/month. Of the 250 adults who consult a physician/month, nine will be admitted to hospital, five will be referred to another physician, and only one will be referred to a university medical center in that same month.

These figures illustrate the importance of primary care in the overall American health care scheme.

8. D. Although family medicine has its roots of origin in general practice, it has definitely established itself as a specialty in its own right. This is especially true in the United States and Canada. Whereas general practice is the practice of medicine in a primary care setting with no specific center or focus, family medicine has as a specific focus the care of the patient in the context of the family. This is in keeping with the previously described biopsychosocial model of illness and the description of that illness in the patient's world. The definition of family is not limited to the typical nuclear family. It is, rather, based on the patient's definition of what, from his or her viewpoint, constitutes his or her family.

9. E. According to the United States Department of Health and Human Services, the 25 most common reasons for visits to family physicians for males include (in descending order of frequency) the following: sore throat, head cold, cough, skin rash, fever, general medical examination, physical examination for employment, earache, chest pain excluding heart pain, nonarticular rheumatism, headache excluding migraine and sinus, abdominal pain, physical examination for school, lacerations of the upper extremity, neck symptoms, foot and toe symptoms, physical examination for extracurricular activities, stomach pain and cramps, prophylactic

immunizations, nasal congestion, shoulder symptoms, leg symptoms, hand and finger injury, knee symptoms, and diarrhea.

There are few differences in this order for females. Pap smears, dizziness, nausea, dysuria, anxiety, and weight gain are among the top 25 reasons female patients visit doctors.

These lists illustrate the nature of primary care: a specialty that is dominated by common, everyday problems. The challenge for the family physician is differentiating serious illnesses from minor illnesses and knowing when to refer the patient to a consultant. This problem includes the wise use of health care resources, an issue that is becoming more important all the time.

10. B. The most common method of reasoning used in family medicine is known as *hypothetical-deductive* reasoning. In this method, a method commonly used in the patient-centered model, the family physician takes cues from the patient, forms hypotheses, and repeatedly and continuously tests these hypotheses against the data being compiled. As more and more information becomes available, hypotheses are rejected and changed until eventually a hypothesis that fits all of the available data is accepted.

The other choices offered in the question, including intuition, pattern recognition, and the use of clinical practice guidelines, are all methods that are used either separately or together by some physicians. Although one might argue that this is a trivial question, it is very important in that it forms the basis of the art of medicine.

SOLUTION TO SHORT ANSWER MANAGEMENT PROBLEM 71

The five most important questions you would ask the patient at this time include the following:
1) What do *you* think is causing the headaches?
2) Describe your mood. Are you anxious? Do you feel irritable or depressed?
3) Describe what is happening in your family. Have there been any recent changes at home with the children, your husband, or in your extended family?
4) Is your husband supportive? Is there anything else going on with your husband that may be contributing to the problem?
5) Do you have any other symptoms?

The case of this 37-year-old mother is typical of the type of problem where knowledge of and use of the biopsycho-

social model of illness is essential. As you have known this patient and her family for some time, and as these very frequent migraine headaches are most unusual, this suggests the likely involvement of other factor(s).

As an opening question, it is often wise to ask the patient what he or she thinks the problem is. This will often produce amazing results!

Some of the potential causes of the headaches that should be considered in this patient include the following:
1) Family or personal stressors: difficulty coping with five young children, potential concerns over other family matters, alcohol abuse in self or husband, unemployment or fear of same in spouse
2) Masked depression
3) Marital disharmony: always consider spousal abuse as a potential cause.

Although none of these may be present, chances are that something in the family has triggered these headaches. Always dig deeper before digging into your pocket for the prescription pad!

SUMMARY

1. Family medicine is a specialty in itself. It is inherently different from general practice in its focus on the family.
2. The biopsychosocial model is the operational model of the patient-centered clinical method in family medicine. It has replaced the biomedical model.
3. There is a difference between illness and disease. Illness is an intensely personal experience that only the patient can describe. It is associated with suffering that can be relieved by family physicians concerned with the art, as well as the science, of family medicine.
4. In family medicine common things are common; uncommon things are uncommon. When you hear hoofbeats, think of horses, not zebras.
5. Family medicine is a specialty of which we can all be proud; family medicine is not just for students who cannot do anything else.

SUGGESTED READINGS

American Psychiatric Association. Diagnostic and Statistical Manual. 4th Ed. Washington, DC: American Psychiatric Association Press, 1994.

McWhinney IR. A textbook of family medicine. 2nd Ed. Oxford: Oxford University Press, 1982.

Medawar PB. The art of the soluble. London: Methuen, 1967.

PROBLEM 72   A 35-YEAR-OLD FEMALE WITH A 4-YEAR HISTORY OF CHRONIC ABDOMINAL PAIN

A 35-year-old female, a well-known patient of yours who has a 4-year history of chronic abdominal pain (diagnosed by you as irritable bowel syndrome), presents to your office for a periodic health examination. During the encounter she mentions that she would like to see a specialist about her condition; although you have completely investigated her symptoms, she continues to have intermittent abdominal pain. She states that she really is not sure that her complaints have been sufficiently investigated and asks you to make a referral to a gastroenterologist that has been recommended to her.

SELECT THE ONE BEST ANSWER TO THE FOLLOWING QUESTIONS

1. Considering the case cited, what should you do now?
   a) explain to the patient that you have completely investigated the condition and that there is no need for a referral
   b) tell the patient that if that is the way she feels she should probably find another family physician
   c) empathize with the patient about her symptoms and refer her to a gastroenterologist of your choice
   d) empathize with the patient about her symptoms and refer her to the gastroenterologist that she mentions unless there is a specific reason not to
   e) tell the patient that you are deeply offended by her request; she has no right to question your competence

2. Considering a patient's request for a second opinion, which of the following statements is true?
   a) a patient does not have the right to ask for a second opinion
   b) a patient who asks for a second opinion is demonstrating lack of trust in you as a family physician
   c) a patient has the right to ask for a second opinion
   d) the request for a second opinion should be granted only if you have some uncertainty about either diagnosis or therapy
   e) it is difficult to answer this question; some patients do have the right to ask for a second opinion, and others do not

3. In considering the relationship of the health care team to the patient, which of the following statements is(are) true?
   a) the health care team must coordinate all patient care; there is no true leader or head
   b) the family physician is the head of the health care team
   c) the attending physician in whatever circumstance is being dealt with at the time is the head of the health care team
   d) the leadership or headship of the health care team depends on the individual situation, the patient, and many other factors
   e) none of the above statements are true

4. What is the primary purpose of consultation or referral to a specialist?
   a) to validate the findings of the family physician
   b) to make sure that you, the family physician, haven't missed anything
   c) to provide reassurance to your patient that you are concerned about his or her welfare
   d) to improve the quality of health care by making available to patients and referring physicians the knowledge and skills of specialist/consultants at appropriate times
   e) to provide protection for you, the family physician, against a malpractice suit

5. It is generally agreed that family physicians, given the proper training, can adequately care for what percentage of the patients they see in their practices without the aid of consultation or referral?
   a) 50%
   b) 60%
   c) 75%
   d) 85%
   e) 95%

6. Which of the following is(are) responsibilities of the physician making the referral to a specialist or consultant?
   a) to ensure that patients understand the need for and purpose of referral and consultation
   b) to demonstrate courtesy and respect for patients and specialists/consultants during the consultation and referral process
   c) to communicate clearly to the specialist/consultant the purpose and problems for which help is needed
   d) to send specialists/consultants (when necessary and possible) the results of findings and investigations, including copies of radiological films, so that they will be available at the time of the consultation
   e) all of the above

7. Examine the five following situations. Indicate whether each is either an appropriate referral or referral in an inappropriate manner.
   a) A family physician has carefully worked up a patient with multiple joint pains by careful history, physical examination, and laboratory testing. He is unable to

find any abnormalities and refers his patient to a rheumatologist. His referral letter contains the essence of his history, his physical examination, copies of the laboratory investigations, and his differential diagnosis and opinion.

b) A family physician sees an elderly patient with multiple medical problems who is on multiple medications. He decides to refer the patient to a general internist and writes her a brief note stating: "Elderly patient with CHF, hypertension, diabetes, and osteoarthritis on multiple medications. PLEASE ASSESS. Thank you."

c) A family physician sees a middle-aged man with what appears to be a chronic fatigue syndrome. She takes a complete history, does a complete physical examination, and does laboratory work to exclude anemia and other blood abnormalities, and hypothyroidism. She also rules out major depression. She refers the patient to an infectious disease specialist for a second opinion.

d) A family physician sees a patient who has the signs and symptoms of a major depressive illness. The patient, however, does not accept this diagnosis and asks to be referred to a general internist for a second opinion. The family physician agrees to this referral.

e) A family physician sees a new patient who has been to four other physicians with complaints of chronic lumbar pain. She requests a referral to a pain clinic. The family physician takes a complete history, does a complete physician examination, and agrees to the patient's request.

8. Regarding the responsibilities of patients in referral to a consultant or specialist, which of the following statements is(are) true?
   a) the patient should understand the need for and purpose of the consultation or referral
   b) the patient should demonstrate respect and courtesy for both the referring and the consulting physician
   c) the patient should understand that, after the consultation or referral, returning to the referring physician for continuing care and advice as a result of the consultation is the preferred practice
   d) the patient should understand the importance of keeping the appointment and make every effort to do so
   e) all of the above

9. Regarding the responsibilities of specialists/consultants in the referral process, which of the following statements is false?
   a) the consultant has the responsibility to provide his or her services in a timely manner depending on the urgency of the condition

b) the consultant has the responsibility to communicate his or her findings in a timely manner to the referring physician
c) the consultant has the responsibility of deciding whether or not the patient should continue to be seen on an ongoing basis by himself or herself or should return to the family physician for ongoing care
d) the consultant has the responsibility to advise referring physicians promptly of their patients' admission to hospital
e) the consultant has the responsibility to participate in peer and system review of the consultation and referral process

10. A 28-year-old female with chronic headaches presents to your office for the specific purpose of seeking referral to a neurologist. She has seen five neurologists already but is not satisfied with what any of them have told her. What is the most appropriate action for you to take at this time?
    a) agree to refer her to another neurologist and get out of the room as quickly as possible
    b) refuse to refer the patient to another neurologist
    c) ask the patient to come back in a few weeks; you have to think carefully about this request
    d) tell the patient that although you will refer her to another neurologist, this is a complete waste of everyone's time and money; there is obviously nothing wrong with her
    e) none of the above

11. Which of the following statements is true regarding the future number of family physicians in the United States relative to specialists/consultants?
    a) the relative proportion of family physicians/specialists is likely to remain the same
    b) the relative proportion of family physicians/specialists is likely to decrease
    c) the relative proportion of family physicians/specialists is likely to increase
    d) it is difficult to predict which way the trend will develop over the next several years
    e) there are likely to be decreases in both the number of family physicians and the number of specialists relative to other health care professionals

12. Regarding the definition of lateral referrals and the ethical implications of same, which of the following statements is true?
    a) lateral referrals are referrals in which a family physician refers a patient from one specialist to another; lateral referrals are completely ethical
    b) lateral referrals are referrals in which a specialist who has been consulted refers the patient to another specialist without the knowledge or consent of the family physician; lateral referrals are completely ethical

c) lateral referrals are referrals in which a specialist who has been consulted refers the patient to another specialist without knowledge of the family physician; lateral referrals without the knowledge of the referring family physician may not be in the patient's best interest and should be discouraged

d) lateral referrals are referrals in which a family physician refers a patient to another family physician with expertise in the particular area; lateral referrals may not be in the best interest of the patient

e) lateral referrals are referrals in which a family physician refers a patient to another family physician with expertise in the particular area; lateral referrals are always ethical and in the best interest of the patient

13. Regarding referrals from one family physician to another, which of the following statements is true?

a) family physicians rarely develop expertise in a specific area; thus referrals from another family physician are rarely appropriate

b) family physicians may develop significant expertise in a specific area; referrals from one family physician to another may well be in the best interest of the patient

c) family physicians who develop specific areas of interest are really straying away from the foundations of their specialty

d) family physicians should always consider referral to a specialist/consultant rather than to another family physician

e) family physicians are not in a position to identify each other's areas of expertise with any degree of knowledge

14. A 35-year-old female with cancer of the colon is admitted for surgery to her local hospital by the surgeon who is going to perform her hemicolectomy. How should the patient's family physician be notified regarding the admission?

a) an admitting slip from the hospital once the patient is admitted

b) through the ward clerk in charge of the ward to which the patient is admitted

c) through the charge nurse who is looking after the patient on the day of the admission

d) through the resident on the surgery service

e) none of the above

15. A patient who was originally seen by an obstetrician for care during pregnancy is subsequently referred to an internist, a neurologist, a dermatologist, and a gastroenterologist for multiple other problems. No family physician is involved in the patient's care. Regarding this type of referral pattern, which of the following statement(s) is(are) true?

a) this pattern of referral is likely to lead to optimal patient care

b) this pattern of referral is likely to be followed by close communication between the various specialists

c) this pattern of referral, without the coordinating role of a family physician, may create significant problems in the care of this patient and her family

d) this pattern of referral is extremely uncommon

e) none of the above are true

Short Answer Management Problem 72

Your patient, a 28-year-old female, is hospitalized for repair and reconstruction of a torn left anterior collateral knee ligament, removal of a torn left lateral meniscus, and a partially torn left medial meniscus. The surgeon performs the operation. The patient is in severe pain after the procedure, but the surgeon tells her that the pain is not severe enough to warrant a strong analgesic. You, her family physician, do not have admitting or order-writing privileges on the surgical floor. You are called by a close friend and informed of the patient's condition. Discuss your approach to helping solve this patient's problem.

ANSWERS

1. D. Unless there is a specific reason not to, you should refer the patient to the gastroenterologist of her choice. Although the family physician may feel offended by the patient's request, he or she should not be. Patients with chronic symptoms are difficult to manage. You may very well find that a second opinion not only validates your findings but also improves the relationship between you and the patient. She may in fact find the chronic abdominal pain to be less of a problem. In this case, it would prove to be less of a problem for both you and her.

2. C. A patient has the right to ask for a second opinion. In this case, you should look on her request as an opportunity to confirm your findings and as an opportunity for the patient to receive the reassurance she needs to manage the abdominal pain more effectively. In the long term, this will turn out to be beneficial to you as well; the patient will likely complain less of the problem and the doctor-patient relationship will likely improve.

3. E. The patient is the head of the health care team. The patient must be fully informed on all matters relating to his or her health and have the opportunity to make decisions with all pertinent information available. The responsibilities of the physicians (both family physicians and specialists/consultants) and the patient will be discussed in subsequent questions.

4. D. The primary purpose of consultation or referral is to improve the quality of health care by making available to patients and referring physicians the knowledge and skills of specialists/consultants at appropriate times.

There may be situations in complicated cases in which you wish to validate your findings or make sure that nothing has been overlooked. There may also be times when additional reassurance is needed that only a specialist can provide.

To refer to specialists for the sole purpose of protecting yourself against malpractice (especially on a regular basis) should give you cause for concern. Perhaps you need to upgrade your skills in one or more areas to help build confidence in your own abilities. Also, in this situation, perhaps you should reconsider the type of practice you are in and make adjustments that will decrease your anxiety level.

5. E. Most authorities have stated that family physicians can well look after the vast majority of patient problems that cross their office doors. A well-trained family physician should be able to look after at least 95% of the patients seen in practice without referral to a specialist or consultant.

6. E. In addition to the four responsibilities listed in the question choices, the other important responsibility of the referring physician is to participate in peer and system review of the consultation and referral process.

7. B. This is not an infrequent occurrence and is really a situation of a family physician "dumping" a complicated patient on a consultant or specialist with little significant information given to the consultant. This type of referral is expensive and time-consuming (the specialist will no doubt have to start from the beginning) and certainly could be labeled as unprofessional.

All of the other situations described are appropriate referrals.

8. E. The important point in this question is that patients, as well as their physicians, have a responsibility to make the consultation process work in an efficient, timely, and cost-effective manner.

9. C. The major responsibilities of a consultant or specialist are as follows:

1) To provide his or her services in a timely manner depending on the urgency of the condition. If the family physician feels that the condition is urgent, he or she should communicate this to the consultant, and the consultant should see the patient as quickly as possible. If he or she cannot personally see the patient, then appropriate arrangements should be made for the patient to be seen by someone else.
2) To communicate clearly and promptly the results of the consultation process to both referring physicians and patients
3) To communicate clearly and promptly the results of laboratory tests to the referring physician; the results can be explained to the patient.
4) To participate in peer and system review of the consultation process in an effort to improve it
5) To notify the referring physician at once when his or her patient has been admitted to hospital

The consultant or specialist should return the patient to the referring physician once the consultation is complete. A consultation is just that: a consultation. It is inappropriate for consultants to take over the care of patients referred from family physicians unless they have been specifically asked to do so. Having said that, it may take a consultant or specialist a number of visits to feel that he or she has adequately dealt with the problem. Also, it may be totally appropriate for the consultant (with the family physician's permission) to see the patient on a periodic basis to maximize quality of care.

10. E. This situation is not as uncommon as may initially be thought. There are many situations in which patients (for various reasons) request to see a number of specialists.

The most appropriate actions to take at this time are to perform a complete history, do a complete physical examination, and attempt to determine why the patient has been unsatisfied with the advice she has obtained previously. It may be that what this patient needs is someone to listen and help her deal with her chronic headaches in a different manner. Conversely, it may be that there is something else causing the headaches that has not yet been discovered.

Most likely, however, no matter what the case, it would appear that this patient needs a good family physician much more than referral to another neurologist.

11. C. The number of family physicians relative to the number of specialists is likely to increase significantly in the next several years in the United States. The primary need in the United States at this time is for well-trained family physicians to balance the number of specialists.

12. C. Lateral referrals are referrals that take place from one specialist/consultant to another. If the original referring family physician is not notified, the ethics of such process is very questionable. If a consultant feels that a

patient requires another specialist/consultant, the referral should be done with the knowledge, input, and involvement of the initial referring family physician.

13. B. Family physicians may well develop areas of expertise in which it is in the best interest of the patient to consider referral to another family physician rather than to a specialist. This acquisition of knowledge and skills on the part of the family physicians involved is especially useful in regional centers where specialists are not always available. The patient, rather than having to travel significant distances and wait a significant length of time to see a specialist, may be served as well or better by a family physician with knowledge and skill in the specific area.

14. E. The surgeon who is going to perform the operation should inform the patient's family physician and seek input and help from him or her. At a time when a patient is about to undergo a major cancer operation, the patient's family physician, whether or not he or she has formal hospital admitting privileges, is still able to make a significant contribution to the care of the patient. One of the most frequent errors is that the family physician of record is not notified at all or notified in a way in which a significant delay occurs. The patient, meanwhile, is often left wondering where his or her family physician is and who to turn to for the answers to the many questions that may arise during a significant medical or surgical procedure.

As a principle, miscommunication is often avoided if the contact and communication is direct from attending physician to attending physician. In most cases, this route of communication will optimize patient care.

15. C. This particular scenario is not at all uncommon and in many cases leads not only to a breakdown in communication between the various specialists but to a lower overall quality of patient care. The role of the family physician in treating patients with multiple medical problems is even more critical than in a patient without such problems. The family physician understands the patient and the patient's family and is likely to be able to significantly improve the overall care delivered because of this knowledge.

SOLUTION TO SHORT ANSWER MANAGEMENT PROBLEM 72

One of the roles of a family physician is to be the patient's advocate. In this particular case, if the patient says she is in severe pain, then it is reasonable to believe that she is. The family physician should communicate directly with the surgeon and offer to undertake the responsibility of managing the patient's pain. If there are difficulties due to the issue of hospital privileges, it may be posssible for the patient to be transferred to the care of the family physician. If not, the fam-

ily physician could offer to write analgesic suggestions on the chart, which could be followed by the nursing staff if the surgeon agrees. As the referral of the patient to the surgeon likely came from the family physician, it would seem probable that the surgeon would agree to allow the family physician to participate in the care of his or her own patient at this time.

SUMMARY

1. The referral or consultation process requires the participation and commitment of the family physician, the specialist or consultant, and the patient. All three have responsibilities.
2. Patients are ethically entitled to a second opinion; a physician should not feel offended when one is asked for.
3. The patient is the head of the health care team.
4. The primary purpose of referral or consultation is to improve the quality of care delivered to patients by making available the knowledge, skills, and experience of someone skilled in the management of a particular problem.
5. Family physicians can manage the vast majority of patient care problems without the need for consultation with specialist colleagues.
6. Family physicians who refer a patient to a specialist have the responsibility of providing a detailed summary of the patient's history, physical findings, and laboratory investigations. To refer a patient to a specialist with a brief one- or two-sentence note is completely inappropriate.
7. Specialists or consultants have the responsibility of seeing patients in a timely fashion; in an urgent situation if they or unable to see the patient, they should make arrangements for someone else to do so.
8. Specialists or consultants who admit a patient to hospital should personally inform the patient's family physician and invite the family physician to participate in the care of the patient in whatever way is possible.
9. Lateral referrals from specialist to specialist without the involvement of the original referring family physician should be discouraged.
10. Patients who go from one consultant to another looking for answers should be listened to and cared for by a compassionate family physician.
11. Patient advocacy is a major responsibility of the family physician.

SUGGESTED READINGS

American Psychiatric Association. Diagnostic and statistical manual. 4th Ed. Washington, DC: American Psychiatric Association Press, 1994.

Report of a joint task force of The College of Family Physicians of Canada and The Royal College of Physicians and Surgeons of Canada. Relationship between family physicians and specialists/consultants in the provision of patient care. Canadian Family Physician 1993; 39:1309-1312.

PROBLEM 73   A 34-YEAR-OLD FEMALE WITH METASTATIC MALIGNANT MELANOMA JUST DIAGNOSED

You have just received the CT scan report on a 34-year-old female, a mother of three, who had a malignant melanoma removed 3 years ago. Originally, it was a Clark's level I, and the prognosis was excellent. The patient presented to your office 1 week ago complaining of chest pain and abdominal pain. A CT scan of the chest and abdomen revealed metastatic lesions throughout the lungs and the abdomen. She is in your office and you have to deliver the bad news of the significant spread of the cancer.

SELECT THE ONE BEST ANSWER TO THE FOLLOWING QUESTIONS

1. Regarding the delivery of bad news to patients who are unsupported during the visit, which of the following statements is true?
   a) the fact that the patient is alone is insignificant
   b) you have no right to interfere with her decision to come alone to the office
   c) you should go into the consultation room and explain that the news you are about to deliver is complex; you would feel better if her husband or significant other were present when the test results were explained
   d) patients don't remember much of anything from the first visit, at which this type of news is delivered, so it does not really matter whether someone else is present or not
   e) having a significant other present will only complicate an already difficult situation

2. Which of the following settings is not acceptable for the delivery of bad news?
   a) a private physician's office
   b) a quiet room in a hospital setting
   c) the patient's home
   d) a private hospital room
   e) a multibed hospital room

3. Following the first step (getting started), what is the next step in breaking bad news?
   a) deliver the bad news all in one blow; get it over with as quickly as is humanly possible
   b) fire a "warning shot" that some bad news is coming
   c) find out how much the patient knows
   d) find out how much the patient wants to know
   e) it doesn't really matter what you do next; the end result will be the same

4. Which of the following statements regarding finding out how much the patient wants to know is true?
   a) it is not very important to find out how much the patient wants to know; everyone really should be told everything
   b) most patients would rather not know all of the details of their illness

   c) most patients can't really make up their minds at the first interview how much they want to know
   d) most patients will want to know the whole truth
   e) in some instances patients shouldn't be told anyway

5. In beginning to deliver bad news we frequently suggest that you "fire a warning shot" first. What would be an appropriate warning shot?
   a) "you have cancer, and unfortunately it is a very bad cancer"
   b) "you have a cancer but we'll do our best to 'zap-zap' it with radiation"
   c) "you have a very aggressive malignancy; fortunately, that means we may be able to kill more cells with the chemotherapy"
   d) "unfortunately, the situation appears to be more serious than we would have hoped for"
   e) "unfortunately, the cancer has spread all over your body; I think it's time you called your lawyer and started to get things wrapped up"

6. There are two languages that physicians use in talking to patients: English and "medispeak." Unfortunately, patients usually only understand English.
   Which of the following is an example of "medispeak"?
   a) blast cells
   b) multiple sclerosis
   c) tumor
   d) cancer
   e) leukemia

7. Which of the following statements is false regarding the involvement of family physicians in the care of a patient with cancer?
   a) ideally, the family physician should be present when the patient is told of a bad diagnosis and/or prognosis
   b) the family physician and the primary consultant should be in constant contact and should be certain that the same message is delivered
   c) family physicians have a limited role to play once the patient is enrolled in a tertiary care cancer treatment center
   d) the family physician has a responsibility to follow up on the care of his or her patients whether or not he or she is actively involved in all aspects of care

e) as cancer becomes more common with an aging population, more and more of the care that is traditionally delivered in a specialty center may be transferred to the family physician

8. Which of the following is(are) descriptive roles played by family physicians in the care of patients with cancer?
   a) coordinating
   b) compassionate
   c) continuous
   d) comprehensive
   e) all of the above

9. Which of the following is(are) true regarding the delivery of bad news to patients with a serious disease?
   a) check the reception of the news frequently
   b) reinforce and clarify the information you are giving frequently
   c) check your communication level frequently
   d) listen for the patient's concerns
   e) all of the above

10. In an interview in which news of a serious disease is presented, which of the following is the thing to do before the patient leaves the office?
    a) make sure the patient understands every word
    b) make sure the patient understands that you are doing everything you can
    c) make sure you leave the patient with a follow-up plan and provide the patient with some hope
    d) make sure the patient understands the dismal prognosis
    e) make sure that you have left no question unanswered

11. A 45-year-old physician, a well-known academic at a prestigious medical school, travels to a world-famous medical center to consult a neurologist regarding symptoms including "stiffness in the legs," very brisk deep tendon reflexes, and fasciculations. The neurologist confirms the physician patient's suspicion of amyotrophic lateral sclerosis. He then goes on to give the physician patient a pamphlet setting out in grim detail the future the patient already knows too well. The neurologist describes the mortality curve of ALS to the physician patient and comments, "Very interestingly, there is a break in the mortality slope after 3 years."

   As a physician, what is your first reaction to this patient's story?
   a) this must be fiction; no physician would treat another physician in this manner
   b) the ALS that the physician patient has acquired has obviously also affected his brain, although confabulation is not characteristic of ALS
   c) these are comments from some off-the-wall case history; in real life this would not happen
   d) something must have triggered the physician patient to completely misinterpret the neurologist's comments
   e) none of the above

12. The physician patient goes back to his home university to continue the pursuit of his academic career to the best of his ability. He purposefully does not tell his colleagues the truth about his condition and continues to teach, write, receive grants, publish, and practice medicine. As his condition deteriorates and he becomes more and more physically disabled, which of the following scenarios is most likely to occur?
    a) he will likely receive more phone calls from concerned colleagues and more inquiries as to whether or not they can be of assistance to him
    b) when his colleagues see him in the hall, they will likely go out of their way to talk to him and offer any assistance they can
    c) once his colleagues are aware of the full extent of his illness they will likely offer not only moral support but support in terms of assistance in teaching, assistance in looking after his patients, and assistance in keeping his research programs viable
    d) all of the above are likely to occur
    e) none of the above are likely to occur

Short Answer Management Problem 73

You are the physician in charge of the care of an 85-year-old woman who you have just diagnosed as having breast cancer. Before you have an opportunity to talk to the patient, the patient's son and daughter come to your office to advise you that they do not wish you to tell their mother anything about her diagnosis. Describe how you would respond to the request.

ANSWERS

1. C. You should go into the patient's room and explain that the news you are about to deliver is complex; you would feel better if her husband or significant other were present when the test results were explained. To have devastating news delivered to a patient in an unsupported environment is absolutely unacceptable. If a

spouse, son, daughter, brother, sister or other significant other cannot be present during the delivery of the news, a social worker, psychologist, or member of the clergy should be present for patient support.

2. E. A multibed hospital room is not an acceptable location for the delivery of bad news. Patients in beds next to your patient will obviously be able to hear all or most of the conversation. Just pulling the hospital curtains is not an acceptable alternative.

The first rule in breaking bad news is getting started, which includes getting the physical context right and starting off the discussion in the presence of a significant other.

The other alternatives in the question are all acceptable.

3. C. The next step is to find out how much the patient knows. The following are questions that may be of help in this regard:[1]
   a) What have you made of the illness so far?
   b) What have you been thinking about this nausea/unsteadiness/breast lump?
   c) Have you been worried about this illness/these symptoms?
   d) What did the previous doctors tell you about the illness/operation?
   e) Have you been thinking that this illness might be serious?
   f) Have you been worried about yourself?
   g) When you first had symptom X, what did you think it might be?
   h) What did Doctor X tell you when he sent you here?
   i) Did you think something serious was going on then?

4. D. Most patients will want to be told the whole truth, but there are some exceptions. Questions that can be asked to determine how much the patient wants to know include the following:
   a) If this condition turns out to be something serious, are you the kind of person who likes to know exactly what's going on?
   b) Would you like me to tell you the full details of the diagnosis?
   c) Are you the kind of person who likes the full details of what's wrong, or would you prefer just to hear about the treatment plan?
   d) Do you like to know exactly what's going on or would you prefer me to give you just a brief outline?
   e) If your condition is serious, how much would you like to know about it?
   f) Would you like me to tell you the full details of your condition, or is there somebody else that you'd like me to talk to?

5. D. A "warning shot" tells the patient that there is going to be more bad news. The most appropriate warning shot in a situation like this would be something like one of the following:
   a) "Unfortunately, the situation is more serious than we would have hoped for."
   b) "The chest X ray shows that there is a tumor on the lung. Does that make you think of anything?"
   c) "When you had those bruises, your blood test showed that you weren't making some components in the blood called platelets. They're made in the bone marrow and that's why your doctor ordered a bone marrow test to see what was wrong. It was that test that showed the problem."

6. A. Most health care professionals are justifiably proud of their own esoteric language. Unfortunately, this understanding does not extend to patients. Using "medispeak" to explain something to a patient makes it less likely that the patient will be able to ask difficult questions. As well, it isolates and alienates the patient who finds it unfamiliar. A comparison of English and "medispeak" is shown in the following list. (from Buckman R. How to break bad news: a guide for health care professionals. Toronto: University of Toronto Press, 1992)

ENGLISH	MEDISPEAK
Leukemia	Blast cells
Multiple sclerosis	Demyelination
Cancer	Abnormal growth
Cancer	Space-occupying lesion
The situation is serious	The prognosis is guarded

7. C. Family physicians must assume and maintain a coordinating role in the care of the cancer patient at all times. Although at a certain time a patient may be receiving treatment in a tertiary care treatment center, the family physician must be seen as coordinating that care. It is the family physician's responsibility to ensure that constant communication between himself or herself and the specialist(s) involved is maintained. As the population ages and more and more patients develop cancer, the care of patients with cancer will be transferred to the family physician.

8. E. The family physician's role can best be described in terms of 5 C's: continuous, comprehensive, compassionate, coordinated and competent care.

9. E. While providing information to the patient, it is imperative that physician keep the following principles in mind:
   1) Provide the information in small chunks—remember the "warning shot."
   2) Use English, not medispeak.
   3) Check reception frequently.
   4) Reinforce and clarify information frequently.
   5) Check communication level frequently.

6) Listen to your patient's concerns.

7) Blend your agenda with the patient's.

10. C. Make sure before the patient leaves your office that you provide him or her with a follow-up plan. This will reinforce the belief that you are indeed in charge of his or her care and will ensure that the care plan is implemented. In addition, be sure to leave the patient with some hope for the future. That hope must be realistic hope, but hope nevertheless.

11. E. None of the above is a correct first reaction. The other choices are reasons for us to believe that things didn't happen that way, in effect believing that one physician wouldn't treat another this way.

12. E. None of the above is likely to occur.

This case is a true story, and was eloquently told by a physician in the *New England Journal of Medicine.*[2] I will summarize the observations made of both the consultation with the neurologist and the reaction and treatment that the physician patient received when he returned to his home university.

My first reaction to the neurologist was one of deep disappointment from his impersonal manner. The neurologist exhibited no interest in me as a person, and did not make even a perfunctory inquiry about my work. He gave me no guidelines about what I should do, either concretely—in terms of daily activities—or, what was more important, psychologically, to muster the emotional strength to cope with a progressive degenerative disease. The only thing my doctor did offer me was a pamphlet setting out in grim detail the future that I already knew about too well.

The reaction of colleagues is illustrated very well in the following description:

By early 1980, however, the limp was worse, and I now held a cane in my right hand. The inquiries ceased and were replaced by a very obvious desire to avoid me. When I arrived at work in the morning I could see, from the corner of my eye, colleagues changing their pace or stopping in their tracks to spare themselves the embarrassment of bumping into me. As the cane became inadequate and was replaced by a walker, so my isolation from my colleagues intensified.

One has to ask why this happened. The author suggests the following:

Perhaps it is because we, as physicians, are the healers. We dispense treatment, counsel, and support; and we represent strength. The dichotomy of being both doctor and patient threatens the integrity of the club. To this fraternity of healers, becoming ill is tantamount to treachery. Furthermore, the sick physician makes us uncomfortable. He reminds us of our own vulnerability and mortality, and this is frightening for those of us who deal with disease every day while arming ourselves with an imaginary cloak of immunity against personal illness. This account is meant to draw attention to our frequent inability as physicians to deal with members of our profession who no longer fit the mold of complete healer.

(From Rabin D. Compounding the ordeal of ALS: isolation from my fellow physicians. New England Journal of Medicine 1982; 307(8):506-509)

The author suggests some very simple steps that we can take to support our colleagues in time of illness, stress, trouble, or other difficulty:

First, do not ignore your ill colleagues. Greet them; inquire about their health; visit them. Offer them support if they are physically handicapped.

Second, be conscious of the physician patient's family and extend support to them. The spouse and children are suffering at least as much as the physician and need support, encouragement, and acknowledgement of their difficulties.

Third, remember that the absence of a magic potion against the disease does not render you impotent. No one can assume the burden, but knowing that you are not forgotten does ease the pain.

This special type of communication and caring among physicians (or any other professional group) is essential as we enter an era of change unlike any other era health care has ever seen. Remember that the word *doctor* is translated from the Latin *"doktor,"* meaning *teacher.* As physicians we are all teachers, some in more diverse ways than others. Medical students, residents, patients, other health care professionals, and most of all ourselves play the role, at one time or another, as *student.*

When the student is ready, the teacher will appear. Confucius

SOLUTION TO SHORT ANSWER MANAGEMENT PROBLEM 73

This is not an infrequent occurrence. In this situation, it is extremely important to remember who the patient is and what rights the patient has and does not have. I would proceed in the following manner:

1) First, I would remember who the patient is: the mother, not the son and daughter.

2) Second, I would attempt to sit down with the son and daughter and explain that as their mother's physician you have an ethical responsibility to talk to her about her disease. I would offer to do it in such a way that their mother had an opportunity to communicate how much information about the disease that she wanted. As described earlier, I would ask the mother (in the presence of the son and daughter) if she was the kind of person who would like to know what the entire picture was or whether she would just as soon get on with treatment. This will usually be as far as you have to go. If the

mother says she wants to know (and the son and daughter hear this) they will usually understand that she has that right. If, on the other hand, she states that she does not wish to know, then the problem is also solved.

3) In the very occasional circumstance, you will have to resort to other procedures such as a hospital ethics committee if the son and daughter still do not agree. This, however, is very unusual.

SUMMARY

1. **The six-step protocol to breaking bad news:**
    a) Getting started:
        1. Get the physical setting right.
        2. Ensure family support at the time of breaking the news.
    b) Find out how much the patient knows.
    c) Find out how much the patient wants to know.
    d) Share the information:
        1. Decide on objectives.
        2. Give the information in small chunks—start with the "warning shot."
        3. Use English, not medispeak.
        4. Reinforce and clarify the information frequently.
        5. Listen for the patient's concerns.
        6. Blend your agenda with the patient's.
    e) Respond to the patient's feelings.
    f) Plan and follow through.

2. **Remember your colleagues:** physicians as patients are just as vulnerable if not more vulnerable than non-physicians and need our friendship, encouragement, help, and hope.

3. **Guidelines and suggestions:**
    a) Always leave the patient with (realistic) hope.
    b) Realize that the patient will not absorb all the information on the first visit; schedule follow-up visits frequently.
    c) Facilitate and coordinate all care from this point on.
    d) Remember the 5 C's of the family physician: continuous, comprehensive, compassionate, coordinated, and competent care.
    e) Try to unlearn medispeak.

SUGGESTED READINGS

Buckman R. How to break bad news: A guide for health care professionals. Toronto: University of Toronto Press, 1992.

Rabin D. Compounding the ordeal of ALS: Isolation from my fellow physicians. New England Journal of Medicine 1982; 307(8):506-509.

American Psychiatric Association. Diagnostic and statistical manual. 4th Ed. Washington, DC: American Psychiatric Association Press, 1994.

Swanson RW: The role of the family physician in the treatment of cancer. Canadian Family Physician 1990; 36:839.

PROBLEM 74   A 45-YEAR-OLD MOTHER OF TWO WHO HAS JUST LOST HER HUSBAND

A 45-year-old mother of two presents to your office the day after her husband was killed in an automobile accident. She is brought to your office by her mother who tells you that she just keeps screaming and wailing uncontrollably. She has been like this since she was informed by the police of her husband's death at 3 PM yesterday afternoon.

SELECT THE ONE BEST ANSWER TO THE FOLLOWING QUESTIONS

1. What would be the best description of this patient's condition?
   a) a normal grief reaction
   b) a pathological grief reaction
   c) an exaggerated grief reaction
   d) an abnormal grief reaction
   e) a masked grief reaction

2. What would you do at this time?
   a) shout at the patient and tell her to "snap out of it"
   b) ask your nurse to get the haloperidol *stat*
   c) ask the patient's mother to bring her back to the office when she is "more controlled"
   d) ask your nurse to get the librium *stat*
   e) none of the above

3. Which of the following *is not* a task of mourning?
   a) accepting the reality of the loss
   b) experiencing the pain of grief
   c) adjusting to an environment in which the deceased is missing
   d) withdrawing emotional energy and reinvesting it in another relationship
   e) attempting to block out all memories of the deceased

4. When is a grief reaction considered complete?
   a) when the individual is able to think of the deceased without pain
   b) when 1 year has passed
   c) when the individual has attempted to complete all of the tasks of mourning
   d) when psychotherapy is complete
   e) none of the above

5. Which of the following is not a pathognomonic characteristic of normal or acute grief?
   a) somatic or bodily distress
   b) preoccupation with an image of the deceased
   c) the inability of the individual to work productively until the grief reaction has been completely resolved
   d) guilt relating to the deceased or circumstances of his death
   e) all of the above are pathognomonic characteristics of normal or acute grief

6. Regarding normal grief reactions, which of the following is not a normal feeling in the bereaved?
   a) sadness
   b) guilt and self-reproach
   c) anxiety
   d) persistent feelings that "life isn't worth living"
   e) fatigue

7. Regarding normal grief reactions, which of the following is not a normal physical sensation in the bereaved?
   a) chest tightness and chest pain
   b) oversensitivity to noise
   c) an inability to move one side of the body in any manner
   d) general muscle weakness
   e) a sense of depersonalization

8. Regarding normal grief reactions, which of the following thoughts or cognitions is(are) not considered normal in the bereaved?
   a) hallucinations
   b) disbelief
   c) confusion
   d) sense of a presence of the deceased
   e) none of the above; all are considered normal thoughts or cognitions

9. Regarding normal grief reactions, which of the following behaviors is not considered normal in the bereaved?
   a) sleep disturbances
   b) persistent aggressive behavior toward other family members
   c) appetite disturbances
   d) social withdrawal
   e) visiting places or carrying objects that remind the survivor of the deceased

10. In comparing and contrasting normal grief behaviors with the manifestations of a major depressive disorder, which of the following statements is true?
   a) normal grief reactions and major depressive illnesses are very difficult to distinguish
   b) the main distinction between a normal grief reaction and a major depressive illness is that in a normal grief reaction there is frequently a loss of self-esteem whereas in a major depressive illness there is not.

c) the main distinction between a normal grief reaction and a major depressive illness is that a major depressive illness is associated with a loss of self-esteem whereas a normal grief reaction is not

d) the major distinction between a normal grief reaction and a major depressive illness is that a normal grief reaction usually has a significant appetite disturbance whereas a major depressive illness does not

e) the major distinction between a normal grief reaction and a major depressive illness is that a normal grief reaction usually has significant hyposomnia whereas a major depressive illness does not

11. Once the shock of the loss has abated, you attempt to provide counseling to the patient described in Question 1. Which of the following is not a principle that you should employ in grief counseling?
a) help the patient to actualize the loss
b) help the patient experience the pain of grief
c) assist the patient in beginning to live without the deceased
d) facilitate the patient in withdrawing emotional energy from the deceased
e) help the patient rid her mind of memories of the deceased

12. Regarding the prescription of mood-modifying drugs to patients who have suffered the loss of a loved one, which of the following statements is true?
a) mood-modifying drugs may be used freely in the acute phase of a grief reaction
b) mood-modifying drugs should never be used in the treatment of symptoms in individuals who have suffered the loss of a loved one
c) of the mood-modifying drugs available, the tricyclic antidepressants are reasonable choices for the acute

phase of the grief reaction; anxiolytics should be avoided
d) of the mood-modifying drugs available, the acute anxiety agents can be used freely in acute grief reactions; tricyclic antidepressants should be avoided
e) under normal circumstances all mood-modifying drugs should be avoided in acute grief; occasionally, and in an effort to give relief from anxiety or insomnia for a short period, an antianxiety agent may be prescribed

13. Which of the following are considered pathological grief reactions?
a) chronic grief reactions
b) delayed grief reactions
c) exaggerated grief reactions
d) masked grief reactions
e) all of the above

14. In which of the following situations is it most likely that anticipatory grieving has already taken place at the time of actual death?
a) death of a patient from a sudden myocardial infarction
b) death of a patient from an automobile accident
c) death of a patient as a result of suicide
d) death of an infant in NICU after a prolonged illness
e) death of a patient following a surgical complication

15. What is the family physician's role in grief counseling?
a) rule out physical disease
b) set up a contract with the survivor and establish an alliance
c) assess which of the formal grief tasks are not completed
d) explore and define linking objects
e) all of the above

Short Answer Management Problem 74

A 51-year-old female presents to your office to discuss her deceased husband. Her husband died 4 years ago, but she continues to believe that he is "still beside her." Discuss your approach to this patient.

ANSWERS

1. A. This is a perfectly normal reaction to the shock of the sudden death of a spouse. There are many behaviors that are considered to be "normal" following the death of a loved one. They include sleep disturbances, appetite disturbances, absent-minded behavior, social withdrawal, dreams of the deceased, avoiding reminders of the deceased, searching and calling out, sighing, visiting places or carrying objects that remind the survivor

of the deceased, and treasuring objects that belonged to the deceased. In this case, the two other common behaviors of crying and restless overactivity are paramount in this patient and should certainly be regarded as normal.

2. E. All of the options presented in this question are inappropriate. The most reasonable tactic to take would be to ask the mother to leave the room and to try and get the patient to talk about her feelings. A reassuring hug

or other gesture may be all that it takes to "break down the barrier" that exists. Above all else, you should tell the patient that you are here to listen, and that anything that she does or says is OK. The patient may very well open up to you in an environment that does not include her mother.

Although medication can be used, it should be used only as a last resort. Medication while calming the patient down momentarily will simply postpone or hinder the inevitable grief reaction.

3. E. The four tasks of mourning are as follows:
   1) Accept the reality of the loss.
   2) Experience the pain of grief.
   3) Adjust to an environment in which the deceased is missing.
   4) Withdraw emotional energy and reinvest it in another relationship.

   The bereaved should not attempt to block out all memories of the deceased; to do so is counterproductive and simply leads to a prolongation of the grief reaction.

4. A. A grief reaction is considered complete when the survivor can think about the deceased without pain. Although we put rough guidelines on how long normal mourning should last, we must realize that this is highly individual and depends on the type of relationship that the survivor had with the deceased, as well as a number of other factors.

5. E. Lindemann and colleagues, following the tragic Grove Nightclub fire in which 500 people lost their lives in 1942, interviewed 101 recently bereaved persons. From these interviews he formulated the pathognomonic characteristics of normal or acute grief:
   1) Somatic or bodily distress of some type
   2) Preoccupation with the image of the deceased
   3) Guilt relating to the deceased or the circumstances of the death
   4) Hostile reactions
   5) The inability to function as one had before the loss

6. D. Normal feelings after the death of a loved one include sadness, guilt and self-reproach, anxiety, loneliness, fatigue, helplessness, shock, yearning, emancipation, relief, and numbness.

   A persistent feeling that "life isn't worth living" is *not* a feature of normal grief reactions and should alert the family physician that suicide is a very real threat.

7. C. Physical sensations that are normal following the loss of a loved one include
   1) Hollowness in the stomach
   2) Tightness in the chest and chest pain
   3) Tightness in the throat
   4) Oversensitivity to noise

5) A sense of depersonalization: "I walk down the street and nothing seems real, including myself"
6) Breathlessness and feeling short of breath
7) Muscle weakness
8) Lack of energy and fatigue
9) Dry mouth

An inability to move one side of the body in any manner could represent a hysterical conversion reaction; on the other hand, it could represent a cerebrovascular accident (especially in an older individual who had just received the news of the loss of a spouse).

8. E. Thoughts or cognitions that are considered normal following the loss of a loved one include disbelief, confusion, preoccupation with an image of the deceased, sense of presence, and hallucinations.

9. B. The only behavior that is not considered normal is persistent aggressive behavior toward other family members. The other normal behaviors have been discussed in the answer to Question 1.

10. C. The major distinction between an acute grief reaction and a major depressive illness is that a major depressive illness is associated with a significant loss of self-esteem or a significant sense of hopelessness; a normal grief reaction is not.

    Disturbances of appetite and/or sleep are common in both normal grief reactions and major depressive illness.

11. E. The only choice that is not a task of normal grieving and the one that the grief counselor should not attempt is to "help the patient rid her mind of memories of the deceased." Exactly the opposite is true. The patient must, with your facilitation, work through the memories of the deceased and in so doing begin to draw away from the deceased. Reliving the happy memories is not only a normal part of grieving, but very much helps the patient withdraw the emotional energy in the manner that they must.

12. E. Although this is still a topic of debate, most authorities would suggest that no mood-modifying drugs be prescribed during the acute phase of a grief reaction. There are occasions in which the symptoms of the grief reaction become so intolerable that the benefit outweighs the risk. In these cases, and in these cases only, the prescription of an antianxiety agent for a short period of time is indicated.

13. E. All of the choices listed are considered to be pathological grief reactions.

    A *chronic grief reaction* is one that is prolonged, is excessive in duration, and never comes to a satisfactory conclusion.

A *delayed grief reaction* is sometimes called inhibited, suppressed, or postponed. In this case, the bereaved may have had an emotional reaction at the time of the loss, but it is not sufficient to the loss. At a future date the bereaved may experience the symptoms of grief over some subsequent and immediate loss, but the intensity of his or her grieving will seem excessive.

An *exaggerated grief reaction* is one in which the bereaved is usually conscious of the relationship of the reaction to the death, but the reaction to the current experience is excessive and disabling enough to seek therapy.

A *masked grief reaction* is one in which patients experience symptoms and behaviors that cause them difficulty, but they do not see or recognize them as related to the loss.

A *prolonged* grief reaction is one in which the bereaved is not able to arrive at a satisfactory grief reaction conclusion. This usually is related to the incompletion of one of the tasks of grieving.

14. D. The term *anticipatory grief* refers to grieving that occurs prior to the actual death of a loved one. The term implies a decrease or absence of overt manifestations of grief at the actual time of the death in survivors. This is associated with significant and often prolonged grieving prior to the actual death.

Death of an infant in the NICU would be the most likely death to be associated with anticipatory grieving. All of the other choices listed involve sudden death, death for which it has not been possible to prepare.

15. E. In performing grief therapy, the following guidelines are recommended for the family physician:
    1) Rule out physical disease.
    2) Set up a contract with the patient and establish an alliance.
    3) Revive memories of the deceased.
    4) Assess which grief tasks are not completed.
    5) Deal with effect or lack of effect stimulated by memories of the deceased.
    6) Explore and defuse linking objects (symbolic objects that the survivor keeps to provide a means through which the relationship with the deceased can be maintained externally).

SOLUTION TO SHORT ANSWER MANAGEMENT PROBLEM 74

This patient is undergoing a prolonged grief reaction. This is likely related to some separation conflict that resulted in an incompletion of one of the tasks of grieving. The therapy in this patient should revolve around ascertaining which of the grief tasks have yet to be completed and what impediments to this completion are. As a beginning it would be wise to go over the loss of the patient's loved one and her perceptions of it, and try to understand where in the grieving process the difficulties began.

SUMMARY OF GRIEF AND GRIEF THERAPY FOR THE FAMILY PHYSICIAN

1. There is no definite time limit for a "normal grief reaction." One can assume, however, that if there are still significant problems at 18 months to 2 years that the bereaved may have entered into a pathological grief reaction.
2. Manifestations of normal grief include feelings, physical sensations, cognitions, and behaviors.
3. Counseling procedures for the family physician revolve around helping the survivor realize the loss, work through thoughts and feelings about the deceased, and to readjust to life without the deceased.
4. Abnormal grief reactions include chronic grief reactions, delayed grief reactions, exaggerated grief reactions, and masked grief reactions.
5. Avoid the use of mood-modifying drugs whenever possible; if a mood-modifying drug has to be used, consider a short-term anxiolytic for the relief of insomnia or anxiety only. Avoid tricyclic antidepressant drugs for acute grief reactions.
6. The key difference between a major depressive illness and an acute grief reaction is the loss of self-esteem or the sense of hopelessness in a major depression.
7. Anticipatory grieving may occur in some situations: a chronic illness and a child in the NICU are prime examples. In these situations much of the grieving occurs before the actual death.

SUGGESTED READINGS

American Psychiatric Association. Diagnostic and statistical manual. 4th Ed. Washington, DC: American Psychiatric Association Press, 1994.

Worden JW. Grief counseling and grief therapy: A handbook for the mental health practitioner. New York: Springer, 1982.

PROBLEM 75   A 6-MONTH-OLD INFANT WHO FELL OFF A SOFA AND FRACTURED HIS HUMERUS

A 6-month-old infant presents to the hospital ER with his mother. She says that he fell off the sofa this evening and injured his right arm.

On examination, the infant has a swollen, bruised right arm. An X ray reveals a spiral fracture of the right humerus. There are also a number of old abrasions and old bruises that appear to be in various stages of healing and evidence of recent trauma to his right eye and also to the right side of his face.

The remainder of the physical examination is normal. The mother says that the child has been well since birth. He has not had any significant medical illnesses.

SELECT THE ONE BEST ANSWER TO THE FOLLOWING QUESTIONS

1. Given the history, the physical examination, and the X-ray report, what should you do now?
   a) obtain an orthopedic consultation
   b) prescribe a sling for the child's arm
   c) investigate the child for possible osteogenesis imperfecta
   d) suggest that the mother purchase a walker instead of laying her child on a sofa
   e) discuss the details of the incident more fully with the mother and contact the hospital social worker

2. After your initial intervention or recommendation, what is the next step you should take?
   a) ask the mother to return with the child for follow-up in 3 weeks
   b) ask the mother to return with the child for follow-up in 1 week
   c) arrange for the family physician to see the child at home the following day
   d) hospitalize the child
   e) none of the above

3. A 1-year-old child is admitted to the hospital for investigation of failure to thrive. The child's weight is below the fifth percentile for age. The child appears scared and clings to anyone who is present in the room. His mother states that "there is something wrong with him," and she can't understand why she "had to get a kid like this."

   Apart from the child being below the fifth percentile for weight, no other abnormalities are found on physical examination.

   A complete blood count, a complete urinalysis, and serum electrolytes are within normal limits.

   What is the most likely diagnosis for this child's behavior?
   a) the "white-coat" syndrome
   b) psychotic depression
   c) child abuse or neglect
   d) childhood schizophrenia
   e) acute paranoia of childhood

4. Which of the following statements regarding the parent(s) of a child with the disorder described in Question 3 is(are) true?
   a) the parent(s) may be overwhelmed
   b) the parent(s) may be depressed
   c) the parent(s) may be isolated
   d) the parent(s) may be impoverished
   e) all of the above statements are true

5. If your diagnosis is correct in the child described in Question 3, you would expect that the child
   a) will not gain significant weight during the initial hospitalization period
   b) will gain weight during the initial hospitalization period only if put on a significant antipsychotic agent
   c) will gain weight quickly during the initial hospitalization period
   d) will lose weight during the initial hospitalization period
   e) none of the above

6. Which one of the following statements most accurately reflects the situation in a family in which there has been documented child abuse?
   a) in most cases the child has to be permanently removed from the family and placed in a foster home
   b) rehabilitation of parents that have been involved in child abuse is almost always unsuccessful
   c) with comprehensive and intensive treatment of the entire family, 80%-90% of families involved in child abuse or neglect can be successfully rehabilitated
   d) in most cases child abuse will leave a permanent scar on the child's personality
   e) in a situation in which one child in a family has been abused, there is usually no increased risk to other children in the same family

7. Which of the following statements concerning child abuse in relation to spousal abuse is true?
   a) women who are abused are unlikely to abuse their children
   b) men who abuse their wives or partners are unlikely to abuse their children

c) men who abuse their wives are much more likely to abuse their children than are men who do not abuse their wives
d) there is no correlation between the various forms of family violence
e) parents who abuse their children are unlikely to have come from families in which they themselves were abused or their mother was abused

8. Regarding the epidemiology of child abuse, which of the following statements is(are) true?
a) in 1992 the National Committee for the Prevention of Child Abuse estimated that 3 million cases of child abuse and neglect were reported to public social service agencies in the United States
b) each year in the United States approximately 2000 to 4000 deaths are caused by child abuse and neglect
c) each year 150,000 to 200,000 new cases of child sexual abuse are reported in the United States
d) it is estimated that by the age of 18 years one out of every three to four girls will be sexually assaulted, and an estimated one out of every seven to eight boys will be sexually assaulted
e) all of the above are true

9. An 8-month-old child presents to the hospital ER with a large blistering burn in the shape of an iron on his buttocks. The child's father states that the child dropped the iron on himself approximately 20 minutes ago as he was reaching for his toys. As the ER doctor in charge, what is(are) your next step(s)?
a) treat the burn and move on to the next patient: time is money!
b) call the police and have the hospital security guards detain and restrain the father
c) obtain a more detailed history of the child's present injury and his previous health; at the same time immerse the child's buttocks in cold water in an attempt to minimize damage from the burn
d) to obtain a more detailed history of the child's present injury and his previous health; try and make the child comfortable with analgesics and apply a burn dressing as soon as possible
e) use a confrontational approach and accuse the father of concealing information and abusing the child; have your resident deal with the immediate burn injury

10. What is the most common form of childhood sexual abuse in the United States?
a) father-son
b) father-daughter
c) mother-son
d) mother-daughter
e) uncle or close relative-daughter

Short Answer Management Problem 75

Consider the following ten environmental, family, and genetic factors or situations. Indicate whether or not each one is or is not related to child abuse or is or is not a risk factor for child abuse.

FACTOR	RELATED? (YES/NO)
1. Parents brought up in harsh family environment	_____
2. A single mother who is socially isolated and unemployed outside the home	_____
3. Alcohol abuse in the father	_____
4. Major depressive disorder in the mother	_____
5. The child himself or herself is mentally retarded	_____
6. The child himself or herself has attention deficit disorder	_____
7. The family lives below the poverty line	_____
8. Both father and mother have inappropriately high expectations of their children	_____
9. Father was brought up in a strictly religious home where lack of immediate obedience meant corporal punishment	_____
10. Mother has just recently lost her job as a waitress	_____

ANSWERS

1. E. Such a child is almost always a victim of child abuse. Child abuse is defined as any maltreatment of children or adolescents by their parents, guardians, or other caretakers. The definition includes physical abuse, sexual abuse, physical neglect, medical neglect, emotional abuse, and emotional neglect.

    The physician must be able to distinguish accidental from nonaccidental injury. Clues to nonaccidental injury include the following:

A. A discrepant history: the explanation given by the parents or significant other does not fit the pattern and severity of the medical findings. Thus the "baby rolling off the sofa" is a totally inadequate explanation for a fractured humerus.

B. A delay in seeking care

C. A current family crisis

D. A triggering behavior such as excessive crying

E. Unrealistic expectations of the child on the part of the parents or guardians

F. Increasing severity of injuries

G. A history of the parent(s) being abused as children

H. Families that are socially isolated

The treatment of the fracture itself, although it must be treated, should not be the focus of attention. An orthopedic consultation may be appropriate depending on the severity of the fracture.

It would be inappropriate to suggest the purchase of a walker at the best of times, as this is associated with an increased incidence of falls and injuries.

There are no associated findings to suggest the diagnosis of osteogenesis imperfecta.

2. D. The most appropriate action at this time is to hospitalize the child. This removes the child to a safe environment and permits time for a complete evaluation.

The complete evaluation must include a complete physical evaluation, a complete laboratory evaluation, a complete radiological evaluation (of which the most important element is a skeletal survey), a complete evaluation by a child psychiatrist, and a complete evaluation of family dynamics including any other problems that are evident in other family members, such as alcohol or drug abuse in the father or mother, other psychiatric problems in either mother or father, and problems in other siblings (such as truancy).

3. C. The most likely diagnosis in this child is failure to thrive due to child abuse or neglect. A maltreated child often presents no obvious evidence of being battered but has multiple signs of minor deprivation, neglect, and abuse. The maltreated child is often taken to a hospital or a private physician and has a history of failure to thrive, malnutrition, poor skin hygiene, irritability, withdrawal, and other signs of psychological and physical neglect.

Children who have been neglected may show overt failure to thrive at less than 1 year of age; their physical and emotional development is drastically impaired. The child may be physically small and not able to show appropriate social interaction. Hunger, chronic infection, poor hygiene, and inappropriate dress may be present. Malnutrition is common.

In a behavioral sense, children who are chronically neglected may be indiscriminately affectionate, even with strangers, or they may be socially unresponsive. Child abuse or neglect is one of the most common causes of failure to thrive, even in familiar social situations. Neglected children may present as either runaways or as children with a conduct disorder.

4. E. Parents who neglect their children are often overwhelmed, depressed, isolated, and impoverished. Unemployment, lack of a two-parent family, and substance abuse may exacerbate the situation.

There are several "prototypes" of neglectful mothers that have been suggested. Again, this term seems to be somewhat disparaging and some may object to it. Some mothers are young, some inexperienced, some are socially isolated, and some cannot comprehend what is going on around them. Others have been portrayed as chronically passive and withdrawn; these women have often been raised in chaotic, abusive, and neglectful homes.

5. C. Once the neglected child is hospitalized and in a safe environment, the child should gain weight rapidly if given unlimited feedings.

6. C. With comprehensive and intensive treatment of the entire family, 80%-90% of families involved in child abuse or neglect (excluding incest) can be rehabilitated to provide adequate and appropriate care for their children. Approximately 10%-15% of such families can only be stabilized and will require an indefinite continuation of support services until the children in the family become independents. In only 2%-3% of cases is termination of parental rights or continued foster care necessary (again excluding incest).

7. C. Men who abuse their wives are more likely to abuse their children than men who do not abuse their wives. In fact, the abuse of a spouse is an absolute red flag to inquire about child abuse. It is estimated that approximately 25%-50% of men who abuse their wives also abuse their children.

Women who are abused presently (as spouses) or who have been abused in the past (as children) are also more likely to abuse their children than women who are not abused or who have not been abused (either as a spouse or as a child).

Parents who abuse their children are much more likely than not to have come from nuclear families in which abuse occurred. Most commonly they were abused themselves as children, although the witnessing of abuse as a child is also a common characteristic.

Thus abuse is very much a family affair and moves not only from generation to generation at different times, but also occurs among different generations at the same time. That is, it may well be that child abuse, spousal abuse, and elder abuse are occurring at the same time in the same family.

8. E. According to the National Committee for the Prevention of Child Abuse, in 1992 about 3 million cases of child abuse and neglect were reported to public social

service agencies; of that number, about 1 million cases were substantiated. Each year in America, between 2000 and 4000 children die as the result of fatal physical injuries from beatings or other physical trauma. Each year, approximately 150,000 to 200,000 new cases of childhood sexual abuse are reported in the United States. It is estimated that one in every three to four girls will be sexually assaulted by the age of 18 years, and an estimated one out of every seven to eight boys will be sexually assaulted. It should be remembered that the actual occurrence rates are likely to be higher than those estimates, because many maltreated children go unrecognized, and many are reluctant to report the abuse.

9. C. The most appropriate (and next) steps at this time are as follows:
   A. Treat the child's burn injury: even though it has been 20 minutes since the burn occurred, it is still very possible that you will be able to alter the extent and degree of thermal injury to the child by immersing the child's buttocks in cold water. This will also serve the dual purpose of acting as an analgesic for the child's pain.
   B. Obtain a more detailed history of the child's present injury and his previous health: even though it seems obvious what has actually happened here, it is important that as complete a history as possible be taken and documented for legal purposes.

10. B. Incest is defined as the occurrence of sexual relations between close blood relatives. A broader definition describes incest as intercourse between participants who are related to one another by some formal or informal bond of kinship that is culturally regarded as a barrier to sexual relations. As an example of the latter, sexual relations between stepparents and stepchildren or among step siblings are usually considered incestuous even though no blood relationship exists.

    The most common forms of incest include father or stepfather abusing his daughter or son, mother abusing her daughter or son, uncle or other relative abusing their niece or nephew, or a close friend abusing the daughter or son.

    Of the relationships cited above, the most common relationship involved in sexual abuse is father-daughter. Father-daughter incest accounts for 75% of the total of reported cases.

    A few general rules:
    1. Mothers abuse their children more often than fathers.
    2. Girls are abused more often than boys.
    3. Strangers are very seldom the perpetrators of the child abuse.
    4. One parent is usually the active batterer, while the other parent passively accepts the battering.

5. Of the perpetrators studied, 80% were regularly living in the homes of the children they abused.

The answer to all 10 scenarios or situations is yes. All of the scenarios and situations cited are associated with an increased risk of child abuse.

SUMMARY OF THE DIAGNOSIS AND TREATMENT OF CHILD ABUSE

1. **Prevalence:** 3 million cases reported each year in the United States; 2000 to 4000 children die every year of injuries incurred from child abuse in the United States.
2. **Definition:** *child abuse* can be defined as any short-term, intermediate-term or long-term situation in a family in which a child is
   a) Physically abused
   b) Sexually abused
   c) Emotionally or psychologically abused
   d) Physically neglected
   e) Emotionally neglected
   f) Medical care neglected by any other member of that family
3. **Characteristics:** Most commonly child abuse is perpetrated by a close relative, usually the parent. Mothers abuse their children more often than fathers; girls are abused more often than boys; one parent is usually the "active batterer" and the other parent is the "passive batterer." Strangers are rarely involved in child abuse.
4. **"Red lights" for child abuse:** Suspect child abuse if
   a) There is a discrepant history (what is said to have happened does not match the injury pattern)
   b) There is a delay in seeking care.
   c) There was a recent family crisis.
   d) There are unrealistic expectations put on the child by the parents.
   e) There is a pattern of increasing severity of so-called accidents.
   f) Families are living under stressful living conditions including overcrowding and poverty, there is a real lack of a support system for the family and the family members, and aggressive behavior is displayed by the child.
   g) You are aware of underlying psychiatric disease in either the father or the mother.
   h) There is either alcohol abuse or drug abuse in the father or mother.
5. **Acute treatment:** the acute treatment (no matter what type of child abuse is being dealt with) is hospitalization of the child. This allows time to subcategorize the type of child abuse that has occurred (often more than one type); observe the child and the child's behavior in a safe envi-

ronment; investigate the child from a physical, psychological, and social perspective; obtain all details necessary to clearly understand this episode of abuse, and any others that have taken place before this; and interview the parents, grandparents, and other family members.

6. **Immediate and long-term treatment:** the ultimate goal in a situation in which child abuse has occurred is to eventually return the child to the home.

The steps necessary, however, before that happens are as follows:
a) Restore the child to a health state.
b) Identify and understand the reason for the abuse.
c) Provide individual and family counseling to the parents and the family.
d) Treat coexisting psychiatric conditions in both parents (alcoholism, drug abuse, depression).
e) Set up an ongoing counseling program for the individuals in the family.

f) Establish a contract with the abusing parents (much like a suicide contract: I will call if I get to a stage where I think I can no longer handle it).

Remember that family violence begets family violence. Where you find one type you will likely find another type: Child abuse—spousal abuse—elder abuse.

SUGGESTED READINGS

American Psychiatric Association. Diagnostic and statistical manual. 4th Ed. Washington, DC: American Psychiatric Association Press, 1994.

Kaplan HI, Sadock BJ, Grebb JA. Problems related to abuse or neglect. Kaplan and Sadock's synopsis of psychiatry. Behavioral sciences/clinical psychiatry. 7th Ed. Baltimore: Williams and Wilkins, 1994.

PROBLEM 76   A 25-YEAR-OLD FEMALE WITH PELVIC DISCOMFORT, LOW BACK PAIN, INSOMNIA, AND FATIGUE

A 25-year-old female presents to the ER with a 6-month history of pelvic discomfort, low back pain, and generalized bone pain, lethargy, and fatigue. On direct questioning, she also notes some dryness of her hair and her nails. These problems have been getting progressively worse over 3 months.

She tells you that she "fell down the stairs last night" when she lost her balance.

She is accompanied by her husband who tells you that he "wants her fixed." He appears to be very agitated.

On examination, she has a bruise on her left eye and a number of bruises on her arms and legs, in various stages of healing. Her blood pressure is 130/85 mm Hg. Her pulse is 108 and regular. She looks very anxious and apprehensive. Examination of the cardiovascular system and the respiratory system is normal. Examination of the abdomen reveals a deep lower abdominal/pelvic tenderness.

SELECT THE ONE BEST ANSWER TO THE FOLLOWING QUESTIONS

1. Which of the following should be considered to be part of the differential diagnosis in this patient?
   a) acute leukemia
   b) hypothyroidism
   c) a bleeding disorder
   d) spousal abuse
   e) all of the above

2. Based on the constellation of findings, and the relative probabilities of the various disease entities, which of the following is the most likely diagnosis?
   a) acute leukemia
   b) hypothyroidism
   c) a bleeding disorder
   d) spousal abuse
   e) none of the above

3. What is the estimated prevalence of spousal abuse in North America?
   a) 1 in 100 women
   b) 1 in 50 women
   c) 1 in 25 women
   d) 1 in 10 women
   e) 1 in 2 women

4. All of the following are characteristics of the disorder described except
   a) the association of violence with alcohol intake by the batterer
   b) violent behavior in the family of origin of both victim and batterer
   c) high risk of suicide attempt or gesture in the victim
   d) high incidence of neurotropic drug use in the victim
   e) association of this disorder mainly with the lower socioeconomic classes

5. What is the psychological term or phrase that is used to describe the profile of women who are abused?
   a) intense intrapersonal and interpersonal conflict status
   b) learned helplessness
   c) inadequate psychological functioning in general
   d) uninhibited anger focus
   e) inadequate personality disorder or thought process

6. Which of the following is the least common presenting symptom or complaint in a victim of spousal abuse?
   a) back pain
   b) headache
   c) dyspareunia
   d) spousal abuse itself
   e) abdominal pain

7. Which of the following terms best describes the relationship that must develop between the patient (client) and physician in this disorder?
   a) understanding
   b) active listening
   c) active sharing
   d) trust
   e) collaboration

8. What is(are) the main fear(s) that women express concerning the condition described?
   a) a fear of escalation of the process
   b) a fear of being unable to function independently
   c) a fear of not being believed when they tell their story
   d) a fear of not being able to support themselves and their children
   e) all of the above

9. What is the most important "medical facility" in the diagnosis of the condition described?
   a) the ER
   b) the gynecologist's office
   c) the family doctor's office
   d) the internist's office
   e) all of the above are equally important

10. A woman who has been abused presents for medical help and receives it. She and her children are removed from a violent home environment and placed in a transition house where intensive counseling takes place. She leaves the transition house in 6 weeks.

What is the most likely next step in this scenario?
a) the woman and her children will establish a new life on their own
b) the woman and her children will soon enter into another abusive relationship
c) the woman will be unable to cope on her own and will go on to welfare; she and her children, however, will keep living on their own
d) the woman and her children will go back to their original violent home with the husband
e) c or d

11. It is currently estimated that what percentage of husbands or partners that abuse their wives also abuse their children?
a) 5%-10%
b) 10%-15%
c) 15%-20%
d) 20%-25%
e) 25%-50%

12. Following an episode of spousal abuse, the husband will usually be in what frame of mind?
a) anger
b) confused
c) conciliatory
d) silent
e) unrepentant

13. A husband physically abuses his wife for the first time on their honeymoon. Following the episode of violence he "promises that it will never happen again." What is the most likely outcome in this situation?
a) he is right: it will never happen again
b) it will happen again but the intensity of the violence will be less
c) it will happen again but the intensity of the violence will be greater
d) it will happen again and the intensity of the violence will be the same
e) nobody really knows for sure; it depends on the situation

14. The state of learned helplessness usually evolves from which of the following?
a) the upbringing of the victim
b) the upbringing of the abuser
c) repeated and escalating psychological abuse of the victim
d) the economic environment (unemployment most often) that the abuser finds himself in
e) none of the above

15. Which pharmacologic drug class is most commonly prescribed to victims of abuse when they present to physicians?
a) tricyclic antidepressants
b) sedative-hypnotics
c) beta blockers
d) antipsychotic agents
e) antimanic agents

Short Answer Management Problem 76

Discuss the interventions and the order of those interventions that should take place for victim, victim's children, and husband or mate in a situation as the one described.

ANSWERS

1. E.

2. D. First, all of the diagnostic entities listed in the question are possibilities.

Although unlikely, the low back pain, generalized pain, bruising, and fatigue and lethargy could represent the signs and symptoms of an acute leukemia.

The symptoms of fatigue and lethargy, along with the dry skin and dry nails, could certainly represent hypothyroidism.

Similar to the explanation for acute leukemia, the signs and symptoms could represent a bleeding disorder.

Although not listed, some of the symptoms could represent a masked depression.

Spousal abuse, however, is the most likely diagnostic entity. The inability to diagnose spousal abuse may be explained by the fact that the profile presented to the clinician in cases of spousal abuse is vague. Women who are victims of spousal abuse visit physicians often, usually with somatic or conversion symptoms or psychophysiologic reactions. The most frequent complaints include headache, insomnia, a choking sensation, hyperventilation, gastrointestinal pain, chest pain, pelvic pain, and back pain. As well, the patient may show signs of suicidal behavior, drug abuse, and noncompliance with medication.

Spousal abuse is one of a number of diagnoses in medicine that is best described as follows: if you don't think of the diagnosis, you won't make the diagnosis.

3. D. The estimated prevalence of spousal abuse in North America is 1/10 women. One study suggests that up to 12 million families in the United States are affected by spousal abuse. The DSM-IV specifies five problems related to abuse or neglect: physical abuse of a child, sexual abuse of a child, neglect of a child, physical abuse of an adult, and sexual abuse of an adult. The first three are covered in other chapters of this book, but remember from this that abuse is a family affair. When abuse occurs between two members of a family, it is very likely to occur between another two members. This will be discussed in detail later.

4. E. Alcohol intake by the batterer is associated with spousal abuse. The majority of men who beat their spouses have an alcohol abuse problem. Sometimes, the batterer uses alcohol as an excuse to disavow his behavior and convince others that "I was not responsible for my actions at the time." The most important point to be made in this regard, however, is that alcohol does not cause spousal abuse. The two problems are separate and must be dealt with separately. As well as alcohol, other drug abuse, including the use of crack cocaine, is frequently associated with spousal abuse.

   A nuclear family of origin in which violence occurred is common in both victims and batterers.

   Spousal abuse occurs in families of every racial and religious background and in all socioeconomic strata of society. Every race and religious background and all socioeconomic groups are represented. It may well be true that psychosocial stressors such as chronic unemployment, welfare status, and other financial problems increase the probability of abuse.

5. B. The psychological term that is used to describe women who are abused is *learned helplessness*. Learned helplessness refers to a situation in which a woman who has been abused and continually told that she is worthless eventually comes to believe just that. Not only do the victims often see themselves as worthless, but they also believe that everything that has happened and is happening is, indeed, their fault. As the abuse (both psychological and physical) continues, this pattern becomes more and more deeply ingrained into the psyche of abuse victims.

6. D. Women who are abused have been shown to visit physicians frequently. Those visits, however, consist mainly of complaints or concerns regarding various "body pains" (back pain, headache, abdominal pain, pelvic pain, and dyspareunia, as well as anxiety and depression). Very rarely, however, do the victims present to a physician's office complaining of being abused. Usually, this information has to be carefully sought, initially through the asking of general, open-ended questions, and later by a more close-ended, direct approach. If you suspect spousal abuse as the cause of the patient's presenting complaints, you could begin with an open-ended question such as, "Describe your marital relationship," and then after obtaining either verbal or nonverbal cues that indicate another agenda you could switch to a direct question regarding abuse: "Does your husband ever hit you?" This questioning approach provides the best opportunity for open dialogue and sharing of the essential information between patient and physician.

7. D. The single most important aspect of the patient-physician communication process that must occur when a woman who has been abused presents to a physician is the development of a trusting relationship between herself and the physician. Without trust, essential information will not be revealed and no significant progress will be made. Although active listening and understanding on the part of the physician are important, they can never take the place of trust.

8. E. All of the fears listed are reasons for victims' choosing to stay in abusive relationships.

   Fear of escalation of violence and even murder are common reasons for staying in the relationship. A significant percentage of the total homicides in the United States are committed by husbands who kill their wives. In fact, this is the single most common type of homicide in this country.

   Fear of being unable to function independently and support both herself and her children is an almost universal fear.

   Perhaps the greatest fear, and the fear that is linked to nondisclosure of spousal abuse, is the fear on the part of the victim that they will not be believed.

9. A. The most important "medical facility" in the diagnosis of spousal abuse is the ER. The reason for this is the cycle of violence. In the cycle of violence there are three distinct phases:
   A. Escalating tension
   B. Violence erupting
   C. Reconciliation
   The victim almost always presents immediately after the eruption of violence. At this time the individual is most vulnerable to suggestion and therapy. Because the abuse often involves significant physical injuries, the ER is the most likely place that the initial contact with health care professionals will take place. This does not mean, however, that the other medical facilities listed are not important; it simply puts the ER at the top of the list. As well, it illustrates the point that the most cost-effective screening with the highest rate of pickup will occur in the ER.

10. D. Leaving an abusive relationship is difficult for many reasons, including fears of the victim that have

already been discussed. On average, a woman will return four times to her residence of origin (that is, go back to her husband) before she permanently separates.

Choice c really is an insult to abused women and women in general. It is a typical stereotype that helps perpetuate the repeated cycle of violence that we witness. Although it is an insult, it is a concern that many of these women do have to seek financial assistance. When child care arrangements are taken into account it is almost impossible for them to work. Cuts that have been made to the financial programs available to help these women (and it appears from the new U.S. political agenda that this will continue) are a tragedy to abused women and their children.

We would hope for choice a. The woman and her children will establish a new and independent life on their own.

Choice b unfortunately occurs all too often. There is a theory termed *the theory of assortive mating*, which states that for reasons unknown (probably reasons at a subconscious level) the victim more often than not will find herself (unknowingly) in another abusive relationship when she forms one.

All of these choices are based on the assumption that the abuser cannot be rehabilitated. Although this was the established view in the past, it is changing somewhat. Current estimates suggest that approximately 25% of abusers can and do seek help to correct behavior. This figure can be rationaled on two premises: the abuser must not only stop the abuse but must also stop and be successfully treated for his other problems (the first of which being alcohol), and the abuser often has other psychiatric difficulties (such as personality disorders) that are difficult to treat.

11. E. This is a very important question and a very important point. It is currently estimated that 25%-50% of husbands and mates who physically abuse their wives also physically abuse thier children. Thus family violence is a family affair. From this, the obvious follows: whenever one form of family violence exists in a family, all other potential types must be considered, evaluated, and proven not to be the case.

Family violence can take many forms:
A. Husband abuses wife
B. Wife abuses husband (uncommon, but it does occur)
C. Husband abuses children
D. Wife abuses children (particularly when the husband has instigated the abuse)
E. Husband abuses grandmother/grandfather (elder abuse)
F. Wife abuses grandmother/grandfather
G. Children (older) abuse grandmother/grandfather (especially when husband or wife has set the example)

12. C. Going back to the cycle of violence described in the answer to Question 9, the husband will usually be in a very conciliatory mood after the episode of violence. He will seek the forgiveness of his wife with words such as, "It will never happen again, Honey; it was just a mistake and a misunderstanding. I'm sorry." Along with this apology will often come flowers or chocolates. The wife, wanting desperately to believe this, will often go back at that time or shortly thereafter. Although in medicine we say "never say never" and "never say always", spousal abuse is an exception: without counseling and help, the abuse will almost surely recur.

13. C. As stated above, the violence will recur. When it does it will likely be more severe. And so the cycle goes, generally more and more frequently and more and more severe. The culmination of this is our worst nightmare; the husband eventually kills his wife. As mentioned earlier, spousal abuse is the single most important and prevalent category of homicide in the United States. In many of these cases, he also kills his children and then himself. This is obviously a very tragic end to a situation that could have been averted with proper diagnosis, assistance for both victim and abuser, and the provision of an ongoing safe environment for the children.

14. C. Learned helplessness is characterized by a deep belief on the part of the victim that she can do nothing to change her environment, and it is she, really, who is ultimately responsible for all the violence that has occurred in the relationship. She is led to believe that she is unable to do anything, that she is, in fact, "a nothing." This is almost always ingrained by the abuser in a situation of repetitive psychological abuse.

15. B. Frequently, when victims of abuse present to their physicians, the victim walks away with a prescription for a sedative-hypnotic agent. Anxiety is almost always a frequent underlying symptom that is "picked up" and treated by the physician. Antidepressants and other neurotropic agents such as antipsychotic drugs are also frequently prescribed.

SOLUTION TO SHORT ANSWER MANAGEMENT PROBLEM 76

The interventions that should take place include the following:

1. Victim and children:
   A. Establish the diagnosis by asking first open-ended followed by more direct, closed-ended questions.
   B. Explain the importance of the removal of both the spouse and her children to a safe environment (preferably a transition house).
   C. Facilitate the placement of victim and children in this safe environment.

D. Use supportive psychotherapy in the safe environment to reestablish the victim's self-esteem and to reverse the ingrained feeling in the victim of learned helplessness.

E. After a period of time (approximately 6 weeks), facilitate the victim and children's reintegration into society and establishment of a new life.

F. Continue contact and supportive psychotherapy for the victim and assist the children with any difficulties that they are having (such as school problems).

2. Abuser (husband or mate):

A. Group psychotherapy appears to work best for abusers. This facilitates the sharing of experiences with other individuals who have had the same experience.

B. Treatment of concurrent psychiatric problems (especially alcoholism and drug abuse) is essential.

C. A long term (1 year) should pass before the victim and abuser are reunited, if ever.

SUMMARY OF THE DIAGNOSIS AND MANAGEMENT OF SPOUSAL ABUSE

1. **Definition:** wife abuse is defined as the physical or psychologic abuse directed by a man against his female partner in an attempt to control her behavior or intimidate her.

2. **Prevalence:** current prevalence is estimated as 10% of American women.

3. **Presenting symptoms:** usually vague somatic or psychophysiologic symptoms

4. **Diagnosis:** first, think of the diagnosis. Proceed from open-ended questions to more direct questions.

5. **Treatment:**

Victim/children: removal to a safe environment and supportive psychotherapy for the victim to reestablish self-esteem and reverse learned helplessness.

Abuser: group psychotherapy to help the abuser accept responsibility for his actions and to help him learn to express anger and frustration in other ways, and treatment of concomitant psychiatric problems (especially alcoholism and drug abuse)

Remember, one form of abuse begets another: where spousal abuse is present, consider the very high probability of child abuse and elder abuse.

SUGGESTED READING

American Psychiatric Association. Diagnostic and statistical manual. 4th Ed. Washington, DC: American Psychiatric Association Press, 1994.

Swanson R. Battered wife syndrome. Canadian Medical Association Journal 1984; 130:709-713.

Swanson R. Recognizing battered wife syndrome. Canadian Family Physician 1985; 31:823-825.

PROBLEM 77   A 72-YEAR-OLD FEMALE WITH A SORE RIGHT SHOULDER AND MULTIPLE BRUISES

A daughter brings her 72-year-old mother to the ER for assessment. The mother has Alzheimer's disease and is unable to communicate with you directly. The daughter tells you that her mother has had Alzheimer's disease for 5 years and has been living with her for the majority of that time.

The daughter tells you that her mother fell on her right shoulder approximately 3 hours ago. As you look at the patient you notice a large bruise in the area of the head of the right humerus.

On examination, there are multiple bruises on her arms, legs, and abdomen. The head of the humerus is tender. The resident who is with you tells you that he "has things pretty well squared away." He has made the diagnosis of a rare inherited bleeding disorder on the basis of (as the nurse that is caring for the patient says) "goodness knows what."

You decide that you aren't quite satisfied with this diagnosis and need to investigate further. Meanwhile, the patient is complaining of pain and holding her shoulder. You order an X-ray of the shoulder and diagnose a fractured head of the humerus.

SELECT THE ONE BEST ANSWER TO THE FOLLOWING QUESTIONS

1. At this time, what should you do?
   a) treat the patient's pain, provide a collar and cuff, and say good-bye to the patient and her daughter
   b) treat the patient's pain, provide a collar and cuff for the patient, and tell the patient that she really should be more careful
   c) treat the patient's pain and contact orthopedic surgery as you are sure they will wish to manage this fracture with internal fixation
   d) order a CBC, clotting time, and all other laboratory tests vaguely associated with the hematologic and clotting system to pacify the resident and get him off your back
   e) none of the above

2. What is the prevalence of elder abuse in the United States population?
   a) 4%
   b) 2%
   c) 10%
   d) 8%
   e) 15%

3. Regarding screening for the condition described, which of the following statements is(are) true?
   a) screening for the condition described above is recommended by the American Medical Association
   b) it is recommended that physicians incorporate routine questions related to the condition above into their daily practice
   c) direct, concrete action should be taken when a situation is identified that confirms the above diagnosis
   d) all of the above
   e) none of the above

4. When comparing the prevalence of this condition in the community setting with the prevalence of the same condition in long-term care institutions, which of the following statements is(are) true?

   a) the prevalence of this condition is much higher in institutionalized elderly patients compared to elders in the comunity setting
   b) the institutionalized elderly patient is at greater risk of this condition because of his(her) physical or psychological status
   c) one of the reasons for the high prevalence of this condition in the institutionalized elderly is lack of staff training and/or institutional under staffing
   d) all of the above
   e) none of the above

5. There are various forms of this condition. Which of the following would be placed in that category of forms?
   a) a physical form
   b) a psychological form
   c) a financial form
   d) a neglect form
   e) all of the above

6. Which of the following is(are) associated with the condition described?
   a) excessive use of restraints
   b) pushing
   c) grabbing
   d) yelling
   e) all of the above

7. What is the most common manifestation of the condition described?
   a) excessive use of restraints
   b) pushing
   c) grabbing
   d) yelling
   e) slapping or hitting

8. Which of the following is not a risk factor for the condition described?
   a) unsatisfactory living arrangements
   b) low educational level of staff
   c) physical or emotional dependence on the caregiver

d) living apart from the victim

e) age greater than 75 years

9. Which of the following is false regarding the condition described?

a) abusive events tend to be one-time-only events

b) abusive events tend to escalate in the same manner in which spousal abuse escalates

c) the situation rarely resolves spontaneously

d) many victims refuse help

e) serious illness, crisis, admission to an institution, or even death are all long-term sequelae of this condition

10. With respect to research priorities and the condition described, which of the following is(are) true?

a) there should be a determination of the cause of the condition in different ethnic and cultural groups in North America

b) there should be a comprehensive assessment of the prevalence of this condition in American long-term care institutions

c) valid, reliable tools should be developed for use in settings such as primary care, hospital ERs, and long-term care institutions

d) all of the above

e) a and c only

11. In which of the following settings is the incidence of the condition described likely to be highest based on screening history and physical examination?

a) the family physician's office

b) the local ER facility

c) the referral-based specialist's office

d) any of the above

e) none of the above

Short Answer Management Problem 77

Discuss a comprehensive plan to manage elder abuse in your community.

ANSWERS

1. E. This patient is much more likely to have injuries inflicted as a result of abuse rather than a rare inherited clotting disorder or anything else.

   Obviously, the patient's pain and her fractured arm have to be treated. This is not, however, the end of the treatment.

   Elder abuse is extremely common and is one of those conditions that will not be diagnosed unless it is included in a differential diagnosis and thought of in all situations in which it may occur.

   In this case, a consult to social services is essential. With the history of physical injury it would seem that the wisest course of action at this time is removal of the patient to a safe environment.

2. A. The prevalence of elder abuse in North America is estimated at 4%. In many cases this abuse is long-term, repeated, or both. In one study 58% of elderly patients had suffered previous incidents of abuse.

   Some studies have estimated the prevalence of elder abuse to be much higher than 4%; 10% appears to be a more realistic figure.

3. D. When a situation arises that confirms elder abuse, direct action should be taken to rectify, improve, or resolve the situation.

   The American Medical Association recommends that physicians screen for elder abuse in their practices, and that they incorporate routine questions related to elder abuse and neglect when seeing elderly patients.

4. D. The prevalence of elder abuse is much higher in institutionalized elderly patients than in elderly patients who live in the community. In one study of nursing home staff, 36% had witnessed physical abuse of residents in the preceding year.

5. E. The simplest definition of elder abuse is "any act of commission or omission that results in harm to an elderly person."

   Elder abuse is distinguished from other crimes against elderly people by the perpetrator's occupying a position of trust. The following definition of elder abuse and neglect is proposed:

   1) *Physical abuse:* assault, rough handling, sexual abuse, or the withholding of physical necessities such as food or other items of personal, hygienic, or medical care

   2) *Psychosocial abuse:* verbal assault, social isolation, lack of affection, or denial of the person's participation in decisions affecting his or her life

   3) *Financial abuse:* the misuse of money or property, including fraud or use of funds for purposes contrary to the needs, interests, or desires of the elderly person

   4) *Neglect:* in active neglect, the caregiver consciously fails to meet the needs of the elderly person; in passive neglect the caregiver does not intend to injure

the dependent person. Neglect can lead to any of the three types of abuse.

Other categories of abuse have been proposed, such as violation of rights and medical abuse (inappropriate treatment, excessive use of restraints, and withholding of treatment). Abuse may be intentional or unintentional.

6. E.

7. A. As mentioned above, a figure of 36% has been quoted as the percentage of institutionalized elderly that have been abused. In this study, the most common forms of abuse were excessive use of restraints (witnessed in the quoted study by 21% of staff), pushing, grabbing, shoving, or pinching (17%), and slapping or hitting (15%).

Psychologic abuse was observed by 81% of the staff; 70% had witnessed a staff member yelling at a patient in anger; 50% had seen someone insulting or swearing at a patient; and 23% had seen a patient isolated inappropriately.

8. D. Living apart from the victim is not a risk factor for elder abuse.

The risk factors for elder abuse are as follows:
I. Situational factors:
  A. Community situational factors:
    1. Isolation
    2. Lack of money
    3. Lack of community resources for additional care
    4. Unsatisfactory living arrangements
  B. Institutions:
    1. Shortage of beds
    2. Surplus of patients
    3. Low staff-to-patient ratio
    4. Low staff compensation
    5. Staff burnout
II. Characteristics of the victim:
    1. Physical or emotional dependence on caregiver
    2. Lack of close family ties
    3. History of family violence
    4. Age > 75 years
    5. Recent deterioration in health
III. Characteristics of the perpetrator:
    1. Stress caused by financial, marital, or occupational factors
    2. Deterioration in health
    3. Bereavement
    4. Substance abuse
    5. Psychopathologic illness
    6. Related to victim
    7. Living with victim
    8. Long duration of care for victim (mean = 9.5 years)

9. A. Elder abuse rarely resolves spontaneously; it tends to escalate in the same way as spousal abuse. Abusive events tend to be repeated and will almost always continue unless there is a major change in the environment. Such an environmental change may not occur because, in 25% to 75% of cases, victims or their families refuse help. This may subsequently result in serious illness, crisis, admission to an institution, or even death.

10. D. The research priorities for elder abuse include the following:
  a. A determination of the causes of this condition in different ethnic and cultural groups in the United States and Canada
  b. A determination of the prevalence of abuse in American and Canadian institutions
  c. The development of valid and reliable assessment tools for use in such settings as primary care, hospital ER departments, and long-term care institutions
  d. An evaluation of the effectiveness of interventions on the prevalence of this condition

11. B. The highest incidence (or pick-up rate) is likely to be at the local ER facility. The reason is that the time that elders are most likely to present is at the time of, or shortly after, an event of abuse. This does not imply that screening should not occur at the other facilities; it should occur in all health care settings all of the time.

SOLUTION TO SHORT ANSWER MANAGEMENT PROBLEM 77

A comprehensive plan to manage elder abuse should include recognition of the condition, comprehensive treatment of the condition, and a significant education component aimed at the following:

1) Increasing public awareness of the magnitude of the problem
2) Increasing public awareness of the signs and symptoms of elder abuse
3) Increasing public awareness of the treatment options available

The actual components of the management of elder abuse include the following:
I. **Detection and risk assessment:**
  a) Documentation of the type of abuse, the frequency and severity of abuse, the danger to the victim, and the perpetrator's intent and level of stress
  b) Involvement of other health care professionals (social worker, visiting nurse, and geriatric assessment team)
  c) Documentation of the injuries (take photographs)
  d) Assessment of the victim's overall health status, the victim's functional status, and the victim's social and financial status

II. **Assessment of decision-making capacity of the victim:** assess the cognitive state and the emotional state of the victim.

III. **Measures to take if the victim is competent:**
   a) Provide information to the victim.
   b) In providing information, outline the choices or possible choices that the victim has, such as temporary relocation, home support, community agencies, and criminal charges
   c) Support the victim's decision.

IV. **Measures to take if the victim is not competent:**
   a) Separate the victim and the perpetrator.
   b) Relocate the victim.
   c) Arrange advocacy services for the victim.

SUGGESTED READINGS

American Psychiatric Association. Diagnostic and statistical manual. 4th Ed. Washington, DC: American Psychiatric Association Press, 1994.

The Canadian Task Force on the Periodic Health Examination. Periodic health examination, 1994 update: 4. Secondary prevention of elder abuse and mistreatment. Canadian Medical Association Journal 1994; 151(10):1413-1420.

PROBLEM 78   A 75-YEAR-OLD MALE WITH NO WILL TO CARRY ON LIVING

A 75-year-old male is brought to the ER by his daughter. She is very distraught and tells you that she arrived at her father's home just when he was about to kill himself.

When you question the patient he says that he has nothing more to live for and starts to cry. He tells you directly that he has just updated his will and purchased a new handgun. He intended on shooting himself (and was just putting the bullets into the gun) when his daughter walked in. He then begins to sob uncontrollably and apologizes for putting you to all this trouble.

His past history is significant for cardiovascular disease. He has a history of "heart attacks and angina" and has also had something he says his doctors referred to as "heart block." He is presently taking nifedipine for "angina," and he was put on "some little pink pills last week" by his family doctor for depression. You determine that the latter is amitriptyline.

As well as ischemic heart disease, his daughter tells you that he has had "other bouts with depression" but none as severe as this.

The patient lives alone in a seniors' housing complex. He does not socialize, nor has he socialized during the past few years (since his wife died).

On examination, his affect is severely blunted. His mini-mental status examination produces a score of 27/30. His blood pressure is 100/70 mm Hg and his pulse is 74 and irregular. No other major abnormalities are found on P/E.

SELECT THE ONE BEST ANSWER TO THE FOLLOWING QUESTIONS

1. Given the history and P/E to this point, what would you do?
   a) increase the amount of amitriptyline he is taking and tell him to call his family doctor in the morning
   b) prescribe diazepam for both the patient and his daughter to try and calm everyone down; make an appointment with a counselor and ask him to report in 2 weeks
   c) try to form a "no-suicide contract" with the patient
   d) hospitalize the patient
   e) prescribe a major tranquilizer for the patient and have him see a psychiatrist (that you will arrange for) in 3 weeks

2. Which of the following psychiatric conditions is(are) associated with a high suicide risk?
   a) major depressive disorder
   b) schizophrenia
   c) alcoholism
   d) a and b
   e) a and c
   f) all of the above

3. Successful suicides are reported to have what male/female ratio?
   a) 1 to 3
   b) 5 to 1
   c) 3 to 1
   d) 1 to 1
   e) 1 to 5

4. Unsuccessful suicide attempts are reported to have what male/female ratio?
   a) 1 to 3
   b) 1 to 4
   c) 4 to 1
   d) 1 to 1
   e) 1 to 10

5. Regarding the neuropsychiatric basis of suicide, which of the following is(are) true?
   a) a serotonin deficiency exists in some depressed patients who attempt suicide
   b) platelet MAO (monoamine oxidase) deficiency is an important risk factor for suicide
   c) high outputs of urinary free cortisol are associated with suicidal behavior among depressed patients
   d) all of the above
   e) none of the above

6. Regarding the total suicide rate and the number of deaths by suicide/year in the United States, which of the following is true?
   a) 12.5 suicide deaths/100,000 population: 30,000 deaths/year
   b) 10.0 suicide deaths/100,000 population: 15,000 deaths/year
   c) 20.5 suicide deaths/100,000 population: 45,000 deaths/year
   d) 5.5 suicide deaths/100,000 population: 7,500 deaths/year
   e) no accurate estimate is available

7. Which of the following countries has the highest total suicide rate/100,000 population?
   a) Russia
   b) Egypt
   c) United States
   d) Spain
   e) Canada

8. The term *chronic suicide* refers to which of the following?
   a) death from alcohol and substance abuse
   b) death from nonadherence to medical regimens for obesity, diabetes, and hypertension
   c) individuals who attempt suicide frequently but never succeed (this may be intentional or unintentional)
   d) a and b
   e) all of the above

9. What is the main determining factor when deciding whether or not to hospitalize a patient with suicidal ideation?
   a) how many attempts he or she has made
   b) the method by which the individual attempted suicide
   c) the ability to form a meaningful suicide contract with the individual
   d) the age of the individual
   e) all of the above are equally important

10. Which of the following is(are) true regarding the emergence of an acute suicidal episode?
    a) the emergence is often superimposed on a pre-existing or concurrent psychiatric illness
    b) feelings of hopelessness, despair, pessimism, and helplessness are more important than depression
    c) the emergence is often precipitated by psychosocial life events
    d) most patients have visited a physician within one month of the acute suicidal attempt
    e) all of the above

11. Which of the following are part of the treatment plan for a patient after the emergence of an acute suicidal episode?
    a) reduction in psychological pain by suggesting modifications to the patient's stressful environment
    b) the offering of alternatives to suicide
    c) providing effective antidepressant or antipsychotic pharmacologic therapy
    d) arranging accommodation in a risk-free environment with constant supervision
    e) all of the above

12. Which of the following aspects of the patient's history plus signs and/or symptoms is(are) important in suicide risk assessment?
    a) previous suicidal attempt or fantasized suicide
    b) anxiety, depression, or exhaustion
    c) a proximal life crisis
    d) a family history of suicide
    e) a, b, and c
    f) all of the above

13. Considering the patient described, which of the following statements is(are) true regarding the use of amitriptyline therapy as first-choice therapy for depression (as was begun by the family doctor)?
    a) there are no contraindications to prescribing amitriptyline in this patient
    b) this patient's cardiac status is a contraindication to prescribing amitriptyline
    c) this patient's suicide risk is a contraindication to prescribing amitriptyline in large supply to this patient
    d) b and c
    e) all of the above

Short Answer Management Problem 78

List the factors associated with increased suicide risk in rank order of importance (list at least 10 factors).

ANSWERS

1. D. You should hospitalize this patient. The patient has just updated his will and bought a new handgun. Suicidal contract or not, this does not bode well. There is clearly enough evidence to conclude that this patient is a serious suicide risk.

   For patients who are acutely suicidal, inpatient evaluation and management is the safest option. It protects the patient from himself and from others. It allows for continuous assessment and assessment of response to treatment. If the patient refuses hospitalization, involuntary commitment may be necessary.

   The question of suicide contracts will be more fully discussed in another question.

2. F. Approximately 95% of all patients who commit or attempt suicide have a diagnosed mental disorder. Depressive disorders account for 80%, schizophrenia accounts for 10%, and dementia or delirium accounts for 5%. Among all mentally disordered persons, 25% are also alcohol dependent and have a dual diagnosis. In patients with major depressive disorder, the risk of suicide is approximately 15%. Up to 15% of all alcohol-dependent persons commit suicide, and up to 10% of schizophrenics commit suicide.

3. C.

4. B. Men commit suicide more than three times as often as do women; this rate is stable over all age groups. Women, however, are four times as likely to attempt suicide as men.

5. D. A serotonin deficiency, measured as a decrease in the metabolism of 5-hydroxyindoleacetic acid, has been

found in a group of depressed patients who committed suicide. Serotonin is the key neurotransmitter that is altered by both the new selective serotonin reuptake inhibitors (SSRIs) (the drugs of choice for depressive illness) and the tricyclic antidepressant agents work on altering levels of both serotonin and norepinephrine.

Blood samples analyzed for platelet (MAO) suggest that those persons with the lowest level of the enzyme in their platelets have eight times the prevalence of suicide in their families as compared with persons with high levels of this enzyme. This expands to suggest strong evidence for an alteration in platelet MAO activity in depressive disorders and for the use of MAO inhibitors in depressive illness.

6. A.

7. A. Each year 30,000 deaths are attributed to suicide in the United States. This figure represents successful suicides; the number of attempted suicides is 8 to 10 times that number. Lost in that reporting number are intentional misclassifications of the cause of death, accidents (especially MVAs), and the so-called chronic suicides, which will be discussed in a later question. The total suicide rate has remained fairly constant over the years. The current rate is 12.5 suicide deaths per 100,000 population.

Currently suicide is ranked as the eighth overall cause of death in this country, after heart disease, cancer, cerebrovascular disease, accidents, pneumonia, diabetes mellitus, and cirrhosis. In the age group 15-24 years, however, suicide is the third leading cause of death after accidents and homicides. Attempted suicides in the United States number between 1 million and 2 million annually.

Suicide rates in the United States are at the midpoint of the national rates reported to the United Nations. Internationally, suicide rates range from highs of more than 25/100,000 people in Scandinavia, Switzerland, Germany, Austria, the Eastern European countries such as Russia (which is known as the "suicide belt"), and Japan to fewer than 10/100,000 in Spain, Italy, Ireland, Egypt, and the Netherlands.

8. D. The term *chronic suicide* refers to the following:
   A. Death from alcohol abuse
   B. Death from substance abuse
   C. Death from nonadherence to medical regimens for treatment of diabetes mellitus, obesity, and hypertension

   It does not include individuals who attempt suicide frequently but never succeed.

9. C. Whether to hospitalize patients with suicidal ideation is the most important clinical decision to be made. Not all such patients require hospitalization; some may be treated on an outpatient basis. To determine whether or not an outpatient approach is feasible, the physician should use a straightforward clinical approach: Is the patient prepared to and does he agree to call whenever he reaches a point beyond which he is unsure he can control his impulses? Patients who can affirm such an agreement reaffirm the belief that they have sufficient strength to control such impulses and seek help. This is known as a *suicide contract*.

Other indications for inhospital management include the following: absence of a strong social support system, a history of impulsive behavior, and a suicide plan.

10. E. The emergence of an acute suicidal episode is often superimposed on a preexisting or concurrent psychiatric diagnosis.

Feelings of hopelessness, despair, pessimism, and helplessness tend to be more predictive of acute suicidal risk than depression.

The emergence of an acute suicidal episode is often precipitated by psychosocial life stressors.

Although most patients who are acutely suicidal have visited a physician recently, most are not receiving treatment for psychiatric illness or complying with the treatment regime prescribed previously.

11. E. The important elements of treatment after the emergence of an acute episode of suicide include the following:
    A. To determine whether or not the patient should be treated as an inpatient or outpatient: suicide contract; presence or absence of a social support system; presence or absence of impulsive behavior; presence or absence of a suicidal plan of action
    B. Preventive measures for dealing with suicidal ideation: reduction of the psychological pain by modification of a stressful environment and offering alternatives to suicide
    C. Psychotherapy: individual psychotherapy, group psychotherapy, and family psychotherapy
    D. Treatment directed toward concurrent disorders: alcoholism and drug abuse
    E. Pharmacotherapy: antidepressant medication, antipsychotic medication, and specific therapy for schizophrenia
    F. Electroconvulsive therapy (ECT) for resistant depression
    G. Safe environment: constant supervision in-hospital if risk is very high

12. F. The history, signs, and symptoms of suicide risk include the following:
    A. Previous suicide attempt or fantasized suicide attempt
    B. Anxiety, depression, or exhaustion

C. Availability of the means of suicide
D. Preparation of a will, resignation after agitated depression
E. Proximal life crisis, such as mourning or impending surgery
F. Family history of suicide
G. Pervasive pessimism or hopelessness

13. D. This patient's history of a "heart block" is at least a strong relative contraindication to prescribing amitriptyline for his depression. Tricyclic antidepressants adversely affect conduction through the AV node and must be used with extreme caution in patients with a history of any type of heart block.

As well, since amitriptyline in large supply may be used as a means of suicide, it is much safer to prescribe one of the new selective serotonin reuptake inhibitors such as fluoxetine, sertraline, or paroxetine.

SOLUTION TO SHORT ANSWER MANAGEMENT PROBLEM 78

The factors associated with an elevated suicide risk in rank order include the following:

RANK ORDER	FACTOR
1	Age (> 45 years)
2	Alcohol dependence
3	Irritation, rage, violence
4	Prior suicidal behavior
5	Male sex
6	Unwilling to accept help
7	Longer-than-usual duration of an episode of depression
8	Prior inpatient psychiatric treatment
9	Recent loss or separation
10	Depression
11	Loss of physical health
12	Unemployed or retired
13	Single, widowed, or divorced

SUMMARY OF THE DIAGNOSIS AND MANAGEMENT OF THE SUICIDAL PATIENT

1. **Prevalence:** 12.5/100,000 in United States/30,000 deaths per year in United States
2. **Risk factors:**
   a) Consider rank order for suicide risk.
   b) Remember three most important concomitant psychiatric diagnoses: depression, alcoholism, and schizophrenia.
   c) Risk factors that indicate that patient should be hospitalized: inability to establish a meaningful suicide contract, lack of a strong social support system, history of impulsive behavior, definite suicide plan of action, and a patient with profound guilt or hopelessness.
3. **Suicide contract:** health professionals must ensure daily contact with the individual during the immediate crisis period.
4. **Treatment:**
   a) Psychotherapy: individual, group, family
   b) Pharmacotherapy: depression, SSRIs/TCAs, respirone for schizophrenia
   c) ECT
   d) Observation/close monitoring

SUGGESTED READINGS

American Psychiatric Association. Diagnostic and Statistical Manual. 4th Ed. Washington, DC: American Psychiatric Association Press, 1994.

Kaplan H, Sadock B, Grebb J. Psychiatric emergencies. Kaplan and Sadock's synopsis of psychiatry: Behavioral sciences/clinical psychiatry. Baltimore: Williams and Wilkins, 1994.

PROBLEM 79   A 26-YEAR-OLD PRIMIGRAVIDA, 4 DAYS POSTPARTUM, WHO IS TEARFUL AND DEPRESSED

A 26-year-old primigravida delivers a healthy male infant at 40 weeks' gestation. She is doing fairly well until the fourth day postpartum. At that time she develops insomnia, fatigue, and feelings of sadness and depression.

The patient has a history of bipolar affective disorder in the past, but has not had an episode of either hypomania or depression for the last 5 years.

In spite of your concern regarding her history of bipolar affective disorder, she begins to improve on the eighth postpartum day and returns to her normal mental state 2 weeks postpartum. When you see her in the office in 6 weeks she is well.

SELECT THE ONE BEST ANSWER TO THE FOLLOWING QUESTIONS

1. What is the most likely diagnosis in this patient?
   a) postpartum depression
   b) postpartum blues
   c) a mild depression, definitely associated with her previous disease
   d) postpartum anxiety
   e) a normal postpartum reaction

2. What is the treatment of choice for the patient presented in Question 1?
   a) a tricyclic antidepressant
   b) lithium carbonate
   c) a MAO inhibitor
   d) a selective serotonin reuptake inhibitor (SSRI)
   e) none of the above

3. Considering this patient's history of bipolar affective disorder (BAD), which of the following statements is true?
   a) the probability of a recurrence of BAD is no greater after pregnancy than in the nonpregnant state
   b) the probability of a recurrence of BAD is actually decreased in the postpartum state
   c) the probability of a recurrence of BAD is increased in the postpartum state
   d) none of the above
   e) nobody knows for sure

4. A 28-year-old primigravida delivers a healthy female infant at 39 weeks' gestation. She is well until the fourth postpartum day, when she develops tearfulness, despondency, guilt, anorexia, depression, insomnia, and feelings of inadequacy in coping with her infant. These feelings continue and she is in marked distress when seen for her 3-week checking.
   What is the most likely diagnosis in this patient?
   a) postpartum depression
   b) postpartum blues
   c) acute adjustment reaction
   d) early bipolar affective disorder
   e) none of the above

5. What is(are) the treatment(s) of choice for the patient described in Question 4?
   a) a tricyclic antidepressant
   b) a MAO inhibitor
   c) a selective serotonin reuptake inhibitor (SSRI)
   d) supportive psychotherapy
   e) a and d

6. A 29-year-old primigravida is found on the fourth postpartum day loudly singing hymns at 4 AM in the hospital corridor. During the next 24 hours she causes significant turmoil on the maternity ward. She is found rushing into other patients' rooms announcing that she is about to start classes in bioenergetics and urges them to participate. She refuses meals and denies any need to sleep because she is "in touch with the source of superior power." She is hyperactive and talkative and invites her obstetrician to make love to her. When the psychiatrist is hastily summoned, she jumps out the window (fortunately she has a first-floor room, so only minor injuries are sustained).
   Which of the following statements is(are) true concerning this patient?
   a) this patient has a postpartum psychosis
   b) this patient probably has schizophrenia
   c) this patient most likely has a history of bipolar affective disorder
   d) a and c
   e) b and c

7. What is(are) the greatest risk(s) at this time for this patient?
   a) suicide
   b) infanticide
   c) homicide
   d) degeneration into a more or less permanent paranoid state
   e) a and b

8. Which of the following is(are) treatment(s) of choice for this patient?
   a) intensive observation
   b) lithium carbonate
   c) a neuroleptic agent in the initial phase
   d) a selective serotonin reuptake inhibitor (SSRI)
   e) all of the above

9. Which of the following statements regarding the effects of maternal depression in older children is(are) true?
   a) behavioral problems are more common in children whose mothers have had a postpartum depression
   b) significant cognitive deficits occur in children whose mothers have an episode of depression in the first postpartum year
   c) there is a significant correlation between reading difficulties in children and depression in their mothers
   d) all of the above are true
   e) none of the above are true

10. What is the single most important risk factor for the development of a postpartum depression?
    a) a history of depression
    b) a history of bipolar affective disorder
    c) a greater than average postpartum drop in the serum progesterone level
    d) a recent stressful life event
    e) the mother's experience as a child in her family of origin

Short Answer Management Problem 79

The relationship between the patient and her physician makes a significant difference when considering the probability that postpartum depression will develop, the early and successful recognition of mood disturbances in the postpartum period, and the successful treatment of same. This will decrease the length and severity of those mood disturbances. Provide specific suggestions to accomplish this goal.

ANSWERS

1. B.

2. E.

3. C. This patient has postpartum blues. Postpartum blues occur in about 50%-80% of puerperal women. The syndrome is transitory, resolving spontaneously within a few days to 2 weeks.

   Postpartum blues usually starts with a brief period of weeping on the third or fourth day after delivery and peaks between the fifth and tenth day after delivery. Symptoms include anxiety, headaches, poor concentration, and confusion. Elation may also occur.

   The etiology of postpartum blues is unknown, but a hormonal basis is suspected. Of the hormones involved, the most likely candidate is progesterone, and the most likely alteration is progesterone deficiency.

   The treatment of choice for postpartum blues includes supportive psychotherapy; family (especially spousal) support, understanding, and reassurance; and patient education (reassuring the patient that this is completely normal). In the patient described, it is especially important to reinforce that there is no connection between the postpartum blues now experienced and her previous bipolar illness; resolution of "the blues" will occur within 2 weeks, but monitoring her condition is necessary to ensure both maternal and fetal health.

   In a patient with a history of bipolar affective disorder there is actually an increased chance of reoccurrence in the postpartum period. As well, if it does reappear it is more likely to be associated with a psychotic phase than normally it would be.

Of the 50%-80% of women who develop postpartum blues, only a fraction will go on to have a true postpartum depression. That figure seems to be remarkably constant at around 10% and varies little.

4. A.

5. E. This patient has a true postpartum depression. Postpartum depression, as discussed above, occurs in approximately 10% of women. In postpartum depression, in contradistinction to postpartum blues, the patient is disabled for a period of time greater than 2 weeks. The major symptoms are a depressed mood, a real concern about the ability to cope with the new infant, and increased guilt. Other symptoms include tearfulness, despondency, worrying about not loving the baby enough, worrying about doing something "irrational" to the baby, anxiety regarding feeding the baby, fear about the baby's sleep, fear about older siblings' jealousy, hypochondriac symptoms, irritability, impaired concentration, poor memory, and extreme fatigue.

   The etiology, although unclear, appears to be multifactorial. The following theories have been proposed as theories of the causation of postpartum depression:
   A. Hormonal deficiency: progesterone
   B. Family history of depression
   C. The conduct and stress of the labor itself
   D. A feeling of having "lost control" of the entire labor process (this included interventions or the lack of same: for example, those patients given an epidural felt "less in control," as did those patients having a cesarian section, and those women who were not well informed by health care providers during the labor.)

E. Vulnerability in terms of the mother's experience as a child (especially regarding nurturing behavior)

F. Lack of an intimate confiding relationship with her partner

G. The degree of commitment of the father to the whole process of pregnancy, labor, and delivery

H. The influence of stressful life events including family crises, bereavement, change in housing, financial problems, and caring for her other children

The treatment of choice for postpartum depression is a combination of supportive psychotherapy and a tricyclic antidepressant. Addressing the components listed will certainly decrease the duration and the severity of the postpartum depression. The best strategy appears to involve the health care professionals (doctor, public health nurse, psychiatric nurse), the patient's immediate family (especially a supportive husband), supportive friends and relatives, and group psychotherapy (where postpartum women with this condition compare their experiences).

6. D.

7. E.

8. E. This patient has a frank postpartum psychosis. Postpartum psychoses occur in 1 to 2 per 1000 postpartum women; they may present as schizophrenic or affective disorders or as confusional states.

Postpartum psychosis is thought to be an atypical psychosis and, in fact, in DSM-IV is discussed relative to diagnostic criteria as "diagnostic criteria for psychotic disorder not otherwise specified."

This patient presents with a hypomanic episode. She most likely has a personal history of bipolar affective disorder, a personal history of major depressive disorder, or a family history of bipolar affective disorder.

With hypomania, reclassification into acute and chronic treatment is necessary. Acute treatment consists of administering an antipsychotic drug. Haloperidol, chlorpromazine, or thioridazine are good first choices. At the same time, the patient should be put under intensive watch. A patient with postpartum psychosis is at risk for suicide and infanticide. In one study, 5% of patients committed suicide and 4% of patients committed infanticide.

Once the psychotic episode is resolved, long-term therapy should be started. This should involve:

A. An antimanic agent: lithium carbonate (dose to be determined by blood level)

B. An antidepressant, preferably a selective serotonin reuptake inhibitor (SSRI) because of very low potential for self-harm from overdose; alternatively, a TCA with sedating properties given in a controlled environment

C. Supportive individual psychotherapy

D. Family psychotherapy

E. Regular visits by mental health worker to measure general day-to-day coping skills in the immediate postpartum and for an extended time

9. D. The effects of postpartum depression extend far beyond the postpartum period and persist and are manifested in older children. Behavioral problems, cognitive defects, and reading difficulties are examples of problems that in older children develop as a result of postpartum depression or maternal depression. In this case, the birth of the new baby himself or herself is a "major life stressor."

10. D. Of all the factors discussed earlier, the single most important risk factor for the development of postpartum depression is a recent stressful life event.

SOLUTION TO SHORT ANSWER MANAGEMENT PROBLEM 79

Specific suggestions to alter the course of postpartum mood disturbances in your patients should include the following:

1. Encouraging the attendance of the husband or significant other at all prenatal visits

2. Questioning the couple about prenatal education received concerning mood changes in pregnancy, during labor, and after pregnancy

3. Providing patient education materials on specific mood disturbances

4. Emphasizing the importance of the husband or significant other in all aspects of the pregnancy, labor and delivery, the puerperium, and the care of the new family member

5. Discussing with both members of the couple your philosophy of childbirth (hopefully indicating to the couple that you believe childbirth to be a normal event, not a disease)

6. Describing all tests, all examination procedures, the reason(s) for all routine questions, and any deviation from normal protocol that may occur during pregnancy

7. Discussing all of the minor (but annoying) physiologically based problems of pregnancy (edema, heartburn, ligament relaxation, hemorrhoids, and so on)

8. Providing clear instructions to the couple regarding when to call you and when to go to the hospital, and reassuring that you "would rather receive a call than not receive a call"

9. Making at least one visit to the patient during early labor and reasons for same

10. Explaining every possible intervention during labor and the reason(s) for same (such as artificial rupture of the membranes, internal fetal monitoring, and augmentation of labor)

11. Encouraging the patient at every opportunity during labor and delivery

12. Assessing the patient immediately postpartum and monitoring her condition carefully. Pay particular attention to a patient history of bipolar affective disorder, a patient history of major depressive disorder, a family history of depression, a family history of any other significant psychiatric disease, and a patient who is going through or recently has gone through a major life stressor.

SUMMARY OF POSTPARTUM DEPRESSION DIAGNOSIS AND TREATMENT

1. **Postpartum blues:**
   a) Incidence: 50%-80%
   b) Evolution: begins on or about third day; resolves by 2 weeks
   c) Treatment: reassurance, supportive psychotherapy; spousal involvement or significant other involvement critical
2. **Postpartum depression:**
   a) Incidence: 10%
   b) Evolution: begins on third to fifth day; lasts longer than 2 weeks
   c) Treatment: psychotherapy plus pharmacologic antidepressant therapy
3. **Postpartum psychosis:**
   a) Incidence: 0.1%-0.2%
   b) Treatment: acute: neuroleptic agent, close observation to prevent self-harm and harm to the infant

Long-term treatment:
1) Lithium carbonate
2) Antidepressant: SSRI may be drug class of first choice; TCAs
3) Psychotherapy: supportive, group, individual; spousal or significant other involvement critical

4. **Prevention:**
   a) Education in the prenatal period: this education must include significant attention to the psychological consequences of pregnancy, labor, delivery, and the impact of the neonate on the family.
   b) Explanation of all procedures and interventions to allow the patient as much control as possible during labor
   c) Significant involvement of the husband or significant other in the process is critical.

SUGGESTED READINGS

American Psychiatric Association. Diagnostic and statistical manual. 4th Ed. Washington, DC: American Psychiatric Association Press, 1994.

Holden J. Postnatal depression: Its nature, effects, and identification using the Edinburgh Postnatal Depression Scale. Birth 1991; 18:4:211-221.

Robinson G, Stewart D. Postpartum psychiatric disorders. Can Med Assoc J 1986; 134(1):31-36.

PROBLEM 80   A 21-YEAR-OLD MALE WITH CHRONIC BACK PAIN

A 21-year-old male presents to your office with a chief complaint of chronic back pain. He states that he fell off a ladder 3 years ago and broke his back. Since that time he has been unable to work and has been able to function only when taking a combination of Talwin (pentazocine) and Demerol (meperidine). He walks slowly and carefully and states that he is unable to flex or extend his lumbar spine because of pain. He points to the lower lumbar area as the point of maximum pain. He states that he doesn't like to take drugs but he has to: taking drugs is the only way he can continue to function.

SELECT THE ONE BEST ANSWER TO THE FOLLOWING QUESTIONS

1. What is the most likely diagnosis in this patient?
   a) congenital vertebral deformity with secondary lumbar fractures
   b) old lumbar fractures with chronic paravertebral muscle spasm
   c) chronic lumbar pain syndrome
   d) narcotic drug abuse
   e) somatoform pain disorder

2. If your history and physical examination confirms your suspicions, what would be your next step?
   a) order a CT scan of the lumbar spine
   b) order an MRI scan of the lumbar spine
   c) refer the patient for an orthopedic consultation
   d) refer the patient for a neurosurgical consultation
   e) none of the above

3. Following the initiation of the most appropriate investigative procedure (or other intervention or nonintervention), what would you do then?
   a) prescribe Demerol and Talwin for 1 month and see the patient for review at that time
   b) prescribe Talwin but not Demerol in an effort to cut down on the amount of narcotic analgesic used
   c) prescribe Tylenol with codeine instead of Talwin and Demerol in an effort to decrease the addiction potential of the drug used
   d) begin to prescribe Demerol or Talwin for short periods of time (1 week) in an effort to monitor drug intake carefully
   e) none of the above

4. Which of the following statements regarding drug abuse and drug dependence is(are) true?
   a) drug dependence is defined as the inappropriate use of a drug in terms of either the medical indications or its dose
   b) drug abuse refers to physical or psychologic dependence on drugs
   c) prescription drug abuse includes legal drugs that find their way into the illicit drug market
   d) drug abuse may or may not lead to drug dependence
   e) none of the above statements are true

5. Which of the following prescription drugs are unlikely to be abused?
   a) narcotic analgesics
   b) sedative-hypnotics
   c) benzodiazepines
   d) amphetaminelike substances
   e) anticonvulsants

6. Which of the following benzodiazepines is(are) unlikely to be associated with rebound anxiety?
   a) triazolam
   b) lorazepam
   c) bromazepam
   d) flurazepam
   e) all of the above may cause rebound anxiety

7. Which of the following groups of physicians are likely to be responsible for drug diversion?
   a) impaired physicians
   b) dishonest physicians
   c) duped physicians
   d) dated physicians
   e) all of the above may be responsible for drug diversion

8. Which of the following drugs may be helpful in the treatment of chronic low back pain?
   a) desipramine
   b) methocarbamol
   c) acetaminophen
   d) naproxen
   e) all of the above

9. Which of the following statements regarding chronic low back pain treated with narcotic analgesics is(are) true?
   a) narcotic analgesics are absolutely contraindicated in all cases of chronic low back pain
   b) narcotic analgesics are likely to add to the patient's problems rather than helping them
   c) narcotic analgesics are rarely used in the management of chronic low back pain
   d) narcotic analgesics are likely to have a significant positive impact on the patient's low back pain
   e) none of the above

10. Which of the following conditions is the most frequent diagnosis in which narcotic analgesics are used for a chronic nonmalignant pain problem?
    a) migraine headaches
    b) rheumatoid arthritis
    c) chronic pelvic pain
    d) abdominal pain
    e) ischemic vascular disease

Short Answer Management Problem 80

Describe a set of conditions under which the use of narcotic analgesics for the management of chronic nonmalignant pain may be considered appropriate.

ANSWERS

1. D. The most likely diagnosis in this patient is narcotic drug abuse. If he himself is not a narcotic abuser, he may very well be a prescription drug trafficker.

   The most common office presentations of opioid abusers are complaints of chronic pain, often related to previous trauma. Chronic back pain or other orthopedic pain related to an old injury and chronic headache are the two most common complaints.

   A valuable clue to narcotic abuse in this patient is his statement that his pain is relieved *only* by taking a combination of pentazocine (Talwin) and meperidine (Demerol). A patient who names his analgesics of choice is almost certainly either a narcotic drug addict or a drug trafficker.

2. E. The ordering of a CT scan, an MRI scan, or the referral to a consultant orthopedic surgeon or neurosurgeon would not be valuable in this patient. In most cases, even if the appointment was made, the patient would not keep it. There is a significant probability that no such injury occurred, and the whole episode is factitious. On the other hand, it is possible that the injury occurred and that the patient has become dependent on and/or addicted to narcotic analgesics.

   The appropriate "investigation" in this case would be to attempt to elicit a more complete history regarding the patient's injury, including initial emergency treatment and other physicians consulted, and to discuss with the patient your serious concerns regarding his use of narcotic analgesics.

   His response to your concerns will, in all likelihood, further elucidate the diagnosis. The chronic pain patient may be too frightened of recurrence or too dependent on narcotic analgesics to consider alternative forms of pain management; the prescription drug trafficker will either increase pressure or become angry or even violent; and the patient who is going through withdrawal may admit to this at this point.

3. E. If the patient is a true narcotic drug addict, the most reasonable course of action is to attempt to convince him to enter an inpatient drug rehabilitation program. In programs of this type, methadone is often available for the slow tapering of the narcotic dosage.

   All of the other options are inappropriate. If the patient is a narcotic addict, you have simply continued to supply his habit. If he is a drug trafficker, you have just supplied him with drugs to peddle to other narcotic addicts.

4. D. Drug abuse is defined as inappropriate use of a drug in terms of either its medical indications or its dose. Drug dependence refers to physical or psychologic dependence on drugs. Drug abuse may or may not lead to drug dependence.

   Prescription drug abuse refers to the abuse of drugs that are obtained by physician prescription. It does not include legal drugs that find their way into the illicit drug market.

5. E. The four main classes of psychoactive drugs that tend to be chronically abused include the narcotic analgesics, the sedative-hypnotics, the benzodiazepines, and the amphetaminelike substances.

   Some of the commonly abused prescription drugs (with their street names) include the following: Tuinal/Seconal (candy); Dilaudid (D's); Fiorinal; Novahistex DH (juice); morphine (Mojo); Percocet/Percodan (percs); Valium (V's); and a combination of Talwin and Ritalin (T's and R's). Some of these drugs have a street value of up to $75/tablet.

   The anticonvulsant medications (such as carbamazepine and valproic acid) are unlikely to be associated with abuse.

6. D. Rebound anxiety following continuation of a sedative-hypnotic can produce severe symptoms. The syndrome, however, is transient and lasts for a relatively short time.

   The risk of rebound anxiety is directly related to the elimination half-life after short-term use. Short-acting agents such as triazolam, lorazepam, and bromazepam carry a greater risk than a longer-acting agent with flurazepam.

7. E. Doctors responsible for drug diversion and the continuation of prescription drug abuse can be divided into the four D's: 1) the "disabled or impaired physicians" who prescribe medications for themselves; the "dishonest doctors" who consciously misprescribe for profit; the "duped doctors" who easily give in to patient demands for drugs; and the "dated doctors" who lack medical knowledge regarding the effects of their prescriptions.

8. E. Patients with chronic low back pain should be treated with anything but narcotic analgesics. Direct analgesics such as acetaminophen, aspirin, and nonsteroidal anti-inflammatory agents such as naproxen can be very helpful. Skeletal muscle relaxants such as methocarbamol may reduce skeletal muscle spasm around the injured or chronic pain area. Adjuvant analgesics such as desipramine (a tricyclic antidepressant) are very useful in chronic back syndromes, especially neuropathic chronic pain syndromes.

9. B. Narcotic analgesics are likely to add to the patient's problems rather than help or diminish them. Essentially, what started out as one problem (the chronic low back pain) has become two problems (the chronic low back pain plus narcotic dependence and/or addiction).

   Although not absolutely contraindicated in the management of low back pain, they should not be used unless all of the following conditions have been fulfilled:

   1. You are absolutely sure that the patient has a "real" chronic pain syndrome that is anatomically and physiologically based (this is quite rare).
   2. You have tried all aspects and types of nonpharmacologic therapy and all other types of pharmacologic management before resorting to narcotic analgesics.
   3. A colleague or specialist in pain management has been consulted.

   A complete list of conditions is covered in the summary at the end of this chapter.

   Narcotic analgesics do not create a positive impact on your patient's life and your patient's pain. Usually you start the patient on a low dose and the dose gradually increases. The patient returns and the pain is no better or only minimally better. Therefore you prescribe an increased dose of the narcotic, and the cycle begins to repeat itself again and again.

   In the general population of patients with chronic pain syndromes, narcotic analgesics are used much more often than they should be. Once the cycle is established, it is very difficult to break.

10. A. The most frequent nonmalignant pain diagnosis leading to the prescription of narcotic analgesics is migraine headache. Patients with chronic migraine headache frequently present to the ER of hospitals seeking injections of meperidine and dramamine. The patient tells you that "this is the only combination that works." The probability of that patient's having a nonmalignant pain syndrome without some degree of narcotic dependence or narcotic addiction is very low.

SOLUTION TO SHORT ANSWER MANAGEMENT PROBLEM 80

The answer includes a summary of rules that may be helpful in the management of patients with chronic nonmalignant pain. These represent the guidelines established by the College of Physicians and Surgeons, Province of Alberta. Guidelines vary from state to state and from province to province.

Note that rules and regulations concerning opioid use vary from state to state in the United States and from province to province in Canada. These rules are widely divergent. The following set of guidelines was developed by the College of Physicians and Surgeons in the province of Alberta, Canada. Please consult your state licensing authority before adhering to these guidelines.

GUIDELINES FOR THE MANAGEMENT OF CHRONIC NONMALIGNANT PAIN

1. Take a complete pain history and do a complete physical examination.
2. Assess the patient for the possibility of coexistent depression, sleep disorder, personality disorder, poorly developed coping skills, and level of social function.
3. Obtain all relevant documentation concerning prior investigations and consultations.
4. Consider ways in which the patient can be empowered to assume responsibility for the problem.
5. Long-term treatment with analgesic medication should be administered only if analgesics result in relief of pain, functional improvement, or both.
6. Opioids are not first-line drugs in management of chronic nonmalignant pain but are *occasionally* helpful. One must carefully weigh the potential problems associated with such medications against possible benefit when considering prescribing them.
7. A multidisciplinary team approach to pain management is essential.

GUIDELINES FOR OPIOID USE IN CHRONIC NONMALIGNANT PAIN

1. Diagnosis of the underlying medical condition causing the pain problem must be established.
2. A history of recent or remote substance abuse is a relatively strong contraindication to the use of any opioid; the available evidence suggests that chronic

opioid therapy in such patients should be considered only under extraordinary circumstances.

3. An adequate trial of nonopioid analgesics and adjuvant analgesics should have been carried out without success.

4. Only one physician should prescribe opioids.

5. In order to start a patient on an opioid, the principles of the World Health Organization's "analgesic ladder" should be employed. Patients should first be started on opioids in combination with nonsteroidal antiinflammatory drugs or acetaminophen. Only after a good trial on a weak opioid should a strong opioid be considered.

6. Treatment of pain with opioids is actually a treatment trial and, like all therapeutic trials, may be effective or ineffective. Effective therapy may be defined as identification of a dose associated with meaningful partial analgesia and no adverse effects severe enough to compromise comfort or function.

7. If a fixed preparation of a weak opioid and nonopioid analgesic is not satisfactory, then the patient may be tried on oral morphine.

8. Parenteral dosing of opioids to treat chronic nonmalignant pain should be strongly discouraged and daily IM injections abhorred.

9. There should be an agreement between the patient and the prescribing physician that clearly delineates that there can be no unsanctioned dose escalation, no selling of the opioids, no seeking of opioids from another physician, and no hoarding of opioids.

10. The patient should be seen and assessed at least every 9 weeks and more frequently if there is a history of previous substance abuse. At each visit the clinician should evaluate the patient for several distinct aspects of therapy, including the following:
    1) Analgesic efficacy
    2) Adverse pharmacologic events
    3) Function (physical and psychological)
    4) The occurrence of apparent drug-abuse–related behaviors

    Documentation is very important with this therapy, and physicians should keep careful records that include reference to the various aspects of therapy.

11. Flares of pain can be treated with small extra doses of opioid by mouth; each monthly prescription should include a few extra doses for this purpose.

    The goal of chronic opioid therapy is not the elimination of pain (which may be impossible) but rather the control of pain to a tolerable level; there is clear emphasis on level of function of the patient in his or her social, work, and personal life.

SUGGESTED READINGS

American Psychiatric Association. Diagnostic and statistical manual. 4th Ed. Washington, DC: American Psychiatric Association Press, 1994.

The College of Physicians and Surgeons of Alberta, Canada. Guidelines for the management of chronic non-malignant pain. Edmonton, Canada, 1993.

Weiss K, Greenfield P. Prescription drug abuse. Psychiatric Clinics of North America 1986; 9(3):475-490.

PROBLEM 81   A PHARMACEUTICAL COMPANY THAT IS PAYING FOR A "WEEKEND GETAWAY" FOR ALL OF THE FAMILY PRACTICE RESIDENTS

ETHICAL PROBLEM 1

A pharmaceutical company has just produced another "marvelous" scientific advance (in their own words) in the treatment of peptic ulcer disease. The local representative advises you, the chief family medicine resident, of their desire to send all 24 of your residents on an "all-expenses-paid weekend" to attend a CME event on peptic ulcer disease. There will, of course, be time for certain "organized and expense-paid recreational activities" following the 1½ hours of lecture/day on a 3-day weekend. Included in the offer are the following:

1) Air transportation for you and a significant other to a "get-away retreat" on the eastern seaboard
2) All hotel accommodations for you and your significant other
3) All meals for you and your significant other
4) Conference registration
5) All recreational activities, including golf at a six-star golf course, whitewater rafting, snorkelling, horseback riding, and a "shopping spree" even for the shoppers in the crowd

As the chief resident you are responsible for making the final decision on whether or not this should take place.
For this case, and for the nine additional case descriptions that follow, please indicate your decision in the following manner.

Place a check beside "A" if you consider the event to be unequivocally ethical and would personally support it.
Place a check beside "B" if you consider the event to be ethical enough that it deserves your support.
Place a check beside "C" if you consider the event to be of a questionable ethical nature that you may or may not support depending on the nature of additional information received concerning it.
Place a check beside "D" if you feel that the event is of sufficient ethical doubt to cause you to seriously consider not supporting it.
Place a check beside "E" if you feel the event to be unequivocally unethical and will not support it in any way.

1. A _____

   B _____

   C _____

   D _____

   E _____

ETHICAL PROBLEM 2

You, a practicing family physician, are invited to attend an "evening under the stars" featuring a 3-hour river cruise and a gourmet meal for you and your "significant other." Of course, a short (1-minute) scientific presentation on the merits of the sponsoring company's drug will be the true highlight of the evening.

2. A _____

   B _____

   C _____

   D _____

   E _____

ETHICAL PROBLEM 3

You, the principle investigator for a phase IV (post-marketing) trial are invited to organize and attend an international 1-day symposium on the preliminary results of the "research." The symposium is being held in a luxury hotel on the French Riviera. Your 10 coinvestigators are also invited.

3. A _____

   B _____

C _____

D _____

E _____

ETHICAL PROBLEM 4

You, the director of CME for a major hospital, are offered the use of an "audience response system" donated to your department (an audience response system allows the responses of a CME audience to be measured one-to-another and compared to the correct response). The cost of the system is $10,000.00. The company representatives insist that "there are no strings attached."

4. A _____

B _____

C _____

D _____

E _____

ETHICAL PROBLEM 5

The representative of a large company specializing in the development of new antihypertensive agents offers to sponsor a "dinner meeting" for 100 physicians. At this dinner meeting, a well-known expert (remember the definition of an expert: someone from out of town with a trayful of slides) will present his views on the "new drug treatments for hypertension." The dinner meeting will be held at a world-class French restaurant and will feature "exquisite French cuisine prepared by a chef flown in from Paris for the specific purpose of preparing the meal."

5. A _____

B _____

C _____

D _____

E _____

ETHICAL PROBLEM 6

A well-known pharmaceutical company offers to donate $1,000.000 for a "resident scholarship" to attend a major scientific meeting. The funds will be made available to the residency program director and the selection made by the department of family medicine itself.

6. A _____

B _____

C _____

D _____

E _____

ETHICAL PROBLEM 7

A pharmaceutical company representative makes an appointment to see you, the chief resident in the department of family medicine, to discuss the sponsoring of "noon rounds" for the next 4 weeks. He apparently has "drug videos" which he wishes to familiarize your resident colleagues with. He, of course, will provide all the necessary refreshments and food for the entire group.

7. A _____

B _____

C _____

D ———

E ———

ETHICAL PROBLEM 8

Fifty pharmaceutical companies agree to "buy booths" at a major national scientific meeting. You are the chairperson of the scientific meeting and are asked to make the final decision in this case.

8. A ———

   B ———

   C ———

   D ———

   E ———

ETHICAL PROBLEM 9

The same situation as described in Ethical Problem 8 occurs in this case. The only difference, however, is that each pharmaceutical company is attempting to outdo the other with "tokens of appreciation." These vary from simple pens and pencils to entire sets of golf clubs.

9. A ———

   B ———

   C ———

   D ———

   E ———

ETHICAL PROBLEM 10

A pharmaceutical company asks you, a family physician with expertise in cancer pain management, to speak at a "dinner meeting." The dinner meeting is being held at a "middle-class" restaurant. You will be paid $2,000.00 for your services.

10. A ———

    B ———

    C ———

    D ———

    E ———

ANSWERS

1. E. The following "acid tests" produced by the American College of Physicians should help you to come to a reasonable conclusion on all of the ethical problems presented.

   The two acid tests that can be used in every case are as follows:
   1. Would this event withstand both public and professional scrutiny?
   2. Would you want these arrangements to be generally known?

   In this case, the payment for airfare, accommodation, meals, recreational events, and apparently everything else is completely contrary to the guidelines established by the American Academy of Family Physicians. In addition, it is extremely doubtful that these arrangement would withstand either public or professional scrutiny, nor would many feel comfortable with their publication in the local newspaper the next day.

   Say, for example, that the event is being sponsored by company X marketing drug Y. You are a heart patient taking company X's drug. Further, assume that the drug is very expensive and you are on a fixed income. On reading about this in your local paper, your response would likely be less than positive.

2. E. You may think that this is a complete exaggeration and that no one would seriously consider only a 1-minute presentation. This, in fact, is a true scenario that attracted 75 physicians and their spouses.

3. D. There are enough serious questions that arise from this description to place the event in the D category.

On the ethical side, you, the principal investigator, and your 10 coinvestigators are being invited to a meeting to discuss "research" results.

On the very questionable side are the following:

First, this is a post-marketing study and cannot in any meaningful way be classified as research. These studies are most often uncontrolled and simply require the "researcher" to fill in a simple form, for which a computer system (which, of course, the "researcher" gets to keep) is provided.

Second, and as another acid test, it has been suggested that you must determine the primary attraction to the event. Is it the scientific meeting itself or the social venue? In this case, the social venue would probably win out.

4. A. In this case, the fiduciary relationship of patient and physician is not compromised. In fact, it could be argued that because the audience response system increases the interactive nature of any CME event, the "probability of learning" among the participants will increase. This should result in improved patient care.

5. E. This case reeks of possible "influence peddling" and "peer selling"; what you might as well refer to as a "hit man" for the company presents his views on why this company's product is superior to anything else produced by mankind to date.

Only if the following conditions were satisfied would an affair of this nature be acceptable to both public and professional scrutiny:

1) The speaker presented an independent, unbiased assessment of hypertensive drug treatment. This must include not only an analysis of new products but a comparison (both efficacy and cost) with older products.

2) The affair was held at a somewhat less elaborate restaurant with a somewhat less elaborate menu.

6. A. This is, it appears, a highly ethical proposal that presents few if any problems. The major consideration in this case is the control of the funds and the selection of the resident by the department of family medicine itself.

7. D. Although "noon rounds" should and usually do have significant educational value, you must be very cautious about the nature of the drug videos. If they portray a reasonable summary of the disease condition and its treatment in a balanced perspective (with the company's product mentioned by generic name only and mentioned as one of the treatment options), then it may be a reasonable request. If the drug videos are, as in most cases, strictly promotional in nature, then on the basis of the importance of maintaining a completely ethical re-lationship with the pharmaceutical industry, you would probably have to refuse the request.

8. A. The fact of the matter is that we, as physicians, must work in close cooperation with the pharmaceutical industry. Continuing medical education would suffer greatly and in many cases be completely eliminated without the support of industry. The buying of booths for a major meeting or the buying of advertising space at national and regional medical publications is common practice and considered to be completely ethical by most concerned.

9. D. There is considerable debate on this subject. The major contention by those who consider this practice to be unethical is that the pharmaceutical companies are, by their actions, attempting to "buy" the physicians. It appears to many, however, to be a matter of degree. In my opinion, a pen is unlikely to buy a physician; a complete set of golf clubs is a different story.

10. D. The ethical difficulty with this problem is not the topic, the speaker, or the restaurant; rather, it is the amount of money that both the public and your professional colleagues would consider to be reasonable for a 1-hour presentation. You could even argue that because cancer pain is an area in which family physicians can use considerable education, this activity should be encouraged. When I was faced with this very issue, I donated the $2,000 to the Residency Trust Fund.

SUMMARY OF ETHICAL CONSIDERATIONS—PHYSICIANS AND THE PHARMACEUTICAL INDUSTRY

1. Primum non nocere—"First do no harm" (including no harm in inflating drug costs by your acceptance of pharmaceutical offerings that are clearly unethical).
2. The acid tests for dealing with industry:
   a) Would you want these arrangements generally known?
   b) Would this withstand public and professional scrutiny?
3. Physicians and the pharmaceutical industry must work together. That working together, however, must be on terms that never compromise the fiduciary relationship between patient and physician or pass the cost for these events onto those who can least afford it.
4. Residents beware: as the prescribers of tomorrow, you are the number-one target of the pharmaceutical industry.
5. Consider the primary purpose of the event in question: is it the event itself or the social venue?
6. Remember to call research and marketing what they are. Be cautious of the real purpose of your involvement in post-marketing research: in most cases it is marketing and not research.
7. Beware of experts from afar: they may be "snake-oil salesmen" in disguise.

SUGGESTED READINGS

American Academy of Family Physicians approves statement on the ethics of proprietary relationship with industry. American Family Physician 1991; 44(6):2233-2239.

Newton W, Goldstein A, Frey J. There is no such thing as a free lunch. Developing policies on pharmaceutical industry support. Journal of Family Practice 1992; 34(1):32-34.

PROBLEM 82 A 38-YEAR-OLD FEMALE WITH SIGNIFICANT CONCERNS REGARDING HER HUSBAND'S UPCOMING OPERATION

A 38-year-old female whom you have cared for for many years, along with her husband and three children, presents to your office in a disturbed state. She is crying and states that she has been up all night worrying about her husband's upcoming operation. Her husband has Crohn's disease and has developed a partial intestinal obstruction requiring surgery. His operation is booked for later today. The patient describes feelings of impending doom and is certain that something is going to go wrong during the operation. You are about to try to reassure her regarding the upcoming surgery.

SELECT THE ONE BEST ANSWER TO THE FOLLOWING QUESTIONS

1. What is the most important prerequisite for effective reassurance in a family physician-patient relationship?
   a) the length of time the family physician has known the patient
   b) the premorbid personality of the patient
   c) a preexisting trusting relationship between the family physician and the patient
   d) the communication style of the family physician
   e) the patient's previous experience with the family physician

2. The patient tells you that ever since her husband was diagnosed with Crohn's disease, she has constantly worried about his future and the future of her family. She has had thoughts she describes as "dark forbodings." During this period of time, she has had a number of viral illnesses that she never was predisposed to previously. Regarding worry and stress and the effect of the mind on bodily health, which of the following statements is true?
   a) there is no relationship between mental stress and physical health
   b) mental stress rarely produces any serious health problems
   c) there is no evidence linking mental stress with hormonal function
   d) there is a phenomenon known as the general adaptation syndrome linking mental stress and bodily function
   e) worry and stress are part of everyone's daily life; nobody can do much about it

3. One of the most important skills in psychotherapy is attentive listening followed by genuine and truthful reassurance. Unfortunately, listening is not something many physicians do well. We frequently interrupt. What is the average time between when the patient speaks his or her first word and the physician first interrupts?
   a) 4 minutes, 30 seconds
   b) 3 minutes, 15 seconds
   c) 2 minutes, 4 seconds
   d) 1 minute, 14 seconds
   e) 0 minutes, 18 seconds

4. What is the most important requirement in making physician reassurance patient specific?
   a) taking a long time and repeating the reassurance several times
   b) concentrating on the patient's verbal and nonverbal responses
   c) determining the patient's specific anxieties
   d) backing up words with diagrams and illustrations
   e) asking the patient to come back several times to repeat the process

5. What is the most important message to leave a patient with at the conclusion of an interview in which you, the family physician, are attempting to reassure the patient?
   a) a message of encouragement; a message reiterating that things could always be worse
   b) a message of frankness and confidence that no matter how bad the situation, toughness and fortitude will "help win the day"
   c) a message of hope
   d) a message of confidence in the patient's ability to withstand the absolute worst-case scenario
   e) a message of inspiration in which you attempt to convince the patient that in most cases all worries and fears are completely unfounded

6. One role that family physicians play in times of illness and family disruption is that of healer. Which of the following best describes this role of the family physician?
   a) a facilitator and encourager of the patient's own inner strengths
   b) a describer of the miracles of modern science
   c) an encourager of the ability of anyone to beat any odds in overcoming illness
   d) a provider of drugs and other therapies that as agents of necessary change to the disease state allow total healing
   e) a provider of new technologies that will eventually turn things around

7. Regarding reassurance of a patient by a family physician, which of the following statements is false?
   a) premature reassurance is ineffective and may be interpreted by the patient as rejection
   b) when reassurance can be given with confidence it should not be delayed

c) some hope (no matter what the situation) should always be given

d) the patient's complaints and his or her perception of them should be taken seriously

e) reassurance of the patient by the physician rarely results in altered clinical outcomes

8. Regarding effective listening, which of the following statements is true?
   a) there is no difference between active listening and passive listening
   b) effective listening is a skill that requires the physician to understand and empathize with the patient
   c) eye-to-eye contact is not a significant factor in establishing effective listening patterns
   d) whether a physician sits or stands beside a patient when listening and discussing a patient's problem doesn't make a great deal of difference
   e) listening, as a skill, can and should often be left to other health care professionals

9. With respect to the patient described in the problem, what would be the most appropriate response by the family physician?
   a) tell the patient not to worry; the operation is routine and there really is no cause for concern
   b) explain to the patient that the surgeon performing the operation is experienced and will make sure that nothing goes wrong
   c) listen to the patient's concerns and establish for certain the exact nature of the concerns; go on to

describe in detail the operative process and the significant opportunity for full recovery and significant remission that may occur

d) ask the patient to talk to the surgeon

e) none of the above

10. A patient (patient A) is being visited by her family physician following an uncomplicated oophorectomy. Her physician comes in, stands by the head of the bed, and describes the details of the procedure to her. Another patient (patient B), in the next bed, who has had the same operation, is visited by her family physician that same morning. That physician comes in, sits down beside the patient, and discusses the details of the procedure. Both physicians are in the room exactly the same amount of time.

    Regarding the length of time that the two patients perceive their family physicians to have been in the room, which of the following statements is most likely to be true?
    a) patient A will most likely perceive the visit to have been longer than patient B
    b) patient B will likely perceive the visit to have been longer than patient A
    c) there will likely be no difference between the perceptions of the two patients regarding the length of the visit
    d) this is an impossible question to answer; it all depends on the individuals concerned
    e) without the input of the respective family physicians, it is extremely difficult to answer this question

Short Answer Management Problem 82

Describe the differences between active listening and passive listening with respect to family doctor–patient communication.

ANSWERS

1. C. The essential basis for effective reassurance is a trusting relationship between the patient and the family physician. A family physician who knows the patient has a significant advantage due to this. Other factors such as the length of time the family physician has known the patient, the patient's premorbid personality, the family physician's communication style, and the patient's previous experience with the family physician are all important. The most important factor, however, is a trusting relationship between doctor and patient.

2. D. There is a phenomenon known as the general adaptation syndrome (GAS) that links bodily health with mental function. The major pathways involved in GAS

are the central nervous system, the endocrine system, and the immune system. The essential features of the GAS are adrenal hypertrophy, thymic involution, and elevated corticosteroid levels. High levels of corticosteroids are immunosuppressive, and physiological levels are required for several normal immune functions. The GAS, in response to a challenge from a number of stimuli, causes the hypothalamus to release a corticotrophin-releasing factor, which in turn causes the pituitary gland to release adrenocorticotrophic hormone (ACTH). Following this, the adrenal cortex produces corticosteroids.

3. E. In general, we as physicians are not particularly good listeners. In one study, the average interval between the patient beginning to tell his or her story and the doctor interrupting was 18 seconds. A busy office that is fre-

quently behind schedule, telephone interruptions, and other distractions make us more likely to interrupt the patient while he or she is telling the story.

4. C. The most important component in making physician reassurance to the patient specific is knowing what the patient's specific anxieties are. Only then can the family physician take the necessary steps to maximize the potential of reassurance, in terms of history, physical examination, and laboratory investigations.

5. C. It is essential that at the conclusion of the interview the patient leave the office with some sense of hope. The hope that is given should be realistic and truthful, and not false. It may only be hope for another pain-free day, hope that a walk around the block is still possible, or some other form of hope that many of us would consider minor. To the particular patient, however, it may very well be the most important thing in his or her world at that time.

6. A. As healer, the family physician can best be described as the individual who helps the patient discover the barriers to wellness and facilitates and encourages the patient to find, within himself or herself, the necessary forces and inner strengths that promote physical, psychological, social, and spiritual healing.

To achieve this the family physician should be a master of the tools and therapeutic agents specific to the disease state. At a physical level this includes drugs, instruments, and manual skills. At a psychological level this includes the skills of communication, attentive listening, and reassurance.

At the highest level, healing is not a matter of technique. Techniques are helpful but not sufficient in themselves. At this high level the art of healing is based primarily on a trusting relationship between the healer and the sufferer.

7. E. Physician reassurance may result in markedly altered clinical outcomes. If the patient has a trusting relationship with the family physician and believes in the validity of the reassurance given by the physician, stress is relieved and an environment of hope is allowed to prevail. We now know that once this occurs, improved clinical outcomes can and will occur.

8. B. Effective listening is a skill that requires the physician to be able to understand and empathize with the patient.

There is a significant difference between active and passive listening.

Effective listening requires eye-to-eye contact between the physician and patient. Whether a physician stands or sits while talking to the patient is extremely important. If the physician is standing, eye-to-eye contact is impossible. Patients, furthermore, perceive a significant difference in the amount of time spent by the physician depending on whether he or she stands or sits. Listening as a skill is something that should not be left to other health care professionals (although it is obviously just as important for you as well); it is something that family physicians must learn how to do well.

9. C. The most appropriate response in this case is for the physician to listen to the patient's concerns, empathize with the concerns, and attempt to reassure the patient that her husband will likely come out of this operation very well, with the significant opportunity for a disease-free remission.

Telling the patient to talk to the surgeon or falsely reassuring the patient that the surgeon will make sure nothing goes wrong (that is, a guarantee of a problem-free result) is dangerous.

10. B. The patient whose physician sat down at the bedside and explained the procedure will almost certainly feel that her physician spent more time with her than the patient whose physician stood by the head of the bed. This actually has been tested; physicians who sat down when they talked to patients were perceived to have spent twice as long with their patients than physicians who stood by the head of the bed, even though the actual times were exactly the same.

SOLUTION TO SHORT ANSWER MANAGEMENT PROBLEM 82

Listening begins with hearing and ends with understanding. Active listening is a phrase that is used to describe two qualities: (1) listening with empathy and with support and (2) communicating to the speaker these two qualities. In empathic listening, the listener attempts to listen from the point of view of the speaker rather than from his or her own viewpoint. Listening supportively means listening openly with a view toward understanding rather than judging or evaluating. Only after you fully understand what the other person is saying should judgment or evaluation be used (if at all).

Active listening also includes hearing and understanding the feelings and emotions that accompany a message. For many listeners, this is the hardest part of listening. Many times speakers will imply (but not state) feelings. A skilled listener will be able to "hear" those implied feelings, reflect on them, and accurately interpret them.

The last step is to ask the patient to paraphrase back to you what you have just said to him/her. If the patient is able to do this with reasonable clarity and accuracy you can be assured that the patient understands the message.

SUMMARY

1. Keys of reassurance in patient–family physician relationship:

   a) The essential basis for effective reassurance is a trusting relationship between patient and doctor.

   b) If reassurance is to be specific, the physician must know what the patient's anxieties are.

   c) Premature reassurance is ineffective and may be interpreted by the patient as a rejection.

   d) When reassurance can be given with confidence, it should not be delayed.

   e) The patient's complaints—and his or her perception of them—should be taken seriously.

   f) Some hope should always be given.

   g) Emphasis should be given to the hopeful aspects of the condition.

   h) When the nature of the disease is explained, everyday language should be used, with checks to see that that patient has understood.

2. Don't interrupt the patient.

3. Remember the general adaptation syndrome linking bodily health with mental function.

4. When listening to the patient, sit down.

5. Remember the importance of leaving a message of hope with the patient.

6. Listen actively, not passively.

SUGGESTED READINGS

American Psychiatric Association. Diagnostic and statistical manual. 4th Ed. Washington, DC: American Psychiatric Association Press, 1994.

Beckman HB, Frankel RN. The effect of physician behavior on the collection of data. Annals of Internal Medicine 1984;101:692.

McWhinney I. A textbook of family medicine. Oxford: Oxford University Press, 1989.

PROBLEM 83   AN 87-YEAR-OLD FEMALE WITH A TERMINAL MALIGNANCY WHO HAS NOT BEEN INFORMED OF HER CONDITION BY HER DOCTORS

An 87-year-old female has just been diagnosed as having inoperable cancer of the colon. The biopsied lesion that was sent to pathology following a flexible sigmoidoscopy came back as "anaplastic adenocarcinoma." A liver scan confirms metastatic disease.

A nurse on the patient's unit has told the patient's daughter and son that "your mother has cancer." The daughter immediately telephones you and insists that her mother not be told. You have been the family physician to this patient for many years.

SELECT THE ONE BEST ANSWER TO THE FOLLOWING QUESTIONS

1. On the basis of the information given, what would you do?
   a) tell the daughter not to interfere; you're the boss, and you will tell the mother as soon as possible
   b) tell the daughter that this is not her decision; you'll decide how the whole affair will be settled
   c) tell the daughter quite firmly that you have every intention of telling her mother when the time is right
   d) call your lawyer
   e) none of the above

2. You are the resident in a ward where a 45-year-old female with metastatic breast cancer has just been admitted. The patient is cachectic and exhibits Cheyne-Stokes respirations upon admission. Your attending physician refuses to write a "Do Not Attempt Resuscitation Order" on the chart. Three hours after admission the patient suffers a cardiopulmonary arrest and the attending physician stops the code 45 minutes after ACLS has been instituted.

   Which of the following statements concerning this case is(are) true?
   a) this is an extremely unusual occurrence
   b) patients in the terminal phase of a malignant disease should rarely, if ever, be subjected to attempted resuscitation
   c) to not attempt resuscitation may be an ethically unacceptable decision
   d) CPR has been shown to save lives in terminal cancer patients
   e) none of the above are true

3. You are the resident in charge of a 24-year-old female who was admitted with nausea and vomiting NYD. The abdominal ultrasound you ordered shows multiple liver metastases from a primary pancreatic cancer. You call the attending physician and he instructs you to "say nothing; it's better that way." The patient questions you that evening about the results of her studies.

   At this time, what should you do?
   a) tell the patient that you know nothing
   b) tell the patient that the ultrasound machine broke
   c) tell the patient that everything will be OK

   d) tell the patient that her attending physician will break the very bad news tomorrow
   e) none of the above

4. You are just completing your plastic surgery rotation. On the last day the results of skin lesion biopsy on a 27-year-old female came back as "malignant melanoma—Clark's level IV." You also note that the patient's liver function tests are grossly elevated and conclude that she most likely already has significant metastatic disease.

   You are with the attending surgeon as he sees the patient in his outpatient clinic in the afternoon. You accompany him into the room. He stands by the door flipping nervously through the chart for about 5 mintues while the patient stares at him hoping that he will eventually say something. He then looks up at the patient and says, "My dear, you have a very bad skin cancer that is probably going to kill you. It appears that it is already in your liver. If I were you I would get my affairs in order and do what you've always wanted to do as quickly as you can." You are speechless and try to console the patient after he quickly departs the room.

   With respect to this case, which of the following statements is(are) true?
   a) this situation is not real in any way; doctors just don't do those sorts of things
   b) the remarks of the doctor described are a reflection of the lack of training physicians receive in dealing with this type of scenario
   c) this situation is more common than we either admit or believe
   d) these remarks are not in any way unethical
   e) physicians are well trained in breaking bad news; something is very wrong in this circumstance

5. You have just established a family practice in the suburban area of a large city. One of your first patients is an 18-year-old girl who presents for a pregnancy test. The test is positive. When you present this result to the patient she bursts into tears and requests an abortion. You have very strong feelings against abortion and are planning on becoming actively involved in your local pro-life chapter.

   Based on this information, and assuming you hold the views stated above, what should you do?

a) tell the patient to leave your office; you are completely opposed to her request

b) ask the patient to find another doctor as quickly as she can; you can have nothing more to do with her care

c) discuss the three options that the patient has: carrying through with the pregnancy and keeping the baby, carrying through with the pregnancy and giving the baby up for adoption, and therapeutic abortion; refer her for counseling and ask her to see you again following that counseling

d) tell the patient that your religious beliefs preclude further discussion of the matter

e) none of the above

6. A male infant born at 26 weeks' gestation has been monitored in the ICU for the last 8 weeks. Unfortunately, the infant suffers a severe intraventricular hemorrhage, and the EEG demonstrates no electrical activity. The infant is thought to be essentially "brain dead." When you, the attending physician, ask the parents for permission to consider discontinuing life support systems, you are accused of "just trying to get rid of our son to save money." The parents inform you that you will hear from their lawyer shortly.

At this time, what would you do?

a) call your own lawyer

b) express your displeasure at this "attitude" directly to the parents

c) disconnect the life-support system anyway

d) arrange a family conference with significant support people for the parents present

e) continue the life-support system and promise yourself that you will not bring up the subject again

7. The right of the patient to express his or her desire for treatment following serious unforeseen complications arising out of a hospitalization is referred to as which of the following?

a) The Patient Self-Determination Act

b) The Desire to Live Act

c) The Patient Emancipation Act

d) The Patient Self-Care Act

e) The Medical Profession Obligation Act

8. The term *advance directive* includes or is best described as which of the following?

a) the legal instrument entitled "Directive to Physicians" in the Natural Death Acts enacted by various states

b) the less formal living will

c) the durable power of attorney

d) all of the above

e) none of the above

9. In the case analysis method of ethical decision making, which of the following categories must be considered?

a) indications for medical intervention

b) preferences of patients

c) quality of life

d) contextual features

e) all of the above

10. In the case analysis method of ethical decision making, the category "Indications for Medical Intervention" include which of the following?

a) the concept of beneficence

b) the concept of nonmaleficence

c) the concept of clinical judgment

d) the concept of realistic understanding of the goals of treatment

e) all of the above

11. In the case analysis method of ethical decision making, the category "Preferences of Patients" includes which of the following?

a) the concept of paternalism

b) the concept of informed consent

c) the concept of medical capacity

d) all of the above

e) none of the above

12. In the case analysis method of ethical decision making, the category "Quality of Life" includes which of the following?

a) the concept of life-supporting interventions

b) the concept of euthanasia

c) the concept of physician-assisted suicide

d) the concept of pain relief

e) all of the above

13. In the case analysis method of ethical decision making, the category "Contextual Features" includes which of the following?

a) the concept of ethical problems and public policies

b) the concept of family, friends, and relatives

c) the concept of the economics of care

d) the concept of managed care plans

e) all of the above

Short Answer Management Problem 83

Using the case analysis approach to ethical decision making, consider the following case and attempt to arrive at an ethical solution:

A 71-year-old female with advanced ovarian cancer that is rapidly progressing, to the point where the patient is extremely cachectic, taking almost nothing by mouth, and beginning to exhibit Cheyne-Stokes respiration, is in the hospital under your care. Her daughter comes to you and confronts you with the following statement: "Doctor, you are under no circumstances to offer my mother anything less than an all-out resuscitative effort in the event that she arrests while undergoing treatment in this hospital."

ANSWERS

1. E. The best response to this kind of request from a member of the patient's immediate family is to ask to meet with the family as soon as possible. At that time you should gently point out the following:
   a) Most patients who have a terminal disease know they have one; to refuse to discuss the patient's condition with the patient is in no one's best interest and in fact violates the Medical Code of Ethics.
   b) Ask the family to be present when you discuss the results of the tests with the patient. Reassure the daughter and the rest of the family that one of the first questions you will ask of the patient is "How much do you know about your disease?" to be followed shortly by "Are you the kind of person who wants to know everything, or are you the kind of person who would rather just leave everything up to us?"

   In most cases a response as described from a member of the immediate family indicates that there is some "unfinished business" that the family would rather not discuss. It is in everyone's best interest for this to be allowed to surface.

2. B. Patients in the terminal phase of a malignant disease should rarely, if ever, be subjected to a CPR attempt. It has been clearly documented in a well-designed scientific study that no patient who arrested from a terminal malignant disease has ever been successfully resuscitated with BLS and ACLS protocols.

3. E. The patient has every right to ask about her results, and you have an ethical responsibility to provide her with as much information as she requests and can handle emotionally. The best plan in the case described is a call to the attending physician to let him know that the patient has "specifically asked you about the results." If the attending physician refuses to discuss the results the next day, you may have to take this to a higher level. Your best approach in this case is a telephone call to the chairman of your local hospital ethics committee for advice and action.

4. C. This type of situation and the remarks associated with it are a lot more common than we admit or believe. This situation can be neither accepted nor condoned. It is at least partially attributable to the physician's lack of training in breaking bad news. That, however, is not the entire picture. It is an example of a complete lack of compassion and understanding on the part of the attending physician. It is both unacceptable and unethical.

5. C. This patient has come to you as a patient because of the fiduciary doctor-patient relationship, and you have a responsibility to discuss her options with her. In this case, referral for counseling would be very appropriate and, depending on her subsequent decision, will allow you to decide how much personal involvement you wish to have. You must, however, separate your personal beliefs from your responsibilities as a physician. Even in cases in which ethical dilemmas are prominent, you can usually provide the medical care necessary for your patient's well-being and at the same time not sacrifice your personal beliefs and convictions.

6. D. The response of the parents to this request is quite typical and common. First, the parents have certainly not completed their grief work (especially if hope for a good outcome was put forward to them). Second, they may well have been exposed to the criticism of their son "taking up valuable resources" potentially usable for an infant with a better prognosis by some overt or inadvertent comment. Third, parents may misinterpret something that you said or the manner which it was said.

   A family conference with significant support available for the parents is the preferred method for resolving this situation. Time will be a key that will enable the parents to see the logic of your arguments as well as the nature and reasons for your suggestions. It is important to recognize anticipatory grieving in situations like this. Anticipatory grieving is grieving that takes place before the actual death. It is important to recognize that this may "blunt" the response of the parents at the time of the death itself.

7. A. Legislation written and passed by the United States Congress requires that patients be informed of their right to decide on life-supporting treatment in the event of a catastrophic complication resulting from hospitalization. This is known as the Patient Self-Determination Act.

8. D. In recent years the concept of "advance directives" has emerged and has been widely promoted as a solution to the dilemma expressed by patients concerning their potential inability to make crucial decisions about their medical care when they become important. The general term *advance directive* covers the following:
   a) The legal instrument entitled "Directive to Physicians" enacted in the Natural Death Acts of various states in the union
   b) The less formal "living will"
   c) The Durable Power of Attorney for Health Care

9. E. Clinical ethics are an intrinsic aspect of medical practice. Like diagnosis, prognosis, and treatment, ethical considerations are essential in clinical care issues. The ethics of any particular case arise out of both the facts and the values embedded in the case itself. This is most easily accomplished by dividing the considerations of the case into four categories:
   a) Medical indications for interventions and treatment
   b) Patient preferences (also referred to as patient autonomy)
   c) Quality-of-life issues
   d) Contextual features
   Details of these categories are considered later in this chapter.

10. E. Indications for medical intervention include the following:
    a) *Beneficence:* the duty to assist patients in need
    b) *Nonmaleficence:* the duty to "first do no harm"
    c) *Clinical judgment:* judgment regarding the purely "clinical facts" of the case. Recognize that clinical judgments are made considering a matrix of facts and values that are susceptible to the influence of negative attitudes. Clinical judgments also reflect tacit inclinations about risk avoidance, skepticism about intervention, enthusiasm for innovation, peer esteem, and other personal values.
    d) *Realistic understanding of the goals of treatment:* what exactly are you attempting to accomplish, and why are you trying to accomplish it?
    e) *Medical futility:* a desire to define when a proposed treatment is, in fact, useless
    f) *The moribund patient:* best defined as "eminent death"
    g) *The terminally ill patient:* most commonly the considerations concerning palliative treatment in a patient with cancer or other irreversible disorder
    h) *Medical indications and contraindications for the performance of CPR*

11. D. Patient preferences and patient autonomy must, by their very nature, include analysis and synthesis of the following concepts:
    a) *Paternalism:* overriding or ignoring a person's preferences when you believe it will benefit them or enhance their welfare
    b) *Informed consent:* informed consent is defined as the willing acceptance of a medical intervention by a patient after adequate disclosure by the physician of the nature of the intervention. Disclosure is judged "adequate" by two standards: (1) information that is commonly provided by competent practitioners in the community or in the specialty, and (2) information that would allow a reasonable person to make prudent choices on their own behalf.
    c) *Mental capacity:* the ability to understand, on the basis of intelligence and comprehension, what is being said or asked of a patient on the part of that patient
    d) *Refusal of treatment:* reasons for refusal of same
    e) *Advance directives/living wills* (discussed earlier)

12. E. Quality of life can best be defined as the subjective satisfaction expressed or experienced by an individual in his or her physical, mental, and social situation.
    Quality-of-life considerations include the following:
    a) The distinction between *quality of life* (as just defined) and *sanctity of life* (the concept that human life is so valuable that it must be preserved at all costs, under any conditions, and for as long as possible)
    b) Subjective versus objective considerations in quality of life: who is defining *quality* in this case, and how does your (or someone else's) definition compare with the definition given by the patient? As well, how does a subjective determination of quality of life compare to objective criteria? These objective criteria include consideration of "restricted quality of life" and "minimal quality of life."
    c) Mental retardation: who defines *quality* here?
    d) Issues concerning nutrition and hydration
    e) Euthanasia with all its implications and definitions (active, passive, physician-assisted suicide, and so on)
    f) Pain and symptom relief (especially in terminal cancer)
    g) Suicide

13. E. Contextual features in ethical decision making are diverse, complicated, and multiple. The most important considerations include the following:
    a) The possible conflict between physician responsibilities to the patient and physician responsibilities to the society. This is most clearly articulated in matters concerning cost.
    b) The multiple responsibilities of physicians and methods of resolving how to resolve conflict between those responsibilities. The responsibility to the patient (first and foremost); the responsibility to

society; the responsibility to other health professionals; and the responsibility to self.

c) The role of the patient's next of kin in ethical decision making

d) The importance of confidentiality of patient information

e) The importance of the public welfare; that is, is the patient a danger to others? If so, how can those "others" be identified without revealing confidential information?

f) The concept of patient safety

g) The economics of care, including ever-decreasing health care resources, health care right versus privilege, emergency care, prospective payments and diagnostic related groups, and managed care plans.

The term *contextual features* is also known as *distributive justice*.

SOLUTION TO SHORT ANSWER MANAGEMENT PROBLEM 83

1. **Indications for medical intervention:**
   • Very serious and aggressive tumor
   • Advanced state of cachexia at present
   • No likelihood that patient will improve
   • Symptoms objectively distressing
   Conclusion to indications for medical intervention issue:
   a) Very reasonable to offer interventions that will increase the comfort and reduce the pain and suffering of the patient
   b) Illogical to offer interventions that will in the long run only prolong death, not life

2. **Patient preferences:**
   • The patient has not been consulted as to her wishes vis-á-vis life-support systems.
   • We have no indication that the wishes of the patient's daughter bear any relationship to the wishes of the patient.
   Conclusion to patient preference issue:
   a) The patient must, in some manner, be asked about her understanding regarding the disease process and wishes that stem from that knowledge.

3. **Quality of life:**
   • Objectively, her quality of life appears to be low and decreasing daily.
   • Again, however, we have no knowledge of how the patient rates her own quality of life.
   Conclusion to quality-of-life issue:
   a) A discussion with the patient must take place. The information that should be discussed includes the patient's knowledge of the condition and its progress, her own assessment of quality of life, and her wishes concerning treatments that are and are not acceptable.

4. **Contextual features:**
   • The main contextual feature is the insistence of the daughter to "pull out all the stops" and "spare no effort—no matter what."
   • No idea as to why the daughter feels this way: is there some unfinished business?
   Conclusion regarding contextual features issue:
   • Talk to the daughter; ask her why she has requested the aggressive interventions.
   • Discuss with the daughter the concept of "medical futility."

SUMMARY OF CASE

This is basically an ethical situation in which the concept of indications for medical intervention indicates that aggressive resuscitative attempts are not only not indicated but completely futile. This is counterbalanced by the concept of contextual features, in which the daughter is insisting that "everything be done."

What is done will be determined by patient preferences, in which the patient outlines to all not only her knowledge of the disease process and its effect on her quality of life but her desires for "heroic measures" to be or not to be undertaken on her behalf.

SUMMARY OF ETHICAL DECISION MAKING

1. Ethical decision making can be based on a case analysis method.

2. Case analysis considers four categories:
   a) Indications for medical intervention
   b) Patient preferences
   c) Quality of life
   d) Contextual (or societal) features

3. The most common disagreements involve indications for intervention; patient preferences; and quality-of-life disagreement between individual patient values or autonomy, indications or lack of same for treatment, and one or another of various societal pressures.

4. Golden Rule 1 of Medical Ethics: *Primum non nocere*—first, do no harm (nonmaleficence).

5. Golden Rule 2 of Medical Ethics: Consider first the welfare of the patient (beneficence)

6. Medical futility: a treatment that has no or an extremely remote chance of doing any good whatsoever should not be undertaken. For purposes of security, that really should mean zero chance (as with CPR in a terminal cancer patient with Cheyne-Stokes respiration).

7. There is absolutely no substitute for good doctor-patient communication and good interprofessional health care communication in biomedical ethics.

SUGGESTED READINGS

American Psychiatric Association. Diagnostic and statistical manual. 4th Ed. Washington, DC: American Psychiatric Association Press, 1994.

Jonsen AR, Siegler M, Winslade WJ. Clinical ethics. 3rd Ed. New York: McGraw-Hill, 1992.

PROBLEM 84   A FAMILY MEDICINE RESIDENT WHO IS RESPONSIBLE FOR MONTHLY GRAND ROUNDS AND WHO HAS NOT PREPARED GRAND ROUNDS BEFORE

A family medicine resident who is a resident in your practice tells you upon his arrival one day that he is responsible for grand rounds next week. Although he has selected the topic (the irritable bowel syndrome) he has not presented grand rounds before. He comes to you seeking advice on the "do's and the dont's" of making an effective grand rounds presentation. He knows that this is very important and is concerned that the undergraduate and postgraduate curriculums have not adequately prepared him for this challenge.

You have considerable experience in medical presentation skills and agree to give him a "whirlwind tutorial."

SELECT THE ONE BEST ANSWER TO THE FOLLOWING QUESTIONS

1. The "typical" presentation of rounds at any hospital or other educational forum usually takes which of the following formats?
   a) a format consisting of an excessive number of slides or overheads in an attempt to cover the maximum amount of material in the minimum amount of time
   b) a format in which active involvement of the audience is the rule
   c) a format in which the audience is pretested prior to the presentation beginning
   d) a format in which the lecturer attempts to make four to six major points and leaves it at that
   e) a format in which there is usually a significant amount of time remaining at the end for questions and discussion

2. What is the average adult attention span?
   a) 120 minutes
   b) 90 minutes
   c) 60 minutes
   d) 40 minutes
   e) 20 minutes

3. Regarding AV aids (including 35-mm slides and overhead transparencies), which of the following statements is true?
   a) the amount of information that a slide or overhead should contain is a matter of personal preference
   b) the ideal slide or overhead follows "the 6 × 6 rule"
   c) slides or overheads should form the bulk of an effective medical presentation
   d) a light-green background with dull pink lettering makes an ideal color contrast
   e) overheads are preferable to slides in medical presentations

4. Which of the following statements are true regarding audience participation in your lecture, seminar, or grand round?
   a) audience participation is really a waste of time and energy; most people would rather just sit and listen
   b) audience participation is best facilitated by the process of asking questions
   c) audience participation is very difficult when a large group is involved
   d) audience participation does not increase the probability of audience learning
   e) audience participation is rarely indicated in a professional and mature setting

5. What is the maximum number of significant points or highlights that can be covered in any medical presentation?
   a) 10-12
   b) 7-9
   c) 4-6
   d) 3-5
   e) 1-2

6. *Teaching* is best defined as which of the following?
   a) the transfer of information from one person to another
   b) the transfer of information from teacher to student
   c) the transfer of information in a highly structured manner
   d) helping students learn
   e) providing the necessary raw material that can be expanded by the student in the format of self-study

7. *Learning* is best defined as which of the following?
   a) the transfer of information from one person to another
   b) the reception of information by the student
   c) behavior change
   d) memorization to the point where everything can be successfully regurgitated three times in a row with less than a 10% error rate
   e) none of the above

8. A practicing family physician attends a CME event. He will maximize his or her learning if which of the following conditions is fulfilled?
   a) the information of note is presented in didactic format
   b) the information of note is presented in lecture format
   c) the information of note is presented in theoretical constructs
   d) the information of note is presented in problem-based, case-history-based format
   e) the information of note is presented in a strictly question-and-answer format

9. A family medicine resident prepares her grand round for the following day. Regarding the time she estimates the presentation will take, which of the following is true?
   a) she is likely to underestimate the actual presentation time
   b) she is likely to overestimate the actual presentation time
   c) she is likely to be very close to the true presentation time
   d) the actual presentation time bears no relationship to the rehearsed presentation time
   e) none of the above are true

10. Which of the following CME events or formats is likely to provide the maximum potential for learning?
    a) large-group didactic lecture at a 3-day CME refresher course
    b) small-group problem-based, case-based, discussion
    c) large-group lecture with accompanying prelecture quiz and post-lecture quiz
    d) large-group demonstration of a new technique or skill
    e) reading the four most popular medical journals from cover to cover

Short Answer Management Problem 84

PART A: Discuss the major headings you would use to organize a grand round in family medicine. These headings should cover the presentation from beginning to end.

PART B: Describe the major characteristics that would maximize the learning of attendees at a grand round that you present.

PART C: Feedback is an extremely important component of medical education. It allows the teacher to highlight the performance of the student in any given area. Feedback is useful across the continuum of medical education, from undergraduate education to postgraduate education to continuing medical education. Discuss briefly how you would give feedback to a medical student on a patient problem that he or she just presented to you.

ANSWERS

1. A. Although this is not the recommended format for the presentation of grand rounds or any other teaching session, it is certainly the most common. The presenter feels, above all else, that he has to "cover the subject." Thus begins a presentation dominated by AV aids (most often ineffective) lasting anywhere from 40 to 60 minutes. Usually the presenter has to "rush to complete the talk." Obviously, no time for questions or discussion remains.

   At the end of the presentation, the most likely comment that the presenter receives is, "That was a very complete presentation." Although this is true, the more important and always unasked question is, "Has the audience learned anything?"

   The skill of giving an effective medical presentation or seminar is as important as (if not more important than) any other skill learned in undergraduate or postgraduate education. Unfortunately, it is seldom taught. The other choices listed in the question will be discussed at later points in this chapter.

2. E. The average adult attention span is 20 minutes. Thus, in any medical presentation, the presenter must ensure that no more than 20 minutes is spent in any one format (for example, no more than 20 minutes is spent lectur-

ing). If the presentation needs to be longer than 20 minutes, it is extremely important to switch methods (for example, a switch from lecturing to asking questions or asking the audience to participate in some other way).

3. B. The 6 × 6 rule states that "no slide or overhead transparency should have more than six words/line, and no slide or overhead transparency should have more than six lines/slide."

   The single biggest mistake made is that too much information is put onto the slide or overhead transparency. In many cases, because of the amount of information contained on the slide or overhead, nothing at all can be read by those individuals unfortunate enough to be at the back of the room.

4. B. Audience participation is crucial to audience retention and audience learning. This is a basic tenet of adult education. Audience participation increases audience attention, increases the active processing of information, and increases the probability of learning.

   The active participation of the audience is best facilitated by questioning. If the audience is questioned in a manner that allows them to relate the question to a practical problem or situation, then the probability of learning will increase.

5. C. The maximum number of significant points or highlights that can be covered in any medical presentation is four to six.

An earlier question discussed the common problem of trying to "cover the subject" in any medical grand round, medical presentation, or medical seminar. The relationship between the presenter's attempting to cover the subject and the attendee's ability to retain only a very limited amount of information is obvious.

6. D. Teaching is best defined as helping students learn. The word *doctor* is derived from the Latin word *doktor,* meaning "teacher." All physicians teach, and in many more ways than they realize. Every doctor-patient encounter involves an element of physician teaching. As well, in addition to medical students, residents, and their fellow physicians, doctors often teach nurses, pharmacists, and other health care professionals.

Upon entry to medical school, physicians embark on a lifelong commitment to learning. The vast majority of learning occurs once a physician has left medical school and residency. Thus one of the goals of medical school and residency must be to prepare physicians to become lifelong, self-directed learners.

7. C. Learning is best defined as behavior change. In other words, after the educational event, the student can do something that he or she could not do before.

There is no association between learning and memorization. All too often, unfortunately, the principle applied at both undergraduate and graduate classes in universities is that of providing the student with incredible amounts of material in excruciating detail, most of which must be memorized to successfully complete the course. Both university teachers and students fail to understand that this in no way defines, relates to, or has any connection to the true concepts of teaching and learning.

8. D. Practicing physicians learn best when the information they are presented with is given in a problem-based, case-history format. In other words, practicing physicians learn best if they can relate what is taught to something or someone in their practice. This is best accomplished by the problem-based, case-history type of approach. Although a question-and-answer format has potential to accomplish the same end, it also runs the risk of being less structured and more prone to a loss of focus or a loss of track.

9. A. Most likely, the presenter will underestimate the amount of time his or her presentation will take. The usual percentage of underestimation is 25%-33%. It is very important, therefore, that the presentation be rehearsed prior to being formally presented. The underestimation of time may be increased by the selection and placing of material (for example, on the overhead projector) and movement of the speaker around the front of the lecture hall.

10. B. Although there is very significant variation from individual family physician to family physician, the CME format most likely to maximize learning is the problem-based, case-based approach where learning is directly related to the real and perceived learning needs of the physicians.

Caveats to this, however, are the recognition that multiple learning events need to take place before a knowledge-based concept, skill, or attitude is incorporated into the practice of a physician; and physicians (and all adults) learn in different ways. This latter point provides support for maintaining group didactic seminars and refresher courses.

Pretest quizzes are helpful in stimulating the audience and establishing a baseline knowledge base. Posttest quizzes summarize and reinforce what has already been learned. Pretests and posttests can be used in both small groups and large groups.

Journal reading remains an important form of CME. There is a real question, however, of the value of reading a journal from cover to cover. Journal reading is also most helpful when linked directly to a patient problem.

Consider the following approach as one highly effective means of maximizing the ability of your CME event to improve the quality of patient care (the ultimate goal): identify an important (to you) patient-based problem; complete a literature search on that problem; read the three or four most recent articles that highlight areas of interest that are associated with your patient's problem; find an appropriate CME refresher course that focuses on your problem; and consolidate your understanding of the pertinent information through discussions with colleagues.

SOLUTION TO SHORT ANSWER MANAGEMENT PROBLEM 84

PART A: The major headings to be used in organizing an effective grand rounds are as follows:
1) Opening set—why the members of the audience should be sitting here listening to you instead of doing something else
2) Objectives—stating the objectives for the session are extremely important. The objectives should be stated as "You are going to learn" statements rather than "I am going to teach" statements.
3) Main body of educational session—the main body of the presentation follows.

Remember that the entire presentation should probably not exceed 30 minutes; as a general rule, one-half of your time should be spent in discussion.
4) Summary—the four to six major points of the presentation should be repeated here.

It is often wise to have the audience summarize these points for you. This will prove that they have in fact learned the material.

5) Conclusion—the "punch line"; what is the most important thing that the audience should take away from this presentation?

PART B: The major characteristics that would increase learning in a grand round that you present in your department of family medicine would be the following:

1) Limit the didactic presentation to 20 minutes.
2) Introduce questioning as a means of changing a passive lecture to an active discussion group.
3) Pretest your audience to assess the baseline level of knowledge.
4) Use a posttest to summarize the four to six most important points of the lecture (or ask your audience to do it for you).
5) Follow the major headings outlined in Part A of the Short Answer Management Problem in constructing your lecture.
6) Remember the 6 × 6 rule in using overheads or transparencies.
7) Remember that the purpose of a round or seminar is not to cover the subject; that is what books and journals are for.
8) Remember that the number-one characteristic of "gold-star" teachers is enthusiasm!
9) Get out from behind the podium—podiums are a barrier between you and your audience.
10) Maintain eye contact with your audience, not with the overhead or slide.

PART C: If, as a family medicine resident, you were asked to give feedback to a medical student following the presentation of a clinical problem, consider the following steps:

1) Obtain a commitment from the student: what does he or she think is going on with this patient?
2) Probe for supporting evidence: what led to his or her diagnosis or decision?
3) Teach general rules: rather than teaching specific details, teach general rules that the student may apply to other situations.

4) Reinforce what was done right: always tell the student what he or she did well before offering suggestions for corrections or mistakes.
5) Correct mistakes: always correct mistakes only after you have given the positive feedback.

SUMMARY

1. Remember the origin of the word *doctor*—"teacher."
2. Follow an established pattern for the delivery of any lecture, seminar, or other presentation. Remember that teaching is an art. Remember the three most important words in successful teaching: delivery, delivery, delivery!
3. Minimize passive learning; maximize active learning.
4. Remember that the maximum attention span of an adult audience is 20 minutes.
5. Remember the 6 × 6 rule in constructing overheads or slides.
6. Remember the definitions of teaching and learning.
7. Remember that learning only begins in medical school and residency; the most important function of a medical school is to make students lifelong learners.
8. Continuing medical education is maximized by a small group, problem-based, case-history-based format.

SUGGESTED READINGS

American Psychiatric Association. Diagnostic and statistical manual. 4th Ed. Washington, DC: American Psychiatric Association Press, 1994.

Manning P, Debakey L. Medicine: Preserving the passion. New York: Springer-Verlag, 1987.

Neber J et al. A five-step microskills model of clinical teaching. Journal of the American Board of Family Practice 1992; 5:419-424.

Newble D, Cannon R. A handbook for medical teachers. 2nd Ed. Lancaster/Boston/The Hague, Dordrecht: MTP Press Limited, 1987.

Pediatrics and Adolescent Medicine

PROBLEM 85   A FULL-TERM NEONATE WITH JAUNDICE

A 3750-g male infant was delivered by you at 40 3/7 weeks' gestation. The prenatal course was unremarkable. The mother's blood type is group A:Rh positive. The neonate's blood type is the same. At approximately 36 hours of age the neonate begins to develop visible jaundice. The baby is being breast-fed and is feeding well, approximately every 2 hours. The baby's hemoglobin is 175 grams/l. His total bilirubin is 171 μmol/L (10 mg/dL) and his indirect bilirubin is 154 μmol/L (9 mg/dL). His direct and his indirect Coombs' tests are negative.

On physical examination the infant looks healthy and happy. There is no lethargy, no difficulties with feeding, and no significant abnormalities apart from the yellow color of his skin and the whites of his eyes. There is no organomegaly.

SELECT THE ONE BEST ANSWER TO THE FOLLOWING QUESTIONS

1. What is the most likely diagnosis in this infant?
   a) undiagnosed neonatal sepsis
   b) breast milk jaundice
   c) normal physiologic jaundice
   d) jaundice due to a minor antigen blood group incompatibility
   e) ABO blood group incompatibility

2. Which of the following characteristics would suggest that the diagnosis established in Question 1 is incorrect?
   a) jaundice beginning in the first 24 hours of life
   b) there is an increase in the serum bilirubin level of greater than 86 μmol/L (5 mg/dL)
   c) the total serum bilirubin exceeds 256 μmol/L (15 mg/dL) at any time
   d) all of the above suggest that the correct diagnosis in Question 1 is, in fact, incorrect
   e) none of the above suggest that the diagnosis in Question 1 is, in fact, incorrect

3. Which of the following causes of jaundice is the least common cause of jaundice in the newborn?
   a) ABO mother-neonate blood group incompatibility
   b) neonatal sepsis
   c) physiologic jaundice
   d) breast milk jaundice
   e) a and b are equally unlikely causes of jaundice in the newborn

4. What is the treatment of choice for the neonate described in Question 1?
   a) grab the neonate from his mother and immediately transfer him to the nearest NICU for emergency exchange transfusions; this is a serious medical situation, and we have no time for this biopsychosocial

stuff and explanations to the parents as to what is going on
   b) intensive phototherapy; this neonate has to be "zapped with UV light right away"
   c) grab the infant from the mother, tell the mother that "breast feeding is out," and take the baby to make sure that she doesn't disobey your orders
   d) gently explain to the mother the need for stopping breast feeding; however, let the infant have "one more feed"
   e) none of the above

5. What is the major pathophysiologic basis for normal physiologic jaundice in the newborn?
   a) glucuronyl transferase deficiency (immaturity basis) in the liver
   b) the breakdown of fetal red blood cells into bilirubin and bilirubin metabolites
   c) gamma glutamyl transferase deficiency (immaturity basis) in the liver
   d) dehydration due to lack of sufficient fluid intake in the first 48 hours of life
   e) none of the above

6. What is the pathophysiologic basis for differentiation of normal physiologic jaundice and exaggerated physiologic jaundice in the newborn?
   a) breakdown of fetal red blood cells into bilirubin plus transient limitation in the conjugation of bilirubin (physiologic jaundice) versus glucuronyl transferase deficiency (immaturity basis) in the liver (exaggerated physiologic jaundice)
   b) the breakdown of fetal red blood cells into bilirubin and bilirubin metabolites
   c) gamma glutamyl transferase deficiency (immaturity basis) in the liver
   d) dehydration due to lack of sufficient fluid intake in the first 48 hours of life
   e) none of the above

7. Which of the following is(are) associated with exaggerated physiologic jaundice in the newborn?
   a) prematurity
   b) Oriental race
   c) Caucasian race
   d) a and b
   e) a and c

8. A full-term infant weighing 3640 g develops jaundice on the fourth day of life. He is being breast-fed and is feeding extremely well (every 2 hours).

   On examination, the child is not lethargic, his temperature is normal, and he is not irritable, nor does he have any other signs or symptoms that would suggest significant disease.

   The mother is blood group A: Rh factor positive. The baby is blood group A: Rh factor positive as well. The infant's hemoglobin is 160 g/L. The direct and indirect Coombs' tests are negative.

   The total serum bilirubin is 256 μmol/L (15 mg/dl). The indirect serum bilirubin is 242 μmol/L (14.15 mg/dL).

   What is the most likely diagnosis in this neonate?
   a) undiagnosed and unsuspected neonatal sepsis
   b) breast milk jaundice
   c) physiologic jaundice
   d) jaundice due to minor antigen blood group incompatibility
   e) exaggerated physiologic jaundice

9. What is the treatment of choice for the neonate described?
   a) phototherapy
   b) exchange transfusions
   c) withdrawal of breast feeding for 2 to 4 days
   d) supplementation of breast feeding with DSW
   e) none of the above

10. A 2900-g infant born at term develops jaundice at approximately 18 hours of life. The infant appears generally well, is not lethargic, and is breast-feeding well. Vital signs are normal, and examination of all systems reveals no abnormalities.

    The infant's bilirubin at 24 hours is 220 μmol/L (12.9 mg/dl). The direct bilirubin is 205 μmol/L (12 mg/dl). The neonate is blood group B: Rh positive. The mother is blood group O: Rh positive. The neonate's hemoglobin is 135 g/L, and the reticulocyte count is 10%.

    What is the most likely cause of jaundice in this neonate?
    a) neonatal sepsis
    b) breast milk jaundice
    c) physiologic jaundice
    d) jaundice due to minor antigen blood group incompatibility
    e) ABO blood group incompatibility

11. What is the treatment of choice for the neonate described in Question 10?
    a) phototherapy
    b) exchange transfusion
    c) withdrawal of breast feeding for 2 to 4 days
    d) supplementation of breast feeding with DSW
    e) none of the above

12. When is blood group ABO incompatibility in the neonate most common?
    a) when the mother is blood group O and the infant is blood group O
    b) when the mother is blood group A and the infant is blood group A
    c) when the mother is blood group O and the infant is blood group A or blood group B
    d) when the mother is blood group A and the infant is blood group B
    e) it doesn't really matter; this ABO business has been overdone

13. Jaundice develops in approximately what percentage of full-term neonates?
    a) 20%
    b) 40%
    c) 60%
    d) 80%
    e) 95%

14. Which of the following statements most accurately reflects the association between physiologic jaundice and kernicterus?
    a) kernicterus is a serious problem and can result from failure to treat physiologic jaundice in the newborn with phototherapy
    b) kernicterus is a serious problem and can result from failure to treat exaggerated physiologic jaundice in the newborn with phototherapy
    c) kernicterus is a serious problem and can result from failure to treat breast milk jaundice in the newborn with phototherapy
    d) all of the above are true
    e) none of the above are true

15. What is the mechanism of action of phototherapy in treating neonatal jaundice?
    a) hemolysis of the fetal red blood cells remaining in the circulation
    b) hemolysis of the fetal hemoglobin F blood cells remaining in the circulation
    c) increase in the activity of the liver enzyme *glucuronyl transferase*
    d) increase in the activity of the liver enzyme *gamma glutamyl transferase*
    e) none of the above

16. Which of the following is(are) associated with breast milk jaundice?
    a) a qualitative deficiency in gamma glutamyl transferase in the neonatal liver
    b) a qualitative deficiency in glucuronyl transferase in the neonatal liver
    c) a nonesterified long-chain fatty acid(s) containing 3-alpha-20-beta-diol in the breast milk of the mother
    d) all of the above
    e) none of the above

17. Neonatal jaundice that appears after what day of neonatal life should suggest the possibility of neonatal sepsis?
    a) the fifth day
    b) the second day
    c) the third day
    d) the eighth day
    e) the tenth day

18. With respect to breast-fed neonates and bottle-fed neonates, which of the following statements is(are) true?
    a) neonatal jaundice is more common in bottle-fed babies
    b) neonatal jaundice is more common in breast-fed babies

    c) supplementation of breast-fed babies with DSW will reduce the serum bilirubin level
    d) a and c
    e) b and c

19. Which of the following statements best explains the bronze baby syndrome?
    a) the bronze baby syndrome is associated with Oriental babies whose mothers breast-feed and do not supplement feedings with DSW
    b) the bronze baby syndrome is associated with Oriental babies whose mothers breast-feed and supplement feedings with DSW
    c) the bronze baby syndrome is associated with Caucasian babies whose mothers breast-feed and do not supplement feedings with DSW
    d) the bronze baby syndrome is associated with Caucasian babies whose mothers breast-feed and supplement feedings with DSW
    e) none of the above

20. What is the lowest level at which kernicterus has been seen to develop in uncomplicated neonates?
    a) 10 mg/dL (171 μmol/L)
    b) 20 mg/dL (342 μmol/L)
    c) 30 mg/dL (511 μmol/L)
    d) 40 mg/dL (684 μmol/L)
    e) nobody really knows for sure

Short Answer Management Problem 85

PART A: Discuss the current recommended guidelines for the use of phototherapy in the treatment of jaundice in the newborn.

PART B: List five complications of phototherapy in the treatment of neonatal jaundice.

ANSWERS

1. C.

2. D.

3. B.

4. E.

5. B.

6. A.

7. D. The most likely cause of jaundice in the neonate described in Question 1 is physiologic jaundice. Physiologic jaundice usually begins on the second or third day of life. It is due to the breakdown of fetal red blood cells into bilirubin and transient limitation in the conjugation of bilirubin. This pathophysiologic mechanism differs from the pathophysiologic mechanism involved in exaggerated physiologic jaundice, which will be discussed later.

Physiologic jaundice would not be the explanation for this neonate's jaundice if any of the following factors were present:

1. The jaundice appears in the first 24 hours of life.
2. Serum bilirubin is rising at a rate greater than 5 mg/dl in the first 24 hours of life.
3. The serum bilirubin reaches a value of greater than 12 mg/dl in full-term infants (especially in the absence of risk factors) or 14 mg/dl in preterm infants.
4. Jaundice persists after the first week of life.

5. Direct reacting bilirubin is greater than 1 mg/dl at any time.

The differential diagnosis of neonatal jaundice (presented in order of prevalence) is as follows:

1. Normal physiologic jaundice
2. Exaggerated physiologic jaundice
3. Breast milk jaundice
4. Jaundice due to ABO incompatibility (mother/neonate)
5. Jaundice due to Rh and other blood group antigens (such as Anti-Kell or Anti-Duffy)
6. Neonatal sepsis

There may be some dispute about the order of numbers 5 and 6 on the list; the prevalence of neonatal sepsis will very much depend on the particular facilities capabilities—a high-risk neonatal nursery will have a substantially higher prevalence of neonatal sepsis.

For this neonate, no treatment should be instituted at this time. First, the levels at which phototherapy should be instituted are controversial (a guideline will be provided later on in this chapter). Second, to the best of our knowledge kernicterus has never developed in the absence of at least one other cause for jaundice.

The terms *exaggerated physiologic jaundice* and *hyperbilirubinemia of the newborn* are used for those infants whose primary pathophysiologic mechanism for hyperbilirubinemia is a deficiency in or inactivity of the enzyme bilirubin glucuronyl transferase rather than an excessive load of bilirubin for excretion.

Exaggerated physiologic jaundice is associated with the following risk factors:

1. Oriental race
2. Prematurity
3. Breast-feeding or excessive weight loss

Physiologic jaundice and exaggerated physiologic jaundice are compared in the following list:

A. Pathophysiology:
   1. Physiologic jaundice: breakdown of fetal RBCs plus transient limitation of conjugation of bilirubin
   2. Exaggerated physiologic jaundice: deficiency or inactivity of bilirubin glucuronyl transferase
B. Type of bilirubin elevated:
   1. Physiologic jaundice: indirect bilirubin
   2. Exaggerated physiologic jaundice: indirect bilirubin
C. Appearance of jaundice:
   1. Physiologic jaundice: 2-3 days of age
   2. Exaggerated physiologic jaundice: 3-4 days of age
D. Disappearance of jaundice:
   1. Physiologic jaundice: 4-5 days of age
   2. Exaggerated physiologic jaundice: 7-9 days of age
E. Peak concentration of bilirubin/age/rate of rise:
   1. Physiologic jaundice: 10-12 mg/dl at 2-3 days with < 5 mg/dl/day
   2. Exaggerated physiologic jaundice: 15 mg/dl at 6-8 days with < 5 mg/dl/day

F. Risk factors for jaundice to appear:
   1. Physiologic jaundice: no risk factors identified
   2. Exaggerated physiologic jaundice: prematurity, Oriental race, breast feeding, and weight loss

Note that there is a distinct difference between exaggerated physiologic jaundice due to breast-feeding and breast milk jaundice. The former is much more common than the latter. The two are very frequently confused.

8. B.

9. E. The most likely diagnosis in this neonate is *breast milk jaundice*. Breast milk jaundice usually begins between the fourth and the seventh days of life. Bilirubin levels range between 171 μmol/L (10 mg/dl) to 520 μmol/L (30.4 mg/dl).

If breast feeding is continued, the maximum concentration of bilirubin is reached during the third week of life and then gradually decreases (but persists) between 3 weeks and 10 weeks.

If breast feeding is discontinued, however, the serum bilirubin falls rapidly, usually reaching normal levels within a few days. Cessation of breast feeding for 2 to 4 days and substitution with formula (not glucose in water) will result in the rapid decline. Following the 2- to 4-day period, breast-feeding can be resumed; there should not be any difficulties in reestablishing breast-feeding.

As with physiologic jaundice, there are no other signs of illness in these infants and kernicterus has not been reported. There used to be a differentiation that classified breast milk jaundice into early breast milk and late breast milk jaundice. It appears that the term early breast milk jaundice (thought to be due to caloric restriction) is really part of what we now call exaggerated physiologic jaundice. Late breast milk jaundice, on the other hand, is thought to be due to the 5-beta-pregnane-3-alpha, 20-beta-diol or nonesteriferfied long-chain fatty acids that competitively inhibit the enzyme glucuronyl transferase conjugating activity.

The treatment of this neonate should consist of careful consideration as to whether or not you would suggest that the mother stop breast feeding.

The infant has a total bilirubin of 256 μmol/L (15 mg/dl). As stated earlier, bilirubin levels secondary to breast milk jaundice may reach levels as high as 520 μmol/L. Although interruption of breast feeding will definitely improve the jaundice, the risk of prematurely terminating breast feeding is theoretically present, even though it usually does not happen. Water supplementation not only does not help but actually appears to worsen breast milk jaundice.

Although phototherapy would be initiated by some clinicians at this level, it is not necessary. As well as with physiologic jaundice and exaggerated physiologic jaundice, breast milk jaundice does not lead to kernicterus.

10. E.

11. A.

12. C. This neonate's jaundice is caused by an ABO blood group incompatibility. In cases of ABO blood group incompatibility, the most likely scenario is the following:
    A. The mother is blood group O
    B. The neonate is blood group A or blood group B
       Possible ABO blood group incompatibility develops in approximately 20% to 25% of all pregnancies; however, only in 10% of these pregnancies does hemolytic disease actually develop.
       The factors suggesting ABO blood group incompatibility in this case are as follows:
    A. The "correct match-up": Mother is group O, infant is group A or group B
    B. Jaundice develops within the first 24 hours of life. Therefore, this is not physiologic jaundice, exaggerated physiologic jaundice, or breast milk jaundice.
       Also, because of the compatible Rh factors it is not Rh incompatibility.
       The only other serious consideration at this time is neonatal sepsis; there is, however, no indication that this is a serious consideration from the physical signs and symptoms.
       Pathophysiologically, maternal antibody may be formed against B cells if the mother is type A or against A cells if the mother is type B; usually, however, as mentioned, we have a mother who is type O and an infant who is type A or type B.
       The treatment of choice for this neonate is phototherapy. Even though the bilirubin has not reached a critically high level, this only represents jaundice in the first 24 hours of life; it will obviously rise without therapy. It is generally accepted that if a neonate with ABO incompatibility develops a significant hemolytic anemia, he or she should be treated with phototherapy (this has already occurred in this patient; the hemoglobin is 135 g/l and the reticulocyte count is 10%). If phototherapy is unsuccessful in keeping the serum bilirubin below 342 μmol/l (20 mg/dl), then exchange transfusions should be considered. Kernicterus can result from untreated hemolytic anemia secondary to blood group incompatibility.

13. C. Jaundice is extremely common in newborn infants. Under normal nursery conditions, jaundice is observed during the first week in approximately 60% of full-term infants and 80% of preterm infants.

14. E. Kernicterus is a neurologic syndrome resulting from the deposition of unconjugated bilirubin in the brain cells and does not occur from the following syndromes:
    A. Physiologic jaundice
    B. Exaggerated physiologic jaundice
    C. Breast milk jaundice

It is related to the following:
    A. ABO blood group incompatibility
    B. Rh blood group incompatibility
    C. Other blood group antigen (> 60) incompatibility
    D. Under conditions of prematurity: the less mature the infant, the greater susceptibility to kernicterus
    E. Associated with neonatal sepsis, perinatal hypoxia, neonatal hypoglycemia, and intracranial hemorrhage
    To the best of our knowledge, kernicterus has never resulted from a simple case of physiologic jaundice, exaggerated physiologic jaundice, or breast milk jaundice.

15. E. Clinical jaundice and indirect hyperbilirubinemia are reduced on exposure to a high intensity of light in the visible spectrum. Bilirubin absorbs light maximally in the blue range (from 420 to 470 nm). Bilirubin in the skin absorbs light energy, which by photoisomerization coverts the toxic native 4Z, 15Z-bilirubin into the unconjugated configurational isomer, 4Z, 15E-bilirubin. The latter is the product of a reversible reaction and is excreted in the bile without the need for conjugation. Phototherapy also converts native bilirubin, by an irreversible reaction, to the structural isomer, which is excreted by the kidney in the unconjugated state.
    Phototherapy is indicated only after the presence of pathologic hyperbilirubinemia has been established. The basic cause(s) of the jaundice should be treated concomitantly.

16. C. See the answers to questions 8 and 9.

17. A. Jaundice appearing after the fifth day should be highly suspect for neonatal sepsis as a cause. Causes of neonatal sepsis include the following:
    1. Neonatal pneumonia
    2. Neonatal meningitis
    3. Neonatal urinary tract infection
    4. Necrotizing enterocolitis
    5. Streptococcal/staphylococcal skin infections
    6. Herpes simplex viremia
    7. Toxoplasmosis

18. B. Neonatal jaundice is more common in breast-fed babies than in bottle-fed babies. Supplementation with DSW increases neonatal jaundice rather than decreases it. The increased incidence of neonatal jaundice in breast-fed babies is thought to be mainly due to decreased intake during the first few days and subsequent weight loss.

19. E. The bronze baby syndrome refers to a dark, grayish, brown discoloration of the skin of neonates sometimes noted in infants undergoing phototherapy. Almost all infants observed with this syndrome have had a mixed type of hyperbilirubinemia with other evidence of obstructive liver disease. The discoloration may last for months.

20. B. The precise blood level above which indirect-reacting bilirubin or free bilirubin will be toxic for an individual infant is unpredictable, but kernicterus is rare in term infants with serum levels under 20 mg/dL (342 μmol/L). The duration of exposure necessary to produce toxic effects is also unknown. There is some evidence that motor disturbances in later childhood are more common among newborn infants whose total serum bilirubin raises above 15 mg/dL. *The less mature the infant, the greater is the susceptibility to kernicterus.*

SOLUTION TO SHORT ANSWER MANAGEMENT PROBLEM 85

PART A: Guidelines for maximal permissible total serum bilirubin concentrations:

Birth Weight	Uncomplicated Course	Complicated Course
< 1250 g	13 mg/dl	10 mg/dl
1250-1499 g	15 mg/dl	13 mg/dl
1500-1999 g	17 mg/dl	15 mg/dl
2000-2499 g	18 mg/dl	17 mg/dl
> 2500 g	20 mg/dl	18 mg/dl

PART B: Complications of phototherapy: complications of phototherapy in treating jaundice in the newborn include the following:
A. Loose stools
B. Skin rashes
C. Overheating
D. Dehydration (insensible water loss, diarrhea); may be associated with electrolyte disturbances, particularly hyponatremia and hypokalemia
E. Chilling from exposure of the infant
F. The bronze baby syndrome

SUMMARY OF THE DIAGNOSIS AND MANAGEMENT OF NEONATAL JAUNDICE

1. **Prevalence:**
   a) Full-term: 60% of infants
   b) Preterm: 80% of infants
2. **Differential diagnosis of neonatal jaundice:**
   a) Physiologic jaundice (most common)
   b) Exaggerated physiologic jaundice
   c) Breast milk jaundice
   d) ABO blood group incompatibility jaundice (hemolytic)
   e) Neonatal sepsis
   f) Minor blood group antigen incompatibility and Rh disease of the newborn
3. **Pathophysiology:**
   a) Physiologic jaundice: breakdown of fetal RBCs plus transient inability to conjugate bilirubin
      Onset on second or third day; disappears by fourth or fifth day

   b) Exaggerated physiologic jaundice: a) plus a risk factor (Oriental race, prematurity, breast-feeding, or excessive neonatal weight loss)
      Onset on third or fourth day; disappears by seventh to ninth day
   c) Breast milk jaundice: mother's milk contains 5-beta-pregnane-3-alpha-20-beta-diol
      Onset between fourth and seventh day; persists for 3-10 weeks
   d) ABO incompatibility: usually arises when mother is type O and neonate is type A or type B; may appear within first 24 hours
   e) Neonatal sepsis: the infective process itself with certain associated risk factors: prematurity and hypoglycemia; suspect if neonatal jaundice appears after the fifth day
   f) Minor blood group incompatibility and Rh disease: remember that there are over 60 different blood group antigens, as well as the Rh system.
4. **Treatment:**
   a) Physiologic jaundice/exaggerated physiologic jaundice: phototherapy is usually not indicated unless bilirubin exceeds 20 mg/dl (342 μmol/L).
   b) Breast milk jaundice: phototherapy is usually not indicated unless bilirubin exceeds 20 mg/dl (342 μmol/L). Consider cessation of breast-feeding for 2-4 days.
   c) ABO incompatibility and other blood group incompatibilities: level at which phototherapy is begun is not agreed on. Suggest initiating phototherapy as soon as the diagnosis is made.
5. **Neonatal hyperbilirubinemia diagnosis and treatment:**
   a) Remember that jaundice in the newborn occurs more frequently than it does not occur.
   b) Remember that phototherapy has its risks: always balance risk against benefit. Remember that physiologic jaundice, exaggerated physiologic jaundice, and breast milk jaundice are not associated with kernicterus.
   c) Remember the differentiation between exaggerated physiologic jaundice due to breast feeding and breast milk jaundice.
   d) Jaundice after the fifth day of life = neonatal sepsis, until proven otherwise.
   e) Jaundice in the first 24 hours of life = pathologic jaundice.
   f) Remember that ABO incompatibility can cause kernicterus. Treat with phototherapy earlier rather than later (follow the guidelines outlined in the Short Answer Management Problem).
   g) When considering discontinuation of breast-feeding in breast milk jaundice, consider risk versus benefit of discontinuing breast-feeding.

SUGGESTED READING

Behrman RE et al., eds. Nelson textbook of pediatrics. 14th Ed. Philadelphia: WB Saunders, 1992.

PROBLEM 86   AN 8-WEEK-OLD INFANT WITH INCONSOLABLE CRYING MANY HOURS/DAY FOR THE LAST 4 WEEKS

A 28-year-old mother of two presents to your office with her 8-week-old infant. Her baby has been "crying constantly" for the last 4 weeks, and she is at her "wit's end."

She is bottle-feeding her baby and is having no significant feeding problems apart from what may be "excessive" gas and burping following feeding. No other symptoms have been identified. The mother also states that her first child had "some crying" spells but it was "nothing like this." The baby has had no other problems, specifically no constipation or diarrhea.

On examination, the infant is afebrile and has no abnormalities of the ears, throat, and lungs. The abdomen is soft, and there are no masses palpable.

SELECT THE ONE BEST ANSWER TO THE FOLLOWING QUESTIONS

1. What is the most likely diagnosis in this infant?
   a) infantile colic
   b) excessive spasm syndrome of infancy
   c) early Crohn's disease
   d) psychosocial stress syndrome of infancy
   e) urinary tract infection

2. Investigations that should be undertaken in the infant described include which of the following?
   a) CBC
   b) CBC/diff/ESR
   c) CBC/diff/ESR/urinalysis
   d) urinalysis
   e) none of the above; no investigations need be done

3. What is the most likely underlying cause of the infant's symptom of excesssive crying?
   a) bottle feeding
   b) hormone abnormalities produced by the newly diagnosed psychiatric condition labeled "baby stress"
   c) gastrointestinal hyperperistalsis
   d) maternal stress
   e) none of the above; the cause of these symptoms is unknown

4. Which of the following definitions correctly identifies infants with the syndrome described?
   a) unexplained fussiness or crying lasting longer than 3 hours per day, 3 days per week, and continuing for more than 3 weeks in infants younger than 3 months of age
   b) unexplained fussiness or crying lasting longer than 6 hours per day, 3 days per week, and continuing for more than 2 weeks in an infant younger than 4 months of age
   c) unexplained fussiness or crying lasting longer than 4 hours, 3 days per week, and continuing for longer than 2 weeks in an infant younger than 6 months of age
   d) unexplained fussiness or crying lasting longer than 6 hours per day, 5 days per week, and continuing for more than 3 weeks in an infant younger than 8 months of age
   e) unexplained fussiness or crying lasting longer than 7 hours per day, 6 days per week, and continuing for more than 7 weeks in an infant younger than 6 months of age

5. At this time, what should you do?
   a) tell the mother to relax and to call you in 4 weeks if the crying has not improved
   b) set up an appointment for the baby with the infant psychiatrist
   c) do nothing
   d) discontinue cow's milk and begin soy formula
   e) none of the above

6. Which of the following statements regarding treatment of the condition described is true?
   a) treatment should be begun and continued until the condition improves
   b) treatment is ineffective; it's not worth the bother
   c) the most effective treatment is reassuring the mother about the benign nature of the condition
   d) treatment with oral analgesics appears to be the most effective therapy that can be offered
   e) treatment with antibiotics should be started

7. Which of the following statements regarding drug therapy for the condition described is true?
   a) antispasmodics are safe and effective
   b) antihistamines given to the infant may be beneficial in sedating the baby and settling everybody down
   c) antispasmodics and antihistamines together offer the best form of drug therapy
   d) aspirin should be considered as a first-line option
   e) none of the above

Short Answer Management Problem 86

Describe the educational approach you would attempt with the infant's mother.

ANSWERS

1. A.

2. D. This infant most likely has infantile colic. Infantile colic is defined as spells of unexplained fussiness or crying lasting longer than 3 hours per day, 3 days per week, and continuing for more than 3 weeks in infants younger than 3 months of age. "Unexplained fussiness or crying" implies that other causes (particularly infection) have been ruled out.

Excessive spasm syndrome of infancy and psychosocial stress syndrome of infancy do not exist. Early Crohn's disease is not possible.

Urinary tract infection, along with otitis media, pharyngitis, pneumonitis, and other infections, should be carefully considered before labeling the child as having infantile colic.

The number-one infection to rule out in infants is urinary tract infection. A urinalysis should be performed to rule it out. In addition, a complete P/E should be performed to rule out any other causes. At this age otitis media, pharyngitis, pneumonia, meningitis, intussusception, or volvulus may present initially only with excessive crying. If your index of suspicion is raised following a physical examination, particularly in the presence of a fever, then a more complete laboratory workup and hospitalization is indicated.

3. E. The cause of excessive crying in infancy is unknown. Although gastrointestinal hyperperistalsis, cow's milk protein allergy, lactose intolerance, disturbances in the parent-infant relationship, and a neurophysiologic response of the immature newborn to external and internal stimuli have all been proposed as potential underlying causes of infantile colic, nobody really knows for sure.

The newly diagnosed psychiatric condition known as "baby stress" does not exist.

4. A. Although you might correctly argue that the only type of person who would ask a question like this is one who was really strapped for good questions in the first place, it does reinforce the Wessel criteria for the diagnosis of infantile colic: unexplained fussiness or crying lasting longer than 3 hours/day, 3 days/week, and continuing for longer than 3 weeks in an infant younger than 3 months of age.

5. E. The most reasonable course of action in this case (after you have ruled out other causes) is as follows:

1) Describe the condition to the mother
2) Explain that the cause is unknown
3) Reassure the mother that the colic will pass by the age of 3 months, or shortly thereafter, and if it does continue longer it will certainly continue to improve
4) Discuss maternal coping strategies with the mother
5) Ask the mother to call you in 2 weeks if the symptoms have not improved, or sooner if any other symptoms develop

6. C. The most effective and important treatment is reassurance, stressing the benign nature of the condition and the assurance of resolution of the condition.

Reassure the mother that there is nothing that she is doing wrong and that there is no reason to switch to a soy-based formula. Although infantile colic is less frequent in breast-fed babies than bottle-fed babies, it is not less common in soy-based feeding compared to ordinary infant formula.

To simply tell the mother to relax is not particularly helpful to anyone and indicates your lack of sensitivity to a very difficult problem.

As with the "baby stress" syndrome, the infant psychiatrist option does not exist.

7. E. Many different pharmacologic treatments have frequently been used to treat infantile colic, including dicyclomine (Bentylol), phenergan (an antihistamine), "grippe water" (which is basically a watered-down alcoholic drink), aspirin, acetaminophen, and codeine. Dicyclomine has been associated with apnea and respiratory difficulties and antihistamines may cause significant CNS difficulties.

An "alcoholic mixture" speaks for itself.

Aspirin, because of the potential association with Reye's syndrome, should not be used.

Although you might consider using simple acetaminophen, even with this drug there are no good data to indicate its safety in very young infants.

SOLUTION TO SHORT ANSWER MANAGEMENT PROBLEM 86

The most important points to be made in discussing the infant's condition with the mother are as follows:

1. There is nothing the mother could have done to prevent the condition, and there is nothing that she is doing wrong at present.
2. There is no association between infantile colic and other, more serious problems in the future.

3. Although bottle-fed babies get colic somewhat more frequently than breast-fed babies, this is no reason to change her current feeding pattern.
4. No specific therapy is more effective than explanation to the parent of the benign, self-limited nature of the condition.
5. The condition will resolve spontaneously and will probably resolve by the age of 3 months.
6. If anything changes or any other symptoms appear, or if the mother is worried about anything else, urge her to call you.

SUMMARY OF DIAGNOSIS AND TREATMENT OF INFANTILE COLIC

1. Infantile colic is extremely common; it occurs in up to 25% of infants.
2. Although there are a number of theories as to etiology, the condition's cause at this time is idiopathic.

3. The most important differential diagnosis is infection: if the ears, throat, and lungs are clear, and if no abnormalities are detected on abdominal examination, then a urinalysis is the only investigation that is necessary.
4. Diagnosis of infantile colic is based on Wessel's criteria: 3,3,3, and 3.
5. Reassurance of the parent is as effective as any other therapy and is the treatment of choice.
6. Medications including dicyclomine (Bentylol), antihistamines, "alcohol containing water," and aspirin should not be used. If anything is going to be used it should be acetaminophen.

SUGGESTED READING

Parkin P, Schwartz C, Manuel B. Randomized controlled trial interventions in the management of persistent crying of infancy. Pediatrics 1993; 92:197-201.

PROBLEM 87 A 2-MONTH-OLD-INFANT WITH A HIGH FEVER 8 HOURS AFTER RECEIVING HER FIRST SET OF IMMUNIZATIONS

A 2-month-old-infant is brought to your office by his mother following his "first set of immunizations" at age 2 months. His mother states that approximately 8 hours after being immunized, the infant developed a temperature of 40.6° C. The child is screaming and irritable. On P/E, no localizing signs of infection are found. Examination of the ears shows hyperemia of both tympanic membranes. You realize, of course, that this is probably due to the crying itself. The throat is normal. The lungs are clear. The cardiovascular system and abdomen are normal.

SELECT THE ONE BEST ANSWER TO THE FOLLOWING QUESTIONS:

1. Which immunization is the most likely cause of the fever and the irritability in this child?
   a) poliomyelitis
   b) pertussis
   c) diphtheria
   d) tetanus
   e) none of the above

2. Considering the adverse reaction that appears to be related to the immunization, what would you do?
   a) hospitalize the child
   b) advise the mother to give the child aspirin to bring down the fever
   c) advice the mother to give the child acetaminophen to bring down the fever
   d) obtain *stat* blood cultures, CBC, and urine for analysis and culture, and perform a lumbar puncture
   e) none of the above

3. Considering the most likely cause of this child's adverse reaction, which of the following statements regarding future immunizations is(are) true?
   a) all future DTP-polio immunizations should be canceled
   b) future immunizations should omit diphtheria toxoid
   c) future immunizations should omit tetanus toxoid
   d) future immunizations should not be affected; DTP-polio should be given as before
   e) none of the above are true

4. Which of the following statements regarding vaccination against poliomyelitis is(are) true?
   a) at this time, although two forms of vaccination against poliomyelitis exist, only one is licensed for use in the United States
   b) oral polio vaccine is a live, attenuated trivalent vaccine known as the Salk vaccine
   c) IPV polio vaccine is an inactivated (killed) trivalent vaccine known as Sabin vaccine
   d) all of the above are true
   e) none of the above are true

5. Which of the following statements is(are) true regarding hepatitis B vaccine in children?
   a) it is not recommended as a routine immunization
   b) it is recommended as a routine immunization, and the first dose should be given at 8 months
   c) it is recommended as a routine immunization, and the first dose should be given at 6 months
   d) it is recommended as a routine immunization, and the first dose should be given at 4 months
   e) none of the above are true

6. Which of the following statements is(are) true regarding reactions that follow the immunization of infants and children with DTP?
   a) there are three different types of adverse reaction that may occur
   b) the fever that may develop from one type of reaction often reaches 40.5° C
   c) reactions against the vaccine occur infrequently
   d) a and b
   e) all of the above

7. Which of the following statements is(are) true regarding adverse reactions to immunization against DTP?
   a) reaction 1: (the most common) includes local swelling, tenderness at the site of the injection, slight fever, and irritability
   b) reaction 2 includes somnolence, protracted inconsolable crying that may last 4 hours or more, and an unusual "shock-like" syndrome that may last for hours; if this reaction occurs, no further doses of DTP should be given
   c) reaction 3 includes neurologic reactions that contraindicate further doses of DTP—these include generalized convulsions and acute encephalopathy
   d) these reactions are all overstated; you should tell your mothers not to worry about anything and leave all the decision making up to you
   e) a, b, and c are true

8. Which of the following statements regarding immunization against *Haemophilus influenzae* type b is(are) true?
   a) the vaccine is known as the Hib vaccine
   b) the first dose of Hib vaccine should be given at age 2 months

c) the Hib vaccine is given to protect the infant only from Haemophilus influenzae type b infections that lead to meningitis

d) all of the above are true

e) a and b only

9. Which of the following vaccines is(are) recommended for first administration at age 12-15 months?
a) hepatitis B
b) Hib vaccine
c) MMR vaccine

d) all of the above

e) a and b only

10. By the time a child reaches the age of 7 years, how many doses of OPV (oral polio vaccine) should have been administered?
a) 1 dose
b) 2 doses
c) 3 doses
d) 4 doses
e) none of the above

Short Answer Management Problem 87

Discuss some of the important causes for the reduction in neonatal, infant, and childhood mortality that have occurred during the last century. Indicate whether or not these causes are still a concern in certain parts of the world.

ANSWERS

1. B.

2. C.

3. E. Pertussis vaccine (whooping cough vaccine) is the most likely cause of this adverse reaction. Pertussis vaccine may produce minor reactions such as local discomfort, induration, and fever in up to approximately 75% of children who receive the vaccine.

Drowsiness, anorexia, persistent crying, screaming, and febrile convulsions may also occur.

Although a possibility, adverse reactions against poliomyelitis (oral polio vaccine), diptheria, and tetanus are much less common than adverse reactions against pertussis.

This child has a normal physical examination, apart from some hyperemia on both tympanic membranes that you assume is due to the child's crying (here is an axiom for crying children in an office setting when you are in a hurry: if a child is crying and the only abnormality is hyperemia of the tympanic membrane itself [no retraction, no air-fluid levels], don't give antibiotics: antibiotics do not alleviate crying in children).

It is reasonable to assume a cause-and-effect relationship between the administration of the pertussis vaccine and the onset of fever.

Hospitalization is not necessary, nor is an intensive septic workup.

Acetaminophen is the analgesic of choice for the treatment of fever in children. Aspirin should not be given because of its possible link with Reye's syndrome.

This child should be reassessed within 24 hours if the symptoms (especially the fever) do not improve with the administration of the antipyretic acetaminophen, or if any other symptoms or signs develop.

Future immunizations should not include the pertussis component. Some authorities would argue that the entire combination (diphtheria-tetanus-pertussis) should be omitted from further immunization consideration. This seems to be both "overkill" and potentially dangerous since we know that the vast majority of adverse reactions are due to pertussis. Obviously, if the adverse reaction occurs again in the absence of the pertussis component, then it is reasonable not to continue with DTP immunization as a whole.

4. E. Two types of vaccine are licensed in the United States for prevention of polio: OPV, a live, attenuated, trivalent poliovirus vaccine known as Sabin; and an IPV, an inactivated (killer) trivalent vaccine known as Salk.

5. The answer is E. None of the above.

Vaccination against hepatitis B is routinely recommended for all children born in the United States.

The easiest schedule for hepatitis B immunization is birth, 2 months, 4 months.

6. D.

7. E. First, if a reaction to childhood immunization is going to occur, it will most likely occur secondary to the pertussis component of DTP.

Second, depending on the severity of the reaction, you need to decide which one of the following courses of actions you will follow in the future. The four possible scenarios are as follows:

1) You can do nothing different and proceed with DTP vaccination as before.
2) You can advise the mother to give the child acetaminophen prophylactically if the child had a previous significantly high fever and proceed with DTP vaccination as before.
3) You can omit the pertussis component and give the diphtheria component and the tetanus component in one vaccine.
4) You can cancel the remainder of the DTP series (all components).

The reactions that follow the vaccination for diphtheria, tetanus, and pertussis fall into three different types with further subtyping. They are as follows:

Type 1A

1. Severity: mild
2. Reaction characteristics: local swelling at the site of the injection, slight fever ($< 39.5°$ C), and irritability
3. Treatment: acetaminophen if fever above 39° C
4. Further vaccinations: proceed as normal with vaccinations at recommended time intervals.

Type 1B

1. Severity: moderate
2. Reaction characteristics: same as 1A except fever greater than 40.0-40.5°C.
3. Treatment: acetaminophen; aspirin should not be used
4. A suggested reasonable recommendation for further vaccinations: omit pertussis component. Vaccinate with DT component in one vaccine at recommended time intervals:

Type 2A

1. Severity: moderate
2. Reaction characteristics: excessive somnolence and/or protracted, inconsolable crying lasting > 4 hours
3. Treatment: acetaminophen; aspirin should not be used
4. A suggested reasonable recommendation for further vaccinations: omit pertussis component. Vaccinate with DT component in one vaccine at recommended time intervals.

Type 2B

1. Severity: severe
2. Reaction characteristics: unusual "shock-like syndrome" that may last for hours
3. Treatment: emergency treatment ASAP
4. A suggested reasonable recommendation for further vaccinations: omit all further DTP vaccinations.

Type 3

1. Severity: severe
2. Reaction characteristics: neurologic reactions within 3 days of DTP vaccination; convulsions and/or acute encephalopathy

3. Treatment: emergency treatment ASAP
4. A suggested reasonable recommendation for further vaccinations: omit all further DTP vaccinations.

8. E. Vaccination against *Haemophilus influenzae* type b is recommended in three doses, at 2, 4, and 12-15 months of age. *Haemophilus influenzae* vaccine is given at that time because of the age at which *Haemophilus influenzae* meningitis affects infants and children. Meningitis due to this organism usually occurs between age 1 month and age 4 years. Other significant infections due to *Haemophilus influenzae* are acute epiglottis; pneumonia; septic arthritis; cellulitis; osteomyelitis; pericarditis; bacteremia without an associated focus; neonatal disease; and miscellaneous infections such as urinary tract infection, cervical adenitis, uvulitis, endocarditis, primary peritonitis, periappendiceal abscess, and otitis media. The Hib immunization should, theoretically, be effective against all of these infections.

9. C. The only vaccination that is given for the first time at 12-15 months is measles, mumps, and rubella (MMR).

10. D. By the time a child reaches the age of 7 years, 4 doses of OPV (oral polio vaccine) should have been administered.

SOLUTION TO SHORT ANSWER MANAGEMENT PROBLEM 87

The reductions in neonatal, infant, and childhood mortality in the developed world during the last century are truly remarkable. These reductions are due to better prenatal care and prenatal assessment of high-risk status; improved perinatal care; immunizations; antibiotics; other diagnostic and therapeutic tools; and public health measures including filtration and chlorination of water, hygienic food handling (especially of milk), mosquito control, and isolation of individuals infected with a communicable disease.

In addition, the health of children has been directly affected by improvements in social conditions, economic conditions, and educational advances in the developed world. Little more can be done to further reduce mortality rates apart from a paradigm shift from acute episodic care of children to primary preventive care on visits that occur for a different reason. For example, if a 6-month-old child presents with his mother to your office for assessment of fever and irritability, it is a perfect opportunity to discuss the inadvisability of walkers in relationship to stairs, child safety seats in automobiles, and locations of potential toxic substances and medicines in the home.

There is, however, a startling contrast between neonatal, infant, and childhood health in the developed world and the health of the same-aged population in the developing world, especially in areas of continual war and strife such as Rwanda. In the developing world neonatal, infant, and childhood mortality is significantly higher today than it was in the United States in the eighteenth century.

SUMMARY OF THE CENTER FOR DISEASE CONTROL AND PREVENTION'S GUIDELINES FOR NEWBORN, INFANT, AND CHILDHOOD IMMUNIZATIONS (SIMPLIFIED)

1. Hepatitis B: birth, 2 months, 6 months
2. DPT: 2 months, 4 months, 6 months, 18 months, 4-6 years
3. Oral polio: 2 months, 4 months, 6 months, 18 months, 4-6 years
4. HiB (hemophilus influenzae Type B): 2 months, 4 months, 6 months, 18 months
5. MMR: 12-15 months, 4-6 years
6. Varicella: 12-15 months

New Information 1995

As discussed extensively in this chapter, widespread immunization programs launched almost 50 years ago in the United States have had a major impact on morbidity and mortality in children. Specifically with respect to diphtheria, the CDC in Atlanta points out that in the year 1993 no cases of diphtheria were reported in the nation.

Compare this to Russia today and 12 years ago. In the entire Soviet Union in 1982 there were 340 cases of diphtheria reported. The number of cases of diphtheria reported in Russia alone in 1994 was greater than 40,000. This is thought to be due to inadequate vaccinations and Russia's economic problems that obviously directly affect the health status of the population.

SUGGESTED READINGS

ACIP recommended immunization schedule. Center for Disease Control and Prevention, Atlanta, November 1993.

Behrman R et al., eds. Nelson textbook of pediatrics. 14th Ed. Philadelphia: WB Saunders, 1994.

Feshbach M. The diphtheria zone. Atlantic Monthly 1995; (2):87

PROBLEM 88   AN ANXIOUS MOTHER WITH A 3-WEEK-OLD INFANT AND MANY QUESTIONS CONCERNING FEEDING

A mother who just delivered her first baby 3 weeks ago presents for her first neonatal visit. She has many questions concerning breast-feeding and has been getting much advice from her friends and especially her mother-in-law.

The infant appears to be growing well and, according to her mother, is happy and content. The mother-in-law has suggested that her daughter-in-law change from breast-feeding to cow's milk because she feels the infant's crying is waking up her son (the baby's father) and preventing him from getting "the rest that he needs."

The mother appears somewhat tired herself. The child is on the 50th percentile for weight and the 50th percentile for length. More importantly, the child has gained an average of 50 g/day since discharge from hospital.

The child is feeding every 2 hours at this time.

SELECT THE ONE BEST ANSWER TO THE FOLLOWING QUESTIONS

1. What is the minimal appropriate weight gain (and a sign of both infant health and maternal-infant bonding with breast feeding) following discharge from hospital?
   a) 15 g/day
   b) 20 g/day
   c) 30 g/day
   d) 50 g/day
   e) 75 g/day

2. What should be your suggestion to the mother in terms of feeding her infant?
   a) ask her mother-in-law; she seems to know all the answers
   b) to decrease the feeds of the infant to every 3 hours
   c) to feed the infant on demand
   d) to switch from breast to bottle—it will end up being less hassle for everyone
   e) a and c

3. Common mistakes in the feeding of infants (especially with first-time mothers) include which of the following?
   a) feeding the infant too little
   b) feeding the infant too often
   c) feeding the infant on a fixed schedule
   d) feeding the infant whole cow's milk
   e) all of the above

4. Regarding the feeding of infants when they cry, which of the following offers the best advice to the mother?
   a) crying = food: no ifs, and, or buts
   b) let the infant cry for at least 37.5 minutes; if the infant is still crying, check things out—it's likely to be either one of a diaper problem or a food problem
   c) stop breast feeding; it's too much hassle and much easier just to stick a bottle in the infant's mouth
   d) crying may or may not indicate hunger; infants need not be fed every time they cry
   e) crying almost always indicates hunger; assume that the baby needs to be fed until proven otherwise (that will eliminate the potential problem of under-feeding)

5. Which of the following statements regarding breast milk flow and maternal anxiety is(are) true?
   a) there is little correlation between breast milk flow and maternal anxiety
   b) maternal anxiety may significantly increase the quantity of breast milk in breast milk flow
   c) maternal anxiety may significantly decrease the quantity of breast milk in breast milk flow
   d) maternal anxiety may significantly decrease the quality of breast milk in breast milk flow
   e) c and d

6. Human colostrum is the precursor to good-quality human breast milk. What is(are) the major components found in colostrum that offer a significant advantage to breast-fed infants?
   a) macrophages that synthesize complement, lyso-zyme, and lactoferrin
   b) bacterial antibodies that protect the infant against bacterial organisms entering through the GI tract
   c) viral antibodies that protect the infant against viral organisms entering through GI tract
   d) b and c
   e) all of the above

7. The substances of importance described in Question 6 are of what subtype?
   a) subtype A
   b) subtype G
   c) subtype M
   d) subtype E
   e) all of the above

8. A 28-year-old primigravida develops an erythematous skin discoloration in the upper outer quadrant of the left breast. You suspect bacterial mastitis.
   At this time, what would you do?
   a) stop breast-feeding; have the mother express her breast milk until the infection is cleared up

b) continue breast-feeding and treat the mother with hot compresses and antibiotics

c) continue breast-feeding and treat both the mother and the infant with antibiotics

d) forget breast-feeding for now; provide the "big gun" antibiotics ("quadruple therapy") just to make sure you "snow" the bacteria

e) operate immediately; you never know what you may find underneath that inflamed tissue

9. What is the organism most likely responsible for the condition described in Question 8?
a) *Streptococcus pneumoniae*
b) *Staphylococcus aureus*
c) *Escherichia coli:* subtype H-57
d) *Bacteroides fragilis*
e) b and d together

10. Which of the following statements comparing human breast milk to cow's milk is false?
a) cow's milk may be responsible for diarrhea, intestinal bleeding, and occult melena
b) "spitting up," "infantile colic," and "atopic dermatitis" are more common in infants fed with cow's milk (or infant formula)
c) human breast milk contains bacterial and viral antibodies, antibodies mainly of the IgA class
d) breast-fed babies do not require iron supplementation until the age of 1 year
e) human breast milk has an adequate amount of vitamin C

11. The mother described in the case history at the beginning has been told that she should be "giving the baby lots of every vitamin under the sun." Her mother-in-law even offers to purchase the 37 different vitamins for the baby.

Although it is difficult to acknowledge, Grandma may be right with respect to which of the following vitamins?
a) vitamin A
b) vitamin C
c) vitamin D
d) b and c
e) all of the above

12. Fluoride supplementation for both breast-fed babies and bottle-fed babies should not be required if the fluoride concentration in the water supply of the community exceeds which of the following?
a) 1.0 ppm
b) 2.0 ppm
c) 5.0 ppm
d) 10.0 ppm
e) 100.0 ppm

13. Human breast milk, in comparison to cow's milk, has which of the following?
a) a higher fat content
b) a lower carbohydrate content
c) a lower protein content
d) a greater concentration of the protein casein
e) a greater number of kcal/g of milk

14. Which of the following statements is false regarding infant feeding?
a) infants establish their own feeding pattern; there is considerable variation from one infant to another
b) for the first 1 or 2 months of life, feedings are regularly taken throughout the 24-hour period
c) breast-fed babies should be fed on an established schedule
d) during the first month of life, feedings average 6-8 feedings/24 hours
e) by 8 months of age, the average number of feedings is 3-4 feedings/24 hours

15. The mother-in-law recommends that solids be introduced on day 8 and that one new solid food be introduced every 4 days until a total of 28 different solids are being regularly consumed.

You have a slightly different recommendation. Your recommendation is that solid foods do not have to be introduced into the infant's diet until what age?
a) 1 month of age
b) 2-3 months of age
c) 4-6 months of age
d) 9 months of age
e) 12 months of age

16. You see the same mother presented in the case history 6 weeks later. She has switched from breast-feeding to infant formula feeding because she had to go back to her full-time job as an accountant. She tells you that her infant is now "constipated." On careful questioning, you determine that the infant is having one hard bowel movement every 4 days.

The P/E is completely normal, including anal sphincter tone. At this time, what should you do?
a) tell the mother to go home, take a Valium, and relax
b) suggest supplementation with extra fluids, extra foods, and prune juice
c) suggest the use of milk of magnesia at bedtime
d) suggest the addition of two teaspoons of bran to the pablum and force-feed the pablum every 3 hours
e) pull out the "old glycerine suppositories" and suggest their regular use four times a day for 6 weeks

17. Another mother presents to your office with her infant. The baby is 6 weeks of age and has been "spitting up all of her formula for the last 3 weeks." She believes the

infant is malnourished and has been told so by another "very helpful mother-in-law."

You weigh the baby; she is 11 lb, 3 oz. Her birth weight was 7 lb, 6 oz. At this time, you should advise the mother to do which of the following:

a) go home and relax; the child will grow out of it
b) increase the time spent burping the infant and put the infant on her abdomen for a nap immediately after the feeding
c) investigate the child for pyloric stenosis
d) suggest the use of a GI tract motility modifier such as metoclopramide (IV push of 4h)
e) refer the child *stat* to a pediatric gastroenterologist

18. Another mother presents to your office with her 8-week-old infant girl. She is tearful and depressed. She has been trying to breast-feed but she tells you that "I'm obviously inadequate; I'm not producing enough milk and the baby is fussy all of the time."

On examination, the infant looks thin. Since her last checkup 3 weeks ago, she has gained only 90 g. The rest of the physical examination is normal.

At this time, what should you do?

a) ask some very direct questions about the mother's feeding technique
b) refer the mother to a "lactation consultant"
c) include the husband or significant other in feeding expressed breast milk to the infant
d) suggest a temporary supplementation with infant formula after breast-feeding
e) all of the above

19. Which of the following statements regarding breast-feeding is(are) true?

a) most breast-fed babies lose weight in the first week of life
b) infants should be encouraged to empty both breasts at each feeding during the first few weeks of life
c) maternal fatigue may impair breast feeding
d) 80%-90% of the breast milk obtained is obtained in the first 4 minutes of breast-feeding on a particular breast
e) all of the above are true

Short Answer Management Problem 88

Compare the composition of human breast milk with infant formula and/or cow's milk.

ANSWERS

1. C. The minimal acceptable weight gain in the neonatal period and infancy is 30 g/day. If weight gain equals or exceeds that, you can be reasonably confident that the infant is thriving.

2. C. It is well accepted that especially during the first few weeks and months of life the ideal feeding schedule is feeding on demand. This will vary from infant to infant but eventually settle into a reasonable schedule averaging 6-8 feedings/day.

3. E. Mistakes that are made frequently in the neonatal and infant period regarding feeding include the following:
   A. Feeding the infant too much
   B. Feeding the infant too little
   C. Feeding the infant on a fixed schedule (rather than on demand)
   D. Feeding the infant cow's milk rather than breast milk or formula (cow's milk tends to be more allergenic and less digestible)

4. D. It is important to appreciate that infants cry for other reasons besides hunger and that they need not be fed every time they cry. Some infants are placid, some are unusually active, and some are irritable. Sick infants are often uninterested in food. Infants who awaken and cry consistently at short intervals may not be receiving enough milk at each feeding or may have discomfort from some other cause such as too much clothing, soiled, wet, or uncomfortable diapers and clothing; swallowed air ("gas"); be in an uncomfortably hot or cold environment; or be ill. Some infants cry to gain sufficient attention, whereas other infants deprived of adequate mothering become indifferent. Some infants simply need to be held. Those who stop crying when they are picked up or held do not usually need food, but those who continue to cry when held and when food is offered should be carefully evaluated for other causes of distress.

5. C. Maternal anxiety, fatigue, postpartum depression, or stress due to other causes are candidates for a decreased quantity of milk that may further compound the problem. It is conceivable that mothers may find themselves in a situation where they are in a vicious cycle: maternal stress leads to maternal fatigue, which results in decreased Quantity of Breast Milk, which causes further maternal stress, and so on. It appears that only the quantity and not the quality of breast milk is affected.

6. E.

7. A. Human colostrum contains macrophages that are able to synthesize complement, lysozyme, and lactoferrin; and the iron binding whey protein that is normally about one-third saturated with iron. In addition, human colostrum contains both bacterial and viral antibodies of the IgA class that protect the infant from bacterial species such as *E. coli* and certain viruses.

8. B.

9. B. Unless exceptional circumstances dictate otherwise, the recommended course of action with maternal mastitis is to continue breast feeding and treat the mother with both symptomatic treatments such as hot compresses and antibiotics effective against *Staphylococcus aureus* (including coagulase-positive *Staphylococcus*). The antibiotic of choice in this case is either cloxacillin or methicillin.

10. D. Breast milk has many advantages over cow's milk for the feeding of infants. These advantages include the following: it is easier to digest; it has the bacterial and viral antibodies just mentioned; it does not produce allergic manifestations such as diarrhea, GI tract bleeding, and atopic dermatitis; it has a lower incidence of feeding problems including regurgitation and constipation; it has a lower incidence of infantile colic; and it is the most important method of establishing maternal-infant bonding. Breast milk usually contains adequate supplies of all vitamins, with the possible exception of vitamin D. Vitamin C is not required for supplementation.

    Although breast milk contains some iron, and the iron that is present is well absorbed, the child will need iron-fortified pablum or foods by 6 months of age to prevent iron-deficiency anemia.

11. C. Vitamin D is the only vitamin that may be required for supplementation in a breast-fed baby. If a baby is not exposed to adequate sunlight or has dark skin, the quantity of vitamin D may not be sufficient. It is recommended that the daily intake of vitamin D be 400 IU/day.

12. A. Fluoride supplementation for infants (both breast-fed and bottle-fed) is not required if the fluoride concentration of the water supply exceeds 1.0 ppm. Additional fluoride given to formula-fed babies in a community with a fluoridated water supply could result in fluorosis.

13. C. In comparison to cow's milk, human breast milk has a higher carbohydrate concentration, a lower protein concentration, different protein composition (lactalbumin and lactoglobulin), a higher percentage of polyunsaturated fat (qualitative difference), and the same caloric content (20 kcal/oz).

14. C. The following statements concerning infant feeding are true:
    A. There is considerable variation in feeding patterns from infant to infant.
    B. During the first month or two of life, feedings are taken regularly during the 24-hour period.
    C. During the first few months of life, feedings average 6-8/24-hour period.
    D. By 8 months of age, feedings have settled down to an average of 3-4/24-hour period.
    As stated earlier, neonates and infants should be fed on demand, not on a strictly imposed schedule.

15. C. Solid foods do not have to be introduced into an infant's diet until 4-6 months of age. Infant pablum is the first food to be introduced. Infant pablum should be followed by vegetables, fruits, and finally meats. New foods should not be introduced more often than one every 1-2 weeks. The order of food introduction appears relatively unimportant. The introduction of one food at a time will allow you to establish an allergic or atopic reaction to any particular newly introduced food.

16. B. Constipation is a common problem in formula-fed infants. It is extremely rare in a breast-fed baby. Constipation in a formula-fed baby may be due to an insufficient amount of food or fluid, a diet too high in fat or protein, or a diet deficient in bulk. Constipation may be alleviated by increasing the amount of fluid or sugar in the formula or by adding or increasing the amounts of cereal, vegetables, or fruit; prune juice ($\frac{1}{2}$ to 1 oz) may also be helpful.

    The use of milk of magnesia and glycerine suppositories as anything but a temporary measure is inappropriate. The addition of 2 teaspoons of bran to the pablum, although theoretically sound as a measure of increasing the bulk in the infant's diet, would be somewhat unpalatable and would result in an irate infant!

    Telling the mother to go home and relax is not appropriate.

17. B. Regurgitation, or spitting up, is a common problem in infants. The mechanism appears to be an incompetent gastroesophageal sphincter. Regurgitation can be reduced by adequate eructation of swallowed air during and after eating, by gentle handling, by avoidance of emotional conflicts, and by placing the infant on the right side or abdomen for a nap immediately after eating. The head should not be lower than the rest of the body during rest periods. Unless the child (especially a male) demonstrates projectile vomiting and has a palpable mass in the pylorus, pyloric stenosis is not likely.

18. E. This is a very common scenario in pediatric family practice.

    The mother should be carefully questioned regarding feeding technique. Before assuming that the mother has insufficient milk, three possibilities should be excluded: errors in feeding technique responsible for the infant's inadequate progress; remediable maternal factors related to diet, rest, or emotional distress; or physical disturbances in the infant that interfere with eating or with weight gain.

    Occasionally infants who seem to be nursing well may not thrive because of milk insufficiency; in this case increased frequency of feedings may be indicated.

    Referral to the La Leche League is an alternative that can be recommended to this mother. The La Leche League is a volunteer organization composed of successfully nursing mothers willing to assist other mothers desiring to nurse.

    If the mother is able to successfully express sufficient milk, the husband or significant other may be able to assist the mother in feeding. This alternative is attractive because it gives the mother time to rest and recover her strength.

    Supplementation with an infant formula is an alternative that should be considered in some cases. In this case, the mother is encouraged to breast-feed and supplement her baby with formula following each feeding. As long as the nipple in the bottle does not have too big a hole in it (making it too easy for the infant to obtain the formula), the infant will probably continue to suck vigorously at the breast. This will allow the mother to continue breast-feeding while ensuring adequate infant nutrition.

    Infant formulas provide excellent nutrition for the infant. They all combine milk, sugar, and water, and modification of a digestible curd protein. As with breast milk, infant formulas provide 20 kcal/oz.

    Although "breast is best," a dogmatic approach to breast-feeding should be avoided.

19. E. Important characteristics of breast-feeding include the following:
    A. Most breast-fed babies lose weight in the first week.
    B. Infants should be encouraged to empty both breasts at each feeding.
    C. Maternal fatigue may impair breast feeding.
    D. 80%-90% of breast milk is obtained by the infant during the 4 minutes of the feeding.

SOLUTION TO SHORT ANSWER MANAGEMENT PROBLEM 88

A succinct comparison between human breast milk and formula or cow's milk is as follows:
A. Breast milk has a higher carbohydrate content than formula or cow's milk.

B. Breast milk has a lower protein content than cow's milk.
C. Breast milk has qualitatively different proteins:
   1. Breast milk has lactalbumin and lactoglobulin.
   2. Formula or cow's milk has casein as a major protein.
D. Breast milk has a different composition of fats; breast milk has a higher percentage of polyunsaturated fat.
E. Breast milk and cow's milk or formula have equivalent caloric content (20 kcal/oz).

SUMMARY OF INFANT FEEDING

1. **Preference of infant feeding:** breast feeding is preferable. Advantages of breast feeding include convenience, digestibility, transfer of antiviral and antibacterial antibodies, lack of allergic phenomena, maternal-infant bonding, low incidence of regurgitation, and no constipation.

   Breast feeding should be encouraged: before assuming that milk production is insufficient for the infant you should consider errors in feeding techniques, remediable maternal factors, and physical disturbances in the infant.

   Feeding should be on demand: although erratic in the first few months, infants tend to regulate themselves after short periods of time.

   Supplementation with formula and formula feeding provide excellent nutrition; a dogmatic approach to breast-feeding should be avoided.

2. **Vitamin/fluoride/iron supplements:** vitamins are unnecessary in all formula-fed infants and probably in most breast-fed babies. If the mother is not exposed to sufficient sunlight or is darkly pigmented, supplemental vitamin D is recommended. Fluoride supplementation is unnecessary if the community water supply is fluoridated; this applies to breast-fed and bottle-fed babies.

   Iron supplements (in the manner of iron-fortified food) should be begun at the age of 6 months in breast-fed babies due to the exhaustion of iron supplied by the mother in utero.

3. **Solid foods:** solid foods need not be introduced until 4-6 months of age; after that time introduce one new food every 1-2 weeks.

4. **Unwarranted assumptions:** don't assume that a crying infant is a hungry infant. Consider all causes of infant crying before making that assumption. Don't assume that information received from other sources (including well-meaning family members) is valid information.

5. **Advantages of human colostrum:**
   a) Macrophages
   b) Viral antibodies
   c) Bacterial antibodies
      Antibody class: IgA

6. **Growth and development:** here is a diagnostic clue: minimum standard for neonate is a weight gain of 30 g/day.

7. **Comparison of human milk and formula/cow's milk:**
   a) Carbohydrate: higher in human milk
   b) Protein content: lower in human milk

c) Protein quality: lactalbumin and lactoglobulin in human milk versus casein in formula/cow's milk

d) Fat: quality/distribution: polyunsaturated fat higher in breast milk

e) Caloric content: identical: 20 kcal/oz

SUGGESTED READING

Nutrition and nutritional disorders. In: Behrman R ed., Nelson textbook of pediatrics. 14th Ed. Philadelphia: WB Saunders, 1992.

PROBLEM 89   AN 18-MONTH-OLD INFANT WHO APPEARS MALNOURISHED

An 18-month-old infant is brought to the ER by his mother for an assessment of an upper respiratory tract infection. He has been coughing for the past 3 days and has had a runny nose.

On examination, his temperature is 37.5° C. He appears malnourished and has thin extremities, a narrow face, prominent ribs, and wasted buttocks. He has a prominent diaper rash, unwashed skin, a skin rash that resembles the skin infection impetigo contagiosum on his face, uncut fingernails, and dirty clothing. His weight is below the third percentile for his age.

SELECT THE ONE BEST ANSWER TO THE FOLLOWING QUESTIONS:

1. What is the most likely diagnosis in the infant described?
   a) nonorganic failure to thrive
   b) organic failure to thrive
   c) child neglect
   d) a and c
   e) b and c

2. What is the most likely cause of this child's condition?
   a) maternal deprivation
   b) cystic fibrosis
   c) constitutionally small for age
   d) infantile autism
   e) congenital bilateral sensorineural hearing loss

3. What is the procedure of choice for this infant at this time?
   a) provision of a high-calorie formula; reassessment of the infant in 1 week's time
   b) initiation of outpatient investigations in the child to exclude serious organic disease
   c) treatment of the respiratory tract infection and instruction to the mother in correct feeding practices
   d) all of the above
   e) none of the above

4. Where is follow-up of this child best performed?
   a) in the hospital outpatient department
   b) in the hospital ER room
   c) in the family physician's office
   d) in the home by the public health nurse
   e) in the social worker's office

5. The initial follow-up plan would suggest the frequency of visits for the child be which of the following?
   a) every month
   b) every 3 months
   c) every week
   d) every 6 weeks
   e) every 6 months

6. The environment that exists for this child should be thoroughly assessed for which of the following?
   a) child abuse/potential for child abuse
   b) spousal abuse/potential for child abuse
   c) level of family income
   d) inappropriate parental coping mechanisms: alcohol and drug use
   e) all of the above

7. A 13-year-old female is brought to your office for assessment of her short stature. On examination the child has a weight below the fifth percentile, a webbed neck, lack of breast bud development, high-arched palate, and a low-set hairline.
   What is the most likely diagnosis in this child?
   a) Noonan's syndrome
   b) trisomy 21
   c) Turner's syndrome
   d) fragile X syndrome
   e) constitutional delay of growth

8. What is the most common cause of short stature in children?
   a) familial short stature
   b) chromosomal abnormality
   c) constitutional delay of growth
   d) hypothyroidism
   e) psychosocial dwarfism

9. Bone age can sometimes be used to differentiate certain causes of short stature in children. With respect to bone age, which of the following statements is true?
   a) bone age is normal in both familial short stature and in constitutional delay of growth
   b) bone age is normal in familial short stature and delayed in constitutional delay of growth
   c) bone age is normal in constitutional delay of growth and delayed in familial short stature
   d) bone age is delayed in both familial short stature and in constitutional delay of growth
   e) bone age is variable in these two situations and cannot be used to differentiate them

10. Psychosocial dwarfism is a situation in which poor physical growth may be associated with an unfavorable psychosocial situation. With respect to psychosocial dwarfism, which of the following statements is false?
   a) sleep and eating aberrations occur in these children

b) growth usually returns to normal when the stress is removed
c) behavioral problems are common in these children
d) all of the above
e) none of the above

11. Which of the following investigations should be performed in a child with failure to thrive or a child in which short stature is unlikely to be familial in nature?
a) CBC
b) complete urinalysis
c) serum BUN/creatinine
d) stool for ova and parasites
e) all of the above

Short Answer Management Problem 89

List 10 physical disorders that may manifest themselves as failure to thrive in infants and children.

ANSWERS

1. D.

2. A. This child most likely has nonorganic failure to thrive secondary to child neglect.

   Failure to thrive (FTT) may be due to organic causes, nonorganic causes, or both. Nonorganic causes predominate. Nonorganic FTT includes psychologic FTT (maternal deprivation), child neglect, lack of education regarding feeding, and errors in feeding.

   Nonorganic failure to thrive is most often attributable to maternal deprivation or lack of a nurturing environment at home.

3. E.

4. D.

5. C. The treatment of choice at this time is to hospitalize the child and to give the child unlimited feedings for a minimum time period of 1 week. At the same time, a careful physical examination and certain routine investigations including complete blood count, complete urinalysis, renal function testing, and serum TSH level can be completed. If the child lives in a poor inner-city neighborhood in the United States, a serum lead level test should also be done.

   The family physician can and should involve social services and should also initiate a detailed assessment of the child's home environment.

   Before the child is discharged home, the home environment must be assessed, and the parents of the child must be given explicit instructions in feeding practices.

   If the child begins to gain weight rapidly and reestablish his health in hospital (which is very likely), reassessment should ideally be done in the environment that allowed the development of the problem in the first place (at least on some occasions). This is obviously the home, and the health care professional in the best position to do this is probably the public health nurse or the community health nurse. The initial follow-up supervision should be close and frequent; every week for the first 6 weeks following discharge from the hospital seems reasonable.

6. E. Maternal neglect resulting in nonorganic failure to thrive should not be just left at that: the reasons need to be investigated. A mother who neglects her child (a form of child abuse) is also at risk for other forms of child abuse. In addition, she herself is at greater-than-average risk for being abused by her husband or partner. Remember that family violence begets family violence, and in this case we already have established that a form of family violence (child abuse: subtype neglect) exists.

7. C. The most likely cause of this child's short stature is Turner's syndrome. Noonan's syndrome (an autosomal dominant trait with widely variable expressivity) also has short stature as its most common presentation. It can be easily distinguished from Turner's syndrome, however, due to its normal chromosome compliment. Turner's syndrome will have either a 45 XO chromosome complement or a mosaic.

   Trisomy 21 will usually be recognized long before the age of 13 years. The fragile X syndrome is a syndrome associated with mental retardation and macro-orchidism in males.

8. A. The most common cause of short stature in children is short parents. When a short child who is growing at a normal rate and has a normal bone age is found to have a strong family history of short stature, familial short stature is the most likely cause. Other causes of short stature include constitutional delay of growth,

chromosomal abnormalities, intrauterine growth retardation, chronic diseases such as renal disease or inflammatory bowel disease, hypothyroidism, adrenal hyperplasia, growth hormone deficiency, bioinactive growth hormone, and psychosocial dwarfism.

9. B. Bone age determination can distinguish between the two most common causes of short stature: familial short stature and constitutional delay of growth. Children with familial short stature have normal bone ages. Constitutional delay of growth, which is really a delay in reaching ultimate height and sexual maturation, presents with delayed bone age and delayed sexual maturation.

10. D. Inadequate growth in children may be associated with an unfavorable psychologic environment. In this situation, the child may show transiently low human growth hormone levels during periods of stress. He or she may also have behavioral, sleep, and eating disturbances. Both growth and growth hormone levels return to normal when the psychologic stressors are removed.

11. E. Recommended investigations in a child with failure to thrive or a child in which short stature is unlikely to be familial in nature should include CBC, complete urinalysis, serum BUN/serum creatinine, ESR, serum thyroxine, serum lead level, stool for ova and parasites, liver enzymes (serum bilirubin, ALT, AST), and X-rays of the hands and wrists.

SOLUTION TO SHORT ANSWER MANAGEMENT PROBLEM 89

Ten disorders that may manifest themselves as failure to thrive in infants and children include the following:
1. Cystic fibrosis
2. Congenital heart disease
3. Hypothyroidism
4. Chronic renal disease
5. Inflammatory bowel disease
6. Juvenile rheumatoid arthritis
7. HIV infection/AIDS
8. Chronic liver disease
9. Anorexia nervosa and bulimia nervosa
10. Bronchiectasis
   Other diseases include the following:
11. Malignancies (neuroblastoma, nephroblastoma, glioma)
12. Tuberculosis
13. Certain metabolic disorders and inborn errors of metabolism
14. Turner's syndrome
15. Down syndrome
16. Hirschsprung's disease

SUMMARY OF THE DIAGNOSIS AND TREATMENT OF FAILURE TO THRIVE AND SHORT STATURE IN INFANTS AND CHILDREN

1. **Failure to thrive:**
   a) Nonorganic: psychologic failure to thrive, maternal deprivation; child neglect; lack of education regarding feeding; errors in feeding. Suspect family dysfunction and monitor carefully in these cases.
   b) Organic failure to thrive: See the solution to the Short Answer Management Problem.
   c) Treatment:
      1. An initial period of hospitalization is indicated in most cases. Unlimited feedings (especially to any infant) should be given in these cases, and a complete investigation should be performed to attempt to elucidate the cause.
      2. When the child goes home, careful and frequent observation is indicated, especially in the initial period of time. Some of these observations should take place in the environment (the home) in which the problems began (for nonorganic failure to thrive). Weekly observation is indicated initially.
2. **Short stature:**
   a) Familial short stature: most common cause
   b) Familial short stature can be differentiated from constitutional delay of growth (the second most common cause) by bone age.
   c) Other causes of short stature include chromosomal abnormalities, intrauterine growth retardation, hypothyroidism, psychosocial dwarfism, bioinactive growth hormone, and true growth hormone deficiency.
   d) Investigations of a child with short stature should include CBC, complete urinalysis, serum BUN/creatinine, liver enzymes and bilirubin, ESR, serum thyroxine, serum lead level, stool for ova and parasites, and X-ray of the hands and wrist for bone age.

SUGGESTED READING

Behrman R et al., ed. Special considerations in the care of sick children. Nelson textbook of pediatrics. 14th Ed. Philadelphia: WB Saunders, 1992.

PROBLEM 90   AN 18-MONTH-OLD INFANT WITH AN UPPER RESPIRATORY TRACT INFECTION

An 18-month-old infant is brought to the ER by his mother. He developed an upper respiratory tract infection 2 days ago and suddenly this evening developed a harsh, barky cough and difficulty breathing.

On examination the child is coughing. His respiratory rate is 40/minute and he is in some respiratory distress. The breath sounds that are heard appear to be transmitted from the upper airway. There are nasal flaring and suprasternal, infrasternal, and intercostal retractions. The child's temperature is 38.5° C.

SELECT THE ONE BEST ANSWER TO THE FOLLOWING QUESTIONS:

1. What is the most likely diagnosis in this child?
   a) viral pneumonia
   b) acute epiglottis
   c) bronchiolitis
   d) croup
   e) bacterial pneumonia

2. The etiologic agent responsible for this child's condition is most likely which of the following?
   a) adenovirus
   b) *Pneumococcus*
   c) parainfluenza virus
   d) *Haemophilus influenzae*
   e) respiratory syncytial virus

3. What is the treatment of choice for mild to moderate cases of the disorder described?
   a) racemic epinephrine
   b) ribavirin
   c) humidification
   d) aerosolized steroids
   e) all of the above

4. You see the same child 6 months later in the ER. On this occasion, he presents with an acute onset of rhinorrhea and cough, which has progressed to wheezing, dyspnea, and irritability. On examination, the child's temperature is 38° C. There are rhonchi heard in all lobes. His respiratory rate is 50, and he exhibits flaring of the alae nasi and use of the accessory muscles of respiration resulting in intercostal and subcostal retractions. Widespread fine rales are heard at the end of inspiration and in early expiration. The expiratory phase is prolonged, and wheezing is audible throughout the lung fields.
   What is the most likely diagnosis in this patient?
   a) viral pneumonia
   b) acute epiglottis
   c) bronchiolitis
   d) croup
   e) bacterial pneumonia

5. The treatment of this child at this time may include which of the following?
   a) humidified oxygen
   b) nebulized bronchodilators
   c) ribavirin
   d) none of the above
   e) all of the above

6. What is the etiologic agent most likely responsible for this child's condition?
   a) adenovirus
   b) *Pneumococcus*
   c) rhinovirus
   d) *Haemophilus influenzae*
   e) respiratory syncytial virus

7. A 5-year-old child is brought to the ER by his mother. The mother tells you that for the past 24 hours the child has been "talking strangely" and drooling. He has had no appetite and has not been drinking. Based on this history, what is the diagnosis of major concern?
   a) viral pneumonia
   b) acute epiglottis
   c) bronchiolitis
   d) croup
   e) bacterial pneumonia

8. What is the diagnostic procedure that can substantiate the diagnosis of the patient described in Question 7?
   a) a WBC count
   b) an ESR
   c) a chest X-ray
   d) a lateral X-ray of the neck
   e) a CT scan of the head and neck

9. What is the treatment of choice for the patient described in Question 7?
   a) IV ampicillin
   b) oral ampicillin
   c) IV/IM ceftriaxone
   d) IV ciprofloxacin
   e) oral ciprofloxacin

10. What is the causative organism responsible for the condition described in Question 7?
   a) parainfluenza virus
   b) respiratory syncytial virus
   c) *Haemophilus influenzae*
   d) rhinovirus
   e) *Pneumococcus*

11. Which of the following statement(s) concerning wheezing in infancy is(are) true?
    a) it is sometimes difficult to differentiate bronchial asthma from bronchiolitis by clinical assessment
    b) children with bronchiolitis who do not develop asthma may be inappropriately labeled as asthmatics
    c) the relationship between bronchiolitis and ongoing airway hyperreactivity is unclear; ongoing bronchial hyperreactivity or asthma may be precipitated by an acute episode of bronchiolitis
    d) none of the above statements are true
    e) all of the above are true

12. A 6-year-old male presents to the ER with an acute asthmatic attack. He developed a respiratory tract infection 3 days ago and began wheezing 24 hours ago. He had his first asthma attack 2 years ago and usually has one attack per month. He is on no prophylactic medications.

    On examination, the child is in severe respiratory distress. His respiratory rate is 48/minute. He has marked indrawing of the accessory muscles of respiration. Generalized wheezes are heard throughout the lung fields.

    What is the treatment of choice in this patient at this time?
    a) intravenous sodium cromoglycate
    b) intravenous corticosteroids
    c) nebulized beta-agonist with or without ipratropium bromide
    d) humidified oxygen
    e) b and c

13. Pulmonary function tests are performed on the patient described in Question 12. Which of the following parameters of pulmonary function would be expected to increase after administration of a bronchodilator?
    a) FVC (forced vital capacity)
    b) FEV$_1$ (forced expiratory volume in 1 second)
    c) MEF 25-75 (maximum expiratory flow between 25% and 75% of the vital capacity)
    d) TLC (total lung capacity)
    e) b and c

14. The patient described in Question 12 is stabilized and you decide to begin prophylactic therapy. Which of the following is the prophylactic agent of choice?
    a) an inhaled beta-agonist
    b) oral theophylline
    c) an inhaled corticosteroid
    d) sodium cromoglycate
    e) an oral corticosteroid

15. A 12-year-old boy presents for assessment of exercise-induced asthma. The child is fine when at rest but develops shortness of breath and wheezing at the end of or during a vigorous exercise session.

    What is the treatment of first choice in this child?
    a) sodium cromoglycate
    b) an inhaled beta-agonist
    c) oral theophylline
    d) an inhaled corticosteroid
    e) an oral corticosteroid

Short Answer Management Problem 90

Defend the following statement: "all that wheezes is not asthma."

ANSWERS

1. D. This child has croup. A child with croup (the most common form being acute laryngotracheobronchitis) usually has a typical upper respiratory tract infection for several days before the brassy cough, inspiratory stridor, and respiratory distress become apparent. As the infection extends downward involving the bronchi and the bronchioles, respiratory difficulty increases and the expiratory phase of respiration becomes labored and prolonged.

    The child often appears restless, agitated, and frightened. The child's temperature may be only slightly elevated or may be as high as 39° to 40° C (102-104° F).

    On examination there are usually bilaterally diminished breath sounds, rhonchi, and scattered rales. Symptoms are characteristically worse at night and often recur with increasing intensity for several days. The child, however, is not seriously ill and often has associated rhinitis, conjunctivitis, or both. Some children, however, develop severe suprasternal, infrasternal, and intercostal retractions with significant dyspnea.

2. C. Most cases of croup (with the most common form being acute laryngotracheobronchitis) are caused by the parainfluenza group of viruses.

3. D. Until very recently, the treatment of choice for mild to moderate cases of croup was simple humidification. A recent landmark study, however, has clearly established that nebulized budesonide (an inhaled steroid) is of significant benefit in young children with mild to moderate croup.

4. C. This child has bronchiolitis. The signs and symptoms of bronchiolitis have been well described in the clinical history just noted.

Roentgenographic examination reveals hyperinflation of the lungs and an increased anteroposterior diameter of the chest on lateral view. Scattered areas of consolidation are found in about one-third of patients and are due either to atelectasis secondary to obstruction or to inflammation of the alveoli. The WBC and the differential are usually within normal limits.

5. E. Humidified oxygen is of benefit in the treatment of infants and children with bronchiolitis.

Ribavirin (Virazole), an antiviral agent, is effective in reducing the severity of bronchiolitis due to RSV infection when administered early in the course of the illness. Its use is indicated in children under 2 years of age who have severe infection documented by fluorescent antibodies or culture or strongly suspected on epidemiologic grounds and whose hospitalization is likely to exceed 3 days. It should also be administered to patients with milder bronchiolitis due to RSV infection who have underlying severe chronic illness due to cardiac disease.

Bronchodilating aerosolized drugs are frequently used empirically. Epinephrine or other alpha-adrenergic agents have a theoretical basis for use, but have not been adequately tested.

Antibiotics have no therapeutic value unless there is a secondary bacterial infection.

6. E. The agent responsible for most cases of bronchiolitis is the respiratory syncytial virus. Other causes include the parainfluenza 3 virus, mycoplasma, some adenoviruses, and occasionally other viruses. Adenovirus-caused bronchiolitis may be responsible for long-term complications including bronchiolitis obliterans and unilateral hyperlucent lung syndrome.

7. B.

8. D.

9. C.

10. C. This child must be suspected of having acute epiglottis until proven otherwise.

Acute epiglottis, a potentially lethal condition, occurs in the age group 2 years to 7 years and peaks at the age of $3\frac{1}{2}$ years. Acute epiglottis is characterized by a fulminating course of fever, sore throat, dyspnea, rapidly progressive respiratory obstruction, and prostration. In hours, epiglottis can lead to complete obstruction of the airway and death unless adequate treatment is administered.

Respiratory distress is the first symptom. The child may be well at bedtime but awakens later in the evening with a high fever, aphonia, drooling, and moderate to severe respiratory distress with stridor. An older child will often complain of a "sore throat."

Severe respiratory distress may ensue within minutes or hours of the onset, with inspiratory stridor, hoarseness, a brassy cough, irritability, and restlessness. Drooling and dyspnea are common.

On physical examination the child is noted as having moderate to severe respiratory distress with inspiratory and at times expiratory stridor; flaring of the alae nasi; and inspiratory retractions of the suprasternal notch, the supraclavicular and intercostal spaces, and the subcostal area. The pharynx is inflamed, and there is often an abundance of mucus and saliva, which may also result in rhonchi. With progression, stridor and breath sounds may become diminished as the patient tires. There may be a brief period of air hunger with restlessness and agitation, which may progress to cyanosis, coma, and death. The other presentation is that of only mild hoarseness and a large, shiny, cherry-red epiglottis.

The child's pharynx should *not* be examined with a tongue depressor. The diagnosis requires direct visualization by laryngoscopy with the ability to intubate immediately at hand.

The diagnosis can be made by a lateral X-ray of the neck, which will clearly show the swollen epiglottis.

The treatment of choice for a child with acute epiglottis is the following:

a) If the child is seriously ill, an artificial airway must be immediately established. Untreated patients have a substantial mortality even when observed in the hospital with appropriate intubation equipment nearby.

b) Ceftriaxone (100 mg/kg/24 hours) OR ampicillin (200 mg/kg/24 hours) plus chloramphenicol (100 mg/kg/24 hours) should be given pending culture and susceptibility reports due to the increasing possibility of ampicillin-resistant strains of *H. influenzae* being the cause of the condition.

c) Supplemental oxygen: the causative organism associated with acute epiglottis is *Haemophilus influenzae*. As mentioned, there are increasing problems with ampicillin-resistant *Haemophilus* species.

11. E. All of the statements are true. It is sometimes difficult to differentiate bronchial asthma from bronchiolitis by clinical assessment. Thus an inappropriate diagnosis of asthma may be made and the child may be labeled as having this disease. The relationship, however, between bronchiolitis and asthma is unclear; young infants with bronchiolitis may be at an increased risk of developing asthma later in childhood. Bronchial asthma may be precipitated by an acute episode of bronchiolitis.

12. E. This child is in severe respiratory distress from the current asthmatic attack and should be treated with a combination of an intravenous corticosteroid (deter-

mined on a mg/kg basis) and a nebulized beta-agonist with or without ipratropium bromide. Early and aggressive treatment will prevent deterioration and possibly even death.

13. E. Pulmonary function testing before and after administration of an aerosol bronchodilator will assess the degree of reversibility of airway obstruction. Normally the administration of a bronchodilator will result in an increase in FEV_{-1} and MEF 25-75. FVC and TLC, which may already be increased in patients with bronchial asthma, will not increase further after administration of a bronchodilator.

14. C. In the last edition of this book, the answer to this question was an inhaled beta-agonist. This has changed. The current recommendation is that an inhaled corticosteroid is now the agent of first choice for the prophylaxis of bronchial asthma. The inhaled steroids that are most commonly used are given either once or twice/day.

15. A. Exercise-induced asthma may be manifested by both an early (in terms of time following exercise) and late bronchoconstriction. Early bronchoconstriction begins 3-8 minutes following exercise and late bronchoconstriction occurs 4-6 hours after exercise. Inhaled sodium cromoglycate will block both early and late bronchoconstriction. An inhaled beta-agonist will block only early bronchoconstriction. Corticosteroids will block only late bronchoconstriction.

SOLUTION TO SHORT ANSWER MANAGEMENT PROBLEM 90

"All That Wheezes Is Not Asthma."

It is important to realize that there are causes for wheezing in infancy and childhood other than asthma. Although asthma remains the most common cause of wheezing, it is by no means the only cause. The second most common cause is bronchiolitis. As described earlier, the association between asthma and bronchiolitis remains unclear. It may very well be the case that an attack of acute bronchiolitis actually predisposes a child to develop asthma at a later date.

In addition to asthma and bronchiolitis as causes of wheezing, remember airway obstruction. This would most commonly be due to the lodging of a foreign body in the trachea or one of its branches.

As a corollary to "all that wheezes is not asthma" we can add "all asthma does not wheeze." This is particularly true with the so-called cough variant asthma, in which the principal manifestation is cough. It is estimated that up to one-third of children with asthma exhibit this variation, a variation that unfortunately all too often goes unnoticed or undiagnosed.

SUMMARY OF THE DIAGNOSIS AND TREATMENT OF SOME COMMON AND SERIOUS RESPIRATORY SYNDROMES IN INFANTS AND CHILDREN

1. **Major worrisome symptoms:**
   a) Harsh, barky cough
   b) Stridor and respiratory distress
   c) Drooling
   d) Wheezing
2. **Croup:** most common form is acute laryngotracheobronchitis. A harsh, barky cough in a young infant is almost pathognomonic of croup. Respiratory distress can be pronounced.
   Causative agent: parainfluenza virus.
   Treatment (which used to consist of humidified oxygen almost exclusively): croup now has been shown to be effectively treated with nebulized corticosteroids even in mild to moderate cases.
3. **Bronchiolitis:** may produce very significant respiratory distress and stridor, rales, and wheezing. Expiratory phase prolonged.
   Causative agent: respiratory syncytial virus
   Treatment: humidified oxygen and ribavirin
4. **Acute epiglottis:** drooling, very sore throat, difficulty swallowing liquids (this can be used as a diagnostic test). Do not attempt visualization of the epiglottis unless you are prepared to intubate.
   Lateral X ray of the neck will help substantiate the diagnosis (swollen epiglottis seen on lateral X ray of the neck).
   Causative agent: *Haemophilus influenzae*
   Treatment: IV/IM ceftriaxone
5. **Asthma:** most common cause of wheezing in infants and children
   Causative agent: often familial; often associated with some extrinsic allergen in children
   Treatment:
   a) Acute, severe cases: IV steroids, nebulized beta-agonists, oxygen
   b) Stable cases: inhaled corticosteroids are drugs of first choice. Inhaled beta-agonists may be used but are no longer drugs of first choice.
   Exercise-induced: sodium cromoglycate

Other Information:
1. Asthma still kills. Asthma should be treated aggressively.
2. Not all that wheezes is asthma.
3. Not all asthma wheezes.

SUGGESTED READINGS

Behrman E, ed. Nelson's textbook of pediatrics. 19th Ed. Philadelphia: WB Saunders, 1992

Klassen TP, Feldman ME, Watters LK, et al. Nebulized budesonide for children with mild-to-moderate croup. N Engl J Med 1994; 331:285-289.

PROBLEM 91   A 24-MONTH-OLD CHILD WHO IS CONSTANTLY CRYING AND WHO COMPLAINS OF A RIGHT-SIDED EARACHE

A mother presents to your office with her 24-month-old daughter. The child developed an upper respiratory tract infection approximately 1 week ago. The infection started with cough, congestion, and rhinorrhea. Two days ago the child began complaining of pain in the right ear.

On examination, the child has nasal congestion and a hyperemic throat. The left tympanic membrane is normal and the right tympanic membrane is bulging and red. There appears to be fluid behind it. The lungs are clear. The child's temperature is 39.5° C.

SELECT THE ONE BEST ANSWER TO THE FOLLOWING QUESTIONS

1. What is the most likely diagnosis in this child?
   a) acute otitis media
   b) otitis media without effusion
   c) chronic otitis media
   d) otitis media with effusion
   e) none of the above

2. An 8-month-old male presents to your office the same day. He too has had an upper respiratory tract infection but has no signs of acute ear infection such as pain, pulling at his ears, or fever.

   On examination there is a middle-ear effusion, and the tympanic membrane is dull but not red.

   What is the most likely diagnosis in this child?
   a) acute otitis media
   b) otitis media without effusion
   c) chronic otitis media
   d) otitis media with effusion
   e) none of the above

3. A 7-month-old child presents to your office with his mother the same day as you saw the other two children. He has had an upper respiratory tract infection for the past 3 days.

   On examination there is erythema of the left tympanic membrane with opacification. There are no other signs or symptoms.

   What is the most likely diagnosis in this patient?
   a) acute otitis media
   b) otitis media without effusion
   c) chronic otitis media
   d) otitis media with effusion
   e) none of the above

4. This is obviously "ear day" in your practice. A fourth child, 9 months of age, presents with a discharge from the left ear that has been present for the last 4 days. The child has a history of frequent ear infections, all of which have been treated with antibiotics.

   What is the most likely diagnosis in this patient?
   a) acute otitis media
   b) otitis media without effusion
   c) chronic otitis media

   d) otitis media with effusion
   e) none of the above.

5. Referring again to the first patient you saw, which of the following statements regarding her condition described is(are) false?
   a) this condition usually begins a few days after the onset of an upper respiratory tract infection
   b) this condition is usually associated with eustachian tube dysfunction
   c) environmental factors such as pollen, dusts, molds, and cigarette smoke are unlikely to be associated with an increase in the incidence of this condition
   d) most cases of this condition are considered to be bacterial in origin
   e) none of the above statements are false

6. What are the most common bacterial organisms responsible for the condition described in the first patient you saw?
   a) pneumococcus, group A streptococci, *Haemophilus influenzae*
   b) pneumococcus, *Haemophilus influenzae*, staphylococcus
   c) pneumococcus, *Haemophilus influenzae*, *Moraxella catarrhalis*
   d) *Haemophilus influenzae*, pneumococcus, group A streptococcus
   e) *Haemophilus influenzae*, pneumococcus, *Moraxella catarrhalis*

7. What is the drug of choice for the condition described in Question 1?
   a) penicillin
   b) amoxicillin
   c) erythromycin-sulfamethoxazole
   d) cefaclor
   e) amoxicillin-clavulinic acid

8. A family practice resident who is working with you describes the condition of a child he has just seen. He describes a R tympanic membrane behind which is significant fluid. He tells you, however, that there are no other symptoms associated with this effusion. He asks you what he should do.

   You should tell him to do which of the following?
   a) forget about it—it's not bothering him

b) perform a myringotomy and suck out all the fluid that is present

c) perform a tympanometry to assess the movement of the tympanic membrane

d) refer the child to an ENT surgeon for myringotomy, tubes, and an adenoidectomy (you might as well suggest a tonsillectomy at the same time and get everything over at once)

e) none of the above

9. Which of the following statements regarding treatment of the condition described in Question 1 is(are) false?
   a) earache and fever should be treated with aspirin
   b) topical decongestants are useful in improving eustachian tube dysfunction
   c) eardrops provide significant relief in children with the condition described in Question 1
   d) systemic antihistamine-decongestants have been shown to improve the symptoms and shorten the course of the condition described
   e) all of the above statements are false

10. The condition described in the first patient has occurred at least once in what percentage of 18-month-old children?
    a) 10%
    b) 35%
    c) 74%
    d) 18%
    e) 29%

11. How is recurrent otitis media defined?
    a) three or more episodes of acute otitis media that occur within 6 months, or four episodes that occur within a year
    b) four or more episodes of acute otitis media that occur within 6 months, or five episodes that occur within a year

    c) five or more episodes of acute otitis media that occur within 6 months, or six episodes that occur within a year
    d) six or more episodes of acute otitis media that occur within 6 months, or eight episodes within a year
    e) two or more episodes of acute otitis media that occur within 6 months, or three or more episodes that occur within a year

12. Which of the following statements regarding recurrent otitis media is(are) true?
    a) recurrent bouts of acute otitis media usually occur in the winter or early spring
    b) recurrent bouts of acute otitis media should be managed by myringotomy and the insertion of ventilation tubes
    c) medical management appears to be less effective and not as safe as myringotomy and tubes in children with recurrent acute otitis media
    d) amoxicillin does not have a major role to play in the management of recurrent acute otitis media
    e) none of the above statements are true

13. Which of the following is(are) possible intracranial complications of otitis media?
    a) meningitis
    b) subdural empyema
    c) brain abscess
    d) all of the above
    e) none of the above

14. Which of the following is(are) possible extracranial complications of otitis media?
    a) mastoiditis
    b) cholesteatoma
    c) labyrinthitis
    d) all of the above
    e) none of the above

Short Answer Management Problem 91

A mother presents to your office with her 18-month-old child following the treatment of an episode of acute otitis media. She states that the child was in considerable pain despite analgesics and antibiotics and asks you to refer her child to an ENT surgeon. She wishes to have "tubes" inserted in her child's ears. She has a number of friends who have had this done to their children following the first episode of otitis media and it has been extremely successful. Discuss how you would approach this problem.

ANSWERS

1. A.

2. D.

3. B.

4. C. The signs and symptoms presented in the first four questions can be matched to the classification of otitis media that is outlined below.

1. Otitis media without effusion: this is also known as myringitis. It indicates the presence of erythema (redness) and opacification of the tympanic membranes without the presence of an effusion. This may be seen in the early stages of acute otitis media or as otitis media resolves.

2. Acute otitis media: this is also known as acute suppurative, acute purulent, or acute bacterial otitis media. The pathophysiology is basically an effusion of the middle ear that becomes infected with viruses and/or bacteria. There is often a rapid onset of signs and symptoms such as fever; ear pain; a red, bulging, tympanic membrane; and fluid behind the middle ear.

3. Otitis media with effusion: this is also known as non-suppurative, serous, or mucoid otitis media. This is manifested as otitis media without signs or symptoms of acute disease but with a middle-ear effusion. Otitis media with effusion may be subdivided into acute, subacute, and chronic based on the duration of the effusion.

4. Chronic otitis media: this is synonymous with chronic suppurative, purulent, or intractable otitis media. There is a presence of pronounced, intractable middle-ear pathology with or without suppurative otorrhea. *Suppurative* refers to an active infection and *otorrhea* refers to a discharge through a perforated tympanic membrane.

5. C. Acute otitis media usually begins a few days after the onset of an upper respiratory tract infection. The upper respiratory tract infection usually produces eustachian tube dysfunction and obstruction. This subsequently leads to the accumulation of fluid in the middle ear. This fluid then becomes infected with a virus, a bacteria, or a virus followed by bacteria.

Environmental factors such as exposure to respiratory tract irritants (cigarette smoke, pollen, dust, molds) may increase the incidence of upper respiratory tract infection and acute otitis media. Supine nursing (habitually putting the infant to bed with a bottle) may also contribute to the incidence of otitis media.

6. C. The bacteriology of acute otitis media suggests that the following bacterial organisms (in this order) are responsible for most cases of acute otitis media:
   1. Pneumococcus
   2. *Haemophilus influenzae*
   3. *Moraxella catarrhalis*
   4. Group A streptococci
   5. *Staphylococcus aureus*

As mentioned above, viruses have also been implicated as primary causative agents. Also, we believe that if a virus produces the primary infection, most of these cases will become secondarily infected with a bacterium.

7. B. The drug of choice for acute otitis media in primary care practice is still amoxicillin. The usual length of treatment is 7-10 days. Although this has been challenged and does not apply to those patients with recurrent otitis, it is true for primary family medicine care.

A patient who does not improve on amoxicillin most likely has an infection with a beta-lactamase-producing organism. In this case, second-line agents including trimethoprim-sulfamethoxazole, erythromycin-sulfamethoxazole, or cefaclor can be used.

8. C. The most reasonable maneuver to perform at this time is tympanometry to assess the movement of the tympanic membrane. This will provide an accurate indication of whether or not there is fluid present in the middle-ear cavity. This easily performed maneuver is often omitted in primary care.

Referral to an ENT surgeon for myringotomy, tubes, adenoidectomy, and tonsillectomy is not indicated at this time. Similarly, the performance of a myringotomy in the office is an invasive and painful procedure. Although this is not an acute otitis media now, it may very well become one. Therefore treatment with amoxicillin is also reasonable in this case.

9. E. Symptoms of earache or fever should be treated with acetaminophen. Aspirin should be avoided because of the possible link to Reye's syndrome.

Ear drops do not provide any symptomatic relief in otitis media and interfere with otoscopic examination and follow-up.

Topical decongestants (sympathomimetic nose drops and sprays), used to relieve obstruction in the eustachian tube, and systemic antihistamine-decongestant combinations have not been shown to be effective in the treatment of otitis media. They affect neither the duration nor the severity of symptoms.

10. C. Studies suggest that 35% of children have at least one episode of acute otitis media by 6 months of age; 74% have at least one episode between the ages of 6 monthes and 18 months.

11. A. Recurrent otitis media is defined as three or more episodes of acute otitis media that occur within 6 months or four episodes within a year.

12. A. Recurrent bouts of acute otitis usually occur in the winter or early spring.

Recurrent episodes of acute otitis media can be managed to some extent with prophylactic antibiotics. Although a myringotomy and the insertion of ventilation tubes may ultimately have to be performed, it is not the first-line option. Medical management with antibiotics has been shown, in most studies, to be just as effective. Half-strength amoxicillin or sulfisoxazole is reasonable prophylactic therapy.

13. D. Otitis media is not an innocuous diagnosis and should be treated aggressively with antibiotics. Intracranial complications associated with otitis media include meningitis, subdural empyema, brain abscess, lateral sinus thrombosis, and focal otitis encephalitis.

14. D. Extracranial complications and sequelae associated with otitis media include hearing loss, tympanic membrane perforation, chronic suppurative otitis media, mastoiditis, cholesteatoma, facial paralysis, tympanosclerosis, and labyrinthitis.

SOLUTION TO SHORT ANSWER MANAGEMENT PROBLEM 91

This is a difficult issue because the mother has come in to your office expecting and wanting a referral to an ENT surgeon. At this time, I would do the following:

1. Discuss the incidence of acute otitis media and point out to the mother that more children have had it than have not had it.
2. Describe the resolution of the symptoms with simple antibiotic therapy in most cases.
3. Describe briefly the anatomy of the eustachian tube and point out that as her child grows, the probability of infections will continue to decrease.
4. Try to establish why she is so concerned and wants a referral at this time. Often (referring back to the biopsychosocial model) there are other issues that need to be addressed with the mother.
5. If the mother, despite all of your reassurance, insists on a referral, then I would give her one. I would, however, point out to the mother that the ENT surgeon is unlikely to want to put in tubes at this time.
6. Offer to discuss the issue of her child's otitis media or any other issues at any time. Provide for the mother a framework in which she can begin to view you, the family physician, as her advocate in health care. She probably needs this more than anything else.

SUMMARY OF THE DIAGNOSIS AND TREATMENT OF OTITIS MEDIA

1. Acute otitis media is common in childhood. By 18 months of age, 74% of children have had at least one infection.
2. When discussing otitis media, use the right terminology. The Panel for the Definition and Classification of Otitis Media suggests the following:
   a) Otitis media without effusion
   b) Acute otitis media
   c) Otitis media with effusion (OME)
   d) Chronic otitis media (COM)
3. Most common etiologic agents in order of frequency: pneumococci, *Haemophilus influenzae, Moraxella catarrhalis,* group A streptococci.
4. Treatment of choice for acute otitis media in the primary care setting is still amoxicillin.
5. Definition of acute otitis: otalgia, fever, and irritability associated with a full or bulging tympanic membrane with effusion.
6. Decongestants-antihistamines and ear drops have not been shown to influence either the severity or duration of the symptoms.
7. Consider prophylactic antibiotics before considering myringotomy and tubes for the treatment of recurrent otitis media.
8. Remember that otitis media can produce complications: treat with an antibiotic for at least 7 full days.

SUGGESTED READINGS

Sagraves R, Maish W, Kameshka A. Update of otitis media. Part I: Epidemiology and pathophysiology. American Pharmacy 1992; 12:27-31.

Sagraves R, Maish W, Kameshka A. Update on otitis media. Part II: Treatment. American Pharmacy 1993; 1:29-35.

Stool S. Otitis media: Update on a common, frustrating problem. Postgraduate Medicine 1989; 85(10):40-53.

PROBLEM 92   A 4-YEAR-OLD CHILD WITH A RUNNY NOSE, A SORE THROAT, AND A NONPRODUCTIVE COUGH

A 4-year-old child with a runny nose, a sore throat, a feeling of "fullness" in his ears, and a nonproductive cough presents with his mother to your office. He has had these symptoms for the last 4 days and is not improving. He has had no fever, no chills, or any other symptoms.

On examination, the child's temperature is 37.6° C. His ears are clear, his throat is slightly hyperemic, and both sides of his nose look congested and red. His lung fields are clear. There is no significant cervical lymphadenopathy. No other localizing signs are present.

The child's past history is unremarkable, and he has had no significant medical illnesses.

SELECT THE ONE BEST ANSWER TO THE FOLLOWING QUESTIONS

1. What is the most likely diagnosis in this child?
   a) early streptococcal pharyngitis
   b) early *Mycoplasma* pneumonia
   c) early acute otitis media
   d) early viral pneumonia
   e) none of the above

2. What is the most likely pathogen responsible for this condition?
   a) *Streptococcus pneumoniae*
   b) rhinovirus
   c) parainfluenza A
   d) adenovirus
   e) respiratory syncytial virus

3. Investigations at this time should include which of the following?
   a) CBC
   b) throat swab
   c) rapid antigen test for *Streptococcus* (ELISA)
   d) all of the above
   e) none of the above

4. Which of the following statements regarding the common cold is(are) false?
   a) adults are affected less than children
   b) the highest incidence of the common cold is among children of kindergarten age
   c) adults with young children at home have an increased number of colds
   d) infants with older siblings have an increased incidence of colds
   e) none of the above are false; all of the above are true

5. Which of the following statements regarding treatment of the condition described is true?
   a) the use of antibiotics in the condition described has been shown to decrease the probability of complications; their routine use is reasonable
   b) vitamin C has been shown to decrease the frequency of occurrences of the condition described
   c) interferon has been shown to prevent the majority of rhinovirus-caused upper respiratory tract infections
   d) rhinoviruses associated with the condition described have not been shown to be temperature sensitive
   e) antihistamines have not been shown to be effective in reducing symptoms in the condition described

6. Children of kindergarten age are subject to how many colds on an average yearly basis?
   a) 12
   b) 7
   c) 3
   d) 6
   e) 8

7. What is the most effective preventive measure against the common cold?
   a) megadoses of vitamin C
   b) meticulous handwashing
   c) extra sleep
   d) avoiding all contact with children and adults who have a cold
   e) none of the above

Short Answer Management Problem 92

A 28-year-old male presents to your office with "a cold." He has had the cold for approximately 10 days and his rhinorrhea, cough, and congestion continue. He tells you that his wife has just seen her family doctor for the same symptoms. An antibiotic was prescribed for his wife, and he asks you to prescribe the same for him. On examination he has nasal congestion and a hyperemic throat. No other abnormalities are found. Discuss your approach to this patient's request.

ANSWERS

1. E. This child most likely has the common cold. Although the fullness in his ears may be associated with fluid in the middle-ear cavity, the absence of fever, pain, and hyperemia on the tympanic membranes makes acute otitis media unlikely. Movement of the tympanic membranes would further clarify the likelihood of fluid collection in the middle ear.

   The presence of a runny nose and a cough significantly diminishes the probability of streptococcal pharyngitis.

   Although viral pneumonia or *Mycoplasma* pneumonia may develop, there is no evidence of either of these now.

2. B. The most common cause of the common cold is a rhinovirus. Rhinoviruses are responsible for approximately 25% of all cases of the common cold. Influenza viruses; parainfluenzae types A, B, and C; respiratory syncytial viruses; and mumps and measles viruses are responsible for many others. Other viruses that cause coldlike symptoms include coronaviruses, adenoviruses, certain ECHO viruses, and coxsackieviruses.

   More than 100 sero-specific rhinovirus types have been established, and many viruses remain untyped.

   The absence of significant fever, cervical lymphadenopathy, and exudates along with the presence of rhinorrhea and cough significantly decrease the probability of *Streptococcus pneumoniae* as a cause of this patient's symptoms.

3. E. At the present time no investigations should be initiated. As the pretest probability of a streptococcal pharyngitis is very low, it is inappropriate to order a CBC, a throat swab, a rapid antigen test for streptococcus, or any other investigations at the present time.

4. E. In general the common cold affects children significantly more frequently than adults. The highest incidence is among children of kindergarten age. Adults with young children in the home do themselves have an increased number of colds, as do infants with older siblings. At times parents often notice the latter (the "second sibling syndrome") and sometimes need reassurance that their children do not have some other constitutional weakness.

5. C. Interferon has been used experimentally as a nasal spray and when studied has been shown to prevent 75% of rhinovirus-caused colds. It may hold promise as a future prophylactic measure.

   Antibiotics have not been shown to reduce the incidence of complications and thus should not be used in a prophylactic fashion.

   Vitamin C, although extremely controversial, has not been shown to be effective in reducing the frequency or severity of symptoms. This is, however, a difficult area to study objectively because of problems associated with measuring improvement in symptoms.

   Rhinoviruses are temperature sensitive. A controlled study testing warm (30°) humidified air against hot (45°) humidified air to provide nasal hyperthermia for 20 to 30 minutes has demonstrated a significant reduction in the severity and duration of common cold symptoms. Thus it may be that this "old-fashioned" remedy has some basis in fact.

   Antihistamines have been found to be helpful in reducing symptoms of the common cold. Antihistamines act through nonspecific sedating or anticholinergic mechanisms rather than through any histamine-releasing action of the virus. As well, pseudoephedrine, alone or in combination with antihistamines, is also effective in reducing symptoms. Analgesics, such as acetylsalicylic acid or acetaminophen, have not been shown to have any significant effect on the duration or the severity of the common cold.

6. A. Children of kindergarten age are subject to an average of 12 colds annually, whereas school-aged children are subject to an average of 7 colds annually. Adolescents and adults are subject to an average of 3 colds annually.

7. B. The most effective preventive measure against the common cold is meticulous handwashing and avoidance of contact with the face or nose. There is increasing evidence that aerosol spread of the cold viruses is less important than indirect spread. Experiments suggest that cold-causing viruses can be spread by self-inoculation from deposits of virus on such surfaces as plastics to the surface of the finger, and then transferred to mucous membranes of the nose and eye. This is particularly true if the inoculum is still moist.

Extra sleep and megadoses of vitamin C have not been shown to be at all effective.

It is unrealistic to suggest avoiding all contact with children and adults who have colds. Cold viruses are everywhere and will continue to be everywhere.

SOLUTION TO SHORT ANSWER MANAGEMENT PROBLEM 92

The prescription of antibiotics for an obviously viral infection (the common cold is probably the best example) is likely the most frequent "mistake" made by family physicians. It is obviously a lot easier to prescribe an antibiotic for the child than to explain to the parent why one is not needed. Considering that upper respiratory tract infections are the most frequent presenting complaint to a family physician's office, this "mistake" may actually happen several times/day in an average practice. A reasonable approach to take to this patient's request may be as follows:

1. Explain the viral nature of the symptoms and your certainty in coming to that conclusion in the patient.
2. Explain the side effects of antibiotics including drug intolerance, drug allergy, and the possibility of creating an environment in the patient's body that promotes the growth of resistant organisms.
3. Carefully go over some alternatives to antibiotic therapy that the patient may pursue. These include the use of steam, the use of antihistamines for symptomatic relief, and the importance of adequate rest.
4. Take the opportunity to discuss how meticulous hand-washing and related hygienic measures can significantly decrease spread of the common cold among family members.
5. Repeat the following age-old edict to the patient: "The symptoms will abate in a week with antibiotics and in 7 days without" (Having said that, remember that 30% of patients with common cold symptoms who had visited a physician still had a cough and a runny nose by the eighth day.)
6. Do not compromise your principles and prescribe an antibiotic when you know it is at best not indicated and possibly harmful. If the patient insists on an antibiotic, consider this an opportunity to discuss your philosophy of care with the patient: have the patient consider whether or not he is comfortable with the advice you are giving. If not, you should ask the patient if he really wishes to continue as a patient in your practice.

This can actually be done in a very pleasant manner. My experience suggests that there is rarely a problem in reaching a mutually agreeable position. It really comes down to a question of trust between the patient and the physician.

SUMMARY OF THE DIAGNOSIS AND TREATMENT OF THE COMMON COLD

1. As the most common presentation of an upper respiratory tract infection, it is the most common problem presenting to the family physician.
2. Viral infections are the major if not the only cause of common colds.
3. Rhinovirus is the most common pathogen (25%); influenza; parainfluenza A, B, and C; and respiratory syncytial virus make up another 15%.
4. No laboratory investigations are necessary: the combination of rhinorrhea, cough, congestion, sneezing, and a sore throat (or some reasonable combination) in the absence of significant fever, cervical nodes, or an exudate virtually rules out streptococcal pharyngitis.
5. Prevention of spread to family members is best accomplished by meticulous hygiene. Self-inoculation is more important than aerosol spread.
6. Treatment is symptomatic: steam and antihistamines. Interferon given prophylactically may hold some hope for the future.
7. Resist the temptation to prescribe antibiotics. Remember, "a week with antibiotics, 7 days without."

SUGGESTED READING

Saroea HG. Common colds: Causes, potential cures, and treatment. Canadian Family Physician 1993; 39:2215-2220.

PROBLEM 93   A 4-YEAR-OLD BOY WITH AN EXTREMELY SORE THROAT

A 4-year-old male presents with his mother to your office. He has had a fever, chills, pain on swallowing, and pain in both ears for the past 3 days.

On examination, the child has a temperature of 39.5° C. He has tender anterior cervical lymphadenopathy and exudates on both tonsils. There is no hepatomegaly or splenomegaly present. He has no rhinorrhea, no cough, and no other respiratory tract symptoms. He is developing a fine macular-papular rash over his body.

He had a similar episode of sore throat 6 months ago, and another episode 15 months ago. He has had no other significant illnesses. He has no allergies.

SELECT THE ONE BEST ANSWER TO THE FOLLOWING QUESTIONS

1. What is the most likely diagnosis in this child?
   a) bilateral otitis media
   b) non-beta-hemolytic streptococcal pharyngitis
   c) group A beta-hemolytic streptococcal pharyngitis
   d) infectious mononucleosis
   e) none of the above

2. At this time, what would you do?
   a) perform a throat culture; wait before treating
   b) perform a throat culture and begin treatment with penicillin
   c) begin treatment with penicillin; no throat culture
   d) do not test and do not treat
   e) nobody really knows for sure

3. Regarding culture-confirmed streptococcal pharyngitis in childhood, which of the following statements is(are) true?
   a) 80% of children with culture-confirmed streptococcal pharyngitis have tonsillar exudates
   b) if pharyngitis is accompanied by exudates, 80% have culture-confirmed streptococcal pharyngitis
   c) of all children with clinically documented pharyngitis, only 15% have culture-proven streptococcal pharyngitis
   d) all of the above are true
   e) none of the above are true

4. Scarlet fever is caused by which of the following organisms?
   a) non-beta-hemolytic streptococcus
   b) group A beta-hemolytic streptococcus
   c) group B beta-hemolytic streptococcus
   d) group D streptococcus
   e) Lancefield group G streptococcus

5. What percentage of children have group A streptococci as part of the normal flora of the mouth and pharynx?
   a) 5%-10%
   b) 10%-15%
   c) 15%-20%

   d) 25%-35%
   e) 35%-50%

6. What is the most common organism responsible for bacterial endocarditis in children?
   a) group A beta-hemolytic streptococcus
   b) group B beta-hemolytic streptococcus
   c) group D streptococcus (*Enterococcus*)
   d) *Streptococcus viridans*
   e) group A non-beta-hemolytic streptococcus

7. What is the most common cause of neonatal septicemia and meningitis?
   a) group B streptococcus
   b) group A beta-hemolytic streptococcus
   c) group D streptococcus (*Enterococci*)
   d) *Streptococcus viridans*
   e) group A non-beta-hemolytic streptococcus

8. Erysipelas is most commonly caused by which of the following?
   a) group A beta-hemolytic streptococcus
   b) *Streptococcus pneumoniae*
   c) group B streptococcus
   d) *Streptococcus viridans*
   e) Lancefield group G streptococcus

9. Which of the following statements concerning impetigo (pyoderma) is(are) true?
   a) deeper skin infections (cellulitis) may complicate impetigo
   b) impetigo is most frequently caused by group A beta-hemolytic streptococcus
   c) colonization of unbroken skin usually precedes impetigo by 7-10 days
   d) all of the above
   e) none of the above

10. Which of the following statements concerning the ELISA streptozyme test is(are) true?
   a) the ELISA streptozyme test has a very high sensitivity
   b) the ELISA streptozyme test has a very high specificity
   c) the ELISA streptozyme test has a very low false positive rate

d) the ELISA streptozyme test has a very low false negative rate
e) b and c
f) a and d

11. Recurrent tonsillitis is usually caused by which of the following?
   a) group A beta-hemolytic streptococcus
   b) parainfluenzae virus
   c) rhinovirus
   d) adenovirus
   e) Epstein-Barr virus

12. Which of the following statements regarding tonsillitis and recurrent sore throat is(are) correct?
   a) tonsillectomy often decreases the frequency of recurrent sore throat in young children
   b) in many cases children who have not undergone a tonsillectomy experience a similar decrease in recurrent sore throat
   c) tonsillectomy often decreases the frequency of recurrent upper respiratory tract infection (colds) in young children
   d) a and b
   e) all of the above
   f) none of the above

13. Regarding tonsillar size and the frequency of tonsillitis, which of the following statements is(are) true?
   a) most hypertrophic tonsils are actually normal in size
   b) in children, tonsils are relatively larger in younger children than in older children
   c) hypertrophic (larger) tonsils are more likely to become infected than nonhypertrophic (smaller) tonsils
   d) a and b
   e) all of the above

14. Which of the following is(are) complications of tonsillectomy?
   a) hemorrhage
   b) postoperative throat infection
   c) pulmonary edema
   d) a and b
   e) all of the above

15. Which of the following is(are) manifestations of adenoidal hypertrophy?
   a) mouth breathing
   b) persistent rhinitis
   c) snoring
   d) a and c
   e) all of the above

Short Answer Management Problem 93

List the definite indications for the performance of a tonsillectomy.

ANSWERS

1. C.

2. B.

3. C. The most likely diagnosis in this child is group A beta-hemolytic streptococcal pharyngitis. The ear pain that the boy is experiencing is most likely referred pain from the throat. The absence of other symptoms (rhinorrhea, cough) favors bacterial pharyngitis over viral pharyngitis, although this is by no means certain. At this time you should do the following:
   A. Make a provisional diagnosis of group A beta-hemolytic streptococcal infection.
   B. Culture the exudates bilaterally.
   C. Begin the child on penicillin V in a mg/kg dose three or four times per day.
   D. Await the results of the throat culture.

There are a number of advantages to performing a throat culture and starting the child on penicillin at the same time:
1. Early treatment with penicillin reduces the severity of symptoms from group A beta-hemolytic *Streptococcus* and decreases the time to resolution of symptoms.
2. Early treatment of group A beta-hemolytic *Streptococcus* infections reduces the incidence of subsequent rheumatic fever; it does, not, however, reduce the incidence of post-streptococcal glomerulonephritis.
3. Early treatment of group A beta-hemolytic *Streptococcus* decreases the incidence of sibling and family colonization, subsequent infection, and the so-called ping-pong effect of colonization and recolonization.

Although 30% of children with a sore throat have a positive throat culture for group A beta-hemolytic *streptococcus,* only 50% of these have a positive antibody response indicative of acute infection rather than colonization. Streptococcal pharyngitis is suggested by age greater than 5 years, tender anterior cervical lymphadenopathy, scarlatiniform rash, and a history of exposure. Only 15% of children with pharyngitis and 25% of children with exudates have streptococcal infection; as well, 30% of those with streptococcal pharyngitis do not have tonsillar exudates.

Throat culture is the most accurate laboratory aid in making a diagnosis of acute tonsillitis or pharyngitis.

4. B. Scarlet fever is caused by group A beta-hemolytic streptococcus.

    The patient described in Question 1 has the characteristic features of scarlet fever, which is described in detail in another chapter of this book.

5. C. In 15%-20% of children with group A beta-hemolytic streptococcus, the group A beta-hemolytic streptococcus is a normal commensal organism. This makes the interpretation of the throat swab difficult due to the false positives produced.

6. D. The causative organism of bacterial endocarditis in children is *Streptococcus viridans.* Bacterial endocarditis due to *Streptococcus viridans* may follow one of three patterns:
    a) A protracted course featuring prolonged fever (often the only manifestation for several months)
    b) An acute course with high fever and prostration
    c) Symptoms that are nonspecific and consist of low-grade fever with afternoon elevations, fatigue, myalgias, arthralgia, headache, chills, nausea, and vomiting

7. A. Group B *Streptococcus* is the most common cause of neonatal septicemia and neonatal meningitis. Group B streptococcus is the organism cultured for in the last trimester of pregnancy, and which the neonate usually acquires as he or she passes through the birth canal. To significantly decrease the probability of neonatal group B streptococcal infection, it is recommended that all pregnant women have a cervical culture performed at 34-36 weeks, and those who test positive be treated.

8. A. Erysipelas is an acute, well-demarcated infection of the skin involving the face (associated with pharyngitis) and extremities (associated with wounds). With erysipelas the skin is erythematous and indurated; the margins of the lesions have a raised, firm, border. Associated symptoms include fever, vomiting, and irritability.

Erysipelas is caused by group A beta-hemolytic streptococcus.

9. D. Impetigo (pyoderma) is the most common form of skin infection due to Group A beta-hemolytic streptococci. Colonization of unbroken skin precedes pyoderma by 7-10 days. Skin lesions including impetigo and cellulitis develop following intradermal inoculation by insect bites, scabies, or minor trauma. Deeper soft tissue infections may occur secondary to impetigo. Streptococcal cellulitis is a painful, erythematous, indurated infection of the skin and subcutaneous tissues. Lymphangitis and regional lymphadenitis are common.

    The other major causative organism of impetigo and other skin infections is *Staphylococcus aureus.*

10. E. The streptozyme slide test is a test designed to detect antibodies against multiple streptococcal extracellular antigens. This test detects more patients with increased antibody titers than any other test. It has a very high specificity and a very low false positive rate. The sensitivity of the test, and therefore the false negative rate, is much higher. In clinical terms, therefore, if a test is positive you can assume the patient has the disease; if it is negative, on the other hand, you cannot assume anything.

    The "gold standard" for the diagnosis of streptococcal pharyngitis remains the throat culture. It should be performed in most patients suspected of having streptococcal pharyngitis.

11. A. Recurrent tonsillitis is almost always caused by group A beta-hemolytic streptococci. We must, however, differentiate between cases of clinically suspected streptococcal tonsillitis and culture-proven streptococcal tonsillitis.

    Often a parent will present to your office with a child, complaining that the child has "continual tonsillitis" or "recurrent tonsillitis." It is very important to document whether or not these cases of tonsillitis are culture-proven group A streptococcal tonsillitis or simply recurrent pharyngitis assumed to be streptococcal. This is especially important when the issue of tonsillectomy for recurrent tonsillitis is raised.

12. D. Tonsillectomy will often decrease the frequency of recurrent sore throats in young children. This same decrease in the frequency of recurrent sore throats, however, often occurs in children as they grow older anyway (in spite of not having had a tonsillectomy). It is difficult, therefore, to suggest a "relative value" of tonsillectomy in this age group and for this reason.

    Tonsillectomy, does not, however, decrease the incidence of recurrent upper respiratory tract infections (colds) in young children. Thus an important distinction exists between recurrent sore throats and recurrent upper respiratory tract infections in relationship to the efficacy (or nonefficacy) of tonsillectomy.

13. D. Most hypertrophic tonsils are actually normal in size; the misinterpretation results from failure to appreciate that normally tonsils are relatively larger in young children than in older children. There is no evidence that hypertrophic (or larger) tonsils become infected any more frequently than nonhypertrophic (or smaller) tonsils.

14. E. Complications of tonsillectomy include minor hemorrhage, postoperative throat infection, severe postoperative hemorrhage, and pulmonary edema.

    Pulmonary edema is not uncommon after the relief of upper airway obstruction with tonsillectomy or adenoidectomy. It seems to be directly related to the relief of airway obstruction.

    The possibility of severe postoperative hemorrhage also makes this operation a risky procedure. The indications for the procedure (that will be discussed in the Short Answer Management Problem) should be followed closely.

15. E. Reasons for adenoidectomy include persistent mouth breathing, persistent rhinitis, chronic otitis, and persistent snoring.

SOLUTION TO SHORT ANSWER MANAGEMENT PROBLEM 93

The definite indications for the performance of a tonsillectomy include the following:
1. One episode of peritonsillar abscess (quinsy)
2. Airway obstruction (as a result of markedly hypertrophied tonsils)
3. Seven episodes of throat-culture-proven streptococcal tonsillitis in 1 year; five episodes of throat-culture-proven streptococcal tonsillitis per year in 2 successive years.

SUMMARY OF THE DIAGNOSIS AND TREATMENT OF STREPTOCOCCAL INFECTIONS IN CHILDREN

1. **Neonates:** group B streptococcus is now the most frequent cause of neonatal septicemia and meningitis.
2. **Streptococcal pharyngitis:**
   a) Only 15% of pharyngitis cases in children have Group A beta-hemolytic streptococcus as the cause.
   b) Streptococcal pharyngitis is suggested by the following:
      1. Age greater than 5 years
      2. High fever
      3. Tonsillar exudates
      4. Tender anterior cervical lymphadenopathy
      5. Scarliniform rash
      6. History of exposure

      7. Absence of cough
      8. Absence of rhinitis
   c) Only 25% of patients with exudates have streptococcal pharyngitis.
   d) Although some authorities believe that the predictive value of physicians in distinguishing streptococcal pharyngitis from viral pharyngitis is at best 50%, in the presence of either cough or rhinitis, the probability of streptococcal pharyngitis is very low.
   e) 15%-20% of children carry group A beta-hemolytic streptococcus as a normal commensal organism.
3. **Erysipelas:** acute well-demarcated infection of the skin caused by group A beta-hemolytic streptococcus
4. **Impetigo:** impetigo is caused primarily by group A beta-hemolytic streptococcus. Impetigo may lead to more serious conditions such as cellulitis. The other significant cause is *Staphylococcus aureus.*
5. **Bacterial endocarditis:** bacterial endocarditis in children is caused by *Streptococcus viridans.*
6. **Tonsillitis and tonsillectomy:** tonsillitis should be performed only when there is one episode of peritonsillar abscess (quinsy), a history of airway obstruction, or seven documented episodes of group A beta-hemolytic streptococcus in 1 year or five documented episodes in each of 2 successive years.
   Remember:
   1. Most hypertrophied tonsils are normal tonsils.
   2. Tonsils grow smaller as the child grows older.
   3. Large tonsils are no more prone to tonsillitis than small tonsils.
   4. Not all tonsillitis is due to beta-hemolytic streptococcus (approximately 25%; the other 75% of causes are viral in origin).
7. **Adenoids and adenoidectomy:**
   a) The only indication that is similar for both tonsillectomy and adenoidectomy is airway obstruction.
   b) The other indications for adenoidectomy are chronic otitis media and chronic rhinitis.
8. **Other streptococcal infections:** human infection with streptococci of groups C, D, E, F, G, H, K, L, M, N, and O has been reported in normal infants and children. Penicillin G provides effective therapy for non-group-A streptococci except for group D (*Enterococci*). This organism is generally susceptible to ampicillin.
9. **Treatment for streptococcal infections:**
   a) Group A beta-hemolytic streptococcal pharyngitis: culture and begin treatment with penicillin V for 10 days. In nonreliable patients use benzathine penicillin G.
   b) *Streptococcus viridans:* bacterial endocarditis: use ampicillin plus an aminoglycoside.
   c) Infection with Lancefield group G streptococci has been recognized as an increasingly serious and frequent cause of human disease. This group can cause endovascular infection, endocarditis, and septic arthritis.

d) Early treatment of group A beta-hemolytic strepto-coccal pharyngitis does the following:
   1. Decreases the virulence and severity of the infection
   2. Decreases the length of symptoms of the infection
   3. Protects against rheumatic fever, an increasing problem once again in the United States.

It does not, however, protect against post-streptococcal glomerulonephritis.

SUGGESTED READING

Behrman R, ed. Streptococcal infections. Nelson textbook of pediatrics. 14th Ed. Philadelphia: WB Saunders, 1992.

PROBLEM 94   A 1-YEAR-OLD BOY WITH A RASH AND A FEVER

A 1-year-old boy is brought to your office by his mother. The child was well until 3 days ago when he developed a fever of 40° C. The child's mother has been trying to keep the fever down with acetaminophen. Today the child's temperature suddenly dropped, and at the same time he developed a skin rash.

On physical examination, the child does not look ill. His temperature has come down to 38° C. He has a fine (in texture) erythematous maculopapular eruption over his entire body. His nose is running and his throat is slightly hyperemic. His lungs are clear. His blood pressure is 75/50 mm Hg and his pulse is 124 and regular. His abdominal, musculoskeletal, and neurological examinations are normal.

SELECT THE ONE BEST ANSWER TO THE FOLLOWING QUESTIONS

1. What is the most likely diagnosis in this child at this time?
   a) exanthem subitem
   b) erythema infectiosum
   c) adenoviral exanthem
   d) rubella
   e) rubeola

2. What is the most outstanding feature of this illness?
   a) the rapid fall in the temperature
   b) the rapid rise in the temperature
   c) the appearance of the rash at the same time as the temperature falls
   d) the absence of physical signs to explain the (usually) extremely high temperature
   e) the complication of Reye's syndrome that is directly linked to the causative agent

3. What is the causative agent of the condition described?
   a) human parvovirus
   b) human papilloma virus
   c) human herpes virus
   d) adenovirus
   e) rhinovirus

4. A 5-year-old boy is brought to your office by his father. He has been running a low-grade fever for the past 24 hours. This afternoon he suddenly developed a bright red rash on both cheeks.
   On physical examination, the child has erythema of the cheeks, as well as the beginning of a maculopapular rash on the trunk and the extremities. No other abnormalities are noted on examination.
   What is the most likely diagnosis in this child?
   a) exanthem subitem
   b) erythema infectiosum
   c) adenoviral exanthem
   d) rubella
   e) rubeola

5. What is the causative agent of the condition described on Question 4?
   a) human papilloma virus
   b) adenovirus
   c) human parvovirus
   d) human herpes virus
   e) rhinovirus

6. The characteristic rash of the condition described in Question 4 is morphologically best linked to which of the following descriptions of facial rash appearance and appearance of the rash on the trunk?
   a) circumoral pallor and sandpaperlike appearance of trunk
   b) slapped-cheek appearance and lacy-reticular pattern
   c) fine pustular appearance and right red maculopapular rash with central clearing
   d) coalesced erythemalike appearance and solid macular rash
   e) none of the above

7. A 4-year-old female presents with her mother to your busy afternoon office for assessment and treatment of fever and a skin rash.
   The child's present illness began with very mild upper respiratory tract symptoms approximately 1 week ago. Then, last night, the child complained to her father of pain behind her ears. This morning a maculopapular rash that began on the face appears to be spreading distally.
   This child has not seen a physician, a nurse practitioner, or a public health nurse or clinic since birth. Her mother basically does not believe in anything the medical profession has to offer. She brought the child in to see you today only because her teacher threatened to keep her out of school until she had a doctor's note that authorized her return.
   On examination, the child's temperature is 38.8° C. Examination of the head and neck reveals a moderately injected pharynx, a "flushed face," a slight reddening of the conjunctiva bilaterally, and coryza.
   The child appears what you would term "slightly ill."
   What is the most likely diagnosis in this child?
   a) exanthem subitem
   b) erythema infectiosum
   c) adenoviral exanthem
   d) rubella
   e) rubeola

8. Which of the following statements is(are) true concerning the condition described in Question 7?
   a) this condition is a self-limiting condition that poses no significant risk to anyone
   b) this condition is caused by human parvovirus B27
   c) this condition is likely to reoccur several times during childhood
   d) there is no protection available for the prevention of this condition
   e) none of the above statements are true

9. The American Academy of Pediatrics recommends which of the following for the treatment and/or prevention of this condition?
   a) no antibiotics; no vaccination in childhood
   b) no antibiotics; yearly vaccination in childhood
   c) no antibiotics; an antiviral agent to prevent complications
   d) no antibiotics; two vaccinations in childhood
   e) antibiotics; no vaccinations in childhood

10. A pregnant woman presents to your office for her first prenatal visit at 8 weeks' gestation. She has her routine blood work done and you determine her rubella titer to be < 1/8. Three weeks later her 18-month-old son (who has not received any immunizations to date) develops rubella. She is aware of the risk of congenital rubella syndrome developing in the fetus but indicates to you that under no conditions would she consider a therapeutic abortion.

    At this time, what should you do?
    a) immunize her with live rubella virus vaccine
    b) immunize her with attenuated rubella virus vaccine
    c) immunize her with inactivated rubella virus vaccine
    d) provide passive protection to her with an injection of immune serum globulin (ISG)
    e) inform her that under the circumstances "your hands are tied"

11. A 4-year-old male, previously unimmunized, presents to your office with a 5-day history of fever, a dry hacking cough, coryza, and conjunctivitis. This morning the child's temperature rose to 40° C and a fine maculopapular rash appeared on his face, his upper arms, and the upper part of his chest. The other significant symptom is photophobia.

    On examination, there is significant posterior cervical lymphadenopathy. There is marked conjunctival injection bilaterally. There is a diffuse maculopapular eruption over the face, arms, and chest that appears to be spreading onto the back and the thighs.

    What is the most likely diagnosis in this patient?
    a) exanthem subitem
    b) erythema infectiosum
    c) adenoviral exanthem

   d) rubella
   e) rubeola

12. Which of the following is(are) characteristic of the disease described in Question 11?
    a) Koplik's spots
    b) coryza
    c) conjunctivitis
    d) cough
    e) all of the above

13. An 8-year-old male presents to your office with his father. The child has been ill for 3 days. The illness began as a fever that reached 39° C. Associated with the fever have been chills, vomiting, and headache.

    On P/E, the child has a hyperemic pharynx and tonsillar areas. The tonsils are covered with exudate. The dorsum of the tongue has a white coat and also appears edematous. There is a generalized, fine maculopapular rash that has the consistency of sandpaper. The child has a flushed forehead and flushed cheeks, and the area around the child's mouth is pale (circumoral pallor).

    What is the most likely diagnosis?
    a) erythema infectiosum
    b) adenoviral exanthem
    c) rubella
    d) rubeola
    e) none of the above

14. What is the causative agent in this child's illness?
    a) human parvovirus
    b) human adenovirus
    c) paramyxoviridae: genus *Morbillivirus*
    d) group A beta-hemolytic *Streptococcus*
    e) togaviridae: genus *Rubivirus*

Questions 15-25 are matching questions. Eleven disease-producing pathogens/disease entities are listed in the left-hand column and 11 disease-defining characteristics in the right-hand column. Beside each disease-producing pathogen/disease entity, put the letter of the disease-defining characteristic to which it corresponds.

15. Herpes varicella	a) discrete, dome-shaped papules
16. Herpes simplex virus	b) Herald patch
17. Coxsackievirus A 16 virus	c) erythema chronicum migrans
18. Kawasaki disease	d) hand-foot-and-mouth disease
19. Adenovirus	e) acute gingivostomatitis
20. Lyme disease	f) ringworm
21. Parainfluenza virus	g) #1 cause: conjunctivitis
22. Tinea versicolor	h) #1 cause: infectious croup
23. Tinea corporis	i) hyper/hypo pigmented lesions
24. Pityriasis rosea	j) coronary vasculitis
25. Molluscum contagiosum	k) "crops of lesions": vesicles

Short Answer Management Problem 94

Define the following terms, which are the primary skin lesions seen in children: a) macule; b) papule; c) nodule; d) vesicle; e) bullae; f) pustule; g) wheal; and h) cyst.

ANSWERS

1. A.

2. D.

3. C. The most likely diagnosis in this child is exanthem subitem (roseola infantum).

   Exanthem subitem is a viral illness of infants and young children that initially presents with a high fever that typically lasts for 3 or 4 days. Usually there are no physical findings to explain the fever, and the child looks generally well. As the child's temperature falls (often rapidly), a fine maculopapular rash appears over the entire body that lasts for approximately 24 hours.

   The causative agent of exanthem subitem is human herpesvirus type 6.

   The treatment of exanthem subitem is symptomatic only. Acetaminophen should be administered if the temperature exceeds 40° C.

   The most outstanding feature of exanthem subitem is the inability to explain to any degree the very high fever that this condition produces. The rapid fall of the temperature and the appearance of the rash at the same time that the fever falls are not as "outstanding" as the inability to explain the high fever. There are sometimes very minor physical signs such as slight reddening of the throat, but nowhere near the degree of signs/symptoms that would explain the high fever.

4. B.

5. C.

6. B. This child has erythema infectiosum. Erythema infectiosum is caused by a human parvovirus—parvovirus B19. The infection begins as a low-grade fever and produces a "slapped-cheek" rash appearance on the face associated with a lacy, reticularlike maculopapular rash pattern on the trunk and extremities. The rash may last from a few days to several weeks. It is frequently pruritic. Recurrences after exercise or after application of heat or emotional upset are not uncommon.

   Constitutional symptoms of this infection include the following: headache, pharyngitis, myalgia, arthritis, GI upset, coryza.

   There are no diagnostic tests for this condition.

The differential diagnosis of erythema infectiosum includes rubella, atypical rubeola, drug-induced rashes, and other viral exanthems.

7. D.

8. E.

9. D. This child has rubella, or German measles, as it is commonly known. Rubella is caused by a pleomorphic, RNA-containing virus currently listed in the family of viruses named Togaviridae, genus *Rubivirus.*

   The American Academy of Pediatrics recommends immunization against rubella twice in childhood: first at 12-15 months, and then again at 4-6 years. With reference to the other part of Question 9, antibiotics are not recommended.

   The statements given in Question 8 are all false, for the following reasons:
   a) This is a self-limiting condition that in no group of patients causes any significant risk.
      False: Pregnant women are at moderately severe risk for rubella if they have no antibodies against it.
   b) This condition is caused by human parvovirus B27.
      False: This condition is caused by Togaviridae virus, genus *Rubivirus.*
   c) This condition is likely to recur several times during childhood.
      False: once rubella has been contacted for sure on one occasion, active immune status is produced. The condition can occur again in the same individual, but it is extremely unlikely.
   d) There is no protection available for the prevention of this condition.
      False: a Rubella live-virus vaccine, RA 27/3, is used extensively in the United States as an immunization against rubella.

   Rubella usually begins with symptoms of a mild upper respiratory tract infection. There is significant tender retroauricular, posterior cervical, and postoccipital lymphadenopathy. In some cases of rubella, an enanthem covering the soft palate and fauces may appear prior to the onset of the rash.

   The exanthem usually begins on the face and spreads to cover the trunk. The rash is maculopapular, with areas of confluence and flushing. Mild pruritus is common. The rash usually clears by the third day. There is no associated photophobia and few complications; unusual complications include neuritis, arthritis, and encephalitis.

10. D. Pregnant women, especially early in pregnancy but also during the entire gestational period, should avoid exposure to rubella regardless of either history of the disease during childhood or history of active immunization. Exposure of pregnant women to infants with congenital rubella syndrome should be especially guarded against because of prolonged shedding of the virus.

Because therapeutic abortion has been rejected by this mother-to-be (you should certainly not advocate TA, but you should inform her of the risk of exposure of congenital rubella syndrome in her infant if she were to acquire the infection with a nonimmune status), you should provide passive protection to her with an intramuscular injection of immune serum globulin (ISG) given in a large dose (0.25-0.50 ml/kg or 0.12 or 0.20 ml/l b) within the first 7-8 days of exposure.

Pregnant women should not be given live rubella virus vaccine (live viral vaccine is the only rubella vaccine available).

11. E.

12. E. This child has rubeola. The prodromal phase of rubeola (red measles) is characterized by a low-grade to moderate fever, a dry hacking cough, coryza, and conjunctivitis. *Koplik spots* are grayish-white dots, usually as small as grains of sand, with slight, reddish areolae that are occasionally hemorrhagic. Their location tends to be opposite the lower molars, but they may spread irregularly over the rest of the buccal mucosa. Thus rubeola can be remembered by the following mnemonic, which refers to a copy of a letter sent to "cpk": cc-CPK.

c = cough
c = coryza
C = conjunctivitis
P = photophobia
K = Koplik spots

The temperature in rubeola rises as the rash appears. The maculopapular rash usually begins on the face and neck and spreads over the entire body from the neck down. By the time the rash reaches the feet, clinical improvement has begun.

Cervical lymphadenopathy may be prominent.

The major complications of rubeola are otitis media, bronchopneumonia, and gastrointestinal symptoms including vomiting and diarrhea.

Prevention against rubeola can be achieved with active immunization at 12-15 months. This is preferable to passive immunization (with gamma globulin) for disease attenuation.

13. E.

14. D. This child has scarlet fever.

Scarlet fever, which is caused by Group A betahemolytic streptococcus, usually begins with the abrupt onset of fever, vomiting, headaches, pharyngitis, and chills. The temperature usually peaks on the second day and gradually returns to normal within 5 to 7 days.

The tonsils are hyperemic and edematous and may be covered with an exudate. The throat is inflamed and may be covered by a membrane. The dorsum of the tongue often initially has a white coat, with projecting edematous papillae.

The exanthem usually consists of a finely papular or punctate group of lesions. It is sometimes described as having the consistency of sandpaper. The rash generally begins in the axillae, the groin, and the neck; within 24 hours it becomes generalized. The forehead and the cheeks may appear to be flushed and the area around the mouth (circumoral) is pale.

Desquamation usually begins on the face and proceeds to the hands and feet, and may continue for up to 6 weeks.

The treatment of choice for all group A betahemolytic streptococcus is penicillin. Amoxicillin is a better-tasting and acceptable alternative for children. If an allergy to penicillin exists, the drug of choice is erythromycin.

Of the other choices listed for causative agents, remember that *Morbillivirus* is the cause of rubeola and *Rubivirus* is the cause of rubella.

15. K. Viral agent: herpes varicella = chicken pox
Disease-defining characteristic: crops of small, red, papules, which develop into oval, "teardrop" vesicles on an erythematous base

16. E. Viral agent: herpes simplex virus
Disease-defining characteristic: acute herpetic gingivostomatitis—the most common cause of stomatitis in children ages 1-3

17. D. Viral agent: coxsackievirus A16
Disease-defining characteristic: hand-foot-mouth disease; an enteroviral exanthem-enanthem with the distribution portrayed by the name

18. J. Disease-entity: Kawasaki disease
Disease-defining characteristic: coronary vasculitis, also known as mucocutaneous lymph node syndrome or infantile polyarteritis. Cardiac involvement is the most important manifestation of Kawasaki disease (10% to 40% of children within the first 2 weeks of illness). Causal agent is either a retrovirus or *Rickettsia*.

19. G. Viral agent: adenovirus
Disease-defining characteristic: adenovirus is the single most common cause of conjunctivitis.

20. C. Disease entity: Lyme disease

    Disease-defining characteristic: erythema chronicum migrans; begins as an erythematous macule or papule at the site of a tick bite (causative organism: *Borrelia burgdorferi*) that develops into an expanding erythematous annular lesion with central clearing and often reaches a diameter of 16 cm.

21. H. Viral agent: parainfluenza virus

    Disease-defining characteristic: most common cause of infectious croup.

22. I. Disease entity: tinea versicolor

    Disease-defining characteristic: hypopigmented or hyperpigmented macules covered with a fine scale; lesions begin in a perifollicular location, enlarge, and form confluent patches, most commonly on the neck, upper chest, back, and upper arms. Causative organism is dimorphic yeast: *Pityrosporon orbiculare (Malassezia furfur)*.

23. F. Disease entity: tinea corporis

    Disease-defining characteristic: ringworm; common name for group of disorders known as dermatophytoses. The three principal genera responsible for dermatophyte infections are *Trichophyton*, *Microsporum*, and *Epidermophyton*. Classical lesion begins as a dry, mildly erythematous, elevated, scaly papule or plaque and spreads centrifugally as it clears centrally to form the characteristic annular lesion responsible for the designation *ringworm*.

24. B. Disease entity: pityriasis rosea

    Disease-defining characteristic: the herald patch. This is a solitary, round or oval lesion that may occur anywhere on the body and is often but not always identifiable by its large size. The herald patch usually precedes the generalized maculopapular eruption of oval or round lesions that crop.

25. A. Disease entity: molluscum contagiosum

    Disease-defining characteristic: describes a disorder characterized by discrete, dome-shaped papules varying in size from 1 to 5 mm. Typically these lesions have a central umbilication from which a cheesy material can be expressed. The papules may occur anywhere on the body, but the face, eyelids, neck, axillae, and thighs are sites of predilection. Causative agent is a DNA virus, the largest member of the poxvirus group.

SOLUTION TO SHORT ANSWER MANAGEMENT PROBLEM 94

A. *Macule:* an alteration in skin color that cannot be felt
B. *Papule:* palpable solid lesions smaller than 0.5-1.0 cm
C. *Nodule:* palpable solid lesions larger than 1.0 cm
D. *Vesicle:* raised, fluid-filled lesions less than 0.5 cm in diameter
E. *Bullae:* raised, fluid-filled lesions larger than 0.5 cm in diameter
F. *Pustules:* raised lesions that contain pustular material
G. *Wheals:* Flat-topped, palpable lesions of variable size and configuration that represent dermal collections of edema fluid
H. *Cyst:* circumscribed, thick-walled lesions that are located deep in the skin; are covered by a normal epidermis; and contain fluid or semisolid material

As so many conditions were described in this chapter, the summary will be limited to a discussion of what are termed the "big five" viral exanthems in children. (Note that *erythema infectiosum* is also known as "fifth disease.")

SUMMARY OF THE "BIG FIVE" VIRAL EXANTHEMS IN CHILDREN

1. **Exanthem subitem (roseola infantum):** high fever followed by defervescence with the appearance of an erythematous maculopapular rash at the same time
2. **Erythema infectiosum:** low-grade fever followed by the appearance of a rash: "slapped-cheek" appearance followed by a generalized lacy-reticular pattern rash
3. **Rubella:** mild fever; significant tender retroauricular, posterior, and postoccipital lymphadenopathy
4. **Rubeola:** prodromal symptoms include the "3 C's": cough, coryza, conjunctivitis. Koplik spots are pathognomonic. Photophobia is common. The temperature rises abruptly as the rash appears. The severity of the disease is directly related to the extent and confluence of the rash.

    Mnemonic: *cc-CPK (c = cough; c = coryza; C = conjunctivitis; P = photophobia; K = Koplik's spots*
5. **Scarlet fever:** group A beta-hemolytic streptococcal infection that presents as fever, chills, headache, vomiting, and pharyngitis. Exanthem has texture of coarse sandpaper. Circumoral pallor is common. Penicillin V is the drug of choice.

SUGGESTED READING

Behrman R, Klegnan RN, Nelson W, Vaughan VC eds. Nelson textbook of pediatrics. 14th Ed. Philadelphia: WB Saunders, 1992.

PROBLEM 95   A 2-DAY-OLD INFANT WITH PNEUMONIA

A 4000-g infant born at 39½ weeks' gestation appeared healthy at birth. His Apgars were 7 and 9. On the second day of life he begins to cough, his temperature increases to 40.5° C, his breathing becomes labored, and he appears ill.

His chest X-ray shows a reticulogranular pattern, a pattern that appears exactly like hyaline membrane disease. You also note the following on physical examination: apnea, tachypnea, grunting, flaring of the nares, and subcostal retractions. There are adventitious breath sounds heard in all lobes of the lungs.

SELECT THE ONE BEST ANSWER TO THE FOLLOWING QUESTIONS

1. Based on the information provided to this point, what is the most likely diagnosis?
   a) group A streptococcal pneumonia
   b) *Klebsiella* pneumonia
   c) adenoviral pneumonia
   d) group B streptococcal pneumonia
   e) staphylococcal pneumonia

2. What is the most likely source of this infant's infection?
   a) airborne droplets
   b) oral-fecal transmission
   c) direct spread from the mother
   d) intrauterine colonization
   e) none of the above

3. What is the treatment of choice in this child at this time?
   a) penicillin G
   b) amoxicillin
   c) trimethoprim-sulphamethoxazole
   d) clavulinic acid
   e) penicillin G plus metronidazole

4. A 3-year-old female presents with a 4-day history of fever, chills, nasal flaring, subcostal indrawing, and a harsh cough. The child is in respiratory distress.

   Prior to the onset of the present symptoms, the child had a recent respiratory tract infection. The child's symptoms were as follows: bilateral conjunctivitis, rhinorrhea, nonproductive cough, and sore throat.

   On physical examination the child's temperature is 39° C. Her respiratory rate is 32/minute. There are rales and rhonchi in all lobes. The child is using her accessory muscles of respiration, especially her intercostal muscles and sternocleidomastoid muscles.

   What is the most likely diagnosis in this case?
   a) *Mycoplasma* pneumonia
   b) adenoviral pneumonia
   c) *Streptococcus pneumoniae* pneumonia
   d) *Hemophilus influenzae* pneumonia
   e) group B streptococcal pneumonia

5. What is the most common etiologic agent responsible for pneumonia in children age 5 years and under?
   a) respiratory syncytial virus
   b) *Mycoplasma* pneumonia
   c) adenovirus
   d) *Streptococcus pneumoniae*
   e) *Haemophilus influenzae*

6. What is the most common bacterial etiologic agent responsible for pneumonia in children under the age of 5 years?
   a) *Streptococcus pneumoniae*
   b) *Staphyylococcus aureus*
   c) group A beta-hemolytic streptococcus
   d) *Haemophilus influenzae*
   e) *Klebsiella pneumoniae*

7. A child who is considered low risk for complications and who develops the clinical picture described in Question 4 should be treated with which of the following?
   a) ribavirin
   b) ampicillin
   c) erythromycin
   d) penicillin
   e) none of the above

8. A child who is considered high risk for complications and who develops the clinical picture described in Question 4 should be treated with which of the following?
   a) ribavirin
   b) ampicillin
   c) erythromycin
   d) hospitalization
   e) a plus d

9. A child who develops pneumonia secondary to the agent described in Question 6 and who is considered at high risk for complications should be treated with which of the following?
   a) ribavirin
   b) ampicillin
   c) penicillin G
   d) hospitalization
   e) c plus D

10. What is the most common pneumonia in children over the age of 5 years?
    a) *Mycoplasma* pneumonia
    b) streptococcal pneumonia
    c) respiratory syncytial virus pneumonia
    d) *Haemophilus influenzae* pneumonia
    e) adenovirus pneumonia

11. What is the most common bacterial agent responsible for pneumonia in children over the age of 5 years?
    a) *Streptococcus pneumoniae*
    b) *Haemophilus influenzae*
    c) *Staphylococcus aureus*
    d) *Klebsiella pneumoniae*
    e) group B streptococcus

12. Which of the following etiologic agents usually evolves into a pneumonia that often includes an empyema or a pleural effusion?
    a) *Streptococcus pneumoniae*
    b) *Staphylococcus aureus*
    c) group B streptococcus
    d) *Haemophilus influenzae*
    e) *Klebsiella pneumoniae*

Short Answer Management Problem 95

With respect to viral, *Mycoplasma*, and viral pneumonias in neonates, infants, and children, list the following:
a) The most common etiologic agent in the age group in question
b) The most common bacterial etiologic agent in the age group in question
c) The recommended treatment for each of the pneumonias in question

ANSWERS

1. D.

2. C.

3. A. This neonate has group B streptococcal pneumonia. This is primarily a disease of newborns who are colonized with the organism by passage through the birth canal, thus a direct spread from the mother.

   The treatment of choice for group B streptococcus is penicillin G. The recommended dose is 300,000 units penicillin G/kg/24 hours.

   The mortality rate from group B streptococcal pneumonia is still quite high: 10%-40%. Thus early diagnosis and treatment are critical.

4. B.

5. A.

6. A. First, considering the child presented in Question 4, the initial presentation of conjunctivitis, nonproductive cough, rhinorrhea, and sore throat is most compatible with adenoviral infection. The real "tipoff" in this case is the conjunctivitis, a symptom much more common with adenovirus infection than with any other virus infection.

   In the case described in Question 4, it appears that the sequence of events is as follows:
   1. Minor adenoviral upper respiratory tract infection proceeding to
   2. Adenoviral pneumonia

   The most common cause of pneumonia in children under the age of 5 years is respiratory syncytial viral pneumonia.

   The typical signs and symptoms of viral pneumonia in children include the following: dry, tight, and non-productive cough; fever/chills absent as frequently as present; and auscultatory findings including rhonchi, fine rales, and audible wheezing.

   In general, the younger the infant, the more severe the disease. Infants are prone to the most severe disease with symptoms that include significant respiratory distress, listlessness, and apnea.

   Radiographic findings are more likely to include air trapping, bilateral fine/fluffy infiltrates, and atelectasis. Secondary bacterial invasion must be considered when consolidation is present.

   In infants and children, the four most common viral agents causing pneumonia are as follows:
   1. Respiratory syncytial virus
   2. Parainfluenza virus
   3. Adenovirus
   4. Influenza virus (in children mostly influenza B)

   The most common bacterial cause of pneumonia in a child under the age of 5 years is *Streptococcus pneumoniae.*

   Bacterial pneumonias usually present with quite a different clinical picture. Signs and symptoms of bacterial pneumonias include fever, chills, cough productive of purulent sputum, pleuritic chest pain, and dyspnea and tachypnea. Also, the use of the accessory muscles of respiration is very common, especially in children.

   The chest X-ray will frequently show lobar consolidation. The CBC will often reveal an extremely high white blood cell count with a shift to the left.

7. E. The treatment of an infant or child with adenoviral pneumonia is symptomatic. No antibiotics or antiviral agents have been shown to be effective for the treatment of this infection. The major decision regarding this child will be whether or not hospitalization is necessary. This will depend on the child's clinical condition and most importantly, on the degree of respiratory distress that the child demonstrates.

If you even think about hospitalizing a child with pneumonia, do it. You will not have made a mistake.

8. D. The treatment of a child with adenoviral pneumonia at high risk for complications (congenital heart disease, cystic fibrosis, malignancy, chronic immunosuppression for another reason, primary immune deficiency) should be hospitalized and treated with supplementary oxygen (with or without a mist tent).

9. E. The treatment of choice for a child at high risk with a streptococcal pneumonia includes antibiotic therapy (penicillin G is still the drug of first choice) and hospitalization with supplementary oxygen and close monitoring. As the child improves, it is not uncommon for the chest X-ray changes to lag significantly behind the clinical improvement. In a child with this picture, arterial blood gases are also a very good way of measuring response to treatment and improvement.

10. A. The most common cause of pneumonia in children over the age of 5 years is *Mycoplasma pneumoniae*. In a child with mycoplasma pneumonia, there is often a significant discrepancy between the clinical findings and the radiological findings. The most important clinical symptom is a persistent, hacking, nonproductive cough that is difficult to treat. Often auscultation of the lungs will be normal. The CXR, on the other hand, may very well be quite revealing (with a significant bilateral infiltrate being the most common picture).

The treatment of choice for *Mycoplasma pneumoniae* in a child is erythromycin.

11. A. As in children under the age of 5 years, in children over the age of 5 years streptococcal pneumonia is the most common cause of bacterial pneumonia. This condition has been reviewed in Question 6.

12. B. The answer is staphylococcal pneumonia. Most patients with staphylococcal pneumonia have roentgenographic evidence of nonspecific bronchopneumonia early in the course of the illness. However, the infiltrate may soon become patchy and limited in extent or, on the other hand, dense and homogenous and involve an entire lobe or hemithorax. The right lung is involved in approximately 65% of cases; bilateral involvement occurs in fewer than 20% of cases. A pleural effusion or empyema is noted during the course of illness in most patients; pyopneumothorax occurs in approximately 25% of patients. Pneumatocele occur frequently and vary considerably in size.

Although no X-ray change can be considered diagnostic, progression over a few hours from bronchopneumonia to effusion or pyopneumothorax with or without pneumatocele is highly suggestive of staphylococcal pneumonia.

The treatment of choice for staphylococcal pneumonia is a semisynthetic, penicillinase-resistant penicillin given intravenously (such as methicillin).

SOLUTION TO SHORT ANSWER MANAGEMENT PROBLEM 95

Age Group 1: Birth to 5 Months
Most common etiologic agent: group B *streptococcus*

Most common bacterial agent: Group B *streptococcus*

Treatment for most common bacterial agent: penicillin G or ampicillin

Age Group 2: 5 Months to 5 Years
Most common etiologic agent: viral pneumonia. Most common cause: respiratory syncytial virus. Other viral agents: parainfluenza virus, adenovirus, influenza (type B)

Most common bacterial agent: *Streptococcus Pneumoniae*

Treatment for most common etiologic agent: symptomatic treatment only for mild to moderate cases; ribavirin for severe respiratory syncytial virus infection

Treatment for most common bacterial agent: penicillin G

Age Group 3: 5 Years and Older
Most common etiologic agent: *Mycoplasma pneumoniae*

Most common bacterial agent: *Streptococcus pneumoniae*

Treatment for most common etiologic agent: erythromycin (Note: tetracycline should not be used in children due to staining of teeth).

Treatment for most common bacterial agent: penicillin G

SUMMARY OF THE DIAGNOSIS AND TREATMENT OF CHILDHOOD PNEUMONIA

This is well summarized in the answer to the Short Answer Management Problem.

SUGGESTED READINGS

Greenberg S. Bacterial pneumonia. In: Rakel R, ed. Conn's current therapy. Philadelphia: WB Saunders, 1994.

Moskal MJ. Mycoplasma and viral pneumonia. In: Rakel R, ed. Conn's current therapy. Philadelphia: WB Saunders, 1994.

PROBLEM 96   A 9-MONTH-OLD INFANT WITH FEVER AND NO LOCALIZING SIGNS

A 9-month-old infant is seen in the ER for evaluation of fever. His mother states that he has had an intermittent fever of 39° C for 24 hours. She has used acetaminophen to treat the fever and has brought the temperature down to 38° C. The child has not been ill and has had no symptoms of upper respiratory tract infection or other symptoms.

The child has no history of serious illnesses, allergies, or other problems. He is on no medications.

On examination, the child is actively playing with his toys. He does not look toxic. His temperature is 39° C rectally. On examination, the head and neck, lungs, cardiovascular system, abdomen, neurological examination, and musculoskeletal system are normal.

Your clinical judgment suggests that this child has no serious illness.

SELECT THE ONE BEST ANSWER TO THE FOLLOWING QUESTIONS

1. What is the diagnosis in this child at this time?
   a) fever without a focus
   b) fever of unknown origin
   c) infantile febrile response
   d) fever of occult bacteremia
   e) none of the above

2. Fever of unknown origin is strictly defined as which of the following?
   a) fever in a child that persists for a time that exceeds 1 week in duration
   b) fever that continues once a child is hospitalized
   c) fever that continues despite at least 1 week of ongoing investigations
   d) all of the above
   e) a and c only

3. What is the most important diagnostic entity to consider in the infant?
   a) drug fever
   b) occult bacteremia
   c) factitious fever
   d) occult viremia
   e) collagen vascular disease

4. In the infant presented in the case history, what would be the most appropriate next step?
   a) obtain a more detailed history
   b) order a WBC count and ESR
   c) start the child on antibiotics
   d) send the child home on antipyretic therapy
   e) obtain a stat consultation with a pediatrician

5. If you are unable to obtain the necessary information based on the most appropriate action taken in Question 4, what is the next step?
   a) to perform a WBC
   b) to perform a lumbar puncture
   c) to perform an ESR
   d) to send the child home on antipyretic therapy
   e) to obtain a stat consultation with a pediatrician

6. In an infant between the ages of 3 months and 24 months, the probability of occult bacteremia is increased if
   a) the temperature is greater than 40° C
   b) the white blood cell count is < 5000/mm³
   c) the white blood cell count is > 15,000/mm³
   d) there is a positive exposure history
   e) all of the above increase probability

7. What is the most common organism responsible for occult bacteremia in infants?
   a) *Neisseria meningitidis*
   b) *Haemophilus influenzae*
   c) *Streptococcus pneumoniae*
   d) *Salmonella* species
   e) *Mycoplasma pneumoniae*

8. What is the most common condition in infants associated with occult bacteremia?
   a) pneumonia
   b) otitis media
   c) cellulitis
   d) gastroenteritis
   e) osteomyelitis

9. Which of the following statements regarding the presumptive use of antibiotic therapy in infants with fever without a focus is(are) true?
   a) presumptive use of oral antibiotics in infants with febrile illnesses decreases morbidity
   b) the earlier an antibotic is used the more significant the effect on morbidity
   c) presumptive oral antibiotics reliably prevent meningitis
   d) all of the above
   e) none of the above

10. A remittent fever pattern in an infant is defined as which of the following?
    a) a daily temperature elevation that returns neither to a baseline level or a normal level
    b) a daily temperature elevation that returns to a baseline but not to a normal level at least once a day
    c) a daily temperature elevation that returns to both a baseline and a normal level at least once/day

d) a daily temperature elevation that returns to a baseline but not to a normal level at least three times/day

e) a daily temperature elevation that returns to both a baseline and normal level three times/day

11. Which of the following statements regarding antipyretic therapy in infants and children is(are) true?
   a) all infants and children with pyrexia should be treated
   b) all high-risk infants and children with pyrexia should be treated
   c) antipyretic therapy alters the course of common infectious diseases in children
   d) antipyretic therapy alters the course of common infectious diseases in children regardless of the height of the temperature
   e) all of the above

12. Which of the following statements concerning antipyretic therapy in infants and children is(are) true?
   a) acetaminophen, aspirin, and NSAIDs are equally effective antipyretics in infants and children
   b) tepid sponge bathing in cool water (not alcohol) is recommended for reducing body temperature in infants and children
   c) aspirin and acetaminophen have an equal safety/efficacy ratio for reducing pyrexia in infants and children
   d) a and b
   e) all of the above

13. Fever, as defined as an elevation in body temperature, is mediated as a final common pathway by which of the following?
   a) endotoxins produced by the invading agent
   b) exotoxins produced by the invading agent
   c) antiendotoxins produced by the body in response to the invading agent
   d) antiexotoxins produced by the body in response to the invading agent
   e) production of endogenous pyrogens, which directly alter the hypothalamic temperature set-point

14. The signal to the hypothalamus to reset the heat regulatory set point is mediated by which of the following?
   a) endogenous-produced cytokines
   b) exogenous-produced cytokines
   c) endogenous macrophages
   d) endogenous monocytes
   e) type B lymphocytes

15. A 2-year-old infant develops a temperature of 39° C. He began complaining of a sore right ear this afternoon. His mother called you and you asked her to meet you at the hospital this evening. On the way to the hospital, the child had a "convulsion."

   When the mother arrived at the hospital, the ictal phase was over. The infant appeared slightly lethargic. His temperature was 39.5° C rectally. His right tympanic membrane was red and bulging. The rest of the P/E was normal.

   Which of the following is(are) characteristics of febrile convulsions in infants and children?
   a) the onset is usually between age 6 months and age 5 years
   b) the convulsion is usually of short duration (< 15 minutes)
   c) the convulsion is usually a generalized tonic-clonic pattern
   d) there is usually no focal or lateralizing features
   e) all of the above

Short Answer Management Problem 96

Describe a reasonable approach to the diagnosis and treatment of fever without a focus in an infant of age 1 year.

ANSWERS

1. A.

2. D. This infant has fever without a focus. Fever without localizing signs and symptoms is a common diagnostic dilemma for pediatricians caring for infants < 24 months of age. Fever is usually of acute onset and present for less than 1 week. Age is a very significant risk factor; the younger the infant, the greater the risk.

   Fever occurs when various infectious and noninfectious processes interact with the infant's defense mechanisms. In most children fever is either due to an identifiable microbiologic agent or subsides after a short time.

   Fever in children is best classified in the following manner:
   1. Fever of short duration with localizing signs in which the diagnosis can be established by clinical history and P/E, with or without laboratory tests
   2. Fever without localizing signs, in which the history and P/E do not suggest a diagnosis but in which laboratory tests may establish a diagnosis
   3. Fever of unknown origin (FUO), which by strict definition only applies to children who

A. Have a fever exceeding 1 week in duration
B. Have a fever that is documented in hospital
C. Have had all possible investigations performed during that week

3. B. Fever without a focus is due to an occult bacteremia until proven otherwise.

4. A. The next step is to obtain a more detailed history, including the fever itself (remittent, intermittent, hectic, or sustained) and a history of exposure to infective agents such as siblings at home with a febrile illness, exposure to other children in day care center, and other exposure to infectious diseases.

5. A.

6. E. The prevalence of occult bacteremia depends in part on the value of the WBC count. Thus this is the most appropriate next step for infants age 3-24 months. The probability of occult bacteremia will be increased if any of the following criteria are met:
A. The fever is > than 40° C.
B. The white blood cell count is < 5000/mm³ or > 15,000/mm³.
C. There is a positive exposure history.

7. C. The most common organism causing occult bacteremia in children is *Streptococcus pneumoniae*. This organism is responsible for approximately 65% of cases of occult bacteremia. Other common causative agents include the following:
A. *Haemophilus influenzae* type b (25%)
B. *Neisseria meningitidis*

8. B. The most common condition in infants and children associated with occult bacteremia is otitis media. This otitis media is most likely to be caused by *Streptococcus pneumoniae*. Remember that *Streptococcus pneumoniae* also causes pneumonia and meningitis in infants and children.

Haemophilus influenzae type b is a very common cause of otitis media and is the second most common cause of occult bacteremia.

9. E. The use of presumptive or prophylactic antibiotics in the prevention of morbidity associated with bacteremia is controversial. Although oral antibiotics may retard the emergence of some less serious focal bacterial disease (streptococcal pharyngitis, otitis media, and pneumonia), they do not reliably prevent meningitis. There is no solid evidence that the sooner a presumptive antibiotic is used, the greater it will affect morbidity and mortality from the disease.

10. B. The diurnal variation of temperature is usually preserved in patients with febrile illnesses. When this circadian rhythm is associated with tachycardia, chills (rigors), and sweating, a true rather than a factitious fever should be suspected. Fever patterns are classified as follows:
A. Remittent fever: daily elevated temperature returning to a baseline but above the normal temperature
B. Intermittent fever: daily elevated temperature returning not only to a baseline level but also to normal
C. Hectic fever: daily elevated temperature of either an intermittent pattern or a remittent pattern with temperature excursion > 1.4° C (2.5° F).
D. Sustained or continuous fever: daily elevated temperature with fluctuation of elevated temperature < 0.3° C (0.5° F).

11. B. Not all children with a fever need antipyretic treatment. In fact, antipyretics do not alter the natural history of the disease. The only children that should be treated with an antipyretic are those who are considered to be a high risk due to chronic cardiac disease, chronic respiratory disease, neurologic disease, febrile/nonfebrile convulsions, and metabolic disorders.

12. D. Although acetaminophen, aspirin, and NSAIDs are equally efficacious antipyretics, they do not have an equal safety/efficacy ratio: aspirin has been associated with Reye's syndrome, and NSAIDs have been associated with gastric side effects and gastric bleeding. The antipyretic of choice is acetaminophen.

Tepid sponge bathing may be just as effective as antipyretic therapy with drugs in reducing an infant's body temperature.

13. E.

14. B. Fever, as defined as an elevation in body temperature, is mediated as a final common pathway by the production of exogenous pyrogens. This directly alters the hypothalamus temperature set-point, resulting in heat generation and heat conservation.

This hypothalamic set-point is mediated by cytokine generation in response to exogenous pyrogens, with subsequent hypothalamic prostaglandin E_2 (PGE_2) production. This supports the drawing of blood for culture prior to fever elevation, when circulating bacteria (exogenous pyrogens) are more likely to be present.

15. E. Febrile convulsions may accompany high fever in a child. Few children with febrile convulsions go on to develop epilepsy in later life.

Febrile convulsions usually develop between the ages of 6 months and 5 years; occur with a rise in temperature above 39° C; last 15 minutes or less; are tonic-clonic in character; have no focal or lateralizing aspects; and do not manifest neurologic deficits postictally.

Treatment of the fever and the underlying condition is usually sufficient.

SOLUTION TO SHORT ANSWER MANAGEMENT PROBLEM 96

A reasonable approach to the diagnosis and management of fever without a focus in an infant of age 1 year is as follows:

1. Remember: a proper history and P/E is both sensitive and specific in determining the prevalence of occult bacteremia.

   Question: does the child appear ill?

   If no, then reassure parent.

   If yes, then consider this a serious sign and continue investigation.

   Consider the following in an infant:
   A. Quality of cry
   B. Reaction to parent stimulation
   C. Color
   D. Hydration
   E. Response (talk, smile) to social overtones

2. Remember: the risks for occult bacteremia:
   A. Fever > 40° C
   B. WBC < 5000
   C. WBC > 15,000
   D. Positive exposure history

3. Remember: the importance of repeated examinations and continuing contact with parents if fever without a focus is diagnosed and the child is allowed to go home.

4. Remember: the most common organisms associated with occult bacteremia.
   A. *Streptococcus pneumoniae*
   B. *Haemophilus influenzae*
   C. group A beta-hemolytic streptococcus
   D. *Neisseria meningitidis*

5. Remember: the most common conditions associated with occult bacteremia.
   A. Otitis media
   B. Bacterial pneumonia
   C. Streptococcal pharyngitis
   D. Meningitis

6. Consider: the possibility of febrile convulsions if the temperature is > 40.0° C.

7. Remember: not all infants with fever have to be treated with antipyretics. Antipyretics do not speed the resolution of the condition. They may, in fact, hide certain symptoms.

8. Remember: symptomatic treatment (tepid sponge baths) may be just as effective as antipyretics.

9. Remember: the importance of repeated reassessment of a child with fever without a focus until either the fever abates or the condition becomes overt.

10. Remember: if you are going to use an antipyretic to treat a child with a fever without a focus that the preferred agent is acetaminophen.

11. Remember: blood cultures should be obtained prior to the rise in temperature.

The Solution to the Short Answer Management Problem adequately summarizes this chapter.

SUGGESTED READING

Behrman R et al., eds. General considerations: Fever. In: Nelson textbook of pediatrics. 14th Ed. Philadelphia: WB Saunders, 1992.

PROBLEM 97   AN 18-MONTH-OLD INFANT WITH DIARRHEA

A mother presents to your office with her 18-month-old infant son who has had "diarrhea" for the past 5 days. When asked about the diarrhea, the mother states that the infant has "six to eight loose bowel movements every day." There has been no blood in the stools. The infant has a mild fever (38° C) and also appears to have some abdominal discomfort. The child vomited several times in the first 3 days of the illness, but this has since subsided. The infant has two siblings; neither one of them has any abnormal symptoms.

On P/E, the child is active and does not appear to be significantly dehydrated. Examination of the ears, throat, lungs, and abdomen are normal. There are no abdominal masses and no tenderness.

SELECT THE ONE BEST ANSWER TO THE FOLLOWING QUESTIONS

1. What is the most likely cause of this infant's diarrhea?
   a) Norwalk agent
   b) rotavirus
   c) coxsackie virus
   d) echovirus
   e) Shigella

2. What is the treatment of choice in this infant at this time?
   a) admission to hospital for IV therapy
   b) observation in hospital and oral rehydration therapy
   c) treatment at home with fluids including fruit juices and uncarbonated beverages
   d) treatment at home with an oral rehydrating solution
   e) none of the above

3. Which of the following statements regarding rotavirus infection in children is(are) true?
   a) upper respiratory tract symptoms frequently precede the gastrointestinal symptoms of rotavirus
   b) upper respiratory tract symptoms of rotavirus include rhinorrhea, pharyngeal erythema, and cough
   c) otitis media frequently precedes the gastrointestinal symptoms of rotavirus
   d) a and b
   e) all of the above

4. Which of the following represents the composition of an ideal rehydrating solution for moderate dehydration (all numbers are represented in mEq/L except CHO, which is given in %)?
   a) $Na^+ = 23$; $K^+ = 3$; $Cl^- = 15$; CHO = 3.0%
   b) $Na^+ = 40$; $K^+ = 10$; $Cl^- = 20$; CHO = 3.0%
   c) $Na^+ = 75$; $K^+ = 20$; $Cl^- = 65$; CHO = 2.0%
   d) $Na^+ = 140$; $K^+ = 50$; $Cl^- = 80$; CHO = 5.0%
   e) $Na^+ = 100$; $K^+ = 40$; $Cl^- = 100$; CHO = 7.5%

5. What is the most common bacterial cause of diarrhea in the pediatric age group?
   a) Salmonella
   b) Shigella
   c) Campylobacter
   d) E. coli
   e) Enterococcus

6. Which of the following infectious agents may produce bloody diarrhea in infants and children?
   a) Shigella
   b) Salmonella
   c) Enteroinvasive E. coli
   d) Enterococcus
   e) a, b, and c
   f) all of the above

7. Which of the following is(are) subtypes of E. coli gastroenteritis in infants and children?
   a) enteropathogenic E. coli
   b) enteroinvasive E. coli
   c) enterohemorrhagic E. coli
   d) a and c
   e) all of the above

8. What is the most common cause of antibiotic-associated diarrhea in infants and children?
   a) ampicillin
   b) clindamycin
   c) erythromycin
   d) penicillin
   e) none of the above

9. An infant age 23 months is brought to the ER by his mother. He has had diarrhea and vomiting for the past 3 days and appears to be at least 15% dehydrated. His eyeballs are sunken and his skin is doughy. The child has no satisfactory veins in which to place an IV line. What should you do now?
   a) attempt oral rehydration therapy
   b) perform a venous cutdown in the ankle
   c) begin an interosseous infusion
   d) begin a subcutaneous infusion
   e) none of the above

10. Which of the following investigations should be performed on all children who present with ongoing diarrhea?
    a) urine specific gravity
    b) stool evaluation for blood

c) stool evaluation for fecal leukocytes
d) all of the above
e) none of the above

11. A mother presents with her 3-year-old boy who has developed severe crampy diarrhea and mild fever. The family has just returned from a camping trip in the Rocky Mountains; the child became sick on the third day. He was apparently drinking water from the local stream.
What is the most likely diagnosis?
a) viral gastroenteritis
b) *Shigella* gastroenteritis
c) *Salmonella* gastroenteritis
d) giardiasis
e) amebiasis

12. What is the most common bacterial cause of mesenteric lymphadenitis in children?
a) *Salmonella*
b) *Yersinia enterocolitica*
c) *Shigella*
d) *E. coli*
e) *Campylobacter*

13. Which of the following pediatric infections often present(s) with diarrhea as the initial symptom?
a) acute appendicitis
b) otitis media
c) urinary tract infections
d) pneumonia
e) all of the above

Short Answer Management Problem 97

Discuss the most common cause of pediatric death from gastroenteritis (worldwide). Comment on community health aspects of this condition.

ANSWERS

1. B. The most common cause of pediatric gastroenteritis is rotavirus. Symptoms of rotavirus infection include low-grade fever, anorexia, nausea, vomiting, diarrhea, and abdominal cramps. Dehydration may occur. The disease typically runs its course in a 4- to 10-day time frame.

    Other causes of viral diarrhea in children include (a) parvoviruses such as the Norwalk agent, (b) coxsackie viruses, (c) echoviruses, (d) adenoviruses, and (e) caliciviruses.

2. D. Because this child does not appear to be significantly dehydrated, hospitalization is not required. The treatment of choice is home oral rehydration therapy. Fruit juices (undiluted) and commercial beverages are not recommended because of high osmolarity and the danger of hypernatremia.

    Details of oral rehydrating solutions are discussed elsewhere in the chapter.

3. E. Viruses are the most common cause of wintertime diarrhea in infants. Rotavirus, as mentioned above, is the most common agent. It is responsible for more than 50% of cases of acute diarrhea in children. The other causes are listed in the answer to Question 1. The majority of infants and children who develop rotavirus develop an upper respiratory tract infection preceding the gastrointestinal symptoms. The respiratory tract symptoms include rhinorrhea, cough, pharyngeal erythema, and otitis media.

4. C. Oral rehydration therapy will effectively treat most cases of pediatric gastroenteritis.

    The World Health Organization standard for oral rehydration therapy recommends the following: Na^+ = 90 mEq/L; K^+ = 20 mEq/L; Cl^- = 80 mEq/L; $HCO3$ = 30 mEq/L; and CHO = 2%.

    Among the common oral rehydration solutions used, gastrolyte has the identical composition to the World Health Organization's formula. Pedialyte is less ideal as it contains only 45 mEq/L of sodium instead of 90 mEq/L and CHO 2.5%.

    Clear-liquid solutions should not be used in infants with diarrhea due to a low sodium content, low potassium content, and high carbohydrate content. These clear-liquid solutions include liquids such as apple juice, carbonated beverages, and other liquids.

5. C.

6. E.

7. E. The most common cause of bacterial gastroenteritis in both the pediatric and adult populations is *Campylobacter jejuni*.

    Campylobacter typically begins with fever and malaise, followed by nausea, vomiting, diarrhea, and abdominal pain. The diarrhea is often profuse, and may contain blood. The illness is self-limited, lasting less than one week in 60% of cases. Recurrences and chronic symptoms can occur, especially in infants.

    Infection with *Campylobacter jejuni* usually occurs due to endotoxin production. Invasive strains also occur and produce disease. *Campylobacter* is effectively treated with erythromycin.

Salmonella gastroenteritis begins with watery diarrhea, accompanied by fever and nausea. As with *Campylobacter,* the diarrhea may be bloody. *Salmonella* produces disease both by mucosal invasion and endotoxin production. Most cases of *Salmonella gastroenteritis* do not require antibiotic therapy.

Shigella gastroenteritis begins with watery diarrhea, high fever, and malaise; this is usually followed in 24 hours by tenesmus and frank dysentery. Mucosal invasion with frank ulceration and hemorrhage often occur. Dehydration is common. *Shigella gastroenteritis* should be treated with trimethoprim-sulfamethoxazole (TMP-SMX).

E. coli gastroenteritis may occur as an enteropathic infection, an enterohemorrhagic infection, an enterotoxigenic infection, or an enteroinvasive infection. Enteropathic *E. coli* usually produces a mild self-limited illness. Enterohemorrhagic *E. coli* produces diarrhea that is initially watery and later becomes bloody. Enterotoxigenic *E. coli* is the most common cause of traveler's diarrhea. Enteroinvasive *E. coli* invades the mucosa and produces a dysentery-like illness.

In infants and children, *Yersinia enterocolitica* may produce acute and chronic gastroenteritis as well as mesenteric lymphadenitis. Mesenteric lymphadenitis is, at times, extremely difficult to distinguish from acute appendicitis. Diarrhea, fever, and crampy abdominal pain are the most common presenting symptoms. Treatment is symptomatic only; antibiotic therapy is unnecessary.

Enterococcus is not a cause of bacterial gastroenteritis in children.

8. A. The most common cause of antibiotic-associated diarrhea is ampicillin. Ampicillin induced diarrhea is probably due to the presence of the toxin associated with *Clostridium difficile.* Most cases are mild and resolve on discontinuation of the drug. Treatment of severe cases consists of vancomycin or metronidazole.

9. C. In a young infant or child who presents with severe dehydration, it is often very difficult to establish good IV access. The skull is a possibility, but even that is difficult. An excellent alternative is an interosseous infusion (usually placed in the tibia). A large bore needle is used after local anesthesia has been infiltrated around the bone. This allows easy access and affords an excellent alternative to venous access.

10. D. The investigations that should be performed on all children who present with ongoing diarrhea include urine specific gravity, stool analysis for blood, and stool analysis for fecal leukocytes. A urine specific gravity below 1.015 suggests adequate hydration.

If a patient presents with bloody diarrhea, high fever, persistent symptoms, tenesmus, or a history of foreign travel, a stool culture and examination of the stool for ova and parasites should be performed. Routine stool culture, however, is not cost-effective.

Other investigations that should be considered in a toxic child include CBC, serum electrolytes, and serum osmolality.

11. D. Gastroenteritis that begins while camping in the Rocky Mountains is most likely due to giardiasis. Giardiasis needs a very low "organism load" to produce a very painful gastroenteritis. The recommended treatment is metronidazole and rehydration.

12. B. See the answer to Question 5.

13. E. Many nonenteric infections may produce diarrhea as the first and most prominent symptom. These include otitis media (rotavirus is most common), urinary tract infection, acute appendicitis (from inflammation extending to involve the ureter on the right side of the body), lower lobe pneumonia, and mesenteric lymphadenitis *(Yersinia enterocolitica).*

SOLUTION TO SHORT ANSWER MANAGEMENT PROBLEM 97

The most common cause of gastroenteritis-produced death in infants and children is cholera.

Cholera is both endemic and epidemic, and both have a seasonal pattern. Contaminated water is the major source of infectivity and transmission and cholera becomes an epidemic when crowded conditions such as refugee camps are established.

The responsible organism is *Vibrio cholerae.* The resulting illness is sudden in onset and produces severe rice-water diarrhea and severe dehydration that can lead to death quickly.

SUMMARY OF THE DIAGNOSIS AND TREATMENT OF PEDIATRIC GASTROENTERITIS

1. **Prevalence:** during the first 3 years of life a child experiences an estimated 1-3 acute, severe episodes of diarrhea.
2. **Most common causes:** rotavirus is the most common cause (> 50%). Rotavirus gastroenteritis is usually preceded by upper respiratory tract symptoms.

   Campylobacter jejuni is the most common bacterial cause. Other viral agents producing gastroenteritis include the following:
   a) Norwalk agent (parvovirus)
   b) Coxsackie viruses
   c) Echoviruses
   d) Adenovirus
   e) Caliciviruses
      Other bacterial agents include the following:

a) *Salmonella*
b) *Shigella*
c) *Yersinia*
d) *E. coli*

Parasites include the following:

a) Giardiasis ("beaver fever")—most common
b) Amebiasis

3. **Diagnosis:** all children should be evaluated by a complete urinalysis including urine specific gravity and a stool examination for blood and fecal leukocytes. Specific gravity < 1.015 suggests adequate hydration.

If bloody diarrhea, persistent symptoms, fever, tenesmus, or recent foreign travel are present, a stool culture should be done. In mild and self-limiting diarrhea, a stool culture is not cost-effective.

4. **Treatment:** most children can be managed by oral rehydration therapy using a solution containing the following:

a) Na^+ (75-90 mEq/L)
b) K^+ (20-30 mEq/L)
c) Cl^- (65-80 mEq/L)
d) $HCO3$ (30 mEq/L)
e) CHO 2%

Antibiotic therapy should be initiated for *Shigella* (TMP-SMX) and *Campylobacter jejuni* (erythromycin).

SUGGESTED READING

Behrman R, ed. Diarrhea and diarrhea-like illness. Nelson textbook of pediatrics. 14th Ed. Philadelphia: WB Saunders, 1992.

PROBLEM 98   A 12-YEAR-OLD FEMALE WITH RECURRENT ABDOMINAL PAIN

A 12-year-old female presents to your office with a history of recurring abdominal pain. She is having episodes of abdominal pain once or twice/week. These episodes last approximately 8 hours. She has been seen on many occasions for the same problem and has been completely investigated. The investigations have included a complete blood count, urinalysis, stool for ova and parasites, a KUB, and an abdominal ultrasound. All of those investigations were normal. The pain is described as umbilical in location with a quality described as a "dull ache." She rates the pain at a baseline quantity of 6/10, with increases to 8/10 and decreases to 4/10. It is not associated with any food intake, and it is not associated with any diarrhea or constipation.

On physical examination, the young girl is in no apparent distress. Her vital signs are normal. On examination of the abdomen, there is slight tenderness in the area of the periumbilical region. There is no hepatosplenomegaly and there are no other masses.

SELECT THE ONE BEST ANSWER TO THE FOLLOWING QUESTIONS

1. What is the most likely diagnosis in this patient?
   a) recurrent abdominal pain syndrome (RAP syndrome)
   b) lactose intolerance
   c) Crohn's disease
   d) mesenteric lymphadenitis
   e) chronic appendicitis

2. What is the prevalence of this condition in children?
   a) 1%
   b) 5%
   c) 10%
   d) 20%
   e) 25%

3. Regarding the physiologic basis for the pain that occurs in the condition described in Question 1, which of the following statements is(are) true?
   a) the pain can be conceptualized as a disorder that provokes pain pathways
   b) the pain can be conceptualized as an alteration in the patient's threshold to pain
   c) there is evidence that an abnormality in the autonomic nervous system is involved in this condition
   d) there is evidence that intestinal motility can be affected along with the occurrence of hyperalgesia
   e) all of the above statements are true

4. Which of the following statements regarding school attendance and the condition described in Question 1 is(are) true?
   a) there is no association between school attendance and the RAP syndrome
   b) School phobia (reluctance to attend school) may be an important etiologic factor in this condition

   c) children with this condition usually achieve higher marks than their counterparts without this condition
   d) there is no association between stressful events at school and this condition
   e) none of the above are true

5. Which of the following investigations should be ordered in the patient described in Question 1 at this time?
   a) urinalysis
   b) complete blood count
   c) KUB
   d) abdominal ultrasound
   e) none of the above

6. Which of the following organisms is most commonly associated with organic recurring abdominal pain in children?
   a) enterotoxigenic *E. coli*
   b) enteropathogenic *E. coli*
   c) *Giardia lamblia*
   d) *Entamoeba histolytica*
   e) *Salmonella*

7. Which of the following conditions is most closely associated with the syndrome described in Question 1?
   a) anorexia nervosa
   b) bulimia
   c) major depressive illness
   d) generalized anxiety disorder
   e) panic disorder

8. Which of the following is the treatment of choice for the condition described?
   a) muscle relaxants
   b) tricyclic antidepressants
   c) narcotic analgesics
   d) nonsteroidal antiinflammatory agents
   e) none of the above

Short Answer Management Problem 98

A mother presents with her 11-year-old son, who has a 3-year history of recurrent abdominal pain. He has been to six different doctors, has had multiple investigations, and has been tried on many different drugs in an effort to alleviate the symptoms. So far nothing has worked. She demands that you find out the cause and fix it. Discuss how you would respond to this mother's request.

ANSWERS

1. A. The most likely diagnosis in this patient is the recurrent abdominal pain syndrome of childhood (RAP syndrome). The signs and symptoms of the RAP syndrome are marked by their lack of specificity. The crucial separation of organic from nonorganic pain can be based on a few important findings, including the specificity and consistency of the pain and the relationship of the pain to meals and movement. The patient with nonspecific recurrent abdominal pain tends to look well, to have pain that is inconsistent in relationship to meals and to movement, and to be free of the occurrence of additional symptoms such as nausea, vomiting, or dysuria.

   Lactose intolerance is often confused with the RAP syndrome in childhood and with irritable bowel syndrome in adults. In fact, these two syndromes can coexist. Lactose intolerance is usually associated with diarrhea.

   Crohn's disease and mesenteric lymphadenitis are usually associated with systemic symptoms. The lack of systemic symptoms in this patient is strong evidence against these diagnoses.

   "Chronic appendicitis," if it exists, is more likely to be associated with pain in the right lower quadrant, as well as with nausea and vomiting.

2. C. The prevalence of the RAP syndrome in childhood is 10%.

3. E. There are many theories related to the RAP syndrome in children. Pain in children is conceptualized as a disorder that provokes pain pathways or an alteration in the patient's threshold to pain. A widely held plausible explanation in these cases is some abnormality in the functioning of the autonomic nervous system. This is thought to result in altered intestinal motility and the occurrence of hyperalgesia as well as altered secretory pathways.

4. B. School phobia (reluctance to attend school) may be an important etiologic factor in the RAP syndrome in childhood. There is a significant association between stressful events at school and the RAP syndrome. Children with this condition, on average, achieve lower marks than their cohorts without this condition. This may actually be more associated with school attendance than anything else. There is a significant association between stressful events at school and exacerbations of this condition.

5. E. Because this child has already had numerous investigations, including all of the investigations described in this question, it is pointless to repeat them unless her condition is markedly different from previous episodes.

   Because the possible mechanisms associated with abdominal pain are so numerous and not completely understood, the investigation and treatment of these cases of recurrent abdominal pain in childhood test not only the physicians' scientific acumen but also their skill in the practice of the art of medicine. There is a great temptation to "overdo" the testing and treatment when reliance on a careful clinical evaluation is the most important first step toward resolving the problem.

6. C. *Giardia lamblia* is sometimes the cause of a recurrent pain syndrome in children. Thus every child with recurrent pain should have an examination of the stool for ova and parasites × 3.

7. A. Anorexia nervosa is the psychiatric condition most commonly associated with recurrent abdominal pain.

   Depression, generalized anxiety disorder, and panic disorder can present with recurrent abdominal pain but are not as clearly associated as is anorexia nervosa.

8. E. Treatment for the RAP syndrome in childhood should not be based on pharmacotherapy, especially pharmacotherapy that may do more harm than good. Therapy should emphasize the patient's response to the pain. In most cases, these efforts should involve the parents.

   First, the patient and parents need to be reassured that the problem is not life-threatening.

   Second, the physician should be realistic and frank and warn the patient and family that the problem may persist for an extended period of time. As mentioned, the physician should avoid prescribing medications and other therapies that may be harmful. Sedatives, antispasmodics, and analgesics are not only not beneficial but actually harmful. These agents, as well as having potentially deleterious effects on the intestinal motility and appetite, may also create dependency.

Laxatives, and at times enemas, may be beneficial. With some evidence of retained stool or, in difficult cases, even a suspicion of constipation, a trial of aggressive targeted treatment with mineral oil or lactulose, with or without enemas, can be effective in relieving the constipation that often goes along with RAP syndrome.

General measures such as the promotion of full activity and a sense of normal health are extremely important. A well-balanced diet, which is not excessive in fiber content, is recommended.

Every attempt should be made to maintain school attendance. In some otherwise physically well patients a cycle of emotional turmoil, school absenteeism, and pain evolve. Identifying the stressors and breaking the cycle by ongoing counseling is the most important first step.

The prognosis for children with recurrent abdominal pain is unclear. There is certainly no increased risk of intraabdominal disease, and in most cases symptoms improve before the age of 20 years. Some children with the RAP syndrome, do, however, go on to develop an irritable bowel syndrome as adults.

SOLUTION TO SHORT ANSWER MANAGEMENT PROBLEM 98

This is an all-too-common problem. It would seem at first glance that perhaps no physician has really sat down to explain the illness to the child and to the mother. The most appropriate thing to do in this case is to spend a fair amount of time describing the syndrome of recurrent abdominal pain and explaining what should and should not be done to treat it. An emphasis on healthy lifestyle, exercise, and decreased stress is probably the best advice you can give the patient and his mother. An explanation as to why you do not think any more tests are indicated and why you do not wish to prescribe additional medication should go a long way both to provide reassurance and to communicate the message that you truly care.

SUMMARY OF THE DIAGNOSIS AND TREATMENT OF RECURRENT ABDOMINAL PAIN IN CHILDHOOD

1. The diagnosis of recurrent abdominal pain (the RAP syndrome) in childhood can usually be made from the history and physical examination, supplemented with a few investigations including complete blood count, urinalysis, ESR, stool for ova and parasites, occult blood, KUB, and abdominal ultrasound.
2. Recurrent abdominal pain in childhood is common; the prevalence is estimated at 10%.
3. Do not overinvestigate or overtreat patients with recurrent abdominal pain in childhood. The vast majority of cases are nonorganic in origin.
4. Treatment should be supportive and should consist of reestablishing a healthy lifestyle, eating a well-balanced diet, exercising daily, and avoiding stress, especially at school.
5. There is a strong association between school phobia (school avoidance) and RAP syndrome. Take a careful history of school performance, school fears, and general feelings about attending school.

SUGGESTED READING

Behrman RE, Kliegman RM, Nelson WE, Vaughan V, eds. The digestive system, recurrent abdominal pain. Nelson textbook of pediatrics. 14th Ed. Philadelphia: WB Saunders, 1992.

PROBLEM 99   A 9-YEAR-OLD BOY WITH LEG PAIN

A 9-year-old boy presents to your office with his mother. He complains of a recurrent (nightly) pain in both legs. The pain is so severe that it wakes him from sleep. It is described as a "deep pain." The pain is bilateral and is usually gone by morning. There is no associated fever, chills, limp, or other symptoms. Occasionally the pain may come on during the day; this usually occurs with excessive or strenuous exercise.

His past history has been excellent. He has had no significant medical illnesses.

On examination, the child has no limp and no leg length discrepancy.

SELECT THE ONE BEST ANSWER TO THE FOLLOWING QUESTIONS

1. What is the most likely diagnosis in this child?
   a) slipped capital femoral epiphysis
   b) Legg-Calvé-Perthes disease
   c) osteogenic sarcoma
   d) Ewing's sarcoma
   e) growing pains

2. What is the preferred treatment for this condition?
   a) surgical fixation
   b) bracing and/or traction
   c) amputation
   d) radiotherapy followed by chemotherapy
   e) none of the above

3. Regarding limb pain in children, which of the following statements is(are) false?
   a) limb pain is a common presenting complaint in children
   b) there is significant association between limb pain, headache, and abdominal pain
   c) there is frequently an association between limb pain in children and pain of other types in family members.
   d) there is frequently an emotional component to limb pain in children
   e) all of the above statements are true

4. The following criteria describe which of the following pediatric orthopedic conditions listed below?
   1) Occurs as a result of acute trauma or in a more subtle fashion over time
   2) The typical patient is a somewhat overweight and sedentary teenage boy.
   3) Pain is located either in the groin or on the medial side of the knee.
   4) The hip is held in abduction and external rotation and there is marked limitation of internal rotation.
   5) Diagnosis is made by X-ray.
   a) slipped capital femoral epiphysis
   b) Legg-Calvé-Perthes disease
   c) osteogenic sarcoma
   d) Ewing's sarcoma
   e) growing pains

5. What is the preferred treatment for the condition described in Question 4?
   a) surgical fixation
   b) bracing and/or traction
   c) amputation
   d) radiotherapy followed by chemotherapy
   e) none of the above

6. The following criteria describe which of the pediatric orthopedic conditions listed below?
   A condition that is also known as aseptic necrosis of the femoral head, is found mainly in children under the age of 10 and is suggested by pain in the area of the hip or knee. Demonstration of a limp and a decreased range of motion on physical examination is most likely.
   a) slipped capital femoral epiphysis
   b) Legg-Calvé-Perthes disease
   c) femoral head abnormality
   d) hypermobile femur
   e) none of the above

7. What is the preferred treatment for the condition discussed in Question 6?
   a) surgical fixation
   b) bracing and/or traction
   c) casting
   d) any of the above may be indicated depending on the case
   e) none of the above are indicated

8. The following criteria describe which of the orthopedic pediatric conditions listed below?
   1) There is localized tenderness and swelling present over the tibial tubercle.
   2) The pain is aggravated by running, jumping, going up and down stairs, and kneeling.
   3) The condition is an overuse syndrome that occurs commonly in physically active males around puberty.
   4) Significant athletic activity plus a recent growth spurt that may result in detachment of cartilage fragments from the tibial tuberosity
   a) chondromalacia
   b) osteochondritis dissecans
   c) Osgood-Schlatter disease
   d) patellofemoral syndrome
   e) lateral diskitis

9. What is the preferred treatment for the condition described in Question 8?
    a) surgical removal
    b) casting
    c) bracing and/or traction
    d) splinting
    e) none of the above

10. The following criteria describe which of the pediatric orthopedic conditions below?
    1) It is characterized by subchondral bone necrosis and complete or partial separation of articular fragments.
    2) It is usually caused by repeated trauma to a segment of the bone with tenuous vascularity.
    3) The clinical manifestations may include episodic knee pain, aching after exercise, stiffness, clicking, muscle atrophy, mild joint swelling, and occasional locking.
    4) The demarcated fragments of subchondral bone are best demonstrated radiographically by a "notch view" of the knee.
    a) chondromalacia
    b) osteochondritis dissecans
    c) Osgood-Schlatter disease
    d) patellofemoral syndrome
    e) lateral diskitis

11. What is the preferred treatment for the condition described in Question 10 in most cases?
    a) surgical removal
    b) casting
    c) bracing and/or traction
    d) splinting
    e) none of the above

A 13-year-old female, a star on the junior high school basketball team, presents with left anterior knee pain and a grating sensation aggravated by activities involving knee flexion such as climbing stairs and running.

On P/E you ask the patient to extend her knee while you compress the patella against the femoral condyle. The patient refuses to extend the femoral condyle due to pain.

12. What is the most likely diagnosis?
    a) chondromalacia patellae
    b) osteochondritis dissecans
    c) Osgood-Schlatter disease
    d) soft patella syndrome
    e) none of the above

13. What is the preferred treatment for most cases of this condition?
    a) surgical removal
    b) casting
    c) bracing and/or traction
    d) splinting
    e) none of the above

14. The following criteria describe which of the following pediatric orthopedic conditions?
    1) It is the most common cause of limb and hip pain in the age group 3-6 years.
    2) It is characterized as an idiopathic, nonspecific, common, unilateral, inflammatory arthritis involving the hip joint.
    3) Symptoms of upper respiratory tract infection often precede hip symptoms in this condition.
    4) This condition is more common in boys than in girls.
    a) toxic synovitis
    b) Legg-Calvé-Perthes disease
    c) slipped capital femoral epiphysis
    d) septic arthritis
    e) osteomyelitis

15. What is the preferred treatment for the condition described in Question 14?
    a) surgical decompression
    b) casting
    c) bracing and/or traction
    d) splinting
    e) none of the above

Short Answer Management Problem 99

The differentiation between organic hip or leg pain and nonorganic hip or leg pain often has to be made. It is sometimes a very difficult problem for the primary care physician.

Compare and contrast eight characteristics and/or distinguishing features of organic limb pain and/or nonorganic limb pain that will help you, the family physician, distinguish serious illness from nonserious illness when presented in your office with a similar problem.

ANSWERS

1. E. This child has typical "growing pains."

The current concept of growing pains is that it describes a very specific symptom complex consisting of deep pain, often in the lower limbs, that is severe enough to wake the child from sleep. The pains occur intermittently, are always bilateral, and are usually completely gone in the morning. The pains can, however, be aggravated by heavy exercise during the day and improved by nonpharmacologic therapies such as heat, massage, and physiotherapy.

There is often a psychological component to growing pains. There seems to be a relationship between limb pains, abdominal pains, and headaches in children, and an inherited or environmentally determined link between siblings with pain and parents with pain.

2. E. No treatment in this situation is vastly superior to many other treatments. Again, following the simple but very important dictum *primum non nocere* (first do no harm), the physician must explain the condition in english (not medispeak) to the patient. (Remember that the patient is the child, not the mother, and thus the physician should, if possible, maintain eye level contact with the child when speaking to him or her.) The patient should be told that heat in the form of hot packs, massage, or warm baths may alleviate pain in the lower extremity, and that the pain will certainly disappear in time. Time can be helped along with mild analgesics/antiinflammatories such as naprosyn or acetaminophen. Although avoidance of activities that aggravate the condition should be advised, this must be balanced against the positive benefits of maintaining some type of exercise program.

3. E. Limb pain is a common presenting complaint in primary care practice. It is estimated to account for 7% of pediatric visits.

With limb pain in childhood, there is frequently an emotional component. As mentioned previously, there is a relationship between growing pains and headache/abdominal pain in children with these symptoms, who often come from "pain prone" families. The parents have often had pain as children that has sometimes persisted into adulthood. In up to 33% of cases, this "childhood pain syndrome" itself persists.

4. A. This child has a slipped capital femoral epiphyses (SCFE). The characteristics of slipped capital femoral epiphyses are listed in the question. Physiologically, SCFE occurs before the epiphyseal plate closes and usually at a time before and during the maximal pubertal growth spurt (13-15 years in males; 11-13 years in females). This condition is the most common adolescent hip disorder and has an incidence of 1-4/100,000. Blacks are affected more than whites. The disease is usually unilateral in 90% of patients and is bilateral in 10%.

5. A. Slipped capital femoral epiphyses is an orthopedic emergency. Immediate hospitalization and operative fixation is indicated. Stabilization of the SCFE is essen-

tial if acute or gradual slipping is to be prevented. Spica hip casting is needed to decrease the risk of femoral neck fracture and to protect the epiphyses for 6-8 weeks. In severe chronic (and poorly aligned) SCFE, osteotomies are required to realign and stabilize the capital femoral epiphyses.

6. B. These criteria describe Legg-Calvé-Perthes disease. As the major criteria have been listed in the question they will not be repeated here. Perthes disease, in pathologic terms, is a juvenile idiopathic avascular necrosis of the femoral head. The etiology is unknown, although trauma, transient synovitis, venous congestion, hyperviscosity, coagulation abnormalities, and other mechanisms have been suggested.

Males are affected more than females (4-5:1). Twenty percent of cases are familial. The incidence is 1:1000 to 1:5000 in the general population but 1:35 in affected females.

7. D. Legg-Calvé-Perthes disease is difficult to treat because of the necessity for long-term treatment and the need to limit activities. The psychologic status of the child during treatment must be monitored. A biopsychosocial approach is often necessary to treat both the psychological and orthopedic aspects of the problem. Braces and casting may be required for up to 1-2 years. Surgery, the other option, will allow the child to return to normal activity in 4-6 months.

The prognosis for Legg-Calvé-Perthes disease is, at best, fair. In the middle years, approximately 50% of patients go on to develop severe degenerative hip disease and require hip replacement.

8. C. Osgood-Schlatter disease results from overuse of the lower extremity. Athletic activity plus/minus a recent growth spurt may lead to cartilage detachment. The diagnosis is made by localizing the point of maximal tenderness over the tibial tuberosity.

9. E. The preferred treatment for Osgood-Schlatter disease is a reduction in physical activity. The disease process itself is usually self-limited with complete remission when there is fusion of the tibial tubercle to the diaphysis. Resolution occurs over a period of months.

In a small percentage of cases, the use of a knee immobilizer splint may be helpful. Excision of the ossicle may eventually be required. Local corticosteroid injections should not be used; injections of this nature may weaken the quadriceps tendon and produce local cutaneous thinning and depigmentation.

10. B. Osteochondritis dissecans is a condition characterized by subchondral bone necrosis and on occasion by complete or partial separation of the articular fragments.

The most common site for osteochondritis dissecans is the lateral aspect of the medial femoral condyle. It may also occur in the patella in the lateral condyle of the femur.

Males are affected more often than females (3:1), and there appear to be two peaks of incidence: children younger than 12 years of age and young adults.

11. E. In most cases of osteochondritis dissecans, the treatment (in the patient with open growth plates) is conservative. Isometric quadriceps exercises, limitation of activities, and time itself lead to resolution of most lesions. Open arthrotomy or arthroscopic surgery is indicated when the fragments are greater than 1 cm in diameter.

12. A. This young girl has chondromalacia patellae.

Chondromalacia patellae is the most common form of the broader group of disorders known as patellofemoral disorders. Chondromalacia patellae is an overuse syndrome occurring in susceptible children before adolescence. Most children show some degree of patellofemoral malalignment.

The principal symptoms (anterior knee pain and a grating sensation aggravated by activities involving knee flexion, such as climbing stairs or running) are reflected by a tender undersurface on the medial side of the patella and some crepitance.

13. E. The treatment for chondromalacia patellae includes an active isometric progressive resistance exercise program to strengthen the quadriceps. During the acute phase, NSAIDs drugs may be of benefit. In a few cases, arthroscopy may be needed to remove bone or cartilaginous fragments, shave the undersurface of the patella, or release the lateral retinacular tethering structures.

14. A. Toxic synovitis, which is also known as irritable hip, is an idiopathic, transient, nonspecific, common, unilateral (5% bilateral) inflammatory arthritis involving the hip joint. It principally occurs in children under the age of 10 years (typically 3-6 years) and is the most common cause of limp with hip pain in this age group. The male-to-female ratio is approximately 4:1.

Toxic synovitis usually follows a viral upper respiratory infection, and begins 3-6 days after the respiratory symptoms abate. In addition to guarded hip rotation, there is pain in the hip, and pain in the anteromedial aspect of the thigh and knee. There also may be constitutional symptoms. These include a low-grade fever (less than or equal to 38°-39° C (101° F) and slight elevation of the ESR.

Aspirated fluid from the hip joint is clear, and X-ray demonstrates normal hips with an increased space between the medial acetabulum and the ossified femoral head. As the bones are normal, the probability of aseptic necrosis, osteomyelitis, and other serious conditions is greatly diminished. Ultrasound of the hips usually demonstrates a joint effusion.

Note that it is extremely important to differentiate toxic synovitis from septic arthritis. In contradistinction to toxic synovitis, septic arthritis demonstrates higher fever, malaise, more pronounced spasm, guarding and fixed positioning, and a sedimentation rate greater than 25 mm/hour.

15. E. The preferred treatment for toxic synovitis is conservative:
   1. Non-weight-bearing on the affected leg
   2. Rest in bed for a few days
   3. Analgesics and/or antiinflammatories

SOLUTION TO SHORT ANSWER MANAGEMENT PROBLEM 99

The differentiation of organic disease from nonorganic disease in a child that limps is a critical skill for the family physician. The family physician must be able to separate the two and refer serious organic conditions to specialty care. Table 99-1 demonstrates the differences

TABLE 99-1: THE LIMPING CHILD: ORGANIC VERSUS NONORGANIC

CHARACTERISTIC	ORGANIC	NONORGANIC
1. Pain: time of day	Day and night	Only at night
2. Pain: timing re: weekends and vacations	Occurs on weekends and vacations	Occurs primarily on school days
3. Severity: pain	Interrupts play and other pleasant activities	Child carries out normal activities
4. Location: pain	Located in joint	Located between joints
5. Location: pain	Bilateral	Unilateral
6. Limp	Child limps or refuses to walk	Child is able to walk normally
7. Description of pain	Fits with logical anatomic explanation	Description is illogical; pattern does not fit any recognizable anatomic pattern
8. Systemic disease	Signs and symptoms present	Signs and symptoms absent

SUMMARY OF THE LIMPING CHILD (AGE 3 AND >) IN FAMILY MEDICINE

1. A child with a limp is a common presentation in family medicine.
2. **Number-one priority of family physician:** distinguish organic from nonorganic.
3. **Number-two priority of family physician:**
   a) If urgent organic, refer.
   b) If nonurgent organic, investigate/diagnose/treat.
   c) If nonorganic, evaluate/treat/reassure.

4. **Common causes of childhood limp:**
   a) Organic
      1. Toxic or transient synovitis
      2. Septic arthritis
      3. Osteomyelitis
      4. Legg-Calvé-Perthes disease
      5. Slipped capital femoral epiphyses
      6. Malignancies (uncommon)

      Remember the proverb of the ancient Chinese philosopher who started an early medical school. He was concerned that if medical students remembered one thing and one thing only from his medical school, it would be this: "common things are common; uncommon things are uncommon."

   b) Nonorganic/benign
      1. Growing pains
      2. School phobias
      3. Osgood-Schlatter disease
      4. Osteochondritis dissecans
      5. Chondromalacia patellae
      6. Other patellofemoral disorders or syndromes

SUGGESTED READINGS

The bones and joints. In: Behrman RE, Kliegman RM, Nelson WE, Vaughan VC, eds. Nelson textbook of pediatrics. 14th Ed. Philadelphia: WB Saunders, 1992.

Eilert R, Georgopoulos G. Orthopedics. In: Hathaway WE, Hay WW, Groothuis JR, Paisley JW, eds. Current pediatric diagnosis and treatment. 11th Ed. Norwalk, CT: Appleton and Lange, 1993.

PROBLEM 100   AN ANXIOUS MOTHER WITH A 3-MONTH-OLD INFANT WITH CROOKED FEET

A 3-month-old infant is brought to your office by his mother. She states that he has "crooked feet." She has been told by her friend that he will "need a number of casts to correct this."

On examination, the infant's feet deviate inward. The heel position as viewed from behind with his feet dorsiflexed is valgus. No other abnormalities are found on examination.

The mother's pregnancy was unremarkable. The birth weight of the infant was 10 lb 8 oz.

SELECT THE ONE BEST ANSWER TO THE FOLLOWING QUESTIONS:

1. What is the most likely diagnosis in this infant?
   a) calcaneovalgus
   b) metatarsus valgus
   c) metatarsus varus
   d) talipes equinovarus
   e) clubfoot

2. What is the treatment of choice in this child?
   a) serial casts
   b) bilateral osteotomies
   c) Denis-Browne splints
   d) immediate referral to an orthopedic surgeon
   e) reassurance and foot exercises

3. A mother brings her 4-week-old infant to the office for assessment of her child's "toeing in." She states that another physician has told her that this will probably require "serial casts" to correct.

   On physical examination, both feet deviate medially. The feet dorsiflex easily and the heel position is dorsiflexion in valgus.

   What is the most likely diagnosis in this patient?
   a) calcaneovalgus
   b) metatarsus varus
   c) metatarsus valgus
   d) talipes equinovarus
   e) clubfoot

4. What is the most likely predisposing factor to the diagnosis described in Question 3?
   a) abnormality at the embryo stage of development
   b) hereditary susceptibility to the condition
   c) in utero position of the fetus
   d) abnormality in the shape of the materal uterus
   e) abnormality in the formation of the fetal legs and feet

5. What is the treatment of choice for the majority of patients with the condition described in Question 3?
   a) serial casts
   b) bilateral osteotomies
   c) Denis-Browne splints
   d) immediate referral to an orthopedic surgeon
   e) reassurance and foot exercises

6. A mother brings her 15-month-old toddler into your office for an assessment of "his bowlegs." She states that he has been "bowlegged" since he began to walk 3 months ago.

   On examination, the toddler's feet point inward while his knees point straight ahead.

   On the basis of the information provided, what is the most likely diagnosis?
   a) internal tibial torsion
   b) internal femoral torsion
   c) metatarsus varus
   d) fixed tibia varum
   e) calcaneovalgus

7. What is the treatment of choice for the child presented in Question 6?
   a) serial casts
   b) bilateral osteotomies
   c) Denis-Browne splints
   d) immediate referral to an orthopedic surgeon
   e) reassurance and leg exercises

8. What is the most common cause of intoeing in children?
   a) internal tibial torsion
   b) excessive femoral anteversion
   c) metatarsus adductus
   d) metatarsus varus
   e) none of the above

9. A mother presents with her 18-month-old infant. She tells you that her child appears to have "both legs twisted inward from the hips." You examine the child and confirm that the mother's impression appears to be correct. What appears in this case is an inward twist of the femur on both sides.

   What is the most likely diagnosis in this case?
   a) internal tibial torsion
   b) excessive femoral anteversion
   c) flexible flat feet
   d) metatarsus adductus
   e) metatarsus varus

10. What is the treatment of choice of the condition described in Question 9 at the present time?
    a) serial casts
    b) bilateral osteotomies

c) Denis-Browne splints
d) immediate referral to an orthopedic surgeon
e) watchful expectation

11. What is the most common method of measuring the degree of the condition described in Question 9?
a) CT scanning of the lower leg
b) ultrasonography of the lower leg
c) biplanar radiography of the lower leg
d) MRI scanning of the lower leg
e) none of the above

12. A mother brings her 6-month-old infant to your office for assessment. She tells you that "her child's feet are completely crooked" and that there is no way she can correct it.

On examination, you are unable to dorsiflex either foot. You notice that the heels are in the varus position (medial deviation) and the sole is kidney-shaped when viewed from the bottom.

What is the most likely diagnosis in this infant?
a) talipes equinovarus
b) metatarsus adductus
c) internal tibial torsion
d) excessive femoral anteversion
e) none of the above

13. Which of the following treatments may be indicated for correction of the condition described in Question 12?
a) Denis-Browne splints
b) posterior medial release of the "heel cords"
c) series casts
d) a and b
e) all of the above

14. Which of the following may be associated with the condition described in Question 12?
a) congenital dislocation of the hip
b) spina bifida
c) myotonic dystrophy
d) a and b
e) all of the above

15. A mother presents with her 21-month-old infant. She tells you that he "slaps his feet when he walks." Her mother-in-law has informed you that he has "flat feet" and instructed her daughter to "make darn sure the doctor does something about it." On examination, you observe the child walking. There certainly does seem to be a difference between the contour of the foot when weight bearing as compared to when not weight bearing.

What is the most likely difference?
a) a difference in "heel lift"
b) a difference in "toe lift"
c) a difference in foot varus
d) a difference in foot valgus
e) a difference in sag versus nonsag weight bearing

16. Assuming that the abnormalities in this child's feet involve arch support and ligamentous laxity, what is the most likely diagnosis?
a) muscular dystrophy
b) cerebral palsy
c) flexible flatfeet
d) osteochondrosis
e) obesity

17. Which of the following coexisting conditions is(are) associated with this condition?
a) muscular dystrophy
b) cerebral palsy
c) congenital heel cord tightness
d) a and c
e) all of the above

18. What is the treatment of choice for the primary condition described in Question 15 and diagnosed in Question 16?
a) corrective orthopedic shoes
b) orthotic inserts
c) flexible, well-fitted soft shoes
d) specially designed shoes
e) none of the above; watchful waiting is more appropriate

Short Answer Management Problem 100

A mother presents with her 6-month-old infant boy who is intoeing. Her mother-in-law has indicated that "a serious problem exists" that needs to be fixed now! Describe in detail how you would handle this situation.

ANSWERS

1. A.

2. E. The calcaneovalgus foot is the most common neonatal foot deformity. It is the result of positional confinement in utero. The foot has a banana-shaped sole (lat-

eral deviation); dorsiflexes quite easily because of a stretched, abnormally long heel cord; and has a heel that deviates laterally.

Prognosis is excellent; most cases improve spontaneously and rapidly. Parents who are uncomfortable with the prescription of observation alone should be encouraged to exercise the child's foot at each diaper change by stretching the ligaments and stretching the dorsal tendons.

Only in the rare instance that the foot remains severely deformed should corrective casts be applied. If the calcaneovalgus foot can be only partially corrected, a flexible flatfoot results.

This calcaneovalgus foot must be differentiated from a congenital vertical talus (congenital convex pes valgus), which is associated with neurologic disorders such as spina bifida or arthrogryposis in about 50% of cases. The vertical talus foot has a "rocker-bottom" appearance with a tight heel cord.

3. B.

4. C.

5. E. This child has metatarsus adductus and metatarsus varus. They are used synonymously in practice, although they describe slightly different variations in the forefoot. In both cases, the heel deviates laterally, the sole is kidney-shaped (medial deviation), and the foot is easily dorsiflexed.

The incidence of this disorder is two cases/1000 live births. Metatarsus adductus (varus) may be either bilateral or unilateral; it is probably secondary to in utero confinement.

Metatarsus adductus usually improves spontaneously; this applies to at least 85% of cases. In the examination the severity of the metatarsus adductus should be documented; severity is classified as follows:

Category A: mild/flexible
Category B: moderate/fixed
Category C: severe/rigid

The vast majority of cases fall into the mild/flexible group (Category A).

Patients should be taught how to stretch the child's foot by firmly holding and stabilizing the heel to prevent more heel valgus and stretching the forefoot laterally, holding it to a count of five (the baby may wince but should not cry). The exercise should be performed five times at each diaper change.

Category B metatarsus adductus may need to be treated by serial casting. Category C: metatarsus adductus may need corrective surgery, sometimes between the ages of 2 months and 4 months.

6. A.

7. E. Internal tibial torsion is a normal finding in the newborn. The mean tibial torsion at maturity is 15 degrees to 20 degrees. At birth, the mean tibial torsion is 5 degrees, that is, 10 to 15 degrees inward compared with adults. Internal tibial torsion usually presents at walking age, and affected children have an inward foot progression angle. When the child walks, it can be observed that the kneecaps point forward but the foot points inward.

Internal tibial torsion is thus a physiologic bowing of the lower extremities produced by the external rotation of the femur and internal rotation of the tibia.

The natural history of internal tibial torsion is spontaneous resolution in more than 95% of children. Internal tibial torsion usually resolves by 7 or 8 years of age, at which time the rotatory conformation of the bones is largely established. Reassurance and leg exercises are important and a key to the management of internal tibial torsion.

8. B.

9. B.

10. E.

11. C. The most common cause of intoeing in children is excessive femoral anteversion. The femoral neck is normally anteverted 15 degrees to 25 degrees with respect to the axis of the femoral condyles in the knee in adults. The femoral neck is more anteverted in children. In one large study, the average degree of anteversion of the femur in children between the ages of 3 months and 12 months was 39 degrees; and in 1-to-2-year-olds, 31 degrees.

A number of techniques have been devised to accurately measure the degree of femoral anteversion. The most commonly used techniques involve biplanar radiography.

In children who have excessive femoral anteversion as the cause of their intoeing, the typical clinical finding is that the child is observed to walk with his or her patellae and feet pointing inward. The clinical diagnosis is made by having the child lie prone or supine with the hips extended, and externally rotating the hip. In children with excess femoral anteversion, most of the arc of rotation of the hip will be inward.

The treatment of choice in children with excessive femoral anteversion is "watchful waiting." In 90%-95% of children, the degree of anteversion will progressively decrease to a level that is both within the normal range and completely acceptable.

12. A.

13. E.

14. E. This child has talipes equinovarus, or "clubfoot." When a child develops clubfoot, you notice the following:
    A. The inability to dorsiflex the clubfoot
    B. The presence of heel varus (medial deviation)
    C. A sole that is kidney-shaped

    Mild cases of clubfoot can be attributed to deformation caused by intrauterine compression, whereas more severe, fixed, cases are usually secondary to underlying anatomic abnormalities, such as an abnormal talus.

    Accompanying deformities with talipes equinovarus include the following: congenital dislocation of the hip, spina bifida, myotonic dystrophy, and arthrogryposis.

    Treatment options for talipes equinovarus include the following:
    A. Corrective serial casts
    B. Denis-Browne splints
    C. Posterior medial release of the heel cords.

    The proportion of children requiring corrective surgery varies from 75% if full anatomic, radiographic, and clinical correction is attempted to less than 50% if mild radiographic and clinical deformity is accepted.

15. E.

16. C.

17. E.

18. E. This child has flexible flatfeet. The flexible flatfoot is extremely common, with an incidence ranging from 7% to 22%. The condition is often hidden by normal adipose tissue and usually becomes noticeable after a child begins to stand. The most common etiology of the flexible flatfoot is ligamentous laxity, which allows the foot to sag with weight bearing. Children often present with accompanying hyperextension of fingers, elbows, and knees, as well as with a family history of flatfeet and ligamentous laxity.

    A child with flexible flatfeet secondary to ligamentous laxity can form a good arch when asked to stand on tiptoe. The heel rolls into a varus position (medial deviation) on tiptoe, and good strength of the ankle and foot muscles is assured.

    When the child walks, the difference that can be seen immediately is that when the child is not weight bearing there is an arch. When the child is weight bearing, there is no arch.

    Although flexible flatfeet are usually not associated with any secondary conditions (that is, primary flexible flatfeet), it must be recognized that flexible flatfeet can be secondary to a tight heel cord, muscular dystrophy, mild cerebral palsy, or congenital tightness of the heel cords.

    Although many treatments have been advocated for flatfeet, including corrective shoes, custom orthotics, corrective inserts, and flexible flatfoot wear, none of them have been shown to be better than "no treatment" or "watchful expectation."

SOLUTION TO SHORT ANSWER MANAGEMENT PROBLEM 100

The single most important aspect of management at this time is to establish a therapeutic alliance with the mother.
1. Begin with a complete history of the pregnancy and birth (pay particular attention to any complications).
2. Carry out a complete physical examination where the following are especially noted:
   A. Foot varus versus foot valgus
   B. Flexibility of varus or valgus deformity
   C. Explanation to the mother of the various causes of intoeing and with the very high frequency with which they self-correct (90%-95%)
3. Ask the mother to return monthly for recheck.
4. Provide a "patient information guide" as was published in the November 1994 issue of *American Family Physician*.
5. Ask the mother to call you if she has any lingering concerns.
6. At the same time, reassure yourself that nothing more serious is causing this deformity.

SUMMARY OF THE DIAGNOSIS AND TREATMENT OF FOOT AND LEG DEFORMITIES IN INFANTS AND CHILDREN

1. **Prevalence of foot and leg deformities:** common: up to 10% of infants
2. **Foot deformities in infants and children:**
   a) Calcaneovalgus foot: most common neonatal foot deformity. It results from the fetal position in utero. The foot has a banana-shaped sole (lateral deviation) and dorsiflexes quite easily because of a stretched, abnormally long heel cord and a heel that deviates laterally. Treatment: watchful waiting.
   b) Metatarsus adductus (metatarsus varus): the heel deviates laterally, the sole is kidney-shaped, and the foot is easily dorsiflexed. Treatment: foot exercises and watchful waiting.
   c) Talipes equinovarus (true clubfoot): this disorder is characterized by the inability to dorsiflex, the presence of a heel varus (medial deviation), and a sole that is kidney-shaped when viewed from the bottom. Most cases are due to intrauterine compression or, in the odd case, an abnormal talus. A tight heel cord is exceedingly common. Treatment: serial casts, Denis-Browne splints, or surgical posterior medial heel cord release in the latter part of the first year.
3. **Other causes of intoeing in young children:**
   a) Internal tibial torsion: in internal tibial torsion, the entire foot points inward while the knee points straight ahead (medial tibial torsion). Treatment: watchful waiting.

b) Excessive femoral anteversion: the entire leg turns in so that both the knee and the foot are facing medially (medial femoral torsion or increased anteversion of the hips). Treatment: watchful waiting.

4. **Flexible flatfeet:** in a child with flexible flatfeet, when the foot is not weight bearing, the arch of the foot is preserved. When the child is weight bearing, it is not. Treatment: watchful waiting.

SUGGESTED READINGS

Churgay C. Diagnosis and treatment of pediatric foot deformities. American Family Physician 1993; 47(4): 883-889.

Dietz F. Intoeing—fact, fiction, and opinion. American Family Physician 1994; 50(6): 1249-1259.

PROBLEM 101 A 16-YEAR-OLD MALE WITH ACNE

A 16-year-old male presents to your office for assessment of "pimples." He tells you that he has had "a lot of pimples for the last 4 years" and "they really aren't getting much worse or much better." You determine that he has never seen a physician for this problem even though it has been a problem for as long as it has. You wonder why he has chosen to seek advice from a doctor at this time.

On examination the patient appears to answer questions slowly, and he never makes eye contact with you. He has grade II acne with some whiteheads, blackheads, and a few papules.

SELECT THE ONE BEST ANSWER TO THE FOLLOWING QUESTIONS

1. With respect to this young man's presentation, which of the following statements most likely best portrays the patient's situation and/or your response at this time?
   a) acne is most likely the only problem this young man has
   b) acne may very well be the "ticket of entry" to your office
   c) acne is the problem; treat his acne and send him on his way
   d) adolescents like this young man are more likely to present with minor problems rather than less likely
   e) it is very difficult to establish rapport with an adolescent patient like this young man

2. Regarding the patient described, you should now do which of the following?
   a) attempt to identify an underlying agenda
   b) call his mother and ask her if she thinks anything is wrong with him
   c) call the social worker and ask that the patient be seen at once
   d) refer the patient to a dermatologist
   e) none of the above

3. In order to facilitate further discussion with this patient at this time, what should you say?
   a) "we'll treat your acne; any other problems?"
   b) "acne is easily treated; don't worry"
   c) "I have a feeling there is something else you'd like to talk about—I'm listening"
   d) "don't look so down; this is easy as pie to treat"
   e) "my nurse will give you your acne medications—see you in a month"

4. What is the most common cause of death in adolescents in North America?
   a) homicide
   b) suicide
   c) motor vehicle accidents
   d) congenital malformations
   e) AIDS

5. What is the psychiatric disorder most common in adolescents?
   a) major depressive disorder—unipolar
   b) bipolar affective disorder
   c) schizophrenia
   d) adjustment disorder
   e) antisocial personality disorder

6. What is the key ingredient to ensure healthy adolescent development?
   a) early graded independence
   b) a prolonged supportive environment
   c) negotiating autonomy
   d) prevention of consequences for failure to perform up to parental expectations
   e) independence dependent on performance

7. Regarding exploratory behavior in adolescence, which of the following statements is(are) true?
   a) exploratory behavior is unnecessary and should be discouraged
   b) exploratory behavior is associated with some risks
   c) much of adolescent exploratory behavior is developmentally appropriate
   d) b and c
   e) all of the above

8. Early adolescence is mostly concerned with which of the following?
   a) a preoccupation with bodily changes
   b) a preoccupation with independence
   c) a preoccupation with becoming an adult
   d) a preoccupation with conforming to the peer group
   e) a preoccupation with distancing from parents

9. What is the second leading cause of death in adolescents in North America?
   a) motor vehicle accidents
   b) cancer
   c) alcohol-related disease
   d) suicide
   e) infectious disease—primarily AIDS

10. Which of the following factors is(are) associated with an increased risk of early adolescent sexual intercourse?
    a) divorce or separation of the parents

b) poor school grades or low future education plans
c) negative parental attitudes
d) none of the above
e) all of the above

11. Regarding the abuse of alcohol and other drugs by adolescents, which of the following statements is(are) true?
   a) cigarette smoking is the "gateway"
   b) the age at which children and adolescents begin experimenting with alcohol and other drugs is decreasing
   c) dimenhydrinate is becoming a "drug of abuse" among adolescents
   d) none of the above
   e) all of the above

12. The risk of adolescent drug abuse is influenced by which of the following?
   a) risky sexual behavior
   b) school performance
   c) physical activity
   d) a and b only
   e) all of the above

13. Regarding visits to family physicians by adolescents, which of the following is(are) true?
   a) the "acute episodic visit" is often the only type of visit adolescents make to physicians
   b) most adolescents making "acute episodic visits" to their family physicians have either an underlying behavior, an underlying social circumstance, or an underlying "myth" that should be explored at this opportunity
   c) 10% of adolescents have chronic conditions necessitating frequent visits to physicians' offices
   d) a and b only
   e) all of the above

14. Which of the following statements regarding teenage pregnancy is(are) true?
   a) teenage pregnancy is associated with poor prenatal care
   b) teenage pregnancy is associated with poor nutrition
   c) teenage pregnancy is associated with the use of illicit drugs
   d) all of the above are true
   e) none of the above are true

15. What is the central task of adolescence generally considered to be?
   a) the formation of a self-image of competency and strength
   b) to develop a way of coping with the major adjustment disorder that goes along with adolescence
   c) the ability to develop an independent ego
   d) the ability to follow the cycle of dependence to interdependence to independence without significant problems
   e) the ability to begin to think independently

Short Answer Management Problem 101

Describe the preventive medicine strategies that should be incorporated into an office visit in which an adolescent presents to his or her physician for acute episodic care.

ANSWERS

1. B. The acne that this young man presents with may very well be the ticket of entry to your office. Although it is possible that acne is the major reason for attending your office at this time, it is unlikely simply because he has acne. He states that his acne is "not much better or not much worse" than it has been for the last 4 years; therefore, more likely than not there is a second, or hidden, agenda.

2. A.

3. C. At this time you should attempt, if possible, to identify exactly what the likely hidden agenda is. An appropriate "opener" would be "I have a feeling there is something else that you would like to talk about—I'm listening." An alternative would be the following "are there any other problems that you wish to discuss at this time with me?" More direct questions would include questions about school (problems at school), questions about the relationship with his parents, questions about relationships (girlfriend problems and so on), and questions about sexual activity.

4. C. Violence has replaced communicable disease as the primary cause of death among youth. In 1985 USA statistics showed that 77% of adolescent deaths were caused by accidents, homicide, and suicide. Many of these deaths are completely preventable.

5. D. Many youths present with emotional symptoms. Unfortunately, some physicians feel uncomfortable or

awkward with these patients, and others deal with them in an awkward manner. The majority of adolescents in this category are suffering from a minor adolescent adjustment disorder and require little more than caring and reassurance. On the other hand, be on the lookout for more serious psychiatric conditions, conditions that would lead you to come up with a diagnosis of major depression, suicidal ideation, or a similar serious condition.

6. B. Experts agree that the key ingredient to ensure healthy adolescent development is a prolonged supportive environment with graded steps toward autonomy. Healthy development is encouraged by a process of mutual positive engagement between adolescents, various adults, and peers. Schools and youth-serving community agencies can also play a major role by engaging youth in meaningful ways.

7. D. Adolescence is characterized by exploratory behavior, much of which is developmentally appropriate and socially adaptive. The adolescent must experiment with new behaviors and relationships, inevitably courting some risks. There is a not a simple distinction between what is normal and what is abnormal in exploratory behavior. It is better to judge a particular behavior in the context of how the adolescent is developing in the family, at school, and among peers and friends.

8. A. Early adolescence brings a preoccupation with body changes. Early adolescents feel uncertain about their appearance, and their interests are directed toward themselves. This is a period marked by high levels of physical activity and mood swings.

9. D. In North America suicide is now the second leading cause of death in the adolescent population. In some parts of the United States, homicide is second and suicide is third.

10. E. Factors associated with initiation of intercourse in adolescence include divorce or separation of parents, poor school grades and low future educational plans, negative parental attitudes (that is, if teens are taught that sex is not healthy or normal), and the use of drugs and/or alcohol.

11. E. First, nicotene is definitely the "gateway drug"—the drug that leads to the use of other and more dangerous drugs, including alcohol, marijuana, and cocaine.

    Second, the age at which adolescents first begin experimentation with alcohol and other drugs is dropping.

    Third, the antinauseant dimenhydrinate (Dramamine, Gravol) has now become a drug of abuse, so much so that many pharmacies have now put this substance behind the counter.

12. E. The use of alcohol and other drugs is one of the many risk factors that contribute to the deterioration in the health of adolescents. Different risk factors are associated with each individual, and these risks vary in accordance with age and sex. The use of drugs and alcohol, risky sexual behavior, school performance, peer pressure, diet, physical activity, socioeconomic status, and parental relationships are all factors that influence and predict the likelihood of risky behavior.

13. E. Acute episodic care or the acute episodic visit is the most frequent reason for an adolescent to visit a physician's office. These visits most frequently involve visits for respiratory tract infections, skin conditions, genitourinary tract concerns, musculoskeletal trauma, and emotional disorders.

    First, an episodic care visit is often the only type of visit that a youth will make to a physician's office.

    Second, most youth have an underlying behavior, a social circumstance, or a myth that may or may not be affecting the presenting condition but has the potential to affect future health.

    Third, youth are establishing health habits for adult life.

    Ten percent of adolescents have chronic medical conditions affecting them, including problems such as diabetes mellitus, asthma and respiratory allergies, epilepsy, inflammatory bowel disease, juvenile rheumatoid arthritis, various cancers (especially leukemia), congenital heart disease, cystic fibrosis, and hemophilia.

14. D. Teenage pregnancy is associated with the following:
    1) Poor prenatal care due to reluctance to seek care
    2) Poor nutrition leading to IUGR
    3) Smoking (one-third of pregnant teens)
    4) Use of illicit drugs
    5) Associated STDs
    6) Poor parenting skills
    All of these may negatively affect the infant.

15. A. It is development in the psychosocial area that gives adolescence its main distinctive characteristics. The adolescent is faced with the resolution of a number of developmental tasks. It is widely accepted that the central task of adolescence is the formation of a self-image of competency and strength. Adolescents who have difficulty establishing an identity are plagued by role confusion. They also have difficulty establishing long-lasting relationships and stable career opportunities. If they enter adulthood without a sense of identity, their further development may be in jeopardy.

SOLUTION TO SHORT ANSWER MANAGMENT PROBLEM 101

Adolescence is a period of time when at least one health maintenance examination should be carried out. Episodic care visits are an ideal time to carry out these health screenings and assessments. Two mnemonics are available that are useful in screening adolescents:

    A. SAFE TIMES

    B. HEADS

A. SAFE TIMES:

    S = sexuality issues

    A = affect (depression) and abuse (drugs)

    F = family (function and medical history)

    E = exam (sensitive and appropriate)

    T = timing of development (body image)

    I = immunizations

    M = minerals (nutritional issues)

    E = education, employment (school and work issues)

    S = safety (vehicle)

B. HEADS:

    H = home

    E = education, employment (school and work issues)

    A = activities, affect, anxieties, ambitions

    D = drugs

    S = sex, stress, suicide, self-esteem

C. **Phases of adolescent development:**

1. Early adolescence: preoccupation with body changes. Early adolescents often feel uncertain about their appearance and their interests are directed toward themselves. This is a period marked by high levels of physical activity and mood swings.

2. Mid-adolescence: in mid-adolescence the major concern is independence. The peer group dominates social life, and risk behaviors become more prevalent. This is the time when sexual matters receive much interest.

3. Late adolescence: in many ways, youth in the late-adolescence phase appear to be adults. They are more capable of future orientation, mutual caring, and internal control. However, most late adolescents also have uncertainties about sexuality, future relationships, and future work possibilities. Allowing them to be adolescents is very important.

SUMMARY OF THE DIAGNOSIS AND TREATMENT OF ADOLESCENT DEVELOPMENT

The solution to the Short Answer Management Problem is an excellent summary of adolescent development.

SUGGESTED READINGS

The College of Family Physicians of Canada. A report of the Task Force on Adolescent Health. 1993.

Bennett D. Understanding the adolescent patient. Australian Family Physician 1988; 17(5): 345-346.

Schubiner HH. Preventive health screening in adolescent patients. Primary Care 1988; 16(1): 211-230.

PROBLEM 102   A 6-YEAR-OLD BOY WHO "WETS THE BED"

A mother brings her 6-year-old boy to your office for a periodic health assessment. The child continues to wet his bed at night (an average is two to three times per week). He is dry during the day.

The child has no history of significant medical problems. Specifically, he has had no urinary tract infections. Labor and delivery were normal, as was the neonatal period.

His growth (both weight and height) has always been on the tenth percentile. He started school last year but did not do well. He had to repeat his first grade.

His blood pressure measured today is 85/60 mm Hg. The examination of all other body systems is normal.

SELECT THE ONE BEST ANSWER TO THE FOLLOWING QUESTIONS

1. What is the most likely diagnosis in this child?
   a) separation anxiety, with or without school phobia
   b) nocturnal enuresis
   c) SBS (small bladder syndrome)
   d) masked childhood depression
   e) none of the above

2. With respect to this condition, which of the following statements is false?
   a) at age 5 years 7% of children have the condition
   b) the condition is more common when one or both parents had the condition
   c) the functional bladder capacity in children with this condition is significantly less than those without
   d) the condition usually implies significant psychopathology in the child
   e) urethral valves, neurogenic bladder, and ectopic ureter may be associated with the condition

3. A child is defined as enuretic if he or she has not attained full bladder control by what age?
   a) 3 years
   b) 4 years
   c) 5 years
   d) 6 years
   e) 8 years

4. Which of the following investigations is the most important to be performed in a child with enuresis?
   a) urinalysis
   b) urine culture
   c) CBC
   d) complete cystometric evaluation
   e) IVP

5. Which of the following is not a consideration in the differential diagnosis of enuresis?
   a) diabetes mellitus
   b) diabetes insipidus
   c) petit mal seizures
   d) separation anxiety disorder
   e) posterior urethral valve syndrome

6. Which of the following is the drug of choice in the pharmacologic treatment of this disorder?
   a) oxybutynin chloride
   b) imipramine
   c) chlorpromazine
   d) diazepam
   e) none of the above

7. Which of the following statements most accurately reflects the treatment of this condition?
   a) most nonpharmacologic therapies have been shown to be no more effective than placebo in the treatment of this condition
   b) behavior modification has been shown to be superior to other nonpharmacologic therapies
   c) pharmacologic therapy is recommended in enuretic children who do not respond to nonpharmacologic therapies
   d) b and c
   e) all of the above

8. What is the most effective form of behavior modification in the treatment of the disorder described?
   a) biofeedback
   b) "electric shock" treatment (spontaneously triggered when the child wets the bed)
   c) a bell or buzzer system
   d) the behavior modification theory of logical consequences
   e) all of the above are equally effective

9. Which of the following is(are) important in the treatment of this condition?
   a) enlisting the cooperation of the child in dealing with the problem
   b) establishing a rule that older children should be expected to launder their own soiled bed clothes and pajamas
   c) elimination of liquids prior to bedtime
   d) voiding just prior to bedtime
   e) all of the above

10. Which of the following should not be used in the treatment of this condition?
    a) punishing the child

b) postponing bedtime in an effort to decrease the frequency of the problem

c) providing the child with a feeling of inferiority for having the problem

d) all of the above

e) a and c

Short Answer Management Problem 102

Discuss the possible relationship between enuresis in a child and psychologic or psychiatric problems in children.

ANSWERS

1. B.

2. D.

3. C. The DSM-IV classification of enuresis (which this child has) is based on the following criteria:
   1. Repeated voiding of urine into bed or clothes (whether involuntary or intentional)
   2. The behavior is clinically significant as manifested by either frequency of twice/week for at least 3 consecutive weeks or the presence of clinically significant distress or impairment in social, academic (occupational), or other important areas of functioning.
   3. Age of at least 5 years
   4. Not due to the direct physiological effect of a substance (such as a diuretic) or a general medical condition (such as diabetes, spina bifida, or a seizure disorder)

   DSM-IV further subclassifies enuresis into the following:
   A. Nocturnal only
   B. Diurnal only
   C. Nocturnal and diurnal

   This child does not meet the criteria for separation anxiety disorder, and there is no information that suggests a diagnosis of masked depression. SBS (small bladder syndrome) does not exist.

   Enuresis is usually defined as the involuntary discharge of urine after the age at which bladder control should usually have been established (age 5). As just classified, this child has nocturnal enuresis (only at night).

   The prevalence of enuresis decreases with increasing age. Thus 82% of 2-year-olds, 49% of 3-year-olds, 26% of 4-year-olds, and 7% of 5-year-olds have been reported to wet beds or clothes on a regular basis.

   Enuresis is definitely more common in children when one or both parents were enuretic as children.

   There appears to be a developmental immaturity leading to a decreased functional bladder capacity in enuretic children.

Uropathies may be associated with enuresis. Urethral valves, neurogenic bladder, and ectopic ureter may occasionally be the cause of primary enuresis.

Urinary tract infections are a common organic cause of enuresis, especially secondary enuresis in girls.

It is estimated that mental disorders are present in only about 20% of enuretic children. They are most common in enuretic girls, in children with symptoms during both day and night, and in children who maintain the symptoms into older childhood. Thus mental disorders are the exception rather than the rule.

4. A.

5. D. The only mandatory laboratory evaluation for enuretic children is a urinalysis. WBCs in urinary tract infection, low specific gravity in diabetes insipidus, proteinuria, or hematuria in renal disease, and glucosuria in diabetes mellitus are all important abnormalities that may be associated with enuresis.

   Urine culture, CBC, IVP, and cystometric evaluation should be performed only if specific indications suggest the need. Posterior urethral valves (especially in boys) may be associated with enuresis.

   The only disorder listed in Question 5 that is not part of the differential diagnosis of enuresis is separation anxiety disorder.

6. E.

7. B.

8. C.

9. E.

10. D. The second edition of this textbook suggested that the pharmacologic therapy of choice for enuresis was imipramine. The current recommendation regarding imipramine is that its administration is generally effective only briefly, and drug tolerance is common. Its use in children with enuresis should be discouraged because

of exacerbation of symptoms after the discontinuation of the drug, and medication side effects.

Because there is usually no identifiable cause of enuresis and the disorder tends to remit spontaneously even if not treated, treatment should be conservative.

The methods approved for the treatment of enuresis include the following:

A. Appropriate toilet training (scheduled voiding times especially in the evening; wake up to urinate in the middle of the night)
B. Behavior modification (bell or buzzer) and pad
C. Positive reinforcement system that charts the child's progress

Although all of the approved methods are effective and should be used together, it appears that the most effective behavior modification method is the "buzzer or bell" and pad system.

Here are some general recommendations that may prove helpful in the treatment of enuresis:

1. Enlisting the support and cooperation of the child in treating the condition
2. Having older children launder their own soiled bedclothes and pajamas (not as a punishment but rather as participation in their own illness)
3. Prohibiting liquids after dinner
4. Making sure the child voids before retiring

Here are some general recommendations to avoid in the treatment of enuresis:

1. Waking the child repeatedly during the night to take him or her to the bathroom; this has negative consequences in most children for the following reasons:
   a) It disturbs sleep
   b) It may further engender or aggravate anger in the child or the parent.
2. Punishing the child for wetting the bed
3. Intimidating the child or lowering his self-esteem
4. Postponing the child's bedtime in an effort to decrease the frequency of bedwetting

SOLUTION TO SHORT ANSWER MANAGEMENT PROBLEM 102

The key points to consider in discussing the relationship between enuresis and psychological or psychiatric problems are as follows:

1) The vast majority of enuretic children (80%) have no associated psychologic or psychiatric pathology.
2) Chronic psychologic stress (unrelated to toilet training experiences) can impair the child's ability to achieve bladder control.
3) A situation in which the child becomes enuretic after a period of dryness is called *regressive enuresis.* This type of enuresis is precipitated by stressful environmental events such as a move to a new home, marital conflict, birth of a sibling, or a death in the family. Such bedwetting is in-

termittent and transitory; the prognosis is better, and management is less difficult than in a child with primary enuresis.

SUMMARY OF THE DIAGNOSIS AND TREATMENT OF ENURESIS IN CHILDREN

1. **Prevalence:** 7% at the age when bladder control should have been fully achieved (that is, 5 years)
2. **Subtypes of enuresis:**
   Two basic classification systems:
   a) Classification based on whether or not child has ever achieved bladder control
   b) Classification based on period when child does not have bladder control
   Classification 1:
   1. Primary enuresis: child has never been dry.
   2. Regressive enuresis: child has been dry for a period but becomes enuretic later.
   Classification 2:
   1. Nocturnal enuresis: enuresis at night only
   2. Diurnal enuresis: enuresis during the day only
   3. Nocturnal and diurnal enuresis: enuresis during both day and night
3. **Pathophysiology:** immaturity of part of autonomic nervous system controlling bladder in vast majority of cases. Infrequently, enuresis is associated with organic problem such as congenital urinary tract system abnormality or urinary tract infection.
4. **Investigations:** urinalysis is the only mandatory investigation.
5. **Treatment:**
   a) Pharmacologic: imipramine is no longer recommended for the treatment of enuresis in most children.
   b) Nonpharmacologic: behavior modification program is treatment of choice.
   1. Buzzer or bell system
   2. Positive reinforcement
   3. Charting progress to increase confidence and self-esteem of the child
   4. Urinating before bed
   5. Avoiding liquids after supper
6. **Relationship to psychopathology:**
   a) Only 20% of children with enuresis have a mental disorder.
   b) Regressive enuresis is usually associated with some stressful environmental event.

SUGGESTED READINGS

American Psychiatric Association. Diagnostic and statistical manual of mental disorders. 4th Ed. Washington, DC: American Psychiatric Association Press, 1994.

Behrman R, ed. Nelson textbook of pediatrics. 14th Ed. Philadelphia: WB Saunders, 1992.

PROBLEM 103   A 6-YEAR-OLD BOY WITH A CONSTANTLY RUNNING NOSE

A mother presents to your office with her 6-year-old son. She states that for the past 15 months the child has been "constantly rubbing his nose and his eyes." She adds that "his nose is constantly running."

He has had no significant upper respiratory tract infections, nor is there any history of wheezing or coughing that might suggest asthma.

There is, however, a family history of both asthma and allergies. There appears to be a temporal association between the onset of the symptoms the mother describes and the acquisition of "Boots", a black cat with white paws.

On examination, there is obvious nasal congestion, hyperemia, and discharge bilaterally. There also appear to be bluish-purple rings around both eyes. On examination of the respiratory system there are a few rhonchi heard, especially on expiration.

SELECT THE ONE BEST ANSWER TO THE FOLLOWING QUESTIONS

1. What is the most likely diagnosis in this child?
   a) vasomotor rhinitis
   b) chronic infectious rhinitis
   c) allergic rhinitis
   d) primary atrophic rhinitis
   e) eosinophilic nonallergic rhinitis

2. The bluish-purple rings around both eyes are best described as which of the following?
   a) abnormal: the diagnosis is most likely a serious coagulation defect
   b) normal: the diagnosis is most likely a mild coagulation defect
   c) normal: the rings are known as allergic shiners
   d) normal: the rings are known as eosinophilic eye syndrome
   e) nobody really knows for sure; we know they have something to do with allergy, but not much more

3. Which of the following immunoglobulins are associated with the condition described in Question 1?
   a) IgA
   b) IgE
   c) IgG
   d) IgM
   e) none of the above

4. Which of the following statements regarding the cause of this child's symptoms is(are) true?
   a) there is likely no association between this child's symptoms and Boots the cat
   b) although there is a temporal relationship between the acquisition of the cat and the symptoms, it is unlikely to be a true cause-and-effect relationship
   c) the temporal relationship between the acquisition of Boots the cat and the symptoms suggests a cause-and-effect relationship
   d) although the cat may be a small part of the answer, there is likely to be some other underlying reason for this child's symptoms

   e) there is likely no significance to this child's symptoms and the family history of allergy

5. What is the single most common cause of seasonal allergic rhinitis in children in the United States?
   a) grasses
   b) tree pollens
   c) tumbleweed
   d) ragweed pollen
   e) mold spores

6. What is the single most common cause of perennial allergic rhinitis in children in the United States?
   a) house dust and house dust mite
   b) cat dander
   c) cat saliva
   d) feathers
   e) mold spores

7. What is the single most important part of the treatment protocol in the condition described?
   a) the use of intranasal corticosteroids
   b) the use of intranasal sodium cromoglycate
   c) the use of systemic antihistamines
   d) the use of systemic adrenergic drugs
   e) none of the above

8. What is the pharmacologic agent of first choice in the treatment of the condition described?
   a) intranasal corticosteroids
   b) intranasal sodium cromoglycate
   c) systemic antihistamines
   d) systemic adrenergic drugs
   e) none of the above

9. What is the single best pharmacologic treatment for the condition described?
   a) intranasal corticosteroids
   b) intranasal sodium cromoglycate
   c) systemic antihistamines
   d) systemic adrenergic drugs
   e) none of the above

10. What is the mechanism of action of sodium cromogly-cate as a treatment for the condition described?
    a) a decongestant
    b) a vasoconstrictor
    c) an antigen-induced mediator inhibitor
    d) a IgE inhibitor
    e) none of the above

11. What is the diagnostic test of choice for the condition described?
    a) serum IgE determination
    b) a nasal smear for eosinophil count
    c) RAST testing
    d) skin prick testing
    e) CT scan of the nose

12. Vasomotor rhinitis is best distinguished from allergic rhinitis by which of the following?
    a) the absence of sneezing, itching, or rhinorrhea in vasomotor rhinitis
    b) the absence of eosinophils on nasal smear in vaso-motor rhinitis
    c) the predominance of nasal obstruction as the pri-mary symptom in vasomotor rhinitis
    d) all of the above
    e) none of the above

13. Which of the following systemic disorders is most closely associated with nasal obstruction?
    a) diabetes mellitus
    b) hyperthyroidism
    c) hyperparathyroidism
    d) hypothyroidism
    e) systemic lupus erythematosus

14. The condition *triad asthma* includes all of the following except
    a) nasal polyps
    b) asthma
    c) aspirin intolerance
    d) persistent nasal rhinorrhea
    e) all of the above are included

15. Allergic conjunctivitis associated with the condition described is best treated with which of the following?
    a) corticosteroid eye drops
    b) sodium cromoglycate eye drops
    c) silver nitrate eye drops
    d) erythromycin eye ointment
    e) chloramphenicol eye drops

Short Answer Management Problem 103

Define and describe the disorder *rhinitis medicamentosa*.

ANSWERS

1. C.

2. C.

3. B. This child most likely has allergic rhinitis. Allergic rhinitis is an inflammatory disorder of the nasal mucosa initiated by an IgE-mediated hypersensitivity. It is the most common disease of the nasal passages.

   The symptoms of allergic rhinitis include nasal de-congestion (stuffy nose), sneezing, pruritus, rhinorrhea, nasal discharge, mouth breathing, and snoring.

   Exposure to cigarette smoke, paint fumes, strong odors, and allergens may precipitate the symptoms.

   Physical examination may show an "allergic solute" (rubbing and dorsal manipulation of the nose resulting in a transverse wrinkle externally), edematous and con-gested nasal mucosa, obstruction of venous drainage in the periorbital region (the allergic shiners just men-tioned), hypertrophy of the tonsils, and hypertrophy of the adenoids. Serous otitis media is commonly observed in association with allergic rhinitis. As well, allergic rhinitis is more common in children who have either atopic dermatitis or asthma.

   Eosinophilic nonallergic rhinitis may manifest the same symptoms as allergic rhinitis but is much less common and may be distinguished by the absence of positive skin tests or radioallergosorbent tests (RASTS).

   Vasomotor rhinitis is a nonallergic, noninfectious rhinitis caused by an imbalance of autonomic nervous system control.

   Chronic infectious rhinitis results in mucopurulent rhinorrhea, often associated with low-grade fever, cough, sore throat, and malaise. Sinusitis and recurrent purulent otitis media may be present.

   Primary atrophic rhinitis, with autosomal dominant inheritance, rarely occurs in children.

4. C.

5. D.

6. A. The symptom of a constantly running nose suggests the subtype of allergic rhinitis classified as *perennial allergic rhinitis*. The causative agents, when identified, are usually allergens to which the patient is exposed more or less continually, although exposure may vary during the year. Indoor inhalant allergens are implicated most often. These include the following:
   a) Components of house dust (house dust and house dust mite are the most common cause)
   b) Feathers
   c) Allergens or danders of household pets
   d) Mold spores

   Because this child did not have symptoms prior to the acquisition of the cat, the temporal relationship certainly is very suspicious and almost certainly the cause of this child's symptoms. The actual allergen may be either cat dander or cat saliva.

   Seasonal allergic rhinitis, on the other hand, is also known as *hay fever*. This is most commonly seen in children who have been exposed to windborne pollens of trees, grasses, and weeds. The single most common cause of seasonal allergic rhinitis is ragweed pollen.

7. E. The single most important part of the treatment protocol for allergic rhinitis is removing, whenever possible, the environmental source responsible for the condition.

   Although it is difficult or impractical to avoid exposure to seasonal pollens, much can be done to avoid indoor inhalant factors such as house dust, house dust mites, animal danders, and molds. Control of house dust, with special attention to the child's bedroom, often significantly improves symptoms. Elimination of exposure to danders and feathers is mandatory for a child with perennial allergic rhinitis when these factors are responsible for the symptoms. Thus, after confirmation by prick testing, Boots will have to go.

8. B.

9. A.

10. C. Intranasal corticosteroids are by far the most effective treatment for allergic rhinitis. Beclomethasone of flunisolide should be used in children whose nasal symptoms are resistant to sodium cromoglycate. The usual dose of metered inhaler is one to two inhalations two or three times/day. Intranasal corticosteroids are considered to be by most authorities the drugs of second choice. Although they have superior efficacy, the possibility of systemic absorption does exist. Sodium cromoglycate, an inhibitor of antigen-induced mediator release, is the drug of first choice in the treatment of allergic rhinitis. It is administered by intranasal inhalation, one or two inhalations three to six times/day.

   Systemic antihistamines are useful in the treatment of allergic rhinitis, especially in the seasonal subtype.

Nonsedating antihistamines such as astemizole and terfenadine are preferred to the more sedating hydroxyzine.

Inhaled or systemic adrenergic agents, such as the decongestant pseudoephedrine or phenylpropanolamine, are best avoided, especially in perennial allergic rhinitis. Nasal sprays containing these agents should be used sparingly if at all due to the possibility of rebound congestion.

11. B.

12. D. Vasomotor rhinitis is a very poorly understood diagnostic entity, related somehow to autonomic nervous system dysfunction. Vasomotor rhinitis has the following features:
    A. Nasal obstruction is the primary symptom.
    B. There is an absence of sneezing, itching, and rhinorrhea.
    C. No eosinophils are seen on nasal smear.

13. D. The systemic disease most closely associated with nasal obstruction is hypothyroidism.

    The drug most closely associated with nasal congestion in the past was reserpine, a drug almost unheard of for pediatric use.

14. D. The triad asthma includes nasal polyps, asthma, and aspirin intolerance. On examination this child demonstrates audible expiratory rhonchi; these rhonchi may well be a sign of bronchial asthma.

    Persistent nasal rhinorrhea is not part of the symptom complex triad asthma.

15. B. Allergic conjunctivitis goes along with allergic rhinitis. The treatment of choice for allergic conjunctivitis at this time is sodium cromoglycate. If severe, corticosteroid eye drops can be temporarily used with caution. A consultation with an ophthalmologist would be advisable.

SOLUTION TO SHORT ANSWER MANAGEMENT PROBLEM 103

Rhinitis medicamentosa is a disorder of chronic nasal congestion and obstruction produced by a rebound effect from the excessive use of vasoconstrictor nose drops. It is imperative to educate patients regarding using nasal decongestant nose drops for a time period not exceeding a few days. Rebound congestion works in much the same manner as rebound headaches from the too-frequent use of analgesics.

SUMMARY OF THE DIAGNOSIS AND TREATMENT OF ALLERGIC RHINITIS

1. **Classification:**
   a) Seasonal allergic rhinitis (also known as seasonal pollinosis and hay fever): causes include tree pollen, weed pollen, grasses; most common cause is ragweed.

b) Perennial allergic rhinitis: the patient has symptoms year-round. The causative agents include house dust and house dust mite (most common), animal saliva, animal dander, feathers, and molds.

2. **Symptoms:**
   a) Nasal congestion
   b) Sneezing
   c) Itching
   d) Rhinorrhea
   e) Nasal discharge
      Clues:
      1. Allergic shiners: due to venous stasis resulting from interference with blood flow through edematous nasal mucous membranes
      2. Allergic salute: rubbing hand in an upward direction

3. **Diagnosis:**
   a) Nasal smear to demonstrate eosinophils
   b) Allergy testing to identify specific allergen

4. **Associated disorders:**
   a) Serous otitis media (acute and chronic)
   b) Adenoid hypertrophy
   c) Tonsillar hypertrophy
   d) Asthma

5. **Treatment:**
   a) Avoidance:

1. Difficult to avoid seasonal allergic pollens in seasonal allergic rhinitis
2. In perennial allergic rhinitis, the causative agent should be minimized wherever possible. Special attention should be paid to the child's bedroom and an electronic air filter installed if possible.

b) Pharmacologic agents:
   1. Inhaled sodium cromoglycate is drug of first choice.
   2. Inhaled corticosteroids are best and most effective drug.
   3. Systemic (nonsedating antihistamines)
   4. Sparing use of decongestants and local vasoconstrictors

6. **Differential diagnosis of rhinitis:**
   a) Allergic rhinitis
   b) Eosinophilic nonallergic rhinitis
   c) Infectious rhinitis: viral/bacterial
   d) Vasomotor rhinitis
   e) Rhinitis medicamentosa

SUGGESTED READING

Behrman R, ed. Nelson textbook of pediatrics. 14th Ed. Philadelphia: WB Saunders, 1992.

PROBLEM 104   A 2-MONTH-OLD INFANT WITH A RASH ON HIS CHEEKS

A 2-month-old infant is brought to your office by his mother. He developed an erythematous, dry skin rash on both cheeks approximately 1 week ago. Although the rash is always present, the mother states that "it seems to be worse after I feed him."

The mother breast-fed for the first 4 weeks of life but returned to work 4 weeks ago and switched the baby from breast to bottle. In addition, she decided to feed him with "whole milk" rather than with infant formula.

On examination, the child appears healthy. He has an erythematous maculopapular eruption that covers his cheeks, and he appears to be developing an erythematous rash on his neck, both wrists, and both hands. The rest of the physical examination is within normal limits.

SELECT THE ONE BEST ANSWER TO THE FOLLOWING QUESTIONS

1. What is the most likely cause of this infant's skin rash?
   a) atopic dermatitis
   b) allergic contact dermatitis
   c) seborrheic dermatitis
   d) infectious eczematoid dermatitis
   e) none of the above

2. What is(are) the recommended treatment(s) of the skin rash in the infant presented?
   a) wet dressings
   b) local corticosteroid therapy
   c) systemic antihistamines
   d) antibiotics (local)
   e) all of the above

3. With which of the following antibodies is the described disorder associated?
   a) IgA
   b) IgG-VCA
   c) IgM-VCA
   d) IgE
   e) none of the above

4. Regarding this child's feeding, what would be the best course of action at this time?
   a) continue feeding the infant with cow's milk
   b) switch from whole milk to a soy-based formula as the first step
   c) switch from whole milk to a non-soy-based formula as the first step
   d) switch from whole cow's milk to 1% cow's milk
   e) switch from whole cow's milk to skimmed cow's milk

5. A 1-month-old infant is brought to your office by his mother. She states that the infant has had a "diaper rash" for the past 2 weeks that has not cleared up on zinc oxide tid. She tells you that "I must be doing something wrong" and is extremely upset.

   On examination, the infant has an erythematous, weeping, oily eruption in the diaper area. As well, he has a scaly eruption on the scalp, the ear, the sides of the nose, and the eyebrows and eyelids. The rest of the physical examination is normal.

   What is the most likely diagnosis in this infant?
   a) atopic dermatitis
   b) allergic contact dermatitis
   c) seborrheic dermatitis
   d) infectious eczematoid dermatitis
   e) none of the above

6. What is(are) the treatment(s) of choice for the condition described in Question 5?
   a) wet compresses
   b) topical corticosteroids
   c) topical ketoconazole
   d) a and b
   e) all of the above

7. An 8-month-old infant presents to your office with his mother for assessment of a "diaper rash." His mother has tried the following remedies: corn starch, talcum powder, vitamin E cream, zinc oxide, three different prescribed corticosteroid creams from three different physicians. She tells you that "I went to three doctors because the first two said, 'Oh, don't worry dear, just a little diaper rash—it will go away; don't worry your pretty little head about it.'"

   On examination, the infant has an intensely erythematous diaper dermatitis that has a scalloped border and a sharply demarcated edge. There are numerous "satellite lesions" present on the lower abdomen and thighs.

   What is the most likely diagnosis in this infant?
   a) atopic dermatitis
   b) allergic contact dermatitis
   c) seborrheic dermatitis
   d) infectious eczematoid dermatitis
   e) candidal diaper dermatitis

8. What is the treatment of choice for the diaper rash of the infant described in Question 7?
   a) a topical corticosteroid
   b) a topical antibiotic
   c) a systemic antibiotic
   d) a topical antifungal agent
   e) none of the above

9. A 4-month-old infant is brought to your office by her mother. Her mother complains that the child has a "diaper rash" that is probably related to her "lack of changing by the babysitter." Apparently, the infant went for long periods of time while the babysitter sat on the couch watching television. Needless to say, the babysitter is no longer in the employ of the mother.

On examination, the infant has an erythematous, scaly, papulovesicular diaper dermatitis with numerous bullous lesions, fissures, and erosions.

What is the most likely diagnosis in this infant?
a) atopic dermatitis
b) primary irritant contact dermatitis
c) seborrheic dermatitis
d) fungal dermatitis
e) allergic contact dermatitis

10. What is(are) the treatment(s) of choice for the infant presented in Question 9?
a) zinc oxide paste
b) topical hydrocortisone
c) systemic antibiotics
d) a and b
e) all of the above

Short Answer Management Problem 104

For each of the following four types of diaper dermatitis, provide a "diagnostic clue" that will help you distinguish one from another.
1. Atopic dermatitis
2. Seborrheic dermatitis
3. Candidal dermatitis
4. Primary irritant dermatitis

ANSWERS

1. A.

2. E.

3. D.

4. C. This child has atopic dermatitis. Atopic dermatitis is an inflammatory skin disease characterized by erythema, edema, pruritus, exudation, crusting, and scaling.

Atopic dermatitis usually begins in infancy. The areas most commonly affected include the cheeks, the neck, the wrists, the hands, and the extensor aspects of the extremities. Spread often occurs from extensor to flexor. Pruritus may lead to intense scratching and secondary infection.

Atopic dermatitis is usually precipitated by or exacerbated by the introduction of certain foods to the infant's diet, particularly cow's milk, wheat, or eggs. Environmental factors such as dust, mold, and cat dander may also trigger the condition.

Atopic dermatitis usually remits by the age of 3-5 years. There is often a family history of allergies, asthma, hay fever, or atopic dermatitis. Atopic dermatitis is mediated and regulated by an IgE antibody response and by antigen-specific T cells that secrete IgE antibody binding factors.

The treatment of atopic dermatitis begins with the avoidance of any environmental factors that precipitate the condition.

Smooth-textured cotton garments eliminated added irritation in this disorder.

The use of soaps, detergents, and bathing without bath oil defat the skin and should be avoided whenever possible. Ideally, the child should be in the tub for at least 15 minutes before the bath oil is added to the water.

Atopic dermatitis is best managed with local therapy. Flare-ups of the condition are treated with wet dressings (such as aluminum acetate: 1/20). These wet dressings, in addition to providing symptomatic relief, immobilize and protect the affected parts of the skin and prevent scratching. To further prevent scratching, the fingernails should be cut short.

Topical corticosteroid creams or lotions can be applied between wet dressing changes. Percutaneous absorption of corticosteroid does occur, and atrophy of the skin should be watched for. This can be managed by using the mildest hydrocortisone preparation available (0.5% hydrocortisone 1%).

Systemic antihistamines such as diphenhydramine, promethazine, and hydroxyzine may have to be used to control pruritus (use with caution).

Infected atopic dermatitis is best managed by antibiotic therapy. Systemic antibiotics, the mainstay of treatment for infected atopic dermatitis, have largely been replaced by the newer, nonsensitizing local antibiotic preparations such as fusidic acid.

This child should be taken off cow's milk and, as a first step, put onto a regular infant formula. If the atopic dermatitis persists despite the regular infant formula, it would then be reasonable to consider switching to a soy-based formula.

5. C.

6. E. This infant has seborrheic dermatitis.

Seborrheic dermatitis is an inflammatory disorder that often begins in the first month of life. The initial manifestation of seborrheic dermatitis is often a diffuse or focal scaling and crusting of the scalp, a condition known as "cradle cap." A dry, scaly, erythematous, papular dermatitis, which is usually nonpruritic, may develop, involving the face, neck, retroauricular areas, axillae, and diaper area. The dermatitis may be patchy or focal, or may spread to involve the entire body.

Wet compresses (saline) are an effective first treatment for seborrheic dermatitis. A soft brush can be used to remove some of the scales associated with cradle cap. Scalp lesions may also be controlled with an antiseborrheic shampoo such as selenium sulfide.

Topical corticosteroids (hydrocortisone 0.5%-1%) may be applied to inflammatory lesions. The use of topical ketoconazole (2%) has been found to be of benefit in the treatment of seborrheic dermatitis.

7. E.

8. D. This infant has candidal diaper dermatitis.

Candidal diaper dermatitis presents as an erythematous confluent plaque formed by papules and vesiculopustules, with a scalloped border and a sharply demarcated edge. Candidal diaper dermatitis can usually be distinguished from other childhood diaper dermatoses by the presence of "satellite lesions" produced at some distance from the primary eruption.

The treatment of choice in candidal diaper dermatitis is a topical antifungal agent. Topical miconazole, clotrimazole, or ketoconazole can be used after soaking the inflamed area with wet aluminum acetate compresses. In an infant with a severe inflammatory reaction, a topical corticosteroid may be mixed 50/50 with a topical antifungal agent and applied on a regular basis for a few days to a week.

The attitude displayed by the first two physicians (condescending and arrogant) is not as uncommon as we think. Doctor-patient communication in something as simple as a diaper dermatitis can significantly affect not only efficacy of treatment but compliance and postdiagnostic attitudes.

9. B.

10. D. This child has a primary irritant contact dermatitis.

Irritant contact dermatitis is a reaction to friction, maceration, and prolonged contact with urine and feces. It usually presents as an erythematous, scaly dermatitis with papulovesicular or bollous lesions, fissures, and erosions. The eruption can be either patchy or confluent. The genitocrural folds are often spared.

Secondary infection with either bacteria or yeast can occur. The infant can be in considerable discomfort due to marked inflammation that is sometimes associated with this type of diaper rash.

Primary irritant diaper dermatitis should be managed by frequent changing of diapers and thorough washing of the genitalia with warm water and a mild soap. Occlusive plastic pants that promote maceration should be avoided. Disposable diapers should be used instead of cloth diapers.

An occlusive topical agent such as zinc oxide or petroleum jelly should be applied after washing. A mild hydrocortisone cream with or without zinc oxide can be applied until healing occurs. Systemic antibiotics are not indicated in the treatment of primary irritant diaper dermatitis.

SOLUTION TO SHORT ANSWER MANAGEMENT PROBLEM 104 AND SUMMARY OF THE DIAGNOSIS AND TREATMENT OF DIAPER DERMATITIS

1. **Atopic dermatitis:**
   Diagnostic clue: usually begins and is more prominent on the cheeks of infants
   Treatment: wet dressings (saline), moisturization, mild topical corticosteroids, systemic antihistamines (with caution), topical antibiotics for secondary infection
2. **Seborrheic dermatitis:**
   Diagnostic clue: cradle cap is often associated with this type of diaper dermatitis.
   Treatment: wet compresses (saline), mild topical corticosteroids, topical ketoconazole
3. **Candidal dermatitis:**
   Diagnostic clue: satellite lesions around the peripheral area of the main area of dermatitis
   Treatment: topical miconazole, topical ketoconazole; mild topical hydrocortisone can be mixed 50/50 when severe inflammation is present.
4. **Primary irritant dermatitis:**
   Diagnostic clue: maceration, often a history of the use of cloth diapers and/or plastic pants
   Treatment: occlusive topical agent such as zinc oxide or petroleum jelly; with severe inflammation, zinc oxide can be applied over hydrocortisone base.

SUGGESTED READING

Behrman R, et al., eds. Eczema and atopic dermatitis. Nelson textbook of pediatrics. 14th Ed. Philadelphia: WB Saunders, 1992.

PROBLEM 105   A 3-YEAR-OLD CHILD WITH A CARDIAC MURMUR

A 3-year-old child is brought to your office by his mother for a periodic health examination. The child has been well and has no history of significant medical illness. He has reached all of his developmental milestones.

On physical examination, the child is on the 50th percentile for weight and height. His blood pressure is 90/70 mm Hg. He has a grade II/VI short ejection systolic murmur heard maximally along the left sternal edge from the midsternum to the lower end of the sternum. There is no radiation of the murmur to either the neck or back. There is no associated thrill with this murmur. The child's pulse is 84/minute and regular. The femoral artery pulses are normal and are not delayed.

The rest of the physical examination is normal.

SELECT THE ONE BEST ANSWER TO THE FOLLOWING QUESTIONS

1. Which of the following statement(s) best reflect(s) the character of this heart murmur?
   a) the location of the heart murmur (mid to low sternum) increases the probability of this murmur being pathologic
   b) the systolic timing of the heart murmur increases the probability of this murmur being pathologic
   c) the grade of the murmur (II/VI rather than I/VI) increases the probability of this murmur being pathologic
   d) all of the above statements are true
   e) none of the above statements are true

2. This murmur is best referred to as which of the following?
   a) Mustard's murmur
   b) Fallot's murmur
   c) Still's murmur
   d) De Bakey's murmur
   e) Framingham's murmur

3. Which of the following signs or symptoms is not associated with "innocent" cardiac murmurs?
   a) low frequency
   b) an associated thrill
   c) short ejection systolic in timing
   d) grade I or grade II in audibility
   e) a and b

4. The murmur described is intensified by which of the following?
   a) the sitting position
   b) increasing the heart rate
   c) fever
   d) anxiety
   e) all of the above

5. At this time, which of the following investigations should be performed on the child?
   a) CXR
   b) ECG
   c) echocardiogram

   d) none of the above
   e) all of the above

6. At this time, what should you do?
   a) call the pediatric cardiologist *stat*
   b) tell the mother that the child has a heart murmur but "not to worry, it probably isn't anything important"
   c) tell the mother that all heart murmurs need to be taken very seriously; therefore, it is probably best to have the pediatric cardiologist do "every test he can"
   d) tell the mother that the heart sound you hear (a very soft murmur) is very common and occurs in at least half of all children
   e) tell the mother nothing; there is no need to cause her unnecessary worry

7. A 6-month-old infant is brought to your office by his mother. It has come in for a periodic health assessment. You have not seen the child before. The mother states that the child has been well and has had no medical problems.

   On examination, the child has a grade III/VI harsh pansystolic heart murmur heard along the lower left sternal edge. There is no radiation of the murmur. The heart rate is 72 beats/minute and regular. There is no thrill. The blood pressure is 80/60 mm Hg.

   No other abnormalities are found in examination. Most importantly, the child is on the 50th percentile for weight and length.

   What is the most likely cardiac diagnosis in this infant?
   a) innocent cardiac murmur
   b) tetralogy of Fallot
   c) pulmonary atresia
   d) ventricular septal defect
   e) coarctation of the aorta

8. At this time, the child described in Question 7 should
   a) have immediate surgery
   b) be managed with digoxin and diuretics
   c) be managed with digoxin, diuretics, and an ACE inhibitor
   d) have an immediate cardiac catheterization performed followed by surgical closure within 3 months
   e) none of the above

9. In the child described in Question 7, what preventive health practices should be followed?
    a) prophylaxis against bacterial endocarditis if dental work is to be done
    b) cardiac catheterizations every 3 months until resolution
    c) echocardiograms every 3 months until resolution
    d) a and c
    e) none of the above

10. What is the prevalence of cardiac murmurs in childhood?
    a) 5%
    b) 10%
    c) 20%
    d) 50%
    e) 90%

11. What is the most common pathologic cardiac murmur in childhood?
    a) atrial septal defect
    b) tetralogy of Fallot
    c) ventricular septal defect
    d) transposition of the great arteries
    e) aortic stenosis

12. Which of the following is(are) common innocent cardiac murmurs in childhood?
    a) neonatal pulmonary artery branch murmur
    b) "venous hum" of late infancy
    c) "Still's aortic vibratory" murmur
    d) pulmonary valve area "flow" murmur
    e) all of the above

Short Answer Management Problem 105

Discuss the relative sensitivity and specificity of an experienced clinician's clinical diagnosis of a childhood cardiac murmur compared to the findings and/or diagnosis suggested by echocardiography.

ANSWERS

1. E.

2. C. This murmur has all the characteristics of an innocent murmur:
    A. It is located at the mid to low sternal border.
    B. It is systolic in timing.
    C. It has no associated thrill.
    This murmur, which is described as "vibratory" or "musical" in nature, is known as Still's murmur. Still's murmur is safely diagnosed clinically, and laboratory studies add nothing to its assessment.

3. B.

4. E. Other characteristics of innocent cardiac murmur include the following:
    A. It is low in frequency.
    B. It is a localized murmur.
    C. It is accentuated by the sitting position, anxiety, fever, and increasing heart rate.
    Note that an innocent cardiac murmur in a child is never associated with a thrill.

5. D. This murmur, a Still's murmur, is safely diagnosed clinically, and laboratory and diagnostic imaging studies add nothing to its assessment.

6. D. In explaining heart murmurs to parents, not just what you say but how you say it is very important. It is very important to be reassuring in your tone and to point out that 50% of children have cardiac murmurs. Make sure that you provide an opportunity for the mother to ask any questions that she may have.
    It is extremely unwise not to tell the parents when you detect a heart murmur in a young child. Sooner or later someone is going to hear it and mention it. At that time it will come back to haunt you. It is far better to tell the parent(s) that a heart murmur exists but that you are positive (if you are) that it is innocent. If you are not positive, an elective referral to a pediatric cardiologist would be reasonable.

7. D. The most likely cardiac diagnosis in this infant is ventricular septal defect. The typical heart murmur associated with a ventricular septal defect is harsh, pansystolic, and best heard at the lower left sternal edge. Even as the VSD becomes smaller, it maintains its regurgitant characteristic of starting off with the first heart sound.

8. E. The treatment recommended at this time is none of the above. Rather, watchful expectation should be pursued. The prognosis is excellent, and the defect will likely close spontaneously. As the VSD becomes smaller, the murmur becomes shorter and (as men-

tioned) maintains its regurgitant characteristics (that is, it starts off with the first heart sound). At least 50% of VSDs will close by the end of the first year or shortly thereafter.

9. A. The only prophylaxis that needs to be followed in this child is protection with antibiotic therapy (penicillin) prior to any dental procedure or any other procedure that would increase the probability of bacterial endocarditis. This can obviously be discontinued when the defect closes.

10. D. The prevalence of cardiac murmurs in the pediatric population is at least 50%, probably considerably higher to the sensitive ear. The vast majority of these murmurs are innocent in nature and do not reflect any cardiac pathology.

11. C. The most common pathologic cardiac murmur in childhood is ventricular septal defect. With a VSD the cardiac murmur is often not present at birth but is first heard on the discharge examination or at the first well-baby checkup. As discussed earlier, the most common outcome of this congenital heart defect is spontaneous closure. In some cases, however, surgical closure is indicated. The most uncommon scenario is the development of congestive cardiac failure secondary to VSD.

The frequencies of pathologic cardiac murmurs in childhood are as follows:
Ventricular septal defect: 38%
Atrial septal defect: 18%
Pulmonary valve stenosis: 13%
Pulmonary artery stenosis: 7%
Aortic valve stenosis: 4%
Patent ductus arthrosis: 4%
Mitral valve prolapse: 4%
Others: 11%

12. E. The common functional or common innocent murmurs of infancy and childhood include the following:
A. Neonatal pulmonary artery branch murmur
B. Venous hum of late infancy and early childhood
C. Still's aortic vibratory systolic murmur
D. Pulmonary valve area "flow" murmur of late adolescence and childhood

SOLUTION TO SHORT ANSWER MANAGEMENT PROBLEM 105

As our health care dollars become stretched to the limit, we need to take a critical look at exactly how much more certain diagnostic tests add to the diagnosis and treatment arrived at by an experienced clinician in all aspects of medicine. The diagnosis of childhood cardiac murmurs is no exception.

A recent study of experienced pediatric cardiologists yielded the following results with respect to their diagnostic acumen.
A. Sensitivity of clinical examination of all childhood cardiac murmurs = 96%
B. Specificity of clinical examination of all childhood cardiac murmurs = 95%
C. Positive predictive value of clinical examination of all childhood cardiac murmurs = 88%
D. Negative predictive value of clinical examination of all childhood cardiac murmurs = 98%

Thus this study showed that the clinical examination by a pediatric cardiologist is the most useful means of initial evaluation of referred pediatric cardiac murmurs.

As supplementary screening tools, the ECG and the echocardiogram were unlikely to reveal clinically unsuspected cardiac disease. Thus there is every reason (clinically and cost-effectively) to go back to the evaluation of patients by physicians rather than by machines. Remember, as doctors we treat patients, not laboratory results.

SUMMARY OF THE DIAGNOSIS AND TREATMENT OF CHILDHOOD CARDIAC MURMURS

1. **Prevalence of murmurs:**
   a) Overall prevalence = 50% of all children
   b) Innocent/pathologic = 10/1
2. **Epidemiology:** clinical assessment is just as sensitive and specific as echocardiography and more sensitive and specific than electrocardiography.
3. **Innocent murmurs:**
   a) Still's murmur (most common)
   b) Venous hum (second most common)
   c) Pulmonary flow murmur
   d) Neonatal pulmonary artery branch murmur
4. **Pathologic murmurs:**
   a) Ventricular septal defect (most common)
   b) Atrial septal defect (second most common)
   c) Pulmonary valve stenosis
5. **Clinical signs and symptoms that are reassuring for the family physician as he or she evaluates a childhood cardiac murmur:**

   Following are the 10 questions a family physician should ask himself or herself about a cardiac murmur:
   a) Is there any evidence of failure to thrive in the child? If *no*, this suggests an innocent murmur.
   b) Are there any signs (shortness of breath, blue lips, lethargy) or symptoms (cyanosis, diastolic murmur, parasternal heave, thrill, loud murmur > II/VI, holosystolic murmur) to suggest pathologic murmur? If *no*, this suggests an innocent murmur.
   c) Is the murmur accentuated by sitting forward? If *yes*, this suggests an innocent murmur.
   d) Is the murmur accentuated by exercise or increased heart rate due to another cause? If *yes*, this suggests an innocent murmur.

e) Is the murmur accentuated by fever? If *yes,* this suggests an innocent murmur.

f) Is the murmur accentuated by anxiety, restlessness, or crying? If *yes,* this suggests an innocent murmur.

g) Is the murmur a murmur without any radiation (that is, to the neck or to the back)? If *yes,* this suggests an innocent murmur.

h) Is the murmur present lower (rather than higher) along the left sternal edge? If *yes,* this suggests an innocent murmur.

i) Did the mother bring the child in for a specific reason that may be associated with cardiac disease (such as having to stop and rest while playing)? If *no,* this suggests an innocent murmur.

j) Do you, an experienced clinician, think this is an innocent murmur? If *yes,* this suggests an innocent murmur.

SUGGESTED READINGS

Behrman R et al., eds. The cardiovascular system. In: Nelson textbook of pediatrics. 14th Ed. Philadelphia: WB Saunders, 1992.

Symthe J et al. Initial evaluation of heart murmurs: Are laboratory tests necessary? Pediatrics 1990; 86(4):497-500.

PROBLEM 106   A 6-MONTH-OLD INFANT WITH AN UPPER RESPIRATORY TRACT INFECTION

A 6-month-old infant is brought to your office by his mother. He has had an upper respiratory tract infection consisting of a runny nose, cough, and a mild fever for the last 4 days. The infant's mother is concerned because his temperature reached 39° C last evening.

On examination, the child looks well. He has nasal congestion as well as a hyperemic pharynx. His lungs are clear; no adventitious breath sounds are heard.

SELECT THE ONE BEST ANSWER TO THE FOLLOWING QUESTIONS

1. Regarding the child's fever, what should you tell the mother?
   a) treat the fever if it reaches 39° C again; use baby aspirin to treat
   b) treat the fever if it reaches 39° C again; elixir of acetaminophen
   c) treat the fever if it reaches 39° C again; use a combination of baby aspirin and elixir of acetaminophen
   d) use only symptomatic treatment: cool clothes, fan in the room, and so on
   e) tell the mother that everyone has a different opinion; as far as you are concerned, she can do whatever she wants

2. What is the analgesic agent of choice in the treatment of childhood fever and mild childhood pain?
   a) elixir of naproxen
   b) elixir of hydromorphone
   c) elixir of acetaminophen
   d) aspirin: 75 mg children's size
   e) elixir of acetaminophen and codeine

3. Regarding the use of aspirin and acetaminophen in pediatric analgesia, which of the following statements most accurately reflects current recommended practice?
   a) aspirin is still the analgesic of choice in the treatment of infant and childhood pain
   b) aspirin is not contraindicated in the treatment of infant and childhood pain associated with upper respiratory tract infections
   c) aspirin is a more potent analgesic than acetaminophen
   d) acetaminophen is the drug of choice for the treatment of infant and childhood pain
   e) acetaminophen should be used in all infants and children

4. Regarding the use of antihistamines in pediatric patients, which of the following statements is(are) true?
   a) antihistamines shorten the duration of respiratory tract illness in children
   b) antihistamines reduce the incidence of otitis media following the beginning of an upper respiratory tract infection in a young child
   c) the prescription of an antihistamine in a child with a viral upper respiratory tract infection is considered good practice
   d) antihistamines may produce seizures in young children who are given antihistamine doses (tablets or suppositories) that are meant for older children (on a kg/kg basis)
   e) none of the above statements are true

5. Regarding the relief of nasal congestion in infants and children, which of the following statements is(are) true?
   a) antihistamines produce excellent relief of pediatric nasal congestion
   b) antihistamines, when compared to cool or warm steam, produce superior relief of nasal congestion in pediatric patients
   c) cool or warm steam, when compared to antihistamines, produce superior relief of nasal congestion in pediatric patients
   d) antihistamines and cool/warm steam are equally efficacious in providing relief of nasal congestion
   e) nobody really knows for sure

6. The child described in the preceding problem returns in 3 days with his mother. She states that despite your treatment the child has not improved. He now has significantly greater nasal congestion and is having a difficult time breathing at night.

   On examination, the ears and throat remain clear. You do not really notice any change in the state of the nasal congestion.

   With respect to treatment of this infant at this time, which of the following statements is(are) true?
   a) a decongestant to relieve nasal congestion is a reasonable therapeutic maneuver now
   b) decongestants have been shown to reduce the duration of viral URI symptoms
   c) topical sympathomimetic agents are unlikely to be systemically absorbed
   d) overstimulation is a common side effect when decongestant preparations are given to children
   e) none of the above statements are true

7. A mother presents to your office with her 6-month-old infant daughter for assessment of a persistent cough. The cough has been present for the past 10 days.

It is nonproductive, and the mother feels it is interfering significantly with the child's sleep. You are considering prescribing an antitussive and/or an expectorant.

Which of the following statements regarding the use of antitussives and/or expectorants in infants and children is(are) true?

a) dextromethorphan suppresses cough and is unlikely to produce any significant adverse reactions in infants and children
b) the combination of a cough suppressant and an expectorant is a logical combination to try in a child with a persistent cough
c) dextromethorphan has been shown to significantly decrease the duration of respiratory tract infection symptoms in children
d) respiratory depression in children has been reported with dextromethorphan
e) none of the above are true

8. A mother brings her 13-month-old infant to the office for assessment of nausea and vomiting. She stopped in at the local ER 24 hours previously and was told to purchase childhood dimenhydrinate suppositories for the nausea. Apparently, the ER physician did a complete workup and there were no other significant findings.

The nausea and vomiting continues. The child appears to be approximately 5% dehydrated. On physical examination, there are no other abnormalities found. The child appears somewhat sedated and lethargic.

You decide to admit the child for observation, re-evaluation, and rehydration.

Which of the following statements regarding the use of antiemetics in children is(are) true?

a) dimenhydrinate is effective for the treatment of nausea and vomiting associated with gastrointestinal infection and is devoid of significant side effects

b) the sedation that is seen in this infant may be secondary to the dimenhydrinate
c) dimenhydrinate toxicity may be difficult to distinguish from worsening of the illness
d) b and c
e) all of the above are true

9. A mother brings her 8-month-old infant to your office for assessment of fever, diarrhea, and "red cheeks" that she attributes to "teething." She was advised by her neighbor to purchase a preparation of topical benzocaine. This has not helped.

On examination, the infant has a temperature of 39° C. There are no other abnormalities on physical examination.

Which of the following statements regarding this infant is(are) true?

a) the symptoms described probably are due to teething
b) topical benzocaine preparations are virtually devoid of side effects
c) acetaminophen is a reasonable treatment for a child that is teething
d) teething often begins at 4-6 months of age and carries on intermittently up to the age of 2 years
e) c and d
f) all of the above statements are true

10. Adolescents have recently adopted the use of a common OTC drug for its CNS properties as a favorite drug of abuse. This has caused many pharmacies to move this drug from the drug store shelf to behind the counter. Which drug is this?

a) chlorotripolon
b) diphenylhydramine
c) dimenhydrinate
d) terfenadine
e) dextromethorphan

Short Answer Management Problem 106

Describe a general rule of thumb for the use of over-the-counter drugs in infants and children.

ANSWERS

1. D. The basic axiom relevant to this question is that "not all fever has to be treated with drugs." In fact, there are good reasons for suggesting that fever per se only be treated when it reaches a level > 39.5° C. Fever is a normal body response mechanism. In children, the major concern with very high fever is the possibility of a febrile convulsion.

2. C. The analgesic agent of choice in the treatment of childhood fever and mild to moderate childhood pain

is acetaminophen. Hydromorphone is a strong narcotic. Naproxen is a nonsteroidal antiinflammatory agent, and aspirin is contraindicated (see the answer to Question 3). Acetaminophen/codeine elixir is available and may be indicated in more severe pain syndromes in childhood.

3. D. Acetaminophen is the analgesic of choice for the treatment of infant and childhood pain. Aspirin use should basically be discouraged; this is by far the safest policy. Aspirin use has been linked to Reye's syndrome

(influenza/aspirin/Reye's syndrome) and it seems wise to avoid this drug in any children with infections of any kind. Not all childhood pain needs to be treated with drugs. Many children will do just as well and feel just as well without drug use.

4. D. Most cough and cold remedies contain antihistamines. Antihistamines, however, have never been shown to be of value in the treatment of viral upper respiratory tract infections (contrary to many authorities, including ENT specialists). Antihistamines do not shorten the duration of respiratory tract illness in children and do not reduce the subsequent incidence of otitis media following the onset of a viral URI. They may, however, produce seizures in children if given in toxic amounts. The younger the child, the easier it is to inadvertently produce antihistamine toxicity.

Treatment of a viral URI in an infant or young child should consist of reassurance and cool steam (if nasal congestion is present).

5. C. Cool or warm steam is actually superior to antihistamines in producing relief of nasal congestion in infants and young children. If steam is being used in a humidifier in the child's room, it is safer to use a humidifier that emits cool steam, due to the risk of burns. However, the use of warm steam (as from turning on the shower in the bathroom) does, as well, produce significant symptomatic relief of nasal congestion.

6. D. Decongestants have not been shown to shorten the duration of viral URI symptoms. Topical sympathomimetic agents are systemically absorbed and may result in elevation of blood pressure, tachycardia, and overstimulation of the central nervous system leading to irritability, insomnia, and sometimes even frank psychosis. Overstimulation is a particularly common side effect in children. Thus, as with antihistamines, the risks of using decongestants in children outweigh any potential benefits.

It may be reasonable to use a very dilute nasal sympathomimetic for a short period of time in this child if all else fails; however, it is still preferable to stick to steam if possible.

7. D. Dextromethorphan is the most common ingredient in OTC cough medicines. As well as producing drowsiness, it has been reported to produce respiratory depression in infants and children as well. As with antihistamines and decongestants, dextromethorphan has not been shown to shorten the duration of respiratory tract illness in children or adults.

Many cough preparations also contain an expectorant. The combination of a cough suppressant and an expectorant in one preparation is beyond comprehension.

Time remains the best cure for the viral URI symptoms. The use of a nasal aspirator (bulb syringe) will help

to clear a young infant's nasal secretions and make feeding easier. Saline nasal drops may also be used. In infants who are irritable and feverish from viral symptoms, the use of acetaminophen is the safest OTC drug to use.

8. D. Dimenhydrinate *should not* be used for the treatment of nausea and vomiting secondary to gastroenteritis in children (especially very young children). Even in adults the use of this agent is questionable; it has been demonstrated to be of value only in the treatment of motion sickness in adults. Dimenhydrinate may produce significant sedation (and even a semicomatose state) in children. The pediatric suppository contains 25 or 50 mg of dimenhydrinate (half the adult oral dose or the full oral adult dose).

It may be difficult for the physician to differentiate dimenhydrinate toxicity from a worsening of the illness itself. This makes the use of this agent in children dangerous.

9. E. Teething usually begins at 4-6 months and continues until the age of 2 years. Although often blamed on teething, there is no good evidence that rash, fever, diarrhea, vomiting, nasal congestion, irritability, or sleeplessness are related to teething.

Although topical benzocaine usually does not produce any side effects, cases of methemoglobinemia have been reported in children who have been treated with this agent.

Teething is best treated with reassurance and appropriate doses of acetaminophen.

10. C. An OTC drug that has recently been adopted by adolescents as a "drug of abuse" is dimenhydrinate. The CNS side effects that the adolescent is looking for are the sedation, drowsiness, and perhaps euphoria. This has caused many pharmacists to move the drug from the drug store shelf to behind the counter.

SOLUTION TO SHORT ANSWER MANAGEMENT PROBLEM 106

A good general rule of thumb for treating infants and children with OTC drugs is as follows:

Over-the-counter drugs should be avoided in almost all cases, especially in young infants and children. The only safe drug that can be routinely used without significant concern (as long as the directions are followed as per dose) is acetaminophen.

SUMMARY OF THE ABUSE OF OTC DRUGS IN INFANTS AND YOUNG CHILDREN

1. **Upper respiratory tract infections:** there is no evidence to suggest that antihistamines, decongestants, cough suppressants, or expectorants are of any value in the

treatment of viral URI symptoms in infants and young children. Potential toxicity is present with all of these agents.

2. **Nausea and vomiting:** dimenhydrinate is not useful and is potentially toxic.

3. **Diarrhea:** kaolin/pectin may change the appearance of stools slightly, but it has no effect on water loss, the major hazard of protracted diarrhea.

4. **Teething:** There is no evidence to suggest that rash, diarrhea, vomiting, nasal congestion, irritability, and sleeplessness are associated with teething. Benzocaine preparations should be avoided. Reassurance and judicious use of acetaminophen may be indicated.

SUGGESTED READING

Goldbloom A. Hazards of over-the-counter medications in children. Medicine North America 1986; 2:392-405.

PROBLEM 107   AN 8-YEAR-OLD FEMALE WITH ACUTE SKELETAL PAIN

An 8-year-old female presents with an acute attack of pain in the back, ribs, sternum, and extremities. The child, of African-American descent, has had previous episodes of the same type of pain in the same areas. On P/E the child is in acute distress and is clutching both lower extremities.

Examination of the head and neck, the respiratory system, the cardiovascular system, and the abdomen are normal. Examination of the musculoskeletal system demonstrates acute tenderness in the areas in which the pain is presently located.

SELECT THE ONE BEST ANSWER TO THE FOLLOWING QUESTIONS

1. Based on the findings described, what is the most likely diagnosis?
   a) sickle-cell trait
   b) sickle-cell disease
   c) metastatic carcinoma
   d) malingering
   e) none of the above

2. What is the pathophysiology of this condition?
   a) replacement of normal hemoglobin A by hemoglobin S
   b) replacement of normal hemoglobin A by hemoglobin C
   c) replacement of normal hemoglobin A by hemoglobin F
   d) osteolytic bone lesions produced by an undifferentiated carcinoma
   e) none of the above

3. An aplastic crisis is often associated with this condition. Which of the following infections is often associated with an aplastic crisis?
   a) human papilloma virus
   b) human parvovirus
   c) herpes zoster
   d) pneumococcus
   e) *H. influenzae*

4. Which of the following immunizations/vaccines should be given to this patient?
   a) hepatitis B vaccine
   b) *H. influenzae* immunization
   c) pneumococcal vaccine
   d) a and c
   e) all of the above

5. The patient described presents to the ER 6 months later. On this occasion the child has a painful swelling of the right foot. What is the most likely cause of this symptom?
   a) the hand-foot syndrome
   b) acute gout
   c) acute juvenile rheumatoid arthritis

   d) bilateral hand and foot osteomyelitis
   e) none of the above

6. What is the pathophysiologic reason for the patient presentation in Question 5?
   a) an autoimmune process
   b) an osseous infection
   c) an acute bacterial infection
   d) a viral infection
   e) none of the above

7. What is the most frequent complication of sickle-cell trait?
   a) splenic rupture
   b) painless hematuria
   c) splenic sequestration
   d) stroke
   e) none of the above

8. In which of the following races is the disease state discussed least common?
   a) African-Americans
   b) Italians
   c) Greeks
   d) Saudi Arabians
   e) Caucasian North Americans

9. Which of the following statements regarding this disease and priapism is false?
   a) priapism is a recognized complication of this condition
   b) priapism in this disorder usually presents in younger men
   c) priapism, when it occurs, is generally self-limited
   d) nifedipine and/or nitroglycerine are the treatments of choice for this priapism
   e) hospitalization is rarely indicated

10. Which of the following is(are) recognized complications of this disorder?
   a) a stroke, a stroke-in-evolution, or a transient ischemic attack
   b) avascular necrosis primarily affecting the hips
   c) acute vaso-occlusion
   d) splenic sequestration and splenic enlargement
   e) all of the above

Short Answer Management Problem 107

List the major complications of the disorder described.

ANSWERS

1. B. This child has sickle-cell disease.

   Sickle-cell disease is an inherited hemolytic anemia that results when all of the normal hemoglobin A is replaced by the mutant hemoglobin S (Hb S). About 1 in 12 people of African descent in the Americas carry the sickle-cell trait (A/S). It is also present in Greeks, Italians, Turks, Saudi Arabians, and members of certain tribes on the Indian subcontinent.

   Subjects who have the sickle-cell trait are not anemic and have a normal life expectancy. Between 25% and 40% of their hemoglobin is hemoglobin S. Under normal circumstances their red blood cells do not hemolyze.

   Sickle-cell anemia (S/S), as this child has, comes about through the inheritance of two Hb S genes, one from each parent. At birth, the red blood cells of the S/S infant contain mainly fetal hemoglobin (hemoglobin F). Within a few months, these red cells are replaced by cells containing mainly Hb S.

   The acute pain that this child is experiencing at this time is due to recurrent vaso-occlusive phenomena. Throughout their lives, sickle-cell patients are plagued by recurrent painful crises. These episodes may occur with explosive suddenness and attack various parts of the body, particularly the abdomen, chest, back, and joints. Approximately 1/4 of these painful crises are preceded by a viral or a bacterial infection. A given patient may have months or even years without a crisis and then have a cluster of frequent, severe attacks. In some patients these crises occur more frequently in cold weather; this may be due to reflex vasospasm. In others the attacks occur in warm weather and are presumably due to dehydration.

   When a sickle cell crisis is localized to the extremities, as in this case, it may induce acute synovitis and joint effusion.

2. A. As mentioned, sickle-cell disease is genetically inherited from both parents, with hemoglobin A being replaced by hemoglobin S. The electrophoretically abnormal hemoglobin S differs from hemoglobin A by the substitution of valine for glutamic acid at the sixth position of the beta-chain.

3. B. In patients with sickle-cell disease, aplastic crises are often precipitated by viral infections, particularly viral infection with the human parvovirus B19. An aplastic crisis usually occurs in a child under the age of 18 who may be recovering from an infection. The child presents with profound anemia and a fall in the reticulocyte count to below 1%.

   Treatment consists of blood transfusions. The child usually recovers spontaneously within 7 to 10 days.

4. E. Patients with sickle-cell disease should be given the usual course of immunizations as recommended by the CDC. In addition, however, it is imperative that the child receive *Haemophilus* B conjugate, hepatitis B immunization, and pneumococcal vaccine.

5. A. This presentation, designated *hand-foot syndrome,* presents as a painful swelling of either the hand or foot and is caused by infarction of bone marrow in metacarpal or metatarsal bones and phalanges. It resolves spontaneously in approximately 1 week.

   As the sickle-cell patient grows older, infarcts in the long bones can cause pain or swelling of an arm or leg. In these cases, osteomyelitis, usually caused by *Salmonella,* should be ruled out.

6. E. The pathophysiology of the hand-foot syndrome is basically a vaso-occlusive process, a process that occurs due to the sickle shape of the red blood cells themselves, a shape that evidently predisposes to vaso-occlusion in the bone marrow.

7. B. The most frequent complication of sickle-cell trait is painless hematuria. The hematuria, which is usually gross hematuria, is produced by necrosis of the tip of the renal papilla and is prolonged by the action of urokinase in the urine. Although the hematuria may continue for several weeks, it seldom requires hospitalization and may cease spontaneously.

   Even considering the frequency of painless hematuria (approximately 20% of patients with sickle-cell trait), it is obviously important to rule out other causes and not automatically assume that it is due to the sickle-cell trait every time it occurs.

8. E. Sickle-cell disease and sickle-cell trait, as discussed in the first question, occur in African-Americans, Greeks, Italians, Turks, Saudi-Arabians, and certain tribes on the Indian subcontinent. They do not, however, occur in white North Americans.

9. E. Attacks of priapism in boys and young men are distressing but can usually be managed conservatively. The attacks, which are self-limited, may occur frequently.

Priapism sometimes responds to nifedipine (10 mg in repeated doses) and to a nitroglycerine patch, 0.2 to 0.4 mg/hour applied at bedtime, to prevent nocturnal attacks. If an attack persists for more than 6 hours, the patient should be admitted to a hospital, and if it continues for more than 24 hours despite conservative treatment measures, a urologist should be consulted.

Many of the patients who develop attacks of priapism have relatively high hemoglobin and hemocrit levels.

A corpora spongiosa/cavernosa shunt through the glans penis is often effective and may need to be repeated. Subsequent erectile function is usually not affected.

Repeated attacks of priapism can result in thickening and gross enlargement of the penis, which may remain semi-erect. Impotence can be effectively treated by penile implants.

10. E. Cerebrovascular accidents (stroke) resulting from blockage of the internal carotid artery or its branches affect approximately 5% of S/S children. The treatment for same is a program of exchange transfusions to lower the proportion of Hb S to less than 50% and maintain it at that level throughout childhood. This facilitates prevention of a recurrence as well as neurologic recovery.

Avascular necrosis, particularly of the head of the femur, is very common in patients with sickle-cell disease and can lead to significant disability. Some patients benefit from surgical intervention; this ranges from core decompression to total hip replacement. Like infarcts in other organs, infection is much more common as a complication of these surgical interventions.

Acute vaso-occlusion, as discussed, is the basic pathophysiologic process underlying many of the complications of sickle-cell disease. Specifically, it is responsible for osseous complications such as the hand-foot syndrome and acute pain crises, which have been discussed previously.

The spleen is usually palpable in infants and small children but may become acutely enlarged due to rapid sequestration of sickled blood. As the acute anemia can be rapidly fatal, this is an emergency requiring admission to the hospital and rapid blood transfusion.

SOLUTION TO SHORT ANSWER MANAGEMENT PROBLEM 107

Sickle-cell disease is characterized by the following complications (although not required for the answer, a detailed explanation of each complication is provided):

1. Hemolytic anemia: sickle-cell disease (genotype S/S) is associated with a severe hemolytic anemia with hematocrit values varying between 18% and 30%. The mean red blood cell survival is between 10 and 15 days.

2. Acute pain crises/chronic organ damage: the morbidity and mortality of sickle-cell disease are due primarily to recurrent vaso-occlusive phenomena. This vaso-occlusive damage can be divided into microinfarcts that produce the painful crisis and macroinfarcts that produce organ damage. Although almost any organ can be involved, the most common organs involved are the lung, kidney, liver, skeleton, and skin.

3. Pulmonary function restriction: impairment of pulmonary function is a common complication of sickle-cell disease. Resting arterial PO_2 is reduced in part due to intrapulmonary arterial-venous shunting. Since SS red blood cells have decreased oxygen affinity, arterial blood is significantly undersaturated. This creates an increased tendency for red cells to sickle when they reach the peripheral circulation.

4. Congestive cardiac failure: SS homozygotes frequently develop overt CHF. The pathophysiology of this CHF is associated with the severe chronic anemia and the hypoxemia (high-output cardiac failure).

5. Cerebrovascular accidents: the primary cause of CVA in sickle-cell patients is cerebral thrombosis. The other cause, however, is subarachnoid hemorrhage. A sickle-cell disease patient has approximately a 25% lifetime chance of developing some type of neurologic complication. Hemiplegia is encountered more frequently than are coma, convulsions, or other visual disturbances. Patients generally make a full recovery, particularly after only one CVA.

6. Ophthalmalogic complications: a variety of ocular abnormalities are encountered in patients with SS disease. These include retinal infarcts, peripheral vessel disease, arteriovenous anomalies, vitreous hemorrhage, proliferative retinopathy, and retinal detachment.

7. Genitourinary complications: patients with sickle-cell disease develop significant and prolonged painless hematuria as a result of papillary infarcts. The amount of blood loss can be so significant that iron deficiency develops.

Longer-surviving SS patients (patients living into the fourth and fifth decades) develop progressive renal failure.

Boys and young men with sickle-cell disease occasionally develop priapism. The treatment of this condition has been discussed.

8. Hepatobiliary complications: sickle-cell patients are icteric due to the hemolytic anemia discussed previously. The hyperbilirubinemia that is associated with sickle-cell disease is nonconjugated hyperbilirubinemia. Sickle-cell patients are also at increased risk of gallstone formation.

9. Skeletal complications: the skeletal complications associated with SS disease develop due to expansion of the red marrow, bony infarcts, and avascular necrosis of joints in hip and shoulder. The biconcave, or "fish-

mouth," vertebrae are virtually pathognomonic for sickle-cell disease.

The previously mentioned hand-foot syndrome is a painful swelling of the hand or foot caused by infarction of the bone marrow in metacarpal or metatarsal bones and phalanges.

10. Skin disease: chronic skin ulcers often occur in the lower extremities. These skin ulcers appear to be associated with SS patients that have more severe hemolytic anemia.

11. Splenic sequestration: the spleen becomes enlarged due to the rapid sequestration of sickled blood. The acute anemia that results may be rapidly fatal and should be treated with emergency blood transfusions.

12. Aplastic crises: the previously mentioned aplastic crises, which usually occur when a child is recovering from an infection, are caused by human parvovirus B19. Profound anemia occurs, and blood transfusions are necessary to treat it.

SUMMARY OF THE DIAGNOSIS AND TREATMENT OF SICKLE-CELL DISEASE

1. **Population at risk:** African-Americans
   a) 1 in 12 carry the sickle-cell trait—A/S (are heterozygous for sickle-cell trait)
   b) Homozygous genotype = S/S
2. **Diagnosis:**
   a) Blood smear: red blood cells sickle and hemolyze
   b) Hemoglobin electrophoresis
3. **Clinical manifestations:** prominent and frequent clinical manifestations include the following:
   a) Severe hemolytic anemia
   b) Recurrent bouts of acute pain crises that arise from vaso-occlusion and microinfarction—also associated with hand-foot syndrome
   c) Chronic organ damage from same pathophysiology: lung, kidney, liver, skeleton, skin
   d) Congestive heart failure
   e) Cerebrovascular accidents
   f) Eye complications: proliferative retinopathy, retinal infarcts, retinal detachment, vitreous hemorrhage
   g) Chronic renal failure, painless hematuria, priapism
   h) Jaundice (unconjugated hyperbilirubinemia), cholelithiasis
   i) Systemic skeletal microinfarction, avascular necrosis
   j) Skin ulcers
   k) Splenic sequestration
   l) Aplastic crises
4. **Treatment:**
   a) Treat and wherever possible prevent complications (recurrent CVA may be prevented by starting the child on a chronic transfusion program).
   b) Nutritional supplements: folic acid, 1 mg/day
   c) Immunizations/vaccines: *Haemophilus influenzae* B, hepatitis B, pneumococcal vaccine, and all other routine vaccinations recommended by the CDC
   d) Prophylactic antibiotics: penicillin V 150 mg bid up to age 3
   e) Pain control for acute pain crises and other painful events: IV fluids and analgesics as needed; do not be afraid to use narcotic analgesics
   f) Painless hematuria: aminocaproic acid (EACA)

NEW INFORMATION—1995

A drug that has been found to reduce painful episodes of sickle-cell anemia (the vaso-occlusive phenomena) has been so successful that the trial in which it was compared to placebo was stopped early. The drug, hydroxyurea, is believed to work in sickle-cell anemia by increasing the production of fetal hemoglobin in red blood cells. The formal results of the trial will be published soon.

SUGGESTED READING

Milner P. Sickle cell disease. In: Rakel R, ed. Conn's current therapy. Philadelphia: WB Saunders, 1994.

General Surgery and Surgical Specialties

PROBLEM 108 A 29-YEAR-OLD FEMALE WITH NAUSEA, VOMITING, AND CENTRAL ABDOMINAL PAIN

A 29-year-old female presents to your office with a 2-day history of nausea, vomiting, and central abdominal pain. The pain has begun to move down and to the right. She also describes mild dysuria. Anorexia began 24 hours ago and the patient also has "felt warm."

Her past health has been excellent. She has no drug allergies and is on no medication.

On P/E, the patient looks ill. Her temperature is 38.1°C. She has significant tenderness in both the right lower quadrant and the left lower quadrant. The tenderness is greatest in the right lower quadrant. Rebound tenderness is present. The rectal examination discloses tenderness on the right side. There is no CVA tenderness.

SELECT THE ONE BEST ANSWER TO THE FOLLOWING QUESTIONS

1. What is the most likely diagnosis in this patient?
   a) pelvic inflammatory disease
   b) twisted ovarian cyst
   c) acute appendicitis
   d) acute cholecystitis
   e) acute pyelonephritis

2. At this time, what would be the most reasonable course of action?
   a) advise the patient to go home and return for follow-up in 24 hours
   b) hospitalize the patient for observation and evaluation
   c) begin outpatient oral antibiotic therapy and see the patient in 48 hours
   d) advise the patient to go home and call you if no improvement occurs within the next 72 hours
   e) none of the above

3. The investigations you perform heighten your suspicion of the primary diagnosis. The white blood cell count is elevated and there is a definite abnormality seen on the abdominal X-ray. At this time, you, the family physician, should do which of the following?
   a) continue to observe the patient for improvement or deterioration
   b) arrange for a CT scan to definitely establish the diagnosis
   c) arrange for an ultrasound to definitely establish the diagnosis
   d) arrange for a barium enema to definitely establish the diagnosis
   e) none of the above

4. A consultant sees your patient and makes an appropriate suggestion. Which of the following is the suggestion likely to be?
   a) perform an abdominal laparoscopy or laparotomy
   b) begin intensive triple-drug IV antibiotics
   c) continue the period of observation
   d) perform further diagnostic tests
   e) none of the above

5. Which of the following is(are) complications of the definitive therapy/and the original condition?
   a) wound infection
   b) subphrenic abscess
   c) pelvic abscess
   d) appendiceal abscess
   e) all of the above

6. In which of the following age groups are the signs and symptoms of the condition described likely not to be classic?
   a) infants
   b) young children
   c) the elderly
   d) all of the above
   e) none of the above

7. In which of the following age groups is the diagnosis of the condition described in Question 1 most likely to be confused with another serious intraabdominal inflammatory condition?
   a) infants
   b) young children
   c) young adult males
   d) young adult females
   e) elderly males and females

8. The condition described has been called which of the following?
   a) the "great imitator"
   b) the "typical condition"
   c) a diagnosis "unable to miss"
   d) a diagnosis "unable to make under the best of conditions"
   e) none of the above

9. Regarding the pathophysiology of the condition described, which of the following is(are) usual components of the pathological process?
   a) obstruction of the organ accounting for early symptoms and signs
   b) rapid invasion of the wall of the organ by bacteria leading to inflammation

c) spreading of the inflammation to involve the whole wall of the organ
d) perforation of the organ
e) all of the above

10. Which of the following is the most important sequelae of delayed treatment of this condition in young women?
    a) tuboovarian abscess formation
    b) chronic low-grade pelvic infection
    c) infertility due to peritonitis and subsequent adhesion formation
    d) chronic inflammatory bowel disease
    e) endometriosis

Short Answer Management Problem 108

Discuss the use of antibiotics in patients with signs and symptoms suggesting peritonitis.

ANSWERS

1. C. The most likely diagnosis in this patient is acute appendicitis.

   The typical history of acute appendicitis is vague central abdominal discomfort followed by anorexia, nausea, vomiting, and indigestion. The pain, which is continuous but often not severe, usually moves into the right lower quadrant. The pain is aggravated by movement, walking, or coughing.

   In patients with retrocecal appendicitis (which this description fits) there are often dysuria and hematuria due to the attachment of the appendix to the ureter and rectal tenderness. With perforation (as in this patient) there is generalized abdominal tenderness and rebound tenderness. Retrocecal appendicitis often produces poorly localized epigastric pain and only mild nausea and vomiting. Thus retrocecal appendicitis can be significantly more difficult to diagnosis than classic appendicitis. Peritonitis can develop very rapidly.

   Temperature elevation is usually mild in appendicitis.

   The most important differential diagnosis in this case is acute pain. The constellation of signs and symptoms, however, favors appendicitis. Acute cholecystitis, acute pyelonephritis, and acute pelvic inflammatory disease will be discussed in separate chapters.

2. B. This patient has an acute abdomen and therefore should be hospitalized for further evaluation. A white blood cell count, a urinalysis, and three views of the

abdomen are all investigations that should be performed in this patient.

In acute appendicitis the average leukocyte count is 15,000/mm³, and 90% of patients have a leukocyte count greater than 10,000/mm³. In 75% of patients, the differential count will show greater than 75% neutrophils.

Three views of the abdomen may show localized air-fluid levels, localized ileus, and an increased soft tissue density in the right lower quadrant. In addition, an altered right psoas shadow or an abnormal right flank stripe may be seen. On the other hand, they may show nothing specific.

With an acute abdomen, definitive treatment should not be delayed. This will be discussed in a subsequent question.

Antibiotics should not be given to this patient as they may mask the signs of peritonitis by reducing the inflammation of the peritoneum without treating the underlying pathology.

3. E. At this time the probability of the diagnosis of acute appendicitis with perforation and peritonitis is very high.

   At this time the most important intervention is a surgical consult ASAP.

4. A. The most appropriate action at this time would be an abdominal laparoscopy or laparotomy to confirm the diagnosis and treat the condition. The laparoscope is now being used for the removal of appendices by

some surgeons. Advantages to laparoscopy include the ability to examine the entire abdomen without the need for extending the operative incision. In addition, there are significantly fewer infectious wound complications.

Once the decision to operate has been made, it is reasonable to consider starting the patient on broad-spectrum antibiotics that are effective against both aerobic and anaerobic organisms. The probability of an anaerobic organism as part of the bacterial process is extremely high.

5. E. Complications of appendectomy include the following:
   1) Wound infection. This complication occurs in less than 1% of patients with unperforated appendicitis but rises to 20% with perforation. With perforation, delayed primary closure of the wound is a good strategy. Treatment is directed at drainage of the infection followed by the administration of appropriate antibiotics.
   2) Subphrenic abscess. The persistence of spiking fevers beginning on day 4 or day 5 without obvious cause should raise the suspicion of an intraabdominal collection of pus. The diagnosis is established by physical examination demonstrating a fixed diaphragm and a pleural effusion. There is often tenderness over the seventh and eighth ribs laterally and edema or erythema of the lower chest wall.
   3) Pelvic abscess. A patient with recurrent fever and diarrhea after appendectomy suggests the formation of a pelvic abscess. Diagnosis is made by rectal examination and is confirmed by ultrasonography or a CT scan.
   4) Appendiceal abscess. Although uncommon, a small percentage of patients seek treatment after the acute infection has become walled off. Under these conditions, it may be preferable to delay appendectomy until the inflammation has settled down.

6. D. Infants, young children, and elderly and frail patients may all present with very unclassic symptoms, making the diagnosis of appendicitis very difficult. In infants and young children the presenting symptoms may be very nonspecific and include only lethargy and irritability, especially in the early stages. In elderly patients, the same situation applies. As well, in elderly patients, the probability of rupture increases from 20% to 70%.

7. D. This question is meant to reiterate both the difficult issue raised previously and the importance of distinguishing acute appendicitis from acute PID and its complications such as tuboovarian abscess. Laparoscopy is definitely indicated in this circumstance.

8. A. Acute appendicitis is often called the "great imitator." This name arises from the different presentations of the disease that are possible, especially at the extremes of life. For example, any elderly patient with signs and symptoms of infection and/or inflammation has appendicitis until proven otherwise. Similarly, young infants and children hardly ever present in a classic manner. Thus appendicitis is one of those conditions in which you often will not make the diagnosis unless you think about the diagnosis.

9. E. The small size of the appendix accounts for its ability to produce symptoms quickly. The pathological process can be divided into stages:

   Stage 1 involves the obstruction of the appendix by a fecalith, a mucous plug, a foreign body, a parasite, or a tumor. This obstruction is associated with the early signs of periumbilical cramping and vomiting due to distention of the appendix.

   Stage 2 involves the rapid invasion of the wall of the organ by bacteria, with secondary inflammation. Gradual onset of systemic signs such as anorexia and malaise, low-grade fever, and leukocytosis then occur.

   Stage 3 involves spreading of the infection/inflammation to involve the entire wall of the organ and neighboring peritoneum, leading to a change in character of the pain to constant and localized. At this stage this differential diagnosis may include pyelonephritis, cholecystitis, or tuboovarian abscess.

   Young women with right-sided ovarian disease are particularly difficult to differentiate from young women with acute appendicitis. One clue may lie in the point of maximal tenderness. In appendicitis, the point of maximal tenderness is McBurney's point (two-thirds of the distance from the umbilicus to the anterior superior iliac spine). In right-sided ovarian disease the point of maximal tenderness is 2 to 3 cm below this point.

   Stage 4 is the last stage and involves perforation of the appendix. All four stages may develop within a very short period of time (24-48 hours).

10. C. The most significant complication of peritonitis following a ruptured appendix is the development of pelvic adhesions and scar tissue. This may significantly decrease the fertility of a young woman. Chronic pelvic pain may also develop.

SOLUTION TO SHORT ANSWER MANAGEMENT PROBLEM 108

Antibiotics should not be used in patients with signs and symptoms suggesting peritonitis. The antibiotic may mask the infectious/inflammatory process that is ongoing in the patient and thus prolong definitive diagnosis and therapy. The patient should be observed, placed on NPO and IV fluids, and observed and monitored both clinically and by laboratory evaluation.

SUMMARY OF THE DIAGNOSIS AND TREATMENT OF ACUTE APPENDICITIS

1. Acute appendicitis is the "great imitator." If you don't think of appendicitis, you won't make the diagnosis. Maintain a high index of suspicion, especially in the young and in the elderly.
2. **Classic symptoms of appendicitis:** central abdominal pain, initially vague, but later localized to the right lower quadrant; anorexia; nausea and vomiting; localized abdominal tenderness; low-grade fever; and leukocytosis
3. **Retrocecal or retroileal appendicitis:** poorly localized abdominal pain, mild nausea and vomiting, mild diarrhea, urinary frequency, and hematuria
4. **Diagnostic tests:** WBC, urinalysis, three views of the abdomen, ultrasonography, and CT scanning (ultrasonography and CT scanning have become important methods of investigation in the last few years.)
5. **Definitive therapy:** laparoscopic appendectomy or laparotomy and open removal (laparoscopic appendectomy is being performed more and more commonly. The procedure itself is associated with fewer postoperative complications, but is still in its development.)
6. **Complications:** wound infection, subphrenic abscess, pelvic abscess (leading to adhesions and fertility problems), and appendiceal abscess (with appendix walled off)

SUGGESTED READING

Gardner B, Stone HH. Acute abdominal pain. In: Basic surgery. 4th Ed. St Louis: Quality Medical Publishing, 1993.

PROBLEM 109   A 43-YEAR-OLD FEMALE WITH RECURRENT RIGHT UPPER QUADRANT PAIN

A 43-year-old female presents to your office with a 3-hour history of right upper quadrant pain. The pain is described as spasmodic and sharp. It radiates through to the back. The patient describes several episodes of this pain within the past 6 months. Nausea and vomiting accompany most of these episodes. Fever and chills are usually absent. The pain usually comes on after a meal.

On examination, there are no abdominal masses or tenderness. The chest is clear and the cardiovascular system is normal. The patient's blood pressure is 140/70 mm Hg.

There are no drug allergies, and the patient is on no medications at the present time.

SELECT THE ONE BEST ANSWER TO THE FOLLOWING QUESTIONS

1. What is the most likely diagnosis?
   a) acute cholecystitis
   b) biliary colic
   c) acute pancreatitis
   d) ileocecal appendicitis
   e) Crohn's disease

2. The patient's symptoms subside before your consultation is complete. You elect a wait-and-see policy. In 3 weeks the patient returns. On this occasion, the patient's symptoms have been present for the last 24 hours. The patient is nauseated and has vomited three times since this pain began. The pain, as well as radiating to the back, is also radiating to the right shoulder.

   On examination, there is tenderness in the right upper quadrant. On deep inspiration and palpation the patient's pain is accentuated and actually interrupts inspiration.

   What is the most likely diagnosis at this time?
   a) acute cholecystitis
   b) biliary colic
   c) acute pancreatitis
   d) ileocecal appendicitis
   e) Crohn's disease

3. Given this patient's signs and symptoms, which of the following investigative procedure is likely to yield the best information?
   a) a WBC
   b) an oral cholecystogram
   c) an abdominal ultrasound
   d) an ECG
   e) three views of the abdomen

4. What is(are) the treatment(s) of choice for the patient described in Question 2 at this time?
   a) intravenous fluids
   b) parenteral cefazolin
   c) nasogastric suction
   d) all of the above
   e) none of the above

5. Regarding the definite procedure to correct this condition, which of the following statements is true?
   a) a definite procedure should not be contemplated at this time; if required it should be performed several months later
   b) a definitive procedure should not be contemplated at this time; if symptoms continue to recur, you can reconsider
   c) a definitive surgical procedure should be performed at this time
   d) a definitive procedure is contraindicated given the signs and symptoms that this patient presents with
   e) a definitive procedure should not be considered until all other methods of treatment have failed

6. Which of the following statements about gallbladder disease in the United States is(are) true?
   a) more than 20 million Americans have gallstones
   b) in the United States more than 300,000 cholecystectomies are performed annually; at least 6000 deaths result from complications
   c) most gallstones are composed predominantly of cholesterol
   d) all of the above
   e) none of the above

7. Regarding the use of oral dissolution therapy in gallstone disease, which of the following statements is(are) true?
   a) oral dissolution therapy is an excellent option for most patients
   b) few if any gallstones that are dissolved with oral dissolution therapy recur
   c) the preferred agent for oral dissolution therapy is ursodiol
   d) oral dissolution therapy should not be combined with extracorporeal shock wave lithotripsy (ESWL)
   e) oral dissolution therapy works best in patients with large gallstones

8. Which of the following statements regarding the treatment of asymptomatic gallstones is most accurate?
   a) asymptomatic gallstones should be treated with cholecystectomy
   b) asymptomatic gallstones should not be treated

c) whether or not asymptomatic gallstones should be treated depends on the presence or absence of comorbid conditions

d) asymptomatic gallstones should or should not be treated; it all depends on who you talk to

e) asymptomatic gallstone treatment has radically changed since the introduction of laparoscopic cholecystectomy

9. What is the most common complication during laparoscopic cholecystectomy?
a) excessive bleeding
b) small bowel perforation
c) injury to the biliary tract system
d) inability to remove the gallbladder through the laparoscope
e) liver laceration

10. Which of the following is(are) true of laparoscopic cholecystectomy?
a) laparoscopic cholecystectomy provides a safe and effective treatment for most patients with symptomatic gallstones; it is the treatment of choice
b) laparoscopic cholecystectomy provides distinct advantages over open cholecystectomy
c) laparoscopic cholecystectomy can be performed at a treatment cost equal to or slightly less than that for open cholecystectomy
d) during laparoscopic cholecystectomy, when the anatomy is obscured due to excessive bleeding or other problems, the operation should be converted promptly to open cholecystectomy
e) all of the above

Short Answer Management Problem 109

The two most common diagnostic conditions associated with gallbladder disease are biliary colic and acute cholecystitis. Describe the differences in presentation and pathophysiology between biliary colic and acute cholecystitis.

ANSWERS

1. B.

2. A. This patient exhibits a typical presentation of biliary colic. Biliary colic is characterized by transient obstruction of the cystic duct. The pain located in the right upper quadrant lasts from minutes to several hours. The pain is best described as spasmodic and constant. Postprandial presentation is common. Nausea and vomiting usually accompany the pain. The major clinical differentiation between biliary colic and acute cholecystitis is the persistence of the pain in acute cholecystitis, the presence of abdominal (RUQ) tenderness, and the continuation of other systemic signs in addition to the pain. In acute cholecystitis there is also voluntary guarding. The pain is sometimes referred to the right scapula, and the gallbladder may be palpable. As well, mild jaundice can occur.

   Acute cholecystitis is manifested pathologically by gallbladder distention (hydrops), serosal edema, and infection secondary to obstruction of the cystic duct. Although the other choices presented can sometimes present atypically with RUQ pain only, the probability is low.

3. C. The diagnostic procedure of choice in this patient is an abdominal ultrasound. Gallstones will be demonstrated in approximately 95% of cases, and the specificity of the procedure is very high.

4. D. In a patient with acute cholecystitis, intravenous fluids should be given to correct dehydration and possible electrolyte imbalance, and an NG should be inserted. For acute cholecystitis of average severity, parenteral cefazolin (2-4 g daily) should be given. Parenteral penicillin (20 million units daily), clindamycin, and an aminoglycoside should be given to patients with severe disease.

5. C. Acute cholecystitis can be managed either aggressively or conservatively. Since the disease resolves spontaneously in approximately 60% of cases, the conservative approach is to manage the patient expectantly, with a plan to perform elective cholecystectomy after recovery, reserving early surgery for those patients with severe or worsening disease.

   The preferred treatment plan at this time, however, is to perform cholecystectomy in all patients following an episode of acute cholecystitis unless there are specific contraindications to performing the operation. The most common contraindication is severe concomitant disease. The reasoning for this approach is as follows:
   1) The incidence of technical complications is no greater with early surgery.
   2) Early surgery reduces the total duration of illness by approximately 30 days, the length of hospitalization by 5-7 days, and direct medical costs by several thousand dollars.

3) The death rate is slightly lower with early surgery.
   In addition, the following factors affect the decision as to when to operate:
   1) The diagnostic certainty
   2) The general health of the patient
   3) Signs of local complications of acute cholecystitis such as perforation or empyema

6. D. More than 20 million Americans have cholelithiasis; approximately 300,000 operations are performed annually for the disease, and at least 6000 deaths result from complications of treatment. The incidence of cholelithiasis increases with age.

   Most gallstones (75%) are composed of predominantly cholesterol (70%-95%). The remainder are pigment stones. The composition of the gallstone affects neither the symptoms associated with biliary colic nor the symptoms associated with acute cholecystitis.

7. C. Oral dissolution therapy with bile acids was first introduced in the early 1970s. The first agent available was chenodiol, which has been replaced by urosdiol.

   Oral dissolution therapy is indicated only in a small minority of patients. The most effective use of bile acids occurs with small gallstones (< 0.5 mm) that are floating, cholesterol in nature, and within a functioning gallbladder. This represents approximately 15% of patients. Patients must be treated between 6 and 12 months, and monitoring is necessary until dissolution is achieved. In such patients 60%-90% of stones will dissolve. Unfortunately, at least 50% of these stones reoccur within 5 years. Dissolution rates are higher and recurrence rates are lower in patients with single stones, nonobese individuals, and young patients. Indications for bile acid therapy are limited to patients with a comorbid condition that precludes safe operation and patients who choose to avoid operation.

   Extracorporeal shock wave lithotripsy (ESWL) may be used along with oral dissolution therapy. In patients with a functioning gallbladder and solitary noncalicified stones < 20 mm in diameter, this technique may be successful in up to 95% of patients. Recurrence is infrequent following therapy with ESWL for a single, small stone but is more common in patients with multiple stones. Again, the gallbladder remains and the probability of further stone formation is high.

8. B. Current opinion suggests that asymptomatic gallstones should not be treated. The vast majority of gallstones remain silent throughout life. Only 1%-4% per year of asymptomatic patients will develop symptoms or complications of gallstone disease. Existing data suggest that 10% of patients will develop symptoms within the first 5 years following diagnosis and approximately 20% within 10 years. Almost all patients will experience symptoms for a period of time before they develop a complication. Therefore, with few exceptions, prophylactic treatment of asymptomatic patients cannot be justified.

9. C. The most common complication of laparoscope cholecystectomy is bile duct injury. The frequency of bile duct injury is dependent on the skills of the surgeon. All of the complications listed are possible, but bile duct injury is the most common.

10. E. Laparoscopic cholecystectomy provides a safe and effective treatment for most patients with symptomatic gallstones. It appears to be the treatment of choice for most patients at this time.

    Laparoscopic cholecystectomy provides distinct advantages over open cholecystectomy. It decreases pain and disability without increasing mortality or overall morbidity. Although the rate of common bile duct injury is slightly increased, this rate is still sufficiently low to justify the use of this procedure.

    Laparoscopic cholecystectomy can be performed at a treatment cost that is equal to or slightly less than that of open cholecystectomy and will result in substantial cost savings to the patient and society due to reduced loss of time from work.

    The outcome of laparoscopic cholecystectomy is influenced greatly by the training, experience, skill, and judgment of the surgeon performing the procedure.

    During laparoscopic cholecystectomy, when anatomy is obscured, excessive bleeding occurs, or other problems arise, the operation should be converted promptly to open cholecystectomy. Conversion under these circumstances reflects sound surgical judgment and should not be considered a complication of laparoscopic cholecystectomy.

SOLUTION TO SHORT ANSWER MANAGEMENT PROBLEM 109

Biliary colic results from transient obstruction of the common bile duct with a small gallstone. The pain associated with biliary colic usually begins abruptly and subsides gradually, lasting from a few minutes to several hours. It is located in the upper right quadrant and may or may not be associated with abdominal tenderness. There is no associated inflammation of the gallbladder with biliary colic because of the very transient nature of the condition.

Acute cholecystitis, on the other hand, is associated pathophysiologically with inflammation of the gallbladder wall, with secondary infection in the gallbladder due to the blockage of the common bile duct.

The first symptom is abdominal pain in the right upper quadrant, with referral of the pain to right scapula. The pain persists and becomes associated with abdominal tenderness. There is nausea, vomiting, and a positive Murphy's sign (arrest of inspiration with palpation in the right upper quadrant). The pain does not resolve spontaneously.

SUMMARY OF THE DIAGNOSIS AND TREATMENT OF BILIARY TRACT DISEASE

1. **Acute cholecystitis:** Symptoms and signs:
   a) Acute right upper quadrant pain and tenderness
   b) Mild fever and leukocytosis
   c) Nausea and vomiting
   d) Palpable gallbladder
   e) Gallstones on ultrasound scan
      Treatment: nasogastric suction, parenteral fluids, analgesics, IV antibiotics, and laparoscopic cholecystectomy as soon as possible.
2. **Biliary colic:** Symptoms and signs:
   a) Recurrent abdominal pain (usually RUQ)
   b) Dyspepsia
   c) Gallstones on ultrasound
      Treatment: laparoscopic cholecystectomy when recurrent episodes occur
3. **Choledocholithiasis/cholangitis:** choledocholithiasis occurs in 15% of patients with gallstones. Controversy exists over whether or not the common bile duct should be explored when cholecystectomy is undertaken.
   Choledocholithiasis is the major cause of cholangitis. Symptoms of cholangitis include biliary colic, jaundice, fever, and chills. Treatment of cholangitis include IV antibiotics followed by cholecystectomy and exploration of the common bile duct.
4. **Laparoscopic cholecystectomy:** Laparoscopic cholecystectomy is now the treatment of choice for the vast majority of patients with biliary tract disease. It is a much more conservative operation, causes much less postoperative pain, and is associated with a much earlier return to work.
5. **Asymptomatic gallstones:** asymptomatic gallstones should be left where they are: don't create a problem where one does not exist.

SUGGESTED READINGS

Gallstones and laparoscopic cholecystectomy. NIH Consensus Conference. JAMA 1993; 269:1018.

Way L. Biliary tract. In Way L ed.: Current surgical diagnosis and treatment. 10th Ed. Norwalk, CT: Appleton and Lange, 1993.

PROBLEM 110   A 37-YEAR-OLD FEMALE WITH A SKIN LESION ON HER BACK

A 37-year-old female presents to your office for assessment of a skin lesion on her back that has been present for the last 3 years. It has recently increased in size, and the patient is concerned about it.

The lesion is pigmented, raised, and dark brown in color. It is approximately 1.5 cm in greatest diameter. There are other, smaller lesions that have a similar appearance on the patient's back, but they have neither increased in size nor changed color.

You decide to remove the skin lesion in your office.

SELECT THE ONE BEST ANSWER TO THE FOLLOWING QUESTIONS

1. In removing the skin lesion from your patient's back, what should you do?
   a) follow Langer's lines
   b) use silk sutures for skin closure
   c) use catgut sutures for subcutaneous tissue closure
   d) all of the above
   e) none of the above

2. In considering the deep subcutaneous tissue on your patient's back and your selection of suture material, you should be aware that it takes approximately how many days for fibroblasts to grow across the wound line and develop enough strength to hold together the deep portion of the wound?
   a) 10 days
   b) 15 days
   c) 21 days
   d) 28 days
   e) 35 days

3. In deciding on the use of needles for suture placement on skin surfaces in deep layers, which of the following statements is true?
   a) a cutting needle should be used for skin closure; a taper needle should be used for deeper tissues
   b) a taper needle should be used for skin closure; a cutting needle should be used for deep tissue
   c) a cutting needle should be used for both skin closure and deep tissue closure
   d) a taper needle should be used for both skin closure and deep tissue closure
   e) both cutting and taper needles may be used for either skin or deep tissue closure

4. What is the local anesthetic of choice for the patient described?
   a) lidocaine with epinephrine
   b) lidocaine plain
   c) bupivacaine plain
   d) bupivacaine with epinephrine
   e) none of the above

5. Which of the following is(are) useful in controlling bleeding from a skin lesion base?
   a) application of pressure
   b) electrocautery
   c) a pressure dressing
   d) hemostatic sutures
   e) all of the above

6. Which of the following techniques is(are) recommended for the removal of pigmented skin lesions?
   a) punch biopsy
   b) shave biopsy
   c) electrocautery
   d) a or b
   e) any of the above

7. What is(are) the treatment(s) of choice for the removal of plantar warts?
   a) cryosurgery
   b) electrocautery
   c) surgical excision
   d) podophyllin application
   e) any of the above

8. The treatment(s) of choice for the removal of venereal warts include which of the following?
   a) electrocautery
   b) cryosurgery
   c) surgical excision
   d) podophyllin application
   e) all of the above

9. A 5-year-old child presents to your office with a small second-degree burn on her right hand. The burn was sustained when she put her hand in a kettle of boiling water. On examination, there is an area of 3 cm × 5 cm on the left hand that has undergone blister formation. Her mother wrapped the burn in a gauze dressing.
   At this time, what would be the most appropriate first course of action?
   a) debride the wound
   b) cool the burn site by immediately immersing the hand in cold water
   c) aspirate the fluid underneath the blister
   d) leave the gauze in place and send the child on her way
   e) debride the wound, aspirate the fluid, and apply an antibiotic cream

10. Following the initial step described in Question 9, what should be the next step(s)?
    a) carefully cleanse the burn site

b) debride the burn site

c) provide tetanus prophylaxis

d) a and c

e) all of the above

11. A 4-year-old boy presents with his mother after having banged his thumb in a door. He is crying and irritated. His left thumb has a purplish discoloration under the nail.
    At this time, what should you do?
    a) reassure the mother and send the child home with a pat on the head
    b) reassure the mother and give the child some plain acetaminophen
    c) under local anesthetic remove the nail
    d) under local anesthetic perform a wedge resection
    e) none of the above

12. A 25-year-old female has had a sore left toe for the past 4 weeks.
    On examination, the lateral aspect of the left toe is erythematous and puffy, with pus oozing from the corner between the nail and the skin tissue surrounding the nail.
    This is the first occurrence of this condition in this patient.
    At this time, what should you do?
    a) do nothing
    b) have the patient soak her toe in hydrogen peroxide three times daily
    c) have the patient apply a local antibiotic cream and prescribe system antibiotics for 7 to 10 days
    d) under local anesthesia, remove the whole toenail
    e) b and c

13. If the treatment advocated in Question 12 is unsuccessful, what should you do then?
    a) still do nothing; these things have a habit of going away if you wait long enough; tell the patient she will only be in pain for another 3 or 4 months at the most
    b) have the patient continue to soak her toe in hydrogen peroxide; tell the pharmacist to mix up a double-strength mixture for her

c) change both the local and the systemic antibiotics to the big, all-inclusive, all-pervasive, kill-everything-in-sight guns

d) under local anesthesia, remove the whole toenail

e) none of the above

14. A 45-year-old male presents to your office with a 4-day history of rectal pain. The pain is dull, constant, and made worse by defecation.
    On examination, there is a 3 cm × 2 cm thrombosed mass present at the 3 o'clock position in the anal area.
    At this time, what should you do?
    a) advise the patient to take five sitz baths per day
    b) advise the patient to apply a local antiinflammatory cream three times/day
    c) under local anesthesia, remove the contents of the mass with a straight incision
    d) under local anesthesia, remove the contents of the mass with an elliptical incision
    e) apply a band to this mass and wait for it to fall off

15. A 28-year-old male presents to your office with rectal bleeding and local burning and searing pain in the rectal area. The patient describes a small amount of bright red blood on the toilet paper. The pain is maximal at defecation and following defecation. The burning and searing pain that occurs at defecation is replaced by a spasmodic pain after defecation that lasts approximately 30 minutes.
    What is the most likely diagnosis in this patient?
    a) adenocarcinoma of the rectum
    b) squamous cell carcinoma of the rectum
    c) internal hemorrhoids
    d) anal fissure
    e) an external thrombosed hemorrhoid

16. What is(are) the treatment(s) of choice for large prolapsing internal hemorrhoids?
    a) excision and drainage
    b) sclerotherapy
    c) internal banding
    d) all of the above are equally effective
    e) none of the above

Short Answer Management Problem 110

Discuss the classification of burns and how that classification affects office or hospital treatment.

ANSWERS

1. A. For skin incision, it is extremely important that the skin lines of tension be followed (Langer's lines). This is especially important on areas such as the face where

Langer's lines tend to run horizontally on the upper face and vertically on the lower face.

2. C. It takes approximately 21 days for fibroblasts to grow across a wound line and for the wound to develop

enough strength to hold deep portions of a wound together. If deep portions of a wound pull apart, a depression on the skin surface may develop, which represents a poor cosmetic outcome.

3. A. Cutting needles should always be used on the skin. Almost all cutting needles now have a reverse cutting design (flat surface is on the inside of the curve). For deeper layers, taper needles are less likely to cut through a blood vessel and start bleeding that is difficult to control.

4. A. The anaesthetic agent of choice for this patient is lidocaine with epinephrine. The epinephrine will decrease the amount of bleeding from the incision site. The prepackaged solution of lidocaine with epinephrine has a very low pH (pH 4.05) and produces much more pain on injection than lidocaine plain. The pain reaction can be avoided by buffering the lidocaine with sodium bicarbonate in a combination of (10/1) lidocaine to one part of sodium bicarbonate. When this combination is used, the pH is near neutral and the stinging sensation is eliminated.

Other measures that lessen the pain of injection include warming the solution to body temperature, injecting the solution extremely slowly and cooling the injection site with ice or ethyl chloride before injection. In addition, very small caliber needles can be used for the initial injection (such as a #30 ½-inch needle) or a local anesthetic such as TAC (tetracaine, epinephrine, and cocaine) or 20% benzocaine liquid or gel can be used.

5. E. Common methods for controlling bleeding after incision include the following:
   1) Application of pressure with a sponge held firmly against the bleeding areas
   2) Electrocautery
   3) Use of local anesthesia containing epinephrine
   4) Topical epinephrine or lidocaine containing epinephrine
   5) Dysol solution (aluminum chloride 20% in alcohol)
   6) Hemostatic sutures
   7) Elevation
   8) Pressure dressings
   9) Various methods of cooling

6. D. A pigmented skin lesion should be removed intact to ensure an "unharmed" specimen for pathologic evaluation. If electrocautery is used to remove the lesion, the lesion will obviously be destroyed in the process.

7. A. The treatment of choice for the removal of plantar warts is cryosurgery with liquid nitrogen. Cryosurgery with liquid nitrogen combined with paring down the callus has been shown to be the most effective method of removal.

The first step is to pare down the excess callus in the area of the wart. This is best done by shaving off thin layers of the callus with a straight-edge razor blade held by hand or a scalpel with a #10 blade. This process should be continued until most of the callus is gone and normal-appearing pliable skin is seen.

The shaving is kept superficial to any bleeding or sensation of pain. The circular plantar wart then becomes much clearer and more evident. Some of the keratin plug can then be excised with the corner of the razor blade or the tip of the scalpel blade. Following that, cryosurgery is performed with liquid nitrogen. A donut-shaped felt pad should be applied. This pad transfers the patient's weight off the hard wart and provides immediate relief of pain during walking. After adequate cryosurgery, the wart should peel off in 1 to 3 weeks. On occasion, a second or third treatment is necessary to ensure complete removal.

8. D. The treatment of choice for venereal warts is 25% podophyllum in tincture of benzoin. Care must be taken to apply the agent only to the wart to avoid damaging the surrounding normal skin. This can be accomplished with the application of petroleum jelly. The patient should be instructed to wash off the podophyllin in 2 to 4 hours to avoid a chemical burn.

9. B. The most important first step in patients who present with burns is to cool the burn site. A patient who telephones should be told to run cold water over the burn and apply cold compresses while on the way to the ER. Ice cubes can be placed in a towel. At the ER or in the office, this same type of cooling is continued during the initial assessment. Cooling serves two important functions: it controls the pain and it limits the extent of damage. Tissues involved in a burn injury contain enough heat to continue the damaging process for a significant period of time—even up to ½ to 1 hour. Thus the cooling process is critical.

10. D. Following cooling the burn site (and while the cooling process continues) the burned area should be gently cleansed with a surgical soap to remove dirt, oil, or other foreign matter. The use of 4 × 4 gauze sponges or cotton balls can facilitate cleansing. If cleansing is done gently together with proper cooling, minimal pain should result.

Tetanus prophylaxis is important in all patients with serious burns. If this child's tetanus is not up to date, it must be brought up to date.

For a second-degree burn as in this child, expert opinion is divided on whether or not debridement should take place. Most experts elect to leave the blister intact for several days. The skin of a natural blister may act as a natural dressing, protecting the wound against infection and also reducing the amount of pain.

After the initial cooling and cleansing, the blistered area is covered with a layer of silver sulfadiazine ointment (Silvadene) or, in patients who are allergic to sulfa, Polysporin. A nonadherent dressing should then be applied. Following that, a conforming protective material, such as Kling or Kerlix, should be applied. Finally, an ABD-type pad may be used to offer more absorbency under the outer dressing.

11. E. This patient has a subungual hematoma that needs to be released. The best method of release is to heat a wire (a paper clip), reassure the patient that this is not going to hurt, and gently press the hot metal tip directly over the central portion of the hematoma. As soon as penetration is complete, blood flows through the opening and relief of pain is immediate. An antibiotic ointment will help protect against infection.

12. E.

13. E. This patient has an ingrown toenail. It is perfectly reasonable to try a conservative approach first. The conservative approach consists of topical and oral antibiotics for infection, hot soaks and/or hydrogen peroxide soaks, good nail care (make sure that the nail is cut straight across), and wearing wider shoes. The corner of the nail that is causing the problem (that is, the corner of the nail that is infected) can often be encouraged to grow out over the skin at the end of the toe by elevation. The corner may be held up by some articles such as a wisp of cotton, a folded piece of Telfa, or a vaseline gauze or other dressing.

This "first try" at conservative treatment has the additional advantage of decreasing the swelling and inflammation and facilitating injections of the local anaesthetic if wedge resection does, in the end, have to be performed. Wedge resection of the nail (the next step) is a procedure whereby the offending curve is cut off at an angle of approximately 30 degrees. Only in recurrent cases is it necessary to completely remove the nail.

14. D. This patient has a thrombosed external hemorrhoid. This condition is painful and causes the patient a great deal of discomfort. With local anesthetic, and using an elliptical incision and a #15 scalpel, the contents (a clot) should be removed. The area should be cleansed and, once bleeding is controlled, an antibiotic ointment and 4 × 4 gauze pads applied.

15. D. This patient has an anal fissure. Anal fissures are common causes of rectal bleeding. A crack or a fissure in the skin of the anal canal results from the passage of large, hard boluses of stool. A small amount of bright red blood is noted on the toilet paper. The bleeding most often occurs after defecation. Pain is an important symptom; it is usually a local burning or searing pain and is often very severe.

Examination reveals a semielliptical defect or crack in the anal skin running in a radial direction.

Initially treatment of anal fissures involves the application of a local steroid cream applied twice daily for 2 or 3 weeks. The use of stool softeners and daily hot sitz baths are recommended. In most cases this treatment will promote complete healing.

16. C. The treatment of choice for internal hemorrhoids is banding. This office procedure should be performed with no more than two hemorrhoids at once. If there are three or more hemorrhoids, wait 3 or 4 weeks before repeating the procedure.

SOLUTION TO SHORT ANSWER MANAGEMENT PROBLEM 110

Burns are classified as follows:

First degree: symptoms/signs include pain and redness but no blistering. Dressing is not necessary. Application of cold packs is useful. Pain from small burn areas can be relieved with the use of topical creams, ointments, and lotions containing a "caine" medication.

In areas of clothing, the burn can be covered, and a medicated ointment followed by the application of a nonadherent dressing is recommended.

Pain can be treated with either acetaminophen, aspirin, or another NSAID.

Second degree: the hallmark of a second-degree burn is blister formation. Second-degree burns may be either superficial or deep. Treatment options include cooling, cleaning, and application of a topical antibiotic and dressing. In most cases, leave the blister intact.

Third degree: these are full-thickness skin burns. Referral to a plastic surgeon as soon as possible is mandatory. Third-degree burns are much more likely to be more serious, be more extensive, have a much greater chance of developing sepsis, and often require an ICU situation if the burn covers a significant portion of the body.

SUMMARY OF COMMON PROCEDURES IN OFFICE SURGERY

1. **Remember the ABCs:** Always have an emergency cart available if you are planning on doing office surgery.
2. **Skin lesion removal:**
   a) Follow Langer's lines.
   b) Use an elliptical incision (long enough to avoid puckering at the ends).
   c) Local: lidocaine with epinephrine except on the fingers and toes
   d) Sutures: skin: monofilament nylon 3-0, 4-0, 5-0, 6-0; Deep: Dexon needle, Cutting for skin, taper for deep

e) Do not fry anything that should rightly go for biopsy or you might end up getting fried yourself in court.

f) Small skin lesion removal: punch biopsy

If you are not absolutely, 150% sure of what a skin lesion is, then biopsy it. If you don't, sometime in your life you will wish you had.

3. **Sebaceous cysts:** these are most frequent on the scalp and back and can be a cause of significant irritation. Try wherever possible to shell out the whole cyst. If you aren't able to remove the entire cyst, there is a significant chance of recurrence.

4. **Incision and drainage of abscesses:** make sure you know exactly what you are incising and draining and why you are doing it. Be very careful of both the vascular supply and the nerve supply if you go deep.

5. **Finger warts:** cryosurgery with liquid nitrogen

6. **Plantar warts:**
   a) Pare down excess callus to bleeding point.
   b) Remove keratin plug if possible.
   c) Cryosurgery with liquid nitrogen

7. **Burns:** described in solution to Short Answer Management Problem

8. **Paronychia:**
   a) Try conservative management first.
   b) Remove proximal segment of fingernail and dress.

9. **Subungual hematoma:** the old, wise, worn, and true heated paper clip

10. **Thrombosed external hemorrhoids:**
    a) Local anesthesia
    b) Elliptical incision and remove clot

11. **Lacerations:** use rules as stated for skin lesion removal.

12. **Anal fissures:**
    a) Prevention of further episodes is mandatory. Prevention is best achieved by preventing constipation.
    b) Conservative treatment includes sitz baths and local steroid cream.

13. **Internal hemorrhoids:**
    a) Make sure you know what you're banding before you band it.
    b) Banding is the preferred method of treatment.

SUGGESTED READING

AAFP Home Study Self-Assessment. Office surgery. Monograph #174, American Academy of Family Physicians, December 1993.

PROBLEM 111   A 44-YEAR-OLD MALE WITH A HISTORY OF VERY HEAVY ALCOHOL INTAKE

A 44-year-male with a 20-year history of heavy drinking presents to your office with his wife. His wife is very concerned about her husband's condition, and specifically about an abdominal pain that began 4 days previously. The pain has been so severe that her husband has been crying at night. Despite this severe pain, the patient managed to make it to his local bar last evening and straggled home at 3 AM.

On examination, you observe a stoic, overweight male who looks much older than his stated years. When you ask him what's wrong, he says, "Nothing, just a little indigestion." As you examine him you clearly smell alcohol on his breath.

On P/E the patient's blood pressure is 90/70 mm Hg. He has a marked tenderness in the epigastric region along with "bruising" in the epigastric area. There is also a sensation of a mass present in the epigastric area. When questioned about the bruising, the patient states that he fell down the stairs yesterday. No other abnormalities are present.

SELECT THE ONE BEST ANSWER TO THE FOLLOWING QUESTIONS

1. Following the history and P/E, which of the following is the next step?
   a) send the patient for blood work
   b) send the patient for X-rays
   c) send the patient for both blood work and X-rays
   d) consult psychiatry to assess his alcohol intake and subsequent family problems
   e) none of the above

2. Following the step taken in Question 1, what would you do now?
   a) order additional blood tests and X-rays if any abnormalities were found
   b) order an ultrasound of the abdomen
   c) call a GI colleague and ask him to see the patient within a few days
   d) do a complete mental status examination to determine suicidal ideation
   e) none of the above

3. What is the most likely diagnosis in this patient?
   a) alcoholic esophagitis
   b) severe alcoholic gastritis
   c) acute pancreatitis
   d) perforated duodenal ulcer
   e) early alcoholic encephalopathy with underlying alcoholic gastritis

4. The "bruising" present in the epigastrium is most likely the result of which of the following?
   a) the patient's wife's floor wax
   b) trauma secondary to a barroom brawl
   c) retroperitoneal bleeding
   d) superior mesenteric artery erosion
   e) disseminated intravascular coagulation

5. What is the most likely disease complication associated with the "bruising"?
   a) a defect in the intrinsic coagulation pathway
   b) a defect in the extrinsic coagulation pathway

   c) DIC as a result of the alcohol intake
   d) pseudocyst formation
   e) hemorrhagic abscess formation

6. What is(are) the essential diagnostic feature(s) of the condition of the patient described in Question 1?
   a) abrupt onset of epigastric pain with radiation to the back
   b) nausea and vomiting
   c) elevated serum amylase
   d) all of the above
   e) none of the above

7. The treatment of this condition may include all of the following except
   a) gastric suction
   b) fluid replacement
   c) calcium replacement
   d) oxygen
   e) an H_2 receptor blocker

8. Which of the following statements about the disease discussed is(are) true?
   a) many cases of this disease are associated with biliary tract pathology
   b) there is very strong evidence to suggest a link between this disease and alcohol
   c) the chronic condition of this disease is more likely to be associated with alcohol abuse rather than biliary tract disease
   d) all of the above statements are true
   e) none of the above are true

9. In approximately ⅔ of cases of this disease, a plain film of the abdomen is abnormal. Which of the following abnormalities is this plain film most likely to show?
   a) a "sentinel loop"
   b) the "colon cutoff sign"
   c) air under the diaphragm
   d) distention in both the small bowel and the large bowel
   e) feces throughout the colon

10. Complications of the condition described in Question 1 include which of the following?
    a) ascites
    b) pleural effusion
    c) abscess formation
    d) all of the above
    e) none of the above

Short Answer Management Problem 111

Describe the four essential features of the diagnosis of chronic pancreatitis.

ANSWERS

1. E.

2. E. This patient is extremely ill and should be hospitalized now. The combination of low blood pressure, abdominal pain, and history of heavy alcohol intake strongly suggest the diagnosis of an acute abdomen. No time should be taken for doing laboratory investigations or X-rays at this time; that can wait until the patient has been assessed and stabilized.

3. C. This patient has acute pancreatitis. His admission to an ICU would be the best course of action. His blood pressure should be stabilized and input and output measurements begun immediately.

4. C. This patient has Cullen's sign. Cullen's sign is a bluish discoloration in the periumbilical area due to the dissection of blood retroperitoneally.

   This also confirms the diagnosis of hemorrhagic pancreatitis.

   Another sign that can sometimes be found in patients with acute pancreatitis is called Grey-Turner's sign. In Grey-Turner's sign there is the same bluish discoloration, only the location is the flank area rather than the periumbilical area.

5. D. The most likely cause of the bleeding is bleeding into a pancreatic pseudocyst that has formed as a complication of acute pancreatitis.

   The bleeding must be stopped. This may be accomplished by embolization of the artery. If the bleeding cannot be stopped by embolization, emergency surgery should be performed. In this patient it may be necessary to open the pseudocyst, ligate the bleeding vessel in the cyst wall, and drain the cyst.

6. D. The essential diagnostic features of acute pancreatitis include abrupt onset of epigastric pain with radiation to the lower lumbar spine, nausea and vomiting, and elevated serum or urinary amylase. Acute pancreatitis usually originates from either cholecystitis or alcoholism.

The essential diagnostic features of pancreatic pseudocyst include an epigastric mass and pain, mild fever and leukocystosis, persistent serum amylase or serum lipase elevation, and demonstration of pseudocyst by CT scan.

7. E. The essentials of treatment of acute pancreatitis include the following:
   a) Gastric suction: to eliminate gastric secretions
   b) Fluid replacement: to replace sequestered fluid in the retroperitoneal space
   c) Replacement of calcium and magnesium: in severe attacks of pancreatitis both hypocalcemia and hypomagnesemia may occur and need to be treated.
   d) Oxygen therapy: severe hypoxemia develops in 30% of patients. The onset is often insidious and can result in ARDS (adult respiratory distress syndrome).
   e) Peritoneal lavage: this is required in severe cases to remove toxins.
   f) Nutrition: NPO and TPN
   g) Blood transfusion: when hemorrhage into either the pancreas or a pancreatic pseudocyst occurs
   The efficacy of H_2 receptor blockers, anticholinergic drugs, glucagon, and antibiotics has not been demonstrated.

8. D. Gallstone disease and alcohol abuse are responsible for approximately 40% of cases of acute pancreatitis. Other causes include hyperparathyroidism, hyperlipidemia, familial pancreatitis, postoperative (iatrogenic) pancreatitis, protein deficiency, certain drugs, and obstruction of the pancreatic duct.

   Chronic pancreatitis is much more likely to be associated with alcoholism than with biliary tract disease. In fact, an alcoholic patient who presents with one attack of acute pancreatitis is very likely to go on to subsequent attacks and to chronic disease.

9. A. In approximately ⅔ of cases, a plain film of the abdomen is abnormal. The most frequent finding is isolated dilatation of a segment of gut (the sentinel loop) consisting of jejunum, transverse colon, or duodenum adjacent to the pancreas. Gas distending

the right colon that abruptly stops in the mid or left transverse colon is called the *colon cutoff sign*. This is due to colonic spasm adjacent to the pancreatic inflammation.

Air under the diaphragm is suggestive of a perforated peptic ulcer.

A completely distended small and large bowel suggest a distal bowel obstruction.

Constipation is not associated with acute pancreatitis.

10. D. In addition to chronic pancreatitis and pancreatic pseudocyst formation, acute pancreatitis may also be associated with pancreatic abscess (fatal if not treated surgically), pancreatic ascites, and pancreatic pleural effusion.

SOLUTION TO SHORT ANSWER MANAGEMENT PROBLEM 111

The four essential features of chronic pancreatitis are as follows:
1) Persistent or recurrent abdominal pain in almost all cases
2) Pancreatic calcification on X-ray in 50% of cases
3) Pancreatic insufficiency in 30% of cases; this may lead to either steatorrhea or diabetes mellitus.
4) Most often due to alcoholism

SUMMARY OF THE DIAGNOSIS AND TREATMENT OF PANCREATITIS

1. Acute pancreatitis is usually caused by either alcohol abuse or biliary tract disease (40% biliary tract-gallstone associated; 40% alcohol intake).
2. **Essential features of diagnosis:** abrupt onset of epigastric pain radiating through to the back; nausea and vomiting; elevated serum amylase, serum lipase or urinary amylase.
3. **Laboratory investigations:** CBC; serum amylase and urine amylase; serum lipase; serum glucose; serum LDH; serum bilirubin; serum AST/ALT; serum calcium; serum magnesium; electrolytes; cholesterol and triglycerides; blood gases; plain film of abdomen or three views; abdominal ultrasound; and CT scan

4. **Ranson's criteria of severity of acute pancreatitis:**
Criteria initially present:
   a) Age > 55 years
   b) WBC > 16,000/mm³
   c) Blood glucose > 200 mg%
   d) Serum LDH > 350 IU/L
   e) AST (SGOT) > 250 IU/L
Criteria developing during first 24 hours:
   a) Hematocrit falling to > 10%
   b) An increase in BUN > 8 mg/dl
   c) Serum Ca + < 8 mg/dl
   d) Arterial PO_2 < 60 mm Hg
   e) Base deficit > 4 meq/L
   f) Estimated fluid sequestration > 600 ml
      Morbidity and mortality rates correlate with number of criteria present:
      0-2 criteria = 2% mortality
      3 or 4 criteria = 15% mortality
      5 or 6 criteria = 40% mortality
      7 or 8 criteria = 100% mortality
5. **Essentials of management:** NPO, nasogastric suction; urine output (a measure of fluid sequestration); fluid replacement of sequestered fluid, replacement of calcium and magnesium if low; oxygen, peritoneal lavage; TPN
6. In most cases resolution occurs within a week.
7. **Complications:** pseudocyst formation, abscess formation, hemorrhage, ascites, pleural effusion, and chronic pancreatitis
8. Chronic pancreatitis is almost always associated with alcohol-induced cases. Complications of chronic pancreatitis include malabsorption (steatorrhea) and diabetes mellitus.

SUGGESTED READINGS

Alridge MC et al: Colonic complications of severe acute pancreatitis. British Journal of Surgery 1988; 76:362.

Burch JM. Acute pancreatitis. In: Rakel R, ed. Conn's current therapy. Philadelphia: WB Saunders, 1993.

Garder B, Stone HH. Acute abdominal pain. In Polk HC, Gardner B, Stone HH, eds. Basic surgery. 4th Ed. St. Louis: Quality Medical Publishing, 1993.

Reber HA, Way L. Pancreas. In: Way L, ed. Current surgical diagnosis and treatment. 10th Ed. Norwalk, CT: Appleton and Lange, 1994.

PROBLEM 112 A 48-YEAR-OLD MALE WITH WEAKNESS, FATIGUE, AND LOWER RIGHT-SIDED ABDOMINAL PAIN

A 48-year-old male presents to your office with a vague lower right-sided abdominal fullness (not pain). He describes to you a general feeling of "not feeling well," fatigue, and a somewhat tender area "down near my appendix." He tells you that "I have no energy; I'm tired all the time." As well, he wonders if his skin has changed color, first to a pale color and then to a slightly yellow color.

On direct questioning he admits to anorexia, weight loss of 30 lb in 6 months, nausea most of the time, vomiting twice, constipation (by that he means a "stringy type of bowel movement", and blood in the stool almost every day for the past 3 months. When you ask him what he makes of all this he tells you, "A very bad flu."

On examination the patient looks very pale. Examination of the abdomen reveals abdominal distention. You record the abdominal girth as a baseline. There is a sensation of "fullness" in the right lower quadrant of the abdomen. This area also is dull to percussion.

As well, the area is slightly tender. There is definite percussion of tympany on both sides of the area of dullness. The liver span is approximately 20 cm. The sclera are yellow.

SELECT THE ONE BEST ANSWER TO THE FOLLOWING QUESTIONS

1. At this time, what would you do?
   a) tell the patient to relax and recheck with your office in 6 months
   b) diagnose the irritable bowel syndrome and start the patient on dietary therapy
   c) tell that patient that he probably is going through a viral illness; relax and come back in 2 months if the symptoms have not improved
   d) order the complete workup on the patient; the good old shotgun approach: every test known to man and then some
   e) none of the above

2. What is the definitive diagnostic procedure of choice in this patient?
   a) CBC
   b) fecal occult blood samples
   c) air-constrast barium enema
   d) colonoscopy
   e) three views of the abdomen

3. What is the most likely diagnosis in this patient?
   a) irritable bowel syndrome
   b) lactose intolerance
   c) adenocarcinoma of the pancreas
   d) adenocarcinoma of the colon
   e) ruptured appendix

4. Considering a correct diagnosis from Question 3, what is the definitive treatment of choice in this patient?
   a) colonic resection
   b) total colectomy
   c) removal of the appendix
   d) abdominoperineal resection of the rectum
   e) Nd:YAG laser photocoagulation of the identified lesion

5. Carcinoma of the colon most commonly originates in which of the following?
   a) an adenomatous polyp
   b) an inflammatory polyp
   c) a hyperplastic polyp
   d) a benign lymphoid polyp
   e) a leiomyoma

6. Adenomatous polyps are found in approximately what percentage of asymptomatic patients who undergo screening?
   a) 5%
   b) 10%
   c) 15%
   d) 20%
   e) 25%

7. A barium enema is performed on a patient with a suspected carcinoma of the descending colon following an unsuccessful colonoscopy. What is the best radiologic description that fits the probable diagnosis in this patient?
   a) a "strawberry cutout" lesion
   b) an "orange dimpled" lesion
   c) an "apple core" lesion
   d) a "cabbage fulfurating" lesion
   e) a "banana peel" lesion

8. Colorectal polyps are thought to be the origin of most colorectal cancers. Which of the following statements regarding colorectal polyps is false?
   a) the larger the colorectal polyps, the greater the chance of malignancy
   b) hyperplastic polyps have the highest malignant potential of all colorectal polyps
   c) adenomatous polyps increase in incidence with each decade after the age of 30 years
   d) routine removal of adenomas from the colon reduces the incidence of subsequent adenocarcinoma
   e) villous adenomas carry the highest malignant potential of all adenomas

9. Which of the following statements best describes the current evidence for fecal occult blood screening and/or sigmoidoscopy as measures to reduce the morbidity and mortality from colorectal cancer?
   a) there is good evidence to include fecal occult blood testing and/or sigmoidoscopy in screening asymptomatic patients over the age of 50 years for colorectal carcinoma
   b) there is fair evidence to include fecal occult blood testing and/or sigmoidoscopy in screening asymptomatic patients over the age of 50 years for colorectal carcinoma
   c) there is insufficient evidence to include or exclude fecal occult blood testing and/or sigmoidoscopy as effective screening tests for colorectal cancer in asymptomatic patients over the age of 50 years
   d) there is excellent evidence to include or exclude fecal occult blood testing and/or sigmoidoscopy as effective screening tests for colorectal cancer in asymptomatic patients over the age of 50 years
   e) none of the above are true

10. Which of the following statements regarding carcinomebryonic antigen (CEA) and colorectal cancer is(are) true?
    a) CEA is a cost-effective screening test for colorectal cancer
    b) preoperative CEA levels correlate well with postoperative recurrence rate in colorectal cancer
    c) CEA is a sensitive test for colorectal cancer
    d) CEA is a specific test for colorectal cancer
    e) CEA has no value in predicting recurrence in colorectal cancer

11. A 78-year-old male presents to your office with acute and severe abdominal pain, left lower-quadrant tenderness, a left lower-quadrant mass, and a temperature of 39° C. As well, the patient has noticed the passage of bright red blood/rectum for the past 4 days.

    The patient has had no significant illnesses in the past. He is a very healthy 78-year-old male. He sees his physician once/year and has had a normal heart, normal blood pressure, and normal "everything else," as he says, for many years.

    On examination, the patient's temperature is 39.5° C. His pulse is 96 and regular. His blood pressure is 210/105 mm Hg. There is significant tenderness in the left lower quadrant. Rebound tenderness is absent. There is a definite sensation of a mass present.

    What is the most likely diagnosis in this patient?
    a) adenocarcinoma of the colon
    b) diverticulitis
    c) diverticulosis
    d) colorectal carcinoma
    e) atypical appendicitis

12. What is the treatment of choice for the patient described in Question 11?
    a) primary resection of the diseased segment with anastomosis
    b) primary resection of the diseased segment without anastomosis
    c) colectomy
    d) abdominal perineal resection
    e) none of the above

13. Which of the following is(are) components of the acute treatment of this patient's condition?
    a) IV fluids
    b) IV (broad-spectrum) antibiotics
    c) NG suction
    d) all of the above
    e) a and c only

14. Which of the following investigations is(are) contraindicated in the patient described in Question 11 at this time?
    a) CT scan of the abdomen and pelvis
    b) MRI scan of the abdomen and pelvis
    c) three views of the abdomen
    d) air-contrast barium enema
    e) none of the above are contraindicated

15. Which of the following statements regarding this patient's blood pressure elevation is(are) true?
    a) this patient most likely has essential hypertension
    b) this patient's abdominal pain is most likely related to his hypertension
    c) this elevation of blood pressure could be due to the pain he is experiencing
    d) this patient's physician (the one he has been seeing every year) obviously has made a very serious mistake in labeling this patient as normotensive
    e) none of the above statements are true

16. What is the analgesic of choice for control of pain in this patient?
    a) morphine
    b) hydromorphone
    c) methadone
    d) pentazocine
    e) codeine

17. Which of the following organism(s) is(are) the most likely cause(s) of the condition described?
    a) *Escherichia coli*
    b) *Bacteroides fragilis*
    c) *Streptococcus pneumoniae*
    d) a and b only
    e) all of the above

18. A 35-year-old male presents with rectal bleeding, mucoid discharge from the rectum, and protrusion of certain structures through the anal canal.

    On protoscopic examination, large internal hemorrhoids are seen.

    At this time, what should you do?
    a) proceed with definitive treatment
    b) proceed with further investigations
    c) prescribe a hemorrhoidal cream
    d) do nothing; ask the patient to return in 6 months for review
    e) none of the above

19. What is the treatment of choice for the condition described in Question 18?
    a) a hemorrhoidal cream
    b) a hemorrhoidal ointment
    c) hemorrhoidectomy
    d) injection of phenol into the hemorrhoidal tissue
    e) rubber band ligation of the internal hemorrhoids

20. Which of the following statements regarding angiodysplasia is(are) true?
    a) angiodysplasia is an acquired condition most often affecting individuals over the age of 60 years
    b) angiodysplasia is a focal submucosal vascular ectasis that has the propensity to bleed profusely
    c) most angiodysplastic lesions are located in the cecum and proximal ascending colon
    d) multiple lesions occur in 25% of cases
    e) all of the above

Short Answer Management Problem 112

Discuss the evidence for dietary modification to reduce the risk of developing colorectal cancer.

ANSWERS

1. E.

2. D.

3. D. The problem list at this point, in this patient, is as follows:
   1. Middle-aged male: nonspecific feelings of "ill health"
   2. Right lower-quadrant mass on P/E—query carcinoma
   3. Enlarged liver—query metastases
   4. Pale appearance—query anemia
   5. Icterus—query conjugated hyperbilirubinemia
   6. Clinically apparent abdominal distention—query ascites

   With this constellation of symptoms and signs the working diagnosis is adenocarcinoma of the cecum with liver metastases.

   The investigations that must be performed at this time include the following:
   I. Laboratory:
      1. CBC
      2. Serum bilirubin
      3. Liver enzymes: AST, ALT, gamma-GT
      4. Alkaline phosphatase
      5. Serum calcium
      6. Serum electrolytes
      7. CEA (carcinoembryonic antigen)
   II. Radiology:
      1. Chest X-ray
      2. Three views of the abdomen
      3. Abdominal ultrasound

   III. The diagnostic procedure of choice in this patient is a total colonoscopy to confirm a mass lesion, determine the location of that lesion, and obtain a biopsy of the lesion if possible.

   For colon carcinoma the essentials of diagnosis are as follows:
   I. Right colon:
      A. Unexplained weakness or anemia
      B. Occult blood in feces
      C. Dyspeptic symptoms
      D. Persistent right abdominal discomfort
      E. Palpable abdominal mass
      F. Characteristic X-ray findings
      G. Characteristic colonoscopic findings
   II. Left colon:
      A. Change in bowel habits
      B. Gross blood in stool
      C. Obstructive symptoms
      D. Characteristic X-ray findings
      E. Characteristic colonoscopic or sigmoidoscopic findings
   III. Rectum:
      A. Rectal bleeding
      B. Alteration in bowel habits
      C. Sensation of incomplete evacuation
      D. Intrarectal palpable tumor
      E. Sigmoidoscopic findings

4. A. The definitive surgical treatment of choice in this patient (if feasible) is colonic resection. The "preliminary location" of the lesion based on P/E is in the area of the cecum. If this proves to be correct, then the

colonic resection will involve the removal of the area from the vermiform appendix to the junction of the ascending and transverse colons.

5. A.

6. E. The vast majority of colonic adenocarcinomas evolve from adenomas. Adenomas are definitely a premalignant lesion, and in the large bowel the sequence adenoma—epithelial dysplasias in the adenomas—adenocarcinoma occurs.

Both adenomas and the subsequent evolved adenocarcinomas increase in incidence with age, and the distribution of adenomas and cancer in the bowel is similar. Adenomatous polyps are found in approximately 25% of asymptomatic patients who undergo screening colonoscopy. The prevalence of adenomatous polyps is 30% at age 50 years, 40% age age 60 years, 50% at age 70 years, and 55% at age 80 years. The mean age of patients with adenomas is 55 years, approximately 5-10 years earlier than the mean age for patients with adenocarcinoma of the colon. Approximately 50% of polyps occur in the sigmoid colon or in the rectum, and about 50% of patients with adenomas have more than one adenoma. Fifteen percent have more than two adenomas. There is an interesting correlation between patients with breast cancer and adenomatous polyps in the colon and rectum. Those patients with breast cancer have an increased risk of adenomatous polyps.

The malignant potential of the adenoma also depends (in addition to the growth pattern) on the size of the polyp and the degree of epithelial atypia or dysplasia. Adenocarcinoma of the colon is found in approximately 1% of adenomas under 1.0 cm in diameter, in approximately 10% of adenomas between 1.0 cm and 2.0 cm in diameter, and in approximately 45% of adenomas with a diameter greater than 2.0 cm.

The potential for cancerous transformations rises with increasing degrees of epithelial dysplasia. Sessile lesions are more apt to be malignant than pedunculated ones. The time period that it takes an adenoma to proceed through the process to frank adenocarcinoma is between 10 and 15 years.

In terms of the types of adenomas and their malignant potential, the following represents the most reliable information:

Neoplastic Polyps

1. Villous adenoma — 40% become malignant
2. Tubulovillous adenoma — 22% become malignant
3. Tubular adenoma — 5% become malignant

7. C. A barium enema (preferably an air-contrast barium enema) of an encircling carcinoma of the descending colon presents what is best described as an apple-core lesion. On the barium enema you will note the loss of mucosal patterns, the "hooks" at the margins of the lesion, the relatively short length of the lesion, and the abrupt ending of the lesion.

8. B. Hyperplastic polyps are polyps that are designated as "unclassified" but are totally benign.

9. A. The recommendation of the United States Preventive Services Task Force on screening for colorectal cancer is currently as follows.

Screening for colorectal cancer is recommended for all persons aged 50 or older for annual fecal occult blood testing or periodic (every 2 to every 3 years) flexible sigmoidoscopy or both.

U.S. Preventive Task Force on the Periodic Health Examination. Guide to clinical preventive services. Baltimore: Williams and Wilkins, 1996.

10. B. Carcinoembryonic antigen (CEA) is a glycoprotein found in the cell membranes of a number of tissues, a number of body fluids, and a number of secretions including urine and feces. It is also found in malignancies of the colon and rectum. Since some of the CEA antigen enters the bloodstream, it can be detected by the use of a radioimmunoassay technique of serum.

Elevated CEA is not specifically associated with colorectal cancer; abnormally high levels of CEA are also found in patients with other GI malignancies and non-GI malignancies. CEA levels are elevated in 70% of patients with an adenocarcinoma of the large bowel, but less than 50% of patients with localized disease are CEA-positive. Thus, because of these difficulties with sensitivity and specificity, CEA does not serve as a useful screening procedure, nor is it an accurate diagnostic test for colorectal cancer at a curable stage.

However, preoperative CEA levels correlate with postoperative recurrence rate, and failure of CEA to fall to normal levels after resection implies a poor prognosis. CEA is helpful in detecting recurrence after curative surgical resection; if high CEA levels return to normal after operation and then rise progressively during the follow-up period, recurrence of cancer is likely. CEA just happens to be one of many chemical markers used for cancer detection. Another future possibility is ras-oncogene products in urine or serum.

11. B.

12. E.

13. D.

14. D.

15. C.

16. D.

17. D. This patient has diverticulitis. Diverticulitis is defined as infection and inflammation of one or more diverticula, a condition that in its noninflammatory state is known as diverticulosis. In the United States and Canada, approximately 50% of patients have diverticula, 10% by age 40 and 65% by age 80. The prevalence of diverticula varies tremendously around the world. Cultural factors, especially diet, play a very important etiologic role. Among dietary factors, the most important one is the fiber content of ingested food.

The essentials of diagnosis of diverticulitis are as follows:
1. Acute abdominal pain (usually left lower)
2. Left lower-quadrant tenderness plus/minus a mass in the same area
3. Fever and leukocytosis
4. Characteristic X-ray findings:
   A. Plain films:
      i) If inflammation is localized: ileus, partial colonic obstruction, small bowel obstruction, or left lower-quadrant mass
   B. CT scans: no perforation: effacement of pericolic fat; plus or minus abscess or fistulas
   C. Barium enema: barium enema is contraindicated during an acute attack of diverticulitis. The risk of perforation and barium escape into the peritoneal cavity is very high.

The treatment of choice for diverticulitis is expectant unless surgical treatment is necessary due to rupture and subsequent peritonitis.

Treatment includes the following:
A. NPO
B. IV fluids with potassium
C. Nasogastric suction
D. Intravenous antibiotics (second- or third-generation cephalosporins plus/minus metronidazole)

The most common organisms involved in the development of diverticulitis are *Escherichia coli* and *Bacteroides fragilis*.

E. Analgesics: the analgesic of choice is pentazocine. The reason for this is that morphine and hydromorphone increase colonic pressure, as does codeine. Methadone is not a first-line analgesic in any situation.

The natural history of the disease includes the following:
1. Approximately 10% to 20% of patients with diverticulosis develop diverticulitis.
2. Approximately 75% of complications of diverticular disease develop in patients with no prior colonic symptoms.
3. Approximately 25% of patients hospitalized with acute diverticulitis require surgical treatment; the operative mortality of primary resection has dropped from 25% to 5%.

Finally, the elevation of blood pressure that this patient presents with is almost certainly directly associated with the pain that he is experiencing. Acute and chronic pain (but especially acute pain) increases the release of the "pressor hormones" such as norepinephrine. This produces vasoconstriction that ultimately results in elevated blood pressure. The patient thus experiences a vicious pain cycle that is circular in dimension: more pain—pressor hormone release—elevated blood pressure—increase in pressor hormone release—more pain, and so on.

18. A.

19. E. This patient has internal hemorrhoids. The treatment of choice for the protruding internal hemorrhoids that this patient has is rubber band ligation. Rubber band ligation is especially useful in situations where the hemorrhoids are enlarged or prolapsing.

To accomplish this procedure, the anoscope is used and the redundant mucosa above the hemorrhoid is grasped with forceps and advanced through the barrel of a special ligator. The rubber band is then placed snugly around the mucosa and the hemorrhoidal plexus. Ischemic necrosis occurs over several days, with eventual slough, fibrosis, and fixation of the tissues. One hemorrhoidal complex at a time is treated, with repeat ligations done at 2- and 4-week intervals as needed.

The major complication of this procedure is pain severe enough to require removal of the band. To avoid this, the band must be placed high and well above the junction of the mucocutaneous region. In this location, few sensory fibers exist. If pain begins and does not resolve, infection should be suspected and investigated immediately. At the time the dead tissue falls off there may be significant bleeding; the patient should be aware of this.

20. E. Angiodysplasia is an acquired colonic condition that mainly affects elderly individuals. Pathophysiologically,

angiodysplasia can be described as a focal submucosal vascular ectasis that has a very significant probability of producing significant bleeding.

The vast majority of angiodysplastic lesions occur in the cecum and in the proximal ascending colon. In at least 25% of patients, multiple lesions are present.

The primary symptom is bright red rectal bleeding that can be extensive and that may require the transfusion of two to four units of packed RBCs.

Diagnosis is made by colonoscopy. The diagnosis is made when two of the following three features are present: (1) an early-filling vein (within 4-5 seconds after injection); (2) a vascular tuft; and (3) a delayed-emptying vein. If searched for carefully, as many as 25% of individuals over the age of 60 have angiodysplasia.

In many cases expectant management is all that is needed. If surgery is required, the operative procedure of choice appears to be hemicolectomy.

SOLUTION TO SHORT ANSWER MANAGEMENT PROBLEM 112

Recently there has been increasing interest in dietary therapy to reduce the risk of developing colonic cancer.

The recommendations of the National Cancer Institute include the following:

1. Drink alcohol only in moderation, if at all.
2. Reduce dietary fat from 40% to 30% of total calories.
3. Include whole grains and vegetables high in carotenoids in the diet.
4. Limit ingestion of smoked, pickled, and cured meats.
5. Increase fiber consumption.
6. Increase vitamin C consumption.
7. Limit consumption of nitrates and nitrites.

The recommendations of the American Cancer Society include the following:
1. Avoid obesity.
2. Reduce total fat intake.
3. Eat high-fiber foods, including foods that are rich in vitamins A and C.
4. Include cruciferous vegetables in the diet such as cabbage.
5. Consume alcohol moderately, if at all.
6. Consume only moderate (at most) amounts of salted, smoked, or nitrate-cured foods.

Thus there appears to be almost universal support for the following:
a) Decreasing the amount of fat in the diet, especially saturated fat (this will also lead to decreased BMI or total body weight)
b) Increasing the amount of fiber in the diet
c) Increasing the intake of cruciferous vegetables and fiber
d) Decreasing alcohol intake
e) Decreasing the intake of salted, smoked, and nitrate-based foods

SUMMARY OF THE DIAGNOSIS AND TREATMENT OF COLORECTAL CANCER AND OTHER COLONIC DISORDERS

1. **Colorectal cancer:**
   a) Incidence:
      1. In North America, cancer of the colon and rectum ranks second after cancer of the lung in incidence and death rates. In the United States in 1993 there were 150,000 new cases of colorectal cancer, and 60,000 people died.
   b) Age and sex:
      1. Age: the incidence of carcinoma of the colon increases with age, from 0.39/1000 persons per year at age 50 to 4.5/1000 persons at age 80.
      2. Sex: carcinoma of the colon, particularly the right colon, is more common in women, and carcinoma of the rectum is more common in men.
   c) Genetic predisposition: genetic predisposition to cancer of the large bowel is well recognized in persons with familial adenomatous polyposis.
   d) Risk factors for carcinoma of the colon:
      1. Ulcerative colitis
      2. Crohn's disease
      3. Exposure to radiation
      4. Colorectal polyps
   e) Essentials of diagnosis: see answer to Question 3.
   f) Distribution of cancer of the colon and rectum:
      1. Rectum = 30% of all colorectal cancers
      2. Sigmoid = 20% of all colorectal cancers
      3. Descending colon = 15% of all colorectal cancers
      4. Transverse colon = 10% of all colorectal cancers
      5. Ascending colon = 25% of all colorectal cancers
   g) Pathophysiology: the vast majority of colorectal cancers originate in colonic polyps.
      1. Types of colonic polyps that are premalignant: tubular adenoma > tubulovillous adenoma > villous adenoma
   h) Treatment of colorectal cancer:
      1. Basic treatment:
         i) Cancer of the colon: the basics of treatment consist of wide surgical resection of the lesion and its regional lymphatic drainage after preparation of the bowel.
         ii) Cancer of the rectum: the basics of treatment consist of abdominoperineal resection of the rectum or a low anterior resection of the rectum.
      2. Adjuvant therapy: radiotherapy and combination chemotherapy do have a role to play in lesions diagnosed at an early stage.
2. **Polyps of the colon and rectum:**
   a) Prevalence: adenomatous polyps are found in approximately 25% of asymptomatic adults who undergo screening colonoscopy. The prevalence of adenomatous polyps is 30% at 50 years, 40% at 60 years, 50% at age 70, and 55% at age 80.

b) Malignant potential: adenomas are a premalignant lesion, and most authorities believe that the majority of adenocarcinomas of the large bowel evolve from adenomas (adenoma-to-carcinoma sequence).

The mean age of patients with polyps is 5-10 years younger than the mean age of patients with colorectal cancer.

Benign polyps include hematomas, inflammatory polyps, and hyperplastic polyps.

c) Essentials of diagnosis: the essentials of diagnosis of polyps of the colon and rectum include the passage of blood per rectum and sigmoidoscopic, colonoscopic, or radiological discovery of polyps.

d) Treatment: adenomatous polyps should be removed: methods include electrocautery, Nd:YAG laser therapy, and laparotomy if removal through the colonoscope is unsuccessful.

e) Prevention: high-fiber diet

3. **Diverticulosis and diverticulitis:**

a) Prevalence: approximately 50% of individuals in the United States develop diverticula. Diverticular disease is much more common in the United States than in Japan or other Eastern countries.

b) Symptomatic versus asymptomatic: diverticulosis probably remains asymptomatic in 80% of individuals.

c) Essentials of diagnosis of diverticulitis:
1. Acute abdominal pain
2. Left lower-quadrant tenderness plus/minus a mass
3. Fever and leukocytosis
4. Characteristic radiologic signs showing diverticula

d) Treatment:
1. Conservative:
i) Some patients can be treated at home with oral antibiotics and analgesics.

ii) In-hospital treatment consists of
1) NPO/NG tube/IV fluids
2) Second- or third-generation cephalosporin plus/minus metronidazole
3) Pentazocine for analgesia

The don'ts of diverticulitis:
1) Don't do a barium enema in the acute phase (potential rupture and peritonitis).
2) Don't give morphine, hydromorphone, or codeine as analgesics, as they increase colonic pressure.
3) Organisms associated with diverticulitis:
a) *Escherichia coli*
b) *Bacteroides fragilis*

2. Surgical: surgical treatment is necessitated when there is a diverticula rupture and peritonitis ensues. Approximately 25% of hospitalized patients need surgery.

3. Prevention: high-fiber diet

4. **Other conditions of note:**

a) Internal hemorrhoids with prolapse: treatment: rubber band ligation

b) Angiodysplasia: consider angiodysplasia as a cause of rectal bleeding in elderly patients.

SUGGESTED READINGS

Committee on Diet, Nutrition, and Cancer. National Research Council. Washington, DC: National Academy Press, 1982.

Schrock TR. Large intestine. In: Way LW, ed. Current surgical diagnosis and treatment. 10th Ed. Norwalk, CT: Appleton and Lange, 1994.

PROBLEM 113   A 41-YEAR-OLD FEMALE WITH A NONPAINFUL BREAST LUMP

A 41-year-old female presents to your office after finding a breast lump during a routine self-examination. She has been examining her breasts regularly for the past 5 years; this is the first lump she has found.

On examination, there is a lump located in the right breast. The lump's anatomic location is in the upper outer quadrant. It is approximately 3 cm in diameter and is not fixed to skin or muscle. It has a hard consistency.

There are three axillary nodes present on the right side; each node is approximately 1 cm in diameter. No lymph nodes are present on the left.

SELECT THE ONE BEST ANSWER TO THE FOLLOWING QUESTIONS

1. At this time, what would you do?
   a) tell the patient that she has fibrocystic breast disease; ask her to return in one month—preferably 10 days after the next period for a recheck
   b) tell the patient to see her lawyer and update her will; death is imminent
   c) tell the patient to go home and relax—we generally get too worked up about breast lumps
   d) order an ultrasound of the area
   e) none of the above

2. What is the first diagnostic procedure that should be performed in this patient?
   a) ultrasound of the breast
   b) mammography of the breast
   c) fine-needle biopsy
   d) any of the above
   e) none of the above

3. What is the definitive procedure that should be performed in this patient?
   a) ultrasound of the breast
   b) mammography of the breast
   c) fine-needle biopsy
   d) any of the above
   e) none of the above

4. A 49-year-old female is shown to have a very suspicious lesion on mammography. Clinically, the lesion is a 3-cm mass present in the left upper outer quadrant. No axillary lymph nodes are palpable. You refer her to a surgeon who books her for a surgical procedure. What should be the first surgical procedure?
   a) a lumpectomy
   b) a modified radical mastectomy
   c) a lumpectomy plus axillary lymph node dissection
   d) modified radical mastectomy plus axillary lymph node dissection
   e) none of the above

5. The risk factors for carcinoma of the breast include which of the following?
   a) a first-degree relative with breast cancer
   b) nulliparity
   c) birth of a first child after age 35
   d) early menarche
   e) all of the above

6. Current estimates by the American Cancer Society suggest that one out of every how many women will eventually develop breast cancer?
   a) 1 out of 8
   b) 1 out of 15
   c) 1 out of 25
   d) 1 out of 50
   e) 1 out of 100

7. The U.S. Preventive Services Task Force on the Periodic Health Examination recommends which of the following as the preferred mammographic screening protocol for breast cancer in women?
   a) screen all women over the age of 40 years every year
   b) screen all women over the age of 40 years every 2 years
   c) screen all women over the age of 50 every 1 or 2 years
   d) screen all women over the age of 40 every 1 to 2 years
   e) screen all women between the ages of 35 and 40 with a baseline mammogram and screen all women over the age of 40 every 1 to 2 years

8. Which of the following statements regarding breast-conserving surgery or lumpectomy is(are) correct?
   a) lumpectomy plus breast irradiation is just as effective as modified radical mastectomy for patients with stage I or stage II disease
   b) lumpectomy has not undergone enough testing to predict its efficacy relative to modified radical mastectomy
   c) most American surgeons are following the NIH recommendations concerning lumpectomy
   d) modified radical mastectomy remains the treatment of choice for most women with breast cancer
   e) nobody really knows for sure

9. What is the most common histologic type of breast cancer?
   a) infiltrating ductal carcinoma
   b) medullary carcinoma
   c) invasive lobular carcinoma
   d) noninvasive intraductal carcinoma
   e) papillary ductal carcinoma

Questions 10-16 consist of seven case histories describing seven patients with seven different combinations of breast cancer, ER status, and axillary lymph nodes. Match the numbered case history to the preferred treatment option. Each preferred treatment option may be used once, more than once, or not at all.

Treatment option A: tamoxifen

Treatment option B: adjuvant combination chemotherapy

Treatment option C: neither tamoxifen nor combination chemotherapy

10. A 37-year-old premenopausal woman with an ER- (estrogen receptor) positive breast cancer and positive axillary lymph nodes
    Treatment option: _____

11. A 34-year-old premenopausal women with an ER-positive breast cancer with negative axillary lymph nodes
    Treatment option: _____

12. A 42-year-old premenopausal woman with a 1.5-cm ER-negative breast cancer with negative axillary lymph nodes
    Treatment option: _____

13. A 61-year-old postmenopausal woman with a 3-cm ER-positive breast cancer with positive axillary lymph nodes
    Treatment option: _____

14. A 63-year-old postmenopausal woman with a 2-cm ER-receptor negative breast cancer with positive axillary lymph nodes
    Treatment option: _____

15. A 58-year-old postmenopausal woman with a 2-cm ER-positive breast cancer and negative axillary lymph nodes
    Treatment option: _____

16. A 72-year-old postmenopausal woman with a 3-cm ER-negative breast cancer with negative axillary lymph nodes
    Treatment option: _____

17. Which of the following statements is true regarding breast self-examination?
    a) breast self-examination has been shown to be an effective tool in reducing breast cancer deaths
    b) breast self-examination has not been shown to reduce death rates from breast cancer; it is, however, a reasonable procedure for all women to follow
    c) breast self-examination is no longer recommended as a self-screening procedure for breast cancer
    d) breast self-examination may do more harm than good
    e) breast self-examination is not specifically recommended as a health screening procedure for women; there is, however, not enough evidence to encourage or discourage its use

18. A 42-year-old female presents with bilateral breast masses that are painful and seem to "come and go" depending on the stage of the menstrual cycle. There is significant pain with these masses during menstruation.

    On examination, there are two areas of dense tissue, one in each breast, each approximately 4 cm in diameter. No axillary lymph nodes are palpable.

    What is the most likely diagnosis in this patient?
    a) carcinoma of the breast
    b) mammary dysplasia (fibrocystic disease)
    c) fibroadenoma
    d) Paget's disease of the breast
    e) none of the above

19. If medical treatment is indicated and prescribed for the condition described in Question 18, which of the following should be considered as the therapeutic agent of first choice?
    a) hormone therapy: the oral contraceptive pill
    b) hormone therapy: danazol
    c) a thiazide diuretic
    d) vitamin E
    e) none of the above

20. A 23-year-old female consults her physician because of a breast mass; the mass is mobile, firm, and approximately 1 cm in diameter. It is located in the upper outer quadrant of the right breast. No axillary lymph nodes are present.

    What is the most likely diagnosis?
    a) carcinoma of the breast
    b) mammary dysplasia (fibrocystic disease)
    c) fibroadenoma
    d) Paget's disease of the breast
    e) none of the above

21. What is the treatment of choice for the condition described?
    a) modified radical mastectomy
    b) lumpectomy
    c) excisional biopsy
    d) radical mastectomy
    e) watchful waiting

22. A 33-year-old female presents with a 2-month history of a bloody unilateral left nipple discharge. She has also noted a very small and very soft lump just beneath the areola on the left side.

    On examination, there is a 4-mm soft mass located just inferior to the left areola. No other abnormalities are present in either breast.

    What is the most likely diagnosis?
    a) carcinoma of the breast
    b) fibroadenoma
    c) intraductal papilloma
    d) fibrocystic breast disease
    e) none of the above

Short Answer Management Problem 113

Discuss the recommendations of the U.S. Preventive Services Task Force on (1) breast self-examination, (2) physical examination of the breast, (3) ultrasound of the breast, and (4) mammography.

ANSWERS

1. E.

2. B.

3. E. The most likely diagnosis in this patient is carcinoma of the breast. The most common presenting symptom in breast cancer is a painless lump. Most breast lumps are discovered by patients themselves. Other symptoms that may occur in patients with breast cancer (usually at a more advanced stage) are breast pain, nipple discharge, erosions, retraction, enlargement of the nipple or itching of the nipple, redness, generalized hardness of the breast, and enlargement or shrinking of the breast.

   The first diagnostic procedure that should be performed in this patient is a mammogram. A mammogram will more clearly outline the characteristics of the mass. This, however, must be followed by an open excisional biopsy. This procedure, when properly performed, will yield no false negative results and no false positive results.

   Fine-needle biopsy, although not contraindicated, would certainly not be the procedure of choice in this patient. The rate of false-negative diagnoses with fine-needle aspiration is as high as 10% in some series.

4. E. Excisional biopsy is the surgical procedure of choice in this patient. In addition to making a definitive diagnosis, an excisional biopsy will allow you time to discuss the therapeutic alternative with the patient. The very important decision of lumpectomy versus modified radical mastectomy needs to be made if this is a breast cancer. This is often a difficult decision and requires considerable thought on the part of both patient and doctor as well as information (education) and time.

5. E. Factors associated with an increased risk of breast cancer include the following:
   1. Race: white
   2. Age: older
   3. Family history: breast cancer in mother or sister (especially high risk if breast cancer was bilateral or premenopausal)
   4. Previous medical history:
      a) Endometrial cancer
      b) Some forms of mammary dysplasia
      c) Cancer in the other breast

   5. Menstrual history:
      a) Early menarche (under age 12)
      b) Late menopause (after age 50)
   6. Pregnancy: late first pregnancy (especially after 35)

6. A. Current estimates indicate that among North American women, approximately one woman in eight will, at some time in her life, develop breast cancer.

7. C. Mammographic screening is recommended for all women over the age of 50 on a time interval basis of one mammogram every 1 to 2 years. Mammographic screening can conclude at approximately age 75 unless pathology has been detected in earlier mammograms.

8. A. The National Surgical Adjunctive Breast Project (NSABP) has concluded that segmental mastectomy (lumpectomy) followed by breast irradiation in all patients and adjunctive chemotherapy in women with positive nodes is appropriate therapy and just as effective (that is, no difference in mortality rates) as modified radical mastectomy in patients with stage I and stage II breast cancer with tumors less than 4 cm in diameter.

9. A. The most common histologic type of breast cancer is an infiltrating ductal carcinoma. This type comprises 70%-80% of all breast cancers. The subtypes of infiltrating ductal carcinoma include the following: medullary, colloid (mucinous), tubular, and papillary.

10. B.

11. A.

12. B.

13. A.

14. B.

15. A.

16. B. The current recommendations for the use of tamoxifen and adjuvant combination chemotherapy based on menopausal status (premenopausal-postmenopausal), estrogen receptor status, and axillary lymph node involvement are summarized as follows:
    1) Premenopausal women with positive axillary lymph nodes and either ER-positive or ER-negative tumors

should be treated with adjuvant combination chemotherapy.

2) Premenopausal women with negative axillary lymph nodes whose tumors are ER-positive benefit from tamoxifen; premenopausal women with negative axillary nodes whose tumors are ER-negative should be treated with combination chemotherapy.

3) Postmenopausal women with positive axillary lymph nodes and positive hormone receptors should be treated with tamoxifen.

4) Postmenopausal women with positive axillary lymph nodes whose tumors are ER-negative should be treated with adjuvant combination chemotherapy.

5) Postmenopausal women with negative axillary lymph nodes whose tumors are ER-positive should be treated with tamoxifen; postmenopausal women with negative axillary lymph nodes whose tumors are also ER-negative should be treated with combination chemotherapy.

In addition, the National Institute of Health has issued the following statement concerning women with early-stage breast cancer: "All patients who are candidates for clinical trials should be offered the opportunity to participate in such trials...[and] all node-negative patients who are not candidates for clinical trials should be made aware of the benefits and risks of adjuvant systemic therapy."

17. E. Breast self-examination has been examined by the U.S. Preventive Services Task Force, and the following conclusions were established:
   1. Breast self-examination is not specifically recommended as a screening tool for breast cancer in women.
   2. Although not specifically recommended, there is not enough evidence either to encourage or to discourage its use among women.
   3. There is no reason for women to change what they are currently doing or not doing with respect to breast self-examination and breast cancer.

18. B. This patient almost certainly has fibrocystic breast changes or mammary dysplasia. All breast tissue contains cysts, and thus the term *fibrocystic breast disease,* as the condition was previously called, is confusing and inappropriate. The most common scenario following this label is that a woman with fibrocystic breast changes believes, in fact, that she has a serious breast disease.

Fibrocystic breast changes are most likely hormonal in origin. This may be either an estrogen/progesterone imbalance or a prolactin excess.

The most common presenting symptom of fibrocystic breast change is pain. The pain usually begins 1 week prior to menstruation and is relieved following menstruation. The pain is usually bilateral and is most commonly located in the upper outer quadrants. It may be associated with breast swelling and yellow-green breast discharge.

19. A. In most women, fibrocystic breast changes do not have to be treated. If they do, the most effective treatments are a low-dose oral contraceptive that contains a potent progestational agent (such as Loestrin 1/20) or medroxyprogesterone acetate 5-10 mg/day from days 15-25 of the calendar month.

Danazol may be used to induce a pseudomenopause in patients with severe fibrocystic breast changes. It is expensive, however, and has significant side effects.

Thiazide diuretics are useful in reducing total body fluid volume and edema. In the case of the type of "localized swelling in an enclosed cyst" that is seen in fibrocystic breast change, they are not useful.

Vitamin E has not been shown to be of value in the treatment of fibrocystic breast changes.

20. C.

21. C. This patient has a fibroadenoma, or "breast mouse." Fibroadenomas are the most common type of solid benign breast tumors. They are most prevalent in women under the age of 25 years. They are usually painless, well-circumscribed, completely round, and freely mobile. The classical description with respect to consistency is "rubbery."

The treatment of choice for a suspected fibroadenoma is either a fine-needle biopsy or an excisional biopsy. Although rare, malignancies have occasionally been found in fibroadenomas.

22. C. This patient has an intraductal papilloma. Intraductal papillomas are small, soft, tumors that are found just below the areola. If a patient presents with a bloody nipple discharge associated with a small, soft mass, there is a 95% probability that this is an intraductal papilloma. If P/E reveals no mass, Paget's disease of the nipple, an adenoma of the nipple, or a breast carcinoma with ductal invasion must be considered in the differential diagnosis.

The treatment of choice is surgical removal. This is often facilitated by mammography or a ductogram.

SOLUTION TO SHORT ANSWER MANAGEMENT PROBLEM 113

The recommendations of the U.S. Preventive Services Task Force regarding screening for carcinoma of the breast include the following:

1. Breast self-examination: there is not enough evidence to either include or exclude breast self-examination in the periodic health examination. It should be neither encouraged nor discouraged.

2. Physical examination of the breast: all women over the age of 40 should receive an annual clinical breast examination.
3. Ultrasound of the breast: there is no evidence to suggest that breast ultrasound is a useful screening tool for women in the early detection of cancer of the breast.
4. Mammography: mammography should be performed every 1 to 2 years beginning at age 50 and stopping at age 75. The only exception is a woman in whom previous pathology has been demonstrated.

SUMMARY OF THE DIAGNOSIS AND TREATMENT OF BREAST DISEASE

1. **Fibrocystic breast changes:**
   a) Etiology: hormonal factors
   b) Symptoms: breast pain and fullness premenstrually, with or without discharge
   c) Diagnosis: breast cyst aspiration supplemented by mammography and ultrasound
   d) Treatment: supportive measures; oral contraceptives with low estrogenic activity and potent progestin; medroxyprogesterone acetate
2. **Fibroadenoma:**
   a) Prevalence: most frequent solid benign tumor of breast; painless, well-circumscribed, round, rubbery, freely mobile lesion; common in young women
   b) Treatment: excisional biopsy
3. **Intraductal papilloma:**
   a) Bloody, unilateral nipple discharge with a soft mass
   b) Treatment: surgical removal

4. **Carcinoma of the breast:**
   a) Symptoms: the most common symptom is a painless lump diagnosed by the patient herself.
   b) Treatment: lumpectomy with radiation for stage I or stage II, or modified radical mastectomy; adjuvant combination chemotherapy or tamoxifen for both premenopausal and postmenopausal patients, as outlined in Questions 10-16
   c) Screening: mammography (50-75) every 1 to 2 years; clinical breast examination (> 40) every year; no evidence for breast self-examination

All women between the ages of 50-75 should have a screening mammogram performed every 1 to 2 years. (The screening interval will vary depending on risk factor status.)

NEW INFORMATION—1995

There is renewed interest in examining the recommendation of screening mammography beginning at age 50. There is some recent evidence that suggests that women in the 40-49-year-old age group may benefit from mammography as much as or more than women over age 50. These suggestions need to be replicated, however, before any change to screening protocols can be recommended.

SUGGESTED READING

Giuliano A. Breast. In: Way L, ed. Current surgical diagnosis and treatment. 10th Ed. Norwalk, CT: Lange, 1994.

PROBLEM 114   A 62-YEAR-OLD MALE WITH ABDOMINAL PAIN

A 62-year-old male presents to your office for a "third opinion." He has seen two other physicians during the last 3 months regarding an abdominal pain that is, according to the patient, getting "worse and worse." It is unrelated in any way to food intake except that the patient has become significantly anorexic since developing the pain. The first physician told him that he had irritable bowel syndrome; the second physician told him that the pain was a psychoneurotic pain: "Basically, sir, that means it is all in your head." The patient tells you that he was very disappointed with the two physicians, especially since the first one had been his family doctor for over 15 years.

You decide to spend your time today on a very focused history. The most important information you gather is the following:
1) The patient has lost 20 lb in 3 months.
2) The pain is constant—it never goes away.
3) The patient has never had abdominal pain before.
4) The patient's mood has definitely changed over this period of time—in fact, the very first symptom was depression (even before the pain started).
5) The pain is central abdominal, radiating through to the back, dull/aching in character, and described as a 10/10 in terms of severity.

On examination, the patient looks "unwell." You can't describe it any more clearly than that. However, he just looks unwell. There is no clinical evidence of anemia, jaundice, or cyanosis.

Examination of the abdomen reveals some tenderness in the midabdominal region. The liver edge is felt 2 cm below the left costal margin.

SELECT THE ONE BEST ANSWER TO THE FOLLOWING QUESTIONS

1. The differential diagnosis in this patient would include all except which of the following?
   a) inflammatory bowel disease
   b) carcinoma of the stomach
   c) carcinoma of the pancreas
   d) irritable bowel syndrome
   e) all of the above

2. If you could order only one investigation at this time, which of the following would you order?
   a) an MRI scan of the abdomen
   b) gastroscopy
   c) a CT scan of the abdomen
   d) a colonoscopy
   e) serum amylase or serum lipase

3. Which of the following statements regarding the relationship between this patient's depressive symptoms and his abdominal symptoms is(are) correct?
   a) the abdominal symptoms are unrelated to the depression
   b) the abdominal symptoms are indirectly related to the depression
   c) the abdominal symptoms are directly related to the depression
   d) the abdominal symptoms and the depressive symptoms usually do not coexist in this disorder
   e) nobody really knows for sure

4. The appropriate investigation is ordered. What is the sensitivity of this investigation in the disorder described?
   a) 70%
   b) 80%
   c) 90%
   d) 95%
   e) 100%

5. The patient had planned a holiday for the week after the investigation was performed. He is persuaded to return when he gets back from his vacation in 6 weeks for further evaluation. You encourage him to take his vacation because of your suspicions regarding his disease. Before he leaves for his vacation, however, you must provide the patient with one other treatment. What is the single most important treatment to be undertaken at this time?
   a) begin the patient on an antiinflammatory
   b) begin the patient on an oral corticosteroid
   c) begin the patient on an antidepressant
   d) begin the patient on an oral chemotherapeutic agent
   e) none of the above

6. Cancer pain is an extremely important medical problem. Which of the following statements regarding the management of cancer pain in the United States is true?
   a) cancer pain is extremely well managed by most American physicians
   b) the overtreatment of cancer pain is much more of a problem than the undertreatment of cancer pain in the United States
   c) the undertreatment of cancer pain is much more of a problem than the overtreatment of cancer pain in the United States
   d) most Americans with cancer pain die in very good control; few have cancer pain that is not well controlled
   e) none of the above are true

7. The patient returns to your office in 6 weeks following an overseas tour. Due to your therapy, he was able to enjoy most of his holiday. He is now taking long-acting morphine in a dose of 180 mg twice daily, with breakthrough short-acting morphine totaling 40 mg/day for a grand total of 400 mg/day. Three days ago, his pain began to become acutely worse.

On examination, the patient now appears jaundiced. He has lost another 15 lb, and there is now a palpable mass in the periumbilical region.

The investigation performed earlier is repeated, and a mass measuring 6 cm × 5 cm is now seen in the appropriate region. At this time, what should you do?
a) explore with a surgeon the possibility of a Whipple's procedure
b) begin aggressive radiotherapy and chemotherapy
c) begin high-dose prednisone to increase his weight
d) explore with a surgeon the possibility of the total removal of the organ in question
e) none of the above

8. What is the most clearly established risk factor for the disease described?
a) alcohol consumption
b) cigarette smoking
c) high fat intake
d) environmental toxins
e) previous exposure to radiation

9. With respect to the molecular biology of this disease, which of the following statements is(are) true?
a) no genetic mutations have been established for this disease
b) there is a gene (the Ki-*ras* oncogene) on codon 12 that is present in 25% of patients with this disease
c) the gene is present in 50% of patients with this disease
d) the gene is present in 75% of patients with this disease
e) the gene is present in 90% of patients with this disease

10. A patient with this disease will demonstrate which of the following physical findings?
a) decreased pain when assuming the supine position
b) increased pain when assuming the supine position
c) decreased pain with flexion of the spine
d) increase pain with flexion of the spine
e) b and c
f) a and d

Short Answer Management Problem 114

Discuss the impact of this disease on the American population under the following headings:
a) Disease prevalence over last 30 years (increase or decrease)
b) Place as a killer of Americans (among all cancers)
c) Risk factors
d) Symptoms/signs
e) Treatment(s)
f) Prognosis

ANSWERS

1. D. From the history and the P/E, you determine that the patient has a serious disease. In forming a differential diagnosis, you should consider diagnostic possibilities in the following categories:
A. Infectious/inflammatory
B. Neoplastic
C. Circulatory
D. Traumatic
From the history, the following are diagnostic possibilities:
A. Infectious/inflammatory:
   1. Inflammatory bowel disease:
      i) Crohn's disease
      ii) Ulcerative colitis
      iii) Pancreatitis
      iv) Cholecystitis
B. Neoplastic:
   1. Carcinoma of the stomach (linitis plastica)
   2. Carcinoma of the head of the pancreas
   3. Carcinoma of the colon
C. Circulatory
   1. Aortic aneurysm (leaking)
   2. Mesenteric ischemia
D. Traumatic
   1. Pancreatic pseudocyst

2. C.

3. C. Obviously, before you decide on which investigation to order, you have to make a commitment to your pri-

mary diagnosis. The most likely diagnosis is adenocarcinoma of the pancreas. The reasons are as follows:
A. The abdominal pain is constant and unrelated to food.
B. The patient has experienced a 20-lb weight loss.
C. The patient has a depression: there is a significant correlation between carcinoma of the pancreas and depression.

In many cases, as in this case, the depression actually precedes the abdominal pain.

The investigation of choice is a CT scan of the abdomen.

4. D. The sensitivity of the CT scan in the diagnosis of adenocarcinoma of the pancreas is 95%. That is, only approximately 1 out of every 20 negative CT scan results will be false negatives.

5. E. Although it is very reasonable to start the patient on an antidepressant, it is the second most important treatment. The most important treatment is to start the patient on an adequate pain relief program. It would seem that, because of the severity of the pain, an oral narcotic analgesic such as morphine sulfate would be the drug of first choice. The initial dose should be between 30 mg and 60 mg. It can be increased by the rate of 25% each day until the pain is controlled. A combination of long-acting and short-acting morphine is the preferable combination. You suggest that while he is on vacation he telephone on a regular basis so you can advise medication changes.

6. C. Cancer pain is an enormous medical problem in the United States and Canada. It is likely to become even more of a problem in the future due to the aging of the population. It is estimated that close to 50% of patients in North America with cancer die in moderately severe to severe pain. The reason appears to be multifactorial and related to inadequate education in medical school, residency, and in CME; reluctance to use narcotic analgesics when they need to be used; and fear of licensure difficulties if "too many narcotics" are prescribed.

7. E. You should do the following:
A. Break the news to the patient with his spouse or significant other present, if possible.
B. Go over, with the patient, his treatment options, including palliative radiotherapy, palliative chemotherapy, and palliative radiotherapy and chemotherapy.
C. Suggest an aggressive pain control program. You could:
1. Consider a celiac plexus block
2. Consider changing narcotic analgesics
3. Consider continuing to increase his dose of morphine
D. In terms of symptoms, you should
1. Maintain control of nausea and/or vomiting
2. Maintain control of constipation
3. Consider an appetite stimulant (Megace)

8. B. The most likely established risk factor for adenocarcinoma of the pancreas is cigarette smoking. There is some controversy regarding alcohol intake, but most authorities consider it a significant risk factor.

9. E. There is insufficient evidence to suggest a particular genetic predisposition for adenocarcinoma of the pancreas. However, over 90% of patients who develop adenocarcinoma of the pancreas have a mutation of the Ki-*ras* oncogene on codon 12. This is simply an example of the powerful influence of genetics on cancer and the explosion of new knowledge that will eventually result in more effective, more precise, and more targeted treatments for most or all cancers in the future.

10. E. One of the most important tests in the physical examination of a patient suspected of having a malignancy is known as a provocative maneuver. A provocative maneuver attempts to reproduce the pain (gently). An example of a provocative maneuver for somatic pain due to bony metastatic disease is to put pressure on the bone in question. The provocative maneuver for a patient with a tumor that is retroperitoneal is to have the patient lie flat or lie with a pillow or other object underneath the small of his or her back. This will reproduce the pain. The same patient will obtain relief from their pain when leaning forward.

SOLUTION TO SHORT ANSWER MANAGEMENT PROBLEM 114

Adenocarcinoma of the Pancreas

1. **Prevalence over last 30 years:** the prevalence of adenocarcinoma of the pancreas among Americans during the last 30 years has been rising rapidly. Until recently, the incidence of the disease was increasing in the United States at an annual rate of 15%. It now appears to have leveled off.
2. **Mortality from this disease:** approximately 28,000 new cases of adenocarcinoma of the pancreas occur each year. After squamous cell carcinoma of the lung and adenocarcinoma of the colon, adenocarcinoma of the pancreas is the third leading cause of death due to cancer in men between the ages of 35 and 54.
3. **Risk factors for adenocarcinoma of the pancreas:**
a) Cigarette smoking (number one risk factor)
b) High dietary consumption of fat and meat (especially fried meat)
c) History of gastrectomy (>20 years ago)
d) Alcohol intake
e) African-American race > Caucasian race
f) Diabetes mellitus
High intake of fruits and vegetables appears to have a protective effect.

4. **Signs and symptoms:**
   a) Abdominal symptoms/signs:
      1. Central abdominal pain radiating through to the back; dull, aching and steady in character; most commonly described as a "deep" pain
      2. Weight loss
      3. Hepatomegaly (>50% of patients)
      4. Palpable abdominal mass (indicates inoperability)
      5. A palpable gall bladder. A palpable nontender gall bladder in a jaundiced patient suggests neoplastic obstruction of the common bile duct (Courvoisier's law)
   b) Nonabdominal symptoms/signs: depression due to general medical condition (DSM-IV); the depression is often the initial symptom appearing before any of the abdominal symptoms.
5. **Treatments:**
   a) Surgical: carcinoma of the pancreas is resectable in only 20% of patients (Whipple's procedure).
   b) Chemotherapy/radiotherapy: palliative chemotherapy and/or radiotherapy can be offered.

   c) Pain control: pain control appears to be the single most important part of therapy.
      1. Celiac plexus block
      2. Narcotic analgesics
   d) Symptom control
      1. Nausea and vomiting: control with combination antiemetics.
      2. Constipation: control with lactulose or stool softener plus a peristaltic stimulant.
6. **Prognosis:** the prognosis for adenocarcinoma of the pancreas is dismal. Five-year survival rate is approximately 5%.

SUMMARY OF THE DIAGNOSIS AND TREATMENT OF PANCREATIC CARCINOMA

See the answer to Short Answer Management Problem 114.

SUGGESTED READING

Reber HA, Way L. Pancreas. In: Way L, ed. Current surgical diagnosis and treatment. 10th Ed. Norwalk, CT: Appleton and Lange, 1994.

PROBLEM 115   A 32-YEAR-OLD FEMALE WITH BILATERAL RED EYES, A SORE THROAT, AND A COUGH

A 32-year-old female presents to your office with a 1-week history of bilateral red eyes associated with tearing and crusting, a sore throat with difficulty swallowing, and a cough that was initially nonproductive but has become productive over the last few days.

The patient displays significant fatigue and lethargy and is having great difficulty performing any of her routine daily chores.

The patient, who is a herbologist and natural health practitioner, looks after herself very well, apart from a renal stone that continues to produce symptoms on and off.

On physical examination, there is bilateral conjunctival injection. There is significant pharyngeal erythema but no exudate or membrane. Cervical lymphadenopathy is not present. Examination of the chest reveals a few expiratory crackles bilaterally.

SELECT THE ONE BEST ANSWER TO THE FOLLOWING QUESTIONS

1. What is the most likely cause of this patient's "red eye" condition?
   a) an autoimmune reaction secondary to the beginning of a severe systemic illness
   b) bacterial conjunctivitis related to her other symptoms
   c) bacterial conjunctivitis unrelated to her other symptoms
   d) allergic conjunctivitis secondary to a severe eosinophilic pneumonia
   e) none of the above

2. Concerning this patient's sore throat, and in relation to the case scenario described and the physical findings provided, what would you do?
   a) perform a throat culture and order antibiotics
   b) perform a throat culture and a rapid ELISA strept test and treat with an antibiotic if the ELISA test is positive
   c) perform a throat culture and await the results
   d) order a CBC and total eosinophil count
   e) none of the above

3. What is the most likely (organism/condition) responsible for the constellation of symptoms in this patient?
   a) endotoxin producing staphylococcus
   b) endotoxin producing streptococcus
   c) exotoxin producing staphylococcus
   d) activation of the autoimmune system
   e) none of the above

4. A 17-year-old female presents to your office with a 1-day history of red eye. She describes a sensation of not being able to open her right eye in the morning because of the discharge. The right eye feels uncomfortable, although there is no pain.

   On examination, she has a significant injection of the right conjunctiva. There is a mucopurulent discharge present. No other abnormalities are present on physical examination.

   What is the most likely diagnosis in this patient?
   a) bacterial conjunctivitis
   b) viral conjunctivitis
   c) allergic conjunctivitis

   d) autoimmune conjunctivitis
   e) none of the above

5. What is the most likely etiologic agent causing this patient's red eye problem?
   a) pneumococcus
   b) *Haemophilus influenzae*
   c) *Staphylococcus aureus*
   d) adenovirus
   e) none of the above

6. A 29-year-old male presents to your office with bilateral red eyes. This symptom came on quite suddenly 2 hours ago while visiting a friend's home. He describes itching and a clear discharge from both eyes. The patient mentions one previous episode, and interestingly enough, it also began while visiting the same friend.

   On examination, the conjunctiva are diffusely injected and edematous. On eversion of the eyelids, there are large papillae present.

   What is the most likely diagnosis in this patient?
   a) chemical conjunctivitis
   b) toxic conjunctivitis
   c) allergic conjunctivitis
   d) bacterial conjunctivitis
   e) none of the above

7. A 29-year-old female presents to your office for assessment of a red eye. She describes a tender, painful, and sore right eye that began yesterday. She has had no other symptoms.

   On examination, the patient has a localized area of inflammation and injection in the area of the right conjunctiva. The inflammation appears to lie beneath the conjunctival surface.

   What is the most likely diagnosis in this patient?
   a) localized bacterial conjunctivitis
   b) acute iritis
   c) acute angle closure glaucoma
   d) acute episcleritis
   e) none of the above

8. A 35-year-old female presents with an acutely inflamed and painful left eye. Her symptoms began 2 days ago. There is some visual blurring associated with the symptoms. The patient wears contact lenses.

On examination, there is a diffuse inflammation of the left conjunctiva. On fluorescein staining, there is a dendritic ulcer seen in the center of the cornea.

What is the most likely diagnosis?
a) corneal abrasion
b) herpetic corneal ulcer
c) contact lens stress ulcer
d) adenoviral ulcer
e) foreign body complicated by a viral ulcer

9. A 36-year-old male with ankylosing spondylitis presents to your office for assessment of a painful, red left eye. His red eye is painful and is associated with photophobia.

On examination, the redness is more pronounced around the area of the cornea. His visual acuity in the left eye has decreased to 20/60.

What is the most likely diagnosis in this patient?
a) bacterial conjunctivitis
b) viral conjunctivitis
c) acute iridocyclitis
d) acute episcleritis
e) acute angle closure glaucoma

10. A 61-year-old male presents to your office with a 12-hour history of an extremely painful left red eye. The patient complains that his vision is blurred and he is seeing halos around lights. He states that he has had similar but milder attacks in the past.

On examination, the eye is tender and inflamed. The cornea is hazy and the pupil is semidilated and fixed. On palpation, the left eye is significantly harder than the right.

What is the most likely diagnosis in this patient?
a) bacterial conjunctivitis
b) viral conjunctivitis
c) acute iridocyclitis
d) acute episcleritis
e) acute angle closure glaucoma

11. A 23-year-old female presents to your office with a painful left eye, conjunctival injection, and blurring of vision. The conjunctival injection is primarily circumcorneal.

What is the most likely diagnosis in this patient?
a) acute conjunctivitis
b) acute iritis
c) acute episcleritis
d) acute angle closure glaucoma
e) acute corneal abrasion

12. In the patient described in Question 11, what will the size of the left pupil be (compared to the right pupil)?
a) larger than the right pupil
b) smaller than the right pupil
c) the same size as the right pupil
d) indeterminate
e) nobody really knows for sure

Short Answer Management Problem 115

PART A: Summarize the major causes of a red eye and how they can be distinguished from one another.

PART B: Summarize the treatment of each of the conditions you described in Part A.

ANSWERS

1. E.

2. E.

3. E. This picture is completely consistent with adenovirus infection and a primary viral conjunctivitis. Viral agents, especially adenovirus, produce signs and symptoms of upper respiratory tract infection, with the presence of the red eye being prominent among those symptoms.

With adenovirus there is often associated conjunctival hyperemia, eyelid edema, and a serous or seropurulent discharge. Although viral conjunctivitis is self-limited, there is some debate as to whether or not a topical antibiotic should be used to prevent superinfection. Empirically, it seems reasonable to wait and see what develops; if a purulent discharge develops from the eye, then topical antibiotics should be used. This isn't usually what happens in practice. Most often a topical antibiotic is prescribed.

There is no indication for performing a throat culture or any other test at this time. The only theoretical concern are the "rales" that present in both lung bases; you could argue that if the patient is sick enough a CXR may be indicated.

Of the organisms listed in Question 3, both *Staphylococcus* and *Streptococcus* are frequent causes of superinfection. They are, however, not the primary agents responsible for the symptoms. Whether there are endotoxins produced, exotoxins produced, both endotoxins and exotoxins produced, or no toxins produced is really of no clinical relevance. The bottom line is that the patient is likely going to be treated for the red eye from the beginning, and the topical agent (such as topical sulfacetamide) is going to take care of either organism nicely.

4. A.

5. C. This patient has a primary bacterial conjunctivitis. In contradistinction to viral conjunctivitis, bacterial conjunctivitis will produce a mucopurulent discharge from the beginning. Also, with a primary bacterial conjunctivitis, associated eye discomfort is common. The infection usually begins unilaterally but almost always spreads to the other eye.

   In bacterial conjunctivitis, normal visual acuity is always maintained. There is usually uniform engorgement of all the conjunctival blood vessels. There is no staining of the cornea with fluorescein.

   Bacterial conjunctivitis should be treated with antibiotic drops such as sodium sulfacetamide, chloramphenicol, or garamycin. Initially, the drops may be used every hour or two; within 24 hours this may be decreased to qid.

   The most common organism responsible for bacterial conjunctivitis is *Staphylococcus*. The second most frequent organism is *Streptococcus*.

6. C. The most likely diagnosis in this patient is allergic conjunctivitis. The most common complaint with allergic conjunctivitis is "itchy, red eyes." Both eyes are affected, and there is usually a clear discharge.

   Examination reveals diffusely injected conjunctiva, which may be edematous (chemosis). The discharge is usually clear and stringy.

   The treatment of choice for acute allergic conjunctivitis is either a corticosteroid drop or sodium cromoglycate drops. Because of the risk of steroid-induced cataracts and glaucoma, corticosteroid drops should be used with extreme caution. Sodium cromoglycate drops, on the other hand, may be used without fear of complication. In this case, oral antihistamines may also be of help.

   In this particular scenario, the situation can quickly change to an acute and severe asthma attack. This requires definite management in the ER with epinephrine, IV corticosteroids, and nebulized beta-agonists.

   The culprit, in this case, is most likely to be the friend's cat.

7. D. This patient has episcleritis. Episcleritis and scleritis differ from conjunctivitis in that they usually present as a localized area of inflammation. Although episcleritis and scleritis may occur secondary to autoimmune disease such as rheumatoid arthritis, most cases of episcleritis are idiopathic. Episcleritis is almost always self-limiting; scleritis, on the other hand, may lead to serious complications such as eye perforation.

   The patient with episcleritis usually presents with a sore, red, and tender eye. Although there may be reflex lacrimation, there is usually no discharge. Scleritis is much more painful than episcleritis, and the signs of inflammation are usually more prominent.

   On examination, there is a localized area of inflammation that is tender to touch. The episcleral and scleral blood vessels are larger than the conjunctival blood vessels.

   A patient with episcleritis should probably be referred to an ophthalmologist. The treatment of choice for episcleritis is corticosteroid eye drops. Any other disease should be identified.

8. B. This patient has a dendritic ulcer that is almost always caused by a herpetic infection, although other viral agents, bacterial agents, or fungal agents may also be responsible. These infections may be primary or secondary to excessive contact lens wear, a corneal abrasion, or the use of corticosteroid eye drops.

   The patient with a herpetic dendritic ulcer usually presents with an acutely painful eye associated with conjunctival injection, discharge, and visual blurring. Visual acuity, however, depends on the location and the size of the corneal ulcer. The discharge may be watery (reflex lacrimation) or purulent (bacterial). Conjunctival injection may be generalized or localized depending on the location of the ulcer.

   Treatment consists of specific antiinfective therapy (idoxuridine for herpes simplex ulcers and topical antibiotics for ulcers suspected of being primarily or secondarily infected by bacteria) and cycloplegic drops to relieve pain due to ciliary muscle spasm. Topical corticosteroids are absolutely contraindicated in patients with a dendritic herpetic ulcer.

   In a patient with a dendritic ulcer, referral to an ophthalmologist should be considered.

9. C. This patient has an acute iridocyclitis or anterior uveitis. Patients at risk for anterior uveitis are those patients with a history of a seronegative arthropathy—particularly if they are positive for HLA-B27 (ankylosing spondylitis). Children with seronegative arthritis are also at high risk.

   Symptoms of acute iridocyclitis include a painful red eye, often associated with photophobia and decreased visual acuity.

   On examination, the affected eye is red; the inflammation is particularly prominent over the area of the inflamed ciliary body (circumcorneal). The pupil is small because of spasm of the sphincter or irregular because of adhesions of the iris to the lens (posterior synechiae). Inflammatory cells may be seen on the back of the cornea (keratitic precipitates) or may settle to form a collection of cells in the anterior chamber of the eye (hypopyon).

   Treatment of anterior uveitis should include topical corticosteroids to reduce the inflammation and prevent adhesions within the eye. Mydriatics should be used to paralyze the ciliary body to relieve pain.

   As with episcleritis and dendritic ulcers, a patient with iridocyclitis should be referred to an ophthalmologist.

10. E. This patient has acute angle-closure glaucoma. Acute glaucoma should always be suspected in a patient over the age of 50 years who presents with a painful red eye.

Acute glaucoma usually comes on rapidly. The most common symptom is severe pain in one eye, which may or may not be accompanied by other symptoms such as nausea and vomiting. The patient complains of impaired vision and halos around lights. This is due to edema of the cornea.

On examination, the eye is tender and inflamed. The cornea is hazy and the pupil is semidilated and fixed. Vision is impaired because of edema of the cornea. On palpation, the involved eye often feels significantly harder than the uninvolved eye.

Intraocular pressure must be reduced immediately. Intravenous acetazolamide (Diamox) 500 mg should be given immediately, along with pilocarpine 4% drops to constrict the pupil. This should be followed by either an iridectomy or a laser iridotomy to restore normal aqueous flow. The other eye should be treated prophylactically in a similar way.

11. B.

12. B. This patient has an acute iritis. Acute iritis is characterized by the following. Incidence: common; eye discharge: none; visual acuity: slightly blurred; pain: moderate; conjunctival injection: mainly circumcorneal; cornea: usually clear; pupil size: smaller than non-affected eye; pupillary light response: poor; intraocular pressure: normal; and gram stain and smear: no organisms.

The treatment of acute iritis is a mydriatic to relieve ciliary spasm and a corticosteroid to decrease inflammation. Again, this patient should be referred to an ophthalmologist.

SOLUTION TO SHORT ANSWER MANAGEMENT PROBLEM 115

There are four major conditions that should be considered when a patient presents with a red eye: acute conjunctivitis, acute iritis, acute glaucoma, and corneal trauma or infection. Their differentiation and treatment are as follows:

A. Incidence:
Acute conjunctivitis: extremely common
Acute iritis: common
Acute glaucoma: uncommon
Corneal trauma or infection: common
B. Discharge:
Acute conjunctivitis: moderate to copious
Acute iritis: none
Acute glaucoma: none
Corneal trauma or infection: watery or purulent

C. Vision:
Acute conjunctivitis: no effect on vision
Acute iritis: slightly blurred
Acute glaucoma: markedly blurred
Corneal trauma or infection: usually blurred
D. Pain:
Acute conjunctivitis: none
Acute iritis: moderate
Acute glaucoma: severe
Corneal trauma or infection: moderate to severe
E. Conjunctival injection:
Acute conjunctivitis: diffuse, more toward fornices
Acute iritis: mainly circumcorneal
Acute glaucoma: diffuse
Corneal trauma or infection: diffuse
F. Cornea:
Acute conjunctivitis: clear
Acute iritis: usually clear
Acute glaucoma: steamy
Corneal trauma or infection: change in clarity related to cause
G. Pupil size:
Acute conjunctivitis: normal
Acute iritis: small
Acute glaucoma: moderately dilated and fixed
Corneal trauma or infection: normal
H. Pupillary light response:
Acute conjunctivitis: normal
Acute iritis: poor
Acute glaucoma: none
Corneal trauma or infection: normal
I. Intraocular pressure:
Acute conjunctivitis: normal
Acute iritis: normal
Acute glaucoma: elevated
Corneal trauma or infection: normal
J. Smear:
Acute conjunctivitis: causative organisms
Acute iritis: no organisms
Acute glaucoma: no organisms
Corneal trauma or infection: organisms found only in corneal ulcers due to infection

SUMMARY OF DIAGNOSIS AND TREATMENT OF RED EYE

1. **Conjunctivitis:**
   a) Infectious conjunctivitis:
      1. Adenovirus is the most common cause of conjunctivitis.
      2. Bacterial conjunctivitis: most commonly caused by *Staphylococcus aureus*
      Symptoms:
      i) Discharge: watery discharge with viral infection; mucopurulent discharge with bacterial infection

ii) Other symptoms as described in Short Answer Management Problem

iii) Treatment: sulfacetamide or gentamicin drops

b) Allergic conjunctivitis:

1. Itching and clear discharge are the main symptoms; conjunctiva are diffusely injected and may be associated with swelling (chemosis).

2. Treatment: sodium cromoglycate or corticosteroid drops

2. **Episcleritis/scleritis:**

a) May be bacterial, viral, or fungal in origin or may also be secondary to a corneal abrasion, contact lens wear, and so on.

b) Visual acuity depends on the location and size of the ulcer. Conjunctival injection may be generalized or localized. Fluorescein must be used to stain the cornea.

c) Treatment: cycloplegic eye drops to relieve ciliary muscle spasm. Idoxuridine for dendritic (herpetic) ulcer; antibiotic drops for suspected bacterial infection. Corticosteroid eye drops are absolutely contraindicated in herpetic ulcers.

3. **Iridocyclitis (anterior uveitis):**

a) Often associated with seronegative arthropathy

b) Inflammation of the iris (iritis) and inflammation of the ciliary body (cyclitis) occur together.

c) The inflammation of anterior uveitis is circumcorneal in location, and the pupil is usually small due to associated spasm.

d) Treatment: mydriatic to relieve ciliary spasm; corticosteroid drops to decrease inflammation

4. **Acute angle closure glaucoma:**

a) Acute, unilateral, painful red eye in a patient over the age of 50 years

b) The attack usually comes on quickly, characteristically in the evening.

c) Impaired vision due to corneal edema and halos around lights are common.

d) Palpation reveals a hard eye.

e) Treatment: IV acetazolamide (Diamox) 500 mg, and pilocarpine to constrict the pupil. This should be followed by iridectomy or laser iridotomy.

SUGGESTED READING

Tabbara K. The eye and ocular adnexa. In: Way L, ed. Current surgical diagnosis and treatment. 10th Ed. Norwalk, CT: Appleton and Lange, 1994

PROBLEM 116   A 28-YEAR-OLD MALE WITH CHRONIC LOW BACK PAIN

A 28-year-old male with chronic low back pain presents to your office for renewal of his medication. He was injured at work five years ago while attempting to lift a box of very heavy tools.

Since that time, he has been off work and has not been able to find a job that does not aggravate his back.

On physical examination, the patient demonstrates some vague tenderness in the paravertebral area around L3 to L5. He has some limitations on both flexion and extension.

SELECT THE ONE BEST ANSWER TO THE FOLLOWING QUESTIONS

1. Which of the following statements regarding the epidemiology of acute low back pain is(are) true?
   a) the annual incidence of acute low back pain is 5%
   b) approximately 2% of all workers injure their backs each year
   c) the lifetime prevalence of low back pain is 80%-85%
   d) all of the above are true
   e) none of the above are true

2. Which of the following statements regarding chronic low back pain is(are) true?
   a) chronic low back pain is the most common cause of disability among people younger than 45 years
   b) back injuries account for the majority of claims to compensation boards
   c) in terms of expense to society, low back pain peaks at approximately 40 years of age
   d) all of the above
   e) none of the above

3. Regarding the pathogenesis of chronic low back pain, which of the following statements is(are) true?
   a) in up to 85% of cases of chronic low back pain, a definite anatomical or pathophysiologic diagnosis cannot be made
   b) approximately 10% of patients with acute low back pain will eventually require surgery
   c) patients with acute low back pain and no previous surgical procedures have a 20%-25% chance of recovering after 6 weeks regardless of the treatment employed
   d) the anatomical structures causing low back pain are clearly identified
   e) none of the above statements are true

4. Regarding the pathogenesis of chronic low back pain, which of the following statements is(are) true?
   a) researchers continue to debate whether the pain originates from the spine or from soft tissues
   b) no diagnostic test can definitely distinguish among discogenic, facetogenic, and musculoligamentous pain
   c) ordinary radiographs and CT scans of the lumbar spine have low specificity
   d) all of the above
   e) none of the above

5. Which of the following is the most common cause of low back pain?
   a) metastatic bone disease
   b) inflammatory back pain
   c) lumbosacral sprain or strain
   d) posterior facet strain
   e) none of the above

6. Which of the following is not indicative of inflammatory back pain?
   a) insidious onset
   b) onset before age 40
   c) pain for more than 3 months
   d) morning stiffness
   e) aggravation of pain with activity

7. Which of the following statements regarding the history and physical examination of a patient with low back pain is(are) true?
   a) the positive predictive value of the history in low back pain is high
   b) the positive predictive value of the physical examination in low back pain is high
   c) the positive predictive value of the radiographic investigations for patients with low back pain is high
   d) the positive predictive value of serum blood and chemistry for low back pain is high
   e) none of the above are true

8. Which of the following is(are) characteristic of a history of mechanical low back pain?
   a) relatively acute onset
   b) a history of overuse or a precipitating injury
   c) pain worse during the day
   d) a and b only
   e) all of the above

9. Which of the following is not a danger signal relative to the diagnosis of low back pain?
   a) bowel or bladder dysfunction
   b) impotence
   c) weak ankle plantar flexion
   d) ankle clonus
   e) significant night pain

10. Which of the following statements regarding plain spinal X-rays of patients with low back pain is false?
    a) at least 3 million plain spinal X-ray examinations are ordered annually in the United States
    b) there is little justification for the extensive use of radiography in low back pain
    c) there is a poor relationship between most radiographic abnormalities and symptoms of low back pain
    d) X-rays of the lumbar spine are associated with relatively low doses of gonadal radiation
    e) there is a low yield of findings that alter management from plain X-rays of the lumbar spine

11. Which of the following statements regarding the use of CT scanning in the diagnosis of disk herniations and spinal stenosis is false?
    a) CT and MRI scanning have largely replaced myelography in the diagnosis of disk herniations
    b) the sensitivity of CT scanning for disk herniations is 95%
    c) the specificity of CT scanning for disk herniations is 95%
    d) if CT scanning is to be employed in the diagnosis of disk herniations and/or spinal stenosis, then surgery should be a serious pretest consideration
    e) none of the above statements are false

12. What is the most cost-effective and crucial aspect of the treatment of chronic low back pain?
    a) patient education
    b) physiotherapy
    c) bed rest
    d) muscle relaxants
    e) nonsteroidal antiinflammatory drugs

13. Regarding the use of exercises in the treatment of chronic low back pain, which of the following statements is false?
    a) flexion exercises tend to be more effective than extension exercises
    b) exercises allow patients to participate in their treatment program
    c) any exercise should follow a graduated progression
    d) following the beginning of an exercise program for low back pain, a temporary increase in pain may occur
    e) stretching exercises are recommended in the initial exercise program; isometric strengthening exercises follow

14. Which of the following treatment modalities have been used in the treatment of chronic low back pain?
    a) traction and supports
    b) spinal manipulation
    c) epidural injections
    d) psychological counseling
    e) all of the above

15. Which of the following drugs have been shown to have the best cost/benefit ratio in the treatment of chronic low back pain?
    a) nonsteroidal antiinflammatory drugs
    b) muscle relaxants
    c) narcotic analgesics
    d) tricyclic antidepressants
    e) acetaminophen

16. What is the most common injury cited for personal litigation in the United States?
    a) work-environment-related headaches
    b) "whiplash injury"
    c) chronic low back pain
    d) physical assault injury claims
    e) chronic thoracic back strain

17. "Whiplash injury" pathophysiologically is equated to which of the following?
    a) cervical sprain
    b) cervical strain
    c) cervical facet joint dysfunction
    d) cervical flexion injury
    e) cervical rotation injury

18. The relationship between the physiological time predicted for a whiplash injury to heal and the actual real time required to heal should be 1:1. In whiplash injury, what is that ratio (when considering the totality of cases)?
    a) 1 to 25
    b) 1 to 5
    c) 1 to 1
    d) 5 to 1
    e) 25 to 1

19. Which of the following have been found to prolong whiplash symptoms?
    a) emotional instability or psychological pathology
    b) overtreatment by physicians
    c) previous illnesses, especially psychophysiological illness
    d) litigation
    e) all of the above

20. Which of the following statements about whiplash symptomatology is(are) false?
    a) whiplash injury is an artificial disease
    b) we have allowed the notion that whiplash is a debilitating condition to become part of our unchallenged belief system
    c) by believing that whiplash is a debilitating condition, we frequently manage to make it so
    d) all of the above are false
    e) none of the above are false

Short Answer Management Problem 116

Compensation benefits appear to prolong disability from low back pain. Describe some of the reasons for this phenomenon.

ANSWERS

1. D. The annual incidence of acute low back pain (LBP) is 5%. Approximately 2% of all workers injure their backs each year. The lifetime prevalence of LBP is 80%-85%. Back pain is considered to be one of the most expensive ailments inflicted on advanced industrial societies. Costs are estimated to be at least $16 billion each year in the United States alone. About 80% of these costs are incurred by those 7% to 10% of patients who go on to develop chronic LBP.

2. D. There is increasing concern (and frustration) expressed about the epidemic of LBP disability in Western industrialized countries, where approximately 1% of the population is considered totally disabled as a result of back problems. Back injuries account for the vast majority of Worker's Compensation Board claims and the highest dollar amount paid out to injured workers. Chronic LBP is the most common cause of disability among people younger than the age of 45 years and the third most common cause of disability among people aged 45 to 64 years. In terms of its expense to society, it peaks at about 40 years of age.

3. A. For up to 85% of cases of LBP a definite anatomic or pathophysiologic diagnosis cannot be made. Low back pain has been described as "an illness in search of a disease." Because of diagnostic uncertainty and our very scarce knowledge of treatment efficacy, specific medical therapy is seldom possible. Only 1% of patients with acute LBP will eventually require surgery. Patients with acute LBP and no previous surgical procedure have an 80% to 90% chance of recovering after 6 weeks no matter what treatment is prescribed.

4. D. The anatomic structures causing LBP are not clearly identified. Researchers continue to debate whether the pain originates from the spine (facet joints and disks) or soft tissues (supporting muscles and ligaments). The well-entrenched axiom that pain on flexion originates in the disk and pain on extension in the facet joints is difficult to prove and does not necessarily hold true. In many of these cases, several spinal conditions may coexist.

   No diagnostic test can definitively distinguish among discogenic, facetogenic, and musculoligamentous pain. At this point, physicians tend to focus more on injured musculoligamentous structures as common causes of chronic LBP, not because of improved diagnostic techniques but because of improved understanding of the limitations of interpreting radiographic features. Radiographs and CT scans, the most commonly employed tests, suffer from poor specificity (many false positives).

   Often the debate over musculoligamentous or spinal LBP is resolved with the diagnosis of "mechanical LBP." This does not suggest a pathologic source but does indicate that back pain is aggravated by the effects of activity or sustained postures on already injured but unidentified structures.

5. C. The most common diagnosis in LBP is lumbosacral sprain or strain, or, (as discussed in Question 4) mechanical LBP. Although some experts would argue that these terms are unacceptable diagnostic realities, they do reflect current diagnostic realities. Injury is thought to result from abnormal stress on normal tissues or normal stress on damaged or degenerated tissues.

6. E. Inflammatory back pain (ankylosing spondylitis) is an important subset of chronic LBP, although it accounts for very few cases of acute or chronic LBP. Diagnostic clues to inflammatory low back pain include the following:
   i) Insidious onset of back pain
   ii) Onset before the age of 40 years
   iii) Pain > 3 months in duration
   iv) Morning stiffness (longer than 30 minutes)
   v) Pain relief with activity
   vi) Pain forcing patient from bed
   vii) History of psoriasis, Reiter's disease, or colitis
   viii) Limitation of lumbar spine in sagittal and frontal planes
   ix) Chest inspiratory expansion less than 2 cm
   x) Evidence of sacroiliitis during physical examination
   xi) Evidence of peripheral inflammatory joint disease

7. E. One of the problems with the diagnosis, physical examination, laboratory investigation, and radiographic investigation of chronic LBP is that the sensitivity, specificity, and positive predictive value of the assessments, procedures, and other diagnostic modalities produce false positives and many false negatives. From that follows that the patient ends up with misinformation that may actually "create" disease (anxiety, worry, and increased pain) where none existed before.

8. E. The history of mechanical back pain is typically one of relatively acute onset of pain, often with known precipitating injury or history of overuse. The pain is worse during the day, is relieved by rest (although the pain might worsen with prolonged rest), and also is made worse with activity.

   In contrast, the history of inflammatory back pain classically presents with an insidious onset of pain and stiffness, worse at rest and improved with activity, and often worse at night and in the morning. Many patients need to get up at night to find a comfortable position to partially relieve the pain and stiffness.

9. C. Danger signals in patients with acute or chronic low back pain include the following:
   - i) Bowel or bladder dysfunction
   - ii) Impotence
   - iii) Weak ankle dorsiflexion
   - iv) Color change in extremities
   - v) Considerable night pain
   - vi) Constant and progressive symptoms
   - vii) Fever and chills
   - viii) Weight loss
   - ix) Lymphadenopathy
   - x) Distended abdominal veins
   - xi) Buttock claudication

   Note that the danger signal in terms of ankle movement is weak ankle dorsiflexion, not weak ankle plantar flexion.

10. D. Plain X-rays of the lumbar spine are frequently ordered for LBP; at least 3 million lumbar spine films are ordered annually in the United States. There is, however, little justification for such extensive use of radiography. A much more cost-effective and selective approach should be undertaken.

    Apart from the cost factor, routine radiographs of the lumbar spine have three important drawbacks: a very low yield of findings that alter management in any way, a poor relationship between most radiographic abnormalities and signs and symptoms of LBP, and relatively high (not low) dose of gonadal irradiation. Abnormalities seen on X-ray, particularly changes such as degenerative osteoarthritis, spondylolysis, and congenital abnormalities seen on the radiographs of the lumbarsacral spine are often as common in asymptomatic individuals as they are in symptomatic individuals. As well, many patients who present with chronic LBP have normal X-ray examination results. Most importantly, radiographs rarely alter treatment plans.

    Specific indications for radiographic studies include the following:
    - i) Ruling out an infectious or malignant process
    - ii) Assessing a patient with objective evidence of neurologic abnormalities in the lower extremities, with loss of bowel or bladder control, or with loss of sexual function unexplained by another cause
    - iii) Identifying a compression fracture
    - iv) Identifying sacroiliitis

11. C. CT scanning and MRI have largely replaced myelography and are valuable for diagnosing disk herniations and spinal stenosis. If the test is to influence management, then surgery must be considered a serious option before the test is performed (that is, there should be sciatica potentially due to intraspinal disease, such as suspected disk herniation or spinal stenosis, that is intractable to conservative management. Myelography has a sensitivity of 92% and a specificity of 64% to 87%. The sensitivity of CT for disk herniations is 95% (only 5% are false negatives), while the specificity is between 68% and 88% (12% to 32% false positives). The major potential problem with CT scanning in disk herniations and spinal stenosis is the relatively lower specificity.

12. A. Patient education is the most crucial and cost-effective aspect of the treatment protocol for low back pain. Many patients are very worried that they have a "serious illness" that is causing their pain and are dissatisfied by what they perceive as an inadequate explanation of their symptoms.

    Most patients with mild to moderate LBP do not even consult physicians, and many symptomatic patients are more interested in seeking information and reassurance (the diagnosis and prognosis) than they are in "finding a cure." It is extremely important to reassure patients that "hurt is not equal to harm" in almost all cases. Activity must be limited during the acute stage of the injury to avoid aggravating motions during the healing process. These limitations can be gradually removed over time, except in cases of chronic LBP where certain demanding activities should be continually avoided.

13. A. A cornerstone of treating LBP is physical exercise. Scientific information about the method of action exerted by physical exercise is limited, which reflects the uncertainty regarding the pathophysiology of LBP. Exercises allow patients to participate in the treatment program and as well serve to prevent contractures, deconditioning, and weakness. Contrary to popular belief, exercise programs can safely begin within days of developing LBP or an exacerbation of chronic LBP, even with the persisting muscle spasm.

    The exercise programs that have been developed tend to emphasize repeated flexion and extension exercises and abdominal and lumbar strengthening exercises. Extension exercises appear to be more effective than flexion exercises or traction and are the treatment of choice for disk herniation and radicular pain.

    Any exercise program that is developed and begun should follow a graduated course. Patients need to be warned about a temporary increase in pain; otherwise they will tend to stop the program when it occurs.

Stretching exercises are recommended first, followed by isometric strengthening exercises. One of the most important aspects of any exercise program is regularity.

14. E. Lumbar traction is commonly used in treating LBP, although the use of this modality appears to be declining. With traction, the force required to alter intradiscal pressure while patients are supine is at least 25% of total body weight. Traction less than that is no better (or perhaps worse) than enforced bed rest or placebo.

    Lumbar braces and corsets are designed to restrict movement and hence to prevent further injury. Because they do not, in fact, achieve full immobilization, they are only marginally effective. There are no convincing data to support their use. Biomechanical studies show that braces can cause unpredictable and often increased movements of the lumbar spine.

    Spinal manipulation is a highly controversial treatment for LBP. It has, in spite of its questionable efficacy, enjoyed great popularity. Most health care professionals equate spinal manipulation with chiropractic management. Although spinal manipulation is part of chiropractic management, chiropractors may also employ physical modalities, massage, physical exercises, and education.

    The physiologic basis of manipulation is still unknown. The general consensus on manipulation for acute LBP is that it often provides more rapid pain relief than other modalities, but the final beneficial effect is short-lived, and the outcome remains unchanged. For chronic LBP, manipulation might provide some temporary relief of pain but, again, it does not appear to affect the long-term outcome.

    Recent studies have suggested that chiropractic treatments could, in fact, be superior to conventional treatments. In one British study it was found that sufferers of acute and chronic LBP found chiropractic treatment, of which manipulation is an important part, to be more effective than the physiotherapy provided by the National Health Service.

    Epidural corticosteroid injections deliver corticosteroids to the level of the nerve root and alleviate any nerve root inflammation that is contributing to pain or sciatica. Epidural corticosteroids appear to be useful for cases of nerve root compression as improvement is usually noted within days. With respect to facet joint pathology, epidural corticosteroids appear to be no more effective than placebo.

    Chronic pain and the disability that accompanies chronic pain always have a significant psychological component. The psychological problems certainly add to the complexity of a problem that even under optimal circumstances often proves intractable to medical intervention. At times, patients may exaggerate their symptoms as a plea for help. Individual reactions and clinical responses vary depending on coping skills, the environment, and the culture. In many cases, patients feel absolutely overwhelmed, and they react with anxiety, depression, and desperation. This often results in maladaptive coping mechanisms and strategies. For these reasons supportive psychotherapy and cognitive psychotherapy may have prominent roles to play in the treatment of chronic LBP.

15. D. Pharmacologic treatment is certainly of some value in treating LBP, both acute and chronic. Nonsteroidal antiinflammatory drugs appear to have some value, but the benefit must be weighed against the side effects, particularly gastric side effects and detrimental effects on hepatic and renal function.

    Antidepressant medications, particularly desipramine, nortriptyline, and amitriptyline, often given in subtherapeutic doses are the most commonly used drugs for chronic pain and appear to have the highest benefit/cost ratio. They have both analgesic and antidepressant effects and may also improve sleep.

    Muscle relaxants have shown some efficacy and should be considered.

    Narcotic analgesics should be used with extreme caution and monitored constantly. For chronic pain, it is best to avoid them completely.

16. B. Currently, alleged "whiplash" injury is by far the most common grounds for personal injury litigation in the United States. More than 1 million whiplash injuries occur each year in the United States; whiplash is the cause of much ongoing disability. In one study, 6% of whiplash patients were off work after 1 year, and in another study 9.6% were permanently disabled.

17. B.

18. B. Whiplash injury is physiologically equated to cervical strain, which, like strains in other parts of the body, can be painful. Most strains, however, heal within a few days, weeks, or at most months, with the pain gradually subsiding. However, in spite of normal findings, the symptoms of whiplash frequently do not remit. In the United States and Canada a medicolegal industry has mushroomed around whiplash injury; this situation undoubtedly fosters disability.

    The average actual time to heal for whiplash injuries is approximately five times the normal physiological time to heal would be. Thus, on average, if a normal strain injury would take 3 weeks to heal, the average whiplash strain injury will take 15 weeks to heal (especially if associated with either an MVA or a work accident).

19. E. The delay in recovery of whiplash injury patients is multifactorial. Reasons include the following:
    i) Emotional instability
    ii) Psychologic pathology

iii) Previous illnesses, especially illnesses involving chronic pain

iv) Overtreatment by physicians; failure to recognize that a whiplash injury can be equated to a cervical strain and as such should heal within the average length of time for a strain injury

v) Medical-legal action or litigation: it has been shown in a number of studies that the injury improves when the legal claim is settled

20. E. Whiplash is, indeed, an artificial disease and is so because we have allowed the notion that whiplash is a debilitating condition to become part of our unchallenged belief system. In believing that whiplash is disabling, we frequently manage to make it so. Unfortunately, we as physicians are often at fault; we have often reinforced this idea by helping our patients make this into a truly remarkable chronic disease state not linked in any way to the reality of the physiologic basis of strain injuries and strain injury healing.

SOLUTION TO SHORT ANSWER MANAGEMENT PROBLEM 116

Current compensation schemes often prolong disability from LBP for many reasons. Those reasons are as follows:

A. Patients must convince doctors that injuries are serious enough to deserve compensation.

B. Medical disbelief hardens patients' defensive attitudes and increases the need to prove pain and disability.

C. Compensation represents a personal vindication for patients who blame third parties (that is, employers) for the injury.

D. Patients could perceive that return to work would compromise their safety.

E. Patients sometimes prolong disability to avoid a difficult or boring job or the threat of being laid off or fired.

F. Insecurity about finances results in anxiety and muscle tension that could increase pain.

G. Disability, with compensation, might be a patient's solution to a variety of difficult situations.

SUMMARY OF THE DIAGNOSIS AND TREATMENT OF LOW BACK PAIN AND WHIPLASH INJURIES

1. **Low back pain:**
   a) Incidence: 5%/year. Lifetime prevalence is 80%-85%.
   b) Importance: back pain (especially low back pain) is considered one of the most expensive ailments in advanced industrial societies. Low back pain in industrialized countries can be labeled an epidemic.
   c) History/physical exam: both the history and the physical examination lack both sensitivity and specificity.
   d) Pathophysiology: LBP has been described as "an illness in search of a disease." Specific medical diagnosis and specific medical therapy are seldom possible. It

is very difficult to specifically identify if chronic LBP is muscular, ligamentous/tendinous, facet joint, or discogenic in origin.
   e) Investigations: radiographs and computed tomography scans, the most commonly used tests, are overutilized and suffer from a lack of specificity. Plain spine X-rays in most cases are virtually useless.
   f) Nomenclature: the debate over musculoligamentous or spinal LBP is resolved with the diagnosis of "mechanical" LBP.
   g) Education of patient and prevention: education is the most crucial and cost-effective treatment. This often alleviates the patient's worry that the pain is caused by a "serious illness."
   h) Treatment:
      1. Rest: for cases of acute nonspecific LBP, a short period of rest will decrease time lost from work by up to 40%-50% and reduce the level of discomfort by 60%. This should not extend past 2 or 3 days.
      2. Drugs: In general, pharmacologic treatment is somewhat beneficial in low back pain.
         i) Muscle relaxants are more effective than placebo.
         ii) NSAIDs have some value early in the course.
         iii) Antidepressants are the most commonly used drugs for chronic pain, including chronic LBP.
      3. Physical treatments: heat, ice, hydrotherapy, massage, and deeper thermal modalities are helpful. They function primarily as counterirritants, reducing pain and decreasing muscle spasm.
      4. Exercises: extension exercises appear to be more effective than flexion exercises or traction.
      5. Traction and supports (including lumbar braces and corsets): marginal effectiveness at most
      6. Manipulation: for acute LBP it often provides rapid pain relief, although the final beneficial effect is short-lived and the outcome is unchanged.
      7. Epidural steroids: no evidence of any long-term benefit
      8. Surgery: surgery is the final resort. It is indicated only for disk herniation and spinal stenosis.
         i) Psychologic sequelae, disability, and compensation: these are major problems that are often compounded, rather than helped, by the physician. Always try and determine whether or not an injury is taking longer to heal than it normally should. In other words, is there a significant difference between predicted physiologic healing time and actual healing time? If the answer is yes, do not become part of the problem. Attempt to help the patient understand the problem, and mobilize the patient in an effort to return to a normal lifestyle as soon as possible.
2. **Whiplash injuries:**
   a) Incidence: more than 1 million whiplash injuries/year in the United States

b) Importance: by far the most common grounds for personal injury litigation; as chronic LBP, can be regarded as an epidemic in North America
c) Pathophysiology: essentially a cervical strain; actual healing time to predicted healing time is 5:1.
d) Physician's role: whiplash is essentially an artificial disease. It is a debilitating condition because we have allowed it to become one.

Here is the role of physician stated succinctly: don't reinforce the problem and become part of the problem. Recently, in *The New York Times*, an incident was reported from New Jersey. In this incident, 10 bus accidents were staged and videotaped throughout the state. Typical of one such sting, a bus was deliberately hit from behind by a car traveling less than 10 miles/hr; 17 people who subsequently claimed injury were filmed scrambling onto the bus before the police arrived. Ultimately, each faked bus crash resulted in between $300,000 and $400,000 in fraudulent claims per individual.

SUGGESTED READINGS

Kerr P. Ghost riders are target of an insurance sting. *The New York Times*, Aug. 18, 1993; Sect. A:A1 (col. 3), C:C2 (col. 3).

Malleson A. Chronic whiplash syndrome: Psychosocial epidemic. Canadian Family Physician 1994; 40:1906-1909.

Teasell RW, White K. Clinical approaches to low back pain. Canadian Family Physician 1994; 40:481-495.

PROBLEM 117   A 30-YEAR-OLD MALE WITH FLANK PAIN

A 30-year-old male presents to the ER with acute onset of severe right-side flank pain. The pain radiates down into the groin and testicle and is associated with hematuria, urinary frequency, urgency, and dysuria.

On examination, the patient is in acute distress. He has significant right costovertebral angle (CVA) tenderness. The rest of the abdominal examination is normal. The patient is afebrile.

SELECT THE ONE BEST ANSWER TO THE FOLLOWING QUESTIONS

1. What is the most likely diagnosis in this patient?
   a) renal colic
   b) acute pyelonephritis
   c) acute pyelitis
   d) atypical appendicitis
   e) none of the above

2. What is the most common composition of a kidney stone?
   a) calcium oxalate
   b) mixed calcium oxalate/calcium phosphate
   c) calcium phosphate
   d) struvite
   e) uric acid

3. Which of the following abnormalities is(are) usually associated with calcium oxalate stones?
   a) hypercalciuria
   b) hyperuricuria
   c) hypocitraturia
   d) all of the above
   e) none of the above

4. What is the drug of choice for the management of idiopathic hypercalciuria?
   a) cellulose sodium phosphate
   b) an orthophosphate
   c) potassium citrate
   d) hydrochlorothiazide
   e) pyridoxine

5. What is the most important component of the diagnostic workup in a patient with a kidney stone?
   a) serum calcium/serum uric acid
   b) serum creatinine
   c) intravenous pyelography
   d) 24-hour urine for volume, calcium, uric acid, citrate, oxalate, sodium, creatinine, and pH
   e) serum parathyroid hormone

6. Which of the following statements regarding uric acid stones is(are) correct?
   a) uric acid stones are formed in patients who are found to have an acid urine
   b) uric acid stones are formed in patients with increased uric acid secretion

   c) the initial treatment for patients with uric acid stones is alkalinization of the urine
   d) patients with recalcitrant uric acid stones should be treated with allopurinol
   e) all of the above statements are correct

7. Which of the following statements regarding the treatment of nephrolithiasis is(are) true?
   a) extracorpeal shock wave lithotripsy (ESWL) has become widely used for the treatment of renal stones
   b) ureteral stones, unless large, are best managed by awaiting their spontaneous passage
   c) ESWL has shown its greatest benefit in patients with stones less than 2 cm in diameter
   d) all of the above are true
   e) none of the above are true

8. Which of the following is(are) part of the differential diagnosis of renal colic?
   a) acute pyelonephritis
   b) renal adenocarcinoma
   c) papillary necrosis
   d) all of the above
   e) none of the above

9. What is the treatment of choice for metabolic stone formation?
   a) hydrochlorothiazide
   b) sodium potassium citrate
   c) pyridoxine
   d) an organophosphate
   e) none of the above

10. Magnesium-ammonium phosphate stones are usually secondary to urinary tract infection with which of the following?
    a) *E. coli*
    b) *Proteus* species
    c) *Klebsiella*
    d) *Enterococcus*
    e) *Enterobacter*

Short Answer Management Problem 117

A 45-year-old male presents to the ER with left-sided flank pain. A KUB suggests a ureteric stone. While straining his urine, the patient discovers a stone. The pain subsides. The stone is analyzed and found to be a calcium oxalate stone.

Describe the general treatment measures that you would use to prevent further stone formation.

ANSWERS

1. A. This patient has renal colic. Renal colic is characterized by the sudden onset of severe flank pain radiating toward the groin. It is usually associated with hematuria, urinary frequency, urgency, and dysuria, and is relieved immediately following the passage of the stone.

   Acute pyelonephritis, which may be associated with similar symptoms, is usually accompanied by fever and chills.

   The sudden onset of severe flank pain is not typical of appendiceal disease.

2. A. Calcium oxalate stones are the most common type of renal stones; they constitute 60% of all stones. They are most commonly idiopathic. Other stones in order of frequency are uric acid, mixed calcium oxalate/calcium phosphate, struvite, and cystine.

3. D. Calcium oxalate stones may be associated with hypercalciuria, hyperuricosuria, and hypocitraturia. Hypercalciuria is most common.

4. D. A thiazide diuretic such as hydrochlorothiazide is the agent of choice for the treatment of idiopathic hypercalciuria. Thiazide diuretics work by lowering urine calcium excretion. Other measures include increasing total daily fluid intake and decreasing total daily calcium intake.

5. D. The basic laboratory evaluation of a patient with renal colic includes urinalysis; urine culture; and blood chemistry profile including serum calcium, phosphorus, uric acid, electrolytes, creatinine, KUB, and IVP. The most sensitive test, however, for the diagnosis of metabolic abnormalities associated with nephrolithiasis is the 24-hour urine collection. The 24-hour specimen should be analyzed for calcium, uric acid, citrate, oxalate, sodium, creatinine, and urine pH.

   When stone composition is unknown, urine should also be obtained for qualitative cystine screening. Serum parathyroid hormone assay should be performed when hypercalcemia is present.

6. E. Uric acid stones, the second most common type of renal stone, are formed in patients with a persistently acid urine and/or a very high uric acid secretion (exceeding 1000 mg/day). The initial treatment of a patient with a uric acid stone involves alkalinization of the urine with either sodium bicarbonate or citrate. Patients with uric acid stones should be treated with allopurinol. A decreased purine intake (that is, decreased red meat intake) is also recommended.

7. D. Extracorporeal shock wave lithotripsy (ESWL) is widely used in the treatment of nephrolithiasis. It is based on the use of shock waves to break up renal stones that then spontaneously pass.

   Lithotripsy is most effective when the stone is < 2 cm in diameter.

   For patients with stones larger than 2 cm, a combination of ESWL and percutaneous lithotripsy produces superior results. Initial percutaneous nephrolithotomy followed by ESWL and a "second look" percutaneous nephrolithotomy gives the best results.

   Patients with staghorn calculi, obstruction, or complex anatomy should be treated with open surgery.

   Ureteral stones are best managed by awaiting spontaneous passage. If spontaneous passage is unlikely or delayed, ESWL is the first choice for stones in the upper two-thirds of the ureter; endoscopic surgery is the best alternative for lower ureteral stones.

   A ureteropelvic or other obstruction, as well as stones deposited in diverticuli, should be managed by endourologic techniques.

8. D. The major differential diagnosis of renal colic includes infection of the upper urinary tract (acute pyelonephritis or acute pyelitis), renal adenocarcinoma, and papillary necrosis. Papillary necrosis (ischemic necrosis of the renal papillae or of the entire renal pyramid) is usually secondary to excessive ingestion of analgesics, sickle-cell trait (associated with hematuria), diabetes mellitus, obstruction with infection, or vesicoureteral reflux with infection.

9. B. Metabolic stones including cystine are best treated by giving the patient a sodium-potassium citrate solution, 4-8 mL qid. In this case, the urine pH should be monitored.

10. B. Magnesium-ammonium-phosphate stones are usually secondary to urinary tract infection with bacteria

that produce urease (primarily *Proteus* species). Eradication of the infection will prevent further stone formation. After calculi removal, prevention of stone growth is best accomplished by urinary acidification, long-term use of antibiotics, and the use of acetohydroxamic acid (a urease inhibitor that maintains an acid urinary pH).

SOLUTION TO SHORT ANSWER MANAGEMENT PROBLEM 117

The treatment of calcium oxalate stones includes the following:
1. Reduce dairy products (milk and cheese) in the diet.
2. Reduce calcium in the diet to under 400 mg/day.
3. Restrict dietary sodium to 100 mEq/day.
4. Limit intake of proteins and carbohydrates.
5. Use oral orthophosphates to decrease stone-forming potential.
6. Use thiazide diuretics to decrease urine calcium content.
7. Use allopurinol and urinary alkalinization to reduce the formation of urate crystals.

SUMMARY OF THE DIAGNOSIS AND TREATMENT OF RENAL STONES

1. **Classical symptoms of renal colic:** sudden, severe, flank pain with radiation to the groin; associated with hematuria, frequency, urgency, dysuria, and relief following stone passage
2. **Types of stones:**
   a) Calcium oxalate:
      1. Most frequent type of stone
      2. Usually idiopathic and associated with hypercalciuria, hyperuricuria, and hypocitruria
      3. See the Short Answer Management Problem for details of treatment.
   b) Uric acid:
      1. Second most frequent type of stone
      2. Associated with persistently acid urine and massively increased urinary uric acid secretion (greater than 1000 mg/day)
      3. Prevention with alkalinization of urine with bicarbonate or citrate; allopurinol may have to be used.
   c) Infective stones:
      1. Caused by urea-splitting organisms—*Proteus* species
      2. Stone should be completely removed and antibiotic therapy prescribed.
   d) Cystine stones: occur with the inherited transport disorder cystinuria
3. **Stone treatment:**
   Ureteral stones: await spontaneous passage. If not forthcoming, then use ESWL (upper two-thirds of ureter) and endoscopic techniques (lower one-third of ureter).
   Renal stones: ESWL is the treatment of choice for stones less than 2 cm and located in the upper pole of the kidney. If stones greater than 1 cm are located in the lower pole of the kidney, a combination of ESWL and percutaneous nephrolithotomy is preferred.

SUGGESTED READING

Donovan JF, Williams RD. Urology. In: Way L, ed. Current surgical diagnosis and treatment. 10th Ed. Norwalk, CT: Appleton and Lange, 1994.

PROBLEM 118   A 75-YEAR-OLD MALE WITH NOCTURIA, HESITANCY, AND A SLOW URINARY STREAM

A 75-year-old male presents to your office with a 6-month history of nocturia × 6, hesitancy, a slow urinary stream, and terminal dribbling. The symptoms have been progressing. Otherwise, he is well and has had no significant medical illnesses.

On examination, his abdomen is normal. He has an enlarged prostate gland, which is smooth in contour, is firm, and has no nodules or irregularities.

SELECT THE ONE BEST ANSWER TO THE FOLLOWING QUESTIONS

1. What is the most likely diagnosis in this patient?
   a) benign prostatic hypertrophy
   b) carcinoma of the bladder
   c) prostatic carcinoma
   d) urethral stricture
   e) chronic prostatitis

2. Which of the following symptoms is(are) associated with the condition described in Question 1?
   a) dysuria
   b) daytime frequency
   c) incomplete voiding
   d) urgency
   e) all of the above

3. Which of the following pharmacologic treatments may be indicated in the treatment of the condition described in Question 1?
   a) finasteride
   b) prazosin
   c) terazosin
   d) all of the above
   e) none of the above

4. Prior to the medical or surgical treatment of the condition described, which of the following should be performed?
   a) digital rectal examination
   b) transrectal ultrasound
   c) CT scan of the pelvis
   d) a and b
   e) all of the above

5. Which of the following surgical procedures is the treatment of choice for severe cases of the condition described in Question 1?
   a) transurethral resection of the prostate (TURP)
   b) open prostatectomy
   c) transurethral incision of the prostate
   d) hyperthermia of the prostate
   e) balloon dilatation of the prostate

6. A 58-year-old male presents with a 3-month history of gradually worsening hesitancy of urinary stream, urgency, nocturia, and terminal dribbling. He also complains of lumbar and pelvic bone pain present for the past 3 weeks.

   On P/E the prostate is enlarged and very hard. There is some tenderness over the pelvic ischium on the left side as well as the fourth and fifth lumbar vertebrae.

   Which one of the following statements regarding this patient's condition is false?
   a) the most likely diagnosis is prostatic carcinoma
   b) radiotherapy has no place in the management of this patient
   c) this patient most likely has metastatic disease
   d) the evaluation of this patient should include a bone scan
   e) combination chemotherapy may be indicated for the treatment of this condition

7. Which of the following regarding carcinoma of the prostate is(are) true?
   a) prostatic cancer is a major public health problem in men
   b) prostatic cancer is now the most commonly diagnosed cancer in men
   c) bone is the most common site of metastatic disease
   d) all of the above are true
   e) none of the above are true

8. Which of the following is(are) risk factors for the disease described in the patient in Question 6?
   a) increased age
   b) African-American men
   c) positive family history for the disease
   d) dietary fat intake
   e) all of the above

9. Which of the following statements is true regarding screening for this disorder according to the U.S. Preventive Services Task Force?
   a) there is strong evidence to recommend the inclusion of the digital rectal examination in the periodic health examination
   b) there is fair evidence to recommend the inclusion of the digital rectal examination in the periodic health examination
   c) there is insufficient evidence to recommend for or against the digital rectal examination in the periodic health examination
   d) there is fair evidence to recommend the exclusion of the digital rectal examination from the periodic health examination

e) there is strong evidence to recommend the exclusion of the digital rectal examination from the periodic health examination

10. Which of the following is the treatment of choice for stage A-1 of this disease in an 81-year-old male?
a) radiation therapy
b) radical prostatectomy
c) hormone therapy
d) combination chemotherapy
e) none of the above

11. What is the most common symptom that a male with prostatic cancer presents with?
a) a feeling of "hardness" in the rectal area
b) obstructive voiding symptoms
c) anorexia
d) weight loss
e) bone pain

12. A 24-year-old male presents with a 2-day history of fever, chills, perineal and suprapubic discomfort, dysuria, and inhibited urinary voiding.

On physical examination the lower abdomen is tender. A digital rectal examination reveals a swollen, boggy, and tender prostate. Examination of the urine reveals pus cells and bacterial rods. The man has no history of similar symptoms.

What is the most likely diagnosis in this patient?
a) acute prostatitis
b) acute cystitis
c) chronic prostatitis
d) acute perineal pain syndrome
e) acute nongonococcal urethritis

13. What is the most likely organism responsible for the condition described in Question 12?
a) *E. coli*
b) *Pseudomonas*
c) *Proteus*
d) *Serratia*
e) *Chlamydia trachomatis*

14. What is the pharmacologic agent of choice for the condition described in Question 12?
a) trimethoprim-sulfamethoxazole (TMP-SMX)
b) erythromycin
c) ampicillin
d) tetracycline
e) gentamicin

Short Answer Management Problem 118

Describe the therapeutic mechanism and the therapeutic effects of the drug *finasteride*, recently marketed for the treatment of benign prostatic hypertrophy.

ANSWERS

1. A.

2. E. The most likely diagnosis in this patient is benign prostatic hypertrophy/hyperplasia (BPH). Hyperplasia of the prostate causes increased outflow resistance.

The symptoms of BPH are described as either obstructive or irritative. Obstructive symptoms are attributed to the mechanical obstruction of the prostatic urethra by the hyperplastic tissue and include the following:
a. Hesitancy
b. Weakening of the urinary stream
c. Intermittent urinary stream
d. Feeling of residual urine (incomplete bladder emptying)
e. Urinary retention
f. Postmicturation urinary dribbling

Irritative symptoms are attributed to involuntary contractions of the vesical detrusor muscle (detrusor instability) and are associated with obstruction in approximately 50% of patients with prostatism. These symptoms include nocturia, daytime frequency, urgency, urge incontinence, and dysuria.

Differential diagnosis includes carcinoma of the prostate, neuropathic bladder, chronic prostatitis, and urethral stricture.

3. D. The pharmacologic treatment of BPH is directed toward relaxation of the prostatic smooth muscle fibers through inhibition of alpha-adrenergic receptors, as well as toward regression of the hyperplastic tissue by hormonal suppression.

The growth of BPH depends on the presence of the androgenic hormone testosterone and its derivative dihydrotestosterone (via conversion by the enzyme 5 alpha reductase). The strategy of antiandrogenic therapy in BPH is to interfere with dihydrotestosterone production. Many antiandrogenic drugs have been tried, but at present the most promising is 5-alpha reductase inhibitor *fi-*

nasteride. Finasteride (Proscar) 5 mg/day results in a 20% reduction in prostatic size and a modest improvement of the urinary flow rate and symptom score. It also has a low incidence of adverse effects. Finasteride significantly decreases the prostate PSA level, and detection of cancer of the prostate becomes difficult. Finasteride treatment should be considered in patients with moderate symptoms of prostatism. If the patient improves and side effects are minimal, continuation of therapy under careful urologic control is appropriate.

The tone of prostatic smooth muscle is mediated by the alpha$_1$, adrenoreceptor stimulation through selective or nonselective antagonists relaxing the smooth muscle, resulting in a diminution of urethral resistance, improvement of uroflow, and a significant improvement in symptoms. The results of double-blind, randomized controlled trials have demonstrated the short-term efficacy of selective alpha$_1$ blockade. Selective alpha$_1$-blocking drugs such as terazosin (Hytrin) and prazosin (Minipres) represent an option for patients with moderate symptoms. The long-term efficacy remains to be established.

4. D. The following should be performed prior to any medical or surgical intervention for benign prostatic hypertrophy:
   A. A complete history
   B. A complete physical examination
   C. A digital rectal examination
   D. Ultrasound (transrectal or abdominal)
   E. Determination of post-voiding residual urine
   F. Routine urinalysis and culture
   G. Electrolytes (especially urea and creatinine)
   H. Prostatic specific antigen (PSA)
   I. Cystoscopy

5. A. In general, transurethral resection of the prostate (TURP) remains both safe and efficacious and is the "gold standard" against which all other treatments, both medical and surgical, must be measured. More than 80% of patients experience subjective improvement, and improvement of urinary flow is significant. Approximately 15%, however, report no benefit 1 year after surgery.
   Other surgical treatment options include the following:
   A. Transurethral incision of the prostate
   B. Open surgery
   C. Transurethral laser-induced prostatectomy
   D. Hyperthermia of the prostate
      i) Transrectally
      ii) Transurethrally
   E. Transurethral balloon dilatation of the prostate
   F. Prostatic stents and coils

6. B. This patient most likely has a prostatic carcinoma with osseous bone metastases. Evaluation of this patient should include a PSA level, a bone scan, plain X-rays of the pelvis and lumbar areas, and a CT scan of the pelvis. If these investigations confirm stage D carcinoma of the prostate (pelvic lymph node metastases or distant metastases), the patient should receive hormonal therapy.

Palliative treatment of cancer pain is discussed in another chapter of this book.

7. D. Prostate cancer represents the most common tumor among men in the United States and is certainly a major public health problem; approximately 165,000 new cases were diagnosed in the year 1993, and more than 35,000 patients died that year of their disease. The single most important risk factor for cancer of the prostate is age; the disease prevalence increases almost exponentially after age 50. The true prevalence is unknown, but estimates can be obtained from autopsy series or from a series of patients undergoing TURP. These series suggest that the prevalence of the disease may be as high as 30% in men over the age of 50 and as high as 80% in men over the age of 80. The most common site of prostatic metastases is bone.

8. E. As mentioned above, increasing age is the most important risk factor for carcinoma of the prostate. Other risk factors include African-American race, dietary fat intake, positive family history for carcinoma of the prostate, and possible exposure to certain chemicals (herbicides and pesticides). Certain occupations such as farming and work in the industrial chemical industry may present an especially high risk.

9. C. The U.S. Preventive Services Task Force on the Periodic Health Examination has indicated that "there is insufficient evidence to recommend for or against routine digital rectal examinations as an effective screening test for prostate cancer in asymptomatic men. Transrectal ultrasound and serum tumor markers are not recommended for routine screening in asymptomatic men." This is termed by the U.S. Task Force a *class C recommendation.*

10. E. Multiple treatment options exist for localized prostate cancer. Studies of the natural history of untreated stages A and B disease attest to the slow progression of these lesions with disease-specific survival rates in excess of 85% at 10 years. For this reason, a watch-and-wait policy for older patients and those with significant other comorbid conditions is a reasonable option. For younger patients with a long life expectancy (>10 years), treatment for cure can be accomplished with radical prostatectomy, radiotherapy, or interstitial radiotherapy (brachytherapy).

11. B. The diagnosis of prostate cancer in 1996 is usually a serendipitous finding. Signs and symptoms of the disease are usually encountered only at an advanced stage. These signs and symptoms include anorexia, bone pain, neurologic deficits, obstructive voiding symptoms, and weight loss. Of these, the most common initial presenting symptom is obstruction to voiding.

12. A.

13. A.

14. A. This patient's symptoms are classic for acute bacterial prostatitis. The symptoms include both systemic symptoms (fever, chills) as well as local urinary symptoms such as perineal and suprapubic discomfort, dysuria, and inhibited urinary voiding.

The digital rectal examination that reveals a swollen, tender, and boggy prostate is probably the most sensitive and specific finding. When performing the rectal examination in a patient with systemic symptoms, it is imperative that the prostate gland not be massaged; this may produce a significant bacteria. Only when systemic symptoms are absent can the prostate gland be safely massaged to obtain a prostatic specimen for culture.

The two bacteria responsible for most cases of bacterial prostatitis are *E. coli* and *Klebsiella*. Nonbacterial prostatitis is most often caused by *Chlamydia trachomatis* or *Ureaplasma urealyticum*.

The drugs of choice for the treatment of acute prostatitis are trimethoprim-sulfamethoxazole, norfloxacin, and ciprofloxacin. Antibiotic treatment should continue for at least 4 weeks.

SOLUTION TO SHORT ANSWER MANAGEMENT PROBLEM 118

The medical treatment of benign prostatic hypertrophy has been revolutionized. The growth of BPH depends on the presence of the androgenic hormone testosterone and its derivative dihydrotestosterone (via conversion by the enzyme 5 alpha-reductase). The strategy of antiandrogenic therapy in BPH is to interfere with dihydrotestosterone production.

As mentioned previously, finasteride results in an approximately 20% reduction in prostatic size and a modest improvement of the urinary flow rate and symptom score and has a very low rate of adverse effects. The main adverse effects are a decrease in libido or erectile dysfunction.

Finasteride significantly decreases the serum prostate specific antigen level and thus reduces the ability to screen for carcinoma of the prostate.

The treatment of BPH with finasteride should be considered in patients with moderate symptoms of prostatism. If the patient improves on the drug and does not experience significant side effects, continuation of therapy under careful physician supervision is reasonable.

SUMMARY OF THE DIAGNOSIS AND MANAGEMENT OF BENIGN PROSTATIC HYPERTROPHY (HYPERPLASIA), PROSTATIC CANCER, AND PROSTATITIS

1. **Benign prostatic hyperplasia:**
   Symptoms: both obstructive symptoms (hesitancy, weak stream, intermittent urinary stream, feeling of incomplete emptying, urinary retention, terminal dribbling) and irritative symptoms (nocturia, daytime frequency, urgency, urge incontinence, dysuria)
   Investigations: complete history, PE, urinalysis, culture, transrectal ultrasound, residual urine, electrolytes, BUN, creatinine, serum PSA, cystoscopy
   Treatment: pharmacologic treatment: 5-alpha reductase inhibitor (finasteride), alpha-receptor blocker (prazosin, terazosin); surgical treatment: TURP (transurethral resection of the prostate)

2. **Carcinoma of the prostate:**
   Prevalence: carcinoma of the prostate is now the most common malignancy in men and the second leading cause of death from cancer.
   Symptoms/signs: same as BPH except abnormalities found on examination of the prostate.
   Treatment:
   Stages A and B-1: age < 65: prostatectomy or radiation
   Stages A and B-1: age > 65: watchful waiting
   Stages B and C: radiotherapy
   Stage D: *asymptomatic:* await the onset of symptoms or hormone therapy. *Symptomatic:* hormone therapy (orchidectomy, antiandrogens, LHRH analogues). Combination chemotherapy can be used in hormone-resistant cases.

3. **Prostatitis:**
   a) Acute bacterial prostatitis:
      Symptoms: fever, chills, perineal and suprapubic discomfort, dysuria, and inhibited urinary voiding
      Treatment: septra, norfloxacin, ciprofloxacin
      Organisms: *E. coli/Klebsiella, Chlamydia trachomatis* is thought to be the major cause of nonbacterial prostatitis.
   b) Chronic bacterial prostatitis:
      Symptoms: either asymptomatic or symptoms less prominent than in acute bacterial prostatitis
      Investigation: three-part urine culture (third after prostatic massage)
      Treatment: same drugs as in acute bacterial prostatitis

SUGGESTED READINGS

Anderson R. Prostatitis. In: Rakel R, ed. Conn's current therapy. Philadelphia: WB Saunders, 1994.

Madsen PO, Sparwasser C, Drescher P. Benign prostatic hyperplasia. In: Rakel R, ed. Conn's current therapy. Philadelphia: WB Saunders, 1994.

Thompson I, Teague J. Genitourinary tumors. In: Rakel R, ed. Conn's current therapy. Philadelphia: WB Saunders, 1994.

PROBLEM 119   A 38-YEAR-OLD FEMALE WITH A FEELING OF DIZZINESS AND IMBALANCE

A 38-year-old female presents to your office with a 1-year history of episodic dizziness, ringing in both ears, a feeling of fullness, and hearing loss. The symptoms come on every 1 to 2 weeks and usually last for 12 hours. Nausea and vomiting are present.

When asked to explain the dizziness, the patient says that "the world is spinning around me."

On P/E, the patient has horizontal nystagmus. The slow phase of the nystagmus is to the left and the rapid phase is to the right. Audiograms reveal bilateral sensorineural hearing loss in the low frequencies.

SELECT THE ONE BEST ANSWER TO THE FOLLOWING QUESTIONS

1. What is the most likely diagnosis in this patient?
   a) vestibular neuronitis
   b) acute labyrinthitis
   c) benign positional vertigo
   d) orthostatic hypotension
   e) Meniere's disease

2. The treatment of this disorder includes which of the following:
   a) D/C caffeine
   b) D/C alcohol
   c) a thiazide diuretic
   d) droperidol for nausea and vomiting
   e) all of the above
   f) none of the above

3. A 23-year-old female presents to your office with a 6-month history of dizziness. She "feels dizzy" when she stands up (as if she is going to faint). The sensation disappears within a minute.

   She has a history of major depression. You placed her on doxepin 6 months ago, and she has been much improved since that time.

   The patient's blood pressure is 140/90 mm Hg sitting and drops to 90/70 mm Hg when she stands. There is no ataxia, no nystagmus, and no other symptoms.

   What is the most likely diagnosis?
   a) vestibular neuronitis
   b) acute labyrinthitis
   c) benign positional vertigo
   d) orthostatic hypotension
   e) Meniere's disease

4. What is the best treatment for the patient described?
   a) an antiemetic
   b) education and reassurance
   c) a thiazide diuretic
   d) a change in the antidepressant
   e) b and d

5. A 30-year-old male presents to your office for assessment of "dizziness." The dizziness occurs when he rolls over from the lying position to either the left side or the right side. It also occurs when he is looking up. He describes a sensation of "the world spinning around" him. The episodes usually last for 10-15 seconds. They have been occurring for the past 6 months and occur on average 1-2 times/day.

   What is the most likely diagnosis in this patient?
   a) vestibular neuronitis
   b) acute labyrinthitis
   c) benign positional vertigo
   d) orthostatic hypotension
   e) Meniere's disease

6. What is the treatment of choice for the patient described in Question 5?
   a) avoidance of alcohol and caffeine
   b) dimenhydrinate
   c) a thiazide diuretic
   d) reassurance and simple exercises
   e) endolymphatic surgery

7. A 29-year-old female presents with a 4-day history of "unrelenting dizziness." The dizziness is associated with nausea and vomiting. There has been no hearing loss, no tinnitus, and no sensation of aural fullness. The patient has just recovered from an upper respiratory tract infection.

   On examination, nystagmus is present. The slow phase of the nystagmus is toward the left, the rapid phase of the nystagmus to the right. There is a significant ataxia present.

   What is the most likely diagnosis in this patient?
   a) vestibular neuronitis
   b) acute labyrinthitis
   c) benign positional vertigo
   d) orthostatic hypotension
   e) Meniere's disease

8. What is the treatment of choice for the patient described?
   a) avoidance of alcohol and caffeine
   b) a thiazide diuretic
   c) endolymphatic surgery
   d) reassurance and antiemetics
   e) none of the above

9. A 26-year-old female presents with a 6-day history of severe dizziness associated with ataxia and right-sided

hearing loss. She had an upper respiratory tract infection 1 week ago. At that time her right ear felt plugged.

On examination, there is fluid behind the right eardrum. There is horizontal nystagmus present with the slow component to the right and the quick component to the left. Ataxia is present.

What is the most likely diagnosis in this patient?
a) vestibular neuronitis
b) acute labyrinthitis
c) benign positional vertigo
d) orthostatic hypotension
e) Meniere's disease

10. What is the treatment of choice for the patient described?
a) avoidance of caffeine and alcohol
b) a thiazide diuretic
c) endolymphatic surgery
d) rest, antiemetics, and antibiotics
e) none of the above

11. What is the most common cause of sensorineural hearing loss in the adult population?
a) Meniere's disease
b) chronic otitis media
c) presbycusis
d) otosclerosis
e) mastoiditis

12. What is the most common cause of conductive hearing loss in adults (who have normal-appearing tympanic membranes)?
a) Meniere's disease
b) chronic otitis media
c) presbycusis
d) otosclerosis
e) mastoiditis

13. A 37-year-old female presents to your office for assessment of hearing loss. She has had problems intermittently for the past 12 months.

On examination, the Weber tuning fork test lateralizes to the right ear and the Rinne tuning fork test is negative in the right ear (bone conduction is greater than air conduction: BC > AC).

This suggests which one of the following hearing losses?
a) a right-sided conductive hearing loss
b) a left-sided conductive hearing loss
c) a right-sided sensorineural hearing loss
d) a left-sided sensorineural hearing loss
e) a or d

14. A 43-year-old male presents to your office for assessment of hearing loss. He has had hearing difficulties for the past 4 years.

On examination, the Weber tuning fork test lateralizes to the left ear. The Rinne tuning fork test is positive (air conduction is greater than bone conduction: AC > BC).

This suggests which one of the following hearing losses?
a) a right-sided conductive hearing loss
b) a left-sided conductive hearing loss
c) a right-sided sensorineural hearing loss
d) a left-sided sensorineural hearing loss
e) b or c

15. Which of the following statements is(are) true regarding the condition of acute mastoiditis?
a) it is a complication of acute otitis media
b) it is most likely caused by *Streptococcus pneumoniae*
c) otalgia, aural discharge, and fever are characteristically seen 2 to 3 weeks after an episode of acute suppurative otitis media
d) none of the above are true
e) all of the above are true

16. Which of the following statements concerning sinusitis is(are) true?
a) the most common causes of sinusitis are allergic sinusitis and viral sinusitis
b) rhinovirus is the most common cause of viral sinusitis
c) viral sinusitis is often accompanied by fever, malaise, and systemic symptoms
d) a and b only
e) all of the above

17. Acute bacterial sinusitis is most commonly caused by which of the following organisms?
a) *Streptococcus pneumoniae*
b) *Haemophilus influenzae*
c) *Moraxella catarrhalis*
d) *Streptococcus pyogenes*
e) *Staphylococcus aureus*

18. Which of the following is the most predictive factor distinguishing viral sinusitis and bacterial sinusitis?
a) thick and greenish nasal discharge
b) facial pain
c) degree of fever
d) location of the pain
e) systemic symptoms

19. What is the drug of first choice for acute bacterial sinusitis?
a) amoxicillin (10-day course)
b) Bactrim/Septra (10-day course)
c) cefuroxime (10-day course)
d) augmentin (10-day course)
e) erythromycin (10-day course)

20. Which of the following anatomic forms of acute bacterial sinusitis is most serious?
    a) maxillary sinusitis
    b) ethmoidal sinusitis
    c) frontal sinusitis
    d) mandibular sinusitis
    e) anterior sinusitis

Short Answer Management Problem 119

Describe the long-term complications of chronic otitis media.

ANSWERS

1. E.

2. E. This patient has Meniere's disease. The classical features of Meniere's disease are recurrent episodes of vertigo, fluctuating sensorineural hearing loss, tinnitus (ringing or buzzing in the ears), and aural fullness in the affected ear.

   Meniere's disease is associated with vertigo typically lasting hours, not minutes or days. Low-tone sensorineural hearing loss also occurs. The fluctuating hearing may not be related temporally to the vertigo. In many cases, the tinnitus and fullness become severe just before the vertigo attack begins.

   To make the diagnosis Meniere's disease, the characteristic pattern of vertigo lasting a matter of hours, as well as sensorineural hearing loss, must be present. One additional factor (low-frequency hearing loss, aural fullness, or buzzing tinnitus) should also be present.

   Some patients with Meniere's disease are acutely sensitive to alcohol, caffeine, or both. In these patients, alcohol and caffeine should obviously be avoided.

   Meniere's disease is also known as endolymphatic hydrops. This suggests that a buildup of fluid in the endolymphatic system may be responsible for the development of the acute attack. Thus the use of a mild diuretic such as hydrochlorothiazide is a reasonable treatment (especially for patients that are having frequent attacks).

   The use of an antinauseant such as droperidol IM, chlorpromazine IM, or dimenhydrinate IM or PO may be extremely effective in the treatment of the acute attack.

   Surgery is reserved for patients that do not respond to medical management.

3. D.

4. E. This patient has orthostatic hypotension. This case description illustrates the importance of obtaining an accurate history in the patient who complains of "feeling dizzy." In any patient who has this complaint, it is very important to ask four specific questions:

   1. Can you describe your dizziness?
   2. If you had "a dollar's worth of dizziness," how much would be a sensation of the "world spinning around you," and how much would be a sensation of "things going black in front of you and a feeling that you're about to pass out"?
   3. How long does the feeling of dizziness last: seconds, minutes, or hours?
   4. Are there any other symptoms present when you feel dizzy, such as deafness, ear fullness, or ringing in the ears?

   Orthostatic hypotension is typically initiated after standing up suddenly or, in many cases, is experienced after the patient has been up for a long time, often in closed quarters or crowded shopping malls. The feeling described is that of a subjective dizziness and is closely related to a simple faint or a syncopal episode. It is often accompanied by nausea. It is not associated with any other neurologic sensations or ear symptoms.

   In this case, the orthostatic hypotension is almost certainly associated with the beginning of the tricyclic antidepressant therapy 6 months ago.

   The most important treatment in this patient is to reassure the patient and explain how the symptom can be minimized by slowly assuming the upright position.

   As the orthostatic hypotension developed after the initiation of the tricyclic antidepressant, doxepin, it would be reasonable to switch to an antidepressant with fewer alpha-adrenergic side effects. A good choice would be one of the new selective serotonin reuptake inhibitors (SSRIs) such as sertraline, fluoxetine, or paroxetine.

5. C.

6. D. This patient has benign positional vertigo. Benign positional vertigo is a disorder that consists of brief episodes (lasting anywhere from 2 to 10 seconds) usually caused by either rolling over toward either the right or the left when supine or looking up such as when searching for something on a shelf.

   The etiology of benign positional vertigo is unknown but is thought to be either due to trauma or idiopathic.

The treatment of choice for the patient discussed in Question 5 is reassurance and the prescription of simple exercises. The exercises involve assuming lateral positions, first with the head hanging to the right or the left and then with the head hanging in the other direction, either left or right. The patient is asked to move quickly into position and hold the position until the feeling of dizziness goes away or for 20 seconds (whichever comes first), and then to move quickly and hold that position in the other direction.

Performance of these exercises three of four times in a row (three or four times a day) often provides dramatic relief, but improvement in symptoms sometimes takes up to 10 days to occur.

Even if the exercises are not prescribed, the condition tends to resolve with time (usually several weeks to a few months).

7. A.

8. D. This patient has a left vestibular neuronitis. This disorder is most commonly associated with a viral infection (such as adenovirus) following a respiratory tract infection and involves some portion of the vestibular system, but with total sparing of the cochlea area.

The disorder consists of severe vertigo with associated ataxia and nausea and vomiting. There is no hearing loss, no aural pain, and no other symptoms. Recovery usually takes 1-2 weeks.

The treatment of choice for a patient with vestibular neuronitis is rest, reassurance, and antiemetics. Antiemetics such as droperidol, chlorpromazine, or dimenhydrinate may be given for symptomatic relief of the vertigo. Rest and reassurance are sufficient in most cases.

9. B.

10. D. This patient has acute labyrinthitis. Acute labyrinthitis usually follows an upper respiratory tract infection accompanied by middle ear effusion. The disorder probably represents a chemical irritation of the inner ear from middle ear fluid. The features of acute labyrinthitis include significant sensorineural hearing loss (with a conductive component if a middle ear effusion is present) and severe vertigo that lasts several days.

The treatment of choice for acute labyrinthitis includes rest, antiemetics, and antibiotics. Bacterial labyrinthitis may complicate serous labyrinthitis if antibiotics are not administered. Amoxicillin would be a good first-line agent for antibiotic prophylaxis. If symptoms do not improve, the addition of clavulinic acid to amoxicillin (Clavulin) would be a reasonable second choice.

11. C.

12. D. In adults and children, hearing loss can be divided into sensorineural hearing loss and conductive hearing loss.

The most common cause of sensorineural hearing loss in adults is presbycusis. Presbycusis is a gradual deterioration that begins after the age of 20 years in the highest frequencies and often involves all speech frequencies by the sixth and seventh decades of life. The impaired hearing associated with presbycusis stems from degenerative changes in the hair cells, auditory neurons, and cochlear nuclei. Tinnitus is a common complaint.

Sound amplication with an electrical hearing aid does benefit some patients with relatively good speech discrimination.

The most common cause of conductive hearing loss in adults (who have normal-appearing tympanic membranes) is otosclerosis. Otosclerosis is a localized disease of the otic capsule, producing ankylosis or fixation of the stapes footplate. The resulting conductive hearing loss starts insidiously in the third and fourth decades of life and progressively involves both ears in 80% of individuals. Otosclerosis, an inherited disease, is more common in whites.

13. A.

Facts for Question 13:
A) BC > AC: therefore, this is a conductive hearing loss.
B) Weber test lateralizes to the right ear: in conductive hearing loss, the Weber test lateralizes to the affected ear.
Therefore, this is a unilateral right-sided conductive hearing loss.

14. C. The characterization of hearing loss can be localized by a combination of the Weber test and the Rinne test.

In the Weber test, placement of a 512-Hz tuning fork on the skull in the midline or on the teeth stimulates both cochleas simultaneously. If the patient has a conductive hearing loss in one ear, the sound will be perceived loudest in the affected ear (that is, it will lateralize). When a unilateral sensorineural hearing loss is present, the tone is heard in the unaffected ear.

The Rinne test compares air conduction (AC) with bone conduction (BC). Normally air conduction is greater than bone conduction (AC > BC). Sound stimulation by air in front of the pinna is normally perceived twice as long as sound placed on the mastoid process (AC > BC). With conductive hearing loss, the duration of air conduction is less than bone conduction (BC > AC—that is, negative Rinne test). In the presence of sensorineural hearing loss, the duration of both air conduction and bone conduction are reduced; however, the 2:1 ratio remains the same (AC > BC—that is, a positive Rinne test).

Facts for Question 14:

A) AC > BC: therefore, this is a sensorineural hearing loss.

B) Weber test lateralizes to the left ear: in sensorineural hearing loss the Weber test lateralizes to the unaffected ear. Therefore, the right ear is the affected ear.

Therefore, this is a unilateral right-sided sensorineural hearing loss.

15. E. Acute mastoiditis is a complication of acute otitis media and develops as a result of the retention of pus in the mastoid area. Acute mastoiditis is most commonly caused by the organism *Streptococcus pneumoniae*. *Streptococcus pyogenes* and *Staphylococcal aureus* are other recognized causes.

The inflammatory process in acute mastoiditis results in the destruction of bony septa (almost an osteomyelitis-like process) and as a result there is a coalescence of mastoid air cells. This leads to subsequent erosion of the mastoid process of the petrous temporal bone.

The symptoms of acute mastoiditis include otalgia, aural discharge, and fever. These symptoms usually appear between 2 and 3 weeks after an episode of acute suppurative otitis media. Examination reveals the following: severe mastoid tenderness, lateral displacement of the pinna, and postauricular mastoid swelling secondary to the periosteal abscess. The treatment of choice is ceftriaxone (with or without metronidazole) and surgical drainage (for a subperiosteal abscess).

16. E.

17. A.

18. A.

19. A.

20. C. Diagnosis and treatment of acute sinusitis are as follows:

The most common causes of acute rhinosinusitis are allergic and viral. It is often extremely difficult to distinguish between the two types, although a seasonal sinusitis points to allergic sinusitis, as do symptoms such as itching and redness of the eyes.

Viral rhinitis and sinusitis may be accompanied by systemic systems including fever, chills, facial pain, malaise, and fatigue. The viruses most commonly responsible for viral sinusitis are (in order of frequency) rhinovirus, adenovirus, parainfluenzae, and influenzae.

Bacterial sinusitis can be distinguished from viral sinusitis by the thick, greenish discharge that accompanies the congestion.

The organisms most commonly implicated in bacterial sinusitis include *Streptococcus pneumoniae* (the most common), *Haemophilus influenzae*, *Moraxella catarrhalix*, and *Streptococcus pyogenes*. Other organisms implicated include *Staphylococcus aureus* and anaerobic organisms.

The treatment of choice for acute bacterial sinusitis is a 10-day course of amoxicillin. Second-line antibiotics include Septra/Bactrim (trimethoprim-sulfamethoxazole), cefaclor (Ceclor), cefuroxime (Ceftin), and amoxicillin-clavulinic acid (Augmentin).

The most serious form of acute sinusitis is frontal sinusitis, which manifests as pain, tenderness, and edema of the anterior cortex of the frontal sinus. Acute frontal sinusitis usually necessitates high-dose intravenous antibiotics and decongestants.

Chronic sinusitis is most often associated with *Staphylococcus aureus*, *Haemophilus influenzae*, and anaerobic organisms. In cases of chronic sinusitis not responsive to antibiotics, endoscopic sinus surgery is necessary.

SOLUTION TO SHORT ANSWER MANAGEMENT PROBLEM 119

The long-term complications of chronic otitis media include the following:

1) Seventh nerve paralysis
2) Labyrinthitis
3) Petrositis
4) Intracranial suppuration
5) Cholesteatoma

The major complication of acute otitis media is acute mastoiditis.

SUMMARY OF THE DIAGNOSIS AND TREATMENT OF COMMON ENT PROBLEMS

1. Vertigo:
   a) Meniere's disease:
      1. Symptoms: vertigo (lasting hours), hearing loss, tinnitus, aural fullness
      2. Treatment: avoidance of caffeine, avoidance of alcohol, low-dose hydrochlorothiazide, antiemetics
   b) Acute labyrinthitis:
      1. Symptoms: vertigo (lasting days); associated hearing loss; usually follows an upper respiratory tract infection in which there is a middle ear effusion
      2. Treatment: rest, antiemetics, antibiotics if middle ear fluid infected
   c) Vestibular neuronitis:
      1. Symptoms: vertigo (lasting days), no hearing loss, no ear pain, no other symptoms; may result from upper respiratory tract infection
      2. Treatment: rest, reassurance, antiemetics
   d) Benign positional vertigo:
      1. Symptoms: vertigo (lasting for seconds)—also associated with rolling over toward the left or the

right when supine or when looking up

2. Treatment: reassurance, simple exercises

2. **Orthostatic hypotension:**

a) Symptoms: not true vertigo (rather a sensation of lightheadedness or faintness) on assuming the upright position; often associated with antihypertensive and antidepressant medications

b) Treatment: reassurance, change in medications to one with fewer alpha-blockade properties and fewer orthostatic side effects

3. **Hearing loss:**

a) Sensorineural hearing loss:

1. Pathology: usually a disorder affecting the cochlea and auditory nerves with the perception of a "distorted sound." The deficit is usually greater in the higher frequencies. There are usually degenerative changes in the hair cells, auditory neurons, and cochlear nuclei.

2. Causation: the most common cause is presbycusis, a gradual deterioration that starts with high-frequency loss and often involves all speech frequencies by the sixth and seventh decades.

3. Treatment: a hearing aid may benefit patients with relatively good speech discrimination.

b) Conductive hearing loss:

1. Pathology/causation: the pathology of conductive hearing loss involves either CSOM (chronic serous otitis media) or otosclerosis. Otosclerosis results as a localized disease of the otic capsule where new spongy bone replaces normal bone, producing ankylosis or fixation of the stapes footplate.

2. Treatment: the treatments for the chronic causes of conductive hearing loss are usually surgical.

c) Interpretation of hearing loss:

1. Audiogram

2. Weber test/Rinne test

4. **Sinusitis:**

a) Pathology:

1. Allergic

2. Viral

3. Bacterial

b) Organisms:

1. Rhinovirus is the most common viral cause, followed by adenovirus.

2. *Streptococcus pneumoniae* is most common bacterial cause, followed by *Haemophilus influenzae* and *Moraxella catarrhalis.*

c) Symptoms: fever, chills, malaise, fatigue, facial pain

d) Bacterial sinusitis is distinguished from viral sinusitis mainly by the presence of thick, greenish, nasal discharge.

e) Treatment: amoxicillin (10 days) is the drug of choice for acute bacterial sinusitis.

SUGGESTED READING

Rowe LD. Otolaryngology—head and neck surgery. In: Way L, ed. Current surgical diagnosis and treatment. 10th Ed. Norwalk, CT: Appleton and Lange, 1994.

Geriatric Medicine

PROBLEM 120 A 78-YEAR-OLD FEMALE WITH INCREASING CONFUSION, IMPAIRMENT OF MEMORY, AND INABILITY TO LOOK AFTER HERSELF

A 78-year-old female is brought to the ER by her daughter. She lives alone in an apartment and her daughter is concerned about her ability to carry on living independently. Her daughter tells you that she began having difficulty with her memory 2 years ago, and since that time has deteriorated in a slow, steady manner.

She is, however, not totally incapacitated. She is able to perform some of the activities of daily living, including dressing and bathing. When she cooks for herself, however, she often leaves burners on, and when she drives the car she often gets lost. She has had four motor vehicle accidents in the past 3 months. Her daughter became alarmed when she learned that her mother had gone to the bank and withdrawn the entire contents of her $80,000 savings account to "give to her new boyfriend." She had asked for the entire amount in $1 bills and argued with the bank teller upon learning that this was impossible.

The daughter states that both her memory and her confusion has been getting worse. Her personality has changed; she now displays periods of both agitation and aggression.

On examination, the patient's "mini-mental status" examination course is 8/30. Her blood pressure is 170/95 mm Hg, and her pulse is 84 and irregular. There is a grade II/VI systolic heart murmur heard along the left sternal edge. Examination of the respiratory system is normal. Examination of the abdomen is normal. Digital rectal examination reveals some hard stool. A detailed neurological and musculoskeletal examination cannot be carried out.

SELECT THE ONE BEST ANSWER TO THE FOLLOWING QUESTIONS

1. Based on this history, what is the most likely diagnosis in this patient?
   a) Alzheimer's disease
   b) multiinfarct dementia
   c) major depressive disorder
   d) hypothyroidism
   e) mixed dementia

2. At this time, what would you do?
   a) order an appropriate cost-effective laboratory investigation
   b) arrange for the patient to be admitted to a chronic care facility and placate the daughter
   c) prescribe diazepam for the daughter and haloperidol for the patient
   d) refer the patient for immediate consultation with a geriatrician
   e) begin a trial of a tricyclic antidepressant

3. Which of the following diseases is the most common treatable disease confused with Alzheimer's disease in elderly patients?
   a) hypothyroidism
   b) multiinfarct dementia
   c) congestive heart failure
   d) major depressive disorder
   e) normal pressure hydrocephalus

4. Which of the following statements regarding Alzheimer's disease is(are) true?
   a) Alzheimer's disease is present to some degree in all persons over the age of 80 years
   b) Alzheimer's disease is a rapidly progressive dementia
   c) Alzheimer's disease is easy to differentiate from other dementias
   d) Alzheimer's disease is a pathological diagnosis
   e) Alzheimer's disease usually has a sudden onset

5. In contrast to dementia, patients with depression often
   a) complain about their cognitive deficits
   b) deny that their cognitive deficits exist
   c) try to conceal their cognitive deficits
   d) try to answer questions even if they don't know the answers
   e) perform consistently on tasks of equal difficulty

6. In contrast to dementia, the cognitive impairment associated with depression often
   a) comes on more slowly
   b) comes on more rapidly
   c) is less of an impairment
   d) is not improved with the administration of an antidepressant
   e) none of the above are true

7. Reversible causes of confusion in the elderly is(are)
   a) drug intoxication
   b) hypothyroidism

c) pernicious anemia

d) hyponatremia

e) all of the above

8. A cost-effective workup of a confused elderly patient does not include
   a) a CBC
   b) an electrolyte profile
   c) a plasma glucose level
   d) a CT scan of the head
   e) all of the above investigations are cost-effective

9. After a complete dementia workup you are unsure whether or not a patient has Alzheimer's disease or a major depressive disorder. At this time, what would you do?
   a) reexamine the patient in 3 months
   b) suggest a trial of ECT
   c) arrange for the patient to be admitted to a nursing home and begin supportive psychotherapy
   d) prescribe a trial of a tricyclic antidepressant
   e) none of the above

10. Which of the following is(are) important aspects of dementia management?
    a) maintenance of a daily routine
    b) making the environment safe
    c) assessment of family support
    d) minimization of external stimuli
    e) all of the above

11. Elderly patients frequently develop "acute confusional states." Acute confusional states are also known as which of the following?
    a) dementia
    b) delusional states
    c) delirium
    d) pseudodementia
    e) pseudodelerium

12. Which of the following is(are) associated with acute confusional states in the elderly?
    a) global cognitive impairment
    b) decreased level of consciousness
    c) increased or reduced psychomotor activity
    d) disorganized sleep-wake cycle (REM and non-REM sleep)
    e) all of the above

13. What is the most common cause of dementia in the elderly?
    a) drug-induced dementia
    b) multiinfarct dementia
    c) pseudodementia
    d) Alzheimer's disease
    e) atherosclerotic dementia

14. What is the most common symptom and finding in patients with Alzheimer's disease?
    a) a progressive decline in intellectual function
    b) memory loss
    c) impairment in judgment
    d) impairment in problem solving
    e) impaired orientation

15. What is the percentage of patients with primary Alzheimer's disease who manifest a secondary depression?
    a) 5%
    b) 15%
    c) 25%
    d) 33%
    e) 75%

16. What is the most important risk factor for a patient acquiring Alzheimer's disease?
    a) place of habitation
    b) H/O head injury
    c) H/O thyroid disease
    d) a family history of dementia
    e) H/O psychiatric disease

17. Which of the following characteristics regarding the epidemiology of Alzheimer's disease is(are) true?
    a) the prevalence of Alzheimer's disease at age 65 varies from a low of 971/100,000 persons in Turku, Finland, to 10,300/100,000 persons in East Boston, USA
    b) the incidence of acute Alzheimer's disease increases acutely with age
    c) in the average American city or town, the prevalence of Alzheimer's disease at age 87 years is 50%
    d) there appears to be some cultural and ethnic variation in incidence and prevalence of Alzheimer's disease in the United States
    e) all of the above statements are true

18. What is(are) the histologic criteria for diagnosing Alzheimer's disease post mortem?
    a) senile plaques
    b) neuronal loss
    c) neurofibrillary tangles
    d) a and c
    e) all of the above

19. What is the treatment of choice for Alzheimer's disease at present?
    a) tetraminoacridine (cholinesterase inhibitor)
    b) phosphatidylcholine
    c) pramiracetam
    d) physostigmine
    e) none of the above

20. The main predisposing factors for delirium include which of the following?

a) age > 65 years
b) brain damage
c) chronic cerebral disease
d) b and c only
e) all of the above

21. The best-documented hypothesis for delirium suggests which of the following?
    a) a serotonin deficiency
    b) a norepinephrine deficiency
    c) an acetylcholine deficiency
    d) a dopamine deficiency
    e) a catecholamine imbalance

22. What is the most important investigation for patients suspected for having delirium?
    a) a CT scan of the head
    b) an MRI scan of the head
    c) an EEG
    d) a PET (positron emission tomography) scan
    e) a CBC

23. Which of the following is(are) prodromal symptoms of delirium?
    a) restlessness
    b) anxiety
    c) difficulty thinking coherently
    d) insomnia
    e) all of the above

Short Answer Management Problem 120

PART A: using the Mnemonic DEMENTIA and selecting at least one cause (but in some cases many causes) for each letter, construct a complete differential diagnosis of confusion in the elderly.

PART B: list and briefly describe the distinct disorders that are part of the diagnosis of delirium.

ANSWERS

1. A. The most likely diagnosis is Alzheimer's disease. The slow, insidious course of the decline is much more characteristic of Alzheimer's disease than of any other dementive process.

   Multiinfarct dementia, on the other hand, tends to produce a stepwise decline, with each step (or each decline) being temporally related to a small infarct.

   Major depressive disorder tends to come on rather abruptly. This is discussed in detail in another chapter. Hypothyroidism must always be considered as a reversible cause of dementia; in this case this is unlikely.

   Dementia is characterized by evidence of short-term and long-term memory impairment with impaired abstract thinking, impaired judgment, disturbances of higher cortical thinking, and personality changes.

2. A. Alzheimer's disease is a diagnosis of exclusion. Before a patient is labeled as having Alzheimer's disease, a complete history, a complete physical examination, and a cost-effective laboratory evaluation need to be performed. It is inappropriate to arrange care in a chronic care facility and also inappropriate to treat patients (even with an antidepressant) until a dementia workup has been done.

   The cost-effective workup of dementia includes a complete history, a complete physical examination (including a neuropsychiatric evaluation), a CBC, a blood glucose, serum electrolytes, serum calcium, serum creatinine, and serum TSH. Other tests should be done only if there is a specific indication (example, vitamin B_{12} and folate if macrocytosis is present). A CT scan should be performed only if there is a specific clinical indication.

3. D. The most common treatable disease confused with Alzheimer's disease in elderly patients is depression. It has been estimated that up to 15% of patients who are labeled with Alzheimer's disease actually have major depressive disorder. Many more patients with Alzheimer's disease have depression as a clinical feature of the disease itself.

   Depression, whether the primary diagnosis or a diagnosis secondary to Alzheimer's disease, will respond to pharmacotherapy plus psychotherapy.

4. D. Alzheimer's disease is a pathologic diagnosis.

   The prevalence of Alzheimer's disease increases with age to a prevalence level of approximately 25% in patients over the age of 80 years. It is certainly not present in all patients over any age.

   The clinical progression of Alzheimer's disease is usually slow and insidious, not rapidly progressive.

   It is not easy to differentiate Alzheimer's disease from other conditions or other entities. Because of the slow and insidious onset of the disease, it often goes unnoticed by both friends and family.

5. A.

6. B. In contrast to dementia, the cognitive impairment associated with depression usually comes on rapidly. Also, in contrast to dementia, patients often complain about their cognitive deficits. They know something is wrong. Other features that suggest depression include the following:
   1. A personal or family history of psychiatric illness (especially major depressive disorder, bipolar affective disorder, and alcoholism
   2. Depressive symptoms preceding cognitive changes
   3. Feelings of hopelessness, guilt, and worthlessness
   4. A poor affect on psychologic testing

7. E. Reversible causes of confusion in the elderly can be grouped under the following headings:
   A. Drug intoxication (including alcohol)
   B. Emotional disorders
   C. Metabolic disorders
   D. Sensory disorders
   E. Environmental changes
   F. Neoplasms (benign and malignant)
   G. Trauma
   H. Infectious disorders
   I. Inflammatory disorders
   J. Atherosclerotic disorders
   K. Cardiovascular disorders (not included under item J)
   L. Dementias
   M. Anemias
   N. Endocrine disorders
   In this scheme (which is expanded in the Short Answer Management Problem), the choices offered in the question fall under the following:
   1. Drug intoxication (item A)
   2. Hypothyroidism (item N)
   3. Pernicious anemia (item M)
   4. Hyponatremia (item C)

8. D. See the answer to Question 2.

9. D. As discussed previously,
   A. It can often be difficult to differentiate a dementia from a depression.
   B. A dementia may have, as part of its symptomatology, depressive symptoms.
   C. Depression is reversible; dementia is not.
   Thus a cautious trial of an antidepressant can be both a diagnostic test and a therapeutic trial.
   In elderly patients, tricyclic antidepressants are still the antidepressants of choice; they have not been overtaken by the SSRIs. In an elderly patient, you want to do the following:
   1. Maximize the benefit from the antidepressant without producing an adverse drug reaction.
   2. Start low and go slow.
   3. Select an agent that has low anticholinergic, alpha-adrenergic, and antihistaminic side effects.

The tricyclic antidepressant of choice in elderly patients is nortriptyline. The starting dosage in an elderly patient should be 10 mg.

10. E. The management of dementia in the elderly involves both behavioral methods and pharmacologic methods.
    Regarding behavioral management, the following four principles apply to all elderly patients with a dementia-like syndrome:
    A. External stimuli (especially external stimuli that may confuse, worry, or upset the elder) should be kept to a minimum.
    B. A daily routine that does not vary by any significant degree should be established and maintained.
    C. The environmental safety of the particular residence or facility should be maximized. This will include attention to the maximization of lighting in the home or facility; the minimization of significant noise or distractions; the installation of hand rails in hallways and rooms and at bathtub edges; and the minimization of stairs in the living accommodations of the patient.
    D. Support the elder's family and offer respite care where and when needed.

11. C.

12. E. Delirium, which is also known as an acute confusional state, represents one of the most common mental disorders seen in the institutionalized elder. Despite its frequency and association with many diseases/disorders, it is frequently misdiagnosed or not diagnosed at all. A uniform definition and terminology follows:
    Delirium is defined as an organic mental syndrome featuring the following diagnostic features:
    A. Global cognitive impairment
    B. Disturbances in attention and attention span
    C. Reduced level of consciousness
    D. Increased or decreased psychomotor activity
    E. Disorganized sleep-wake cycles
    The onset of delirium is acute (a matter of hours or a few days at the very most) and seldom exceeds 1 month.
    The severity of symptoms of delirium fluctuates unpredictably over the course of a day and seem to be most marked during a sleepless night. Delirium can occur at any age, but is most common in those individuals over the age of 65 years.

13. D. The most common cause of dementia in the elderly is Alzheimer's disease.
    The wording is very important in this question. Drugs do not cause dementia; they cause delirium. The only other cause of dementia listed in the ques-

tion is multiinfarct dementia, a term equivalent to atherosclerotic dementia. The latter term is not commonly used.

The other choice in the question, pseudodementia, is really a misnomer. Pseudodementia really represents depression that has been incorrectly diagnosed as an irreversible dementia.

14. B. Memory loss is the most common presenting feature of Alzheimer's disease, but a personality change or an impairment in the ability to perform intellectual tasks such as calculations may herald the onset.

The five major clinical manifestations of Alzheimer's disease are as follows:

1. Memory loss: initially the memory loss is a loss for recent events only and is associated with an inability to learn new information. Recall of past events and previously acquired information becomes impaired at a somewhat later stage. Memory loss is the most common presenting feature of Alzheimer's disease.

2. Language impairment: language impairment is also very common among Alzheimer's patients. The term *anomia,* or "word-finding difficulty," often begins with the onset of dementia. This feature usually progresses to a transcortical, sensory-like aphasia.

Severe language disturbance is a poor prognostic feature of Alzheimer's disease.

3. Visuospatial disturbance: patients with Alzheimer's disease are often characterized by a difficulty in getting around the neighborhood or house. Practical examples of visuospatial disturbances in Alzheimer's patients include difficulty following directions and getting lost in a familiar place or in familiar surroundings.

4. Loss of interest in activities: the loss of interest in activities such as personal habits or community affairs parallels the intellectual decline already discussed. This may be Alzheimer's disease first and an accompanying depression second or a primary depression manifesting itself as Alzheimer's disease.

5. Delusions and hallucinations: delusions and hallucinations are prevalent in patients with Alzheimer's disease and tend to indicate a poor prognosis.

15. D. Thirty-three percent of patients who develop Alzheimer's disease develop a depressive illness secondary to the Alzheimer's disease.

16. D. The five most important risk factors for Alzheimer's disease are as follows:

1. A family history of dementia (especially Alzheimer's type dementia in a sibling)
2. Down syndrome (trisomy 21)
3. Maternal age
4. Personal history of a head injury
5. Personal history of thyroid disease

Apart from item 1 (a history of Alzheimer's disease in a first-degree relative), little is known about the etiology of the disorder.

17. E. The epidemiology of Alzheimer's disease is fascinating.

Because the cumulative incidence of Alzheimer's disease increases rapidly, the prevalence at age 87 in the United States averages 50% of the population (this figure includes both institutionalized elderly and community-based elderly). There is obviously a significant difference depending on the individual's capacity to look after himself or herself, but this really becomes a circular argument.

One excellent review of the literature indicates a very significant difference in prevalence depending on geographic location. For example, Turku, Finland, has a prevalence of only 971/100,000 population. East Boston has an estimated prevalence of 10,300/100,000 population. This is extremely difficult to explain, and one wonders whether or not there was a very significant difference in diagnostic criteria and/or a very significant difference in case assessment criteria.

Although details are sketchy, there also appears to be some significant differences depending on the cultural environment and the ethnic background. For a number of reasons, it is best to leave the discussion at that.

18. D. The diagnostic criteria for Alzheimer's disease proposed by the National Institute on Aging (as discussed earlier, Alzheimer's disease really is a pathological diagnosis) are as follows:

A. The quantity of senile plaques (age-specific): senile plaques are microscopic lesions composed of a significant percentage of amyloid.

B. The quantity of neurofibrillary tangles (age-specific): neurofibrillary tangles (NFTs), initially described in 1907, are neuronal cytoplasmic collections of tangled filaments present in abundance in the neocortex, hippocampus, amygdala, basal forebrain, substantia nigra, ocus ceruleus, and other brainstem nuclei.

Although A and B are the two diagnostic criteria on which the diagnosis of Alzheimer's disease is based, the following is a complete list of all of the microscopic lesions seen in the brain of a patient with Alzheimer's disease:

1. Neuritic plaques
2. Neurofibrillary tangles (NFTs)
3. Amyloid degeneration
4. Neuronal loss

Most patients with Alzheimer's disease have a slight reduction in total brain weight, with the majority ranging from 900 to 1100 g. Mild to moderate cerebral atrophy is often present.

19. E. A number of experimental therapies have been tried for the expressed purpose of restoring neurotransmitter imbalances that may be associated with Alzheimer's disease. The classes of agents that have been tried have included the following:
    A. Loading patients with the precursors necessary to increase acetylcholine synthesis in the brain
    B. Providing a cholinesterase inhibitor to decrease the breakdown of acetylcholine
    C. To enhance the survival and function of neurons that are prone to degeneration by providing acetyl levocarnitine hydrochloride (an agent that stimulates natural scavenger functions to reduce oxidized free radicals). So-called neurotrophic factors (proteins that have a role in neuronal growth and survival) have been the focus of increasing attention. The first and best-characterized of these trophic factors is nerve growth factor (NGF).

    Thus the management of Alzheimer's disease remains symptomatic. Some of the useful therapies that have proven their benefit include the following:
    1. Low-dose neuroleptic agents to reduce hallucinations and delusions
    2. Low-dose benzodiazepines to reduce anxiety, insomnia, and especially agitation
    3. Tricyclic antidepressants and MAO inhibitors to treat coexisting depression

20. E. Delirium (acute confusional state) is caused by one or more organic factors that bring about widespread cerebral dysfunction. The factors associated with delirium can be divided into the following subcategories:
    I. Predisposing factors
    II. Facilitating factors
    III. Precipitating (organic) causal factors

    I. Predisposing factors: the predisposing factors for delirium in the elderly are as follows:
       A. Age greater than 65 years
       B. Brain damage
       C. Chronic cerebral disease (such as Alzheimer's disease)

    II. Facilitating factors: the facilitating factors for delirium in the elderly are as follows:
       A. Psychological stress
       B. Sleep loss or sleep deprivation
       C. Sensory deprivation or sensory overload

    III. Precipitating (organic) causal factors:
       A. Primary cerebral diseases
       B. Systemic diseases affecting the brain secondarily
          1. Metabolic encephalopathies
          2. Neoplasms
          3. Infections
       4. Cardiovascular diseases
       5. Collagen vascular diseases
       C. Intoxication with exogenous substances
          1. Medical drugs
          2. Recreational drugs
          3. Poisons of plant, animal, and industrial origin
       D. Withdrawal from substances of abuse
          1. Alcohol
          2. Sedative-hypnotic drugs

    One of the most common causes of delirium in the elderly is intoxication with anticholinergic drugs, such as tricyclic antidepressants given in doses that would be appropriate for a younger adult but not for a frail elderly patient.

    Other common causes are as follows:
    1. Congestive cardiac failure
    2. Pneumonia
    3. Urinary tract infection
    4. Cancer
    5. Uremia
    6. Hypokalemia
    7. Dehydration
    8. Hyponatremia
    9. Epilepsy
    10. Cerebral infarction (right hemisphere)

    Risk factors for delirium in hospitalized elderly patients include the following:
    1. Urinary tract infections
    2. Low serum albumin levels
    3. Elevated white blood cell count
    4. Proteinuria
    5. Prior cognitive impairment
    6. Limb fracture on admission
    7. Symptomatic infective disease
    8. Neuroleptic drugs
    9. Narcotic drugs
    10. Anticholinergic drugs

21. C. The best-documented hypothesis for delirium in the elderly suggests that the syndrome results from a widespread imbalance of neurotransmission. It is postulated that there is a reduction in brain metabolism that results in diminished cortical function. Impairment of cerebral oxidative metabolism results in reduced synthesis of neurotransmitters, especially acetylcholine, whose relative deficiency in the brain is a common denominator in metabolic-toxic encephalopathies. Hypoxia and hypoglycemia impair acetylcholine metabolism and bring about changes in mental function. The inhibition of acetylcholine metabolism may be due to calcium-dependent release of the neurotransmitter. Thus the cholinergic deficit is currently the most convincing pathogenic hypothesis of delirium. Numerous experimental studies have shown that the syndrome can be readily induced by anticholinergic agents.

22. C. Diagnosis of delirium is based on the following:
    1. A complete history (NB—include a complete drug review)
    2. A complete physical examination
    3. An electroencephalogram on all patients
    4. Tests based on 1 and 2

    The disorder of delirium will be discussed in greater detail in a Short Answer Management Problem.

23. E. Delirium is associated with many different abnormalities. One of the most important is a disordered sleep-wake cycle. In an elderly patient with delirium, either wakefulness is abnormally increased and the patient gets little or no sleep, or the patient suffers from insomnia at night and displays drowsiness and periods of sleep during the day. Thus the sleep-wake cycle is usually fragmented, and the patient tends to be restless and agitated and suffers from hallucinations while awake during the night.

SOLUTION TO SHORT ANSWER MANAGEMENT PROBLEM 120

PART A: What follows is an all-inclusive mnemonic on confusion in the elderly. This includes both reversible causes and nonreversible causes.

The mnemonic is spelled DEMENTIA.

D = (A) Drug intoxication (especially anticholinergic agents)
  = (B) Alcohol abuse
E = (A) Eyes and ears (especially cataracts, diabetes mellitus, and sensorineural hearing loss)
  = (B) Environment (a new environment is a sure trigger for acute confusional state.)
M = (A) Metabolic
    1. Hyponatremia
    2. Hypokalemia
    3. Hyperkalemia
    4. Hypercalcemia
    5. Elevated blood urea nitrogen
    6. Elevated serum creatinine
    7. Elevated gamma-GT
E = (A) Emotional
    1. Major depressive disorder
    2. Bipolar affective disorder
    3. Schizoaffective disorder
    4. Chronic schizophrenia
    5. Pseudodementia (depression masking as dementia)
    6. Adverse drug reaction (propranolol causes depression)
  = (B) Endocrine
    1. Hypothyroidism
    2. Hyperthyroidism
    3. Hyperglycemia
    4. Hypoglycemia

N = (A) Neoplasms
    1. Benign neoplasms (rare)
    2. Malignancies
        i) Breast cancer
        ii) Lung cancer
        iii) Colon cancer
        iv) Prostate cancer
        v) Lymphomas
        vi) Multiple myeloma
  = (B) Normal pressure hydrocephalus
T = (A) Trauma
        Chronic subdural hematoma is most common. Burr holes can be life-saving in a rural center if recognized.
I = (A) Infections (in order of frequency as a cause of delirium in three groups of elderly patients)
    1. Infections predominating in hospitalized patients with delirium
        i) Urinary tract infection
        ii) Bacterial pneumonia
        iii) Surgical wound infections
    2. Infections predominating in nursing home patients who develop delirium
        i) Bacterial pneumonia
        ii) Urinary tract infection
        iii) Decubitus ulcer
    3. Independent, previously healthy individuals living in the community
        i) Bacterial pneumonia
        ii) Urinary tract infection
        iii) Intraabdominal infections (appendicitis, diverticulitis)
        iv) Infective endocarditis
  = (B) Inflammatory
    1. New onset/recurrent inflammatory bowel disease (ulcerative colitis or regional enteritis)
    2. Collagen vascular disorders
        i) Rheumatoid arthritis
        ii) Systemic lupus erythematosus
    3. Musculoskeletal system
        i) Polymyalgia rheumatica (If not treated properly this can lead to serious consequences, such as blindness.)
        ii) Polymyositis/dermatomyositis
    4. Pericarditis
    5. Pleuritis
    6. Acute appendicitis
    7. Biliary colic
    8. Renal colic
    9. Chronic pancreatitis
    10. Diverticulitis
A = (A) Anemia
    1. Iron-deficiency anemia
    2. Anemia of chronic disease
    3. Macrocytic anemia (vitamin B_{12} deficiency)

= (B) Atherosclerotic vascular disease/cardiovascular disease
1. Myocardial infarction
2. Pulmonary embolism
3. Cerebrovascular accident (stroke)
4. Congestive cardiac failure
= (C) Alzheimer's and other dementias
1. Alzheimer's disease
2. Multiinfarct dementia

PART B: The distinct disorders that are part of the complex called delirium include the following:

1. Global disorder of cognition: this constitutes one of the essential features of delirium. In this sense, the word *global* refers to the main cognitive functions, including the following:
   A. Memory
   B. Thinking
   C. Perception
   D. Information acquisition
   E. Information processing
   F. Information retention
   G. Information retrieval
   H. Utilization of information

   These cognitive deficits and abnormalities constitute an essential diagnostic feature of delirium.

2. Global disorder of attention: disturbances of the major aspects of attention are invariably present. Alertness (vigilance), that is, readiness to respond to sensory stimuli, and the ability to mobilize, shift, sustain, and direct attention at will are always disturbed to some extent.

3. Reduced level of consciousness: this implies a diminished awareness of oneself and one's surroundings, to respond to sensory inputs in a selective and sustained manner, and to be able to relate the incoming information to previously acquired knowledge.

4. Disordered sleep-wake cycle: disorganization of the sleep-wake cycle is one of the essential features of delirium. Wakefulness is abnormally increased and the patient sleeps little or not at all, or it is reduced during the day but excessive during the night.

5. Disorder of psychomotor behavior: a disturbance of both verbal and nonverbal psychomotor activity is the last essential feature of delirium. A delirious patient can be predominantly either hyperactive or hypoactive.

Some patients shift unpredictably from abnormally increased psychomotor activity to lethargy and vice versa.

NEW INFORMATION—1995

In early 1995 a breakthrough in the identification of Alzheimer's disease was confirmed. Up to this point in time, it had been impossible to positively "diagnose" Alzheimer's disease without a brain biopsy.

Breakthrough 1: neuritic plaques and neurofibrillary tangles can be identified in a matter of minutes by a modification of MRI technology. This technology, called *frequency-shifted burst imaging,* offers a method of detecting these changes noninvasively. Scans from individuals with Alzheimer's disease show areas where blood flow is lower than in healthy individuals. The region that corresponds to both neuritic plaques and neurofibrillary tangles shows up as a different color from normal brain tissue.

Breakthrough 2: using a simple test, with a few drops of a very dilute solution of tropicamide, a synthetic relative of atropine, individuals with Alzheimer's disease will show pupillary dilatation with the very dilute solution, whereas individuals without Alzheimer's disease will not show this dilatation. The compound blocks the action of the neurotransmitter acetylcholine.

Breakthrough 3: individuals with a certain type of apolipoprotein, apolipoprotein E—Type 4, are much more likely to acquire Alzheimer's disease than are individuals with other forms of apolipoprotein.

The answer to Part A of the Short Answer Management Problem (the mnemonic for confusion in the elderly) will serve as the summary for this chapter.

SUGGESTED READINGS

Beardsley T. Putting Alzheimer's to the tests. Scientific American 1995; 272(2):12-13.

Lipowski ZJ. Delirium (acute confusional states). In: Hazzard WR et al., eds. Principles of geriatric medicine and gerontology. 3rd Ed. New York: McGraw-Hill, 1994.

Mayeux R, Schofield PW. Alzheimer's disease. In: Hazzard WR et al., eds. Principles of geriatric medicine and gerontology. 3rd Ed. New York: McGraw-Hill, 1994.

PROBLEM 121 AN 82-YEAR-OLD FEMALE WITH ACHING AND STIFFNESS IN THE SHOULDER AND HIP GIRDLES

An 82-year-old female presents to your office with a 6-month history of "stiffness" and "aching" in the shoulders and hips present for the last 3 months. The onset was quite abrupt. The stiffness and aching are bilateral in both upper and lower limbs. The symptoms are especially severe in the morning. The patient says that it is very difficult to get out of a chair and very difficult to move her arms above her head.

The patient also mentions significant malaise and fatigue and has experienced a 20-lb weight loss. She mentions a mild fever and also a feeling of "depression."

On examination, the patient's blood pressure and pulse are normal. Although the patient describes "significant weakness," there are no objective findings.

SELECT THE ONE BEST ANSWER TO THE FOLLOWING QUESTIONS

1. What is the most likely diagnosis in this patient?
   a) osteoarthritis
   b) rheumatoid arthritis
   c) polymyalgia rheumatica
   d) polymyositis
   e) acute degenerative arthritis

2. Which of the following disorders is most closely associated with the geriatric population?
   a) polymyalgia rheumatica
   b) osteoarthritis
   c) rheumatoid arthritis
   d) degenerative arthritis
   e) polymyositis

3. Which of the following statements regarding the condition described is(are) true?
   a) the etiology of the disease is unknown
   b) this disease is autoimmune in origin
   c) the overall prevalence of this condition is approximately 17/100,000 patients
   d) family aggregation of this disorder has been described
   e) all of the above are true

4. Which of the following statements regarding this condition is(are) true?
   a) there are no significant complications or related disorders of concern
   b) hypothyroidism, hyperthyroidism, and hyperparathyroidism are part of the differential diagnosis
   c) systemic lupus erythematosus must be considered a potential diagnostic possibility
   d) b and c
   e) all of the above

5. What is(are) the major difference(s) between this disorder and polymyositis?
   a) marked proximal muscle weakness in polymyositis
   b) marked proximal muscle tenderness in polymyositis
   c) elevated muscle enzymes such as creatine kinase (CK) in polymyositis

   d) a and b
   e) all of the above

6. Which of the following is the investigation of choice in this condition?
   a) muscle creatine kinase (CK)
   b) erythrocyte sedimentation rate (ESR)
   c) antinuclear antibody titer (ANA)
   d) rheumatoid factor titer (RA)
   e) CT scan of the shoulders and hip girdle

7. Which of the following is(are) neurologic manifestations of giant cell arteritis?
   a) depression
   b) deafness
   c) amaurosis fugax
   d) paralysis
   e) all of the above

8. Of the symptoms listed in Question 7, which is the most worrisome?
   a) depression
   b) deafness
   c) amaurosis fugax
   d) paralysis
   e) all of the symptoms are equally worrisome

9. The symptom identified in Question 8 as most worrisome can lead to which of the following (greatly feared) complication of giant cell arteritis?
   a) permanent hemiplegia
   b) permanent bilateral and complete sensorineural hearing loss
   c) permanent monocular or binocular total blindness
   d) permanent bilateral and complete sensorineural and conductive hearing losses
   e) permanent quadriplegia

10. What is the treatment of choice for both polymyalgia rheumatica and giant cell arteritis?
   a) intravenous pulsed steroids
   b) oral prednisone: 20 mg/day for PMR and 60 mg/day for GCA
   c) oral methotrexate

d) cyclosporine IV every third day for 4 weeks

e) intravenous dihydroergotamine

11. What is the pathophysiological cause of giant cell arteritis?

a) inflammation of the middle meningeal artery

b) inflammation of the temporal artery

c) inflammation of the common carotid artery

d) inflammation of the internal carotid artery

e) inflammation of the external carotid artery

Short Answer Management Problem 121

An 82-year-old female presents to your office with a history of shoulder girdle pain and hip pain progressing to involve other joints of the upper and lower extremities. Provide a differential diagnosis for this patient's pain.

ANSWERS

1. C.

2. A. The diagnosis in this patient is polymyalgia rheumatica. This is a very important diagnosis to make in the elderly. Of all of the musculoskeletal conditions, none is so closely identified with the geriatric population.

   Polymyalgia rheumatica is a diagnosis that is often missed, a diagnosis in which vague symptoms are present, and a diagnosis that is often characterized by the patient's seeing multiple doctors without being correctly diagnosed.

   Polymyalgia rheumatica is characterized by aching and stiffness in the shoulder and hip girdles. Profound morning stiffness is especially suggestive of this disorder and should be specifically sought out. The diagnosis of polymyalgia rheumatica is seldom seen before the age of 50 years; its mean age of onset is 70 years. The onset may be either very abrupt or very gradual. The stiffness that is present in the hips and the shoulders may become generalized, involving the neck and knees and even extending into the wrists and fingers.

   There are also prominent constitutional symptoms. These include symptoms such as malaise, weight loss, low-grade fever, and depression.

3. E. The etiology of polymyalgia rheumatica is unknown, although an autoimmune process appears to be related to the condition. The overall prevalence of polymyalgia rheumatica is 17/100,000 people. In addition, family aggregation is common.

4. D.

5. E. The single most important feature of polymyalgia rheumatica is its association with giant cell arteritis. Giant cell arteritis will be discussed in subsequent questions.

The differential diagnosis of polymyalgia rheumatica in the elderly includes hypothyroidism, hyperthyroidism, hyperparathyroidism, systemic lupus erythematosus, rheumatoid arthritis, osteoarthritis or degenerative arthritis, and polymyositis. The differences between polymyalgia rheumatica and polymyositis on clinical examination are as follows: (1) there is marked weakness associated with proximal muscle pain in polymyositis; (2) there is marked muscle tenderness associated with the proximal muscle pain in polymyositis; and (3) laboratory examination reveals elevated muscle enzymes in polymyositis.

6. B. The only characteristic laboratory abnormality in polymyalgia rheumatica (and giant cell arteritis) is elevation of the ESR. Elevations to levels greater than 100 mm/hr may be seen in either disease; elevations to greater than 50 mm/hr are almost universal.

7. E.

8. C.

9. C. Neurologic manifestations of giant cell arteritis include the following: depression, deafness, diabetes insipidus, diplopia, paralysis, stroke, seizures, transient ischemic attacks, syncope, ataxia, neuropathies, tinnitus, vertigo, headache, tremor, dementia, psychosis, confusion, aseptic meningitis, transverse myelopathy, and amaurosis fugax.

   Of the neurologic symptoms listed, the most worrisome symptom is amaurosis fugax. Amaurosis fugax (which is defined as brief visual loss) is related to ischemia of the posterior ciliary artery or diplopia due to compromised blood flow to the nerves of the extraocular muscles. These transient symptoms foretell by days, weeks, or sometimes even months the most dreaded complication of permanent monocular or binocular blindness. If it appears as strictly a monocular loss, watch out: blindness in the second eye will follow within days of the first.

10. B. Oral prednisone is the treatment of choice for both polymyalgia rheumatica and giant cell arteritis. The dosage is as follows:
    A. Polymyalgia rheumatica: 20 mg/day orally for 4 weeks with gradual reduction thereafter but maintained for at least 1 year
    B. Giant cell arteritis: 60 mg/day orally for 4 weeks with gradual reduction beginning at 4 weeks but with maintenance therapy for 1 to 2 years. Dosage should be adjusted by monitoring the ESR.

11. B. From a pathological point of view, the cause of giant cell arteritis is inflammation of the temporal artery. Thus giant cell arteritis is also known as temporal arteritis. From a local anatomic standpoint, this results in temporal headache (generally unilateral and accompanied by temporal artery swelling and tenderness). Temporal artery biopsy is the definitive diagnostic procedure for giant cell arteritis.

SOLUTION TO SHORT ANSWER MANAGEMENT PROBLEM 121

Differential diagnosis:
  I. Nonmusculoskeletal problems:
     A. Hypothyroidism
     B. Hyperthyroidism
     C. Hyperparathyroidism
 II. Musculoskeletal problems:
     A. Systemic lupus erythematosus
     B. Rheumatoid arthritis
     C. Osteoarthritis or degenerative arthritis
     D. Polymyalgia rheumatica
     E. Polymyositis
III. Other important systemic conditions:
     A. Metastatic bone cancer
     B. Multiple myeloma

SUMMARY OF THE DIAGNOSIS AND TREATMENT OF POLYMYALGIA RHEUMATICA AND GIANT CELL ARTERITIS

1. **Polymyalgia rheumatica:**
   a) Epidemiology: of all the musculoskeletal conditions, none is so closely identified with the geriatric population as polymyalgia rheumatica.
   b) Prevalence rate: a prevalence rate of 17/100,000 persons over the age of 50 has been established.
   c) Symptoms:
      1. Either sudden onset or gradual onset (if gradual, then months and not years)
      2. Pain, aching, and stiffness in the shoulder girdle and hip girdle is the initial manifestation.
      3. Profound morning stiffness
      4. Pain, aching, and stiffness progress to other joints in the upper and lower extremities
      5. Clue: the patient tells you that suddenly he or she can no longer get out of bed in the morning.
   d) Diagnosis: elevated ESR (almost always greater than 50 mm/hr; frequently greater than 100 mm/hr)
   e) Complication: giant cell arteritis with eventual blindness
   f) Treatment: prednisone, 20 mg/day for 1 month and taper; maintain for 1 year.
   g) Differential diagnosis: see the Short Answer Management Problem.

2. **Giant cell arteritis:**
   a) Presenting signs and symptoms:
      1. The pain, aching, and stiffness in the shoulder and hip girdles as just described.
      2. Additional systemic signs and symptoms of inflammation:
         i) Fever
         ii) Weight loss
         iii) Malaise
         iv) Jaw claudication
         v) Transient visual complaints and blindness if not treated
         vi) Extremity claudication
         vii) Aortic aneurysm
      3. Significant local signs and symptoms:
         i) Temporal headache (unilateral)
         ii) Temporal artery swelling and tenderness
      4. Significant neurologic symptoms: see the answers to questions 7-9.
   b) Diagnosis:
      1. Erythrocyte sedimentation rate (as mentioned earlier)
      2. Temporal artery biopsy
         If you suspect temporal arteritis, do not wait for a surgeon to perform a biopsy. Treat the condition with prednisone now.
   c) Complication: permanent monocular or binocular blindness
   d) Treatment: high-dose prednisone: 60 mg/day for 4 weeks; taper slowly; maintain for 1 to 2 years.

SUGGESTED READING

Eisenberg G. Polymyalgia rheumatica and giant cell arteritis. In: Hazzard WR et al., eds. Principles of geriatric medicine and gerontology. 3rd Ed. New York: McGraw-Hill, 1994.

PROBLEM 122 AN 80-YEAR-OLD MALE WITH HYPERTENSION

An 80-year-old white male, previously healthy, presents for a periodic health examination. He was last seen by a physician 20 years ago. His blood pressure is recorded as 215 mm Hg/95 mm Hg.

A complete history reveals no other cardiovascular risk factors. A complete physical examination reveals no evidence of end organ damage or secondary causes of hypertension.

Basic laboratory investigations, including a CBC, urinalysis, electrolytes, serum calcium, fasting blood sugar, plasma cholesterol, uric acid, and ECG are all normal.

The patient is on a fixed income and is trying to keep up with payments for his wife's nursing home care.

SELECT THE ONE BEST ANSWER TO THE FOLLOWING QUESTIONS

1. Based on the information given, what would you do now?
   a) begin therapy with a thiazide diuretic
   b) begin therapy with a calcium-channel blocker
   c) begin therapy with an ACE inhibitor
   d) begin therapy with a beta blocker
   e) none of the above

2. Following further investigation and two further visits, appropriate therapy is prescribed for the patient described, and he returns in 1 month for follow-up. His blood pressure remains elevated at 205/92 mm Hg. A further visit in 1 week yields the same blood pressure reading.

   You also discuss nonpharmacologic treatment with him, and it appears obvious to you that he is not really prepared to alter his "hamburgers and chips (fried in pure lard)" diet, and he further states that "exercise would kill me." What would you do now?
   a) prescribe a thiazide diuretic
   b) prescribe a calcium-channel blocker
   c) prescribe a beta blocker
   d) prescribe an ACE inhibitor
   e) prescribe a vasodilator

3. Appropriate therapy is prescribed for the patient, and he returns in 1 month for follow-up. His blood pressure is 185/90 mm Hg. His serum potassium level has decreased from 4.0 mEq/L to 3.0 mEq/L. At this time, what would you do?
   a) substitute an ACE inhibitor for the present medication
   b) substitute a calcium-channel blocker for the present medication
   c) substitute a beta blocker for the present medication
   d) substitute a vasodilator for the present medication
   e) review the type and dose of the drug class being prescribed

4. The patient described has the necessary change to his medication treatment regime made. When he returns next month for follow-up, his blood pressure is 175/90 mm Hg.
   At this time, what would you do?
   a) add an ACE inhibitor

   b) add a calcium-channel blocker
   c) add a beta blocker
   d) add a vasodilator
   e) maximize the dose of a beta blocker

5. Which of the following statements regarding the treatment of hypertension in the elderly is(are) true?
   a) elderly patients with hypertension should not be treated
   b) the benefits of treating elderly hypertensives have not been established
   c) no change in morbidity or mortality has been demonstrated for elderly patients treated with antihypertensives
   d) elderly patients treated for hypertension are likely to benefit only from a reduction in cerebrovascular morbidity and mortality, not cardiac morbidity or mortality
   e) none of the above is true

6. Regarding the epidemiologic importance of elevations in systolic versus diastolic blood pressure in elderly patients, which of the following statements is true?
   a) elevation of systolic blood pressure is not as important as elevation of diastolic blood pressure
   b) elevation of systolic blood pressure, although important, does not correlate well with cardiovascular morbidity and mortality
   c) elevations of systolic and diastolic blood pressure are equally important
   d) elevated systolic blood pressure is a greater risk for subsequent cardiovascular morbidity and mortality than diastolic pressure
   e) the relative importance of elevations in systolic blood pressure in terms of cardiovascular morbidity and mortality remains unclear

7. With respect to morbidity and mortality and treatment of systolic hypertension in the elderly, which of the following epidemiologic categories show(s) a significant decrease (compared to placebo) when systolic blood pressure is treated?
   a) total stroke morbidity
   b) total stroke mortality
   c) total coronary artery mortality

d) a and b only

e) all of the above

8. Which of the following drug combinations should be avoided in elderly hypertensive patients (Note: hydrochlorothiazide = HCT)?
   a) HCT/amiloride plus enalapril
   b) HCT/amiloride plus nifedipine
   c) HCT/amiloride plus atenolol
   d) HCT/amiloride plus hydralazine
   e) HCT/amiloride plus reserpine

9. A 75-year-old African-American male with angina pectoris is found, on P/E, to have a BP of 170/100 mm Hg. His angina is controlled on isosorbide dinitrate 30 mg qid. His blood pressure reading is repeated on several occasions and remains unchanged. At this time, what is the most reasonable treatment for this patient's blood pressure?
   a) a calcium-channel blocker
   b) a beta blocker
   c) a thiazide diuretic
   d) an ACE inhibitor
   e) a peripheral alpha receptor blocker

10. A 72-year-old white female with a previous MI and mild CHF (controlled with furosemide 40 mg qid) presents for a routine assessment. She is found to have a blood pressure of 190/100 mm Hg. This reading is repeated on two occasions.

Considering the CHF, what would be the most appropriate treatment for her hypertension?
   a) an ACE inhibitor
   b) a calcium-channel blocker
   c) a beta blocker
   d) a thiazide diuretic
   e) none of the above

11. A 72-year-old white male with a 20-year history of type II diabetes mellitus (NIDDM) is found to have a blood pressure of 170/105 mm Hg. He has no history of angina pectoris or other significant vascular disease.

His blood pressure is repeated on two further occasions and the reading remains the same.

Laboratory evaluation reveals microalbuminuria.

At this time, what would be the most appropriate treatment for this patient's blood pressure?
   a) a thiazide diuretic
   b) a beta blocker
   c) a calcium-channel blocker
   d) an ACE inhibitor
   e) a vasodilator

12. What is the recommended dosage of hydrochlorothiazide for the treatment of hypertension in the elderly?
   a) 12.5-25 mg
   b) 25-50 mg
   c) 50-75 mg
   d) 75-100 mg
   e) whatever you want

Short Answer Management Problem 122

PART A: An 80-year-old African-American male with systolic hypertension (210/85 mm Hg) is a new patient to your practice. He says he has been "healthy all of my life." From three consecutive readings you determine that the patient is truly hypertensive.

Discuss your approach to this patient with respect to education and counseling regarding his hypertension. Include lifestyle advice, medication advice, and other pertinent advice that you consider important.

PART B: Discuss the medication efficacy differences that have been demonstrated with respect to race and age in the following patients:
1. Young African-American patients
2. Young Caucasian patients
3. Elderly African-American patients
4. Elderly Caucasian patients

ANSWERS

1. E. Even though this patient has a systolic blood pressure of 215 mm Hg, you should consider the following: this is only one reading and can not be assumed to represent his "true blood pressure"; and even if you were able to make the diagnosis of hypertension at this time, you would still want to begin with nonpharmacologic therapy.

This patient should have his blood pressure rechecked on two further occasions before the diagnosis of hypertension is made.

2. A. Recent studies have very clearly demonstrated the importance of treating systolic hypertension in the elderly, treating it, in fact, with the same rigor and aggressiveness as diastolic hypertension.

Because of his fixed income, and the proven efficacy of thiazide diuretics in reducing morbidity and mortality from cardiovascular disease, a low-dose thiazide diuretic would be the agent of choice.

3. E. At this time, the most reasonable alternative would be to review both the dose and the drug class.

On the positive side, this patient's systolic blood pressure has dropped significantly (from 205 to 185 mm Hg).

On the negative side, so has his potassium (from 4.0 mEq/L to 3.0 mEq/L). This is a significant drop and furthermore puts this patient into the danger zone for hypokalemia—the level at which dysrhythmias begin to be a serious concern.

The most reasonable strategy in this case would likely be the following:
1. Reduce the dose of the thiazide diuretic to an absolute minimum (12.5 mg).
2. Add a beta blocker (such as atenolol) in a dose of 25-50 mg/day. This combination of drugs is being selected (thiazide plus beta blocker) because of recommendations made by the recent publication of JNC-V (discussed elsewhere in this book) and the issue of documented reduction in cardiovascular morbidity and mortality from thiazides and beta blockers.

4. E. The most appropriate strategy at this time would seem to be an increase in the dose of the beta blocker to its maximum.

At this time, even though the systolic blood pressure has been further reduced (to 175 mm Hg), further lowering of his blood pressure must take place.

5. E. There is ample evidence to show that antihypertensive therapy prevents cerebrovascular accidents, congestive cardiac failure, and other blood-pressure–related complications. Recently, the Systolic Hypertension in the Elderly Program (SHEP) showed a reduction in myocardial infarction and other coronary events in older patients with moderate to severe ischemic heart disease. Other studies confirm this.

6. C. The single most important advance in the treatment of hypertension in the elderly is the clear and unequivocal recognition that systolic hypertension is as important as diastolic hypertension as a risk factor for cardiovascular morbidity and mortality and should be aggressively treated. The goal of systolic blood pressure reduction is a reading not exceeding 160 mm Hg.

7. E. See the critique of Question 5.

8. A. Of the choices provided, the drug combination that should clearly be avoided in elderly patients is HCT/amiloride and enalapril. Both amiloride and enalapril are potassium-sparing drugs. In an elderly patient with decreased renal function, this can lead to profound and rapid hyperkalemia with subsequent complications.

9. A. Calcium-channel blockers have been shown, in elderly African-American patients, to be more effective than beta blockers in controlling of hypertension; thus a calcium-channel blocker (particularly diltiazem) would appear to be the agent of choice.

10. A. Considering that this elderly female has congestive heart failure as well as hypertension, the treatment of choice is an ACE inhibitor. ACE inhibitors reduce both preload and afterload in hypertensive patients and thus are the drug class of choice for the management of CHF.

11. D. Patients with diabetes mellitus and resulting renal impairment or microalbuminuria should definitely be treated with ACE inhibitors as the drug class of choice. There is some evidence that ACE inhibitors can be "renal protective agents" in patients with diabetes mellitus, and can even be indicated as a prophylactic measure.

12. A. The recommended, or "right," dose of hydrochlorothiazide or other thiazide diuretic is the lowest dose that effectively controls the blood pressure and at the same time minimizes all of the metabolic side effects associated with thiazide diuretics.

SOLUTION TO SHORT ANSWER MANAGEMENT PROBLEM 122

Summary of case: an 80-year-old African-American male with documented systolic hypertension
Question: provide advice for this patient at this time.

1. Review the patient's diet with him. Attempt to have the patient's spouse present (if available) while discussing this.
2. Encourage the patient to adopt the general recommendations of the American Heart Association's type I diet. This includes no more than 300 mg of cholesterol/day, no more than 30% of calories from fat, and no more than 10% of calories from saturated fat.
3. Encourage the patient to begin a "gentle" aerobic exercise program. The most reasonable exercise for a man of this age would be a walking program.
4. Advise the patient to decrease his alcohol intake to no more than two drinks/day.
5. Encourage the patient to stop smoking (cutting down might be more reasonable) if he is a smoker.
6. It would seem reasonable to start with these "nonpharmacologic maneuvers" even in a man of this age. Starting a patient on a medication at this time is probably not indicated (unless he quite categorically tells you that he has no intention of following the nonpharmacologic regimen, as the presenting patient did).

The differentiation of efficacy of antihypertensive drugs based on age is extremely interesting. Interdrug differences are particularly apparent in black subjects. The following results are from a major review article on hypertension in the elderly published in *Geriatrics* in April 1994.

The agents used in this study included atenolol, captopril, clonidine, diltiazem, hydrochlorothiazide, and prazosin.

1. African-American patients <60 years: diltiazem was shown in one major study to be superior to all other agents.
2. African-American patients >60 years: diltiazem and hydrochlorothiazide were the most effective agents. Captopril and atenolol were the least effective.
3. White patients <60 years: all of first-line agents (thiazides, beta blockers, calcium-channel blockers, and ACE inhibitors) were equally effective.
4. White patients >60 years: atenolol is the most effective agent.

SUMMARY OF THE DIAGNOSIS, TREATMENT, AND OUTCOME OF HYPERTENSIVE MANAGEMENT IN ELDERLY PATIENTS

1. **Single most important point:** systolic hypertension in the elderly (and in the young as well) is as important as diastolic hypertension.
2. **Diagnosis of hypertension in the elderly:** new criteria established by JNC_1-V (see the chapter on hypertension)
3. **Treatment of hypertension in the elderly reduces all of the following:**
   a) Cerebrovascular morbidity
   b) Cerebrovascular mortality
   c) Cardiovascular morbidity
   d) Cardiovascular mortality
4. A substantial proportion of patients with mild and moderate hypertension can be controlled with a single agent, and in most this control will be maintained in the long term.
5. Overall, and with specific reference to the study just quoted, the calcium-channel blocker produced the greatest number of positive responses. This should be balanced against the recommendation of JNC_1-V that therapy be started with a thiazide diuretic or a beta blocker.
6. Captopril was quite ineffective in African-American patients in this study.

SUGGESTED READINGS

The fifth report of the Joint National Committee on Detection, Evaluation, and Treatment of High Blood Pressure (JNC-V). Arch Intern Med 1993; 153:154-183.

Massie B. First-line therapy for hypertension: Different patients, different needs. Geriatrics 1994; 49(4):22-30.

PROBLEM 123   A 75-YEAR-OLD MALE WITH A SLOW, SHUFFLING GAIT, TREMORS, AND DEPRESSION

A 75-year-old male is brought to your office by his wife. She states that he has just been "staring into space" for the last 2 months. He has been unable to move around the house without falling over. Also, his movements appear to be very slow. According to his wife, he has been very depressed.

On examination, the patient has a slow, shuffling gait and walks in a "stooped-over" position. His blood pressure (lying) is 140/90 mm Hg. His standing blood pressure is 100/70 mm Hg. He has marked rigidity of his upper extremities. He also has a tremor that appears to be present only at rest.

SELECT THE ONE BEST ANSWER TO THE FOLLOWING QUESTIONS

1. What is the most likely diagnosis in this patient?
   a) Alzheimer's disease
   b) major depressive disorder with psychomotor retardation
   c) degenerative orthostatic hypotension
   d) Parkinson's disease
   e) multiple sclerosis

2. What is the most common presenting symptom in this disorder?
   a) orthostatic hypotension
   b) depression
   c) gait disturbance
   d) tremor
   e) rigidity

3. Where is the lesion associated with the described disorder located?
   a) the caudate nucleus
   b) the substantia nigria
   c) the hypothalamus
   d) the putamen
   e) the globus pallidus

4. The disorder described is associated with a CNS neurotransmitter deficiency. What is that neurotransmitter?
   a) acetylcholine
   b) serotonin
   c) gamma-aminobutyric acid
   d) dopamine
   e) norepinephrine

5. Many drugs are associated with side effects that mimic some of the symptoms of the described disorder. Which of the following drugs would not produce these symptoms?
   a) diazepam
   b) haloperidol
   c) chlorpromazine
   d) perphenazine
   e) reserpine

6. Which of the following statements regarding the condition described is false?
   a) there is marked heterogeneity in disease presentation
   b) there are at least two major subgroups of this disorder
   c) patients who present with marked postural instability have a better prognosis than those who present with tremor
   d) personality changes commonly appear in the course of this disorder
   e) significant depression and dementia appear in one-third to one-half of patients with this condition.

7. What is(are) the drug(s) of choice for mild cases of the condition described (*mild* meaning that the main or only symptom is tremor)?
   a) amantadine
   b) trihexyphenidyl
   c) levodopa
   d) carbidopa
   e) c and d
   f) a or b

8. If the symptoms progress to the point where another agent is needed, dose-limiting side effects develop from the drugs being used, or the drugs being used begin to lose their effectiveness, what is the next step in the treatment of the disorder described?
   a) selegiline
   b) trihexyphenidyl
   c) amantadine
   d) all of the above
   e) none of the above

9. Which of the following drugs may be indicated in the treatment of the disorder described?
   a) bromocriptine
   b) pergolide
   c) amitriptyline
   d) all of the above
   e) none of the above

10. Which of the following symptoms is not characteristic of this disorder?
   a) unilateral onset of tremor

b) unilateral onset of bradykinesia
c) impaired balance
d) muscle rigidity
e) psychomotor agitation

11. Which of the following statements regarding levodopa is false?
    a) levodopa in combination with carbidopa remains the drug of first choice for the treatment of most patients with the condition described
    b) levodopa is unlikely to lose its effectiveness over time when being used to treat the disorder described
    c) levodopa is likely to produce an "on-off" phenomenon during treatment of the disorder described
    d) nausea is a frequent side effect of levodopa
    e) centrally mediated dyskinesia, hallucinations, dystonia, and motor fluctuations are common in levodopa-treated patients

12. Which of the following conditions is most closely associated with the condition described?
    a) major depressive disorder
    b) cerebrovascular disease
    c) epilepsy
    d) schizophrenia
    e) schizo-affective disorder

13. Which of the following statements regarding benign essential tremor is(are) correct?
    a) benign essential tremor is often familial
    b) a nodding head and tremulousness of speech are often observed with benign essential tremor
    c) benign essential tremor is a resting tremor rather than an action tremor
    d) a and b only
    e) all of the above

14. Benign essential tremor is frequently treated with which of the following agents?
    a) propranolol
    b) alcohol
    c) atenolol
    d) all of the above
    e) none of the above

15. What illicit drug produces symptoms closely resembling the symptoms of the condition described?
    a) a meperidine analog—MPTP
    b) crack cocaine
    c) LSD
    d) apomorphine
    e) diamorphine (heroin)

Short Answer Management Problem 123

Discuss the therapeutic choices available to treat the condition described in the patient presentation in this chapter. Describe a logical approach to instituting these therapeutic choices in a patient with this disorder.

ANSWERS

1. D. This patient has Parkinson's disease. The most common presenting symptoms in Parkinson's disease include tremor, bradykinesia, rigidity, impaired postural reflexes, gait disturbance, autonomic dysfunction (causing orthostatic hypotension), and depression. A "masked facies" expression is typical of the disease.

   Other presenting symptoms can be constipation, vague aches and pains, paresthesia, decreased smell sensation, vestibular symptoms, pedal edema, fatigue, and weight loss.

   The other choices listed in this question do not explain the constellation of presenting symptoms.

2. D. The most common presenting symptom in Parkinson's disease is a resting tremor. This symptom is seen in 70% of patients with the disease. It may initially be confined to one hand, but it usually extends to involve all limbs.

3. B. The principal pathologic feature in Parkinson's disease is degeneration of the substantia nigra. Degenerative changes are also found in other brain stem nuclei.

4. D. Parkinson's disease is associated with a depletion of dopamine in the substantia nigrostriatal pathway system.

5. A. Parkinsonian-like side effects are common side effects of the neuroleptic drug class. This drug class includes the following agents: chlorpromazine, haloperidol, and perphenazine. In addition, the prokinetic agent metoclopramide can also produce this side effect.

   Reserpine, an older antihypertensive agent, may also produce these extrapyramidal symptoms. This is relevant because many elderly individuals who were started on reserpine are still on it.

   Diazepam does not produce any such side effects.

6. C. There is marked heterogeneity in Parkinson's disease. There are at least two major subtypes of Parkinson's disease. In one group the symptom of tremor is the most predominant clinical symptom. In the second group, postural instability and gait difficulty (PIGD) are the predominant symptoms. There is some overlap, but most patients fit into only one subgroup. Patients with tremor-predominant Parkinson's disease have slower progression of disease and have fewer problems with bradykinesia. They are also less likely to develop significant mental symptoms.

   Personality changes usually occur in the early stages, and patients often become withdrawn, apathetic, and dependent on their spouses. Significant depression occurs in one-half of patients, and dementia occurs in one-third of patients. As mentioned earlier, these personality and mental changes are more common in patients who present with the PIGD subtype of Parkinson's disease.

7. F. In mildly affected patients (especially patients who present only with the symptom of tremor) the drugs of choice are trihexyphenidyl (Artane) 2 mg to 6 mg/day and amantadine (Symmetrel) 100 mg to 300 mg/day.

8. E. The next step in the pharmacological treatment of Parkinson's disease is the combination of levodopa-carbidopa. Levodopa is a precursor for dopamine synthesis in the basal ganglia. The drug is usually administered in combination with carbidopa, which is a decarboxylase inhibitor. Obviously, treatment must be individualized: a good general rule to follow is "start low and go slow."

9. D. Bromocriptine and pergolide are two dopaminergic agonists. Pergolide and bromocriptine can be useful for sudden episodes of hesitancy or immobility, which Parkinsonian patients describe as "freezing." This can be an intermittent event or a regular event. The freezing often occurs when Parkinsonian patients begin to walk or they pass through a structure such as a doorway. Dyskinesias and other types of involuntary movements are also treated by these drugs.

   Amitriptyline is useful in the treatment of Parkinson's disease both as an anticholinergic agent and an antidepressant.

10. E. The unilateral onset of tremor or bradykinesia is common in Parkinson's disease. Muscle rigidity and impaired balance are other important symptoms. Psychomotor agitation (although one of the characteristic symptoms of major depressive disorder) is very rare. Parkinsonian patients present instead with psychomotor retardation.

11. B. Levodopa does lose its effectiveness over time in the treatment of Parkinson's disease. That is why, in patients who have mild symptoms, it is best to begin therapy with either a mild anticholinergic agent or amantadine.

   Levodopa does exhibit a marked "on-off" phenomenon during treatment of Parkinson's disease. This is characterized by periods of "drug working" and "drug not working."

   Side effects of levodopa include nausea and vomiting, dystonias, hallucinations, dyskinesias, and motor fluctuations.

12. A. Depression is a very common problem in patients with Parkinson's disease. The association between the two generally follows this pathway: when depression occurs, the symptoms of Parkinson's disease become worse; the patient then believes that his or her disease has progressed (quickly). This leads to a cycle that is difficult to break.

13. D.

14. D. Benign essential tremor is the major differential diagnostic possibility when considering tremor. Benign essential tremor is familial. Typical features include generalized tremulousness, including tremulousness of speech, and a "head-nodding" motion. Benign essential tremor is, in contradistinction to the tremor of Parkinson's disease, an action tremor. The treatments of choice for benign essential tremor are as follows:
    A. Propranolol
    B. Atenolol
    C. Alcohol (in moderation)
    D. Diazepam

15. A. The illicitly made meperidine analog (MPTP) produces symptoms that are Parkinson-like in presentation. It appears that this agent acts as a poison on the substantia nigra. Also, the symptoms appear to be irreversible, and the individual is left with a lifetime disability.

SOLUTION TO SHORT ANSWER MANAGEMENT PROBLEM 123

A reasonable therapeutic approach to the treatment of Parkinson's disease is as follows:
   I. Patients with minor symptoms (not significantly impairing function):
      A. No pharmacologic treatment
      B. Anticholinergic medications (such as trihexyphenidyl, benztropine)
      C. Amantadine
  II. Patients with moderate symptoms: levodopa-carbidopa (Sinemet) is the drug of choice. Levodopa is a precursor of dopamine synthesis/combination of carbidopa decarboxylase inhibitor.

III. Patients with moderate to severe symptoms (or patients in whom the effect of levodopa has worn off):
   A. Deprenyl (an MAO "B" inhibitor); in patient with a significant depressive component because of the MAO activity
   B. Bromocriptine and pergolide (dopamine agonists); in patients in whom dyskinesias and other involuntary movements are prominent
IV. Parkinson's patients with significant depression: amitriptyline or another TCA with or without anticholinergic properties (balance the benefits of the anticholinergic properties of amitriptyline against the risks of increased orthostatic disturbance and imbalance)

SUMMARY OF THE DIAGNOSIS AND TREATMENT OF PARKINSON'S DISEASE

1. **Epidemiology:** after stroke and Alzheimer's disease, Parkinson's disease is the most commonly encountered neurological disorder in the elderly population.
2. **Pathology:** depigmentation of the substantia nigra, which results in decrease in brain synthesis of dopamine
3. **Major symptoms:**
   a) Resting tremor
   b) Bradykinesia
   c) Rigidity
   d) Impaired postural reflexes
   e) Gait disturbance
   f) Autonomic dysfunction
   g) Depression
4. **Major subtypes:**
   Parkinson's Disease (Group A): this group exhibits tremor (resting) as the major symptom and sign.
   Parkinson's Disease (Group B): this group exhibits postural instability and gait disturbance (PIGD) as the major symptoms. Progression of the disease is usually more rapid in this group; neurobehavioral changes are also more common in this group.
5. **Treatment:** see the answer to Short Answer Management Problem 123.
6. **Other disease entity: benign essential tremor:** Benign essential tremor is an action tremor (as opposed to the resting tremor of Parkinson's disease). It is most often seen in the extremities and is sometimes associated with head nodding and tremulousness of speech. It is familial. The drug treatment of this entity includes, a beta blocker, diazepam, or alcohol (in moderation).

SUGGESTED READING

McDowell FH. Parkinson's disease and related disorders. In: Hazzard WR et al., eds. Principles of geriatric medicine and gerontology. 3rd Ed. New York: McGraw-Hill, 1994.

PROBLEM 124   A 78-YEAR-OLD FEMALE WITH CONSTIPATION

A 78-year-old female presents to your office with a 5-year history of "constipation." The patient, who has had significant difficulties with ischemic heart disease, is currently on atenolol and verapamil.

On examination, the patient's blood pressure is 180/95 mm Hg. Her pulse is 72 and regular. Examination of the head and neck, the lungs, the cardiovascular system and the abdomen is normal. Digital rectal examination reveals impacted stool.

SELECT THE ONE BEST ANSWER TO THE FOLLOWING QUESTIONS

1. Constipation is best defined as:
   a) only one bowel movement in 7 days
   b) only two bowel movements in 7 days
   c) only three bowel movements in 7 days
   d) only four bowel movements in 7 days
   e) none of the above

2. What is the most accurate elderly patient definition of constipation?
   a) anything less than one bowel movement/day
   b) any defecation difficulty
   c) anything less than two bowel movements/day
   d) any straining at stool
   e) any of the above: *constipation* to the elder means almost anything vaguely associated with bowel movements

3. Which of the following is(are) associated with constipation in the elderly?
   a) impaired general health status
   b) increased medication use
   c) decreased level of exercise
   d) all of the above
   e) none of the above

4. Which of the following drug classes is(are) associated with constipation?
   a) tricyclic antidepressants
   b) anticholinergic agents
   c) calcium-channel blockers
   d) all of the above
   e) none of the above

5. Concerning the history and physical examination of elderly patients with constipation, which of the following should be performed?
   a) a digital rectal examination
   b) a complete medication review
   c) a functional inquiry of the gastrointestinal system
   d) all of the above
   e) a and b only

6. Which of the following is(are) complications associated with constipation in the elderly?
   a) fecal impaction
   b) diarrhea
   c) anal fissures
   d) sigmoid volvulus
   e) a and c
   f) all of the above

7. Which of the following is not a recommended treatment for constipation in the elderly?
   a) a bowel training regime
   b) an exercise program
   c) chronic laxative use
   d) a high-fiber diet
   e) an above-average consumption of fluids

8. Which of the following drugs is most closely associated with constipation in the elderly?
   a) hydrochlorothiazide
   b) verapamil
   c) atenolol
   d) acetaminophen
   e) fluoxetine

9. Constipation in the elderly is most closely associated with which of the following?
   a) fecal impaction
   b) diarrhea
   c) crampy back pain
   d) a and c
   e) all of the above

10. What is the self-reported percentage incidence of constipation in elderly Americans?
    a) 10%
    b) 20%
    c) 30%
    d) 40%
    e) 50%

11. What is the laxative group most closely associated with long-term side effects in the elderly?
    a) the stimulant laxatives
    b) the hyperosmolar laxatives
    c) the saline laxatives
    d) the emollient laxatives
    e) the stool softeners

12. An 86-year-old male with stage IV carcinoma of the prostate presents to you seeking "pain relief." He has bony metastatic disease and his pain was well controlled on a combination of diclofenac and morphine sulfate.

With the morphine his pain decreased from 9/10 to 2/10. However, 5 days after morphine was started he began to experience more severe pain. You decide to increase the morphine dose and see him in a week. He refers after that week with worse pain than before. Now 13/10. You increase the morphine dose even further and ask him to return in another week. He returns a week later doubled over in pain that he describes as 15/10.

At this time, what would you do?
a) switch the patient to hydromorphone
b) switch the patient to methadone
c) switch the patient to fentanyl (patch)
d) switch the patient to oxycodone
e) none of the above

13. Your physical examination maneuver of choice in this patient at this time is which of the following?
a) none; you don't believe in the sensitivity, specificity, and positive predictive value of physical examination techniques any more
b) palpation of the abdomen
c) percussion of the abdomen
d) auscultation of the abdomen for bowel sounds
e) none of the above

14. What is the investigation of choice in this patient at this time?
a) an MRI
b) a repeat bone scan
c) a CT of the pelvis
d) a serum calcium level to "look for that ever-elusive entity, hypercalcemia"
e) none of the above

15. What is the single most common cause of abdominal pain in the elderly?
a) angiodysplasia
b) diverticulitis
c) SCOES (newly named, spastic colon of the elderly syndrome)
d) TAGS (newly named, the aging gut syndrome)
e) none of the above

Short Answer Management Problem 124

Fill in the blanks with the name of the drug in each of the drug classes listed that is most commonly responsible for constipation in the elderly.
1. antihypertensive agent: _____
2. Antianginal agent: _____
3. Medical diagnostic agent: _____
4. Antacid: _____
5. Nutritional supplement: _____
6. Analgesics: _____
7. Antipsychotics: _____
8. Antidepressants: _____
9. Anticholinergics: _____
10. Osteoporotic therapy agents (hint—inexpensive osteoporotic therapy): _____

ANSWERS

1. C.

2. E. *Constipation* is usually medically defined as fewer than 3 bowel movements/week. That is, physicians tend to define constipation on the basis of the frequency of stooling and the consistency of stooling. To the elder, on the other hand, constipation can mean almost anything, including any difficulties in defecation such as straining at stool, anything less than one to two completely-normal-in-every-way (shape, caliber, diameter, length, color) bowel movements, anything else vaguely related to the bowel movement. The point is, you must ask the elder what he or she means by constipation. It's almost a guarantee that the patient's definition will not match yours.

Constipation is a major problem for elderly patients in developed countries of the world. This is substantiated by the rise in the use of laxative therapies. Approximately 30% of patients over the age of 65 are regular laxative users.

Again, it is important to realize that there is a very significant discrepancy between what physicians define as *constipation in the elderly* and what the elderly themselves define as *constipation*. For many elderly patients, the daily bowel movement is somehow a significant mark of health.

3. D. The factors that appear to be associated with constipation in the elderly include an impaired general health status, an increased number of medications other than laxatives, diminished mobility, and diminished physical activity.

It is quite unclear what the true effect of diet on bowel habits is. There is epidemiologic evidence from the developed countries that greater amounts of crude dietary fiber are associated with a lesser prevalence of various gastrointestinal disorders, including diverticular disease, colorectal cancer, and constipation. There may be, however, intervening variables that account for some of this difference.

4. D. There are a significant number of drug classes that are associated with constipation, and especially constipation in the elderly. They are as follows:
    I. Antacids:
        A. Aluminum hydroxide
        B. Calcium carbonate
    II. Anticholinergic agents: trihexyphenidyl
    III. Antidepressants:
        A. Tricyclic antidepressants
        B. Lithium carbonate
    IV. Antihypertensive–antiarrhythmics: calcium-channel blockers, especially verapamil
    V. Metals:
        A. Bismuth
        B. Iron
        C. Heavy metals
    VI. Narcotic analgesics: any narcotic analgesic, but especially codeine
    VII. Nonsteroidal antiinflammatory drugs: all NSAIDs may produce constipation in the elderly.
    VIII. Sympathomimetic: pseudoephedrine

5. D. When an elderly patient complains of constipation, a careful history is the most important aspect of the evaluation. Sometimes, all that is required is reassurance from the physician that there is a broad range of normal bowel frequency.

    Symptoms of disorders that impair the motility of the large bowel should be sought. These general medical conditions include hypothyroidism, hyperparathyroidism, scleroderma, Parkinson's disease, cerebrovascular accidents, and diabetes mellitus.

    Localized colorectal diseases, such as tumors or other constricting lesions that may cause constipation, are often accompanied by other symptoms. Thus the history must include questions concerning abdominal pain and bleeding per rectum. In idiopathic, dietary, and drug-related constipation, there are usually no symptoms other than constipation, although a complaint of an abdominal bloating sensation is common with severe constipation.

    A digital rectal examination is a very sensitive screening tool in detecting anal lesions, although fissures and hemorrhoids, unless they are thrombosed or large, are found more reliably on anoscopy. Anoscopy should be performed routinely in constipated elderly patients. Digital rectal examination of the anal canal and rectum is useful in assessing the tone of the internal anal sphincter and also the strength of the external sphincter and the puborectalis muscle.

    The amount and the consistency of stool felt in the rectum may, in fact, indicate what type of constipation is present. Patients with a failure of the defecation mechanism tend to have much stool in the rectal vault, whereas those patients with colonic atony or irritable bowel syndrome have little or no stool in the rectum between defecations.

6. F. Although for most elderly patients, constipation is just a minor annoyance, for some elders it is much more than that. The elders that are most susceptible to constipation are institutionalized, bedridden elders.

    The complications of constipation in the elderly are as follows:
    A. Fecal impaction: heralded by crampy, lower abdominal and lower back pain.
    B. Stercoral ulcer: common in the bedridden patient. It is caused by pressure necrosis of the rectal or sigmoid mucosa due to a fecal mass. In some cases the ulcer may present as rectal bleeding.
    C. Anal fissures: anal fissures may result from excessive straining at stool and the subsequent complications that develop, including tears and passive congestion of the tissues near the dentate line. The problem is enhanced by the irritating effect of hard stools and toilet paper. Intraabdominal pressures of up to 300 mm Hg are generated during straining. Excessive straining at stool may cause prolapse of the anal mucosa, venous distention, and internal hemorrhoids.
    D. Megacolon: megacolon in the elderly is almost always idiopathic. Chronic use of cathartics over a period of years may lead to an acquired degeneration of the colonic myenteric plexus and subsequent megacolon. Bacterial overgrowth may occur and further complicate matters.
    E. Volvulus: volvulus, especially of the sigmoid colon, occurs most commonly in institutionalized, bedbound, elderly patients and carries a high mortality rate.
    F. Carcinoma of the colon: there is some evidence that chronic constipation is a risk factor for the development of carcinoma of the colon, particularly in women. This might be related to increased exposure time of susceptible mucosa to potentially carcinogenic substances.

7. C. The treatment of constipation is based, in large part, on the generally accepted principles that we understand constitute a "healthy lifestyle." This includes a bowel training regime (a schedule of regular times for attempting defecation), regular exercise (bedfast patients are at great risk of constipation and often respond poorly to treatment), dietary adjustment to increase the amount of fiber in the diet (the foods that are highest in

fiber may surprise you; they include 100% bran cereal, beans (baked, kidney, lima, navy), canned peas, raspberries, and broccoli), and an increased consumption of liquids, particularly water.

It is not recommended that a regular or chronic laxative regime be part of a routine prophylactic and treatment protocol for constipation.

8. B. The drug that is most closely associated with the development of constipation in the elderly is verapamil. Verapamil is a calcium-channel blocker commonly used to treat angina. Constipation develops in approximately 16% of patients who take verapamil for any length of time, and this percentage may be significantly higher in the elderly, especially in institutionalized and bedridden patients. The development of constipation-related complications that have already been discussed may well follow.

Constipation can occur as a side effect of hydrochlorothiazide, atenolol, and fluoxetine, but it does not appear to be what would be called a major side effect with those drugs.

9. E. Constipation is often associated with fecal impaction, diarrhea, and crampy lower abdominal and lower back pain.

Fecal impaction is the result of prolonged exposure of accumulated stool to the absorptive forces of the colon and rectum. The stool may become rocklike in consistency in the rectum (70%), in the sigmoid colon (20%), and in the proximal colon (10%).

Symptoms of crampy lower abdominal and lower back pain are common. Diarrhea may paradoxically follow the constipation, which leads to the impaction (watery material making its way around the impacted mass of stool). The impaction can sometimes be evacuated by the patient after the oral administration of polyethylene glycol (Golytely), but manual disimpaction is usually required.

10. C. A recent survey in the United States of community-dwelling persons over age 65 found that 30% of men and 29% of women considered themselves constipated. Twenty-four percent of the men and 20% of the women had used laxatives in the month preceding the survey.

11. A. The laxative group used to treat constipation can be divided into five major categories:
    A. The bulk-forming laxatives
    B. The emollient laxatives
    C. The saline laxatives
    D. The hyperosmotic laxatives
    E. The fiber-containing laxatives

    A. The bulk-forming laxatives: the bulk-forming laxatives include the various fiber-containing preparations and are thought to act in two major ways. First,

they are hydrophilic and tend to increase the stool mass and soften the stool consistency. They are the safest laxatives and are generally well tolerated by elderly patients when introduced gradually.

B. The emollient laxatives: emollients, or stool softeners, include mineral oil, as well as the newer docusate salts such as dioctyl sodium sulfosuccinate (Colace). Mineral oil is generally not recommended because safer, more effective agents are available. The newer agents lower surface tension, allowing water to enter the stool more readily. They are generally well tolerated and may be particularly useful in bedbound elderly patients who are at risk for fecal impaction.

C. The saline laxatives: The saline laxatives and enemas are salts of magnesium and sodium. Those in most common use are oral milk of magnesia, oral magnesium citrate, and sodium phosphate (Fleet's enema). All of these agents function as hyperosmolar agents and cause net secretion of fluid into the colon. Colonic motility is increased by these agents via release of the hormone cholecystokinin. Chronic use of magnesium-containing saline laxatives in elderly patients may contribute to hypermagnesemia (especially when there is associated impaired renal function). The phosphate-containing preparations may also induce hypocalcemia when high doses are used. The phosphate-containing enemas may cause damage to the rectum; this may occur via the nozzle part of the instrument itself, or a direct toxic effect exerted by the hypertonic saline on the rectal mucosa.

D. The hyperosmolar laxatives: hyperosmolar laxatives such as lactulose draw water into the gut lumen by an osmotic action. Lactulose is an undigestible agent that is metabolized by bacteria to hydrogen and organic acids. This causes acidification of the colon, and this, in addition to its osmotic effect, may alter electrolyte transport and colonic mobility.

E. The stimulant laxatives: the stimulant laxatives include the anthraquinone derivatives cascara, senna, and aloe; phenophalein; and bisacodyl (Ducolax) tablets.

Complications of the stimulant laxatives include the following: from the anthraquinone group, melanosis coli, and from the phenophalein group, complications such as Stevens-Johnson syndrome, dermatitis, and photosensitivity reactions. Although bisacodyl tablets probably are safer than the rest of the stimulant laxatives, all of the agents can cause electrolyte imbalance and precipitate hypokalemia, fluid and salt overload, and diarrhea. Thus the stimulant laxatives are the laxatives most closely associated with long-term side effects.

F. The lavage laxatives: The newest group of laxatives are known as the lavage laxatives. They include the agents Golytely and Colyte. They work by stimulating neither secretion nor motility but by passing unimpeded through the GI tract. They are the most commonly used agents for bowel preparation prior to flexible sigmoidoscopy and colonoscopy.

12. E.

13. E.

14. E.

15. E. In this patient the increasing and different abdominal pain was caused by constipation. This patient had actually not had a bowel movement for 34 days. Thus the increasing severe abdominal pain (due to increasing doses of morphine) completely overshadowed his previous pain (the pain due to metastatic bone disease).

   The physical examination maneuver of choice in this patient is a digital rectal examination to confirm impacted stool.

   The investigation of choice is a KUB to confirm stool throughout the colon.

   Remember, constipation is the single most common cause of abdominal pain in the elderly.

   In the patient described the problem was treated by manual disimpaction, tap water enemas, and lactulose.

Treating Patients with Narcotic Analgesics

1. Start a bowel regimen at the same time as you start the narcotic.
2. Maintain the bowel regimen for as long as you maintain the patient on the narcotic.

SOLUTION TO SHORT ANSWER MANAGEMENT PROBLEM 124

The drug classes and their most common offenders are as follows:

DRUG CLASS	MOST COMMON OFFENDER
Antihypertensives	Verapamil
Antianginal agents	Verapamil
Medical diagnostic agent	Barium sulfate
Antacids	Aluminum hydroxide
Nutritional supplement	Iron
Narcotic analgesics	Codeine
Antipsychotics	Thioridazine
Antidepressants	Amitriptyline
Anticholinergics	Trihexyphenidyl
Cheap osteoporosis therapy	Calcium carbonate (TUMS)

SUMMARY OF THE DIAGNOSIS AND TREATMENT OF CONSTIPATION IN THE ELDERLY

1. **Prevalence of constipation:** the reported prevalence of constipation in the elderly is 30%.

2. **Definition:** constipation is usually defined as fewer than three bowel movements/week.

3. **Etiology of constipation:** the etiology of constipation includes declined or impaired general health status in the elder, increasing number of medications (remember verapamil), and diminished mobility and physical activity.

4. **Diagnosis and investigation:** the patient's complete medical history is the most important part of the evaluation (remember to include complete functional inquiry of the GI tract). Digital rectal examination is the most importat part of the physical examination; anoscopy should accompany DRE. DRE and anoscopy may detect fissures, fistulas, strictures, carcinoma, or hemorrhoids.

5. **Complications:** the complications of constipation in the elderly include the following:
   a) Fecal impaction/crampy abdominal and back pain/ and overflow diarrhea
   b) Stercoral ulcers
   c) Anal fissures/anal fistulas
   d) Hemorrhoids (internal and external)
   e) Megacolon
   f) Sigmoid volvulus
   g) Risk factor for carcinoma of the colon

6. **Treatment:**
   a) Nonpharmacologic:
      1. Bowel training
      2. Exercise
      3. High-fiber diet
      4. Increased fluid intake
   b) Pharmacologic: the laxatives:
      1. Bulk laxatives: recommended
      2. Emollient laxatives
         i) Mineral oil: not recommended
         ii) Colace: recommended
      3. Saline laxatives and enemas: not recommended on long-term basis
      4. Hyperosmolar laxatives: recommended
      5. Stimulant laxatives: not recommended

7. **Golden rule summary section:**
   1. Always ask yourself the question, "why?" Why is the patient constipated? Constipation is not part of the normal aging process.
   2. Cancer is a common diagnosis in elderly patients. Most elderly patients with cancer will eventually require a narcotic analgesic. When that time comes, always start a constipation-correcting bowel regime at the same time.

SUGGESTED READING

Cheskin L, Schuster M. Constipation. In: Hazzard WR et al., eds. Principles of geriatric medicine and gerontology. 3rd Ed. New York: McGraw-Hill, 1994.

PROBLEM 125 AN 81-YEAR-OLD MALE WITH INCREASING CONFUSION AND SHORTNESS OF BREATH

A previously healthy 81-year-old male is brought to the ER by his daughter. He lives by himself. He was well until 3 days ago. At that time, he became somewhat confused and began wandering aimlessly around the house and muttering incoherently.

For the last 3 days he has had both nausea and anorexia. In addition, he became short of breath last night.

On physical examination his BP is 100/70 mm Hg. His pulse is 96 and regular. His respiratory rate is 28/minute and his respirations appear slightly labored. On auscultation of his lung fields there are a few rales bilaterally but no other abnormalities.

His WBC is 11,000/mm³. His CXR reveals right lower lobe consolidation. His P_{O_2} is 65 mm Hg and his P_{CO_2} is 40 mm Hg.

SELECT THE ONE BEST ANSWER TO THE FOLLOWING QUESTIONS

1. What is the most likely diagnosis in this patient?
   a) bacterial pneumonia
   b) viral pneumonia
   c) fungal pneumonia
   d) aspiration pneumonia
   e) obstructive pneumonia

2. What is the most likely pathogen in this patient's pneumonia?
   a) *Klebsiella pneumoniae*
   b) *Haemophilus influenzae*
   c) influenza type B
   d) *E. coli*
   e) *Streptococcus pneumoniae*

3. A presentation with almost identical symptoms and signs occurs in an 84-year-old female who is currently residing in a long-term care facility and who has many chronic medical conditions.

   When comparing her presentation to the presentation of the patient just described, which of the following statements is true?
   a) the prognosis is likely to be similar in both individuals
   b) the responsible organism is likely to be the same
   c) the treatment is likely to be the same
   d) all of the above
   e) none of the above

4. What is the treatment of choice for the patient described in Question 1?
   a) amoxicillin
   b) trimethoprim-sulfamethoxazole
   c) gentamicin
   d) cefixime
   e) amphotericin B

5. Which of the following is(are) risk factors for the development of urinary tract infections in elderly patients?
   a) advanced age
   b) decreased bladder emptying
   c) prostatic hypertrophy
   d) decreased host defense mechanisms
   e) all of the above

6. What is the most common pathogen in urinary tract infections in noncatheterized elderly patients?
   a) *Serratia*
   b) *Proteus mirabilis*
   c) *Klebsiella*
   d) *E. coli*
   e) *Pseudomonas aeruginosa*

7. An 81-year-old female presents with a 5-day history of dysuria, frequency, urgency, and incontinence. She has no other symptoms, including no CVA tenderness or other symptoms.

   The patient lives at home by herself and has had no major medical problems.

   On examination, her temperature is 37° C. Her blood pressure is 150/80 mm Hg and her pulse is 84 and regular. No other abnormalities are found on physical examination.

   Which of the following statements concerning this patient is(are) true?
   a) the most likely diagnosis is acute bacterial cystitis
   b) the most likely organism is *Pseudomonas aeruginosa*
   c) ciprofloxacin is a reasonable first-choice antibiotic
   d) this patient should be treated for 14 days
   e) all of the above statements are true

8. Concerning chronic prostatitis in elderly patients, which of the following statements is(are) true?
   a) chronic prostatitis is the most common cause of relapsing urinary tract infections in elderly males
   b) prostatic massage is not helpful in establishing a diagnosis
   c) *Klebsiella* is the most common pathogen in this condition
   d) with prolonged therapy relapse becomes unlikely
   e) all of the above statements are true

9. A 75-year-old female presents with a 2-day history of fever, chills, confusion, dysuria, and diarrhea. There are no other symptoms, including no back pain.

On examination, the patient's temperature is 38.5° C. Her blood pressure is 120/75 mm Hg, and her pulse is 96 and regular. There is no demonstrable CVA tenderness.

What is the most likely diagnosis in this patient?
a) acute bacterial cystitis
b) viral gastroenteritis
c) acute pyelonephritis
d) bacterial gastroenteritis
e) none of the above

10. Regarding the use of antibiotics in elderly patients with indwelling catheters, which of the following statements is(are) true?
a) indwelling urinary catheters are the leading cause of nosocomial infections
b) indwelling urinary catheters are the most common predisposing factor in hospital-acquired fatal gram-negative sepsis
c) by the time a urinary catheter has been in place for 2 weeks, 50% of catheterized patients have significant bacteriuria
d) all of the above
e) none of the above

11. What is the leading cause of death due to infection in hospitalized elderly patients?
a) bacterial pneumonia
b) urinary tract infection
c) pressure ulcers
d) diverticulitis
e) septic arthritis

12. What is the leading cause of death due to infection in institutionalized elderly patients?
a) bacterial pneumonia
b) urinary tract infection
c) pressure ulcers
d) diverticulitis
e) septic arthritis

13. What is the leading cause of death due to infection in elderly individuals living in the community?
a) bacterial pneumonia
b) urinary tract infection
c) pressure ulcers
d) diverticulitis
e) septic arthritis

14. In considering acute appendicitis in elderly patients, which of the following statements is(are) true?
a) the presenting signs and symptoms are similar to younger patients
b) gangrene of the appendix is uncommon
c) morbidity and mortality are much higher than in younger patients
d) all of the above
e) none of the above

15. Which of the following statements concerning tuberculosis in elderly patients is(are) true?
a) 25%-50% of all cases of TB occur in the elderly
b) the incidence of tuberculosis in the United States is increasing
c) 60% of deaths from tuberculosis occur in patients over the age of 65 years
d) all of the above
e) none of the above

16. Which of the following statements concerning fever in elderly patients is(are) true?
a) fever in elderly patients is more likely to be due to serious pathology than in younger patients
b) when compared to younger patients, older adults often fail to show a temperature elevation despite having a serious infectious disease
c) in elderly patients with fever of undetermined origin (FUO), a localized infection (such as an abscess) is often found
d) all of the above are true
e) none of the above are true

Short Answer Management Problem 125

Consider the following functional states or levels of care in elderly patients and the following primary considerations in infectious or inflammatory disease. Fill in the three most common primary infectious diseases in each group, in order of frequency.

For example, the most common infectious disease in independent healthy elderly individuals living in the community might be acute appendicitis.

1. Independent healthy elderly individuals living in the community:
    1. _____
    2. _____
    3. _____
2. Hospitalized elderly patients:
    1. _____
    2. _____
    3. _____
3. Elderly nursing home residents:
    1. _____
    2. _____
    3. _____

Primary considerations in infectious diseases in the elderly:

1. Bacterial pneumonia
2. Urinary tract infection
3. Intraabdominal infection
    a) Cholecystitis
    b) Diverticulitis
    c) Appendicitis
    d) Surgical wound infections

ANSWERS

1. A. The most likely diagnosis in this patient is a bacterial pneumonia.

   The presentation of bacterial pneumonia in elderly patients is usually much more subtle and nonspecific than in younger patients. As illustrated in this case presentation, confusion is a very common early sign. Other nonspecific early signs include disorientation and a change (decrease) in the elder's interest level. As in this patient, a fall is often part of the presenting symptoms and signs of elder infectious illness.

   Findings on physical examination are also nonspecific. Signs of consolidation are often absent. Rales are common, but not very specific. An increased respiratory rate (as in this patient) may precede other signs and symptoms.

   The specificity of laboratory abnormalities found in elders with bacterial pneumonia is low. An increased white blood cell count (WBC > 10,000 mm³) is commonly found, but as well as being nonspecific the WBC also suffers from low specificity. Hypoxemia is a common finding. In elderly patients with bacterial pneumonia, the correlation between clinical findings and radiologic findings is poor.

2. D. The most likely pathogen associated with community-acquired pneumonia is *Streptococcus pneumoniae*. *Haemophilus influenzae, Klebsiella pneumoniae,* and gram-negative bacilli are much less common unless there is associated COPD or other immune-compromising condition.

   In summary, the difference between younger adults and older adults in community-acquired bacterial pneumonia is that *Streptococcus pneumoniae* is the responsible organism in 60% to 80% of younger patients but only 40% to 60% of elderly patients.

3. E. The most important differences between the two presentations are as follows:
   1. Patient 1: the patient presented in the case presentation resides in the community. Patient 2: the patient presented in Question 3 resides in a long-term care facility.
   2. Patient 1 is otherwise healthy and has no significant medical problems. Patient 2 has many other chronic health problems.
   3. The organism in patient 1 is likely to be the commonest cause of bacterial community-acquired pneumonia. The organism in patient 2 is likely to

be a pathogen that attacks patients with some form of immune compromise. The most likely candidates in patient 2 would be *Haemophilus influenzae, Klebsiella pneumoniae,* or another gram-negative organism such as *E. coli* or *Enterococcus.*

4. Because the organisms in patients 1 and 2 are likely to be different, so are the treatments.

5. The virulence of the organism on the host in patient 2 is likely to be significantly greater than the virulence of the organism in patient 1. Thus the prognosis in patient 2 is significantly less favorable than the prognosis in patient 1.

4. D. The treatment of choice for a community-acquired bacterial pneumonia in an elderly patient is an agent that is active against beta-lactamase-producing organisms. Of the drugs listed, cefixime, a second-generation oral cephalosporin, would probably be the best choice. Amoxicillin-clavulinic acid would be an excellent alternative.

In summary, the difference between younger adults and older adults with respect to therapy for community-acquired pneumonia, is that the treatment of choice for community-acquired pneumonia in younger adults is penicillin g or ampicillin. In older adults, a beta-lactamase agent should be used.

5. E. Urinary tract infections in the elderly are second only to respiratory tract infections as causes of febrile illness in patients over the age of 65 years. The risk factors for urinary tract infections in the elderly include the following:
A. Advanced age: the older the patient, the greater the risk (this appears to be immune-system dependent).
B. Decreased functional ability: resulting from cardiovascular accidents, dementia, neurologic deficits, functional ability, and other chronic underlying illness
C. Decreased bladder emptying: results from neurogenic bladder, bladder-outlet obstruction (such as prostatic hypertrophy), and drugs with anticholinergic side effects
D. Nosocomial spread of organisms: spread from hospitalized patients with asymptomatic bacteriuria, the use of indwelling urinary catheters
E. Physiologic changes: decreased vaginal glycogen and increased vaginal pH in women, decreased prostatic secretions and increased prostatic calculi in men

6. D. The most common organism responsible for urinary tract infections in elderly patients who do not have indwelling urinary catheters is *E. coli.* Other gram-negative organisms responsible include *Klebsiella, Enterococcus, Pseudomonas* and *Proteus mirabilis.* However, in the absence of a complication (such as an indwelling catheter), *E. coli* still predominates

In summary, the difference between younger adults and older adults with respect to etiology of uncompli-

cated urinary tract infections is that although *E. coli* is the most common agent in both younger adults and older patients, the percentage of infections due to *E. coli* is lower in older patients; that is, in older patients with an acute uncomplicated urinary tract infection there is more of a chance of an infection due to *Klebsiella, Enterococcus, Proteus mirabilis* and *Pseudomonas.*

7. A. Regarding this case presentation, the following facts can be stated:
A. This appears to be an uncomplicated urinary tract infection.
B. The most likely infecting organism is *E. coli.* As well, the following organisms must also be considered: *Klebsiella, Proteus mirabilis,* and *Pseudomonas aeruginosa.*
C. The most likely diagnosis is acute bacterial cystitis. Acute bacterial cystitis is confirmed when there are no signs or symptoms of upper urinary tract infection, and the bacterial count is greater than 10^5 organisms per milliliter of urine. The most common symptoms encountered in acute bacterial cystitis are lower abdominal and/or pelvic pain, dysuria, increased frequency of urination, and recent episodes of urinary incontinence.
D. First-line drugs in this case would be trimethoprim-sulfamethoxazole and ampicillin. Ampicillin would, in the absence of contraindications, probably be the first choice. A cephalosporin would also be reasonable first-line therapy. Although treatment with a single dose of ampicillin is reasonable for younger adults, it cannot be recommended for the elderly. For elders in the same situation, a 7-day course (250 mg qid) would be the best choice.

8. A. Chronic bacterial prostatitis is the most common cause of relapsing urinary tract infection in elderly males.

The diagnosis of chronic bacterial prostatitis is established by culturing prostatic secretions obtained by prostatic massage.

The most common causative organism is *E. coli. Klebsiella pneumoniae, Proteus,* and *Enterococci sp.* are other organisms associated with the condition.

The preferred antibiotic treatment is trimethoprim-sulfamethoxazole or a quinolone antibiotic such as ciprofloxacin or norfloxacin. Relapses are common, even with prolonged therapy.

This condition may be ameliorated by transurethral resection of the prostate (TURP).

In summary, the difference between younger adult males and older adult males with respect to prostatitis is that acute bacterial prostatitis is much more common in younger males, and chronic bacterial prostatitis is much more common in older patients.

9. C. This patient has acute pyelonephritis. Elderly patients who develop a syndrome of fever, chills, and irritating

voiding symptoms likely have acute pyelonephritis in spite of the absence of CVA tenderness. In fact, not more than one-half of elders who develop pyelonephritis have the back pain and CVA tenderness so classic in younger patients with the disease (such as cough). Some elders do not even have fever. Geriatric patients also often present with GI symptoms such as diarrhea or pulmonary symptoms.

Bacteremia is much more common in elderly patients who develop pyelonephritis, and the urinary tract is the source of bacteremia in over one-third of elders admitted to hospital with generalized sepsis. Thus blood cultures are mandatory before initiating treatment. From sepsis follows septic shock in up to 20% of elders with acute pyelonephritis.

As with lower urinary tract infections, the most common organisms involved are *E. coli, Klebsiella, Proteus,* and *Pseudomonas.*

For elderly patients, the best initial antibiotic choice for suspected pyelonephritis is a combination of a beta-lactamase-resistant cephalosporin and an aminoglycoside (the latter to be used with extreme caution and with careful monitoring of serum levels).

In summary, the difference between younger adults and elderly patients with respect to complicated urinary tract infections such as acute pyelonephritis is that older patients frequently do not manifest the same symptoms and signs of complicated urinary tract infections as do younger adults. Specifically, they are less likely to manifest CVA tenderness and even fever and chills. This infection must be suspected in elderly patients who are immune compromised and incapacitated (hospitalized patients and long-term care facility patients).

In addition, the probability of septicemia/generalized sepsis is greatly increased in elderly patients who develop urinary tract infections.

10. D. By 2 weeks 50% of catheterized patients have significant bacteriuria, and after 1 month virtually all patients do.

Indwelling urinary catheters are the leading cause of nosocomial infection and the most common predisposing factor in hospital-acquired gram-negative sepsis.

Patients who have asymptomatic bacteriuria should not be treated with antibiotics. This applies to catheterized patients as well.

11. B.

12. A.

13. A. The leading infective causes of morbidity and mortality in elderly patients vary depending on location of the elder's habitation.

In elderly patients living in the community and long-term care facilities, the most common cause of death from an infective source is bacterial pneumonia. This serves to illustrate the importance of preventive services designated for this age group. The United States Task Force on the Periodic Health Examination recommends the following:

1. All individuals over the age of 65 years should receive annual influenza vaccinations.
2. All individuals over the age of 65 years should receive the pneumovax vaccination once.

Although we discuss bacterial pneumonia as the primary cause of morbidity and mortality, we have to understand that viral pneumonia frequently predates bacterial pneumonia (that is, influenza produces a viral pneumonia that leads to a secondary bacterial pneumonia).

In the hospitalized elder, the most common cause of morbidity and mortality is septicemia from a urinary tract infection.

14. C. Acute appendicitis is primarily a disease of younger patients in the second and third decades of life. However, it also occurs with increasing frequency in males over the age of 80 years. The mortality in this age group is 10%.

As with other abdominal infections such as acute cholecystitis, the increased severity of disease is largely due to the atypical presentation of the signs and symptoms of acute inflammation (or more appropriately the lack of signs and symptoms of acute inflammation). Instead of the classic time sequence of periumbilical pain; anorexia, nausea, and vomiting; and movement of the pain to the right lower quadrant seen in younger patients, the elderly male with acute appendicitis usually presents with a prolonged period of vague abdominal discomfort. There may be mild nausea and anorexia, but vomiting is unusual. As localized peritonitis develops, pain may appear in the right lower quadrant. Rebound tenderness and abdominal guarding, so common in younger adults, are very uncommon in the elderly.

Perforation of the appendix is much more common in the elderly because of the narrowing of the lumen and the atherosclerotic changes in the artery supplying the appendix. In elderly patients, approximately 70% of cases of acute appendicitis rupture, compared to 20% in younger patients.

In summary, critical differences between younger adults and older adults with appendicitis are that the elderly present with atypical symptoms, have a very high rate of perforation, and have a high mortality rate (10%).

15. D. The incidence of tuberculosis is on the rise in the United States. Tuberculosis in the elderly is a particular problem because of decreased immune function in general and a relative decrease in the ability to resist the spread of infection. Between 25% and 50% of all new cases of TB in the United States occur in elderly patients

(age > 65 years). As well, over 60% of total deaths from TB and complications of TB occur in patients over the age of 65 years.

In summary, the difference between younger adults and older adults with tuberculosis is that elders have a relatively depressed immune system and are less likely to be able to contain the TB bacillus into a localized area, and this relatively depressed immune system is also responsible for the relatively high percentage of new cases in elders (50%) and the higher mortality rate (60% of deaths from TB in the United States are in elders).

16. D. In children and in young and middle-aged adults, fever is often due to a relatively benign disease. Such is not the case with the elderly. The rapid development of an elevated body temperature in an older adult is almost invariably due to a serious infection such as pneumonia, urinary tract infection, or an intraabdominal abscess.

Although the presence of fever in an older adult usually indicates a serious infection or other serious disease process (such as neoplasia and connective tissue disorders), elderly patients are two to three times as likely to demonstrate a lack of febrile to the presence of serious disease.

In older adults who present with fever of undetermined origin (FUO), the probability of a localized infection such as an abscess is high.

In summary, elders with a fever usually have a serious rather than a benign disease process going on. Always take this seriously.

SOLUTION TO SHORT ANSWER MANAGEMENT PROBLEM 125

Primary considerations in infectious diseases in the elderly depending on the habitation status of the elder are as follows:
A. Elders living in a community setting:
   Primary considerations:
   1. Bacterial pneumonia
   2. Urinary tract infections
   3. Intraabdominal infections
      a) Cholecystitis
      b) Diverticulitis
      c) Appendicitis
   Secondary considerations should include the following:
   1. Infectious endocarditis
   2. Tuberculosis
   3. Septic arthritis
   4. Meningitis
B. Hospitalized elders:
   Primary considerations:
   1. Urinary tract infections
   2. Bacterial pneumonia
   3. Surgical wound infections
   Secondary considerations should include the following:
   1. Septic thrombophlebitis
   2. Drug reactions
   3. Pulmonary emboli
   4. Hepatitis
C. Nursing home or other institutionalized elders:
   Primary considerations:
   1. Bacterial pneumonia
   2. Urinary tract infection
   3. Decubitus ulcers
   Secondary considerations should include the following:
   1. Tuberculosis
   2. Drug reactions
   3. Intraabdominal infections
   4. Gastroenteritis

Because of the summaries provided throughout the answers, a detailed summary will not be repeated for this chapter.

SUGGESTED READING

Yoshikawa TT. Approach to the diagnosis and treatment of the infected older adult. In: Hazzard WR et al., eds. Principles of geriatric medicine and gerontology. 3rd Ed. New York: McGraw-Hill, 1994.

PROBLEM 126   AN 88-YEAR-OLD INSTITUTIONALIZED FEMALE WITH URINARY INCONTINENCE

An 88-year-old female patient whom you care for and who resides in a chronic care facility is having increasing difficulties with "bedwetting." She is very embarrassed to talk about this, but the nurses inform you that it is a problem and is getting progressively worse.

On your last weekly visit, the charge nurse requested permission from you to insert an indwelling urinary catheter. At that time, the patient had been incontinent continuously for 6 days. The charge nurse clearly tells you, "I haven't got enough staff to keep changing sheets 10 times a day—please do something."

SELECT THE ONE BEST ANSWER TO THE FOLLOWING QUESTIONS

1. At this time, what should your instructions to the charge nurse be?
   a) insert the indwelling catheter; call me if there are any more problems
   b) begin intermittent 4-hour catheterization to avoid the necessity of inserting an indwelling catheter
   c) wait and see what happens over the next couple of weeks
   d) order some routine blood work to attempt to determine the cause of the problem
   e) clearly indicate that you will begin investigation of this problem now; ask the charge nurse, in return, to attempt to manage the current situation for only a short time longer

2. Regarding urinary incontinence in the elderly, which of the following statements is false?
   a) 50% of elderly patients in nursing homes have established urinary incontinence
   b) 5%-15% of elderly patients in a community setting have developed urinary continence
   c) women are twice as likely as men to have urinary incontinence
   d) humiliation and embarrassment are significant life problems for the patient with urinary incontinence
   e) none of the above statements are false

3. What is the most common type of urinary incontinence in elderly patients?
   a) urge incontinence
   b) stress incontinence
   c) complex incontinence
   d) overflow incontinence
   e) functional incontinence

4. Which of the following statements regarding incontinence in the elderly is(are) true?
   a) stress incontinence is usually manifested by loss of small amounts of urine with intraabdominal pressure increases
   b) overflow incontinence occurs through bladder distention
   c) prostatic obstruction is a common cause of overflow incontinence

   d) functional incontinence is characterized by an involuntary loss of urine despite normal bladder and urethral functioning
   e) all of the above are true

5. Which of the following is(are) contributing factors to urinary incontinence in the elderly?
   a) a loss of the ability of the elderly to concentrate urine
   b) a decreased bladder capacity
   c) decreased urethral closing pressure
   d) decreased mobility
   e) all of the above

6. Which of the following classes of drugs has not been implicated in the pathogenesis of urinary incontinence in the elderly?
   a) thiazide diuretics
   b) neuroleptics
   c) sedatives
   d) antibiotics
   e) hypnotics

7. Which of the following nonpharmacologic treatments may be effective in the management of urinary incontinence in the elderly?
   a) Kegel's exercises
   b) biofeedback
   c) behavioral toilet training
   d) clean intermittent catheterization
   e) all of the above

8. Which of the following cause acute (reversible) urinary incontinence in the elderly?
   a) delirium
   b) restricted mobility
   c) infection
   d) drugs
   e) all of the above

9. Anticholinergic and narcotic drugs are most commonly associated with which of the following types of urinary incontinence?
   a) urge incontinence
   b) stress incontinence
   c) overflow incontinence
   d) complex incontinence
   e) functional incontinence

10. Which of the following components of the diagnostic evaluation of urinary incontinence is not necessary in every elderly patient with the disorder?
    a) complete history
    b) focused physical examination
    c) renal ultrasound
    d) complete urinalysis
    e) postvoiding residual urine determination (PVR)

11. A postvoiding residual urine (PVR) is considered definitely abnormal when it exceeds which of the following?
    a) 50 mL
    b) 200 mL
    c) 75 mL
    d) 100 mL
    e) 150 mL

12. What is(are) the drug(s) of choice for the pharmacologic management of stress incontinence?
    a) supplemental estrogen
    b) alpha-adrenergic agonists
    c) cholinergic agents
    d) a and b
    e) all of the above

13. Which of the following types of urinary incontinence is most amenable to surgical intervention?
    a) urge incontinence
    b) stress incontinence
    c) overflow incontinence
    d) complex incontinence
    e) functional incontinence

14. Which of the following are indications for the use of a chronic indwelling catheter in elderly patients with incontinence?
    a) urinary retention causing persistent overflow incontinence
    b) chronic skin wounds or pressure ulcers that can be contaminated by incontinent urine
    c) terminally ill or severely impaired elderly patients for whom bed and clothing changes are uncomfortable
    d) urinary retention that cannot be controlled medically or surgically
    e) none of the above
    f) all of the above

15. Alzheimer's disease, Parkinson's disease, and cerebrovascular disease are usually associated with which of the following types of urinary incontinence?
    a) urge incontinence
    b) stress incontinence
    c) overflow incontinence
    d) complex incontinence
    e) functional incontinence

Short Answer Management Problem 126

List the patient-dependent (four) and caregiver-dependent (two) behaviorally oriented training procedures that may be beneficial in the management of urinary incontinence in the elderly.

ANSWERS

1. E. In an elderly patient who has just become incontinent, it is inappropriate to insert a Foley catheter or do anything else until you have established the cause. The pathophysiology of urinary incontinence in the elderly population is complex, even among patients with dementia. Elderly patients deserve the same intensive investigation of incontinence etiology as you would perform in a younger individual.

2. E. Fifty percent of elderly patients in nursing homes, and 5% to 15% of elderly patients in the community, have urinary incontinence.

   Women are twice as likely as men to develop urinary incontinence.

   Humiliation and embarrassment are important consequences of urinary incontinence in elderly patients.

This embarrassment leads to social isolation and subsequent anxiety and depression. Incontinence is the second leading cause of admission of elderly patients to long-term care facilities.

   In North America it is estimated that the total health care costs associated with urinary incontinence are over $8 billion per year.

   Physical consequences, such as predisposition to skin irritations and subsequent skin ulcers and infections, are also a major problem.

3. A. The most common type of urinary incontinence in the elderly population is urge incontinence. Urge incontinence (also known as detrusor hyperreflexia) is characterized by leakage of urine due to strong and sudden sensations of bladder urgency. Patients with urge incontinence may also experience frequency, urgency, and nocturia. Urge incontinence is also called unstable blad-

der, uninhibited bladder, and hyperreflexic bladder. Many conditions may predispose to urge incontinence; these include cerebrovascular accidents, Parkinson's disease, Alzheimer's disease, spinal cord injury or tumor, multiple sclerosis, prostatic hypertrophy, and interstitial cystitis.

Urge incontinence may also be present in patients in whom no neurologic or genitourinary abnormality is present.

4. E. Stress incontinence (urethral incompetence) is characterized by loss of small amounts of urine secondary to increases in intraabdominal pressure.

Stress incontinence is most commonly associated with pelvic floor weakening through childbirth, obesity, injury, menopause and aging, and sphincter damage.

Overflow incontinence occurs with bladder overdistention. Overdistention results in a constant leakage of small amounts of urine or "dribbling," a physiologic situation in which the intracystic pressure exceeds the intraurethral resistance. Bladder overdistention is usually caused by an enlarged prostate, urethral stricture, or fecal impaction. A hypotonic bladder secondary to diabetes mellitus, syphilis, spinal cord compression, or anticholinergic medications may also result in overflow incontinence.

Complex incontinence refers to incontinence that has both urge and stress components.

Functional incontinence refers to involuntary loss of urine despite normal bladder and urethral functioning. This is most commonly seen with severe dementia and closed head injuries.

5. E. Many factors are associated with the development and maintenance of urinary incontinence in the elderly. These include a loss of the ability of the kidney to concentrate urine, a decreased bladder capacity, decreased urethral closing pressure following menopause, decreased mobility, decreased vision, depression and secondary inattention to bladder cues, and an inadequate environmental setting.

The importance of drugs in the causation of elderly incontinence is discussed in a subsequent question.

6. D. Drugs are a very common cause of elder incontinence. The major drugs that have been implicated in the pathogenesis and causation of urinary incontinence in the elderly include the following:

DRUG CLASS	MANIFESTATIONS OF CONTINENCE
1. Diuretics	Polyuria, frequency, urgency
2. Anticholinergics	Urinary retention, overflow incontinence, impaction
3. Antidepressants	Anticholinergic actions, sedation
4. Antipsychotics	Anticholinergic actions, sedation, rigidity, immobility
5. Sedative-hypnotics	Sedation, delirium, immobility, muscle relaxation
6. Narcotic analgesics	Urinary retention, fecal impaction, sedation, delirium
7. Alpha-adrenergic blockers	Urethral relaxation
8. Alpha-adrenergic agonists	Urinary retention
9. Beta-adrenergic blockers	Urinary retention
10. Calcium-channel blockers	Urinary retention
11. Alcohol	Polyuria, frequency, urgency, sedation, delirium, immobility

7. E. Nonpharmacologic treatments are both very available and very useful in the treatment of all forms of urinary incontinence in the elderly. The treatments include the following:
    I. Stress incontinence:
        A. Pelvic muscle (Kegel) exercises
        B. Biofeedback
        C. Behavioral therapies: prompted voiding, habit training, and scheduled toileting
        D. Transcutaneous electrical nerve stimulation (TENS)
    II. Urge incontinence:
        A. Biofeedback
        B. Behavioral therapies (as just listed)
        C. Transcutaneous electrical nerve stimulation (TENS)
    III. Overflow incontinence:
        A. Intermittent catheterization
        B. Indwelling catheterization (if no other options possible)
    IV. Functional incontinence:
        A. Behavioral therapies (as just listed)
        B. Environmental manipulations
        C. Incontinence undergarments and pads
        D. External collection devices
        E. Indwelling catheters (if necessary)
        F. Transcutaneous electrical nerve stimulation (TENS)

In the past, transcutaneous electrical nerve stimulation (TENS) has been used successfully to treat chronic pain syndromes. An exciting new development provides us with another opportunity to avoid both surgery and pharmacologic agents in treatment of incontinence. The use of a pessary TENS unit has recently been shown to be effective for stress incontinence and urge incontinence. More trials need to be carried out before definitive conclusions can be made, but initial results are promising.

8. E. Causes of acute and reversible forms of urinary incontinence are provided by the following mnemonic: DRIP.
    1. Delirium
    2. Restricted mobility, retention
    3. Infection (urinary tract), inflammation (urethritis or atrophic vaginitis), impaction (fecal)
    4. Polyuria (diabetes mellitus, diabetes insipidus, congestive heart failure, and venous insufficiency), pharmaceuticals

9. C. Urinary retention with overflow incontinence must be considered when any patient, who was previously completely continent, suddenly becomes incontinent. The causes include the following:
    A. Immobility
    B. Anticholinergic drugs
    C. Narcotic analgesic drugs
    D. Calcium-channel blockers
    E. Beta blockers
    F. Fecal impaction
    G. Spinal cord compression resulting from metastatic cancer

10. C. The evaluation of urinary incontinence in the elderly should be undertaken with the same precision and care as evaluation and investigation of other urinary problems in younger patients.

    All elderly patients who present with urinary incontinence should have the following procedures performed:
    A. A complete history
    B. A complete medication review (ideally, every elderly patient on more than one drug should have this done every 3 months)
    C. An age-specific focused physical examination (U.S. Preventive Services Task Force)
    D. A complete urinalysis
    E. A urine culture
    F. A postvoiding residual (PVR) urine determination

    A renal ultrasound need only be done if you suspect problems such as urinary obstruction (a renal tumor), uremia, or the inability of the kidneys to concentrate urine.

11. B. A postvoiding residual urine should be performed on every elderly patient with incontinence to exclude significant degrees of urinary retention. Neither the history nor the physical examination is sensitive or specific enough for this purpose in elderly patients. The postvoiding residual urine can be done either by itself as a simple one-test procedure or in conjunction with other simple urodynamic investigations.

    To maximize the accuracy of PVR, the measurement should be performed within a few minutes of voiding. A postvoiding residual volume of 100 mL or less in the absence of straining reflects adequate bladder emptying in elderly patients; a PVR value of > 200 mL, on the other hand, is definitely abnormal.

12. D. The ideal combination of pharmacologic agents for certain patients with stress incontinence involves supplemental estrogen and an alpha-adrenergic agonist.

    For patients with stress incontinence, pharmacologic management is appropriate if:
    1. The patient is motivated.
    2. The degree of stress incontinence is "mild to moderate."

3. There is no major associated anatomical abnormality (such as a large cystocele).
4. The patient does not have any contraindications to the use of these drugs.

    Pharmacologic treatment of stress incontinence is as efficacious as but not more efficacious than non-pharmacologic treatment. Approximately 75% of patients improve with each. Combining the two modalities improves the efficacy of treatment.

    Supplemental estrogen has not been found, by itself, to be as effective as when used in combination with an alpha-adrenergic agonist. If either oral or vaginal estrogen is used for a prolonged period of time (greater than a few months), then cyclic progesterone should be added to protect the endometrium. A combination of oral premarin (0.3 mg/day) plus oral pseudo-ephedrine (Sudafed) 30-60 mg tid would be a good starting point for pharmacologic treatment of stress incontinence.

13. B. The type of incontinence that is most amenable to surgical intervention is stress incontinence. The indication for surgery in stress incontinence is continued significant bothersome leakage that occurs after attempts at nonsurgical treatment and patients who, along with their stress incontinence, also have a significant degree of pelvic prolapse.

    The second most amenable subtype of incontinence that may be significantly improved with surgery is outflow obstruction caused by prostatic hypertrophy or prostatic carcinoma in men. With benign prostatic hypertrophy it would be prudent to reduce the size of the prostate and decrease obstruction by use of a 5-alpha-reductase inhibitor before contemplating surgery.

14. F. The indications for chronic indwelling catheter use include the following:
    A. Urinary retention
        i) That is causing persistent overflow incontinence
        ii) That is causing symptomatic infections
        iii) That is producing renal dysfunction
        iv) That cannot be corrected surgically or medically
        v) That cannot be managed practically with intermittent catheterization
    B. Skin wounds, pressure sores, or irritations that are being contaminated by incontinent urine
    C. Care of terminally ill or severely impaired patients for whom bed and clothing changes are uncomfortable and/or disruptive
    D. Preference of patient or caregiver when a patient has failed to respond to more specific treatments

15. A. Central nervous system disorders such as cerebrovascular accidents (stroke), dementia, Parkinson's disease, and suprasacral spinal cord injury are associated with detrusor motor and/or sensory instability.

SOLUTION TO SHORT ANSWER MANAGEMENT PROBLEM 126

Following are examples of behaviorally oriented training procedures for urinary incontinence.

I. Patient dependent:
   A. Pelvic muscle (Kegel) exercises
   B. Biofeedback
   C. Behavioral training
   D. Bladder retraining
II. Caregiver dependent:
   A. Scheduled toileting or prompted voiding
   B. Habit training

SUMMARY OF THE DIAGNOSIS AND MANAGEMENT OF URINARY INCONTINENCE IN THE ELDERLY

1. **Definition:** the involuntary loss of urine in sufficient amount or frequency to be a social and/or health problem
2. **Subtypes of urinary incontinence:** acute (reversible) versus persistent urinary incontinence
3. **Acute (reversible) urinary incontinence:**
   DRIP mnemonic:
   D = Delirium
   R = Restricted mobility, retention
   I = Infection, inflammation, impaction
   P = Polyuria, pharmaceuticals
4. **Persistent urinary incontinence:**
   S = Stress: involuntary loss of urine (usually small amounts) with increases in intraabdominal pressure (such as cough, laugh, or exercise)
      Common causes: weakness and laxity of pelvic floor musculature and bladder outlet or urethral sphincter weakness
   U = Urge: leakage of urine (often larger volumes, but variable) because of inability to delay voiding after sensation or bladder fullness is perceived; also known as detrusor hyperreflexia
      Common causes: detrusor motor/and or sensory instability, isolated or associated with one or more of the following: cystitis, urethritis, tumors, stones, diverticula, or outflow obstruction; also central nervous system disorders such as stroke, dementia, Parkinson's disease, and suprasacral spinal cord injury.
   O = Overflow: leakage of urine (usually small amounts) resulting from mechanical forces on an overdistended bladder or from other effects of urinary retention on either bladder and/or sphincter function
      Common causes: anatomic obstruction by prostate, stricture, and cystocele; hypotonic bladder associated with diabetes mellitus or a spinal cord injury; neurogenic (detrusor-sphincter dyssynergy) associated with multiple sclerosis or supraspinal cord lesions
   F = Functional: urinary leakage associated with the inability to toilet due to impairment of cognitive and/or physical functioning, psychological unwillingness, or environmental barriers
      Common causes: severe dementia and other neurological disorders, or psychological factors such as depression, regression, anger, and hostility
5. **Prevalence of urinary incontinence in the elderly:**
   a) Institutionalized elderly: 50%
   b) Elderly patients living in the community: 5%-15%
6. **Investigations:**
   a) Basic investigations for all elderly patients with urinary incontinence:
      1. Complete history
      2. Complete physical examination
      3. Complete medication review (every 3 months)
      4. Complete urinalysis
      5. Urine for culture and sensitivity
      6. Postvoiding residual urine determination
7. **Primary treatments for different types of geriatric urinary incontinence:**
   a) Stress incontinence:
      1. Pelvic muscle (Kegel) exercises
      2. Alpha-adrenergic agonists
      3. Supplemental estrogen (oral or vaginal)
      4. Biofeedback, behavioral training
      5. Surgical bladder neck suspension
      6. Periurethral injections
   b) Urge incontinence:
      1. Bladder relaxants
      2. Estrogen (if vaginal atrophy present)
      3. Behavioral procedures (such as biofeedback and behavioral therapy)
      4. Surgical removal of obstructing or other irritating pathologic lesions
   c) Overflow incontinence:
      1. Surgical removal of obstruction
      2. Intermittent catheterization (if practical)
      3. Indwelling catheterization
   d) Functional incontinence:
      1. Behavioral therapies (such as prompted voiding, habit training, or scheduled toileting)
      2. Environmental manipulations
      3. Incontinence undergarments and pads
      4. External collection devices
      5. Bladder relaxants (selected patients)
      6. Indwelling catheters (selected patients)

SUGGESTED READING

Ouslander JG: Incontinence. In: Hazzard WR et al., eds. Principles of geriatric medicine and gerontology. 3rd Ed. New York: McGraw-Hill, 1994.

PROBLEM 127   AN 85-YEAR-OLD FEMALE NURSING HOME RESIDENT WHO SIMPLY "STARES INTO SPACE" AND CRIES ALMOST ALL OF THE TIME

You are called to see an 85-year-old patient who moved into a nursing home 9 months ago. Previously, she was living on her own and had managed by herself since the death of her husband 6 years ago. During the past year she has become increasingly disabled with congestive heart failure and osteoarthritis.

During the past 9 months the patient has lost 15 lb, has not been hungry, has lost interest in all of her social activities, and has been crying almost every day.

You are aware that prior to moving into the nursing home she was quite active.

Her mental status examination is difficult. She does, however, describe her mood as being worse in the morning. Her short-term memory, according to the staff, is also impaired. She is currently taking furosemide and enalapril for her congestive heart failure and plain acetaminophen for the pain associated with osteoarthritis.

SELECT THE ONE BEST ANSWER TO THE FOLLOWING QUESTIONS

1. What is the most likely diagnosis in this patient?
   a) major depressive illness
   b) Alzheimer's disease
   c) multi-infarct dementia
   d) hypothyroidism
   e) none of the above

2. Regarding the diagnosis of the patient described, which of the following statements is(are) false?
   a) this condition occurs less often in older patients than in younger patients
   b) elderly patients are less likely to recover from this illness than younger adults
   c) this condition is more common among institutionalized elders than elders living at home
   d) this condition may be related to physical illness
   e) this condition may be related to the move into the nursing home itself

3. Which of the following investigations and/or assessments should be performed in the patient described?
   a) a medication review
   b) a CBC
   c) a serum TSH
   d) all of the above
   e) none of the above

4. Which of the following antidepressants is considered an agent of first choice for the treatment of depression in the elderly?
   a) imipramine
   b) nortriptyline
   c) desipramine
   d) amitriptyline
   e) fluoxetine

5. Which of the following antidepressants specifically blocks serotonin reuptake?
   a) imipramine
   b) desipramine

   c) nortriptyline
   d) amitriptyline
   e) fluoxetine

6. You decide to treat the patient described on nortriptyline. In a patient of this age, at what daily dosage would you start?
   a) 10 mg
   b) 25 mg
   c) 50 mg
   d) 75 mg
   e) 100 mg

7. Regarding the treatment for the condition described, which of the following statements is(are) true?
   a) ECT (electroconvulsive therapy) is unlikely to be of any benefit in the treatment of this condition
   b) socialization, music therapy, and pet therapy have no role to play in the treatment of this condition
   c) cognitive and behavioral therapy may significantly improve this condition
   d) all of the above
   e) none of the above

8. Which of the following features is most commonly associated with this diagnosis in geriatric patients?
   a) acute mania
   b) hypomania
   c) extreme anxiety
   d) psychomotor agitation or retardation
   e) hypersomnia

9. The signs and symptoms of the condition described include all except which of the following?
   a) impaired concentration
   b) guilt
   c) hopelessness
   d) suicidal ideation
   e) violent or aggressive behavior

10. The length of time recommended for the pharmacologic treatment of this condition with the drug selected is at least
   a) 1 month

b) 3 months
c) 6 months
d) 12 months
e) 18 months

11. An elderly institutionalized patient is put on nortriptyline. The dose is increased up to 100 mg but no improvement is noted. You decide to substitute fluoxetine. Which of the following side effects might you anticipate?
a) constipation
b) blurred vision

c) urinary retention
d) dry mouth
e) agitation

12. If the side effect selected in Question 11 occurred, which of the following courses of action would be the most reasonable?
a) increase the dose of the drug
b) decrease the dose of the drug
c) stop the drug
d) elect ECT as your next option
e) c and d

Short Answer Management Problem 127

PART A: Discuss the differential diagnosis of depressive symptoms in the elderly.

PART B: List the three most common physical illnesses that present or manifest depression in the elderly.

PART C: Name the most common drug associated with depression in the elderly.

PART D: Name the most common drug class associated with depression as a psychoactive substance use disorder.

ANSWERS

1. A. This patient has a major depressive illness. The criteria for major depressive illness are summarized in another section of this book. A mnemonic that is very helpful for diagnosing depression is A SIG = E CAPS:
   A = Affect—at least a 2-week period of a depressed mood or a depressed affect
   S = Sleep disturbance (hyposomnia, insomnia, hypersomnia)
   I = Interest (lack of interest of life)
   G = Guilt or hopelessness
   E = Energy level (decreased) or fatigue
   C = Concentration decreased
   A = Appetite disturbance (decreased or increased) plus/minus weight gain or weight loss
   P = Psychomotor retardation or agitation
   S = Suicidal ideation

   Major depressive illness is diagnosed when there are 4/8 criteria present plus at least a 2-week period of a depressed mood or depressed affect.

   Despite these criteria, depression in elderly patients is more likely to present with weight loss and less likely to present with feelings of worthlessness and guilt. Elderly patients are no more likely than persons in midlife to report cognitive problems, although they do have more difficulties with cognition during an episode of depression.

   The other choices listed in this question are discussed in other sections of this book.

2. B. Elderly patients are just as likely to recover from a major depressive illness as are younger adults.

   Major depression is less prevalent among those aged 65 and older than in younger groups. Suicide, however is not; it continues to rise in elderly patients at a rather alarming rate.

   The prevalence of major depression in elderly patients in the community is between 1% and 2%. The majority of depressed elderly patients, however, do not fit the DSM-IV criteria but rather have depressive symptoms that are associated with an adjustment reaction (as in this patient who has just had to leave her own home) or that are associated with significant physical illness (as this patient also demonstrates).

   In chronic long-term care facilities, the prevalence of major depressive illness may be as high as 10%-20%.

3. D. The elderly patient who presents with depressive symptoms should have the following evaluation: a complete history, a complete physical examination, and a complete medication review (both prescribed and OTC medications). Some of the most common pharmacologic agents that contribute to depression include antihypertensive agents such as propranolol and methyldopa as well as cimetidine and sedative hypnotic drugs.

   In addition to the complete history and P/E the elderly patient should also have the following laboratory investigations: CBC, vitamin B_{12}, serum folate level, serum TSH, CXR, ECG, complete urinalysis, and serum electrolytes.

4. B. Nortriptyline is the tricyclic of choice in treating geriatric depression because of its relatively low risks of orthostatic hypotension (low alpha blockade) and low anticholinergic side effects (dry mouth, urinary retention, blurred vision, constipation, and sedation). As well, it has a high therapeutic window.

The serotonin reuptake inhibitors such as fluoxetine are not yet considered the drugs of first choice in elderly patients, even though they may well be the agents of first choice in younger patients. As well, some of these agents, especially fluoxetine, actually increase the probability of or state of agitation in the elderly.

5. E. The new group of antidepressant agents known as selective serotonin reuptake inhibitors (SSRIs) include fluoxetine (Prozac), sertraline (Zoloft), and paroxetine (Paxil). These drugs, as indicated, are not the agents of first choice for the treatment of depression in the elderly. They do, however, offer some significant theoretical advantages in that the common tricyclic antidepressants side effects such as dry mouth, blurred vision, tachycardia, constipation (anticholinergic), orthostatic hypotension (alpha-adrenergic blockade), and weight gain may be averted by their use. As well, they do not increase the cardiac risk due to blockade of impulse conduction through the AV node.

As experience is gained with the selective serotonin reuptake inhibitors in younger patients, they may very well "move up the ladder" and become drugs of first choice for treating depression in the elderly.

6. A. The patient described in this case, an 80-year-old female, should be started on as low a dose of tricyclic as possible. A dose of 10 mg would be an ideal starting dose. This dose could be increased slowly as needed (suggested at 25% per week).

7. C. Elderly patients with depressive illness may be significantly improved with cognitive or behavioral psychotherapy.

Attempts at increased socialization (especially in chronic care facilities), music therapy, pet therapy, and other therapies that serve to redirect the attention of the elderly patient appear to be very effective in the treatment of depression in the elderly.

Electroconvulsive therapy (ECT) may be the only effective therapy for severe depression in elderly patients, especially in patients with psychotic depression. ECT is well tolerated in geriatric patients and lacks the side effects associated with the tricyclic antidepressants.

8. D. Although acute mania, hypomania, extreme anxiety, and hypersomnia may all be associated with depression in elderly patients, by far the most common symptom of those listed in elderly patients is psychomotor agitation or retardation. Psychomotor agitation is the more common presentation of the two.

9. E. The diagnostic symptoms of depressive illness have been covered in the answer to Question 1. They do not include violent or aggressive behavior. If violent or aggressive behavior is found in a patient who has an underlying depression, there is likely another major diagnosis that would explain the symptom. In an elder the most common diagnosis in this case would be Alzheimer's disease.

10. C. Geriatric patients should be treated with antidepressants for at least 6 months. After 6 months, if the patient is improved the drug can be tapered and eventually discontinued.

11. E.

12. E. The side effects of blurred vision, dry mouth, urinary retention, and constipation are all anticholinergic side effects that do not occur with the new SSRI agents. Agitation, however, is a side effect that may be anticipated with these drugs, especially with fluoxetine. The most reasonable course of action would be to discontinue the drug and to use ECT. Two failed drug courses (with drugs of different classes) would be a very reasonable indication for the use of ECT.

SOLUTION TO SHORT ANSWER MANAGEMENT PROBLEM 127

PART A: The differential diagnosis of depressive symptoms in the elderly is lengthy. It includes four major categories: mood disorders, adjustment disorders, psychoactive substance-use disorders, and somatoform disorders.

I. Mood disorders:
   1. Major depression (single episode or recurrent)
   2. Dysthymia (or depressive neurosis)
   3. Bipolar affective disorder, depressed
   4. Depressive disorder NOS (atypical depression with mild biogenic depression)
II. Adjustment disorders:
   1. Primary degenerative dementia with associated depression
   2. Organic mood disorder, depressed
   3. Secondary to physical illness:
      a) hypothyroidism
      b) carcinoma of the pancreas
      c) stroke
      d) Parkinson's disease
   4. Secondary to pharmacologic agents: methyldopa, propranolol
III. Psychoactive substance-use disorders:
   1. Alcohol use and/or dependence
   2. Sedative, hypnotic, or anxiolytic abuse and/or dependence

IV. Somatoform disorders:
1. Hypochondriasis
2. Somatization disorder

PART B: The three most common physical illnesses that present or manifest depression in the elderly are hypothyroidism, carcinoma of the pancreas, and cerebrovascular accident (stroke).

PART C: The most common drug associated with depression in the elderly is propranolol.

PART D: The most common drug class associated with depression as a psychoactive substance-use class is the drug class that includes all of the sedative-hypnotics.

Sedatives and hypnotics are vastly overused in the elderly; this appears to be especially true in institutionalized elderly. It is much easier for nursing home staff to prescribe a sedative/hypnotic or both than to recognize and help an elder adjust to altered sleep patterns.

SUMMARY AND DIAGNOSIS OF DEPRESSION IN THE ELDERLY

1. **Diagnosis:** follow DSM-IV criteria, except recognize that the elderly are more likely to present with weight loss and cognitive problems and less likely to present with feelings of guilt and hopelessness.
2. Recognize that depression is often an adjustment reaction to life stress, environment change (especially having to leave home), and the realization of the effects of aging itself.
3. **Prevalence:** 1%-2% in community environment; 10-20% in institutional environment
4. **Differential diagnosis:** includes mood disorders, adjustment disorders, organic mental disorders, psychoactive substance-use, and somatoform disorders

5. **Investigations:** include mini-mental status examination; complete medication review; and laboratory evaluation including CBC, electrolytes, TSH, vitamin B_{12}, serum folate, ECG, and CXR
6. **Treatment strategies:**
   a) Nonpharmacologic strategies:
      1. Relaxation techniques and mind-occupying techniques such as frequent visitors, pet therapy, and music therapy
      2. Cognitive, supportive, and behavioral psychotherapy
   b) Pharmacologic strategies:
      1. Drugs of first choice: tricyclics
         i) Drug of choice: nortriptyline
         ii) Starting dosage of choice: 10 mg
      2. Drugs of second choice: SSRIs
         i) Use fluoxetine with caution because of potential side effect of agitation.
      3. Drugs of third choice: MAO A inhibitors
      4. ECT: if two drug classes fail, ECT should be considered. ECT has much more of a role to play in geriatric depression than it does in depression associated with younger patients.
      5. Most importantly, depression in the elderly must not be treated with pharmacologic agents only; treatment should, instead, include an equal contribution from nonpharmacologic treatments and pharmacologic agents.

SUGGESTED READING

Blazer D. Depression. In: Hazzard WR et al., eds. Principles of geriatric medicine and gerontology. 3rd Ed. New York: McGraw-Hill, 1994.

PROBLEM 128 AN 80-YEAR-OLD FEMALE NURSING HOME RESIDENT WITH A PRESSURE ULCER

You are called to a nursing home to see an 80-year-old female with a fever of 40°C. The patient is disoriented and confused. The nursing home staff has had difficulty treating her pressure ulcers, especially one on her sacrum.

On physical examination, the patient's blood pressure is 110/80 mm Hg and her pulse is 72 and regular. There is a large 10 cm by 5 cm pressure ulcer present on her sacrum. As well, from that ulcer there is a purulent, foul-smelling discharge.

SELECT THE ONE BEST ANSWER TO THE FOLLOWING QUESTIONS

1. Which of the following diseases/conditions is(are) risk factors for the development of pressure ulcers?
   a) immobility
   b) dementia
   c) Parkinson's disease
   d) congestive heart failure
   e) a, b, and c
   f) all of the above

2. Which of the following nutritional/physiologic variables increase the risk of pressure ulcers?
   a) hypoalbuminemia
   b) dry skin
   c) decreased blood pressure
   d) a and b
   e) all of the above

3. Regarding the pathophysiology of pressure ulcers, which of the following factors has(have) been implicated in their cause?
   a) the pressure of the body weight itself
   b) shearing forces
   c) friction
   d) moisture
   e) a, b, and d
   f) all of the above

4. Which of the following statements concerning the prevention and etiology of pressure ulcers is false?
   a) pressure ulcers are impossible to prevent in immobilized elderly patients
   b) good nutrition in the elderly will help prevent pressure ulcers
   c) anemia in the elderly patient predisposes to the formation of pressure ulcers
   d) incontinence in the elderly increases the risk of pressure ulcers by a factor of five
   e) patients who sit for long periods of time are just as likely to develop pressure ulcers as bedridden patients

5. Concerning the patient described, what amount of time would it take the large ulcer to develop from a small, untreated ulcer?
   a) > 28 days
   b) 21-28 days

c) 14-20 days
   d) 7-10 days
   e) 1-2 days

6. Which of the following anatomic sites is the least common site for the development of a pressure ulcer?
   a) the ischial tuberosity
   b) the lateral malleolus
   c) the medial malleolus
   d) the sacrum
   e) the greater trochanter

7. With respect to pathophysiology, which of the following factors contributes to the formation of pressure ulcers?
   a) blood and lymphatic vessel obstruction
   b) plasma leakage into the interstitial space
   c) hemorrhage
   d) bacterial deposition at the site of the pressure-induced injury
   e) muscle cell death
   f) all of the above

8. Which of the following statements concerning pressure ulcers and mortality in elderly patients is(are) true?
   a) there appears to be no increase in mortality among elderly individuals who develop pressure ulcers
   b) failure of a pressure ulcer to heal or improve has not been associated with a higher death rate in institutionalized elderly
   c) in-hospital death rates for patients with pressure ulcers range from 23% to 36%
   d) all of the above
   e) none of the above

9. Patients at high risk for the development of pressure ulcers should be repositioned how frequently?
   a) every 2 hours
   b) every 4 hours
   c) every 6 hours
   d) every 8 hours
   e) every 12 hours

10. What are the best initial antibiotic treatments for an infected pressure ulcer?
    a) tetracycline and gentamicin
    b) clindamycin and gentamicin
    c) cephalexin and doxycycline

d) penicillin and gentamicin
e) trimethoprim and sulfamethoxazole

11. Which of the following descriptions best illustrates the nature of bacteria usually found in an infected pressure ulcer?
    a) gram-positive aerobic cocci alone
    b) gram-negative aerobic rods alone
    c) anaerobic bacteria alone
    d) a and c
    e) all of the above

12. What is the most common and serious complication of pressure ulcers in elderly patients?
    a) anemia
    b) hypoproteinemia
    c) infection
    d) contracture
    e) bone resorption

13. Bacterial sepsis leading to septic shock in pressure ulcers is most closely associated with which of the following bacteria?
    a) *Bacteroides fragilis*
    b) *Pseudomonas aeruginosa*
    c) *Proteus mirabilis*
    d) *Staphylococcus aureus*
    e) *Providencia* spp.

14. A 78-year-old immobilized male is seen with a small 1-cm area of erythema and bruising on his left heel. Which of the following is the most important aspect of the treatment of this pressure ulcer at this time?
    a) application of a full-thickness skin graft
    b) extensive debridement of the area and cleansing with an iodine-based solution
    c) application of a foam pad to protect the heel from further damage
    d) application of microscopic beaded dextran to the lesion
    e) elevation of the left leg by 30 degrees

15. Which of the following statements concerning the use of pressure-reducing devices in the prevention and treatment of pressure ulcers is(are) true?
    a) with the proper use of pressure-reducing devices, all pressure ulcers can be prevented
    b) there is consensus regarding the pressure-reducing devices of first choice
    c) sheepskin can be considered a pressure-reducing device of first choice

d) there appears to be little difference between the products indicated for the prevention and treatment of pressure ulcers
    e) none of the above are true

16. Which of the following factors have been associated with a more favorable outcome in the prevention and treatment of pressure ulcers?
    a) educational programs for health professionals
    b) educational programs for families and caregivers
    c) multidisciplinary health care
    d) b and c
    e) all of the above

17. Concerning local wound care in superficial pressure ulcers, which of the following is(are) acceptable for cleaning the ulcer and disinfecting the ulcer?
    a) povidone-iodine
    b) hydrogen peroxide
    c) hypochlorite solutions
    d) all of the above
    e) none of the above

18. Which of the following pressure-reducing devices should not be used for the prevention and treatment of pressure ulcers?
    a) an air-fluidized bed
    b) a sheepskin mattress
    c) a conventional foam pad
    d) an air mattress
    e) a water mattress

19. The debridement of moist, exudative wounds originating from the formation of pressure ulcers may be augmented by the use of which of the following?
    a) hydrophilic polymers
    b) enzymatic agents
    c) acetic acid
    d) a and b
    e) all of the above

20. Which of the following statements concerning the use of occlusive dressings for treating pressure ulcers is(are) true?
    a) hydrocolloid dressings and transparent films improve the healing rate of superficial pressure ulcers
    b) hydrocolloid has proven to be effective in treating deep pressure ulcers as well as superficial pressure ulcers
    c) hydrocolloid dressings and transparent films may remain in place for several days
    d) a and c only
    e) all of the above

Short Answer Management Problem 128

Pressure ulcers can be classified into four stages dependent on the degree of thickness of penetration of the epidermis and deeper tissues. As the therapy varies depending on the stage of the ulcer, it is important to understand the difference between the four stages. Provide the definitions of stages I, II, III, and IV pressure ulcers.

ANSWERS

1. F.

2. E. Risk factors for pressure ulcers include the following:
   A. Any disease process leading to immobility and limited activity levels, such as a spinal cord injury, dementia, Parkinson's disease, severe congestive heart failure, and COPD.
   B. Other factors including urinary incontinence and nutritional factors, such as a decreased lymphocyte count, hypoalbuminemia, inadequate dietary intake, decreased body weight, and a depleted triceps skin fold thickness
   C. Potential risk factors identified in prospective studies include dry skin, increased body temperature, decreased blood pressure, increased age, and an altered level of consciousness.

3. F. The pathophysiology of pressure ulcers include the interaction of all of the following:
   A. Pressure: contact pressures of 60 to 70 mm Hg for 1 to 2 hours lead to degeneration of muscle fibers. Repeated exposures to pressure will cause skin necrosis at lower pressures.
   B. Shearing forces: shearing forces are tangential forces that are exerted when a person is seated, or the head of the bed is elevated and the person slides toward the floor or the foot of the bed. Shearing forces lower the amount of pressure required to cause damage to the epidermis.
   C. Friction: friction has been shown to cause intra-epidermal blisters.
      When unroofed, these lesions result in superficial erosions. This kind of injury can occur when a patient is pulled across a sheet or when the patient has repetitive movements that expose a bony prominence to such frictional forces.
   D. Moisture: intermediate degrees of moisture increase the amount of friction produced by the rubbing interface, whereas extremes of moisture or dryness decrease the frictional forces between the two surfaces rubbing against each other.

4. A. Pressure ulcers are not impossible to prevent in immobilized elderly patients. It is true that it is difficult to prevent all pressure ulcers, but many of those that do develop in immobilized elderly patients are, in fact, preventable.
   Good nutrition in elderly patients will help prevent pressure ulcers.
   Anemia and incontinence are predisposing factors to the development of pressure ulcers.
   Elderly patients who sit for long periods of time are just as likely to develop pressure ulcers as bedridden patients.

5. E. Erythema may progress to ulceration quickly. A small ulcer can progress to a large ulcer within 24-48 hours. The progression is due to local edema and/or infection, the former being the most important factor. As in the patient described in the case history, severe infection can lead to septicemia, which must be recognized and treated with appropriate systemic antibiotic therapy.

6. C. The most common sites for pressure ulcers to develop are as follows:
   A. The sacrum
   B. The trochanters
   C. The heels
   D. The lateral malleoli
   E. The buttocks over the ischium
   The least common site of those listed for the formation of pressure ulcers is the medial malleoli.

7. F. The ultimate chain of pathophysiologic events involved in the formation of pressure ulcers are as follows:
   A. Ischemia associated with the occlusion of blood and lymphatic vessels
   B. As plasma leaks into the interstitium, diffusing substances between the cellular elements of skin and blood vessels increase.
   C. Ultimately hemorrhage occurs and leads to non-blanchable erythema of the skin.
   D. Bacteria are deposited at sites of pressure-induced injury and set up a deep suppurative process.
   E. The accumulation of edema fluid, blood, inflammatory cells, toxic wastes, and bacteria ultimately and progressively lead to the death of muscle, subcutaneous tissue, and finally epidermal tissue.
   F. The damage caused by shearing forces probably is mediated by pressure-induced ischemia in deep tissues as well as by direct mechanical injury to the subcutaneous tissue.

8. D. Increased death rates have been consistently observed in elderly patients who develop pressure ulcers. In addition, failure of an ulcer to heal or improve has been associated with a higher rate of death in nursing home residents. In-hospital death rates for patients with pressure ulcers range from 23% to 36%. Most of these deaths are in debilitated patients; in many cases it is difficult to separate what contribution the actual pressure ulcer makes to the process.

9. A. Data support the recommendation that high-risk patients should be repositioned every 2 hours to prevent pressure ulcers from forming and minimizing the size, thickness, and infectivity rate of pressure ulcers that have already formed.

10. B.

11. E. Infected pressure ulcers are usually associated with the following organisms: *Pseudomonas aeruginosa, Providencia, Proteus* spp., *Staphylococcus aureus,* and anaerobic bacteria (particularly *Bacteroides fragilis*). The best combination of antibiotics, therefore, is one that will treat gram-positive aerobic cocci (present in 39% of isolates), gram-negative aerobic rods, and aerobic bacteria.

One realizes the risk of using a powerful agent such as gentamicin in a debilitated elder; on the other hand, the debilitated elder has most likely by that time acquired a very serious bacteremia/septicemia.

12. C. Sepsis is the most common and most serious complication of pressure ulcers in elderly patients. Contraction and bone resorption are also complications of pressure ulcers.

Anemia and hypoproteinemia are risk factors for the formation of pressure ulcers.

13. A. With respect to infection, bacteremia, septicemia and death:
A. Most infected pressure ulcers are polymicrobial.
B. Most infected polymicrobial pressure ulcers have *Bacteroides fragilis* as one of the major organisms involved.
C. Infected pressure ulcers also lead to other infectious complications, such as bacterial cellulitis, osteomyelitis, and septic arthritis.

14. C. The very short time interval between the formation of a small area of erythema and a true pressure ulcer has already been described.

The single most important therapy at this time in this patient is to try and protect the patient's heel from progressing to any further stage of damage. This is best done by using a foam pad or other piece of protective apparatus.

15. B. Regarding the formation of pressure ulcers, the prevention of pressure ulcers, and the pressure-reducing devices available, the following facts have emerged:
A. Despite nurses' best efforts, the use of proper positioning alone is not sufficient to prevent all pressure ulcers. Even with pressure-reducing devices, this is not always possible.
B. The use of water mattresses or alternating air mattresses decreased the incidence of pressure ulcers by 50% compared with the conventional hospital mattresses.
C. Although sheepskin products are very popular, it has been demonstrated that sheepskins and 2-inch convoluted foam pad products do not have the capability of decreasing pressure enough to eliminate the risk of cutaneous injury.
D. The following have been demonstrated to have superior efficacy in preventing pressure ulcers: a foam, a static air mattress, an alternating air mattress, a gel, or a water mattress. In addition, the use of air-fluidized and low-air-loss beds are recommended.

16. E. Several studies have demonstrated a significant decrease in pressure-ulcer incidence after an educational program and a multidisciplinary team approach to the problem of pressure ulcers. Such educational programs should be directed at all levels of health care professionals, patients, and family and caregivers.

17. E. Topical antiseptics such as hypochlorite solutions, povidone-iodine, acetic acid, and hydrogen peroxide should be avoided in cleaning and debriding a pressure ulcer because of the potential of these compounds for inhibiting wound healing. The preferred alternative is normal saline.

18. B. A sheepskin mattress should not be used for the prevention and treatment of pressure ulcers. See the critique in Question 15 for further details.

19. D. The debridement of moist, exudative wounds may be augmented by using hydrophilic polymers such as dextranomer. Enzymatic agents such as collagenase, fibrinolysin, deoxyribonuclease, streptokinase, and streptodornase may be helpful in aiding debridement.

20. D. Once an ulcer is clean and granulation or epithelialization begins to occur, then a moist wound environment should be maintained without disturbing the healing tissue. Superficial lesions heal by migration of epithelial cells from the borders of an ulcer; deep lesions heal as granulation tissue fills the base of the wound. Controlled studies have shown that the use of occlusive dressing such as transparent films and hydrocolloid dressings improves healing of stage 2 pressure ulcers. These dressings remain in place for several days and

allow a layer of serous exudate to form underneath the dressing. This facilitates the further migration of epithelial cells. Although these dressings have not been shown to improve the effective healing rate of deep ulcers, they do reduce the nursing time needed for treatment.

Clean stage 3 and clean stage 4 uclers should be dressed with a gauze dressing kept moistened with normal saline. Moist dressings should be kept off surrounding skin to avoid macerating normal tissues. Unless there are symptoms or signs of infection, these dressings can stay in place for several days.

SOLUTION TO SHORT ANSWER MANAGEMENT PROBLEM 128

The classification of pressure ulcers in elderly patients is as follows:

1. Stage I: stage I pressure ulcers present as nonblanchable erythema of intact skin.
2. Stage II: stage II pressure ulcers involve partial thickness skin loss involving the epidermis and/or the dermis.
3. Stage III: stage III pressure ulcers extend from the subcutaneous tissues to the deep fascia and typically show undermining.
4. Stage IV: stage IV pressure ulcers involve muscle and/or bone. Full-thickness injury is often manifested by eschar frequently involving muscle and bone but cannot be staged until the eschar is removed.

SUMMARY OF THE DIAGNOSIS AND TREATMENT OF PRESSURE ULCERS

1. **Terminology:**
   a) The term *pressure ulcer* is the preferred term at this time.
   b) Previous terms included the following:
      1. Decubitus ulcers
      2. Bedsores
      3. Pressure sores
2. **Prevalence:**
   a) The prevalence of stage II and greater pressure ulcers among patients in acute care hospitals ranges from 3% to 11%.
   b) Among patients expected to be hospitalized and confined to bed or chair for at least 1 week, the prevalence of stage II and greater pressure ulcers is as high as 28%.
   c) The prevalence of pressure ulcers in nursing homes is very similar to that reported in acute care hospitals. As many as 20% to 33% of patients admitted to nursing homes have stage II or greater pressure ulcers.
3. **Complications:**
   a) Sepsis is the most serious complication of pressure ulcers.
   b) Other complications include local infections, cellulitis, and osteomyelitis. As well, infected pressure ulcers may be deeply undermined and lead to pyoarthritis or penetrate into the abdominal cavity and cause peritonitis or secondary amyloidosis. Infected pressure ulcers lead to nosocomial reservoirs for antibiotic-resistant bacteria.
   c) Pressure ulcer infections have the following characteristics:
      1. They are polymicrobial.
      2. Gram-positive aerobic cocci, gram-negative aerobic rods, and aerobic bacteria are the most common organisms found.
      3. Specific organisms commonly found include the following:
         i. *Pseudomonas aeruginosa*
         ii. *Providencia* spp.
         iii. *Proteus* spp.
         iv. *Staphylococcus aureus*
         v. *Bacteroides fragilis*
4. **Mortality:**
   a) Failure of a pressure ulcer to heal is associated with a higher rate of death in nursing home residents.
   b) In-hospital death rates for patients with pressure ulcers range from 23% to 36%. Most of these deaths are patients with severe underlying disease.
5. **Risk factors:**
   a) Disease processes leading to immobility/reduced activity
   b) Spinal cord injury
   c) Dementias
   d) Parkinson's disease
   e) Congestive cardiac failure
   f) Incontinence
   g) Nutritional factors: inadequate intake of protein, vitamins, minerals, calcium, or calories leading to cachexia, hypoalbuminemia, decreased body weight, and decreased triceps skin fold thickness
6. **Pathophysiology:** four factors have been implicated in the pathogenesis of pressure ulcers:
   a) Pressure
   b) Shearing forces
   c) Friction
   d) Moisture
7. **Pathophysiologic series of events in pressure-ulcer formation:**
   1. Pressure on tissues overlying bone prominence
   2. Ischemia produced by occlusion of blood vessels and lymphatic vessels
   3. Endothelial cell swelling and vessel leak
   4. Plasma leakage into the interstitium
   5. Increased distance between cellular elements of skin and blood vessels
   6. Hemorrhage
   7. Nonblanchable erythema of the skin
   8. Continued accumulation of edema fluid, blood, inflammatory cells, toxic wastes, and bacteria
   9. Death of muscle, subcutaneous tissue, and epidermal skin

8. **Prevention of pressure ulcers:**
   a) Formal risk assessment: a formal "risk assessment" for the development of pressure ulcers should be done on all patients.
   b) Frequent repositioning:
      1. Patients at highest risk should be repositioned every 2 hours.
      2. Lower risk patients should be repositioned two to four times/day.
   c) Technique of repositioning: repositioning should be performed so that a person at risk is repositioned without pressure on vulnerable bony prominences. Most of these sites are avoided by positioning patients with the back at a 30-degree angle to the support surface, alternatively from the right to left sides and the supine positions.
   d) Pressure reducing devices:
      1. Although sheepskins and 2-inch convoluted foam pads are very popular, they do not have the capability to decrease pressure enough to eliminate risk of cutaneous injury.
      2. Preferred devices include a foam doughnut, static air mattresses, alternating air mattresses, gel mattresses, and water mattresses
      3. Lifting devices or bed linen movement (not bed linen drag) will minimize friction and shear-induced injuries during transfers and position changes.

9. **Education:**
   a) There is a significant decrease in pressure ulcer incidence after an educational program and a multidisciplinary team approach to the problem of pressure ulcers is implemented.
   b) Educational interventions should be targeted to all levels of health care providers, patients, families, and caregivers.

10. **Assessment of patients with pressure ulcers:**
    a) Appropriate assessment and treatment of underlying diseases and conditions that have put the person at risk for developing pressure ulcers
    b) Nutritional assessment is of particular importance.
    c) Assessment of associated infections (as discussed)

11. **Treatment of pressure ulcers:**
    a) Systemic treatment:
       1. Vitamin C 500 mg bid (84% reduction in pressure ulcer surface area on this vitamin)
       2. Drug combination of choice: clindamycin plus gentamicin; monitor and watch renal function extremely carefully while the patient is on gentamicin.
       3. Air-fluidized bed therapy is much of an improvement over the conventional bed.
    b) Local wound care:
       1. Normal saline is agent of choice for cleaning and gentile debridement. Avoid povidone-iodine, hypochlorite, mild acetic acid, and hydrogen peroxide.
       2. Surgical debridement is augmented with wet-to-dry dressings using normal saline.
       3. The debridement of moist, exudative lesions is facilitated by using hydrophilic polymers such as dextranomer. Enzymatic agents should be used only until the ulcer bed becomes clean.
       4. Once clean and granulation or epithelialization begins to occur, a moist wound environment should be maintained. Occlusive dressings and hydrocolloid dressings improve healing rates for stage II ulcers. Stage II and stage IV ulcers should be dressed with a gauze soaked in normal saline.
       5. Surgical therapies should be used to remove necrotic tissue that cannot be removed any other way and that if not removed will cause septicemia and death. Surgical flaps (a more elective procedure) should be carefully considered, especially on debilitated, cachetic patients.

SUGGESTED READING

Allman R. Pressure ulcers. In: Hazzard WR et al., eds. Principles of geriatric medicine and gerontology. 3rd Ed. New York: McGraw-Hill, 1994.

PROBLEM 129 A 75-YEAR-OLD FEMALE WITH A BAGFUL OF PILLS

A 75-year-old female presents to your office with her daughter. Her daughter describes her mother as having undergone "a marked personality change." Apparently, her elderly mother began seeing "pink rats coming out of the wall" and she began "hearing and seeing people from outer space" floating down into her field of vision.

The patient's daughter brings in her mother's medications in a bag. She describes a visit to her mother's physician 1 week ago. At that time the doctor prescribed a number of medications including pills for her blood pressure, pills for her heart, pills for her arthritis, pills for her stomach, pills for her anxiety, pills for her depression, and pills for her insomnia.

On further questioning the daughter states that her mother had been fairly well before the physician visit but had (unfortunately) mentioned "a few minor ailments." In response to the patient's complaints the physician prescribed the following: hydrochlorothiazide, propranolol, nifedipine, digoxin, ibuprofen, cimetidine, Maalox, amitriptyline, and traizolam.

You are well aware of the fact that medications in the elderly can often produce significant side effects. You conclude that there is a connection between the pink rats, the space men, and the pills.

On examination, the patient is agitated and confused. She points to the ceiling and yells "pink rats, spacemen, pink rats, spacemen."

Her blood pressure is 100/70 mm Hg and her pulse is 54 and regular. She has a bruise on her head from a fall 3 days ago.

Examination of the cardiovascular system reveals a normal S1 and S2 with a grade VI systolic murmur heard along the left sternal edge.

There are no other abnormalities on physical examination.

SELECT THE ONE BEST ANSWER TO THE FOLLOWING QUESTIONS

1. Which of the following statements regarding this patient's acute medical problem is(are) true?
   a) this patient's problem is unlikely to be related to her medications
   b) this patient's presentation is unusual following the initiation of medications in the elderly
   c) this patient's problem is unlikely to lead to hospitalization
   d) this patient's problem is likely to be transient
   e) none of the above statements are true

2. Which of the following statements regarding the use of drugs in the elderly is(are) true?
   a) elderly patients should be treated the same way as younger patients with respect to drug initiation
   b) elderly patients generally need the same dose of medications as younger patients
   c) psychotropic drugs are unlikely to produce significant side effects in elderly patients
   d) elderly patients on multiple medications should be reassessed on a yearly basis
   e) none of the above are true

3. Regarding elderly patients in chronic care facilities, which of the following statements regarding medication use is(are) true?
   a) elderly patients in chronic care facilities are usually on fewer medications than elderly patients living on their own
   b) elderly patients in chronic care facilities are usually on between 12 and 20 different medications at any one time

   c) elderly patients in chronic care facilities are more likely than not to experience iatrogenic side effects from medications at one time or another
   d) b and c
   e) all of the above are true

4. An 85-year-old female patient of yours was placed on a combination of hydrochlorothiazide and clonidine because of a "dangerously high" blood pressure of 150/95 mm Hg.

   When you hear this story you are concerned about possible adverse side effects. Your worst fear comes true when you find yourself attending her in the ER with a serious adverse event you believe is directly related to the medications she was placed on.

   Which of the following specialists will you be calling to manage this adverse event?
   a) a rheumatologist
   b) a general surgeon or a general internist
   c) a gerontologist
   d) an orthopedic surgeon
   e) a psychiatrist

5. The patient becomes acutely short of breath. The adverse effect that you feared has now lead to a feared complication. What is that complication?
   a) a deep venous thrombosis leading to a pulmonary embolus
   b) a splenic infarct
   c) a cerebrovascular accident
   d) aplastic anemia
   e) a drug-induced psychosis

6. What is the most likely medication causing the pink rats and the people from outer space?
   a) propranolol

b) hydrochlorothiazide
c) ibuprofen
d) cimetidine
e) digoxin

7. Consider the possibility that the adverse event and its complication just described did not occur. Considering the rapid introduction of multiple medications that took place on the visit to the other physician, what would be the most appropriate course of action at this time?
   a) discontinue the digoxin
   b) discontinue the hydrochlorothiazide
   c) discontinue the propranolol
   d) discontinue the triazolam
   e) discontinue all medications, observe in a geriatric day hospital environment, and reevaluate the patient continuously for the first few weeks

8. Of the drug combinations listed, which is the most likely to result in a drug-drug interaction in the elderly?
   a) cimetidine and propranolol
   b) digoxin and hydrochlorothiazide
   c) ibuprofen and captopril
   d) triazolam and amitriptyline
   e) haloperidol

9. What is the most common potentially serious side effect of tricyclic antidepressants in elderly patients?
   a) dry mouth
   b) constipation
   c) bladder spasm
   d) orthostatic hypotension
   e) sedation

10. Which of the following combinations of pharmacologic agents is most commonly associated with adverse drug reactions (ADRs) in the elderly?
    a) cardiovascular drugs, psychotropics, and antibiotics
    b) cardiovascular drugs, psychotropics, and analgesics
    c) gastrointestinal drugs, psychotropics, and analgesics
    d) gastrointestinal drugs, psychotropics, and antibiotics

11. Which of the following pharmacologic parameters may be associated with ADRs in the elderly?
    a) altered free serum concentration of drug

b) altered volume of distribution
c) altered renal drug clearance
d) altered tissue sensitivity of the drug
e) all of the above

12. Which of the following is(are) examples of adverse drug reactions in the elderly?
    a) drug side effects
    b) drug toxicity
    c) drug-disease interaction
    d) drug-drug interaction
    e) all of the above

13. What is the recommended starting dose of a tricyclic antidepressant in an elderly patient?
    a) 10 mg-25 mg
    b) 50 mg-75 mg
    c) 100 mg-150 mg
    d) 150 mg-225 mg
    e) 250 mg-300 mg

14. Some pharmacologic agents are excreted virtually unchanged by the kidney. The dosages of these drugs must be carefully titrated in any elderly patient with renal impairment or potential renal impairment. Drugs in this category include the following:
    a) cimetidine
    b) gentamicin
    c) lithium
    d) all of the above
    e) none of the above

15. Regarding antipsychotic drug therapy in the elderly, which of the following statements is(are) true?
    a) antipsychotic drugs are often prescribed for behavior that chronic care staff find objectionable
    b) tardive dyskinesia is a frequent side effect of antipsychotic drug use in the elderly
    c) antipsychotic drugs are prescribed much more frequently in institutionalized patients than in non-institutionalized patients
    d) all of the above
    e) none of the above

Short Answer Management Problem 129

List 10 rules that will minimize adverse drug reactions in the elderly.

ANSWERS

1. E. This patient's problem can be characterized in the following manner:
   A. It is very likely to be related to the bagful of medications that she was started on.
   B. It is very common following the initiation of medication in the elderly—especially multiple medications.
   C. It is very unlikely to be transient unless some or all of the medications are discontinued.
   D. It will very commonly lead to hospitalization. It is believed that up to 20% of hospitalizations, and perhaps significantly more in the elderly, are due to iatrogenic disease. Iatrogenic disease is almost always associated with multiple medication use.

2. E. Some helpful thoughts on the initiation of drugs in the elderly follow:
   A. Drug initiation in the elderly should be done extremely cautiously. The general rule should be "start very low and go very slow."
   B. The elderly patient usually needs a considerably lower dose of drug than does the young adult. This is, of course, especially true of drugs that are renally excreted. The general rule on drug initiation in elderly patients is the following: "no more than 50% of the usual adult dose; no more than one drug at the time. Increases not any more quickly than once/week.
   C. Psychotropic drugs should be used with special caution. The most frequently misused drug class in the elderly is the sedative-hypnotics.
   D. All elderly patients should have a formal drug review performed at least every 3 months. At that time, all drugs and the drug doses should be seriously considered for reduction or discontinuation, especially if the elderly patient has symptoms that suggest an ADR (adverse drug reaction) to one or more of the drugs that he or she is presently taking.

3. D. Patients in chronic care facilities have the following characteristics with respect to medication use:
   A. They are usually on multiple medications. The average number of medications being used by the chronic care facility elder is anywhere from 12 to 20.
   B. It has been found that the most usual scenario is that medications always are added but never subtracted. Thus the number simply continues to increase.
   C. Iatrogenic side effects from medication use in chronic care facilities is extremely common. Considering the number of medications that these seniors are on, they are actually far more likely to experience at least one ADR per year than not.
   D. In comparison to seniors living on their own in the community, the number of medications used by institutional-based elderly patients is approximately three times that of community-based seniors.

4. D.

5. A. The combination of hydrochlorothiazide and clonidine is very likely to produce significant orthostatic hypotension in the elderly patient. The most "adverse effect of the adverse effect" is a fall in the elder leading to a fracture of the neck of the femur. Thus the specialist that you most likely will call will be an orthopedic surgeon.

   The most serious complication from a hip fracture is immobility leading to deep venous thrombosis. The development of a DVT is, of course, directly correlated with a subsequent pulmonary embolus.

   The mortality of elders in the first year following a hip fracture approaches 25%. Prevention is the best treatment.

   Prevention is best accomplished by significantly limiting the number of medications an elder is on, especially medications that tend to produce orthostatic hypotension.

6. A. The most common medication-induced cause of hallucinations in elderly patients is propranolol. Many elderly patients who are started on propranolol develop visual or auditory hallucinations. Unfortunately, many of these patients are then started on antipsychotic medications to treat the hallucinations.

7. E. The most reasonable course of action at this time is to stop everything and start again. The rapid introduction of the nine medications listed was a recipe for disaster. In an attempt to counteract the imminent disaster, this logically should take place in the supervised setting of at least a geriatric day hospital. Many geriatric assessment units do exactly that when an elder is admitted for the assessment of any medical problem. With elders who have been on multiple medications for long periods of time, the safest place to accomplish this is in the hospital under close observation.

8. B. Patients who develop adverse drug reactions (ADRs) are more likely to be taking six or more drugs then those

who do not develop an ADR. The most commonly identified combination likely to result in a drug-drug interaction is digoxin with a diuretic. In this case, the ADR most likely to be produced is hypokalemia. The hypokalemia produced will often lead to digoxin toxicity in the susceptible elder.

9. D. All of the side effects listed are common side effects of tricyclic antidepressant medications. The side effects that are due to an anticholinergic mechanism include dry mouth, blurred vision, constipation, bladder spasm and urinary retention, and sedation.

The orthostatic hypotension is due to an alpha-adrenergic blockade and is potentially the most serious due to the association described above between the following series of events:
1) Orthostatic hypotension
2) Falls in the elder
3) Fractured neck of the femur
4) Deep venous thrombosis
5) Pulmonary embolism
Excess morbidity and mortality is associated with events 3, 4, and 5 in the chain.

10. B. The three most common drug classes associated with ADRs in the elderly are cardiovascular drugs, psychotropic drugs, and analgesics (especially the nonsteroidal antiinflammatory drugs). Unfortunately, many of the drugs used in the treatment of geriatric patients are prescribed for symptoms related to the effects and the diseases of aging, and not necessarily for a specific acute disease where function can be restored. This results, of course, in the elder's being on the particular agent for a longer period of time.

11. E. Many physiologic and social variables increase the incidence of ADRs in elderly patients. They include the number of drugs, compliance, absorption of drug, concentration of free drug in the serum, volume of distribution, tissue sensitivity, metabolic clearance, renal drug clearance, general homeostasis, and concentration of serum albumin.

12. E. An ADR is defined as any unintended or undesired effect of a drug in a patient. This may include abnormal laboratory values, patient symptoms, and signs on physical examination.

ADRs can be divided into side effects (dry mouth: tricyclic antidepressants; hypokalemia: diuretics), drug toxicity (daytime sedation: hypnotics; diarrhea: laxatives; syncope: antihypertensive agents), drug-disease interaction (benzodiazepine and drugs with anticholinergic properties may exacerbate Alzheimer's disease), drug-drug interaction (digoxin: diuretics), and secondary effects (haloperidol causing drug-induced Parkinsonism).

13. A. The recommended starting dose for a tricyclic antidepressant in elderly patients is 10-25 mg. The older and more frail the elder, the lower the dose that should initially be used. We recommend nortriptyline be started on a dose of 10 mg.

14. D. The kidney is the major source of elimination of many commonly prescribed drugs. Drugs that undergo extensive renal clearance and that are therefore likely to accumulate in the elderly include digoxin, gentamicin and other aminoglycosides, lithium, cimetidine, cotrimoxazole, disopyramide, nadolol, procainamide, and sulfonamides.

15. D. Psychotropic drugs are commonly prescribed for geriatric patients. Indications for the use of these drugs are not well established. In nursing home situations, psychotropic drugs are often prescribed for behaviors that staff members find objectionable (that is, for the benefit of the staff, not the patient); the patient may, in fact, remain on this (these) drug(s) for long periods of time. The institutionalized elderly are 10 times as likely to receive antipsychotic agents as age-matched noninstitutionalized controls.

Double-blind, randomized, controlled trials have not established the efficacy of antipsychotic drug use in Alzheimer's disease. Tardive dyskinesia, rigidity, and excessive sedation are frequent side effects of antipsychotic drug use.

SOLUTION TO SHORT ANSWER MANAGEMENT PROBLEM 129

The following are a good set of rules for prescribing medication in geriatric patients:
1. Recognize that there is no drug to treat senescence.
2. Recognize that mere prolongation of life is not a valid reason for using medications that decrease the quality of life.
3. Make sure that the effects of treatment outweigh the risks.
4. Establish a priority order for treatment.
5. Keep the number of drugs administered concurrently to a minimum.
6. Know your patient well. Consider renal and hepatic impairment. Consider what else (including over-the-counter medications) is being taken, and who else is prescribing drugs.
7. Always begin with nonpharmacologic therapy first.
8. If you decide to prescribe a drug, know it well. Consider using a few drugs often rather than a lot of drugs infrequently.
9. Select the dose carefully: start very low and go very slow.
10. Anticipate and minimize ADRs by considering side-effect profiles.
11. Determine whether or not the patient needs help using the medication.

12. Educate the patient and family.
13. Continually reevaluate whether or not your patient needs a specific drug.
14. Perform a drug review every 3 months on every elder on more than one medication.

SUMMARY OF THE DIAGNOSIS AND MANAGEMENT OF DRUG REACTIONS IN THE ELDERLY

1. **Prevalence:** very common, especially in institutionalized elderly who are on an average of 12-20 medications. ADRs are at least twice as common in elderly patients as in younger patients.
2. **Types of adverse drug reactions:**
   a) Side effects
   b) Drug toxicity
   c) Drug-disease interaction
   d) Drug-drug interaction
3. **Most common drugs associated with ADRs:**
   a) Cardiovascular drugs
   b) Psychotropic drugs
   c) Analgesics
4. **Set of reasonable rules:** follow the set of rules listed in the answer to Short Answer Management Problem 129.

SUGGESTED READING

Hazzard WR et al., eds. Principles of geriatric medicine and gerontology. 3rd Ed. New York: McGraw-Hill, 1994.

PROBLEM 130 AN 81-YEAR-OLD FEMALE WHO IS REPEATEDLY FALLING

An 81-year-old female is brought to your office by her daughter. The elderly mother has been falling repeatedly for at least 3 months. The falling has been getting progressively worse, and the patient's daughter is very concerned about the possibility of her mother "breaking her hip."

On examination, the patient is a frail, elderly female in no acute distress. She appears somewhat depressed, but her mini-mental status examination score is 27.

The patient's blood pressure is 180/75 mm Hg. Her pulse is 84 and irregular. No other abnormalities are found.

SELECT THE ONE BEST ANSWER TO THE FOLLOWING QUESTIONS

1. What is the prevalence of falls among community-based elderly patients?
   a) 5% per year
   b) 10% per year
   c) 20% per year
   d) 30% per year
   e) 50% per year

2. Which of the following statements regarding falls in the elderly is(are) true?
   a) the prevalence of falling in the elderly increases with advancing age
   b) elderly patients who are physically active may be at greater risk of falling than those who are not
   c) approximately 50% of elderly patients who fall once will fall again
   d) falling in the elderly may not necessarily be a marker of functional decline
   e) all of the above statements are true

3. Which of the following is the most feared morbid outcome of falling among elderly patients?
   a) fracture of the hip
   b) fracture of the radius
   c) subdural hematoma
   d) epidural hematoma
   e) cervical fracture

4. Which of the following conditions is most closely associated with falls in the elderly?
   a) sensorineural hearing loss
   b) glaucoma
   c) Parkinson's disease
   d) hypertension
   e) ischemic heart disease

5. Which of the following are predisposing risk factors for falls in the elderly?
   a) visual impairment
   b) cerebrovascular accidents
   c) Alzheimer's disease
   d) normal pressure hydrocephalus
   e) all of the above

6. Regarding the incidence of falling and medication use in the elderly, which of the following statements is(are) true?
   a) multiple drug use is associated with an increased incidence of falling in the elderly
   b) the higher the drug dosage, the greater the probability of falling
   c) drug interactions are a major contributing factor to an increased incidence of falling in the elderly
   d) a and b only
   e) all of the above statements are true

7. Falling in the elderly is most commonly associated with which of the following pathophysiologic factors?
   a) orthostatic hypotension
   b) decreased left ventricular output
   c) decreased cerebral circulation
   d) increased left ventricular output
   e) none of the above

8. Which of the following medications is(are) most likely to lead to a serious fall in an elderly patient?
   a) amitriptyline
   b) hydrochlorothiazide
   c) enalapril
   d) nifedipine
   e) fluoxetine

9. What is the prevalence of falling among institutionalized elderly patients?
   a) 50% per year
   b) 40% per year
   c) 30% per year
   d) 20% per year
   e) 10% per year

10. Which of the following statements regarding the use of restraints in elderly patients as a means to prevent falls is true?
    a) restraints have been shown to reduce the incidence of falling in the elderly
    b) no study has every shown a decrease in falls with restraint use in the elderly
    c) potential complications of restraint use in the elderly include strangulation, vascular damage, and neurologic damage
    d) a and c
    e) b and c

Short Answer Management Problem 130

Describe the preventive measures that may result in a reduction in falls in the elderly.

ANSWERS

1. D.

2. E. According to several community-based surveys, about 30% of persons over the age of 65 experience falls each year in situations where there are no overwhelming intrinsic causes (such as syncope). Approximately 50% of these elders have multiple falling episodes. The likelihood of falling increases with age. As illustrated by this very high prevalence of 30% among community-based persons, falling is not just confined to the frail elderly; healthy elderly patients fall as well during ordinary daily activities. This suggests that falling is not merely a marker of functional decline in the elderly. While the elder we all picture as falling is the "frail elder" with multiple medical problems, it may well be the case that falling is more prevalent among the more "healthy" elders who are more, not less, physically active.

3. A. The most feared outcome of falls in the elderly is a fracture of the hip.

   This is especially common among elderly women who have significant osteoporosis.

   The escalating cost of health care has resulted in increased expectations and demands concerning cost-effective health care. In the case of hip fracture, one study reports that age-specific mortality among the elderly from accidental falls, which result in the death of at least 12,000 elderly Americans per year, actually declined 50.2% in men and 56.2% in women during the period 1962-1988. This decline in mortality from accidental falls in elderly persons appears to reflect the effects of improved trauma management rather than injury control.

4. A.

5. E. Vision, hearing, vestibular function, and proprioception are the major sensory modalities related to stability. Thus declines in vision, hearing, imbalance leading to vertigo and dizziness, and peripheral neuropathies and cervical degenerative disease are the most common causes of falls in elderly patients.

   Other associated diseases or conditions associated with falls in the elderly include cerebrovascular accidents, Parkinson's disease, normal-pressure hydrocephalus, dementia (Alzheimer's disease), severe osteoarthritis or rheumatoid arthritis, and medications causing orthostatic hypotension (discussed in another chapter).

6. E. Iatrogenic disease is a major cause of falls in the elderly. This iatrogenic disease, which is almost completely related to medication use, is a serious problem in elders. As discussed in another chapter, the average number of medications per elder (especially in the institutionalized setting) is anywhere from 12 to 20.

   Multiple drugs, increased drug dosage, and drug-drug interactions are all reasons for orthostatic hypotension (an alpha-blockade phenomenon) and sedation (the two most common predisposing pathophysiologic mechanisms associated with falling in the elderly).

7. A. Decreased left ventricular output, most closely associated with congestive heart failure, may also play a prominent role in some cases of falling.

8. A. Four of the medications listed in the question are medications that may produce falls in the elderly. Amitriptyline, hydrochlorothiazide, enalapril, and nifedipine may all be associated with falling in the elderly. Enalapril and hydrochlorothiazide are more likely to be associated with falling when given concomitantly. As well, the first-dose hypotensive effect of an ACE inhibitor should be remembered; that is, it is much safer to give the first dose of an ACE inhibitor to an elder in your office, where this possible side effect can be monitored.

   Of the four medications listed, however, the most prominent predisposing to falls in the elderly is amitriptyline, a tricyclic antidepressant used frequently in the elderly. Amitriptyline predisposes to falls by a combination of two mechanisms: its anticholinergic mechanism and its alpha-blockade mechanism.

   "Starting very low and going very slowly" will minimize falling in elderly patients due to drugs.

9. A. Over one-half of ambulatory nursing home patients fall each year. The estimated annual incidence is 1600 falls per 1000 beds. The higher frequency of falling among institutionalized elderly patients results both from the greater frailty of these patients compared to community-based elderly patients and the greater reliability of reporting in an institutional setting.

10. E. No study has confirmed or suggested that the risk of falling in the elderly is lessened because of the use of restraining devices. Restraining devices have, on the other hand, been shown to result in significant morbidity and

mortality from strangulation, neurologic damage, and vascular damage.

In some countries in the world (such as the United Kingdom), restraints are almost forbidden. In North America the situation appears to be the opposite. In some institutions they are completely routine.

Restraints have other side effects, including anxiety, anger, agitation, and paranoia.

SOLUTION TO SHORT ANSWER MANAGEMENT PROBLEM 130

A preventive program for minimizing falls in the elderly should include the following:

I. Identification of intrinsic risk factors:
1. A thorough clinical evaluation aimed at identifying all contributing risk factors for falling is the first, most important step. Directly observing balance and gait has proved to be effective in identifying residents at risk for falling.
2. A careful review of all situations may identify problem situations to be avoided in the future.
3. A complete medication review with elimination of all medications not necessary and a decrease in the dose of all others

II. Environmental prevention:
1. General environmental measures include ensuring adequate lighting without glare; having dry, non-slippery floors that are free of obstacles and contamination; having high, firm chairs; and having raised toilet seats.
2. Restraints should be used only when there appears to be no other alternative. Restraints should not take the place of close supervision and attention to the risk factors discussed earlier. Alternatives to restraints, including wedges in chairs for maintenance of position and organized walking and grid barriers for prevention of wandering, may afford the necessary protection.

SUMMARY OF THE DIAGNOSIS AND PREVENTION OF FALLS IN THE ELDERLY

1. **Prevalence:**
   a) 30%/year in community-based elders
   b) > 50%/year in institutionalized elders
2. **Major complication:** fracture of the femur: resulting morbidity and mortality from surgery, deep venous thrombosis, and pulmonary embolus

3. **Major predisposing conditions precipitating major complication:**
   a) Vision, hearing, vestibular function, and proprioception impairments
   b) Other conditions associated with increased risk include Alzheimer's disease, Parkinson's disease, and iatrogenic disease (mainly medication use, including the psychotropic agents and the cardiovascular agents, the agents with the greatest probability of producing sedation and other anticholinergic side effects and alpha-blockade side effects [orthostatic hypotension]).
   c) a or b associated with significant osteoporosis increases the risk.
4. **Elder populations at greatest risk:**
   a) Active elderly patients who are at increased risk because of significant activity levels in whom even a minor impairment may be enough to cause significant problems
   b) The "frail elderly" who have concomitant chronic medical conditions
   c) The institutionalized elderly
   (This list may, in fact, include most elders.)
5. **Prevention:**
   a) Prevent the development of osteoporosis in postmenopausal women whenever possible (estrogens, calcitonin, calcium).
   b) Look carefully at identifying intrinsic risk factors and environmental protection methods in helping to prevent falls.
   c) Medications:
      1. Provide a medication review to every elder every 3 months.
      2. Keep the number of medications to a minimum.
      3. In starting medications, start very low and go very slow.
      4. To minimize falls, minimize ADRs (adverse drug reactions). This is covered extensively in another chapter in this book.

SUGGESTED READINGS

Riggs J. Mortality from accidental falls among the elderly in the United States, 1962-1988: Demonstrating the impact of improved trauma management. Journal of Trauma 1993;35(2):212-219.

Tinetti M. Falls. In: Hazzard W et al., eds. Principles of geriatric medicine and gerontology. 3rd Ed. New York: McGraw-Hill, 1994.

Epidemiology and Public Health

PROBLEM 131 A 24-YEAR-OLD MEDICAL STUDENT WHO WISHES TO REVIEW THE RECOMMENDATIONS OF THE U.S. PREVENTIVE SERVICES TASK FORCE ON THE PERIODIC HEALTH EXAMINATION

A 24-year-old medical student presents to your office to discuss the recent recommendations of the U.S. Preventive Services Task Force on the Periodic Health Examination. You are the preceptor of this student. You decide to discuss the recommendations using multiple-choice questions.

SELECT THE ONE BEST ANSWER TO THE FOLLOWING QUESTIONS

1. A 55-year-old male presents for a periodic health assessment. He has no specific complaints or concerns. Which of the following is(are) definitely indicated in the periodic health assessment that you would perform on this individual?
   a) measurement of blood pressure
   b) measurement of body mass index
   c) electrocardiogram
   d) a and b
   e) all of the above

2. Considering the individual described in Question 1, which of the following is(are) indicated in this individual's periodic health assessment?
   a) serum cholesterol
   b) auscultation for carotid bruits
   c) palpation of peripheral pulses
   d) serum triglycerides
   e) all of the above

3. A 66-year-old male presents for a periodic health examination. In this patient, which of the following is(are) definitely indicated as part of this patient's clinical examination?
   a) rectal examination
   b) sigmoidoscopy
   c) fecal occult blood testing
   d) all of the above
   e) b or c

4. A 26-year-old female presents for a periodic health assessment. She is asymptomatic. Which of the following is(are) indicated in this young lady's periodic health examination?
   a) palpation of the ovaries
   b) Pap smear
   c) breast examination

   d) all of the above
   e) b and c only

5. A 53-year-old male with a 20-year history of smoking two packs of cigarettes/day presents for a periodic health examination. Which of the following is(are) definitely indicated in this patient's examination?
   a) ultrasound of the abdomen to screen for pancreatic cancer
   b) chest X-ray to screen for carcinoma of the lung
   c) glaucoma screening
   d) all of the above
   e) none of the above

6. A 32-year-old male presents for a periodic health examination. Which of the following is(are) definitely indicated in this man's assessment?
   a) body mass index
   b) inquiry about smoking
   c) inquiry about alcohol intake
   d) inquiry into regular aerobic exercise activity
   e) all of the above

7. Which of the following statements regarding estrogen prophylaxis is(are) true?
   a) routine post-menopausal estrogen replacement is recommended for all women
   b) estrogen therapy should be recommended for asymptomatic women who are at increased risk for osteoporosis
   c) spinal compression fractures are uncommon in women over the age of 60 years
   d) estrogen replacement therapy should be started at 0.3 mg/day
   e) all of the above are true

8. Which of the following statements concerning prenatal screening is(are) true?
   a) all pregnant women should receive at least one ultrasound

b) all pregnant women should be screened for pre-eclampsia periodically throughout pregnancy with sophisticated tests
c) all pregnant women should be screened at least once for gestational diabetes
d) all of the above are true
e) none of the above are true

9. Which of the following is(are) true regarding the performance of a routine urinalysis to detect the presence of protein in adults?
   a) there is good evidence to support the recommendation that the condition be specifically considered in a periodic health examination
   b) there is fair evidence to support the recommendation that the condition be specifically considered in a periodic health examination
   c) there is poor evidence regarding the inclusion of the condition in a periodic health examination, but recommendations may be made on other grounds
   d) there is fair evidence to support the recommendation that the condition be excluded from the periodic health examination

e) there is good evidence to support the recommendation that the condition be excluded from the periodic health examination

10. Regarding counseling to prevent motor vehicle injuries, which of the following statements is(are) true?
    a) all patients should be encouraged to use safety belts for themselves and others
    b) all patients should be urged to wear safety helmets when riding bicycles
    c) all patients should be urged to refrain from driving while under the influence of alcohol or other drugs
    d) all of the above are true
    e) none of the above are true

11. Screening for infection with human immunodeficiency virus (HIV) should be offered periodically to which of the following groups?
    a) persons seeking treatment for sexually transmitted diseases
    b) intravenous drug users
    c) homosexual and bisexual men
    d) all of the above groups
    e) none of the above groups

Short Answer Management Problem 131

Summarize the 60 major recommendations of the U.S. Preventive Services Task Force on the Periodic Health Examination for a routine screening.

ANSWERS

1. D.

2. A. This patient's periodic health examination should include measurement of body mass index and measurement of blood pressure. An ECG is not routinely recommended as part of the periodic health examination of a 55-year-old male.

   The U.S. Preventive Services Task Force recommends the following screening procedures in a 55-year-old male:
   A. History: dietary intake, physical activity, tobacco/alcohol/drug use, and sexual practices
   B. Physical exam: height and weight (BMI) and blood pressure measurement
   C. Laboratory/diagnostic procedures: nonfasting total blood cholesterol
   D. Counseling:
      1) Diet and exercise: fat (especially saturated fat and cholesterol), complex carbohydrates, fiber, sodium, calcium, caloric balance,
      2) Selection of exercise program

   3) Substance use: tobacco cessation, alcohol and other drugs—treatment for abuse
   4) Sexual practices: sexually transmitted diseases; partner selection, condoms, and intercourse; unintended pregnancy and contraceptive options
   5) Injury prevention: safety belts; safety helmets; smoke detector; and dental health, including regular tooth brushing, flossing, and dental visits
   6) Immunizations: tetanus-diptheria booster every 10 years

3. E. There is now sufficient evidence to recommend either annual fecal occult blood testing or periodic (q2 to q3 years) flexible sigmoidoscopy or both for the screening of the American population for colorectal cancer. Screening with either method is recommended to begin at age 50.

4. B. The only intervention that is recommended by the U.S. Preventive Services Task Force as a screening test in a patient of this age is the Pap smear.

   Regular Pap testing is recommended for all women who are or who have been sexually active. Pap smears should begin at the onset of sexual activity and should be repeated every 1 to 3 years at the physician's discretion. They may be discontinued at age 65 if the previous smears have been consistently normal.

In summary: low-risk patient, 3 normals in a row and then every 3-5 years; high-risk patient, every 6 months of every year depending on the specific or degree of risk

5. E. There is insufficient evidence to recommend routine performance of tonometry by primary care physicians as an effective test for glaucoma. It may be clinically prudent, however, to advise patients aged 65 and older to be tested periodically by an eye practitioner.

6. E. A 32-year-old male, who is otherwise healthy, should have his periodic health assessment concentrate on lifestyle issues. The same issues that were raised in the 55-year-old male should be raised in the 32-year-old male with the lifestyle emphasis being placed on the following: diet (cholesterol, saturated fat); regular aerobic exercise; and inquiry and counseling regarding smoking, regular aerobic exercise, and alcohol and drug use.

The only physical examination maneuvers that have been recommended by the U.S. Preventive Services Task Force in a 32-year-old male include body mass index and blood pressure measurement.

7. B. Although routine postmenopausal estrogen replacement is not recommended, estrogen therapy should be considered for asymptomatic women who are at increased risk for osteoporosis, who lack known contraindications, and who have received adequate counseling regarding the potential benefits and risks. There is also most certainly a role for increased aerobic exercise and dietary calcium supplementation.

Estrogen therapy should be considered in asymptomatic women who are of Caucasian or Asian decent with a low bone mineral content, have a history of early menopause or bilateral oophorectomy prior to menopause and who do not have any known contraindications, have poor skeletal musculature, have a sedentary lifestyle, smoke cigarettes, and have an excessive alcohol intake.

8. A. The recommendations that follow are the latest recommendations of the Canadian Task Force on the Periodic Health Examination rather than the U.S. Preventive Services Task Force. The reason for this is that the Canadian Task Force has just published a new book that contains updated recommendations on the choices offered in this question.

On the basis of the recommendations of the Canadian Task Force on the Periodic Health Examination,

it is clear that on balance, every pregnant woman should receive one prenatal ultrasound in the second trimester of pregnancy. Although trials of a single prenatal ultrasound (PNU) in the second trimester have not shown a statistically significant effect on the rate of live births or on the Apgar score, the clinical trials that have been conducted have indicated that a single PNU early in pregnancy results in lower rates of induction (presumably through better estimates of gestational age), earlier detection of twin pregnancies, increased birth weight in singletons, and higher rates of therapeutic abortion for fetal abnormalities. Based on these clinical effects there is fair evidence to include a single PNU examination in routine prenatal care (recommendation B).

The available evidence does not support a recommendation for or against universal screening for gestational diabetes mellitus (GDM). Women have varying degrees of glucose intolerance during pregnancy and a certain proportion will have adverse outcomes. The value of screening is unclear given potential clinical and financial costs. Women with risk factors for GDM should be carefully followed and prudently screened throughout their pregnancies.

Screening for preeclampsia is not associated with any "sophisticated tests." The accepted screening method is the routine assessment by blood pressure measurement, which in itself should be consistent. Although some studies have documented the efficacy of aspirin prophylaxis as a primary preventive measure, there is not enough evidence to recommend it on a routine basis, even among women at high risk for preeclampsia and intrauterine growth retardation.

9. E. There is good evidence to recommend that routine urinalysis not be performed to detect the presence of proteinuria.

A successful screening program is predicated on the principle that efficacious, nonharmful treatment is available early in the disease course. Thus it is not recommended that dipstick screening for proteinuria in the general adult population for the prevention of end-stage renal disease be part of a routine periodic health examination.

10. D. Safety is a major focus of the periodic health examination. All patients should be encouraged to use seat belts in motor vehicles at all times, use safety helmets for bicycles and motorcycles at all times, and refrain from operating any kind of motor vehicle while under the influence of alcohol or drugs.

These seem very reasonable and self-explanatory, but the third point deserves emphasis. When we talk about drugs, we are talking about all drugs, not just illicit drugs. There are many prescription medications that can impair concentration and reaction time, and patients should always be cautioned about driving while using these medications. A good example of the latter would be antihistamines. Antihistamines are commonly prescribed, but seldom do we caution patients about operating motor vehicles while taking them.

11. D. Patients who should be offered screening for HIV infection include all of the high-risk groups for the infection. This includes homosexual or bisexual men, intravenous drug users, hemophiliacs, and heterosexual patients with multiple sexual partners.

SOLUTION TO SHORT ANSWER MANAGEMENT PROBLEM 131

Summary of the Periodic Health Examination: The 60 recommendations of the U.S. Preventive Services Task Force on the Periodic Health Exam

1. The periodic health examination is replacing the routine complete examination as the most cost-effective regular examination.

2. The task force began by preparing a list of important diseases and injuries in the United States that might be prevented through clinical intervention. The 60 target conditions were selected on the basis of the following important criteria:

   A. Burden of suffering from the target condition: consideration was given to both the prevalence and the incidence of the condition.

   B. Potential effectiveness of the preventive intervention: conditions were excluded from analysis if the task force panel could not identify a potentially effective preventive intervention that could be performed by clinicians.

   C. Selection of preventive services: for each target condition, the task force used two criteria to select the preventive services to be evaluated. First, in general, only preventive services carried out on asymptomatic persons were reviewed. Thus only primary and secondary preventive measures were addressed.

   D. The maneuver had to be able to be performed in the clinical setting.

   E. The criteria for determining effectiveness included the efficacy of the screening test, including the sensitivity and specificity of the maneuver; the reliability (reproducibility) of the test; and the effectiveness of early detection.

3. The task force emphasizes prevention, counseling, and lifestyle changes. It deemphasizes routine history, routine physical examination, and routine laboratory testing. Only procedures that have shown to make a difference are included. The major procedures include measurement of body mass index, measurement of blood pressure, Pap smear, mammography, nonfasting serum cholesterol, lifestyle counseling, and immunizations.

4. A summary of the 60 recommendations of the U.S. Preventive Services Task Force follows.

Recommendation 1: Screening for Asymptomatic Coronary Artery Disease

Clinicians should emphasize the primary prevention of coronary artery disease (CAD) by periodically screening for high blood pressure and high serum cholesterol and by investigating behavioral risk factors for CAD such as tobacco use, dietary fat, cholesterol intake, and inadequate physical exercise. Secondary prevention of CAD (screening) by performing a routine ECG to screen asymptomatic persons is not recommended. It may be clinically prudent to perform screening ECGs in certain high-risk groups. Routine resting or exercise ECG screening before entering athletic programs is not recommended for asymptomatic children, adolescents, or young adults.

Recommendation 2: Screening for High Blood Cholesterol

Periodic measurement of total serum cholesterol is most important for middle-aged men, and it may aso be clinically prudent in young men, women, and the elderly. All patients should receive periodic counseling regarding dietary intake.

Recommendation 3: Screening for Hypertension

Blood pressure should be measured regularly in persons aged 3 and above.

Recommendation 4: Screening for Cerebrovascular Disease

There is currently insufficient evidence to recommend for or against auscultation for carotid bruits or noninvasive testing for carotid artery stenosis as effective screening strategies to prevent cerebrovascular disease in asymptomatic persons. It may be clinically prudent to include cervical auscultation in the physical examination of patients with established risk factors for cerebrovascular or cardiovascular disease. All patients should be screened for hypertension and some persons should be tested for high blood cholesterol. Clinicians should also provide counseling about smoking, exercise, and dietary fat consumption.

Recommendation 5: Screening for Peripheral Vascular Disease

Routine screening for peripheral arterial disease in asymptomatic persons is not recommended. Clinicians should be alert to signs of peripheral arterial disease in persons at increased risk and should thoroughly evaluate those patients for clinical evidence of vascular disease.

Recommendation 6: Screening for Breast Cancer

All women over age 40 should receive an annual clinical breast examination. Mammography every 1 to 2 years is recommended for all women beginning at age 50 and concluding at approximately age 75 unless pathology has been detected in previous mammograms. It may be prudent to begin mammography at an earlier age for women at high risk for breast cancer. Although the teaching of breast self-examination is not specifically recommended at this time, there is insufficient evidence to recommend any change in current breast self-examination practices.

Recommendation 7: Screening for Cervical Cancer

Regular Pap testing is recommended for all women who are or have been sexually active. Pap smears should begin with the onset of sexual activity and should be repeated every 1 to 3 years at the physician's discretion. They may be discontinued at age 65 if previous smears have been consistently normal.

Recommendation 8: Screening for Colorectal Cancer

There is now sufficient evidence to recommend either annual fecal occult blood testing or periodic (every 2 to every 3 years) flexible sigmoidoscopy or both for the screening of the American population for colorectal cancer. Screening with either method is recommended to begin at age 50.

Recommendation 9: Screening for Prostate Cancer

There is insufficient evidence to recommend for or against digital rectal examination as an effective screening test for prostate cancer in asymptomatic men. Transrectal ultrasound and serum tumor markers are not recommended for routine screening in asymptomatic men.

Recommendation 10: Screening for Lung Cancer

Screening asymptomatic persons for lung cancer by performing routine chest X-rays or sputum cytology is not recommended.

Recommendation 11: Screening for Skin Cancer

Routine screening for skin cancer is recommended for persons at high risk. Clinicians should advise all patients with increased outdoor exposure to use sunscreen preparations and other measures to protect their skin from UV rays. Currently there is not evidence for or against counseling patients to perform skin self-examination.

Recommendation 12: Screening for Testicular Cancer

Periodic screening for testicular cancer by testicular examination is recommended for men with a history of cryptorchidism, orchiopexy, or testicular atrophy. There is insufficient evidence of clinical benefit or harm to recommend for or against routine screening of other asymptomatic men for testicular cancer. Clinicians should advise adolescent and young males to seek prompt medical attention for testicular symptoms such as pain, swelling, or heaviness.

Recommendation 13: Screening for Ovarian Cancer

Screening of asymptomatic women for ovarian cancer is not recommended. It is prudent to examine the uterine adnexa when performing gynecologic examinations for other reasons.

Recommendation 14: Screening for Pancreatic Cancer

Routine screening for pancreatic cancer in asymptomatic persons is not recommended.

Recommendation 15: Screening for Oral Cancer

Routine screening of asymptomatic persons for oral cancer by primary care clinicians is not recommended. It may be prudent for clinicians to perform careful examinations for cancerous lesions of the oral cavity in patients who use tobacco or excessive amounts of alcohol, as well as in those with suspicious symptoms or lesions detected through self-examination. All patients should be counseled to receive regular dental examinations, and to limit consumption of alcohol. Persons with increased exposure to

sunlight should be advised to take protective measures to protect their lips and skin from the harmful effects of UV rays.

Recommendation 16: Screening for Diabetes Mellitus

There is insufficient evidence to recommend for or against routine screening for GDM. If screening is to be performed, it should be performed between 24 and 28 weeks of gestation with a 50 gram glucose load.

Recommendation 17: Screening for Thyroid Disease

Screening for congenital hypothyroidism is recommended for all neonates during the first week of life. Routine screening for thyroid disorders is otherwise not warranted in asymptomatic adults or children. Persons with a history of upper-body radiation may benefit from regular physical examination of the thyroid gland.

Recommendation 18: Screening for Obesity

All children and adults should receive periodic height and weight measurements (body mass index).

Recommendation 19: Screening for Phenylketonuria

Screening for phenylketonuria is recommended for all newborns prior to discharge from the nursery. Infants who are tested before 24 hours of age should receive a repeat screening test before the third week of life. Routine prenatal screening for maternal PKU is not recommended.

Recommendation 20: Screening for Hepatitis B

All pregnant women should be tested for hepatitis B surface antigen at their first prenatal visit. The test may be repeated in the third trimester in women at increased risk of exposure during pregnancy. Vaccination against hepatitis B is recommended for high risk groups.

Recommendation 21: Screening for Tuberculosis

Tuberculin skin testing of asymptomatic persons should be performed on those at high risk of acquiring tuberculosis.

Recommendation 22: Screening for Syphilis

Routine screening for syphilis in asymptomatic persons is recommended for those in high-risk groups and for pregnant women.

Recommendation 23: Screening for Gonorrhea

Routine screening for gonorrhea in asymptomatic persons is recommended for persons at high risk and for pregnant women. An ophthalmic antibiotic should be applied topically to the eyes of all newborns after birth to prevent ophthalmia neonatum.

Recommendation 24: Screening for HIV Infection

Screening for HIV infection should be offered periodically to persons seeking treatment for other sexually transmitted diseases, intravenous drug users, homosexual and bisexual men, and others at increased risk of infection. Testing should also be offered to pregnant women (or women contemplating pregnancy) who are at increased risk of the infection.

Recommendation 25: Screening for Chlamydial Infection

Routine testing for Chlamydia trachomatis is recommended for asymptomatic persons at high risk of infection. Pregnant women in high-risk categories should be tested at the first prenatal visit. Ophthalmic antibiotics should be applied topically to the eyes of all newborns immediately after birth to help prevent ophthalmic neonatorum.

Recommendation 26: Screening for Genital Herpes Simplex

Screening for genital herpes simplex virus (HSV) infection is recommended for pregnant women with active lesions.

Recommendation 27: Screening for Asymptomatic Bacteriuria, Hematuria, and Proteinuria

Periodic urine testing of asymptomatic persons is recommended for those with diabetes mellitus and for pregnant women. It is not recommended routinely for asymptomatic adults in the absence of DM.

Recommendation 28: Screening for Anemia

All infants and pregnant women should be tested for anemia. Routine screening of other asymptomatic persons is not recommended in the absence of clinical indications.

Recommendation 29: Screening for Hemoglobinopathies

Hemoglobin analysis is recommended for all newborns at risk for hemoglobin disorders. Hemoglobin analysis should also be discussed and offered to adolescents and young adults at risk for hemoglobinopathies and should be performed routinely at the first prenatal visit on all pregnant black women. All screening efforts should be accompanied by comprehensive counseling and treatment services.

Recommendation 30: Screening for Lead Toxicity

Annual lead screening is recommended for all children aged 9 months to 6 years who are at risk for lead toxicity, especially those who live in or frequently visit older housing that is dilapidated or undergoing renovation.

Recommendation 31: Screening for Diminished Visual Acuity

Vision screening is recommended for all children once before entering school, preferably at age 3 or 4. Routine vision testing is not recommended as a component of the periodic health examination of asymptomatic schoolchildren. Clinicians should be alert for signs of ocular misalignment when examining all infants and children. Vision screening of adolescents and adults is not recommended but may be appropriate in the elderly. Screening for glaucoma is discussed in another recommendation.

Recommendation 32: Screening for Glaucoma

There is insufficient evidence to recommend routine performance of tonometry by primary care physicians as an effective screening test for glaucoma. It may be clinically prudent, however, to advise patients at high risk, such as those aged 65 and older, to be tested periodically for glaucoma by an eye specialist.

Recommendation 33: Screening for Hearing Impairment

Screening should be performed on all neonates at high risk for hearing impairment. High-risk children not tested at birth should be screened before age 3, but there is insufficient evidence of accuracy to recommend routine audiologic testing of all children in this age group. There is also insufficient evidence of benefit to recommend for or against hearing screening of asymptomatic children beyond the age of 3 years. Screening is not recommended for asymptomatic adolescents or adults not exposed routinely to excessive noise. Elderly patients should be evaluated regarding their hearing, counseled regarding the availability and use of hearing aids, and referred appropriately when abnormalities are detected.

Recommendation 34: Screening for Intrauterine Growth Retardation

Women at increased risk for delivering a growth-retarded infant should receive ultrasound examinations early in the second trimester to determine gestational age and in the third trimester to measure the size of critical fetal structures. Routine ultrasound screening is otherwise not recommended in normal pregnancies, although physicians may wish to consider ultrasound dating in pregnant women with uncertain menstrual histories. All pregnant women should receive appropriate counseling regarding smoking, alcohol, and other drug use.

Recommendation 35: Screening for Preeclampsia

All pregnant women should receive systolic and diastolic blood pressure measurements at the first prenatal visit and periodically throughout the pregnancy.

Recommendation 36: Screening for Rh Incompatibility

All pregnant women should receive ABO/Rh blood typing and testing for anti-Rh(D) antibody at their first prenatal visit. Unsensitized Rh-negative women should receive Rh(D) immune globulin at 28-29 weeks' gestation and within 72 hours of delivery. Other indications for giving Rhogam include spontaneous or therapeutic abortion, ectopic pregnancy, amniocentesis, antepartum placental hemorrhage, or transfusion of Rh-positive blood products.

Recommendation 37: Screening for Rubella

Serial testing for rubella antibodies should be performed at the first clinical encounter with all pregnant and nonpregnant women of childbearing age lacking evidence of immunity. Susceptible nonpregnant women who agree not to become pregnant for 3 months following immunization can be vaccinated. Susceptible pregnant women should not be vaccinated until immediately after delivery.

Recommendation 38: Screening for Congenital Birth Defects

Amniocentesis for karyotyping should be offered to pregnant women aged 35 and older. Maternal alpha-fetoprotein should be measured on all pregnant women during weeks 16-18 in centers that have adequate counseling and follow-up services. Ultrasound examination is not recommended as a routine screening test for congenital defects.

Recommendation 39: Screening for Fetal Distress

Fetal heart rate should be measured by auscultation in all women in labor to detect signs of fetal distress. Electronic fetal monitoring should not be performed routinely on all women in labor. It should be reserved, instead, for pregnancies at increased risk of fetal distress.

Recommendation 40: Screening for Post-menopausal Osteoporosis

Routine radiologic screening to detect low bone mineral content is not recommended in post-menopausal women.

Estrogen replacement therapy is discussed in another recommendation.

Recommendation 41: Screening for Risk of Low Back Injury

Screening asymptomatic persons for risk of low back injury is not recommended. Routine spinal radiographs of asymptomatic persons are also not recommended.

Recommendation 42: Screening for Dementia

Screening for cognitive impairment among asymptomatic elderly persons is not recommended.

Recommendation 43: Screening for Abnormal Bereavement

Clinicians aware of the impending or recent death of a patient's loved one should assess potential risk factors for abnormal grieving and should provide emotional support for mourning. Clinicians should also remain alert for the signs and symptoms of pathological bereavement. Suicide is a major problem that is on the increase in U.S. elders (especially men).

Recommendation 44: Screening for Depression

The performance of routine screening tests for depression in asymptomatic persons is not recommended. Clinicians should maintain an especially high index of suspicion for depressive symptoms in those persons who are believed to be at increased risk of suicide.

Recommendation 45: Screening for Suicidal Intent

Routine screening for suicidal intent is not recommended. Clinicians should be alert to signs of suicidal ideation in persons with established risk factors. Persons suspected of suicidal intent should be questioned regarding the extent of preparatory actions and referred for further evaluation if evidence of suicidal behavior is detected. Clinicians should be alert to symptoms of depression and should routinely ask patients about their use of alcohol and other drugs.

Recommendation 46: Screening for Violent Injuries

Routine screening interviews or examination for evidence of violent injuries are not recommended. Children and adults presenting with unusual injuries should be examined with attention to possible abuse or neglect, and efforts should be made to prevent subsequent violent injury. Counseling and referral should be offered to those persons at high risk of becoming victims or perpetrators of violence.

Recommendation 47: Screening for Alcohol and Other Drug Abuse

All adolescents and adults should be asked to describe their use of alcohol and other drugs. Routine measurement of biochemical markers and drug testing are not recommended as the primary method of detecting alcohol and other drug abuse in asymptomatic persons. Persons in whom alcohol or other drug abuse or dependence is confirmed should receive appropriate counseling, treatment, and referrals. All persons who use alcohol, especially pregnant women, should be encouraged to quit drinking alcohol, and all persons who use alcohol or other intoxicating drugs should be counseled about the dangers of operating a motor vehicle or performing other potentially dangerous activities while intoxicated.

Recommendation 48: Counseling to Prevent Tobacco Use

Tobacco cessation counseling should be offered on a regular basis to all patients who smoke cigarettes, pipe, or cigars, and to those who use smokeless tobacco. The prescription of nicotine gum or nicotine patches may be an appropriate adjunct for some patients. Adolescents and young adults who do not currently use tobacco products should be advised not to start.

Recommendation 49: Exercise Counseling

Clinicians should counsel all patients to engage in a program of regular physical activity, tailored to their health status and personal lifestyle.

Recommendation 50: Nutritional Counseling

Clinicians should provide periodic counseling regarding the dietary intake of calories (especially saturated fat), cholesterol, complex carbohydrates (starches), fiber, and sodium. Women and adolescent girls should receive specific information on nutritional guidelines during pregnancy. Parents should also be counseled about nutritional requirements of infancy and early childhood. Counseling regarding alcohol consumption has already been discussed.

Recommendation 51: Counseling to Prevent Motor Vehicle Accidents

All patients should be urged to use occupant restraints (safety belts and safety seats) for themselves and others, to wear safety helmets when riding motorcycles and bicycles, and to refrain from driving under the influence of alcohol or other drugs.

Recommendation 52: Counseling to Prevent Household and Environmental Injuries

Patients who use alcohol or other drugs should be warned about engaging in potentially dangerous activities while intoxicated. It may also be clinically prudent to provide counseling on other measures to reduce the risk of unintentional household or environmental injuries from falls, drownings, fires or burns, poisoning, and firearms.

Recommendation 53: Counseling to Prevent HIV Infection and Other Sexually Transmitted Diseases

Clinicians should take a complete sexual and drug use history on all adolescent and adult patients. Sexually active patients should be advised that abstaining from sex or maintaining a mutually faithful monogamous sexual relationship with a partner known to be uninfected are the most effective strategies to prevent infection with the HIV virus or with other STDs. Patients should also receive counseling regarding the indications and proper methods for the use of condoms and spermicides in sexual intercourse and about the health risks associated with anal intercourse. Intravenous drugs users should be encouraged to enroll in drug treatment programs and should be warned about sharing drug equipment or using unsterilized needles and syringes. All patients should be offered testing in accordance with recommendations on screening for the STDs previously discussed.

Recommendation 54: Counseling to Prevent Unintended Pregnancy

Clinicians should obtain a complete sexual history from all adolescent and adult patients. Sexually active women who do not want to become pregnant and men who do not want to have a child should receive detailed counseling on methods to prevent unintended pregnancy. Sexually active patients should also receive information on measures to prevent STDs.

Recommendation 55: Counseling to Prevent Dental Disease
All patients should be encouraged to visit a dental care provider on a regular basis. Primary care clinicians should counsel patients regarding daily tooth brushing and dental flossing, the appropriate use of fluoride for caries prevention, avoiding sugary foods, and risk factors for developing baby bottle tooth decay. Children living in communities with inadequate water fluoridation should receive appropriate dietary fluoride supplements. While examining the mouth, clinicians should be alert for the obvious signs of oral disease.

Recommendation 56: Childhood Immunizations
All children should receive immunizations that are currently recommended by the American Academy of Pediatrics and the Center for Disease Control in Atlanta. These recommendations have been updated significantly since the U.S. Preventive Services Task Force published its book, and I have included the latest recommendations in the chapter on childhood immunizations.

In brief, the immunizations that are currently recommended in children are the following:

1) Hepatitis B × 3
2) OPV × 3 (early) with one booster
3) DTP × 3 (early) with one booster
4) Hib × 3 (early)
5) MMR at 12-15 months and at 4-6 years (Rubella again at age 12)
6) Td every 10 years thereafter

Recommendation 57: Adult Immunizations
Pneumococcal vaccine should be administered at least once and influenza vaccine should be administered to all persons aged 65 and older in addition to persons in other high-risk groups on a yearly basis. Hepatitis B vaccine should be offered to homosexually active men, intravenous drug users, and others at high risk of infection. All adults should receive tetanus-diptheria toxoid boosters at least once every 10 years. Vaccination against measles and mumps should be provided to all adults who lack evidence of immunity.

Recommendation 58: Postexposure Prophylaxis
Postexposure prophylaxis should be provided to selected persons with exposures to *Haemophilus influenzae* type b, meningococcal infection, hepatitis A, hepatitis B, tuberculosis, and rabies.

Recommendation 59: Estrogen Prophylaxis
Although routine postmenopausal estrogen replacement is not recommended, estrogen therapy should be considered for asymptomatic women who are at increased risk for osteoporosis, who lack known contraindications, and who have received adequate counseling about potential benefits and risks. The role of exercise and dietary calcium supplementation in preventing osteoporosis has been discussed.

Recommendation 60: Aspirin Prophylaxis
Low-dose aspirin should be considered for men over age 40 who are at significantly increased risk of myocardial infarction and who lack contraindications to the drug. Patients should understand the potential benefits and risks of aspirin therapy before beginning treatment.

SUGGESTED READINGS

ACIP recommended immunization schedule. Atlanta: Center for Disease Control, November 1993.

Report of the Canadian Task Force on the Periodic Health Examination. Health and Welfare Canada, 1994.

U.S. Preventive Task Force on the Periodic Health Examination. Guide to clinical preventive services. Baltimore: Williams and Wilkins, 1996.

PROBLEM 132   A 51-YEAR-OLD MALE WHO PRESENTS FOR A COMPLETE PHYSICAL EXAMINATION

A 51-year-old male presents to your office for a complete physical examination. He has been in the habit of "coming in for the once-over" every year. The patient has been told that "a complete physical—head to toe" is the best method of ensuring good health.

SELECT THE ONE BEST ANSWER TO THE FOLLOWING QUESTIONS

1. With regard to the relative effectiveness of the routine complete physical examination, which of the following statements is most accurate?
   a) the effectiveness of the routine complete physical examination has been confirmed in clinical trials
   b) the effectiveness of the routine complete physical examination has been confirmed with anecdotal evidence
   c) the effectiveness of the routine complete physical examination has been demonstrated in case-control trials
   d) the effectiveness of the routine complete physical examination has been confirmed in some studies but not in others
   e) none of the above are true

2. Which of the following is(are) criteria for effective periodic health screening?
   a) the condition tested must have a significant effect on quality of life
   b) the disease must have an asymptomatic phase during which detection and treatment significantly reduce morbidity and mortality
   c) acceptable treatment methods must be available
   d) tests must be available at a reasonable cost
   e) all of the above are true

3. Good reasons to consider performing a physical examination on an asymptomatic adult independent of routine screening include which of the following?
   a) the establishment of a good doctor-patient relationship
   b) to augment history taking
   c) to maximize your income
   d) a and b
   e) all of the above

4. Which of the following statements regarding the performance of a routine physical examination is(are) true?
   a) physical examination may in itself be therapeutic
   b) physical examination may provide the patient with reassurance
   c) physical examination may produce benefit to the patient through therapeutic touch
   d) physical examination may play an important role in development and maintenance of the clinical skills in the physician
   e) all of the above are true

5. Which of the following statements regarding the sensitivity and specificity of the routine physical examination is(are) true?
   a) routine physical examination is neither highly sensitive nor highly specific
   b) routine physical examination is both highly sensitive and highly specific
   c) routine physical examination is high in sensitivity but low in specificity
   d) routine physical examination is high in specificity but low in sensitivity
   e) none of the above are true

6. Which of the following is(are) valid reasons not to rely significantly on physical examination in asymptomatic adults?
   a) routine physical examination may offer a false sense of security
   b) routine physical examination is an inefficient use of time
   c) routine physical examination reinforces misperceptions about physician capabilities
   d) routine physical examination may detract from time that could be spent on other preventive interventions
   e) all of the above are true

7. Which of the following statements is(are) true regarding false positive findings on routine physical examination?
   a) false positive findings create needless patient anxiety
   b) false positive findings often initiate an "intervention cascade"
   c) false positive findings place a substantial burden on the entire health care system
   d) a and b
   e) all of the above

8. A 65-year-old male with a history of angina pectoris presents to his physician for a routine physical examination. The physician, upon auscultation of the cardiovascular system, declares that he "has the heart of a 20-year-old."
   Which of the following statements is(are) true regarding the physician's statement?
   a) this statement may reinforce misperceptions regarding physician capabilities
   b) this statement may result in patient anger if the patient later has a heart attack
   c) this statement may result in legal action if the patient later has a heart attack
   d) a and c
   e) all of the above are true

9. Which of the following statements is(are) true regarding patient perceptions of the routine complete physical examination and related laboratory tests?
   a) patients have come to understand that a routine physical examination, along with a complete laboratory profile, will diagnose the great majority of illness
   b) most patients understand the meaning of the term *periodic health examination*
   c) patients have come to understand the importance of a focused, regional examination and are much less likely to ask for a routine complete physical examination at this time
   d) patients are generally sensitive to the costs of routine physical examinations and routine laboratory tests
   e) none of the above statements are true

10. A 35-year-old female has presented to your office for a routine physical examination. The physician does a complete examination of the skin in an effort to identify dysplastic nevi, other unusual nevi, or other skin lesions.

Which of the following statements regarding examination of the skin during the physical examination of a patient is true?
   a) the examination for skin cancer in a routine physical examination is highly sensitive and highly specific
   b) the examination for skin cancer in a routine physical examination is highly sensitive but of low specificity
   c) the examination for skin cancer in a routine physical examination is neither sensitive nor specific
   d) the examination for skin cancer in a routine physical examination is highly specific but of lower sensitivity
   e) the examination for skin cancer is of variable sensitivity and specificity; it depends very much on the examiner

Short Answer Management Problem 132

A 51-year-old male presents to your office in an acutely agitated state. He presented to your partner last week for a "checkup." Instead of his regular checkup, he tells you he was given a "very cursory examination." He tells you that his heart was not checked, his lungs were not checked, his reflexes were not tapped, a light was not shone in his eyes, and so on.

You determine that your partner performed a focused periodic health examination, a concept that you believe in as well. You have just begun to introduce this concept into your practice. Discuss how you would respond to your patient at this time.

ANSWERS

1. E. Although the routine physical examination has been a primary diagnostic tool throughout the twentieth century, there is little, if any, evidence in the literature to support the efficacy of the routine checkup.

   It has been determined that the procedures that constitute the complete physical examination have not been held up to the same level or intensity of scientific scrutiny as other diagnostic tests, even though the evidence for the effectiveness of the complete physical examination has been found to be entirely lacking.

2. E. The criteria for effective periodic health screening are as follows:
   1. The condition tested for must have a significant effect on quality of life.
   2. Acceptable treatment methods must be available for that particular condition.
   3. The disease must have an asymptomatic phase during which detection and treatment significantly reduce morbidity and mortality.
   4. Treatment during the asymptomatic phase must yield a result superior to that obtained by delaying treatment until symptoms appear.
   5. Test must be available at a reasonable cost.
   6. Tests must be acceptable to the patient.
   7. The incidence of the condition must be sufficient to justify the cost of screening.

3. D.

4. E. Reasons to perform physical examinations in asymptomatic adults, independent of routine screening, include the following:
   1. To establish a good doctor-patient relationship
   2. To augment history taking
   3. To fulfill patient expectations
   4. To provide the therapeutic benefit of touch
   5. To maintain the physician's clinical skills
   6. To reinforce patient education, especially self-examination
   7. To realistically reassure the patient (and the physician)
   8. To establish the patient's baseline health status

9. To determine if the patient is indeed asymptomatic
10. To avoid giving the patient the impression that he or she must have symptoms in order to be examined

One of the choices provided in Question 3 ("to maximize the physician's income") seems like a contraindication to the performance of a physical examination to me.

5. A.

6. E. The procedures entailed in the routine physical examination are neither sensitive nor specific. Because of this, physicians may provide false reassurance on the basis of the findings. Consider statements such as "Your heart sounds great" or "You've got a complete, 100% perfect bill of health." Next week you hear from the ER doctor that your patient has just had a heart attack. Your next phone call probably will come from his lawyer. Such grandiose statements reinforce misperceptions regarding physicians' capabilities and may certainly result in legal action.

Several other considerations are very relevant to the performance of a routine physical examination. First, in their zeal to be complete, physicians sometimes forget the discomfort and the embarrassment caused by certain procedures and end up poking, prodding, and invading spaces that are both tender and very private. This may have a very negative consequence in that previous examination discomfort and embarrassment may keep patients from obtaining routine and very necessary health care.

Excessive concentration on physical examination detracts from time that could be spent in more productive pursuits, such as patient education and counseling about health risk behaviors.

7. E. The same excessive compulsiveness that serves as a survival skill in medical training is often dysfunctional in medical practice. False positive findings are common in the face of low test sensitivity and specificity and low prevalence of the condition in the population tested. Even if a test has a high sensitivity and specificity, the more tests or maneuvers that are performed on the same individual, the higher the likelihood of a false-positive result. Also, the likelihood that a positive test is true positive (positive predictive value) is directly related to the prevalence of the condition in the target population. Performing examinations in populations in which the condition has a low prevalence will thus generate a high false-positive rate.

False-positive test results create needless anxiety in both patients and physicians. More important, such results often lead to an "intervention cascade," initiating further testing of greater invasiveness, which increases the potential for iatrogenic harm. A good example of this is the finding of a slightly enlarged ovary (you think) on pelvic bimanual examination, a situation in which a benign cause is much more likely than a malignant cause. From that may result routine ultrasound, followed perhaps by laparoscopy to rule out a malignant tumor of very low prevalence.

We must all ask ourselves the following question: has this procedure really done the patient any good?

8. E. The explanation to this question is covered completely in the answer to Question 6.

9. A. Most patients have come to believe that a complete history and physical examination, along with a complete laboratory profile, will diagnose the great majority of illnesses. This is obviously a mistaken impression and should be corrected as soon as we begin to move toward a new partnership in health care, a partnership in which the patient (or client) is much more active than previously was the case.

Patients have not come to understand the concept of the periodic health examination or of focused regional examination; it does not appear that there is any more willingness at this time on the part of patients to abandon their conception of the complete or routine health examination.

As well, patients are still not very sensitive about costs of routine examinations and routine tests. A major patient education effort will be necessary to inform patients regarding these very important issues.

10. E. The clinical examination of the skin has significant variability in terms of sensitivity and specificity. The major reason for that variability is the variability in the expertise of the examiner. The greater the training and expertise in skin lesion diagnosis and treatment, the higher the sensitivity and specificity of the examination. Another excellent example of this phenomenon is radiologists reading mammograms. The more training the radiologist has, and the more mammograms the radiologist reads, the higher the sensitivity and specificity of mammograms.

SOLUTION TO SHORT ANSWER MANAGEMENT PROBLEM 132

This is a relatively difficult situation and requires both patience and diplomacy. The following may be a reasonable manner in which to approach this problem.

1. Listen to the patient. Have the patient articulate his concerns regarding the nature and performance of the examination to you.
2. Explain the rationale for the change in examination technique and procedure. Explain to the patient that the probability of producing a better outcome from this new process (the focused periodic health examination) is actually significantly higher than with the old process.

3. If the patient appears receptive to the new approach, then it is reasonable to follow up the conversation with some appropriate literature.

4. If the patient does not appear receptive to the new approach, it is important to convey the message that the "old way" may, in fact, be the best for this particular patient and that you will respect his wishes and continue to carry out your assessments for him in the manner of the complete routine checkup. The answer to Question 4 expands on the reasons why this approach may be preferable for other patients as well.

SUMMARY OF THE ROUTINE COMPLETE CHECKUP VERSUS THE FOCUSED PERIODIC HEALTH EXAMINATION

1. There is little, if any, evidence that the routine complete checkup is effective or addresses the issues and conditions that can be prevented or can be addressed or treated while in an asymptomatic phase.

2. In addition to the lack of established efficacy, there are significant risks to performing a routine complete checkup, not the least of which is labeling someone as healthy when, in fact, he or she is not healthy.

3. There are, however, reasons and situations in which it may be very reasonable to perform a routine complete checkup, reasons that, when balanced against the reasons not to perform the same, come out in favor of doing routine physical. These are outlined in Question 4.

4. There are significant misperceptions concerning the routine physical examination, which often result in excess procedures and excess laboratory tests. If carried to the extreme, this is a sure-fire way to end up on a wild goose chase. This wild goose chase may very well end up in a previously well person now becoming ill, from worry regarding a false positive test result, for example. Thus on many occasions one would not be overstating the case by stating that "everything was fine until the patient went to the doctor."

5. Remember, a normal patient is defined as a patient who has not been sufficiently investigated.

SUGGESTED READING

Frank SH, Stange KC, Moore P, Smith CK. The focused physical examination. Postgraduate Medicine 1992; 92(2):171-184.

PROBLEM 133 A 26-YEAR-OLD MEDICAL STUDENT WHO IS HAVING PANIC ATTACKS REGARDING HIS UPCOMING EPIDEMIOLOGY EXAMINATION

A 26-year-old medical student presents to your office in a state of extreme anxiety manifested by panic attacks throughout the previous week. His physical symptoms include sweating and palpitations.

On physical examination his blood pressure is 120/70 mm Hg, and no thyroid enlargement is noted. You order a T4 to exclude hyperthyroidism.

In an attempt to deal with his symptoms, you decide to spend some time tutoring the student regarding basic epidemiologic concepts. As a beginning you explain the basics of a 2 × 2 table (Table 133-1), which relates positive and negative test results to the presence or absence of disease in a specific population.

TABLE 133-1: RELATIONSHIP BETWEEN A TEST (TEST A) AND A DISEASE (DISEASE B)

	DISEASE B PRESENT	DISEASE B ABSENT
Test A positive	30	50
Test A negative	10	80

SELECT THE ONE BEST ANSWER TO THE FOLLOWING QUESTIONS

1. What is the sensitivity of test A for disease B?
   a) 25%
   b) 37.5%
   c) 75%
   d) 62.5%
   e) 11%

2. What is the specificity of test A for disease B?
   a) 25%
   b) 37.5%
   c) 75%
   d) 61.5%
   e) 11%

3. What is the positive predictive value of test A in the diagnosis of disease B?
   a) 37.5%
   b) 25%
   c) 75%
   d) 61.5%
   e) 11%

4. What is the negative predictive value of test A in the diagnosis of disease B?
   a) 37%
   b) 89%
   c) 25%
   d) 75%
   e) 61.5%

5. What is the likelihood ratio for test A in disease B?
   a) 0.39
   b) 1.95
   c) 3.80
   d) 0.79
   e) 1.51

6. What is the prevalence of disease A in this population?
   a) 15.5%
   b) 23.%
   c) 40.0%
   d) 10.5%
   e) 18.4%

Consider the data in Table 133-2 illustrating the prevalence of disease X in various populations. Based on this information about disease prevalence and assuming the sensitivity of test A for disease X is 80% and the specificity of test A for disease X is 90%, answer Questions 7-9.

TABLE 133-2: PREVALENCE OF DISEASE X IN CERTAIN POPULATIONS

SETTING	PREVALENCE (CASES/100,000)
General population	50
Women, aged 50 and older	500
Women, aged 65 and older with a suspicious finding on clinical examination	40,000

7. What is the positive predictive value of test A in the diagnosis of disease X in the general population?
   a) 0.4%
   b) 1.3%
   c) 5.4%
   d) 15.7%
   e) 39.6%

8. What is the positive predictive value of test A in disease X in women aged 50 and older?
   a) 0.4%
   b) 3.9%
   c) 10.7%
   d) 23.6%
   e) 52.7%

9. What is the positive predictive value of test A in disease X in women greater than 65 years of age with a suspicious finding on clinical examination?
   a) 0.4%
   b) 5.6%
   c) 34.7%
   d) 84.2%
   e) 93.0%

10. If the positive predictive value of a test for a given disease in a given population is 4%, how many true positive test results are there in a sample of 100 positive test results?
    a) 4
    b) 10
    c) 40
    d) 96
    e) none of the above

11. Consider the data in Table 133-3 concerning the sensitivity and specificity in the diagnosis of diabetes mellitus in the population.

TABLE 133-3: THE SENSITIVITY AND SPECIFICITY OF BLOOD SUGAR LEVELS IN THE DIAGNOSIS OF DIABETES MELLITUS

BLOOD SUGAR LEVEL 2 HOURS AFTER EATING	SENSITIVITY	SPECIFICITY
140 mg/100 (7.8 mmol/L)	57.1%	99.4%

Given that the data are correct, if the sensitivity of the test for a given blood sugar level was 38.6%, which of the following would be the most likely value for specificity?
   a) 99.2%
   b) 98.7%
   c) 92.4%
   d) 87.3%
   e) 100.0%

12. The validity of a test is best defined as which of the following?
    a) the reliability of the test
    b) the reproducibility of the test
    c) the variation in the test results
    d) the degree to which the results of a measurement correspond to the true state of the phenomenon
    e) the degree of biological variation of the test

13. Which of the following terms is synonymous with the term *reliability*?
    a) reproducibility
    b) validity
    c) accuracy

   d) mean
   e) variation

14. Which of the following is not a measure of central tendency?
    a) mean
    b) median
    c) mode
    d) standard deviation
    e) none; all of the above are measures of central tendency Gaussian distribution

15. Consider the following experimental data: in a trial of the effect of reducing multiple risk factors on the subsequent incidence of coronary artery disease, high-risk patients were selected for study. Elevated blood pressure was one of the risk factors that caused people to be considered. People were screened for inclusion in the study on three consecutive visits. Blood pressure at those visits, before any therapeutic interventions were undertaken, were as listed in Table 133-4.

TABLE 133-4 BLOOD PRESSURE READINGS VS. VISIT NUMBER

VISIT NUMBER	MEAN DIASTOLIC BLOOD PRESSURE (MM/HG)
1	99.2
2	91.2
3	90.7

Which of the following statements regarding these data is true?
   a) these results are very strange; consider publication in any journal specializing in irreproducible results
   b) this is an example of regression to the mean
   c) this is an example of natural variation
   d) the most likely explanation is either interobserver or intraobserver variation
   e) we are likely dealing with faulty equipment in this case; the most likely reason for this would be failure to calibrate all of the blood pressure cuffs

16. Consider the following experimental data: a population of heavy smokers (men smoking greater than 50 cigarettes/day) is divided into two groups and followed for a period of 10 years. Group 1 (the experimental group) consists of 490 individuals who have an annual chest X-ray performed. Group 2 (the control group) consists of 510 individuals who have no annual chest X-ray. After 10 years the mortality data are obtained:

Experimental group: 37 men diagnosed with lung cancer in that 10-year period; average survival time from diagnosis = 14 months.

Control group: 39 men diagnosed with lung cancer in that 10-year period; average survival time from diagnosis = 8 months.

Regarding these results, which of the following statements is true?

a) these results prove that screening chest X-rays improve survival time in lung cancer

b) these results prove that screening chest X-rays should be considered on all smokers

c) these results are most likely an example of lead-time bias

d) these results are most likely an example of length-time bias

e) these results don't make any sense; the experiment should be repeated

17. Length-time bias with respect to cancer diagnosis is defined as which of the following?

a) bias resulting from the detection of slow-growing tumors during screening programs more often than fast-growing tumors

b) bias resulting from the length of time a cancer was growing before any symptoms occurred

c) bias resulting from the length of time a cancer was growing before somebody got on the ball and started to ask some questions and perform some laboratory investigations

d) bias resulting from the length of time between the latent and more rapid growth phases of any cancer

e) none of the above

18. Concerning population and disease measurement, prevalence is defined as which of the following?

a) the fraction (proportion) of a population possessing a clinical condition at a given point in time

b) the fraction (proportion) of a population initially free of a disease but that develop the disease over a given period of time

c) equivalent to incidence

d) defined mathematically as $a + b/a + b + c + d$ in a 2×2 table relating sensitivity and specificity to positive predictive value

e) none of the above

19. Concerning population and disease measurement, incidence is defined as which of the following?

a) the fraction (proportion) of a population possessing a clinical condition at a given point in time

b) the fraction (proportion) of a population initially free of a disease but that develop the disease over a given period of time

c) equivalent to prevalence

d) of little use in epidemiology

e) none of the above

20. Regarding clinical epidemiology in relation to the practice of family medicine, which of the following statements is true?

a) clinical epidemiology is higher mathematics that bears little relation to the world in general, much less the specialty of family medicine

b) clinical epidemiology was invented to create anxiety and panic attacks that mimic hyperthyroidism in medical students and residents

c) clinical epidemiology is unlikely to contain any useful information for the average practicing family physician

d) clinical epidemiology is a passing fad; fortunately for all concerned, its time has passed

e) none of the above statements about clinical epidemiology are true

Short Answer Management Problem 133

A medical resident, who really isn't the least bit interested in clinical epidemiology, admits an 86-year-old woman to the hospital with congestive cardiac failure. He decides that "we'd better make sure we're complete here—we sure don't want to miss anything" and orders almost every laboratory test listed on the nursing station computer screen as available. You, the young medical student following behind him, regard him as a truly excellent role model and desire to practice like him when you become a resident. Thus, on your next admission (a 37-year-old male with acute gastroenteritis), you "throw the book at him— the 100% complete laboratory workup, no if's, and's, or but's, and no test missed."

Unfortunately for yourself, the attending physician in charge of the patient's care is less than impressed by your attentiveness to detail and completeness and asks you to explain yourself. As it turns out, you have ordered a total of 100 different laboratory tests (many of them disguised in chemistry panels to give the appearance of only a few brief panels). He asks you if you are aware of the probability of labeling someone who is truly normal as normal if you order 100 tests. Discuss your answer to this question.

ANSWERS:

1. C.

2. D.

3. A.

4. B.

5. B.

6. B. The 2×2 table in Table 133-5 will illustrate the answers to Questions 1-6.

TABLE 133–5: DISEASE X

	DISEASE X PRESENT	DISEASE X ABSENT
Test A positive	30 (a)	50 (b)
Test A negative	10 (c)	80 (d)

Sensitivity is defined as the proportion of people with the disease that have a positive test result. A sensitive test will rarely miss patients who have the disease. In Table 133-5, sensitivity is defined as the number of true positives/the number of true positives plus false negatives. That is,

$$\text{Sensitivity} = \text{TP/TP} + \text{FN}$$
$$\text{Sensitivity} = a/a + c = 30/40 = 75\%$$

A sensitive test (one that is usually positive in the presence of disease) should be selected when there is an important penalty for missing the disease. This would be so, for example, when you had reason to suspect a serious but treatable condition, such as a chest X-ray in a patient with suspected tuberculosis or Hodgkin's disease. In addition, sensitive tests are useful in the early stages of a diagnostic workshop of disease, when several possibilities are being considered, in order to reduce the number of possibilities. Thus, in situations like this, diagnostic tests are used to rule out diseases.

Specificity is defined as the proportion of people without the disease who have a negative test result. A specific test will rarely misclassify people without the disease as having the disease. In Table 133-5, specificity is defined as the number of true negatives/the number of true negatives plus the number of false positives. That is,

$$\text{Specificity} = \text{TN/TN} + \text{FP}$$
$$\text{Specificity} = d/d + b = 80/130 = 61.5\%$$

A specific test is useful to confirm, or rule in, a diagnosis that has been suggested by other tests or data. Thus a specific test is rarely positive in the absence of disease, that is, it gives very few false positive test results. Tests with high specificity are needed when false positive results can harm the patient physically, emotionally, or financially. Thus a specific test is most helpful when the test result is positive.

There is always a trade-off between sensitivity and specificity. In general, if a disease has a low prevalence, choose a more specific test; if a disease has a high prevalence, choose a more sensitive test.

Positive predictive value is defined as the probability of disease in a patient with a positive (abnormal) test result. In Table 133-5 the PPV is

$$\text{Positive predictive value} = a/a + b = 30/80 = 37.5\%$$

Negative predictive value is defined as the probability of not having the disease when the test result is negative. In Table 133-5 the NPV is

$$\text{Negative predictive value} = d/c + d = 80/90 = 89\%$$

The likelihood ratio of a positive test result is the probability of that test result in the presence of disease divided by the probability of the test result in the absence of disease. In Table 133-5,

$$\text{Likelihood ratio} (+) = \frac{a/a + c}{b/b + d} = 1.95$$

The prevalence of a disease in the population at risk is the fraction or proportion of a group possessing a clinical condition at a given point in time. Prevalence is measured by surveying a defined population containing people with and without the condition of interest (at a given point in time). Prevalence can be equated with pretest probability. In Table 133-5, prevalence is defined as

$$\text{Prevalence} = \frac{a + c}{a + b + c + d}$$

As prevalence falls, positive predictive value must fall along with it, and negative predictive value must rise.

7. A.

8. B.

9. D. The respective positive predictive values for test A in the diagnosis of disease X in the general population, women greater than 50 years, and women older than 65 with a suspicious finding on clinical examination are 0.4%, 3.9%, and 84.2%, respectively.

To perform the calculations necessary to arrive at these answers the following steps are recommended:

Step 1: identify the sensitivity and specificity of the sign, symptom, or diagnostic test that you plan to use. Many of these are published. If you are not certain, consider asking a consultant with special expertise in the area.

Step 2: using a 2×2 table, set your total equal to an even number (consider, for example, 1000 as a good choice). Therefore,

$$a + b + c + d = 1000$$

Step 3: using whatever information you have about the patient before you apply this diagnostic test, estimate his or her pretest probability (prevalence) of the disease in question. Next, put appropriate numbers at the bottom of the columns (*a* + *c* and *b* + *d*). The easiest way to do this is to express your pretest probability (or prevalence) as a decimal three places to the right. This result is *(a + c)*, and 1000 minus this result is *(b + d)*.

Step 4: start to fill in the cells of the 2 × 2 table. Multiply sensitivity (expressed as a decimal) by *(a + c)* and put the result in cell a. You can then calculate cell c by simple subtraction.

Step 5: similarly, multiple specificity (expressed as a decimal) by *(b + d)* and put the result in cell d. Calculate cell b by subtraction.

Step 6: you can now calculate positive and negative predictive values for the test with the prevalence (pretest probability) used.

TABLE 133-6: CALCULATIONS INVOLVED IN A GENERAL 2 × 2 TABLE

	TARGET DISORDER	
	Present	**Absent**
Test positive	Cell a sensitivity $x(a + c)$	Cell b $(b + d) - d$
Test negative	Cell c $(a + c) - a$	Cell d specificity $x(b + d)$
	Total $= a + b + c + d$	

For example, to calculate the positive predictive value for test A in the diagnosis of disease in women aged greater than 65 years with a suspicious finding on clinical examination,

Prevalence = 40,000 cases/100,000 = 400/1000
Setting the total number equal to 1000,

$$\frac{a + c}{a + b + c + d} = \frac{400}{1000}$$

Therefore, $a + c = 400$ and $b + d = 600$. Thus,

$$\text{Cell a} = \text{Sensitivity} \times 400$$
$$= 0.8 \times 400 = 320$$

and

$$\text{Cell c} = 400 - 320 = 80$$

Similarly,

$$\text{Cell d} = \text{Specificity} \times 600$$
$$= 0.9 \times 600 = 540$$

Therefore,

$$\text{Cell b} = 600 - 540 = 60$$

Positive predictive value $= a/a + b$
$$= 320/320 + 60 = 84.2\%$$

Similar calculations can be made for the general population (prevalence = 50/100,000) and for women greater than 50 years (prevalence = 500/100,000).

10. A. If the positive predictive value of a test for a given disease is 4%, then only 4 of 100 positive test results will be true positives; the remainder will be false positives. Further testing (often invasive) and anxiety will be inflicted on the 96% of the population with a positive test result but without disease.

Thus careful consideration should be given to the positive predictive value of any test for any disease in a given population before ordering it.

11. E. Remember the inverse relationship between sensitivity and specificity: if the sensivity goes down, the specificity goes up, and if the sensitivity goes up, the specificity goes down.

100.0% is the only value that is greater than the previous specificity of 99.4%; therefore it is the most likely correct value of the values listed for the cospecificity of the test. This is actually the case at a cutoff blood sugar level of 180 mg/100 mL 2 hours after eating; if we use this value for the cutoff, there will be even more false negatives than at 140 mg/100 mL (that is, we will incorrectly label more individuals who actually have diabetes as being normal), whereas we will not label anyone who does not have diabetes as having diabetes.

12. D. Validity is the degree to which the results of a measurement of a test actually correspond to the true state of the phenomenon being measured. Another word for validity is *accuracy*.

13. A. Reliability is the extent to which repeated measurements of a relatively stable phenomenon fall closely to each other. Reproducibility and precision are other words for this characteristic.

14. D. A normal or Gaussian distribution is characterized by the following measures of central tendency:
    1. A mean: the sum of values for observations/number of observations
    2. A median: the point where the number of observations above the mean equals the number of observations below the mean
    3. A mode: the most frequently occurring value
    In the same normal or Gaussian distribution, expressions of dispersion are the following:
    1. The range: from the lowest value to the highest value in a distribution
    2. The standard deviation: the absolute value of the average difference of individual values from the mean
    3. The percentile: The proportion of all observations falling between specified values
    The most valuable measure of dispersion in a normal or Gaussian distribution is the standard deviation.
    It is defined as follows:

$$\text{Standard deviation} = \sqrt{\frac{\Sigma(x - \bar{x})^2}{n - 1}}$$

In a normal or Gaussian distribution 68.26% of the values lie within $+/-1$ standard deviation from the mean; 95.44% of values lie within $+/-2$ standard deviations from the mean; and 99.72% of values lie within $+/-3$ standard deviations from the mean.

15. B. As can be seen in this trial, there was a substantial fall in mean blood pressure between the first and third visits. The explanation for this is called *regression to the mean*. The best explanation of regression to the mean is the following:

Patients who are singled out from others because they have a laboratory test that is unusually high or low can be expected, on the average, to be closer to the center of the distribution (normal or Gaussian) if the test is repeated. Moreover, subsequent values are likely to be more accurate estimates of the true value (validity), which could be obtained if the measurement were repeated for a particular patient many times.

16. C. This is an example of lead-time bias. *Lead time* is the period of time between the detection of a medical condition by screening and when it ordinarily would have been diagnosed due to symptoms.

In lung cancer, there is absolutely no evidence that chest X-rays have any influence on mortality. However, if, as in this case, the experimental group had chest X-rays done, then their lung cancers would have been diagnosed at an earlier time and it would appear that they were longer survivors. The control group would most likely have had their lung cancers diagnosed when they developed symptoms. In fact, however, the survival time would have been exactly the same; the only difference would have been that men in the experimental group would have known that they had lung cancer for a longer period of time.

17. A. Length-time bias occurs because the proportion of slow-growing lesions diagnosed during a cancer screening program is greater than the proportion of those diagnosed during usual medical care. The effect of including a greater number of slow-growing cancers makes it seem that the screening and early treatment program are more effective than they really are.

18. A. *Prevalence* is defined as the fraction (proportion) of a population possessing a clinical condition at a given point in time. Prevalence is measured by surveying a defined population in which some have, and some do not have, the condition of interest at a single point in time. It is not the same as incidence, and, as previously discussed in relation to sensitivity, specificity, and positive predictive value in a 2 × 2 table, it is defined in mathematical terms as $a + c/a + b + c + d$.

19. B. Incidence in relation to a population is defined as the fraction (proportion) initially free of a disease or condition that go on to develop it over a given period of time.

20. E. Clinical epidemiology is a specialty that will assume more and more importance in the specialty of family medicine. Clinical epidemiology allows us to understand disease, to understand laboratory testing, and to understand why we should do what we should do and why we shouldn't do what we shouldn't do. More importantly, as family physicians in the future are called on by governments, patients, licensing bodies, and boards to justify clinical decisions and treatments, it will allow us to understand the difference between defensive medicine and defensible medicine (the latter being what we are trying to achieve) in the interest of optimizing the health care of our patients.

SOLUTION TO SHORT ANSWER MANAGEMENT PROBLEM 133

Although 100 may be a bit of an exaggeration, it may not be. At some hospitals, patients have CBCs done routinely every second or third day. With a few chemistry panels thrown in for good measure every week or so, it doesn't take that long to add up to 100 individual tests. The relationship between the number of tests ordered and the percentage of normal people with at least one abnormal test result is shown in Table 133-7.

TABLE 133-7 TESTING AND POSITIVE PREDICTIVE VALUE: AN EXAMPLE OF FALSE POSITIVITY

NUMBER OF TESTS	PEOPLE WITH AT LEAST ONE ABNORMALITY (%)
1	5
5	23
20	64
100	99.4

Thus, if you did order 100 laboratory tests, and the patient was truly well (no evidence of disease), there is less than a 1% chance that you would come to that conclusion. Using the fundamentals of Logic 100 we could quite justifiably say that a normal patient is defined as someone who has not been sufficiently investigated.

The answer to this short answer management problem is to say as little as possible. Offer to read a short textbook on epidemiology before you see your attending physician again.

SUMMARY

1. Remember the importance of sensitivity, specificity, and especially positive predictive value; understand that the lower the prevalence (or likelihood) of a condition in

the patient about to be tested, the lower the positive predictive value of the test.

2. Understand the importance of false negatives and especially false positives in the laboratory tests that you order.

3. Be prepared to draw a 2 × 2 table and calculate the positive predictive value of a test given the sensitivity, specificity, and prevalence of the condition in the population.

4. Misinterpretations that may result in survival statistics in cancer are due to lead-time bias and length-time bias.

5. Apply the principle of regression to the mean in the diagnosis of certain conditions, hypertension being a prime example.

6. Remember the dictum *primum non nocere:* first do no harm.

7. Sensitivity and specificity are inversely related: as sensitivity of a test goes up, the specificity of the test goes down.

8. Sensitive tests should be used to rule out disease; specific tests should be used to rule in disease.

9. Although a test may be reliable, it may not have any validity.

10. Remember the definition of a normal patient: someone who has not been sufficiently investigated.

SUGGESTED READINGS

Fletcher R, Fletcher S, Wagner E. Clinical epidemiology: The essentials. 2nd Ed. Baltimore, MD: Williams and Wilkins, 1988.

Sackett D, Haynes R, Tugwell P. Clinical epidemiology: A basic science for clinical medicine. Boston: Little, Brown, 1985.

PROBLEM 134   A 40-YEAR-OLD EXECUTIVE WHO SMOKES THREE PACKS OF CIGARETTES A DAY

A 40-year-old executive who smokes three packs of cigarettes/day presents for his routine health assessment. He states that he would like to quit smoking but is having great difficulty. He has tried three times before, but "pressures at work mounted up and I just had to go back to smoking."

The patient has a history of mild hypertension. His blood cholesterol level is normal. He drinks only 1 or 2 oz of alcohol/week.

His family history is significant for premature cardiovascular disease and death.

SELECT THE ONE BEST ANSWER TO THE FOLLOWING QUESTIONS

1. Current evidence suggests that coronary artery disease is strongly related to cigarette smoking. What percentage of deaths from CHD are thought to be due directly to cigarette smoking?
   a) < 5%
   b) 10%
   c) 20%
   d) 25%
   e) 30%-40%

2. Which of the following diseases has not been linked to cigarette smoking?
   a) carcinoma of the larynx
   b) hypertension
   c) abruptio placenta
   d) carcinoma of the colon
   e) Alzheimer's disease

3. Which of the following statements with respect to passive smoking is false?
   a) spouses of patients who smoke are not at increased risk of developing carcinoma of the lung
   b) sidestream smoke contains more carbon monoxide than mainstream smoke
   c) infants of mothers who smoke absorb measurable amounts of their mothers' cigarette smoke
   d) children of parents who smoke have an increased prevalence of bronchitis and pneumonia
   e) the most common symptom arising from passive smoking is eye irritation

4. Of the following factors listed, which is the most important factor in determining the success of a smoking-cessation program in an individual?
   a) the desire of the patient to quit
   b) a pharmacologic agent as a part of the smoking-cessation program
   c) the inclusion of a behavior-modification component to the program
   d) physician advice to quit smoking
   e) repeated office visits

5. Which of the following agents is now the pharmacologic agent of choice for inclusion in a smoking-cessation program?
   a) clonidine
   b) propranolol
   c) nicotine-containing chewing gum
   d) transdermal nicotine
   e) mecamylamine (a nicotine antagonist)

6. Which of the following smoking-cessation methods results in the highest percentage of both short-term and long-term success?
   a) transdermal nicotine
   b) a patient education booklet
   c) physician counseling and advice
   d) a contract for a "quit date"
   e) a combination of all of the above

7. What is the percentage of patients who relapse following successful cessation of smoking, approximately?
   a) 10%
   b) 50%
   c) 75%
   d) 85%
   e) 99%

8. What is the most modifiable risk factor for increased morbidity and mortality in the United States in 1994?
   a) hypertension
   c) hyperlipidemia
   c) cigarette smoking
   d) occupational burnout
   e) alcohol consumption

9. Nicotine replacement is especially important in which group of cigarette-smoking patients?
   a) those patients who smoke when work-related stressors become unmanageable
   b) those patients who smoke more than 20 cigarettes/day
   c) those patients who smoke within 30 minutes of awakening
   d) those patients who experience withdrawal symptoms
   e) all of the above
   f) b, c, and d

10. Which of the following statements regarding the economic burden of smoking is(are) true?
    a) the economic burden of smoking is placed not only on the individual but also on society
    b) in the United States in 1985 the costs related to cigarette smoking (directly and indirectly) exceeded $65 billion
    c) smoking has no significant effect on work-related productivity
    d) a and b
    e) all of the above

Short Answer Management Problem 134

A 41-year-old presents to you with an expressed desire to quit smoking. He is smoking three packs of cigarettes/day and has done so for the past 20 years. Discuss your use of nicotine replacement (how, for how long, specific instructions) along with other possible pharmacologic interventions in helping this patient achieve his goal of complete smoking cessation.

Although this question asks you specifically to discuss pharmacologic management, it must be emphasized that this is only one component of a multicomponent program.

ANSWERS

1. D. Twenty-five percent of deaths from CHD are directly attributable to smoking. The incidence of myocardial infarction and death from CHD is 70% higher in cigarette smokers than in nonsmokers. In the United States, 18% of all deaths are due to cigarette smoking.

2. D. The health consequences of smoking are enormous. The major processes involved include active smoking, passive smoking, addiction, and accelerated aging.

    The following disease categories have been directly linked to smoking: cancer, respiratory diseases, cardiovascular diseases, pregnancy and infant health, and other conditions.

    The actual diseases involved include the following:
    I. Cancer:
       A. Carcinoma of the lung
       B. Carcinoma of the larynx
       C. Carcinoma of the mouth
       D. Carcinoma of the pharynx
       E. Carcinoma of the stomach
       F. Carcinoma of the liver
       G. Carcinoma of the pancreas
       H. Carcinoma of the bladder
       I. Carcinoma of the uterine cervix
       J. Carcinoma of the breast
       K. Carcinoma of the brain
    II. Respiratory diseases:
       A. Emphysema
       B. Chronic bronchitis
       C. Asthma
       D. Bacterial pneumonia
       E. TB pneumonia
       F. Asbestosis
    III. Cardiovascular diseases:
       A. Coronary artery disease
       B. Hypertension
       C. Aortic aneurysm
       D. Arterial thrombosis
       E. Stroke
    IV. Pregnancy/infant health:
       A. Intrauterine growth retardation
       B. Abortion
       C. Fetal/neonatal death
       D. Abruptio placenta
       E. Bleeding in pregnancy NYD
       F. Placenta praevia
       G. Premature rupture of the membranes
       H. Prolonged rupture of the membranes
       I. Preterm labor
       J. Preeclampsia
       K. Sudden infant death syndrome (SIDS)
       L. Congenital malformations
    V. Other miscellaneous conditions:
       A. Peptic ulcer disease
       B. Osteoporosis
       C. Alzheimer's disease
       D. Wrinkling of the skin ("crow's feet" appearance on the face)

    The mechanisms whereby the linkage between smoking and the aforementioned diseases occur are multifactorial and are beyond the scope of this chapter. What is striking, however, is the number of medical disease categories that smoking affects and the number of diseases within each category that smoking affects. Carcinoma of the colon has not been causally associated with cigarette smoking.

3. A. Tobacco smoke in the environment is derived from either mainstream smoke (exhaled smoke) or sidestream smoke (smoke arising from the burning end of a cigarette). As well, there is an increased prevalence

of bronchiolitis, asthma, bronchitis, and pneumonia in infants and children whose parents smoke.

The most common symptom arising from exposure to passive smoking is eye irritation. Other significant symptoms include headaches, nasal symptoms, and cough. Exposure to tobacco smoke also precipitates or aggravates allergies.

Spouses of patients who smoke are at increased risk of developing lung cancer and coronary artery disease. For lung cancer, the average relative risk is 1.34 compared to persons not exposed to passive smoke. This risk, in comparison, is more than 100 times higher than the estimated effect of 20 years' exposure to asbestos while living or working in asbestos-containing buildings.

4. A. The most important factor in determining the success of a quit-smoking program is the desire of the individual to quit. If the individual is not interested in quitting, the probability of success is very low. Physician advice to quit, behavior-modification aids, nicotine replacement, and repeated office visits are all important. However, without the will to quit, they will not be effective.

5. D. The pharmacologic agent of choice for inclusion in a smoking-cessation program is transdermal nicotine. Until a transdermal system was developed for the delivery of nicotine, the agent of choice was nicotine-containing chewing gum (Nicorettes). Although the gum is still recommended by some physicians, the transdermal nicotine delivery system has both fewer adverse physiological effects and fewer side effects. The unpleasant side effects that are avoided by prescribing nicotine in a transdermal system rather than in a gum include bad taste, nausea, dyspepsia, and singultus. In addition, there is no unsightly chewing or the inconvenience of the need for frequent administrations.

Clonidine has proven efficacy in the relief of symptoms of opiate and alcohol withdrawal. It has, in some studies, been shown to be superior to placebo in helping patients to remain abstinent from smoking for periods up to 1 year. Thus it may still be considered to be a useful adjunct. It has significant side effects, however, and is certainly not routinely recommended.

Mecamylamine is a nicotine receptor antagonist that is analogous to naloxone for the treatment of opiate abuse. Mecamylamine may be useful as a method of smoking cessation in the recalcitrant smoker. It has not been extensively studied in such a population.

Propranolol has been shown to relieve some of the physiological changes associated with alcohol-withdrawal–induced anxiety, but it has been shown to be ineffective in smoking cessation and has no effect on reducing subjective satisfaction and extinction of smoking behavior.

6. E. A meta-analysis of controlled trials of smoking cessation compared the effectiveness of smoking cessation counseling, self-help booklets, nicotine replacement, and establishing a contract and setting a quit date. The study found that each modality was effective, but no single modality worked significantly better than the others. When treatment modalities were combined, however, the following results were obtained:
   A. Two treatment modalities were more effective than one.
   B. Three treatment modalities were more effective than two.
   C. Four treatment modalities are more effective than three.

   A mnemonic for the smoking-cessation protocol that you should employ with patients is "bad nicotine":
   B = Education booklet
   A = Advice, counseling, specific suggestions for patient behavior modification
   D = Date of quitting (establish a contract and a date that is convenient for the patient)
   NICOTINE = Nicotine replacement (transdermal nicotine)

7. D. Arranging follow-up appointments for the patient is extremely important. This, in effect, prepares the patient for the support and surveillance of the physician. At the follow-up visits there is an opportunity to review concerns, review continuing plans, and discuss lapses. This last issue is extremely important, as lapses occur in 85% of those who quit. The reaction and counseling of the physician following a lapse is crucial and should be framed in the context of a positive learning experience. One of the key points that needs to be reinforced by the physician is that learning to live without cigarettes is like learning any new skill—you learn from mistakes until your action becomes a new habitual behavior.

8. C. Cigarette smoking is the most prevalent modifiable risk factor to decreased morbidity and mortality in the United States, and perhaps also the world. Not only does the smoker incur medical risks attributable to cigarette smoking, but passive smokers and society also bear the ill effects and the increased economic costs attributable to the smoker's habit.

Hypertension and hyperlipidemia have already been modified to some degree (hypertension more than hyperlipidemia).

Alcohol consumption and abuse is also an important problem and is addressed in another chapter in this book.

Although this chapter is focused on smoking, its risks, and the importance and means to quit, one of the choices in Question 8 offers a short detour to stress and burnout. Occupational stress and burnout might, to some, seem like a lightweight compared to the other choices listed. While, relatively speaking, that may be true, one should not underestimate the effect that the move to a global economy is having on the workers in our countries. Although the terms *downsizing* and *rightsizing* make good business talk and are reasonable business jargon (as far as anything in business is reasonable in this age), health care professionals may contend that *wrongsizing* is the more appropriate word, in the sense of what the new economy is doing to employment (or, more correctly, unemployment), relative standard of living, and the family. In health (as defined by the World Health Organization as "not just the absence of disease but the presence of physical, emotional, and social well-being"), one could argue that the effect of this entity on morbidity in North America is underestimated and should always be addressed by primary care physicians when the opportunity arises.

9. F. Nicotine replacement is especially important for the following smokers:
   1. Smokers who smoke more than 20 cigarettes/day.
   2. Smokers who smoke within 30 minutes of waking up.
   3. Smokers who experience withdrawal symptoms.
      Smokers who smoke when exposed to extremely stressful work situations should be managed mainly by behavior modification techniques.

10. D. The individual smoker and society in general incur enormous economic costs due to smoking. The health care costs attributable to cigarette smoking were estimated to exceed $17 billion/year in 1984 and surely significantly exceed that figure today. Lost work and productivity are very important and often forgotten hazards of smoking. With the inclusion of the last two factors, the costs associated with cigarette smoking are estimated to exceed $65 billion/year in the United States.

SOLUTION TO SHORT ANSWER MANAGEMENT PROBLEM 134

This patient is one who certainly will potentially benefit (*potentially* because we aren't sure whether he will be successful in quitting altogether and maintain that status) from a pharmacologic component to his smoking cessation program.

The agent of choice, as described earlier, is transdermal nicotine. I will select a specific agent and describe the method in which it could best be used.

Agent: Habitrol

Dosage: 21 mg nicotine/day, 14 mg nicotine/day, 7 mg nicotine/day

1. Before starting the nicotine replacement, the patient must quit smoking completely (not just cut down). If the patient has been unable to maintain or otherwise reestablish abstinence with the aid of Habitrol after 1 month, then treatment should be discontinued.

2. Begin with one patch/day of the 21 mg nicotine Habitrol. Instruct the patient to apply one system (patch) daily and have him leave it on the skin for 24 hours.

3. Continue with the 21 mg nicotine system for at least 4 weeks (the greater the previous amount/day smoked, the longer you should treat with the transdermal nicotine). The preferred range seems to be from about 8 weeks to about 16 weeks.

4. Switch after 4 weeks to the 14 mg/day nicotine system. Continue for 4 weeks.

5. Switch after a total of 8 weeks to the 7 mg/day nicotine system. Continue for at least another 4 weeks.

6. Discontinue the Habitrol at that time or shortly thereafter. As of the time of writing of this book, clonidine has not been approved by the Food and Drug Administration for use in smoking cessation. You may wish to consider this agent if that status changes, or consider discussing the issue with a physician who has expertise in smoking cessation. If clonidine were to be used, the dosage would be between 0.2 mg/day and 0.4 mg/day.

7. See the patient at least once every 2 weeks while he is maintained on Habitrol.

8. Following cessation of Habitrol, see the patient every 4 weeks to follow up his continued cessation.

SUMMARY OF PHYSICIAN INTERVENTION IN SMOKING CESSATION

1. Identify all patients in your practice who smoke.
2. Present all the health consequences of smoking.
3. Present the health benefits of smoking cessation.
4. Assess and develop the desire to modify smoking behavior.
5. Develop and formalize a patient-centered plan for change.
6. Establish a quit date and have the patient sign a contract.
7. Utilize transdermal nicotine as an adjunct, especially in patients who smoke more than 20 cigarettes/day, smoke within 30 minutes of awakening, and experience withdrawal symptoms.
8. Utilize behavior-modification techniques as part of counseling and advice.
9. Consider using all of the following to improve the chance of quitting permanently: obtain smoking-cessation patient education booklets from the American Lung Association or the American Cancer Society and give one to every patient; establish a quit date and a contract; advise and counsel the patient at regular intervals and incorporate behavior-modification techniques; and use a transdermal nicotine replacement for 8-12 weeks.
10. Have the patient consider times at which he or she may relapse (which will happen in 85% of patients); for ex-

ample, triggers such as having a drink with friends at the end of a stressful week should be avoided for the first few months.

11. Continue surveillance for relapse prevention and plan modifications as needed.

SUGGESTED READINGS

Brosky G. Smoking cessation counselling: A practical protocol. Canadian Journal of CME 1994; January:43-60.

Jayanthi V, Probert K, Sher S, Mayberr J. Smoking and prevention. Respiratory Medicine 1991; 85:179-183.

Kottke T, Battista R, DeFriese G et al.: Attributes of successful smoking cessation interventions in medical practice. Journal of the American Medical Association 1988; 259:2882.

Lee E, D'Alonza G. Cigarette smoking, nicotine addiction, and its pharmacologic treatment. Archives of Internal Medicine 1993; 153:34-48.

PROBLEM 135 A 74-YEAR-OLD FARMER WITH ABDOMINAL PAIN

A 74-year-old grain farmer presents to your office for assessment of abdominal pain of 6 months' duration. The pain is located in the central abdomen with radiation through to the back. It is a dull, constant pain with no significant aggravating or relieving factors. It is not affected in any way by food. It is rated by the patient as 5/10 baseline, with occasional increases to 7/10. It has been getting worse for the last 2 months.

On examination, the abdomen is scaphoid. There is the suggestion of hepatomegaly, with the liver palpated 2 cm below the right costal margin. No other masses are felt.

Abdominal ultrasound reveals a solid mass lesion in the area of the head of the pancreas measuring 4 cm × 3 cm. There are also two or three small areas (< 1 cm) in the liver that are suspicious for metastatic carcinoma.

SELECT THE ONE BEST ANSWER TO THE FOLLOWING QUESTIONS

1. What is the most likely diagnosis in this patient?
   a) benign pseudocyst of the pancreas
   b) adenocarcinoma of the pancreas
   c) squamous cell carcinoma of the pancreas
   d) pancreatitis
   e) malignant pseudocyst of the pancreas

2. With regard to the diagnosis in this patient, which of the following statements is true?
   a) the death rate from this disease has remained constant over the last 20 years in the United States
   b) the death rate from this disease has decreased slightly over the last 20 years in the United States
   c) the death rate from this disease has increased slightly over the last 20 years in the United States
   d) there are no accurate data on death rates from this disease in the United States over the last 20 years
   e) none of the above are true

3. With regard to all cancer deaths in the United States over the last 20 years, which of the following statements is true?
   a) during the last 20 years, the death rate from all cancers has increased by 7%
   b) during the last 20 years, the death rate from all cancers has decreased by 20%
   c) during the last 20 years there has been no significant change in the death rate from all cancers
   d) during the last 20 years, the death rate from all cancers has increased by 1%
   e) during the last 20 years, the death rate from all cancers has decreased by 15%

4. With respect to the reason(s) for the death rates discussed in Question 3, which of the following statements is true?
   a) the major cause of the increased death rate is an increase in the American life span
   b) the major cause of the increased death rate is likely improved diagnostic techniques

   c) the major cause of the decreased death rate is better treatments for the majority of cancers
   d) the major cause of the decreased death rate is increased prevention
   e) there is no clear answer as to the cause of the change in cancer death rates

5. With respect to pesticide application and the patient described in Question 1, which of the following statements is true?
   a) there is no link between this disease and environmental carcinogens
   b) there is some suggestion of a link between pesticide application and the disease described in Question 1
   c) there is clear evidence that there is a link between pesticide application and the disease described in Question 1
   d) environmental carcinogens are not thought to play a role in the disease described in the patient in Question 1
   e) there is no evidence either way to suggest a link between environmental carcinogens and the disease described in the patient in Question 1

6. With respect to the disease described in the patient in Question 1, which of the following statements is the most accurate?
   a) cigarette smoking has been implicated as a cause of the disease
   b) alcohol abuse has been implicated as a cause of the disease
   c) both cigarette smoking and alcohol abuse have been implicated as causes of the disease
   d) neither cigarette smoking nor alcohol abuse have been implicated as causes of the disease
   e) nobody really knows for sure

7. The death rate from which of the following cancers has increased to the greatest extent over the last 20 years?
   a) breast cancer
   b) lung cancer
   c) pancreatic cancer
   d) stomach cancer
   e) malignant melanoma

8. What is the most common cause of cancer death in women in the United States today?
   a) breast cancer
   b) colon cancer
   c) lung cancer
   d) brain cancer
   e) liver cancer

9. Regarding chemotherapy and radiotherapy given to American patients during the past 20 years, which of the following statements is correct?
   a) the use of aggressive chemotherapy has significantly cut the overall death rate from cancer in the United States
   b) the use of therapeutic and prophylactic radiotherapy has significantly increased the overall death rate from cancer in the United States
   c) the use of both aggressive chemotherapy and thera-
   peutic and prophylactic radiotherapy has significantly decreased the overall death rate from cancer in the United States
   d) neither aggressive chemotherapy nor radiotherapy have decreased the overall death rate from cancer in the United States
   e) no data are available on which to comment regarding cancer death rates and the use of chemotherapy and radiotherapy

10. Which of the following cancers have demonstrated a decreased death rate in the last 20 years?
    a) cancer of the stomach
    b) cancer of the ovary
    c) cancer of the lung
    d) cancer of the liver
    e) cancer of the brain

Short Answer Management Problem 135

Discuss the preventive measures that your patients may undertake to lower their risk of cancer from all causes.

ANSWERS

1. B. The most likely diagnosis in this patient is adenocarcinoma of the pancreas.

   With the clinical history of progressive pain, the finding of hepatomegaly (which suggests liver metastases), and the finding of a mass lesion on ultrasound, the diagnosis is almost certainly confirmed.

   None of the other choices are reasonable. Pseudocysts do not show solid mass lesions. Squamous cell carcinoma does not occur in the pancreas. The history, physical findings, and ultrasound findings are not compatible with a diagnosis of pancreatitis.

2. C. Over the last 20 years, the death rate from carcinoma of the pancreas has increased slightly in patients over the age of 65 in the United States. In patients under the age of 65 it has decreased slightly. Overall, there appears to be a slight increase in the death rate from this disease.

3. A. During the last 20 years, the overall death rate from all cancers has increased by 7% in the United States. This is despite all of the work funded and organized through the National Cancer Institute and despite then-

president Richard Nixon's "Declaration of War" on cancer signed on December 23, 1971.

4. E. There is no clear answer as to reason(s) for the increase in cancer death rates in the last 20 years. It has, however, been determined that it is not because the population is living longer. It likely is a combination of increased diagnostic ability and an actual increase in the susceptibility to some cancers in the American population. The possibility of a link to dietary fat, a failure to adequately address lifestyle issues on the part of most Americans, and links to environmental carcinogens may all play a role in this increased death rate.

5. A. There is no suggestion of a link between pesticide application and pancreatic cancer in farmers. The types of cancer that are more common in farmers include Hodgkin's disease, multiple myeloma, leukemia, malignant melanoma, cancer of the lip, and cancer of the prostate.

6. C. Both cigarette smoking and alcohol abuse have been implicated as causes of pancreatic cancer.

7. B. Death rates from lung cancer, especially among women, have increased significantly over the past 20

years. This is mainly due to a significant increase in smoking among women during the early part of this time period.

8. C. Lung cancer is now the most common cause of cancer death in American women. This is primarily associated with the significantly increased risk due to smoking previously discussed.

9. D. Despite a significant increase in both the number and cancer cell toxicity of chemotherapeutic drugs used and a significant increase in the frequency with which radiotherapy is used, there has been no significant effect on the overall cancer death rate. If anything, the use of these forms of therapy may have actually caused more cancers than they have cured.

10. A. Cancers that have shown a decreased death rate over the past 20 years include cancer of the larynx, cancer of the colon, cancer of the mouth and pharynx, cancer of the thyroid, cancer of the bladder, cancer of the stomach, cancer of the uterus, cancer of the cervix, Hodgkin's disease, and cancer of the testes.

   Cancers that have shown an increased death rate in the last 20 years include cancer of the lung, malignant melanoma, multiple myeloma, cancer of the prostate, cancer of the esophagus, cancer of the breast, cancer of the brain, and cancer of the ovary.

SOLUTION TO SHORT ANSWER MANAGEMENT PROBLEM 135

The most important preventive measures that your patients may undertake to lower their risk of cancer from all causes are as follows:
1) Discontinue cigarette, pipe, and cigar smoking.
2) Decrease the amount of alcohol consumed.
3) Decrease the amount of dietary fat, especially saturated fat.
4) Maintain a normal weight (to be accomplished by a decrease in dietary fat, a decrease in overall caloric intake, and an exercise program).
5) Decrease exposure to environmental carcinogens whenever possible (protect yourself when applying pesticides, herbicides, and related chemicals).
6) Avoiding sun exposure without a sunscreen with a SPF (sun protective factor) $\geq$ 20.
7) Follow the recommendations of the U.S. Preventive Services Task Force on the Periodic Health Examination.

SUMMARY OF TRENDS IN CANCER EPIDEMIOLOGY

1. The overall death rate from all cancers has increased by approximately 7% in the United States over the past 20 years.
2. Lung cancer is now the number one cause of cancer deaths among women (overtaking breast cancer).
3. The increase in overall incidence has not been completely explained but may have resulted from a combination of better diagnostic techniques, smoking, alcohol use, and pesticides/herbicides and other environmental carcinogens.
4. Chemotherapy and radiotherapy have, in the overall context, not resulted in any significant decrease in cancer death rate despite their increased use.
5. Prevention remains the best strategy. The most important preventive measures include discontinuing cigarette smoking, discontinuing or significantly decreasing alcohol consumption, decreasing the amount of dietary fat in the diet, avoiding exposure to the sun without a sunscreen, and avoiding exposure to other environmental carcinogens.

SUGGESTED READING

Fletcher RH, Fletcher SW, Wagner E. Clinical epidemiology: the essentials. Baltimore: Williams and Wilkins, 1991.

PROBLEM 136   A 52-YEAR-OLD MALE WITH CAD WHO HAS HAD BOTH A CABG PROCEDURE AND PCTA

A 52-year-old male with a history of CAD treated by a CABG procedure following three PCTA procedures and who currently is on "triple angina therapy" presents to your office for a discussion of his condition and of the implications of his condition for his children. He has recently read that family history is a strong risk factor for coronary artery disease.

SELECT THE ONE BEST ANSWER TO THE FOLLOWING QUESTIONS

1. During the past 15 years, the death rate from cardiovascular disease in the United States has
   a) increased by 15%
   b) decreased by 15%
   c) decreased by 35%
   d) increased by 10%
   e) remained unchanged

2. During the past 15 years, the death rate from coronary artery disease in the United States has
   a) increased by 15%
   b) decreased by 40%
   c) decreased by 25%
   d) increased by 20%
   e) remained unchanged

3. During the past 15 years, the death rate from stroke in the United States has
   a) decreased by 50%
   b) decreased by 25%
   c) increased by 15%
   d) increased by 25%
   e) remained unchanged

4. What has been the major reason for the change in death rate from cardiovascular disease in the United States?
   a) new technology
   b) improved pharmacology
   c) better surgical techniques
   d) risk factor reduction
   e) nobody really knows for sure

5. The risk of developing cardiovascular disease in patients with hypertension compared to nonhypertensive patients is
   a) three to four times as high for CAD and seven times as high for stroke
   b) twice as high for CAD and five times as high for stroke
   c) six times as high for CAD and eight times as high for stroke
   d) the same for CAD and twice as high for stroke
   e) the same for CAD and the same for stroke

6. Regarding cigarette smoking and risk of developing CAD, which of the following statements is true?
   a) cigarette smokers have a 70% greater risk of developing CAD than nonsmokers
   b) cigarette smokers have a 50% greater risk of developing CAD than nonsmokers
   c) cigarette smokers have a 25% greater risk of developing CAD than nonsmokers
   d) cigarette smokers have a 10% greater risk of developing CAD than nonsmokers
   e) there is no difference in the risk of developing CAD between smokers and nonsmokers

7. Regarding serum cholesterol and the incidence of CAD, which of the following statements is true?
   a) for each 1% reduction in serum cholesterol there is a 6% reduction in the risk of heart disease death
   b) for each 1% reduction in serum cholesterol there is a 4% reduction in the risk of heart disease death
   c) for each 1% reduction in serum cholesterol there is a 2% reduction in the risk of heart disease death
   d) for each 1% reduction in serum cholesterol there is a 1% reduction in the risk of heart disease death
   e) there is no established relationship between serum cholesterol and the risk of heart disease death

8. Which of the following statements regarding the influence of race on mortality from CAD, stroke, and end-stage renal failure due to hypertension is true?
   a) the death rate in blacks from CAD and stroke is higher than whites; conversely, the death rate from end-stage renal failure secondary to hypertension is higher in whites than blacks
   b) the death rate from CAD and end-stage renal failure due to hypertension is higher in blacks than whites; conversely, the death rate from stroke is higher in whites than in blacks
   c) the death rate in blacks due to stroke and end-stage renal failure due to hypertension is higher than in whites; conversely, the death rate from CAD is higher in whites than blacks
   d) the death rate in blacks from CAD, stroke, and end-stage renal failure secondary to hypertension is higher than in whites
   e) the death rate in whites from CAD, stroke, and end-stage renal failure due to hypertension is higher than in blacks

9. Regarding the risk of obesity in relation to cardio-vascular disease, which of the following statements is(are) true?
   a) obesity is a risk factor for hypertension
   b) obesity is a risk factor for hypercholesterolemia
   c) obesity is a risk factor for diabetes
   d) obesity is an independent risk factor for CAD
   e) all of the above

10. What is the definition of *obesity?*
   a) a weight > 40% above normal weight for height
   b) a weight > 30% above normal weight for height
   c) a weight > 20% above normal weight for height
   d) a weight > 15% above normal weight for height
   e) a weight > 10% above normal weight for height

11. Body mass index (BMI) is defined as which of the following?
   a) the weight in pounds divided by the square of the height in meters
   b) the weight in kilograms divided by the square of the height in meters
   c) the square of the height in meters divided by the weight in pounds
   d) the square of the height in meters divided by the weight in kilograms
   e) none of the above

12. With respect to physical inactivity and the risk of cardiovascular disease, which of the following statements is true?
   a) physical inactivity (sedentary lifestyle) is an independent risk factor for cardiovascular disease
   b) physical inactivity (sedentary lifestyle) is associated with an increased death rate from cardiovascular disease

   c) physical inactivity (sedentary lifestyle) may be as strong a risk factor for cardiovascular disease as several other risk factors combined
   d) physical inactivity (sedentary lifestyle) is strongly correlated with obesity
   e) all of the above statements are true

13. With regard to the level of serum cholesterol in the American population, which of the following statements is true?
   a) serum cholesterol levels are increased in the United States
   b) serum cholesterol levels are decreasing in the United States
   c) serum cholesterol levels are higher in blacks than in whites
   d) serum cholesterol levels are higher in whites than in blacks
   e) the "target" serum cholesterol for the U.S. population for the year 2000 is 240 mg%

14. What is the percentage of hypertensive Americans whose blood pressure is under good control estimated to be?
   a) 50%
   b) 75%
   c) 25%
   d) 10%
   e) 5%

15. What is the percentage of total calories consumed as fat by the average American?
   a) 10%
   b) 20%
   c) 25%
   d) 30%
   e) 36%

Short Answer Management Problem 136

A 63-year-old male presents for his periodic health examination. You check his serum cholesterol and find it to be 225 mg%. Describe what you would do at this time considering what you know about standardization of serum cholesterol levels in clinical laboratories in the United States.

ANSWERS

1. C.

2. B.

3. A. During the past 15 years, the death rate for cardiovascular disease in the United States has decreased very significantly. Overall, for all cardio-vascular disease, there has been a 35% decrease in the death rate. The death rate from CAD has decreased by 40% and the death rate from stroke has decreased by 50%.

4. D. The major reasons for the very significant decrease in cardiovascular mortality in the United States are changes in lifestyle and risk factor reduction. Other contributing reasons include new technology, improved

pharmacology, better surgical techniques, and more effective medical managements.

5. A. Americans with hypertension have three to four times the risk of developing CAD and as much as seven times the risk of stroke as do those with normal blood pressure.

6. A. Cigarette smoking is a major risk factor for cardiovascular disease. Cigarette smokers are at increased risk for fatal and nonfatal myocardial infarctions and for sudden cardiac death. Smokers have a 70% greater CAD rate, a twofold to fourfold greater incidence of acquiring CAD, and a twofold to fourfold greater risk for sudden death than nonsmokers.

7. C. Elevated serum cholesterol levels are associated with an increased risk of coronary artery disease. Epidemiologic work in this area has suggested that for each 1% reduction in serum cholesterol there is an associated 2% reduction in the risk of heart disease death.

8. D. Death rates from CAD, stroke, and end-stage renal disease due to hypertension are higher in blacks than in whites.

   In 1987 the age-adjusted CAD death rate for black males was 208/100,000, compared to 185/100,000 for white males. As well, while the CAD death rate has declined steadily over the past 20 years for white men, the decline has slowed significantly over the past 10 years for black men, black women, and white women.

   In 1987 the age-adjusted death rates for black men and black women from stroke were 57.1/100,000 and 46.7/100,000, respectively, compared to 30.3/100,000 and 26.3/100,000 for white men and white women.

   End-stage renal failure due to hypertension is significantly higher in blacks than in whites. Overall, during 1983-1986, blacks had a rate of renal failure attributed to hypertension of 10.5/100,000, a figure that was almost six times the rate for whites.

9. E. Being obese is a risk factor for hypertension, hypercholesterolemia, and diabetes mellitus. It is also an independent risk factor for CAD. Being obese and being physically inactive increase all risks.

10. C. The definition of *obesity* is a weight > 20% that expected for (or defined as normal) for height.

11. B. BMI (body mass index) is defined as the weight of a person in kilograms over the height of the person in square meters. Tables are available that allow the calculation of BMI to be made easily in the office.

12. E. Physical inactivity, or a sedentary lifestyle, is becoming quickly recognized as a very powerful risk factor for cardiovascular disease. It is recognized as an independent risk factor for cardiovascular disease and cardiovascular death. There is some evidence that a vigorous exercise program may, in fact, counteract some or all other risk factors when it comes to both the cardiovascular death rate and the cardiovascular disease prevalence rate.

   Physical inactivity is also associated with being obese, and these two risk factors are additive.

   Weight-reduction programs are rarely successful in the absence of a reasonable exercise program. Most authorities suggest that to make a significant difference to the cardiovascular system, vigorous aerobic exercise must occur three times per week and last at least 30 minutes/session.

13. B. Mean serum cholesterol levels in the United States are declining. Values for men and women in the period 1960-1962 averaged 217 mg% and 233 mg%, respectively. By 1980 the same mean serum cholesterol levels were 211 mg% and 215 mg%, respectively. By the year 2000 the U.S. Department of Health and Human Services has targeted a value of no more than 200 mg% for both men and women in the United States.

14. C. The percentage of hypertensive Americans whose blood pressure is under good control is estimated to be no more than 25%. One of the major targets for the years to come is to increase that figure to at least 50%. The U.S. Department of Health and Human Services has set that 50% target for the year 2000.

15. E. At the present time, the average percentage of calories derived from fat in the typical American's diet is 36%. Of this 36%, 13% is saturated fat. The American Heart Association has set the upper limit of fat intake calories at 30% and the upper limit of saturated fat intake calories at 10%.

   A significant reduction in the intake of total fat and saturated fat will be necessary if the 200 mg% of total serum cholesterol is to be met by the year 2000.

SOLUTION TO SHORT ANSWER MANAGEMENT PROBLEM 136

The College of American Pathologists has determined that no more than 53% of American clinical laboratories have established an accuracy standard of plus/minus 5% for total serum cholesterol. Thus one reading of a serum cholesterol that is high is certainly not enough to act on. First, the serum cholesterol should be repeated. If at all possible, inquiries should be made that will allow you to determine whether or not the laboratory to which you are sending your serum cholesterol has established the plus/minus 5% accuracy standard.

If, in this patient, the total serum cholesterol level on repeat is found to be high, then a fractionation is indicated.

To rely on and base your judgment and advice to a patient on a single reading of the total serum cholesterol level is unwise. You may, in fact, be giving the patient misinformation that could contribute to cardiac neurosis or other serious problems. Make sure you know what the true value of serum cholesterol is before you share this information with the patient.

SUMMARY OF IMPORTANT CONCEPTS IN CARDIOVASCULAR EPIDEMIOLOGY

1. Unlike the mortality from cancer, there has been a very significant decrease in cardiovascular mortality in the United States during the last 15 years.
2. Death rates from CAD and stroke, the two major causes of cardiovascular mortality, are down by 40% and 50%, respectively, in the last 15 years.
3. The major reasons for the decrease in cardiovascular mortality rates in the United States are lifestyle modification and risk factor reduction.
4. Lifestyle modification, particularly weight loss and physical activity, are particularly important in efforts to further reduce cardiovascular mortality.
5. Hypertension, hypercholesterolemia, cigarette smoking, obesity, and physical inactivity are all independent risk factors for cardiovascular disease.
6. A vigorous exercise program may be enough to counteract several other cardiovascular risk factors and prevent cardiovascular morbidity and mortality.
7. Death rates from all forms of cardiovascular disease are significantly higher in blacks than in whites. The rate of decline in death rates has also significantly decreased.
8. Cigarette smoking is estimated to account for 40% of deaths from CAD in Americans under the age of 65.
9. The U.S. Department of Health and Human Services has set a number of objectives, or targets, for the year 2000. Most of these targets include a further decrease in modifiable risk factors for cardiovascular disease.
10. The continuing education of the American population with respect to what they can do themselves to decrease risk from cardiovascular disease remains our number-one priority. Aggressive intervention with risk factors through lifestyle modification, education, and counseling will remain one of the greatest and most rewarding challenges for family physicians in the next century.

SUGGESTED READING

U.S. Department of Health and Human Services. Heart disease and stroke. The *healthy people 2000*. National Health Promotion and Disease Prevention Objectives. Boston: Jones & Bartlett, 1992.

PROBLEM 137   A 45-YEAR-OLD "HIGH-POWERED EXECUTIVE" WHO REQUESTS "THE COMPLETE LABORATORY WORKUP—EVERY TEST KNOWN TO MAN"

A 45-year-old "high-powered executive" (self-described) presents to your office for "the old once-over." He further tells you that he would like "every test known to man."

From the history and physical examination of this gentleman you construct the following problem list:

1. Obesity (body mass index = 36)
2. Nicotine addiction (two packs of cigarettes/day)
3. Workaholic: married to his work
4. Essential hypertension (last BP = 175/95 mm Hg)
5. Sedentary lifestyle
6. History of gouty arthritis

You get the feeling that one day soon you will be testing his "cardiac enzymes" in a coronary care unit.

You recall some of the basic principles regarding routine laboratory screening procedures—their usefulness, cost-benefit ratio, and positive predictive value.

SELECT THE ONE BEST ANSWER TO THE FOLLOWING QUESTIONS

1. On the basis of the information provided, what would you do now?
   a) order a complete battery of investigations in order to get rid of the patient
   b) order selected investigations
   c) tell the patient that you don't specialize in his type of problems and give him the name of one of your physician friends down the street
   d) discuss the advantages and disadvantages of screening for various conditions with the patient
   e) none of the above

2. What is the most common reason given by physicians for ordering routine laboratory investigations in asymptomatic patients?
   a) patient expectations
   b) the litigation-prone climate in which we all practice
   c) because we have always done it
   d) quality-of-care reasons—routine laboratory investigations on asymptomatic patients often reveal abnormalities that can be addressed before the patient becomes symptomatic
   e) the inclusion of many routine laboratory tests in clinical practice guidelines

3. The percentage of routine laboratory tests performed in asymptomatic persons that result in a change in management strategy is estimated to be which of the following?
   a) 0.3%
   b) 3.0%
   c) 13.0%
   d) 33.3%
   e) 63.3%

4. The measure of the ability of a test to discriminate between normal and diseased states is known as which of the following?

   a) the sensitivity of the test
   b) the specificity of the test
   c) the likelihood ratio of the test
   d) the positive predictive value of the test
   e) the negative predictive value of the test

5. Which of the following reasons is(are) justifiable reasons for ordering a laboratory or radiologic investigation?
   a) screening
   b) confirmation of clinical findings
   c) disease treatment and follow-up
   d) patient and doctor reassurance
   e) all of the above

6. Which of the following questions is(are) important to ask before implementing a screening program for a particular disorder?
   a) does the current burden of suffering justify a screening program?
   b) has the program's effectiveness been demonstrated in a clinical trial?
   c) can the health care system cope with the screening program?
   d) will people who screen positive accept advice and intervention for the condition?
   e) all of the above are important

7. Which of the following is(are) disadvantages of some screening laboratory tests?
   a) the direct costs of the tests
   b) the direct costs of physician visits at the time of screening
   c) the direct costs of the repeat physician visits to discuss the results of the screening tests
   d) the direct costs of the consultant's fees when a patient is referred to him or her
   e) all of the above

8. In one large Canadian city, there are 45 walk-in clinics. The walk-in clinic phenomenon has spread through

many areas of North America. Walk-in clinics do not maintain, in many situations, the fundamental principles of family medicine.

Which of the following best describes the prevailing opinion regarding patient philosophy of care regarding treatment at a walk-in clinic?
a) convenient care
b) comprehensive care
c) compassionate care
d) continuous care
e) coordinated care

9. Regarding the walk-in clinics described in Question 8, which of the following statements appears to reflect the majority physician philosophy of care at a walk-in clinic?
a) primary prevention
b) secondary prevention
c) tertiary prevention
d) acute, episodic care
e) comprehensive preventive care

10. Cost-effectiveness in the delivery of medical care services is becoming a crucial issue for health care providers, health care consumers, and health care funders (government, private insurance plans, and so on).

Which of the following statements regarding routine laboratory testing in asymptomatic individuals and the standard measure of quality of care (QALY—quality of adjusted life years) best describes the contribution of diagnostic laboratory services in this situation?
a) routine laboratory testing in asymptomatic patients improves QALY
b) routine laboratory testing in asymptomatic patients decreases QALY
c) in a randomized asymptomatic population where 50% receive routine testing and 50% did not, there was no difference in QALY
d) in the same randomized asymptomatic population, a larger proportion of the laboratory screened group ended up in a hospital
e) c and d

11. One of the reasons for significant confusion among physicians regarding routine laboratory test ordering is that there are so many different and contradictory recommendations from many different societies and organizations.

A case in point is screening of the male population over the age of 40 with PSA for the detection of cancer of the prostate. The recommendations of various groups on this issue follow.
1. The United States Preventive Services Task Force: PSA is *not recommended* for routine screening.
2. The Canadian Task Force on the periodic health examination: PSA is *not recommended* for routine screening.

3. The United States National Cancer Institute: there is insufficient evidence to recommend PSA for routine screening.
4. A certain expert American association: annual PSA determination should be performed on all men over the age of 50 years.

You have just started out in practice and are trying to establish your guidelines and protocols for practicing medicine. Based on what you are presented with, which of the following would you recommend for an asymptomatic 55-year-old male at the time of this periodic health examination?
a) follow the recommendation of the certain expert American association; they are the experts, and they should know
b) follow the recommendation of the United States National Cancer Institute; it gives you a little more leeway in what you order in this patient
c) follow the recommendations of the U.S. Preventive Services Task Force and The Canadian Task Force on the Periodic Health Examination
d) flip a coin: heads—do level of PSA; tails—do not do level of PSA
e) forget the whole thing; this is far too complicated

12. *Screening* is defined as which of the following?
a) any health service attempt to measure a variable that may be linked to primary prevention of a disorder
b) any health service attempt to measure a variable that may be linked to secondary prevention of a disorder
c) any health service attempt to measure a variable that may be linked to tertiary prevention of a disorder
d) all of the above
e) none of the above

13. *Case finding* is defined as which of the following?
a) the presumptive identification of an unrecognized disease or defect by the application of tests, examinations, or other procedures in patients who happen to be in your clinical setting
b) the presumptive identification of an unrecognized disease or defect by the application of tests, examinations, or other procedures in a non–health care setting
c) the presumptive identification of an unrecognized disease or defect by use of a screening test among patients who are consulting the physician for unrelated symptoms
d) a or b
e) a and b

14. Which of the following routine laboratory tests is(are) indicated in an asymptomatic 54-year-old male who presents for his periodic health examination?
a) routine urinalysis
b) routine CBC

c) serum PSA
d) nonfasting cholesterol
e) a, b, and d

15. Which of the following routine laboratory tests is(are) indicated in the periodic health examination of an asymptomatic 23-year-old female?
   a) serum BUN
   b) serum creatinine
   c) serum glucose
   d) serum uric acid
   e) none of the above

16. For purposes of laboratory medicine, and in recognition of the "zealous overtesting syndrome" that many physicians seem to have acquired, a *normal patient* is defined as which of the following?
   a) a patient who has had "the works"
   b) a patient who has had all of the laboratory tests performed that he or she has specifically requested
   c) a patient who has not been sufficiently investigated
   d) a patient who has only had the absolute minimum number of tests
   e) it all depends

Short Answer Management Problem 137

As a primary care physician, you see the laboratory services extensively. Discuss the difference between *defensive medicine* and *defensible medicine*.

ANSWERS

1. D. Routine laboratory testing and the costs associated with same are increasing at an alarming rate. Although one individual test is not expensive, when taken together laboratory tests are responsible for an ever-increasing percentage of the total health care budget.

   There is no evidence that physicians' increased use of laboratory testing has improved the care of their patients. There is also no evidence to suggest an increase in quality of adjusted life years (QALY), a measurement that at present is the "gold standard" for macro cost-effectiveness.

   We must introduce and emphasize the concepts of appropriate use of the laboratory at all three levels of medical education: in the undergraduate curriculum through small group discussions with case vignettes, in the postgraduate curriculum with competence and performance assessments in our outpatient clinics and in the wards, and in continuing medical education events geared toward health care resource management.

2. C. The most commonly cited reason for routine laboratory testing being performed on patients by their physicians is simply "because we have always done it." The most common scenario and the reasons behind this explanation (however poor a reason it is) are as follows:
   A. Physicians were trained in residency training to "order the workup." Often, if they failed to perform one test, they were criticized and castigated by their attending physicians. This pattern continued when they completed their residencies, and in addition, they began to pass on their debatably reasonable habits to their students and residents.
   B. Physicians order routine laboratory tests in asymptomatic patients for the following primary reason: "because I have always done it."
   C. Physicians may be unaware of the definition and meaning of the following terms:
      1. Sensitivity
      2. Specificity
      3. Positive predictive value
      4. Negative predictive value
      These terms and the calculations involving them are detailed in Chapter 133.
   D. Physicians (especially family physicians, because of the uncertainty associated with the broad scope of the specialty) are extremely concerned about "missing something" in their patients and thus tend to overinvestigate when there is no real reason for doing so.
   E. The litigation-prone climate that exists in the United States to a startling degree (lawyer advertisements seem more common on television than laundry detergent commercials) encourages the public to file lawsuits. Although lawsuits against physicians occur in Canada, they are certainly significantly less frequent. The Canadian Medical Protective Association, the flagship carrier of insurance for all physicians in Canada, paid out a total of only $115 million in settled claims and court-adjudicated awards on behalf of all physicians in Canada in 1994.

      In addition, under the British system of justice, after which the Canadian system is modeled, there is a very significant difference between a mistake and malpractice for negligence. In Canada, the plaintiff must prove the following:

1. An adverse outcome resulted in which the physician was involved.
2. The adverse outcome was detrimental to present or future health.
3. There was a direct cause-and-effect relationship between the adverse outcome and the physician's management.
4. The adverse outcome was potentially preventable.
5. The physician's judgment was clearly a judgment that the majority of his or her peers would not have made.

F. The patient requests or demands a test and will not be satisfied until he or she receives it. In many cases, this is repeated.

Routine laboratory testing in asymptomatic patients rarely has anything to do with either quality of care or clinical practice guidelines. The latter are produced, in a very real sense, to help the physician provide QALY while at the same time minimizing unnecessary and possibly "disease-producing" testing. The following case history illustrates this point well.

Case History

A 53-year-old male presents for his annual checkup. He has the following tests performed:

A. CBC
B. Electrolytes
C. BUN/creatinine
D. Liver enzymes
E. Proteins and fractionation of same
F. Cholesterol (fractionated) and triglycerides
G. PSA (prostate-specific antigen)
H. Blood sugar
I. Serum calcium, serum phosphate
J. Serum uric acid

The patient finds out that one of his liver function tests (serum bilirubin) is very slightly elevated and starts to worry about it. His physician then orders the following:

A. Abdominal ultrasound
B. CT scan of the abdomen
C. Repeat liver enzymes testing
D. Consult with a gastroenterologist

As he is waiting for these tests, having these tests performed, and waiting to see the gastroenterologist, he becomes more and more anxious. When he finally sees the specialist the consultant states, "Well, I can't really find anything wrong. It's probably of no consequence, but we probably should check it every six months."

The results of this series of events can be summarized as follows:

1. Because of the number of laboratory tests ordered, there was approximately a 40% chance that a positive test result (if found) would be a false positive result rather than a true positive result.

2. The patient who was previously healthy has now lost that status because of anxiety-creating psychologic distress.
3. Even after the testing and consultations are complete, the patient will still be worried (that is, his health is negatively affected) due to the rather inconclusive remarks by the consultant.
4. The testing and consultation process was:
   A. Very expensive
   B. Very costly in terms of patient health

3. A. The percentage of routine laboratory tests performed in asymptomatic patients that result in a change in management strategy is estimated to be between 0.3% and 0.5%. Thus 99.5% to 99.7% of routine laboratory tests are a complete waste of both time and money and may (as just illustrated) actually produce disease.

4. C. The likelihood ratio (LR) is a measure of the ability of a test to discriminate between a normal and a diseased state. The LR ratio is the likelihood of finding a positive test result in a person with, rather than in a person without, the disease. The higher the LR, the more likely is the case that the disease is present if the test result is positive.

5. E. Screening for disease, case-finding for disease, confirmation of clinical findings, and patient and doctor reassurance are all valid reasons for ordering a laboratory or radiologic investigation, to some extent. However, the last reason (patient and physician reassurance) must only be taken so far. If, for example, you believe that by not ordering the test, the patient will suffer from significant anxiety and worry, and the request is reasonable, then you may choose to order the test. A good example of this would be a serological test for HIV in a man who had unprotected intercourse with at least eight different women in a 3-week period. If, on the other hand, this is a repeat request or the request is not reasonable, then it should not be done.

6. E. When trying to decide whether a screening program does more harm than good, you should consider asking the following questions:
   A. Has the program's effectiveness been demonstrated in a clinical trial? Was this trial double-blind?
   B. Are there effective treatments or effective preventive measures for the disorder?
   C. Does the current burden of suffering warrant screening?
   D. Is there a good screening test available?
   E. Can the health care system cope with (afford in terms of financial and nonfinancial resources) the screening program?
   F. Will individuals who screen positive accept advice and intervention for the condition?

If you decide to perform a screening test, the following criteria must also be met:

A. The condition must have a significant effect on the quality or quantity of life in the population.

B. Treatment for the condition must be available.

C. The condition should have an asymptomatic period during which detection and treatment significantly reduce morbidity and mortality.

D. Treatment in the asymptomatic period should result in an outcome that is superior to delaying treatment until symptoms occur.

E. Tests to detect the condition in the asymptomatic period must be readily available.

F. Tests to detect the condition in the asymptomatic period must be acceptable to patients.

G. Tests to detect the condition in the asymptomatic period must not be excessively costly.

H. There must be a high enough incidence of the condition to justify screening.

7. E. There are many direct and indirect costs to the performance of laboratory tests for screening purposes:

I. Direct costs of laboratory tests:

A. The direct cost of the laboratory test as determined by the laboratory charges

B. The direct cost of the physician's visit at which time the test is ordered

C. The direct cost of the repeat office visit to discuss the results of the tests

D. The direct cost of the repeat laboratory test if an abnormal result is obtained

E. The direct cost of additional laboratory and radiologic tests that are ordered due to the presence of one false-positive test result

F. The direct cost of a referral to a consultant in the area of concern

G. The direct cost of repeat and additional laboratory and radiologic tests that are ordered by the consultant

H. The direct cost of the repeat office visit to either the consultant or the family physician following the completion of consultant-ordered tests

II. Indirect costs of laboratory tests:

A. The patient stress and anxiety caused by an abnormality found on routine laboratory testing

B. The patient stress and anxiety of waiting to complete the diagnostic testing and consultations

C. The patient's family stress and anxiety caused by the thought of "what it could be"

D. The lost time from productive employment caused by physician appointments and waiting in physician offices

E. The possible inability to obtain life insurance or disability insurance following one abnormal and probably meaningless result

8. A.

9. D. The walk-in clinic phenomenon has spread across North America like an epidemic. Although it is established much more so in Canada, it is growing in the United States as well.

The reason that patients seem to seek treatment for health-related conditions in a walk-in clinic is, in most cases, convenience. The walk-in clinic phenomenon is geared, from a physician's perspective, to acute, episodic care rather than preventive medical care in most cases. It, again, generally speaking, does not offer the five "C" principles of family medicine:

A. Continuous care

B. Comprehensive care

C. Coordinated care

D. Compassionate care

E. Competent care

10. D. Routine laboratory screening is, for all intents and purposes, completely devoid of any benefits to quality of adjusted life years. It does, however, result in a significantly higher percentage of people who end up in community and secondary care hospitals.

11. C. The most solid, most scientific sources of evidence regarding PSA screening are the United States Preventive Services Task Force and the Canadian Task Force on the Periodic Health Examination. It is very rare, as well, that these two very important task forces disagree on any recommendation.

12. E.

13. C. The distinction between screening, on the one hand, and case finding, on the other, is the following:

A. Screening: screening is defined as the presumptive identification of tests, examinations, or other procedures that can be applied rapidly. Screening tests sort out apparently well persons who have a disease from those who probably do not. A screening test is not intended to be diagnostic. Persons with positive or suspicious findings must be referred to their physician for diagnosis and treatment.

B. Case finding: case finding is defined as the identification by testing following the clinician's search for disease with screening tests among patients who are consulting them for unrelated reasons.

The distinction between screening and case finding is subtle.

14. D. The only test that is indicated from those listed is the nonfasting cholesterol in a middle-aged male. This recommendation is made by the U.S. Preventive Services Task Force and the Canadian Task Force on the Periodic Health Examination.

15. E. None of serum creatinine, BUN, serum glucose, and serum uric acid are indicated in the periodic health examination of a 23-year-old female.

16. C. Although somewhat tongue-in-cheek, it was recently suggested by the scientific editor of a prominent North American family medicine journal that "a normal patient is defined as someone who has not been sufficiently investigated."

    The point is that the zealous overtesting syndrome is a very serious and costly problem. The major problem appears to be that physicians are not aware of the epidemiologic implications of what they are doing. Epidemiologic principles will confirm that if 20 laboratory tests are done, there is a very high probability that at least one of those will be abnormal and that will most likely be a false positive (> 99%). What happens from there, of course, really amounts to a wild goose chase. The goose is never caught, the patient (who was previously well) is now unhealthy due to worry caused by the condition, and the physician is frustrated (in not being able to diagnose something that isn't there).

    This could all be avoided if every time you ordered a laboratory test you asked yourself two simple questions:
    1. "Why am I doing this test?"
    2. "Is there a reasonable chance that the result of this test may change my patient management?"

    If the answer to the first question is valid and able to be substantiated by scientific evidence and the answer to the second question is yes, then do the test. If not, do not do the test.

SOLUTION TO SHORT ANSWER MANAGEMENT PROBLEM 137

The major difference between defensive medicine and defensible medicine is the following:
1. Defensive medicine: a physician who practices defensive medicine practices in a manner in which he or she is afraid of possible litigation and thus orders every possible test (to avoid missing something, however esoteric). The problems with defensive medicine are as follows:
   1) It does not offer you the protection you think it does.
   2) It results in a pathway of decision making that has really nothing to do with hypothetical-deductive reasoning or inductive reasoning. Rather, it is really a blind shot in the dark with a tremendously big gun.
   3) Because of all of the false-positive test results that are generated, you end up spending most of your life chasing geese that you will never catch.
   4) It is a tremendously expensive and wasteful process.
2. Defensible medicine: a physician who practices defensible medicine practices medicine that is based on a sound approach to clinical reasoning and an inherent knowledge of the following concepts:
   i) Sensitivity

   ii) Specificity
   iii) Negative predictive value
   iv) Positive predictive value
   v) Prevalence

Each decision that the physician makes will be a well-thought-out, reasoned decision that you could, with the help of your local epidemiologist, defend from the point of optimal patient outcome.

The advantages of defensive medicine are as follows:
   A. Improved quality of care
   B. Improved physician and ultimately patient satisfaction (although the latter may be somewhat more difficult to attain)
   C. A sense of being in the "innovative group" of physicians who feel confident enough to believe in themselves and in their clinical diagnosis and clinical management

SUMMARY OF USE AND ABUSE OF LABORATORY MEDICINE FOR ROUTINE SCREENING OF ASYMPTOMATIC PATIENTS

1. **Estimate of abuse of laboratory medicine:**
   a) Conservative estimate of abuse: at least 50% of all laboratory tests performed in a primary care setting are unnecessary and cost-ineffective.
   b) Estimates suggest that only 0.3% to 0.5% of all laboratory tests make any difference to the patient or have any chance of changing the patient's management.
2. **Appropriate use of the laboratory:**
   a) Must follow the criteria described in the answer to Question 6
   b) Key questions: the following two questions must be answered in the affirmative or with a specific answer:
      1. "Why am I doing this test?"
      2. "Is there reasonable chance that the result of this test will change my patient's management?"
3. **Laboratory medicine and epidemiology:**
   a) Screening versus case finding:
      Screening: testing a non self-identified population (random testing)
      Case finding: testing a self-identified population in a health care setting
   b) Major epidemiologic concepts:
      1. Prevalence: the lower the prevalence in the population in question, the lower the positive predictive value and the higher the number of false positives
      2. Positive predictive value: the percentage of all positive test results that are actually true positives
4. **Guidelines to follow:**
   a) Task force recommendations: the best guidelines to follow with respect to screening and case finding for all disorders are contained in the following two task force recommendations:
      1. The United States Preventive Services Task Force
      2. The Canadian Task Force on the Periodic Health Examination

5. **The dangers of inadequate knowledge of the epidemiologic principles of effective laboratory testing**

   a) The wild goose chase
   b) The definition of a normal patient as a patient who has not been sufficiently investigated
   c) The complete wasting of resources in an already difficult-to-manage (costwise) health care system
   d) The creation of disease in patients who were previously well before their physician visit
   e) In one controlled study of routine screening versus nonroutine screening, the only difference in the two populations was the excessive hospitalizations in the screened group. There was no effect on QALY (quality of adjusted life years).

SUGGESTED READING

Feldman W. On ordering tests. Annals of The Royal College of Physicians and Surgeons of Canada 1993; 26(5):269-270.

PROBLEM 138   A 24-YEAR-OLD MALE WITH A NONPRODUCTIVE COUGH

A 24-year-old male presents to your office with a 2-month history of a dry, nonproductive cough accompanied by shortness of breath. He has felt tired and has had intermittent fevers for the past 6 weeks.

On P/E, the patient appears pale. He has significant cervical, axillary, and inguinal lymphadenopathy. Examination of the respiratory system reveals rales bilaterally. His respiratory rate is 32/minute.

You suspect HIV infection and question him carefully. He states that he is bisexual. He has a wife and one child but also has two other regular male partners.

His chest X-ray reveals a significant bilateral infiltrate. His HIV serology comes back positive.

SELECT THE ONE BEST ANSWER TO THE FOLLOWING QUESTIONS

1. What is the most likely diagnosis in this patient?
   a) AIDS-related complex
   b) AIDS
   c) HIV-positive status with underlying pneumonia
   d) generalized lymphadenopathy syndrome
   e) none of the above

2. What is the most likely diagnostic possibility based on the limited information provided?
   a) viral pneumonia
   b) streptococcal pneumonia
   c) *Klebsiella* pneumonia
   d) *Mycoplasma* pneumonia
   e) *Pneumocystis carinii* pneumonia

3. What is the treatment of choice for this patient's respiratory tract infection (based on a correct diagnosis in Question 2)?
   a) IV tetracycline
   b) IV ampicillin
   c) IV trimethoprim-sulfamethoxazole
   d) IV cephalexin
   e) none of the above

4. What is the drug of choice for the prevention of respiratory tract infection due to this organism?
   a) dapsone
   b) aerosolized pentamidine
   c) pyrimethamine plus sulfadiazine
   d) trimethoprim-sulfamethoxazole
   e) none of the above

5. Prophylaxis against this respiratory condition should be initiated when the CD-4+ lymphocyte count is reduced to which of the following values?
   a) 1000 cells/mm³
   b) 750 cells/mm³
   c) 500 cells/mm³
   d) 200 cells/mm³
   e) 100 cells/mm³

6. What is the most common life-threatening opportunistic infection in patients with AIDS?

   a) *Pneumocystis carinii* pneumonia
   b) *Toxoplasma gondii* CNS infection
   c) cryptosporidium gastroenteritis
   d) *Isospora belli* gastroenteritis
   e) *Enterocytozoon bieneusi* gastroenteritis

7. What is the most common malignancy associated with the condition described in Question 1?
   a) Kaposi's sarcoma
   b) non-Hodgkin's lymphoma
   c) primary lymphoma of the brain
   d) acute lymphoblastic leukemia
   e) Hodgkin's disease

8. A 31-year-old patient with full-blown AIDS presents to your office with a 10-day history of severe dysphagia. The dysphagia has been getting progressively worse, and the patient's oral intake is limited to liquids. Based on the history, what is the most likely cause of this patient's dysphagia?
   a) herpes simplex esophagitis
   b) Kaposi's sarcoma of the esophagus
   c) esophageal candidiasis
   d) *Pneumocystis carnii* esophagitis
   e) none of the above

9. What is the treatment of choice for the patient described in Question 8?
   a) ketoconazole
   b) acyclovir
   c) trimethoprim-sulfamethoxazole
   d) aerosolized pentamidine
   e) clarithromycin

10. The patient described in Question 8 recovers from his severe dysphagia. He presents to your office 3 weeks later with a new problem: a corrugated white plaque on both lateral borders of the tongue. This plaque does not scrape off.
    What is the most likely diagnosis of this condition?
    a) oral hairy leukoplakia
    b) lichen planus
    c) oral thrush
    d) atypical herpes simplex
    e) cryptococcosis

11. What is the treatment of choice for this condition (Question 10)?

a) α-interferon
b) ketoconazole
c) amphotericin B
d) trimethoprim-sulfamethoxazole
e) none of the above

12. What is the most common cause of sight-threatening infectious disease in patients with AIDS?
a) cytomegalovirus
b) herpes simplex
c) cryptococcosis
d) toxoplasmosis
e) histoplasmosis

13. The point at which AZT (zidovudine) should be initiated in the asymptomatic HIV patient is when the CD-4+ count declines to which of the following?
a) 750 cells/mm³
b) 500 cells/mm³
c) 400 cells/mm³
d) 300 cells/mm³
e) 250 cells/mm³

14. The point at which AZT (zidovudine) should be initiated in the symptomatic HIV patient is when the CD-4+ count reaches which of the following?
a) 750 cells/mm³
b) 500 cells/mm³
c) 400 cells/mm³
d) 300 cells/mm³
e) 250 cells/mm³

15. Which of the following is(are) common side effects of AZT?
a) nausea
b) headache
c) dyspepsia
d) myalgias/myositis
e) all of the above

16. Which of the following statements regarding suggested indications for switching from AZT to ddl (dideoxycytidine) in patients with HIV infection is (are) true?
a) for patients who began AZT with counts between 250 and 500 cells/mm³ and who suffer a 50% decline in CD-4+ count or a decline to less than 200 cells/mm³ (repeated once at least 4 weeks after the first test)
b) for patients who have a CD-4+ count of between 100 cells/mm³ and 250 cells/mm³ and who suffer a 50% decline in CD-4+ count or a decline to less than 50 cells/mm³ repeated once
c) both of the above
d) neither of the above
e) the indications for switching from AZT to ddl are unclear

17. Neurological manifestations of AIDS include which of the following?
a) peripheral neuropathy
b) meningitis
c) encephalitis
d) cognitive impairment
e) all of the above

18. In the transmission of AIDS from mother to newborn, which of the following statements is(are) true?
a) the baby may test negative and continue to test negative throughout its life
b) only 20%-30% of babies born to HIV-positive mothers seroconvert to an HIV-positive state
c) HIV infection in infants and children has a better prognosis than HIV infection in adults
d) all of the above
e) none of the above

19. What is the test most frequently used to screen for HIV infection?
a) CD-4+ count
b) CB-4+ count
c) ELISA test
d) Western blot test
e) none of the above

20. A 39-year-old male tests positive for HIV infection during a routine insurance medical examination. What should be your next step in testing?
a) to do nothing
b) to perform ELISA testing for HIV
c) to perform a Western blot test for HIV
d) to perform a p-24 antigen level for HIV
e) to perform a CD-4+ count

21. Which of the following statements is(are) true concerning HIV infection?
a) toxoplasmosis is the most common infectious etiologic agent associated with CNS AIDS involvement
b) meningitis in patients with AIDS is most commonly caused by cryptococcus
c) CNS infection remains uncommon in patients with AIDS
d) a and b are true
e) all of the above are true

22. Which of the following subsets of lymphocytes is commonly followed as an indicator of disease progression in patients with AIDS?
a) suppressor B cells
b) helper T cells
c) helper B cells
d) suppressor T cells
e) nobody really knows for sure

23. A patient with AIDS begins ganciclovir. This patient most likely has which of the following?
    a) mycobacterium avium intracellulare
    b) cytomegaloviral retinitis
    c) *toxoplasmosis gondii*
    d) enterotoxigenic *E. coli*
    e) herpes simplex

24. What is the most common neoplasm involving the CNS in patients with AIDS?
    a) non-Hodgkin's lymphoma
    b) Hodgkin's disease
    c) glioblastoma multiforme
    d) Kaposi's sarcoma
    e) medulloblastoma

25. What is the antiretroviral agent of choice in the treatment of AIDS?
    a) dideocytosine (ddl)
    b) azidothymidine (AZT)
    c) dideoxycytidine (ddC)
    d) difluclioncizole
    e) acyclovir

26. A patient is begun on appropriate antiretroviral therapy. She is taking AZT in a dosage of 600 mg/day. Her CD-4+ count has decreased from 350 to 225 in 6 weeks. You reconfirm the test result and it comes back the same (CD-4+ count = 225). At this time, what would you do?
    a) switch from AZT to ddI
    b) switch from AZT to ddC
    c) add ddI to AZT
    d) add ddC to AZT
    e) either a or d

27. A 34-year-old male with AIDS presents with a painful, pruritic eruption on his right forehead and right cheek. What is the most likely diagnosis?
    a) herpes simplex
    b) streptococcal cellulitis
    c) herpes zoster
    d) staphylococcal cellulitis
    e) none of the above

28. In patients with AIDS, aerosolized pentamidine is used to treat which of the following?
    a) herpes zoster
    b) coccidiomycosis
    c) toxoplasmosis
    d) *Pneumocystis carinii*
    e) histoplasmosis

29. What is the average length of time from first infection with the HIV virus (the primary infection) to death from AIDS-related complications?
    a) 18 months

b) 6 years
c) 8 years
d) 10 years
e) 12 years

30. What is the most important factor preventing the development of an effective vaccination against AIDS?
    a) the virus is difficult to replicate
    b) effective replication is difficult to sustain
    c) the retroviral nature of the virus increases the probability of and ease of spontaneous viral genome mutation
    d) the virus resists growing in tissue culture
    e) none of the above

31. The prophylaxis against MAC (mycobacterium avium intracellulare) is currently recommended to begin when the CD-4+ count reaches what level?
    a) 1000 cells/mm³
    b) 800 cells/mm³
    c) 500 cells/mm³
    d) 200 cells/mm³
    e) 100 cells/mm³

32. The prophylaxis against toxoplasmosis is currently recommended to begin when the CD-4+ count reaches what level?
    a) 1000 cells/mm³
    b) 800 cells/mm³
    c) 500 cells/mm³
    d) 200 cells/mm³
    e) 100 cells/mm³

33. What is the normal CD-4+ count in patients who are free from HIV infection?
    a) 1000-1500 cells/mm³
    b) 800-900 cells/mm³
    c) 700-759 cells/mm³
    d) 600-650 cells/mm³
    e) nobody really knows for sure

34. What is the drug of choice for AIDS patients who present with serious and life-threatening fungal infections?
    a) ganciclovir
    b) amphotericin B
    c) ciprofloxacin
    d) sulfamethoxazole-trimethoprim
    e) high-dose ampicillin

35. In which of the following body areas are KS (Kaposi's sarcoma) lesions not found?
    a) the scalp
    b) the back
    c) the arms
    d) the thighs
    e) KS lesions are found in all of the above sites

36. Which of the following organisms is least likely to produce diarrhea in patients with AIDS?
    a) enterotoxigenic *E. coli*
    b) toxoplasmosis
    c) *Campylobacter jejuni* infection
    d) *Shigella* species
    e) giardiasis

37. Which of the following statements regarding helper T cells in patients with AIDS is true?
    a) there is a quantitative deficiency of helper T cells in AIDS
    b) there is a qualitative deficiency of helper T cells in AIDS
    c) there is a quantitative deficiency syndrome of suppressor T cells in AIDS
    d) a and b only
    e) all of the above statements

38. Which of the following statements regarding the CD-4+ count in patients with AIDS is(are) true?
    a) during the acute infective period, there is a rapid decrease in the CD-4+ count
    b) from the acute retroviral syndrome heralding

the transmission of HIV virus to the recipient to the time of death, there is a fairly stable, but gradual, decrease in the CD-4+ count
    c) in a patient on AZT who is switched to ddl, it is uncommon to see an increase in CD-4+ count
    d) a and b only
    e) all of the above

39. Which of the following is(are) among the three leading causes of death in AIDS patients?
    a) esophageal candidiasis
    b) AIDS wasting syndrome
    c) *Pneumocystis carinii* capneumonia
    d) all of the above
    e) b and c only

40. Which of the following patient groups are considered high risk for the transmission of the HIV virus?
    a) male homosexuals
    b) IV drug users
    c) heterosexual females with many male sexual partners
    d) a and b only
    e) all of the above

Short Answer Management Problem 138

PART A: Discuss the general principles of HIV counseling and testing services in terms of the general goals and objectives and the important aspects of counseling patients prior to HIV testing.

PART B: Discuss the recommended immunizations and associated tests recommended in the HIV-positive patient.

PART C: Discuss the most cost-effective strategy for using the limited money available to the CDC for prevention of further cases of HIV infection and AIDS in the United States.

ANSWERS

1. B. This patient has AIDS.

    Although recent changes to the classification of AIDS and HIV-related illnesses have been proposed, the old classification system remains. Changes that would consider the CD-4+ count as a much more important part of the working definition have not been formally adopted (at this time) by the Centers for Disease Control. The classification system currently in place is as follows:
    Group I: Acute HIV infection
    Group II: Asymptomatic infection
    Group III: Persistent generalized lymphadenopathy
    Group IV: AIDS (with other diseases)
    Subgroup A: Constitutional disease
    Subgroup B: Neurologic disease

    Subgroup C: Secondary infectious disease
    Subgroup D: Secondary neoplasms
    Subgroup E: Other conditions

    Although it remains speculation at this point, the most likely cause of the "bilateral infiltrates" is *Pneumocystis carinii* pneumonia (PCP). Thus the patient would be considered, in a diagnostic sense, Group IV: Subgroup C: Diagnosis: AIDS.

2. E. As just mentioned, *Pneumocystis carinii* is the most likely cause of this patient's symptoms based on the limited diagnostic information that we have.

    The most characteristic symptoms of *Pneumocystis carinii* pneumonia are the following: a dry cough, dyspnea, fever, and night sweats. The most characteristic signs are increased respiratory rate, acute shortness of breath at rest, rales or rhonchi heard in both lung fields, and a general look of ill health.

Diagnostically, apart from a chest X-ray, which will reveal bilateral diffuse interstitial infiltrates and/or airspace infiltrates, a P_{O_2} and P_{CO_2} saturation level should also be done. Optional investigations depending on the patient include a transbronchial biopsy and a CT scan of the chest.

3. C.

4. D. The drug of choice for acute PCP treatment is IV trimethoprim-sulfamethoxazole. The IV dose is trimethoprim 20 mg/kg/day plus sulfamethoxazole q6h × 14-21 days. Alternatives include (1) pentamidine 4 mg/kg/day IV daily over 1-3 hours × 5 days followed by 3 mg/kg/day for the duration of therapy (14-21 days) or (2) clindamycin 900 mg IV q8h plus primaquine 30 mg po daily.

The prophylactic regime for PCP should ideally consist of 1 tablet of trimethoprim-sulfamethoxazole double strength (DS) daily. Alternatives include diaphenylsulfone (Dapsone) 100 mg 2-3 times/week or aerosolized pentamidine 60 mg q 2 weeks via Fisoneb nebulizer following 5 loading doses in 2 weeks or 300 mg q month via Respirgard II nebulizer.

5. D. Prophylaxis against PCP should be initiated when the CD-4+ count decreases to 200 cells/mm³. The evidence is clear that after that point in the disease process, the probability of the occurrence of at least one episode of PCP provides a favorable risk-benefit ratio for prophylaxis.

6. A. The most common, most serious life-threatening opportunistic infection in patients with AIDS is, again, *Pneumocystis carinii* pneumonia. It is directly responsible for more deaths from AIDS than any other single complication.

7. A. The most common malignancy associated with patients with AIDS is Kaposi's sarcoma. The characteristics of Kaposi's sarcoma are reddish/purplish skin lesions anywhere and complications including GI obstruction causing nausea and vomiting, dyspnea from intrapulmonary lesions, or lymphatic system lesions causing lymphedema and swelling of the extremities.

The second most common malignancy is lymphoma (usually non-Hodgkin's). The non-Hodgkin's lymphoma may occur as a primary tumor in the CNS or as a primary non-CNS tumor (frequently beginning in the gut).

8. C.

9. A. This patient, on the basis of the history alone, has esophageal candidiasis. This is a common opportunistic infection that often progresses from pharynx to esophagus.

Although thrush that is limited to the pharyngeal area is well treated with a relatively simple remedy such as nystatin or clotrimazole, esophageal candidiasis should be treated aggressively with either ketoconazole 200-400 mg po/day for 2-3 weeks or fluconazole 100-200 mg po daily × 2-3 weeks.

Esophageal candidiasis should be considered for maintenance therapy because of the significant risk of recurrence. Ketoconazole 200-400 mg po/day or fluconazole 50-100 mg po/day should be titrated to the minimum effective dose and frequency of administration.

10. A.

11. E. This patient now has oral hairy leukoplakia. Oral hairy leukoplakia is associated with the Epstein-Barr virus and is very uncommon in patients not HIV positive. It is, according to some authorities, diagnostic of AIDS itself.

In most cases oral hairy leukoplakia will not require treatment. If it is treated, oral acyclovir is the drug of choice. Either treated or not treated, however, it will almost certainly recur.

The classic position for oral hairy leukoplakia is on the sides of the tongue; it is characterized by a white-grey membrane that does not rub off.

12. A. The major infectious disease that produces loss of sight in patients with AIDS is cytomegalovirus. Symptoms include blurring of vision or altered vision. Sight can, however, be lost quickly with this disease.

The treatment of cytomegalovirus retinitis is ganciclovir 5 mg/kg IV (infuse over 1 hour) × 14-21 days or Foscarnet 60 mg/kg IV bolus (infuse over 1 hour) q8h × 14-21 days.

13. D.

14. B. Antiretroviral therapy should be initiated as follows:
   1. The asymptomatic patient: CD-4+ count = 300 cells/mm³ (between 500 cells/mm³ and 300 cells/mm³ AZT is an option that should be discussed with the patient)
   2. The symptomatic patient: CD-4+ count = 500 cells/mm³. The initial recommended dose of AZT in HIV-positive patients is between 500 mg/day and 600 mg/day. The only exception to this is an AIDS patient with a significant AIDS-related neurologic disease. In this case therapy may be as high as 1200 mg/day.

15. E. Zidovudine (AZT) has both early and late side effects. The early side effects of AZT are frequent but are usually limited to the first 12 weeks of therapy. They include headache, nausea, and dyspepsia. The late side effects (which occur in < 5% of patients on 600 mg/day

of AZT) include hepatic dysfunction, bone marrow suppression, neutropenia, and myositis and myopathy.

Potential drug interactions include AZT and ketoconazole and AZT and high-dose Septra.

16. C. In general, the reason for switching from AZT to ddl is the development of HIV viral resistance. Viral resistance is manifested by precipitous drops in the CD-4+ count, drops that may be ≥ 50% of the total count. In addition, a patient who has been on AZT from the beginning and in whom the CD-4+ count is becoming very low (50-100) should change antiretroviral agents.

17. E. Neurological complications of AIDS include cognitive impairment AIDS dementia, encephalitis, meningitis, primary lymphoma formation, and peripheral neuropathy.

In general, the last complication (peripheral neuropathy) is more often associated with the treatment of AIDS (particularly ddl and ddC) than the primary disease process itself.

18. D. The transmission of HIV infection from pregnant mother to infant is certainly not universal. It is extremely important that all health care personnel involved in delivery of the infant take meticulous precautions to avoid the transfer of blood and blood products to themselves.

From the point of view of the newborn, several scenarios may occur, and some of those scenarios are positive.
1. The transmission rate from infected mother to infant is thought to be in the range of approximately 20%-30%. Thus 70% to 80% of infants born to mothers infected with the HIV virus will never, we believe, become infected themselves. They will continue, we hope, to test negative for the rest of their lives.
2. In those infants who do eventually test positive (and this may take up to 1 year to occur), the prognosis for HIV infection progression and the development of AIDS and AIDS-related complications is somewhat more favorable than in adults who develop the infection.

19. C.

20. C. HIV testing is based on an ELISA (enzyme-linked immunosorbent assay) test. This is the initial screening test. If a patient has a positive ELISA test, a confirmation test known as the Western blot needs to be carried out to confirm positivity.

21. D. Toxoplasmosis (a protozoal infection) is the most common CNS infection system in patients with AIDS.

22. B. Human immune deficiency virus and AIDS are characterized by both a qualitative and quantitative defect in a specific lymphocyte subpopulation known as the helper T cells. This subpopulation of lymphocytes is responsible for the coordination of the entire immune system response. This population of helper T cells is best followed by declining CD-4+ cell counts.

23. B. See the answer to Question 16.

24. A. The most common neoplasm involving the central nervous system in patients with AIDS is a primary non-Hodgkin's lymphoma.

Meningitis in patients with AIDS is most commonly caused by the fungal agent *Cryptococcus*.

25. B. The antiretroviral agent of choice in the treatment of HIV disease or AIDS is zidovudine (AZT).

26. E. The major indications for switching from one antiretroviral agent to another have already been discussed. Generally, with a declining CD-4+ count, there are two major options:
1) Add ddC to AZT. The dosage of AZT should probably remain the same (500 mg-600 mg). The recommended dosage of ddC is 0.375-0.750 mg po tid.
2) Switch AZT to ddI. The determination of recommended dosage of ddI is made according to body weight. The recommendations are as follows:
   a) 125 mg bid (35 to 45 kg)
   b) 200 mg bid (50 to 75 kg)
   c) 300 mg bid (> 75 kg)

27. C. This is a classic case of herpes zoster involving dermatomal segments of the ophthalmic and the maxillary branches of the trigeminal (fifth cranial) nerve.

In patients with AIDS, the treatment for this condition is acyclovir 800 mg po × 5/day or 10 mg/kg IV q8h for at least 7 days or until the lesions crust over.

The most significant potential complication of this dermatomal eruption is blindness secondary to worsening of and involvement of the eye itself.

28. D. Aerosolized pentamidine is one of the treatment alternatives for *Pneumocystis carinii* pneumonia. It is discussed in Question 4.

29. D. The average length of time from the transmission of the HIV virus and the subsequent acute infection to death from AIDS-related complications is approximately 10 years.

30. C. The major reason for the difficulty encountered to date in the development of an AIDS vaccine is the retroviral nature of the viral genome and the subsequent ease of mutation allowed.

31. E.

32. E. Prophylaxis against MAC *(Mycobacterium avium intracellulare)* should begin when the CD-4+ count reaches 100 cells/mm³. The prophylactic agent of choice is rifabutin 300 mg po daily.

Prophylaxis against toxoplasmosis should begin when the CD-4+ count declines to 100 cells/mm³. The prophylactic agent of choice is the same agent that is recommended for *Pneumocystis carinii* (trimethoprim-sulfamethoxazole DS) 1 tablet daily.

33. A. In patients who are free from AIDS or HIV infection, the normal CD-4+ count is usually in the range of 1000-1500 cells/mm³.

34. B. In AIDS patients who present with serious, life-threatening systemic fungal infections, the drug of choice is still amphotericin B.

Two excellent oral agents, ketoconazole and difluconazole, can effectively treat many serious fungal infections in AIDS patients (such as esophageal candidiasis). These agents, however, have not replaced amphotericin B in cases of overwhelming fungal sepsis.

35. E. Kaposi's sarcoma lesions are found both on the skin and in internal organs. The face, the neck, the arms, the back, and the thighs are the most common external sites. Internally, the GI tract, the lungs, and the lymphatic system are common sites.

36. B. The infective agent least likely to be associated with diarrhea among the listed agents is toxoplasmosis.

Infective diarrhea in patients with AIDS may be cuased by any of the following agents: *Mycobacterium avium*, cytomegalovirus, *cryptosporidiosis*, *Clostridium difficle* (toxin), *Chlamydia*, Norwalk-like viruses, rotaviruses, enterotoxigenic *E. coli*, *Giardiasis*, *Entamoeba histolytica*, *Strongyloides*, *Amebiasis*, *Campylobacter*, *Shigella*, *Salmonella*, *Microsporidia*, *Isospora*, adenovirus and related viruses, and herpes simplex.

37. D. In patients with AIDS and HIV infections, there is both a qualitative and a quantitative deficiency in helper T cells. These are the cells that essentially control the immune system.

38. D. During the phase of acute infection (the acute retroviral syndrome), there is a sharp decrease in the CD-4+ count.

Following that sharp decrease (which eventually returns to baseline level), over many years there is a fairly stable but gradual decrease in the CD-4+ count.

When switching from AZT to ddI, it is not uncommon to see a transient increase in the CD-4+ count. This increase is, however, only transient and lasts for at most a period of a few months.

39. D. The three leading causes of both morbidity and mortality in patients with AIDS are *Pneumocystis carinii* pneumonia, the AIDS wasting syndrome, and esophageal candidiasis.

At the time of this writing major new threats are developing. These include infections such as *Mycobacterium avium intracellulare*, cytomegalovirus, and tuberculosis.

40. E. At the last writing of this book the high-risk groups were homosexual males, IV drug users, Haitians, hemophiliacs, and bisexual males.

At this writing, the heterosexual female with many male sexual partners has been added to that list.

SOLUTION TO SHORT ANSWER MANAGEMENT PROBLEM 138

Part A
HIV counseling and testing are extremely important. HIV counseling and testing services are meant to do the following:
1) Provide an opportunity for individuals to determine their current HIV serostatus
2) Provide behavioral counseling to prevent infection in those who are not infected, in a continued effort to avoid infection, and those who are infected but can transmit the infection to others
3) Help those who are infected to obtain appropriate services
4) Help partners of infected individuals to receive proper preventive services

Individuals have various degrees of understanding and knowledge about HIV transmission, testing, and risky behaviors. The physician should view all requests for HIV testing as an educational opportunity, an opportunity that cannot be missed.

Among the important issues that all health care professionals associated with the counseling, testing, diagnosis, and treatment of HIV-positive patients face are sensitivity to sexual identity, sensitivity to culture, sensitivity to socioeconomic conditions, and an awareness of the individual's previous mental and physical conditions. The language used by the health care professional should be appropriate to the patient. An example of this last issue is the term *HIV-positive*. Frankly, patients who have the HIV virus see nothing "positive" about this at all.

Once risk factors have been identified, the decision to test for HIV seropositivity should be made by the patient. The physician has an ethical responsibility to explain the following tests:
1) Nominal test: this test will directly use the patient's name.
2) Nonnominal test: the patient identifier is known only to the physician and to the patient.
3) Anonymous: this has an identifier known only by the patient.

Given the biological, psychological, and economic consequences of HIV disease, it is essential that the patient be made aware of the reasons for the test and the consequences of the test.

The following should be done prior to the test:

1) Ask the patient directly why he or she wants to be tested.
2) Explain the test. Explain the "window period." The body takes time to produce antibodies, usually 6 to 12 weeks. During this time the individual will continue to test negative.
3) Explain that a positive test means that the patient has been infected and that sexual contacts need to be notified by the patient, the doctor, or the public health authorities. Requirements vary from state to state.
4) Clarify the difference between HIV infection and AIDS.
5) Discuss the benefits of testing.
6) Discuss the risks and disadvantages of testing, including insurance issues, false positives, false negatives, and indeterminate test results.
7) Obtain informed consent before testing.
8) Discuss confidentiality and the circumstances under which the result must be disclosed by law or ethical obligation.

Part B

For HIV-positive patients, the following immunizations and tests are recommended:

1. Regular immunizations:
   a) IPV (inactivated polio vaccine) q 10 years
   b) Td (tetanus toxoid + diptheria) q 10 years
2. Yearly immunizations and tests:
   a) Influenza vaccine
   b) TB testing
3. Once-only immunizations and tests:
   a) Pneumococcal vaccine
   b) Hepatitis B for susceptible patients (3 Energix or Recombinax inoculations)
4. Optional immunizations and tests:
   a) Hib (*Hemophilus influenzae* b vaccine)
   b) Determination of MMR (measles/mumps/rubella) immunity and immunization in susceptible patients

Part C

With decreasing health care dollars, it becomes very difficult to develop a preventative medicine strategy that reaches most of the individuals who are at high risk for acquiring the human immunodeficiency virus. This high-risk group includes those engaging in certain hizgh-risk behaviors (homosexual males, bisexual males, individuals who practice unprotected heterosexual intercourse with no precautions, IV drug users), those living in certain areas of the United States, and those belonging to various demographic population groups.

Examples include targeting the following:

First, those areas with high concentrations of homosexual or bisexual men who have regular homosexual contact with multiple partners, and those areas with high concentrations of IV drug users (these two targets make up 80% of AIDS cases in the United States)

Second, areas with high concentrations of African-Americans and Latinos (48% of AIDS cases in the United States are in these groups in spite of the fact that they make up only 19% of the population)

Third, areas with high concentrations of pregnant IV drug users (over 50% of the heterosexual transmission of HIV occurs among IV drug users)

Similarly, there is a dramatically high seroprevalence of HIV among users of crack cocaine who have not injected drugs: among inner-city women the rates of HIV infection and AIDS are 29.6% in New York and 23% in Miami. This high seroprevalence is apparently not due to the use of crack cocaine in itself or to unprotected sex in itself but rather to a combination of factors: a large number of sexual partners, high rates of unprotected sex (often for money), and a high background HIV seroprevalence among injection drug users in those communities.

By using strategies like these to provide the HIV/AIDS preventative message to those most likely to become infected, the cost-effectiveness of each dollar will be maximized.

This chapter needs no summary section.

NEW INFORMATION—1996

1. According to the recent international HIV conference held in Vancouver, B.C., Canada, it appears that the use of 2 reverse transcriptase inhibitors (AZT + 3TC) along with a protease inhibitor will dramatically decrease the number of HIV viral particles in the body. This appears to be the direction of the future in HIV treatment.
2. AIDS is now the number one cause of death (all deaths) in men up to the age of 44 years in the United States. The five most common causes of death in the male age group up to age 44 years are as follows (in order):
   1. Acquired immune deficiency syndrome
   2. Accidents (primarily motor vehicle accidents)
   3. Heart disease
   4. Malignancies
   5. Suicide

SUGGESTED READINGS

The College of Family Physicians of Canada. A comprehensive guide for the care of persons with HIV disease. Health Canada, 1993. (This is an outstanding reference and can be obtained by writing to the College of Family Physicians, 2600 Skymark Avenue, Mississauga, Ontario, Canada.)

Connor EM et al. Reduction of maternal-infant transmission of human immunodeficiency virus type I with zidovudine treatment. New England Journal of Medicine 1994; 331(18):1174-1180.

Drugs for non-HIV viral infections. The Medical Letter on Drugs and Therapeutics 1994; 36(919):27-32

PROBLEM 139 A 51-YEAR-OLD MALE WHO IS PLANNING ON TRAVELING TO AFRICA

A 51-year-old male presents to your office for a periodic health examination. He is planning on traveling to equatorial Africa in the near future and wishes to discuss immunizations and prophylaxis against malaria.

He is feeling well. He has had no major medical problems in the past, nor has he had any surgeries. He has no known allergies.

SELECT THE ONE BEST ANSWER TO THE FOLLOWING QUESTIONS

1. What is the prophylactic agent of choice for the prevention of malaria in most areas of the world?
   a) chloroquine
   b) mefloquine
   c) pyrimethamine
   d) dapsone
   e) proguanil

2. The drug of choice you selected in Question 1 should be given for the following length of time:
   a) 1 week before travel and for at least 1 month after return from travel
   b) 1 month before travel and for at least 1 month after return
   c) 2 weeks before travel and for at least 2 weeks after return
   d) 1 week before travel and for at least 1 week after return
   e) 6 weeks before travel and for at least 4 weeks after return

3. The drug of choice you selected in Question 1 was chosen for its activity against which of the following?
   a) *P. falciparum*
   b) *P. vivax*
   c) *P. ovale*
   d) *P. malariae*
   e) none of the above

4. Which of the following symptoms is(are) common in clinical malaria?
   a) fever and/or chills
   b) malaise
   c) headache
   d) myalgias
   e) all of the above

5. What is the most common cause of traveler's diarrhea?
   a) *Campylobacter jejuni*
   b) *Shigella*
   c) enterotoxigenic *E. coli*
   d) *Clostridium difficile*
   e) rotavirus

6. What is(are) the prophylactic drug(s) of choice for the prevention of traveler's diarrhea?

   a) bismuth subsalicylate
   b) trimethoprim-sulfamethoxazole
   c) ciprofloxacin
   d) any of the above
   e) none of the above

7. What is the treatment of choice for symptomatic traveler's diarrhea?
   a) bismuth subsalicylate
   b) trimethoprim-sulfamethoxazole
   c) ciprofloxacin
   d) any of the above
   e) none of the above

8. A 43-year-old farmer presents to the ER after having punctured his foot on a rusty pitchfork while cleaning out a pig barn. You consider tetanus immunization. The patient is unsure of his tetanus immunization status at this time. Which of the following regimes should be administered to this patient for the prevention of tetanus?
   a) a single dose of tetanus toxoid
   b) two doses of tetanus toxoid
   c) three doses of tetanus toxoid
   d) three doses of tetanus toxoid and a single dose of tetanus immunoglobulin
   e) three doses of tetanus toxoid and three doses of tetanus immunoglobulin

9. Diptheria and tetanus boosters should be a routine part of preventive health care in adults. How often should diptheria and tetanus boosters be administered?
   a) every year
   b) every 2 years
   c) every 3 years
   d) every 5 years
   e) every 10 years

10. Pneumococcal vaccine is an effective agent for prophylaxis against pneumococcal pneumonia. Which of the following is(are) indication(s) for the administration of pneumococcal vaccine?
   a) chronic cardiopulmonary disease
   b) chronic renal disease
   c) chronic alcoholism
   d) Hodgkin's disease
   e) all of the above

11. A recent outbreak of bubonic or pneumonic plague (the Black Death reported in the Middle Ages) has occurred

in India. If you are traveling to India, especially to areas where the plague has been reported, you should provide prophylaxis for yourself.

Which of the following regimens is (are) recommended for prophylaxis against bubonic or pneumonic plague?
a) amoxicillin 3.5 g plus 1.0 g probenecid *stat* 2 days before travel

b) doxycycline 100 mg once/day 2 to 3 days prior to travel with continuation until 3 or 4 days following return home
c) tetracycline 500 mg qid on landing in India and until 2 weeks following return home
d) TMP-SMX double strength for 1 week before and continuing until 2 weeks following return home
e) all of the above are equally effective

Short Answer Management Problem 139

List the immunizations and other prophylactic measures and treatments that a patient traveling from the United States to Central Africa should receive prior to departure.

ANSWERS

1. B.

2. A.

3. A. Mefloquine 250 mg once/week is the drug of choice for travel to areas with chloroquine-resistant malaria. Because chloroquine-resistant malaria is now found throughout the world, mefloquine has become the preferred drug. The usual recommendation is that treatment begin 1 week prior to traveling to the malaria-infected area and continue for 6 weeks after the return home.

There are several strains of malaria: *Plasmodium falciparum, Plasmodium ovale, Plasmodium vivax,* and *Plasmodium malariae.* Most of the concern arises over *Plasmodium falciparum;* it is crucial that treatment be directed to the most virulent and morbidity-producing strain.

4. E. Typical symptoms of malaria include fever, chills, myalgia, arthralgias, and headache. Abdominal pain, cough, and diarrhea may also occur.

Frequent clinical and laboratory findings include hepatosplenomegaly, anemia, and thrombocytopenia. Pulmonary or renal dysfunction (in the absence of dehydration) and changes in mental status may complicate *P. falciparum* malaria.

5. C.

6. E.

7. D. The most common cause of traveler's diarrhea, usually a self-limited illness lasting several days, is enterotoxigenic *E. coli. Campylobacter, Shigella, Salmonella,* viruses, and parasites are less common causes of this condition. In areas where hygiene is poor, travelers should be advised to avoid foods that are not steaming hot, raw vegetables, and fruit they have not peeled themselves, as well as tap water and ice.

It is generally not recommended to prescribe drugs to provide prophylaxis against traveler's diarrhea, but rather to begin treatment with drugs promptly when symptoms occur. On the rare occasions when prophylaxis is indicated, the prophylactic agent of choice is ciprofloxacin.

Treatment of traveler's diarrhea should consist of oral rehydration solutions, loperamide hydrochloride (a synthetic opioid), and, when diarrhea is moderate or severe, any of the choices given in question 7.

8. D. Because this wound is classified as a dirty wound, the patient should receive both tetanus toxoid and a single dose of tetanus immunoglobulin. Because his primary immunization status is unsure, three doses of tetanus toxoid should be administered. Two doses can be administered 1 month apart and a third dose 6-12 months later. Tetanus immunoglobulin should be administered intramuscularly (250 units).

9. E. Adults should be given a booster dose of Td (tetanus-diptheria) every 10 years unless contraindicated.

10. E. A single dose of pneumococcal vaccine is recommended in the following patients: patients with asplenia, patients with splenic dysfunction, patients with sickle-cell disease, patients with hepatic cirrhosis, patients with chronic cardiorespiratory disease, patients with chronic alcoholism, patients with chronic renal disease, patients with Hodgkin's disease, and conditions associated with immunosuppression.

Because mortality due to bacteremic pneumococcal disease increases with age, elderly patients with or without chronic illnesses should be considered for immunization.

11. B. The recent outbreak of bubonic plague in India is considered serious enough to recommend prophylaxis when traveling to parts of India where plague has been reported. The recommended regimen is doxycycline 100 mg once/day 2 or 3 days prior to travel and continuing until 3 to 4 days following returning to the United States. If the individual is pregnant or under the age of 9 then TMP/SMX DS should be used.

SOLUTION TO SHORT ANSWER MANAGEMENT PROBLEM 139

The immunizations and other prophylactic measures and treatments include the following:

I. **Immunizations:**
   A. Immunization with hepatitis A vaccine
   B. Oral polio (if immunization status not up to date)
   C. Tetanus-diphtheria (if immunization status not up to date)
   D. The new live oral typhoid vaccine
   E. Yellow fever vaccine
   F. Measles vaccine (if not up to date)

II. **Prophylactic measures and treatments:**
   A. Traveler's diarrhea:
      1) Enterotoxigenic *E. coli* is the most common cause.
      2) Prophylaxis is not indicated in most cases: treatment with oral rehydration, loperamide (2 mg orally after each loose stool up to maximum of 16 mg), and ciprofloxacin or another quinolone is indicated if the diarrheal illness is severe.
   B. Malaria:
      1) Mefloquine is now the drug of choice for the prevention of malaria in most areas of the world. Treatment begins 1 week before travel and continues for 6 weeks after returning.

SUMMARY OF ADVICE FOR TRAVELERS

See the answer to Short Answer Management Problem 139.

SUGGESTED READINGS

Advice for travelers. The Medical Letter on Drugs and Therapeutics 36(922):41-44.

McCarthy A. Malaria. In: Rakel R, ed. Conn's current therapy. Philadelphia: WB Saunders, 1994

PROBLEM 140 A 24-YEAR-OLD FEMALE WITH ABDOMINAL PAIN, PELVIC PAIN, AND ADNEXAL TENDERNESS

A 24-year-old female presents to the ER with a 2-day history of lower abdominal pain, pelvic pain, fever, chills, and malaise. Associated with these symptoms, the patient has also felt nauseated for the last 48 hours and has vomited twice.

On physical examination, there is bilateral adnexal tenderness, bilateral lower abdominal tenderness, and tenderness on cervical motion.

The patient has a temperature of 40° C. Her last menstrual period was 5 weeks ago, but she has had a small amount of spotting during the last few days. She had one previous episode of these symptoms, 15 months ago.

SELECT THE ONE BEST ANSWER TO THE FOLLOWING QUESTIONS

1. What is the most likely diagnosis in this patient?
   a) acute appendicitis
   b) chronic salpingitis
   c) acute salpingitis
   d) ectopic pregnancy
   e) endometritis

2. Which of the following statements regarding the relationship between the OCP and the disease described is true?
   a) the OCP protects against all forms of this condition
   b) the OCP protects against one form of this condition but not another
   c) the OCP protects against none of the forms of this condition
   d) the OCP has nothing to do with this condition
   e) nobody really knows for sure

3. Which of the following organisms is not associated with this condition?
   a) *N. gonorrhea*
   b) *Chlamydia trachomatis*
   c) *Mycoplasma hominis*
   d) *peptostreptococcus*
   e) beta-hemolytic streptococcus

4. Which of the following is not a risk factor for this condition?
   a) age < 25
   b) multiple sexual partners
   c) a barrier contraceptive method
   d) a history of previous episodes of the same condition
   e) time of the last menstrual period

5. What is the most appropriate intervention and treatment of this patient?
   a) hospitalize the patient and begin treatment
   b) begin treatment as an outpatient, but recheck the patient's condition within 24 hours
   c) begin treatment as an outpatient and make an appointment for her to see a gynecologist

   d) begin treatment as an outpatient but recheck her if the condition worsens
   e) nobody really knows for sure

6. If hospital management was chosen for this patient, which of the following treatment options would be the most appropriate first-line treatment?
   a) IV ampicillin and gentamicin
   b) IV cefoxitin and doxycycline
   c) IV ampicillin and tobramycin
   d) IV ciprofloxacin
   e) IV ampicillin

7. If outpatient management was chosen for this patient, which of the following treatment regimes would be the most appropriate first-line treatment?
   a) cefoxitin, probenecid, and doxycycline po
   b) ceftriaxone IM, probenecid po, and doxycycline po
   c) aqueous procaine penicillin G IM plus probenecid po and doxycycline po
   d) any of the above
   e) none of the above

8. What is the current United States Public Health Service recommendation for the treatment of uncomplicated genital, rectal, or pharyngeal gonococcal infection?
   a) ampicillin po and probenecid po
   b) ciprofloxacin po
   c) ceftriaxone IM followed by doxycycline po
   d) cefiximine orally followed by doxycycline po
   e) c or d

9. A 24-year-old male presents with a mucoid urethral discharge. This was preceded by a 2-day history of urgency and frequency. He has no other symptoms. What is the most likely diagnosis in this patient?
   a) gonorrhea
   b) acute prostatitis
   c) epididymitis
   d) nongonoccal urethritis
   e) bacterial cystitis

10. What is the most likely organism causing the condition described in the patient in Question 9?
   a) *Chlamydia trachomatis*

b) *Ureaplasma urealyticum*
c) *Trichomonas vaginalis*
d) *Neisseria gonorrhea*
e) nobody really knows for sure

11. What is the treatment of first choice for nongonococcal urethritis?
    a) ciprofloxacin po
    b) doxycycline po
    c) erythromycin po
    d) ampicillin po and probenecid po
    e) none of the above

12. Which of the following statements regarding *Neisseria gonorrhea* infections is false?
    a) the spectrum of illness caused by *N. gonorrhea* ranges from uncomplicated urethritis to septicemia
    b) a gram stain of a tissue or secretion sample with *N. gonorrhea* infection will show gram-positive intracellular diplococci
    c) many *N. gonorrhea* strains have become resistant to penicillin
    d) many *N. gonorrhea* strains have become resistant to tetracycline
    e) all of the above statements are false

13. Many patients presenting with gonococcal genital infections have concomitant infections with Chlamydia trachomatis. To what percentage of patients does this statement apply?
    a) 10%
    b) 20%
    c) 45%
    d) 30%
    e) 25%

14. Which of the following is(are) common symptoms of *N. gonorrhea* in males?
    a) dysuria
    b) frequency
    c) urgency
    d) a and b
    e) all of the above

15. Which of the following is(are) complications of disseminated gonococcal infection?
    a) arthritis
    b) tenosynovitis
    c) bacteremia
    d) b and c only
    e) all of the above

16. A 24-year-old male presents with a mucoid urethral discharge. This was preceded by a 2-day history of urgency and frequency. He has had no other symptoms. He has no previous history of sexually transmitted diseases.

What is the most likely diagnosis?
    a) *C. trachomatis* urethritis
    b) *N. gonorrhea* urethritis
    c) nonspecific urethritis
    d) *E. coli* urethritis
    e) none of the above

17. A 24-year-old female presents with a 2-day history of dysuria accompanied by painful genital lesions that have coalesced to form ulcers. The patient also describes systemic symptoms including fever, malaise, myalgias, and headache. There is no previous history of same. Which of the following statements concerning this patient is false?
    a) the most likely diagnosis is herpes simplex type II
    b) this patient is unlikely to experience a recurrence of these symptoms at a later date
    c) the duration of viral shedding may be reduced by treatment with acyclovir
    d) the time to heal these lesions may be reduced by treatment with acyclovir
    e) severe or frequent recurrences can be treated by the administration of acyclovir prophylactically

18. A 25-year-old female presents with a 2-week history of "growths" in the vulvar region. On examination you find multiple verrucous lesions on the labia majora and the labia minora.

What is the most likely diagnosis in this patient?
    a) condyloma lata
    b) condyloma acuminatum
    c) herpes simplex type I
    d) herpes simplex type II
    e) none of the above

19. What is the treatment of choice for the patient described in Question 17?
    a) podophyllin in benzoin
    b) trichloracetic acid
    c) carbon dioxide laser
    d) 5-fluorouracil cream
    e) acyclovir

20. Which of the following statements regarding syphilis is true?
    a) *Treponema pallidum,* the causative organism of syphilis, is becoming resistant to penicillin
    b) syphilis has become an extremely uncommon STD
    c) treatment of incubating syphilis with ceftriaxone and doxycycline is usually not effective
    d) the Jarsch-Herxheimer reaction is a very common reaction in patients with syphilis who are effectively treated with antibiotics
    e) none of the above

21. What is the treatment of choice for incubating syphilis?
    a) benzathine penicillin G IM

b) ciprofloxacin po
c) ceftriaxone IM
d) trimethoprim-sulfamethoxazole (TMP-SMX) po
e) tetracycline po

22. A patient presents to your office with a mucoid urethral discharge for 3 days. He has associated dysuria, frequency, and urgency.

    You decide to treat him with TMP-SMX po.

    He returns in 3 days with a tender scrotum, and with scrotal skin that is red, warm, and tense, and with partial obstruction of the rugal folds. The upper part of the scrotal structure appears to be acutely tender.

    What is the most likely diagnosis at this time?
    a) *Chlamydia trachomatis* urethritis with complicating orchitis
    b) *Chlamydia trachomatis* urethritis with complicating epididymitis
    c) *E. coli* epididymitis
    d) *E. coli* orchitis
    e) *Mycoplasma hominis* urethritis with complicating epididymitis

23. What is the treatment of choice for the patient just described?
    a) doxycycline po
    b) TMP-SMX po
    c) ampicillin plus probenecid po
    d) benzathine penicillin G IM
    e) ceftriaxone IM

Short Answer Management Problem 140

List the risk factors and the complications of acute PID in women.

ANSWERS

1. C. This patient meets the diagnostic criteria for acute salpingitis. Acute salpingitis is diagnosed when there is a history of lower abdominal pain, lower abdominal tenderness, cervical motion tenderness, and adnexal tenderness that is accompanied by one of elevated temperature, elevated WBC and/or ESR, positive culdocentesis, an inflammatory mass on pelvic examination or sonography, or a positive gram stain or smear.

   The differential diagnosis of acute PID includes the following:
   a) acute appendicitis
   b) acute endometritis
   c) corpus luteum bleeding
   d) ectopic pregnancy
   e) pelvic adhesions
   f) benign ovarian tumor
   g) chronic salpingitis

   The patient described in this question, however, is more likely to have acute salpingitis than any other diagnosis. Although the patient has had one previous episode of these symptoms, a diagnosis of chronic salpingitis cannot be made without laparoscopy.

   An infection confined to the endometrium (endometritis) is unlikely in this patient. The adnexal tenderness is much more compatable with acute salpingitis. Endometritis usually occurs postpartum (retained products of conception) or after a procedure such as a suction D & C for therapeutic abortion.

2. B. The OCP protects against gonococcal PID. The incidence of genital tract infection with *Chlamydia trachomatis* may actually be increased on the OCP.

   The protective effect against gonococcus may be associated with a decreased average amount of menstrual blood flow, with menstrual blood acting as a culture medium; a decreased permeability of cervical mucus to the infective organism; a decreased cervical dilatation at mid-cycle and menstruation; and a decrease in the strength of uterine contractions.

3. E. The most common organisms associated with acute PID are *Neisseria gonorrhoeae, Chlamydia trachomatis,* and *Mycoplasma hominis.* Many episodes of PID are polymicrobial and involve anaerobic organisms such as *Bacteroides fragilis* and *Peptostreptococcus,* in addition to the three most common organisms listed at the beginning of this answer. Beta-hemolytic streptococcus (the streptococcus associated with bacterial pharyngitis) is not associated with acute PID.

4. C. Barrier contraceptive methods (such as a condom or diaphragm) are protective against, rather than contributory to, acute PID. Risk factors for acute PID include age (< 25 years), multiple sexual partners, nonbarrier contraceptive methods (especially the intrauterine device [IUD]), time of the last menstrual period (the closer the time of onset to the last menstrual period, the greater the risk), a history of a previous episode of documented PID, and symptoms of urethritis in a sexual partner.

5. A. Early treatment of acute PID will decrease the probability of tubal scarring and subsequent infertility. Hospitalization and inpatient treatment are preferred in the following situations:
   a) The patient is an adolescent.
   b) The diagnosis is uncertain.
   c) Surgical emergencies such as appendicitis and ectopic pregnancy cannot be excluded.
   d) A pelvic abscess is suspected.
   e) Severe systemic illness precludes outpatient management.
   f) The patient is pregnant.
   g) The patient is unable to follow or tolerate an outpatient regimen.

6. B.

7. B. The recommended regimen for inpatient management of PID is one of the two following regimens:
   Regimen A: cefoxitin (Mefoxin), 2.0 g IV q6h or cefotetan (Cefotan), 2 g IV q12h plus doxycycline, 100 mg q12h PO or IV
   This regimen must be given for at least 48 hours after the patient improves clinically. After discharge from the hospital, continuation of doxycycline, 100 mg PO bid for a total of 10-14 days.
   Regimen B: clindamycin (Cleocin), 900 mg IV q8h, plus gentamicin (Garamycin), loading dose IV or IM (2 mg/kg) followed by a maintenance dose (1.5 mg/kg) q8h
   This regimen must be given for at least 48 hours after the patient improves clinically. After discharge from the hospital, continuation of doxycycline, 100 mg PO bid for 10-14 days total. The recommended treatment regime for patients treated on an outpatient basis includes the following:
   1. Ceftriaxone IM 250 mg.
   2. Probenecid po
   3. Doxycycline po
   The probenecid can be given as a one-time dose (250 g); the doxycycline should continue po for 14 days (100 mg bid).

8. E. The preferred treatment of uncomplicated adult gonococcal urethritis, adult gonococccal cervicitis, and adult gonococcal proctitis is as follows:
   A. Ceftriaxone 250 mg IM or Cefixime 400 mg po once plus
   B. Doxycycline 100 mg po, bid for 7 days

9. D.

10. A. The most likely diagnosis in this patient is nongonococcal urethritis. The most likely organism causing this condition in this patient is *Chlamydia trachomatis* urethritis. *Chlamydia trachomatis* is the most common cause of nongonococcal urethritis (NGU).

Symptoms in men include dysuria, frequency, and mucoid to purulent urethral discharge. Some men have asymptomatic infections. Female partners of men with *Chlamydia trachomatis* NGU are likely to have a mucopurulent discharge. Next in order of frequent causative agents to *C. trachomatis* for NGU is *Ureaplasma urealyticum*.

Men with typical clinical symptoms are presumed to have NGU when their urethral (gram-stained) smear shows WBCs with no gram-negative diplococci and/or their rapid antigen-detection test is positive. As well, cultures for *N. gonorrhea* should confirm the absence of this organism.

11. B. The recommended regimen for treating uncomplicated urethral *C. trachomatis* infections is doxycycline, 100 mg orally bid for 7 days. A good substitute is tetracycline 500 mg orally qid for 7 days. In addition, it is imperative that all recent sexual contacts be treated.
   Alternative regimens include erythromycin base 250 mg orally qid for 7 days, or erythromycin ethylsuccinate 400 mg orally qid for 7 days. If erythromycin is not tolerated, sulfisoxazole 500 mg orally qid for 10 days may be effective.
   A recent controlled trial of a single dose of azithromycin for the treatment of chlamydial urethritis has been shown to be as effective as a 7-day course of doxycycline.

12. B. *Neisseria gonorrhea* has become, in many parts of the world, resistant to both penicillin and tetracycline. Thus, even in areas where there is a relatively low incidence of antibiotic-resistant gonorrhea, the treatment of choice has become ceftriaxone 250 mg IM or cefixime 400 mg po once.
   The spectrum of disease created by *N. gonorrhea* ranges from a mild urethritis to septicemia with many systemic complications, including septicemia and arthritis.
   The gram stain of a WBC containing *N. gonorrhea* shows gram-negative intracellular diplococci, not grampositive intracellular diplococci.

13. C. As many as 45% of patients presenting with gonococcal genital infection have concomitant infection with *Chlamydia trachomatis*. Because current diagnostic tests for chlamydial infection do not permit a timely or reliable diagnosis, patients should be treated presumptively for that organism as well as for gonococcus. Sexual partners of infected patients should be evaluated, have cultures taken, and be treated presumptively for gonococcal and chlamydial infection, regardless of their symptom status.

14. E. *Neisseria gonorrhea* in males may produce dysuria, frequency and urgency. Gonococcal arthritis-dermatitis

syndrome is the most common clinical manifestation of disseminated gonococcal infection (DGI) and consists of tenosynovitis, arthritis, and a pustular or papular rash. Meningitis and endocarditis may complicate bacteremic gonococcal infection.

Gonococcal infection at other sites in adults includes gonococcal conjunctivitis and gonococcal epididymitis.

15. E.

16. A. This patient most likely has *Chlamydia trachomatis* urethritis. It is the most common cause of nongonococcal urethritis (NGU). Symptoms in men include dysuria, frequency, and mucoid to purulent urethral discharge. Some men have asymptomatic infections. Female partners of men with *Chlamydia trachomatis* are likely to have chlamydial mucopurulent cervicitis.

The second most common etiologic agent in NGU is *Ureaplasma urealyticum*.

Men with typical clinical symptoms are presumed to have NGU when their urethral (gram-stained) smear shows WBCs with no gram-negative diplococci and/or their rapid antigen-detection test is positive. As well, cultures for *Neisseria gonorrhea* should confirm the absence of this organism.

17. B. This patient has a primary genital herpes infection.

The most common symptom of genital herpes infection is a cluster of painful genital lesions. With primary infection, the multiple vesicles that are initially present coalesce to form intensively painful ulcers. Most lesions are found on the vulva and vaginal mucosa. Other symptoms include fever, malaise, myalgias, and headache. Dysuria and vaginal discharge are also common. Recurrences are common; the severity of the primary disease symptoms bears no relationship to the chance of acquiring recurrent disease. The diagnosis of genital herpes should always be confirmed by culture.

The treatment of choice for primary herpes simplex genital viral infection is acyclovir. Acyclovir has been shown to shorten the duration of viral shedding and to shorten the time to lesion healing. The recommended dose is 200 mg po × 5/day for 10 days.

Patients with severe or frequent recurrences can be treated with acyclovir prophylactically. General supportive measures including povidone-iodine will often provide relief. Bacterial superinfection can be treated with a topical antibiotic such as fusidic acid ointment or cream.

18. B. This patient has condyloma acuminatum. This is caused by the human papilloma virus.

Condyloma lesions may appear on the introitus, the labia majora, the labia minora, the perineal area, and the urethra.

Patients with condyloma are four times more likely to develop cervical carcinoma in situ and subsequent invasive cervical cancer. These women must have frequent Pap smears (yearly). If any abnormalities are found, colposcopy should be performed.

Patients with condyloma acuminatum should also be carefully screened for other sexually transmitted diseases.

An association has been demonstrated between condyloma acuminatum and laryngeal papillomas in the newborn.

19. C. The treatment that has been reported to have the highest cure rate in patients with condyloma acuminatum is the carbon dioxide laser. Cure rates with this form of therapy approach 90%. Other treatment options include:
a) cryosurgery,
b) trichloroacetic acid,
c) 5-fluorouracil, and
d) podophyllin resin.

20. E. *Treponema pallidum,* the causative organism of syphilis, is not becoming resistant to penicillin. This is an exception to the increasing prevalence of usual antibiotic resistant organisms.

Syphilis is not going away; there were, in fact, alarming increases in incidence rates for new cases of syphilis in the late 1980s. Although this has declined somewhat now, syphilis has, in a very real sense, grown along with AIDS.

Although benzathine penicillin G remains the drug of choice for the treatment of syphilis, a combination of doxycycline and ceftriaxone is effective.

The Jarisch-Herxheimer reaction is a reaction that occurs within several hours of initiating therapy in patients with syphilis. It consists of constitutional symptoms (headache, fever, myalgia), mild hypotension, and worsening of specific syphilis manifestations. This phenomenon should be treated with salicylates (acetaminophen in pregnant women) or, in severe cases, with prednisone.

A localized Jarisch-Herxheimer reaction also may manifest as transient worsening of neurologic, otic, or ophthalmologic symptoms soon after therapy and should be treated with prednisone. Patients should be warned of the possibility of the Jarisch-Herxheimer reaction before therapy begins and instructed with regard to self-medication and the need for contacting the physician.

21. A.

22. B. This patient almost certainly has a primary NGU (a non-gonococcal urethritis) caused by *Chlamydia trachomatis* with a complicating epididymitis.

The symptoms of acute epididymitis include scrotal skin that is red, warm, and tense, with partial or total obliteration of the rugal folds. The epididymis is tender to the touch, indurated, and enlarged.

23. A. If a patient presents with what appears to be an acute epididymitis or an acute orchitis and the inflammation/swelling does not improve on antibiotic therapy, a neoplasm should be suspected and an ultrasound of the testicle performed.

The most common bacterial cause of acute epididmyitis is *E. coli*. The most common pathogens in general are *Chlamydia trachomatis* and *Mycoplasma hominis*.

SOLUTION TO SHORT ANSWER MANAGEMENT PROBLEM 140

I. Risk factors for pelvic inflammatory disease:
   A. Age (women between the ages of 18 and 25)
   B. Multiple sexual partners
   C. Initial sexual encounter at an early age
   D. Black and other nonwhite women have a greater risk than whites.
   E. Instrumentation of the endometrial cavity (that is, insertion of an IUD)
   F. Nonbarrier contraceptive methods
   G. Relationship of infection to LNMP (the closer the time of organism infection to the LNMP, the greater the risk)
   H. History of PID
   I. Symptoms of urethritis in a sexual partner
II. Complications of pelvic inflammatory disease:
   A. Advancement of the infection unchecked to point of tubo ovarian abscess and subsequent peritonitis
   B. Bacteremia secondary to item A
   C. Resultant tubal scarring. This leads to the following:
      1. Chronic pelvic adhesions
      2. Chronic pelvic pain syndrome
      3. Ectopic pregnancy
      4. Subsequent infertility

SUMMARY OF THE DIAGNOSIS AND TREATMENT OF PELVIC INFLAMMATORY DISEASE AND OTHER SEXUALLY TRANSMITTED DISEASES

1. **Pelvic inflammatory disease:**
   a) Signs and symptoms of acute salpingitis:
      1. Lower abdominal pain
      2. Lower abdominal tenderness
      3. Cervical motion tenderness
      4. Adnexal tenderness
   Accompanied by
      5. One of elevated temperature, elevated WBC, elevated ESR, positive culdocentesis, an inflammatory mass on pelvic examination or ultrasound, or a positive gram stain or smear
   b) Differential diagnosis:
      1. Acute appendicitis
      2. Endometritis
      3. Corpus luteum bleeding
      4. Benign ovarian tumor
      5. Chronic salpingitis

   c) Laboratory evaluation/procedures: CBC, ESR, ultrasound, beta-HCG, laparoscopy
   d) Pathophysiology:
      Microbiology: polymicrobial infection most likely; an anaerobic organism is almost always involved.
      Major anaerobic organisms include *Bacteroides fragilis* and *Peptostreptococcus*.
      Pathophysiology involves inflammation of the fallopian tubes (acute salpingitis) with extension in either direction (into uterus) or into ovaries. An extension into the ovaries may lead to the formation of a tubo ovarian abscess.
   e) Treatment of PID:
      1. Inpatient treatment:
         i) Cefoxitin IV plus doxycycline IV
         ii) Clindamycin IV plus gentamicin IV followed by doxycycline orally
      2. Outpatient treatment: cefoxitin or ceftriaxone IM plus proben-ecid PO plus doxycycline PO or tetracycline PO
   f) Risk factors for PID: see the solution to Short Answer Management Problem 140.
   g) Complications of PID: See the solution to Short Answer Management Problem 140.
   h) Key issue in PID: to hospitalize or not hospitalize. See the answer to Question 6.
2. **Gonococcal urethritis:**
   a) Organism: *Neisseria gonorrhea*
   b) Symptoms: dysuria, frequency, discharge (initially serous or milky that changes to a yellow, creamy discharge with significant urethral pain); may be asymptomatic in women
   c) Treatment: ceftriaxone IM (one dose) plus doxycycline po or cefixime po (one dose) plus doxycycline po
3. **Nongonococcal urethritis:**
   a) Organism: *Chlamydia trachomatis* or *Ureaplasma urealyticum*
   b) Symptoms: dysuria, frequency, mucoid to purulent urethral discharge; may be asymptomatic in men as well as in women, although more common in women
   c) Laboratory diagnosis: urethral/cervical/rectal/pharyngeal swab to demonstrate co-existing gram-negative intracellular diplococci
   d) Treatment: doxycycline or tetracycline PO
4. **Epididymitis:**
   a) Organisms:
      1. Most common cause: *Chlamydia trachomatis*
      2. Most common bacterial cause: *E. coli*
      3. Other organism that may be involved: *Ureaplasma urealyticum, Mycoplasma*
   b) Symptoms: painful and red scrotum, tenderness in epididymis and scrotum
   c) Differential diagnosis: testicular tumor, testicular torsion
   d) Treatment: doxycycline po, NSAID (Indocin), scrotal elevation, ice packs

5. **Syphilis:**
   a) Organism: *Treponema pallidum*
   b) Sign: painless ulcer in genital region (primary syphilis)
   c) Laboratory diagnosis: Darkfield examination for *Treponema pallidum*
   d) Treatment: benzathine penicillin IM

6. **Herpes genitalis:**
   a) Organism: herpes simplex type II
   b) Symptoms/signs: painful ulcers in genital area, associated swelling/lymphadenopathy
   c) Laboratory diagnosis: viral culture
   d) Treatment: Acyclovir
   e) Recurrences: recurrences are common.

7. **Condyloma acuminatum:**
   a) Organism: human papilloma virus
   b) Sign/symptom: cauliflower-like lesion in genital area
   c) Treatment: Cryosurgery

Remember, sexually transmitted diseases go together; where one is gathered, others may also be found. The major public health initiatives involve prevention (education) and contact tracing.

SUGGESTED READINGS

Althausen A. Epididymitis. In: Rakel R, ed. Conn's current therapy. Philadelphia: WB Saunders, 1994.

Lynn S. Pelvic inflammatory disease. In: Rakel R, ed. Conn's current therapy. Philadelphia: WB Saunders, 1994.

Mata J. Nongonococcal urethritis. In: Rakel R, ed. Conn's current therapy. Philadelphia: WB Saunders, 1994.

Michael R. Gonorrhea. In: Rakel R, ed. Conn's current therapy. Philadelphia: WB Saunders, 1994.

Tyring S. Viral diseases of the skin. In: Rakel R, ed. Conn's current therapy. Philadelphia: WB Saunders, 1994

PROBLEM 141 A 73-YEAR-OLD MALE WITH FEVER, HEADACHE, AND MYALGIAS

You are called to see a 73-year-old nursing home resident with a temperature of 103°F, headache, myalgias, cough, rhinorrhea, sore throat, and malaise. In this case, seven other nursing home residents have come down with similar symptoms. It is December, and there has been a significant outbreak of respiratory illness in the community.

On examination, the patient appears acutely ill. Apart from the aforementioned fever, the patient also has prominent pharyngeal erythema. There are a few expiratory rhonchi heard and the occasional bilateral rales.

SELECT THE ONE BEST ANSWER TO THE FOLLOWING QUESTIONS

1. What is the most likely diagnosis in this patient?
   a) influenza A
   b) bronchiolitis
   c) bacterial pneumonia
   d) septicemia secondary to an unknown focus of infection
   e) peritonsillar abscess

2. Which of the following investigations may be indicated in this patient?
   a) CBC
   b) blood cultures
   c) CXR
   d) all of the above
   e) none of the above

3. Which of the following statements regarding the influenza virus(es) is(are) true?
   a) influenza epidemics occur annually and are of major public health importance worldwide
   b) influenza viruses are subclassified as influenza A, influenza B, and influenza C
   c) excess morbidity and mortality are reported consistently during influenza epidemics
   d) all of the above
   e) none of the above

4. Concerning the use of antibiotics in influenza infection in the elderly, which of the following statements most accurately describes a high practice standard?
   a) no elderly patients with influenza should receive prophylactic antibiotics
   b) all elderly patients with influenza should receive prophylactic antibiotics
   c) the benefit of prescribing prophylactic antibiotics must be weighed against the risk: in most cases of uncomplicated influenza the risk/benefit ratio favors withholding antibiotics
   d) basically, give the patient antibiotics if they ask for them; if they don't ask, don't give them
   e) nobody really knows for sure

5. What is the most common complication of the illness described in this patient?
   a) meningitis
   b) pneumonia
   c) serum sickness
   d) agranulocytosis
   e) brain abscess

6. Which of the following types of influenza is responsible for most of the world pandemics?
   a) influenza A
   b) influenza B
   c) influenza C
   d) influenza D
   e) influenza E

7. What is the drug of choice for treating the symptoms of the patient described?
   a) acetylsalicylic acid
   b) acetaminophen
   c) amantadine
   d) meperidine
   e) ibuprofen

8. What is the primary mode of transmission of the illness described?
   a) transfer via blood and blood products
   b) oral-fecal contamination
   c) sneezing and coughing
   d) fomites
   e) kissing

9. What is the most reliable method for preventing influenza?
   a) gamma globulin
   b) α-interferon
   c) activated influenza vaccine
   d) inactivated influenza vaccine
   e) amantadine hydrochloride

10. Regarding influenza vaccine, which of the following statements is(are) true?
    a) influenza vaccine is effective only against influenza A
    b) the efficacy of influenza vaccine is approximately 95%
    c) influenza vaccine should be administered every 2 years
    d) the ideal time for administration of influenza vaccine is in the late spring
    e) none of the above are true

11. Regarding influenza vaccination, which of the following statements is(are) true?
    a) influenza vaccination typically produces no ADRs (adverse drug reactions)
    b) the recommended dosage of influenza vaccine is 0.5 mL for adults
    c) influenza vaccination reduces the severity of illness in vaccinated persons who become infected
    d) b and c
    e) all of the above are true

12. Which of the following statements regarding amantadine prophylaxis of influenza is(are) false?
    a) amantadine prophylaxis is effective against both influenza A and influenza B
    b) amantadine prophylaxis has been shown to reduce the duration of fever and other symptoms
    c) amantadine has been shown to reduce the duration of viral shedding
    d) amantadine prophylaxis should be used in high-risk individuals in whom vaccine is contraindicated
    e) all of the above statements are false

13. Amantadine should be administered for how long in unvaccinated individuals?
    a) 1 week
    b) 2 weeks
    c) 3 weeks
    d) 4 weeks
    e) for the duration of the particular outbreak

14. Which of the following groups should be considered for vaccination against influenza on a yearly basis?
    a) healthy adults over the age of 65 years
    b) children and adolescents receiving chronic aspirin therapy
    c) health care workers
    d) adults and children in chronic care facilities
    e) all of the above

15. Which of the following diseases shares a therapeutic agent with influenza?
    a) bronchial asthma
    b) congestive cardiac failure
    c) ulcerative colitis
    d) Parkinson's disease
    e) pulmonary thromboembolism

Short Answer Management Problem 141

You have just assumed the role of medical director of a long-term care facility. It is now the end of November and it appears that the residents were not vaccinated when they should have been.

Two residents come down with symptoms suggestive of influenza. Discuss your management of the long-term care facility residents and staff.

ANSWERS

1. A. This patient most likely has influenza A. Influenza A strains usually predominate in adults; influenza B strains tend to infect children.

   Bacterial pneumonia and a secondary septicemia may follow influenza, but at this time, with the history and P/E reported, the most likely diagnosis is influenza.

   The most common symptom of influenza is a severe generalized or frontal headache, often accompanied by retroorbital pain. Other early symptoms of influenza include diffuse myalgias, fever, and fever and chills. Respiratory symptoms especially tend to follow the occurrence of the early symptoms.

   The term *flu* is used very loosely by both physicians and patients. True influenza has a very specific set of symptoms that can usually be used to differentiate it clinically from other viral infections.

   In children, the signs and symptoms of influenza are more subtle; they may simply appear as another upper respiratory tract infection or "cold."

2. D. At this time, it would be very reasonable to perform a CBC, blood cultures, and a CXR. The CXR is indicated as rales are heard in the lung fields. A CBC and blood cultures, along with the CXR, will rule out a secondary bacterial pneumonia, most often caused by *Streptococcus pneumoniae* and the bacteremia that may accompany it.

3. D. Influenza epidemics occur annually and are of major public health importance worldwide. The epidemics are usually associated with a less serious antigenic drift or a more serious antigenic shift. The antigenic drifts (a shift in the hemagglutinin and neuraminidase antigens) provide, in most cases, the next year's challenge for public health practitioners. The antigenic shifts are responsible

for the major "pandemics" that have occurred with influenza. The are also responsible for the major epidemics seen each year. Influenza epidemics and influenza pandemics are almost always associated with influenza A.

Both morbidity and mortality are definitely associated with influenza epidemics. This is true especially of the very old and the very young. Those with chronic disease are at even greater risk.

There are three major influenza viruses, designated influenza A, influenza B, and influenza C. By far the most virulent and most significant is the influenza A virus.

4. C. In uncomplicated influenza viral infections, as in uncomplicated viral infections in general, there is no indication for the prescription of antibiotics. One could argue that those patients at high risk for the development of complications, such as those patients with chronic bronchitis, should be treated. This, and any other chronic cardiopulmonary condition, may very well be a reasonable exception to the no-antibiotics rule.

5. B. The most common complication of influenza is pneumonia. This pneumonia is initially a viral pneumonia but often develops, especially in susceptible elderly patients, into a double pneumonia, with *Streptococcus pneumoniae* as the most common pathogen. This is the reason for the recommendations of the U.S. Preventive Services Task Force on the Periodic Health Examination with respect to influenza:
   1. Immunize all patients over the age of 65 each year with influenza vaccine.
   2. Immunize all patients at high risk once with pneumococcal vaccine.

6. A. All of the world's pandemics (major antigenic shift) are associated with influenza A.

   Influenza B and influenza C are associated with neither epidemics or pandemics.

7. C. Amantadine is the only drug approved in the United States for the specific prophylaxis and treatment of influenza A.

   Amantadine can be used during the influenza season as an adjunct to late vaccination, as a supplement to preseason vaccination in immunodeficiency persons, and as chemoprophylaxis in the absence of vaccination.

   Amantadine can also be used to reduce the spread of the virus and to minimize disruption of patient care both in the community and in the institutional setting. It can be prescribed as prophylaxis for healthy unvaccinated persons who simply want to avoid illness during an outbreak.

   Amantadine is 70% to 90% effective in preventing influenza A infections. It is also the treatment of choice once influenza A is contracted. When given 24-48 hours after the onset of infection, amantadine reduces both the severity and duration of symptoms.

   The standard dose of amantadine is 200 mg daily. Elderly patients should receive 100 mg.

8. C. The influenza virus is transmitted through respiratory secretions and thus is easily spread to susceptible persons. Sneezing, coughing, and close contact while talking are thought to be the major modes of transmission.

9. D. The most effective method for preventing influenza A is by immunizing patients before the influenza season begins with inactivated (or killed) influenza vaccine. Influenza vaccine confers approximately 70% protection against the development of influenza and an even greater rate of protection against death from influenza.

10. E. Influenza vaccine is effective against both influenza A and influenza B, has an efficacy rate of approximately 70%, and should be administered yearly and ideally 1-2 months before the influenza season begins.

11. D. Influenza vaccine typically produces some minor side effects such as a sore arm, redness at the injection site, and low-grade fever. A history of anaphylactic hypersensitivity to eggs or egg products is a contraindication to receiving influenza vaccine.

    Details of vaccine dose are discussed in a later question, but the usual dose of whole virus vaccine for adults is 0.5 mL.

    In those patients in whom immunization fails and in whom influenza does develop, influenza vaccine still reduces both the severity and the duration of symptoms.

12. A. Amantadine is effective only against influenza A.

    Amantadine reduces viral shedding, reduces the duration and severity of influenza A symptoms (such as headache, fever, chills, myalgias, and cough) once the virus is established, and should be used as treatment in high-risk patients in whom the influenza vaccine is contraindicated.

13. E. Patients who cannot take vaccine can be protected by using amantadine prophylactically during the local outbreak. The drug should be started as soon as possible after the outbreak is recognized and continued until it ends, usually in about 6 weeks. The usual dosage is 200 mg/day, but this depends on renal function. In many elderly patients a dosage of 100 mg/day is safer.

14. E. Individuals who should receive influenza vaccine include the following:
    1. Persons of any age with cardiovascular or pulmonary conditions that necessitate regular medical follow-up

2. Residents of nursing homes and other chronic care facilities regardless of age
3. Medical personnel who have contact with and can therefore transmit the influenza virus to high-risk patients
4. Healthy adults over age 65
5. Children with chronic diseases (diabetes mellitus, renal dysfunction, anemia, immunosuppression, or asthma) or those on aspirin therapy

Split-dose vaccine should be used in children; the dose is 0.5 mL for children ages 3 to 8 years and 0.25 mL for those 6 to 35 months old. A second dose 4 weeks or more after the first is needed if the child has never received influenza vaccine. Children 9-12 years of age should receive one 0.5-mL dose of split-virus vaccine. Adults can be given either whole- or split-virus vaccine as a 0.5-mL dose.

15. D. Parkinson's disease shares a therapeutic agent with influenza. The therapeutic agent is, of course, amantadine. The treatment of Parkinson's disease is discussed in another chapter of this book.

SOLUTION TO SHORT ANSWER MANAGEMENT PROBLEM 141

As the new medical director of the chronic care facility, it is your job to minimize through immunization both the morbidity and mortality from influenza and from the influenza outbreak that appears to be hitting your facility.

First, in those patients who have come down with influenza, amantadine should begin immediately in a dosage of between 100 mg/day and 200 mg/day depending on the renal function. Although those patients are unlikely to benefit from vaccine with respect to the current illness, vaccination should be undertaken in any case to prevent against further infections that year.

All other residents of the nursing home should be vaccinated immediately and also placed on amantadine prophylaxis until the local in-house outbreak is over.

All health care workers who work in your facility should also receive the influenza vaccine immediately.

SUMMARY OF THE DIAGNOSIS AND TREATMENT OF INFLUENZA

1. **Epidemiology:** influenza A is responsible for all epidemics and pandemics of influenza. It is also the most virulent of the influenza types, which include A, B, and C. Yearly outbreaks result mostly from antigenic drift in the H and N antigens.

   Influenza outbreaks begin in the late fall and can last until early into the new year.
2. **Signs and symptoms:** headache is the first symptom. Other symptoms include fever, chills, and myalgias, followed by the symptoms of cough and congestion.
3. **Prevention:** Influenza vaccine should be given to all high-risk groups discussed. Ideally, immunization should take place in September or October. Vaccine efficacy averages around 70% and is effective for both influenza A and influenza B.
4. **Prophylaxis:** amantadine is a prophylactic agent that can be used as an adjunct to vaccination in high-risk situations (especially chronic care facilities). Amantadine is 70%-90% effective in preventing influenza A. It is not effective against influenza B.

   Amantadine not only prevents influenza A but also reduces the severity and duration of symptoms in persons who have already contracted the virus.

SUGGESTED READING

Ruben F. Influenza. In: Rakel R, ed. Conn's current therapy. Philadelphia: WB Saunders, 1994.

Emergency Medicine

PROBLEM 142   A 55-YEAR-OLD MALE FOUND COLLAPSED IN THE STREET

A 55-year-old male is found collapsed in the street by a passerby. The passerby begins CPR and is joined shortly by another citizen. 911 is called and CPR is continued until the paramedics arrive and initiate ACLS.

Despite complete ACLS maneuvers, the patient remains pulseless and breathless as the paramedics hand over care to the ER doctor on duty at the closest hospital.

SELECT THE ONE BEST ANSWER TO THE FOLLOWING QUESTIONS

1. What is the most common rhythm initially responsible for cardiac arrest?
   a) ventricular tachycardia
   b) ventricular fibrillation
   c) ventricular standstill
   d) asystole
   e) complete heart block

2. What is the most common rhythm leading directly to death in cardiac arrest?
   a) ventricular tachycardia
   b) ventricular fibrillation
   c) second-degree heart block-Mobitz type II
   d) ventricular asystole
   e) complete heart block

3. A "quick-look paddles" is performed on the patient above. You diagnose ventricular fibrillation. What should be your first step?
   a) defibrillate with 200 joules
   b) administer sodium bicarbonate 50 mEq IV bolus, epinephrine 10 cc 1:1000 solution and follow by countershock
   c) administer sodium bicarbonate 500 mEq IV bolus and calcium chloride 500 mL of a 10% solution IV bolus; countershock after drug infusion
   d) defibrillate with 400 joules
   e) administer atropine 1.0 mg IV bolus and epinephrine 10 cc 1:10000 solution; wait for the response

4. What is the antiarrhythmic of choice in the management of ventricular arrhythmias?
   a) bretylium
   b) lidocaine
   c) procainamide
   d) verapamil
   e) aminrone

5. The patient above is successfully converted to sinus rhythm. Unfortunately, on the way to the coronary care unit he arrests again. The rhythm strip reveals asystole. CPR is restarted. Which of the following is the next logical step in treatment?
   a) administer epinephrine 1:10,000-1.0 mg IV push
   b) administer calcium chloride-10 cc of a 10% solution-IV push
   c) administer sodium bicarbonate 1 mEq/kg IV push
   d) administer isoproterenol 2-20 ug/kg/min
   e) administer lidocaine 75 mg IV push

6. With appropriate treatment the patient again converts to sinus rhythm. He is stabilized in the coronary care unit. Unfortunately, 2 hours later he develops a ventricular dysrhythmia. His blood pressure is 100/60 mm Hg and he has a palpable pulse. Your next step should be to administer which of the following?
   a) lidocaine 75 mg IV bolus
   b) procainamide 20 mg/min up to a maximum of 1000 mg
   c) bretylium 5 mg IV bolus
   d) verapamil 5 mg IV bolus
   e) none of the above

7. Sinus rhythm is restored again and his condition returns to satisfactory. Unfortunately, he develops a second-degree AV block (Mobitz type II). His pulse is 40 beats/minute and his blood pressure drops to 70/40 mm Hg. Given this change, what would you do now?
   a) observe the patient only
   b) administer isoproterenol 2-10 μg/min
   c) administer atropine 0.5-1.0 mg
   d) administer epinephrine 0.5-1.0 mg
   e) none of the above

8. What is the definitive therapy for the dysrhythmia described in the previous question?
   a) a constant infusion of isoproterenol 2-20 μg/min

b) a constant infusion of lidocaine 2-4 mg/min
c) a constant infusion of procainamide 2-4 mg/min
d) a transvenous pacemaker
e) none of the above

9. CPR is in progress on a 70-kg man who collapsed in the street (witnessed arrest). BLS was begun, as was ACLS, when the paramedics arrived. He was brought immediately to the ER and a blood gas sample was drawn. The results were as follows:
   pH = 7.10
   P_{CO_2} = 60 mm Hg
   P_{O_2} = 75 mm Hg
   H_{CO_3} = 15 mEq/L
   This represents which of the following:
   a) metabolic acidosis with respiratory alkalosis
   b) respiratory acidosis with metabolic alkalosis
   c) pure metabolic acidosis
   d) pure respiratory acidosis
   e) mixed respiratory and metabolic acidosis

10. What is the most appropriate treatment of the patient described in Question 9?
    a) sodium bicarbonate 1 mEq/kg
    b) sodium bicarbonate 0.5 mEq/kg
    c) increased ventilation
    d) both a and c
    e) both b and c

11. Which, metabolic or respiratory, should be treated first in this patient?
    a) respiratory acidosis
    b) metabolic acidosis
    c) respiratory alkalosis
    d) metabolic alkalosis
    e) all of the above

12. A 53-year-old male presents to your ER with a 2-hour history of a "rapid heartbeat," nausea, and dizziness. A 12-lead ECG shows atrial flutter with variable AV conduction. As you are taking his history he becomes disoriented. You are only able to obtain his systolic blood pressure (40 mm Hg). At this time, what should you do?
    a) administer epinephrine 1.0 mg IV
    b) administer isoproterenol 2-20 μg/min IV
    c) defibrillate with 300 joules
    d) cardiovert with 300 joules
    e) cardiovert with 75-100 joules

13. What is the first step in initiation of resuscitation following a witnessed or unwitnessed cardiac arrest?
    a) begin rescue breathing
    b) begin rescue compression
    c) initiate a call to 911

d) check pulse
e) go for help

14. Which of the following statements concerning basic life support (BLS) is false?
    a) BLS is felt to be very successful public health initiative
    b) mouth-to-mouth resuscitation is the recommended method of respiratory exchange in performing BLS
    c) BLS is most commonly used in family situations, one family member resuscitating another
    d) BLS succeeds no more frequently than in 15% of out-of-hospital attempts
    e) infectious diseases such as AIDS and serum hepatitis pose little, if any, risk to rescuers

15. What is the recommended BLS compression/ventilation rescue sequence in one-person CPR?
    a) 15/2
    b) 15/1
    c) 20/4
    d) 10/1
    e) 10/3

16. For optimal survival from out-of-hospital cardiac arrest, BLS and ACLS resuscitation should be initiated, respectively, by
    a) 2 minutes/4 minutes
    b) 3 minutes/6 minutes
    c) 4 minutes/8 minutes
    d) 8 minutes/12 minutes
    e) 10 minutes/15 minutes

17. The National Heart, Lung, and Blood Institute in the United States recommends that in order to minimize permanent cardiac muscle damage the maximum upper limit of time from onset of symptoms (either prodronal or pain symptoms) to hospital admittance should be no more than which of the following?
    a) 30 minutes
    b) 60 minutes
    c) 90 minutes
    d) 120 minutes
    e) 240 minutes

18. The National Heart, Lung, and Blood Institute in the United States recommends that in order to minimize permanent cardiac muscle damage, the "ER door to needletime" for clot dissolving drugs should not exceed which of the following?
    a) 30 minutes
    b) 60 minutes
    c) 90 minutes
    d) 120 minutes
    e) 240 minutes

Short Answer Management Problem 142

PART A: Describe the importance and sequence for performing a "critical incident debriefing" among emergency room personnel or emergency rescue staff involved in an unsuccessful resuscitation. This "critical incident debriefing" is especially important if there is an unusual feature to the case such as a patient of young age, a victim known to some or all of the rescuers, or rescue personnel who are not accustomed to failure.

PART B: Explain the importance of the "chain of survival" in out-of-hospital cardiac arrest.

ANSWERS

1. B.

2. D. The most common initial rhythm diagnosed in patients who suffer a cardiac arrest is ventricular fibrillation. The usual course of events is as follows: coarse ventricular fibrillation to fine ventricular fibrillation to ventricular asystole. If BLS and ACLS are available within the recommended 4- and 8-minute time intervals, the probability of successfully converting ventricular fibrillation before ventricular asystole occurs is significantly increased. Even in the best of community coronary care units, the survival rate of out-of-hospital cardiac arrest rarely exceeds 15%. Higher rates have been reported but are extremely rare. Once ventricular asystole develops, the probability of successful resuscitation is virtually zero. Thus, while ventricular fibrillation is the most common initial rhythm, ventricular asystole is the most common arrhythmia leading directly to death.

3. A. The first step in the treatment of ventricular fibrillation is defibrillation with an energy level of 200 joules. If the first attempt is unsuccessful, two further defibrillations (200-300-360 joules) should follow immediately (before pharmacologic therapy is initiated). If defibrillation is not successful, IV access should be established, epinephrine given, intubation performed, and antiarrhythmic drugs administered. The role of sodium bicarbonate in the management of cardiac arrest is limited. Atropine is indicated in the management of asystole, not ventricular fibrillation. Calcium chloride is no longer recommended for the management of any arrhythmia or dysrhythmia.

4. B. The antiarrhythmic agent of choice is lidocaine. Lidocaine should be administered in a dosage of 1 mg/kg IV push up to a maximum of 3 mg/kg. In addition, a lidocaine infusion in a dose of 2-4 mg/kg should be started in a patient with a ventricular arrhythmia.

   Bretylium and procainamide are equally good second-line agents. Bretylium is administered in a dose of 5 mg/kg IV and repeated at 15-30 min intervals in a dose of 10 mg/kg to a maximum dose of 30 mg/kg.

   Procainamide is administered in a dose of 50 mg every 5 minutes until one of the following is observed:
   (1) The arrhythmia is suppressed.
   (2) Hypotension ensues.
   (3) The QRS complex is widened by 50% of its original width.
   (4) A total of 1 g of drug has been given.

   Bretylium and procainamide levels can be maintained by IV infusion at a dose of 2-4 mg/min.

   Verapamil is indicated in the treatment of supraventricular arrhythmias. It has, however, been replaced by adenosine, as the drug of first choice.

   Amrinone is a rapid acting inotropic agent that is useful in the treatment of patients with severe congestive heart failure refractory to diuretics, vasodilators, and conventional inotropic agents.

5. A. The next step in the management of the original patient is the administration of epinephrine 1:10,000 1.0 mg IV push. This should be repeated every 5 minutes. If intubation has not been performed it should be. Atropine in a dose of 1.0 mg IV push should be given as well and repeated every 5 minutes. If the patient's arrest has been unwitnessed, sodium bicarbonate may be considered if the patient does not respond to other treatments.

   The only other possible treatment is cardiac pacing, but this is really a treatment of last resort.

6. A.

7. E. The use of verapamil in supraventricular dysrhythmias has been discussed. Adenosine has essentially replaced verapamil as the drug of first choice.

   The treatment of choice for patients with ventricular tachycardia who are hemodynamically stable is lidocaine 1 mg/kg. This can be repeated in a dose of 0.5 mg/kg every 8 minutes until the ventricular tachycardia resolves or until a total of 3 mg/kg has been given.

The second-line drug in this case is procainamide in a dose of 20 mg/min until the ventricular tachycardia resolves or a total of 1 g has been given.

DC countershock is recommended only in hemodynamically unstable patients. Bretylium can be used but is recommended for use after procainamide in stable ventricular tachycardia.

When hemodynamically unstable ventricular tachycardia is diagnosed (pulseless or hypotensive) the treatment of choice is synchronized cardioversion. The initial energy recommended is 50 joules. This should be followed by repetitive shocks of 100 joules, 200 joules, and finally 360 joules. If recurrent, lidocaine should be given as an IV bolus and cardioversion again attempted (at the energy level that was previously successful).

8. E. Second-degree heart block (Mobitz type II) occurs below the level of the AV node either at the bundle of His (uncommon) or bundle branch level (more common). It is usually associated with an organic lesion in the conduction pathway. Its usual progression is to a third degree (complete) heart block.

Initial treatment is aimed at increasing the heart rate in an attempt to increase cardiac output. Thus atropine in a dose of 0.5-1.0 mg is the drug of choice. The maximum dose of atropine is 2.0 mg. If signs or symptoms persist, an external pacemaker can be placed or an isoproterenol infusion begun in a dose of 2-10 μg/min. Epinephrine or observation are not appropriate treatment options for this patient. The definitive treatment in this patient is a transvenous pacemaker.

9. A.

10. C.

11. C. Most patients who have arrested and who are undergoing CPR have a mixed respiratory and metabolic acidosis. Normal P_{CO_2} is 40 mm Hg.

The patient in this case has a markedly elevated P_{CO_2} of 60 mm Hg and thus is being hypoventilated. The patient's bicarbonate level of 15 mEq/L is below the normal range of 21-28 mEq/L and thus he has a metabolic acidosis as well.

Recent recommendations, however, suggest that bicarbonate should be used with caution. Although cardiac function is depressed by acidosis, the determining factor is intracellular pH, not extracellular pH, as is measured by arterial pH. Hypoxia, not acidosis, accounts for most of the cardiac depression. Respiratory acidosis, however, produces immediate and profound depression. Thus increasing ventilation should be used as the primary means of correcting acidosis, and respiratory acidosis should be treated first.

By contrast, the use of bicarbonate has long been known to present risks that are not limited to alkalosis but include hypernatremia and hyperosmolarity. All of these conditions are easily and commonly brought about by the typical ACLS-recommended doses and are predictors of an unsuccessful outcome.

12. E. The treatment of choice for acute unstable atrial flutter is synchronized cardioversion. The initial energy chosen should be 75-100 joules. If unsuccessful, this should be followed by cardioversion at 200 and 360 joules. If the patient is stable, vagal maneuvers can be attempted first, followed by verapamil.

13. C. When witnessing a collapse or seeing an unresponsive victim, the first step in the adult BLS protocol is to access the Emergency Medical Service (EMS) system by dialing 911 or the emergency number in your area. This now precedes opening the airway by the head-tilt-chin-lift or the jaw-thrust maneuver.

In children, however, 1 minute of CPR should follow initial assessment before calling EMS.

14. B. Until recently, the recommended method of BLS ventilation was mouth-to-mouth. However, due to increased fear of contact of infectious diseases (especially AIDS), the recommendation has been changed to a primary recommendation of mouth-to-mask ventilation. (However, if masks are not available, mouth-to-mouth resuscitation *must* be immediately begun.) The risk of contacting an infectious disease through mouth-to-mouth resuscitation is extremely remote.

15. A. For one-rescuer CPR, the compression/ventilation ratio recommended is 15/2 (compressions to ventilations). When a second rescuer arrives, a 5/1 compression/ventilation ratio should begin. The compression rate for one-rescuer and two-rescuer CPR remains at 80-100/minute.

16. C. To optimize survival from out-of-hospital cardiac arrest BLS must be begun within 4 minutes and ACLS must be begun within 8 minutes. This has been documented in many studies.

17. B.

18. A. The National Heart, Lung, and Blood Institute in the United States has made very specific recommendations of the maximum time intervals that should not be exceeded to ensure a zero to minimal chance of permanent cardiac muscle death from a myocardial occlusion by a dissolvable clot-inhibiting drug such as T-PA or streptokinase.

The maximum times are as follows:
1. Onset of cardiac symptoms (including prodromal symptoms of nausea, vomiting, and dizziness) to admission to ER = < 60 minutes

2. Time of admission to ER to injection of thrombolytic agents IV = < 30 minutes

If these guidelines are followed, the greatest probability for preserving cardiac muscle will be attained (that is, ischemia and injury, not infarction).

Time = Muscle

SOLUTION TO SHORT ANSWER MANAGEMENT PROBLEM 142

PART A: Following an unsuccessful resuscitation attempt, a therapeutic intervention should be undertaken. This is known as a *critical incident debriefing*.

Critical incident debriefing allows the facilitation of rescuer grief work, reviews critical responsibility, and provides continuing health professional education. Suggested guidelines include the following:

1. The debriefing should occur as quickly as possible after the cardiac arrest with all team members present.
2. Call the group together, preferably in the resuscitation room. State that you want to have a code debriefing.
3. Review the scenario and conduct of the code. Include the contributory pathophysiology leading to the code, the decision tree followed, and any variations present.
4. Analyze the things that were done wrong and especially the things that were done right. Allow free discussion.
5. Ask for recommendations/suggestions for future resuscitations.
6. Encourage all team members to share their feelings of anxiety, anger, and possible guilt.
7. Any team member not able to be present should be informed of the process followed, the discussion generated, and the recommendations made.
8. The team leader should encourage any team member to contact him or her if unanswered questions arise later.

PART B: The effectiveness of community with emergency cardiac care depends very much on what is called the *chain of survival*.

The chain of survival, in simplest terms, requires four basic steps being performed in a specific order. If these four steps are instituted quickly, the probability of a successful outcome is increased:

1. Early access to EMS personnel
2. Early CPR (maximum = 4 minutes from victim down)
3. Early defibrillation
4. Early advanced care (maximum = 8 minutes)

SUMMARY OF THE TREATMENT OF THE CARDIAC ARREST PATIENT

1. **Ventricular fibrillation:**
   a) Defibrillation: 200-300-360 joules
   b) Epinephrine 0.5-1.0 mg IV push (repeat q 5 min)
   c) Defibrillate again

d) Lidocaine 1.0 mg/kg IV push
e) Second-line antiarrhythmic (procainamide/bretylium)

2. **Asystole:**
   a) Epinephrine 0.5 mg-1.0 mg IV push (repeat q 5 min)
   b) Atropine 1.0 mg IV push (repeat in 5 min)
   c) Consider pacing
   d) Consider bicarbonate

3. **Ventricular tachycardia:** stable ventricular tachycardia:
   a) Lidocaine 1.0 mg/kg (repeat at dose of 0.5 mg/kg every 8 minutes until resolution)
   b) Procainamide 20 mg/min until VT resolves or 1 g is given
   c) Cardiovert as in unstable patients unstable ventricular tachycardia:
      1. Consider sedation
      2. Cardiovert 50-100-200-360 joules: if recurrent, add lidocaine and cardiovert again starting at energy level previously successful; then procainamide or bretylium

4. **Heart block (second-degree Mobitz II and third degree):**
   a) Atropine 0.5-1.0 mg IV (maximum 2.0 mg)
   b) Isoproterenol 2-10 μg/min/external pacemaker
   c) Transvenous pacemaker

5. **Supraventricular tachycardia**
   a) Vagal maneuvers
   b) Adenosine 6-12 mg (alternative: verapamil 5 mg IV)
   c) Cardioversion, digoxin, beta blockers, pacing as indicated

SUMMARY OF AMERICAN HEART ASSOCIATION CHANGES ON THE BASIS OF THE 1992 NATIONAL CONFERENCE ON CARDIOPULMONARY RESUSCITATION AND EMERGENCY CARDIAC CARE:

1. BLS: dial 911 first.
2. Chain of survival in CPR:
   a) Early access to EMS
   b) Early CPR
   c) Early defibrillation
   d) Early ACLS
3. Esophageal obturator airway: no longer recommended
4. Increased restrictions on use of sodium bicarbonate
5. Use of calcium chloride: essentially eliminated
6. Adenosine: 6-12 mg—now drug of choice for paroxysmal supraventricular tachycardia in adults
7. Interosseous administration of drugs in infants and children is recommended up to age of 6 years.
8. Glucose-containing fluids should be discouraged in resuscitation attempts due to deleterious effects on cerebral perfusion.
9. Thrombolytic agents: t-PA and streptokinase should be administered within 6 hours of onset of chest pain in patients under age of 70 who have an ECG pattern indicative of acute myocardial infarction.

10. Ethical issues and critical incident debriefing is now considered as part of ACLS courses.

SUGGESTED READINGS

American Heart Association. Guidelines for cardiopulmonary resuscitation and emergency cardiac care. Recommendations of the 1992 National Consensus Conference. JAMA 1992; 16:2125-2302.

Swanson RW. Psychological issues in CPR. Ann Emerg Med 1993; 22(pt.2):350-353.

PROBLEM 143   A 27-YEAR-OLD FEMALE INJURED IN A MOTOR VEHICLE ACCIDENT

A 27-year-old female is injured in a head-on two-car collision. She is transported to your ER in critical condition. You are the duty doctor in a small, rural hospital. The nearest trauma center is 180 miles away.

On examination, the patient is in acute respiratory distress. Her respiratory rate is 32/minute. Breath sounds are absent in the right lung field. She is pale and her blood pressure is 90/60 mm Hg. Her pulse is 106/minute. Her heart sounds are distant and muffled. Her JVP appears elevated.

When you touch her abdomen she pulls back in pain. This appears to be maximal over the left upper quadrant.

Her right hip is in a posture of external rotation.

As she is wheeled through the ER doors, her C-spine appears to be adequately immobilized.

Her neurological examination reveals a dilated right pupil. She is responsive to deep pain and pressure, as well as deep palpation of the abdomen. There is blood and pink-tinged fluid leaking from her nose.

There is blood present at the urethral meatus, and her pelvis appears to be in an "odd position."

A large scalp laceration is present.

SELECT THE ONE BEST ANSWER TO THE FOLLOWING QUESTIONS

1. At this time, what should be your first priority?
   a) carry on with the rest of the complete assessment
   b) establish an intravenous infusion
   c) send the patient to X-ray for a stat chest X-ray
   d) send the patient to X-ray for a lateral X-ray of the cervical spine
   e) none of the above

2. What is the most likely cause of this patient's respiratory distress?
   a) flail chest
   b) tension pneumothorax
   c) acute pulmonary embolus
   d) pericardial tamponade
   e) none of the above

3. After establishing an airway and dealing with the patient's respiratory status, what should you do?
   a) complete the neurological examination
   b) perform a Glasgow coma scale
   c) establish a CVP line or two large peripheral IVs
   d) perform a diagnostic paracentesis
   e) perform a *stat* ECG

4. What is the most likely cause of this patient's dilated (R) pupil?
   a) a middle meningeal artery tear
   b) a chronic subdural hematoma
   c) an acute subdural hematoma
   d) a or c
   e) none of the above

5. The patient's neurological status is as follows:
   Eyes: closed; no response to verbal commands but a response to pain
   Best verbal response: none
   Best motor response: flexion withdrawal to pressure on the brachial plexus

What is the patient's Glasgow coma scale?
   a) 12
   b) 8
   c) 7
   d) 4
   e) 2

6. A paracentesis is performed and draws bloody fluid. On examination, pain is maximal in the left upper quadrant. What is the most likely cause of this patient's abdominal pain?
   a) liver laceration
   b) duodenal rupture
   c) renal hematoma
   d) splenic rupture
   e) pancreatic tear

7. A 31-year-old male is brought to the ER after having been involved in a car-motorcycle accident.

   On examination, he is drowsy but conscious. His respiratory rate is 32/minute. His blood pressure is 70/50 mm Hg. His heart sounds are muffled. He has significant elevation of the JVP. He has a large contusion over the sternal area. There is a laceration seen over the precordial region. No other significant abnormalities are noted on primary survey.

   What is the most likely diagnosis in this patient?
   a) myocardial contusion
   b) pericardial tamponade
   c) aortic rupture
   d) pulmonary contusion
   e) pneumothorax

8. What is the treatment of choice for the patient described in Question 7?
   a) regular observation
   b) increased rate of crystalloid infusion
   c) crystalloid infusion plus blood
   d) pericardiocentesis
   e) chest tube insertion

9. What is the minimal gauge of a peripheral IV catheter that should be inserted in a patient in shock?
   a) #25 gauge
   b) #22 gauge
   c) #18 gauge
   d) #16 gauge
   e) #12 gauge

10. What is the most common error in ER trauma stabilization?
    a) inadequate airway management
    b) inadequate C-spine immobilization
    c) failure to recognize or decompress pneumothorax
    d) inadequate shock therapy
    e) distracting visually impressive but not life-threatening maxillofacial trauma

Short Answer Management Problem 143

PART A: List the major mandatory interventions that should be immediately undertaken in someone who presents with traumatic shock.

PART B: Describe, in order of frequency, the major mistakes in treating patients with trauma.

ANSWERS

1. E. Your first priority is to attend to the ABCs of resuscitation. Thus the establishment of an airway is first. Following that, breathing should be assessed (this includes assessment of breath sounds in both lung fields as well as respiratory rate). Finally, the patient's circulatory status must be attended to with the establishment of either a CVP line or two large bore IV lines.

2. B. The most likely cause of this patient's respiratory distress is a tension pneumothorax. Tension pneumothorax is a common life-threatening injury that needs to be assessed and treated immediately. In this patient, the clue to the high probability of this being a tension pneumothorax is the complete absence of breath sounds in the right lung field.

   The most common error in this situation would be to transport the patient to X-ray without a physician. In fact, with the history and physical findings it would be entirely appropriate to treat the patient on the basis of your presumed diagnosis without an X-ray. A needle can be inserted into the chest wall cavity to decompress the potentially life-threatening tension pneumothorax. A "rush of air" will confirm the diagnosis. A chest-tube connected to underway drainage can then be inserted.

3. C. As mentioned above, the priority following A and B is C, that is, circulation. A CVP line or two large bore (#16 gauge IV catheters) should be inserted to maximize the ability to replace intravascular volume.

4. D. The dilated (R) pupil is most likely caused by an initial skull fracture producing tearing of either veins (subdural hematoma) or the middle meningeal artery (epidural hematoma). A "burr-hole" procedure in this

situation (especially if the patient is received in a rural center where transport to a tertiary care facility will take time) can be lifesaving.

5. C. This patient's Glasgow coma scale is 7.
   The Glasgow coma scale rating is as follows:

   1. Eyes
Open:	Spontaneously	4
	To verbal command	3
	To pain	2
No response:		1

   2. Best verbal response:
Orientated and converses	5
Disoriented and converses	4
Inappropriate words	3
Incomprehensible sounds	2
No response	1

   3. Best motor response:
To verbal command:	Obeys	6
To painful stimulus:	Localizes pain	5
	Flexion withdrawal	4
	Abnormal flexion (decorticate rigidity)	3
	Extension (decerebrate rigidity)	2
	No response	1
	Total =	3-15

6. D. A paracentesis that draws bloody fluid suggests an intraabdominal bleed most likely due to organ laceration or organ rupture. Pain maximal in the left upper quadrant suggests that this is most likely due to splenic rupture.

   Splenic rupture is one of the most common abdominal injuries seen in multiple trauma victims.

7. B.

8. D. This patient has a pericardial tamponade. Pericardial tamponade is an injury that is often missed. It also is a frequent injury in MVAs in which multiple injuries are sustained. For some reason, it appears to be particularly common in car-motorcycle accidents where the motorcyclist is often thrown a significant distance.

   Pericardiocentesis (the removal of fluid from around the heart) is the treatment of choice. Pericardiocentesis will remove the constriction that is impeding the ability of the heart to pump blood.

9. D. The minimum gauge of an IV catheter that should be inserted in a patient in shock is #16 gauge. It is recommended that if a CVP line cannot be secured, two #16 gauge catheters be inserted, one in each arm.

10. A. The most common error in ER trauma stabilization is inadequate airway management. The common errors that arise from diagnosis and treatment of trauma victims will be completely discussed in one of the short answer management problems.

SOLUTION TO SHORT ANSWER MANAGEMENT PROBLEM 143

PART A: The major interventions that should be undertaken when a patient presents with traumatic shock are as follows:

a) Remember the ABCs (airway, breathing, circulation) and assess and treat those priorities first.

   Airway: establish a patent airway with endotracheal intubation if possible.

   Breathing: ensure breath sounds heard in all lobes (assume patient has tension pneumothorax until proven otherwise.) Institute supplementary oxygen with nasal prongs or a Venturi mask.

   Circulation: establish CVP line or two large bore IV lines. Intraarterial catheter is preferable for monitoring vital signs but if not, continuous monitoring by other means necessary.

b) Begin fluid resuscitation with Ringer's lactate or normal saline. X-match for immediate blood.

c) Input and output: urinary catheter, NG tube

d) Perform primary survey of all systems-pay particular attention to the following:

   i) Neurological status—the Glasgow coma scale: is there any sign of increased ICP? Consider IV Mannitol and possibly burr holes if dilated pupil suggests epidural hematoma or subdural hematoma.

   ii) Cardiovascular system—low BP, elevated JVP, muffled heart sounds = pericardial tamponade; consider other myocardial injuries, such as contusion.

   iii) Respiratory system—is there any evidence of pneumothorax? Is a flail chest present? Any other injuries?

   iv) Abdomen—is there any abdominal tenderness or bruising? Any tenderness in the RUQ (possible liver laceration) or LUQ (splenic laceration or rupture)? Any other injury? Do you have a real-time ultrasound available in the ER?

   v) Reassess ABCs at this time. Consider MAST trousers; antishock trousers.

   vi) Musculoskeletal: any obvious fractures, especially open? Any evidence of pelvic fracture? Is there blood at the urethral meatus?

   vii) Maxillary-facial trauma: do not let injuries that look worse than they are detract your attention from more serious injuries.

   viii) Perform secondary survey.

   ix) Contact tertiary care facility and arrange transfer to a tertiary care facility if this has not already been done.

   x) Order investigations: CBC, electrolytes, CXR, C-spine X-ray, skull X-ray, ECG, amylase, urinalysis, KUB, three views of the abdomen, abdominal ultrasound, and any other appropriate investigations deemed necessary for the individual patient (X-rays of long bones, and so on). If CT or MRI facilities are available, other investigations may be ordered.

   xi) Treat non-life-threatening injuries when the patient has been stabilized.

PART B: The major mistakes (in order of frequency) in treating patients with trauma are as follows:

a. Inadequate airway management

b. Inadequate shock therapy

c. Inadequate C-spine mobilization

d. Failure to recognize and decompress pneumothorax

e. Distracting visually impressive but not life-threatening injuries (maxillofacial trauma, compound fractures)

f. Delay in transfer to tertiary care facility

g. Failure to transfer patients to tertiary care center at all

SUMMARY OF THE DIAGNOSIS AND MANAGEMENT OF TRAUMA

An excellent summary of the diagnosis and management of trauma is found in the answers to the Short Answer Management Problem, particularly Part A.

Presented in place of the summary is a probable problem list for this patient.

1. Motor vehicle accident—patient in critical condition
2. Cervical spine injury until proven otherwise
3. Hypovolemic shock
4. Tension pneumothorax
5. Pericardial tamponade
6. Skull fracture—acute epidural or subdural hematoma
7. Cerebrospinal fluid leak secondary to item 6
8. Probably splenic rupture or tear
9. Probable pelvic fracture
10. Probable femoral fracture
11. Probably urethral tear secondary to item 9
12. Scalp laceration

SUGGESTED READING

Tintinalli JE, Krome R, Ruiz E. Emergency medicine: A comprehensive study guide. New York: McGraw-Hill, 1992.

PROBLEM 144 A 17-YEAR-OLD MALE WITH ABDOMINAL PAIN

A 17-year-old male presents to the ER with acute abdominal pain. He describes the pain as follows: quality: dull, aching; quantity: baseline-8/10, incremental increases to 10/10, decreases to 6/10; location: central abdominal; chronology: began approximately 4 days ago, has been getting progressively worse, especially over last 18 hours; constancy/intermittency: constant; aggravating factors: aggravated by movement; relieving factors: relieved by rest; associated manifestations: nausea, vomiting, and significantly increased thirst; radiation: some radiation through to the back; previous pain history: no similar episodes of same; provocative maneuver: superficial palpation to the abdomen reproduces the pain.

On examination, he appears dehydrated. His skin and his tongue are dry. His blood pressure is 140/70 mm Hg, and his pulse 84 and regular. He is hyperventilating and his respiratory rate is 32/minute. His abdomen is tender to touch. The tenderness is generalized. There is no rebound tenderness.

SELECT THE ONE BEST ANSWER TO THE FOLLOWING QUESTIONS

1. The laboratory tests that you should perform at this time include which of the following?
   a) CBC/diff
   b) electrolytes
   c) urinalysis
   d) serum lipase
   e) spot blood sugar
   f) all of the above

2. Of the laboratory tests just listed, which one is likely to be abnormal to the greatest degree?
   a) CBC/diff
   b) serum potassium
   c) serum sodium
   d) serum lipase
   e) spot blood sugar

3. The laboratory investigations ordered produce the following results:
   CBC = 17,500 with 20% bands
   Potassium = 5.7mEq/L
   Chloride = 76 mEq/L
   Sodium = 156 mEq/L
   HCO3− = 10 mEq/L
   Urinalysis = pH 4.5; leukocytes ++, sugar +++, ketones +++
   Lipase = pending
   Blood sugar 450 mg/dL
   Blood pH = 7.1
   What is the most likely diagnosis at this time in this patient?
   a) diabetic hyperosmolar state
   b) diabetic ketoacidosis
   c) acute pancreatitis
   d) acute peritonitis
   e) none of the above

4. At this time, what would you do?
   a) rehydrate the patient in the ER with oral fluids and discharge him
   b) rehydrate the patient in the ER with IV fluids and discharge him
   c) observe the patient for 2 hours before discharge
   d) admit the patient for active treatment
   e) it depends on the patient's condition

5. In the condition described, which one of the following situations regarding the serum/body potassium is usually true?
   a) the serum potassium is low; total body potassium is low
   b) the serum potassium is elevated; total body potassium is low
   c) the serum potassium is low; total body potassium is high
   d) the serum potassium is low; total body potassium is high
   e) neither the serum potassium nor the total body potassium are usually altered

6. Electrolyte and fluid replacement in the condition described should initially be which of the following?
   a) dextrose 5% H$_2$O
   b) hypertonic saline
   c) Ringer's lactate
   d) one-half normal saline
   e) normal saline

7. In this condition, which of the following pathophysiologic abnormalities usually does not occur?
   a) elevated serum potassium
   b) depressed pH
   c) elevated serum insulin level
   d) elevated blood sugar
   e) depressed serum bicarbonate level

8. Insulin is usually administered in this condition in a recommended dosage of approximately
   a) 0.1 units/kg IV/hour
   b) 1.0 units/kg IV/hour
   c) 1.5 units/kg IV/hour
   d) 2.5 units/kg IV/hour
   e) 0.5 units/kg IV/hour

9. In this condition, glucose is usually added to the intravenous solution when the serum glucose is lowered to which of the following?
   a) 600 mg/dL
   b) 500 mg/dL
   c) 400 mg/dL
   d) 250 mg/dL
   e) 125 mg/dL

10. Which of the following is not characteristic of the condition described?
    a) Kussmaul's respirations
    b) significant dehydration
    c) decreased respiratory rate
    d) acetone breath
    e) increased sweating

Short Answer Management Problem 144

Describe the basic therapeutic principles of treating the condition described in this problem.

ANSWERS

1. F. This patient was presented to the ER with acute abdominal pain. In addition to either a KUB or three views of the abdomen, this patient should have a complete blood chemistry workup, including at least CBC and diff, electrolytes, spot blood sugar, serum amylase or serum lipase, BUN and creatinine, serum calcium, serum uric acid, and arterial blood gases.

2. E. This patient has the signs and symptoms compatible with diabetic ketoacidosis. Although the CBC and diff, the serum electrolytes (sodium, potassium, HCO_3, and BUN), and the pH and the P_{CO_2} may be abnormal, the plasma glucose is likely to be the test that is abnormal to the greatest degree.

3. B. This patient most likely has diabetic ketoacidosis. Diabetic ketoacidosis, in its initial presentation to the ER, often presents with abdominal pain being the major symptom. Diabetes may often be overlooked in this situation and the patient not assessed sufficiently. This may result in the patient being discharged without the correct diagnosis being made. Ultimately, this could be catastrophic.

4. D. This patient needs to be hospitalized now. He needs acute, active treatment in a highly monitored area, if not an intensive care unit. At the present time he has severe disturbances of his intravascular volume (he is significantly dehydrated), his electrolyte balance, his arterial blood gases, his blood sugar, and his serum insulin level.

5. B. The serum potassium in a patient with diabetic ketoacidosis is often significantly elevated. This, however, is deceptive. Although the serum potassium is usually elevated the total body potassium is usually low and the patient needs potassium added to the IV fluids.

This is true for the basic reasons. First, there exists a general total body potassium deficit because of urinary losses. Second, the hyperglycemia exerts an osmotic effect, drawing water into the intravascular space and diluting the potassium further. The expected decrease in serum potassium is about 1.6 mEq per liter for every 100 mg per dL increase in plasma glucose.

6. E. The requirements of fluid resuscitation can usually be met if therapy begins with normal saline at a rate of 10 to 20 mL/kg/hour for the first 2 hours. Amounts at the higher end of this range are used in cases with hypotension or severe acidosis. The subsequent rate is calculated from the estimated deficit; a rate of 3 to 6 mL/kg/hr will usually suffice. After the first 2 to 4 hours, saline can be replaced by 1/2 normal saline (NS).

   When the serum glucose approaches 250 mg/dL, the normal saline can be changed to dextrose 5% glucose or dextrose 5%, $\frac{1}{2}$ NS.

7. C. The serum insulin level in diabetic ketoacidosis is depressed. The basic principles of therapy are to replace deficits of fluid, replace deficits of electrolytes, replace CHO deficits, and to reverse the catabolic state with insulin.

   Criteria for grading the severity of diabetic ketoacidosis are given in Table 144-1.

TABLE 144-1 CRITERIA FOR GRADING THE SEVERITY OF DIABETIC KETOACIDOSIS

SYMPTOMS	DEHYDRATION	PH	HCO₃
Severe	7%-10%	<7.1	<8 mEq/L
Moderate	5-7	7.1-7.25	8-12 mEq/L
Mild	<5%	>7.25	<16 mEq/L

8. A. There are many alternative methods for delivering insulin during the treatment of DKA; probably any method that delivers a dose of at least 0.1 units/kg/hour

is acceptable. A constant intravenous insulin infusion offers many advantages, including simplicity of dosing, predictable insulin effect, and ease of dose adjustment. A convenient way to achieve a dose of 0.1 units/kg/hour in a constant infusion is to add 100 units of reguar insulin to 100 mL of saline (1 unit per mL). This solution should be piggybacked onto replacement fluids so that each can be adjusted independently. Before the insulin infusion begins, 10 to 20 mL of insulin-saline mixture should be run through the tubing to saturate insulin binding on the plastic; the infusion is then begun at 0.1 mL/kg/hour.

9. D. As mentioned above, when the serum glucose level approaches 250 mg%, the fluid replacement can be changed from saline to dextrose 5% water.

10. C. The respiratory rate in diabetic ketoacidosis is increased, not decreased.

Kussmaul breathing is a rapid, deep, breathing pattern that is usually associated with metabolic acidosis.

Increased sweating and dehydration are common.

Acetone breath, as a result of the production of acetone as a byproduct of the pathophysiologic process that produces diabetic ketoacidosis, is also common.

SOLUTION TO SHORT ANSWER MANAGEMENT PROBLEM 144

The basic therapeutic principles of treating the condition described are as follows:
1) Replacement of intravascular fluid volume (often several liters due to dehydration)
2) Replacement of electrolytes (potassium, magnesium, phosphate, calcium), even though electrolyte panel suggests elevated potassium and sodium levels
3) Replacement of insulin (beginning at 0.1 unit/kg/IV/hour)
4) Correction of metabolic acidotic state (by actions above the metabolic acidotic state will be corrected in most cases by itself; however, if the pH <7.1, the bicarbonate is indicated to enhance the correction.)
5) Begin IV solution with normal saline; after the first 2 to 4 hours, this can be changed to 1/2 normal saline. When

the blood sugar reaches 250 mg%, 1/2 normal saline can be switched to dextrose 5% water or dextrose 5%, ½ NS.

SUMMARY OF THE DIAGNOSIS AND MANAGEMENT OF DIABETIC KETOACIDOSIS

1. **Diagnosis:** most often a young person presents to the ER with the most common complaints being polyuria, polydipsia, abdominal tenderness and rigidity, increased sweating, and in severe cases altered levels of consciousness.

   The most common error in diabetic keotacidosis is not thinking of the diagnosis because of a "concentration on the abdominal pain" and a failure to associate abdominal pain with diabetes: if you do not think of the diagnosis, you will not make the diagnosis.

2. **Pathophysiology:** diabetic ketoacidosis is caused by insulin deficiency. Its development is promoted by an excess of counter-regulatory hormones, including glucagon, catecholamines, cortisol, and growth hormone; these hormones act synergistically with insulin deficiency to reduce glucose utilization, increase hepatic glucose production, and increase lipolysis and hepatic ketogenesis.

3. **Laboratory evaluation:** investigations should include the following CBC/diff, electrolytes (potassium, magnesium, phosphate, calcium) /BUN/creatinine/bicarbonate, serum amylase or lipase, plasma glucose, urinalysis, and arterial blood gases.

4. **Management:** see the Solution to Short Answer Management Problem 144.

5. **Complications:**
   a) Cerebral edema: most frightening and potentially devastating complication of diabetic ketoacidosis. Subclinical cerebral edema may exist in all patients during process of correction. If this complication becomes symptomatic, treatment with IV mannitol is indicated.
   b) Pancreatitis
   c) Arterial or venous thrombosis or embolism
   d) Hypoglycemia
   e) Hypokalemia

SUGGESTED READING

Lorenz R. Diabetic ketoacidosis. In: Rakel R, ed. Conn's current therapy. Philadelphia: WB Saunders, 1994.

PROBLEM 145 AN 84-YEAR-OLD MALE WITH ABDOMINAL PAIN

An 84-year-old male presents with a 6-hour history of severe abdominal pain. The pain is described as follows: quality: dull, aching; quantity: severe, baseline 9/10, increases to 10/10 and decreases to 8/10; location: epigastric; chronology: began suddenly after supper 6 hours ago; radiation: radiates through to the back; aggravating factor: movement; relieving factor: rest; provocative maneuver: deep palpation to abdomen; pain history: no previous episodes like this, no history of similar pain; previous significant history: angina pectoris; continuous/intermittent: continuous; associated manifestations: "faintness and dizziness" along with nausea.

On examination, the patient's blood pressure is 90/70 mm Hg, and his pulse is 96 and regular. His respiratory rate is 16. He is breathing normally. Examination of the abdomen reveals no distention and normal bowel sounds. There is, however, marked central abdominal tenderness to palpation.

SELECT THE ONE BEST ANSWER TO THE FOLLOWING QUESTIONS

1. What is the major differential diagnosis in this patient's case?
   a) ruptured aortic aneurysm
   b) intestinal ischemia or infarction
   c) perforated peptic ulcer
   d) splenic infarction
   e) all of the above

2. Given the history and physical examination findings, which of the following diagnostic possibilities is most likely?
   a) ruptured aortic aneurysm
   b) intestinal ischemia or infarction
   c) perforated peptic ulcer
   d) splenic infarction
   e) myocardial infarction

3. The diagnosis of the condition described can best be confirmed by which of the following?
   a) real-time ultrasound
   b) CT scan of the abdomen
   c) MRI scan of the abdomen
   d) 12-lead ECG
   e) laparotomy

4. What is the most important diagnostic clue that leads you to arrive at the diagnosis?
   a) the patient's hypotension
   b) the location of the abdominal pain
   c) the symptom of faintness and dizziness associated with hypotension
   d) the periumbilical tenderness
   e) none of the above

5. What is the most critical early intervention that must take place in this patient?
   a) the placement of an endotracheal tube
   b) the establishment of IV access for fluid and blood replacement
   c) an abdominal paracentesis
   d) the administration of a thrombolytic agent
   e) the establishment of an arterial line

6. In which of the following conditions do pharmacotherapy and the adverse effects of same (that is iatrogenic disease) play the greatest role?
   a) ruptured aortic aneurysm
   b) intestinal ischemia or infarction
   c) perforated peptic ulcer
   d) splenic infarction
   e) diverticulitis

7. What is the therapeutic agent most closely associated with a perforated peptic ulcer?
   a) ibuprofen
   b) piroxicam
   c) naprosyn
   d) aspirin
   e) suldinac

8. What is the treatment of choice for the patient described in the problem?
   a) ICU monitoring, thrombolytic therapy, aspirin, beta blockers, and antiarrhythmic therapy
   b) laparotomy—oversew perforation
   c) laparotomy—removal of ischemic bowel
   d) laparotomy—replacement of aortic aneurysm with a dacron graft
   e) laparotomy and splenectomy

9. Which of the following statements is(are) true regarding ruptured aortic aneurysm?
   a) over 80% of abdominal aortic aneurysms are asymptomatic when first diagnosed
   b) the diagnosis is often missed because physicians do not consider it
   c) most abdominal aortic aneurysms are atherosclerotic in nature
   d) all of the above are true
   e) none of the above are true

10. What is the key to reducing morbidity and mortality in the condition described?
    a) enhanced tertiary prevention
    b) enhanced secondary prevention
    c) regular yearly check-ups
    d) early diagnosis and intervention
    e) early administration of thrombolytic agents

Short Answer Management Problem 145

Describe the major differential diagnosis of the elderly patient presenting to the ER with a diagnosis of abdominal pain.

ANSWERS

1. E. The differential diagnosis of abdominal pain in the elderly is extensive. In this case the sudden onset of the pain and the severity of the pain strongly suggests an acute abdomen. At the top of the list would be ruptured aortic aneurysm, perforated peptic ulcer, intestinal ischemia or infarction, a perforated diverticulum, and pancreatitis.

2. A. Given the history and physical findings, the most likely diagnosis is ruptured aortic aneurysm. The tip-off to ruptured aortic aneurysm in this case is the dizziness associated with pain and hypotension that the patient experienced very early in the symptomatology. The dizziness, hypotension, and pain suggest at least a leaking aneurysm.

3. B. The working diagnosis can best be confirmed by the performance of a CT scan of the abdomen. The common presentation of abdominal pain in the elderly is a very good argument for having an ultrasound machine in very close proximity to the ER.

4. C. See the answer to Question 2.

5. B. Remember the ABCs. Since this patient is breathing normally, the next most important step is circulation. You should immediately place either a central venous pressure line or two large bore IV lines (that is, two lines of at least #16 gauge).

6. C.

7. D. Iatrogenic disease (in the form of NSAID prescription) is closely associated with perforated peptic ulcer. Many thousands of Americans (estimated to be >20,000) die each year from perforated and bleeding peptic ulcers caused by the prescription of NSAIDs.

    The NSAID (and it really is a nonsteroidal antiinflammatory) that causes more peptic ulcers and is associated with more perforated peptic ulcers than any other agent (on a prevalence/administration rate basis) is ordinary acetylsalicylic acid (aspirin).

8. D. The treatment of choice in this patient is removal of the segment of the aorta affected by the aneurysm and replacement by a Dacron graft.

9. D. Over 80% of aortic aneurysms are asymptomatic when first diagnosed. As previously stated, the diagnosis is often missed because the possibility is not considered.

    The vast majority of aortic aneurysms are atherosclerotic in nature and result from a generalized (total body) atherosclerotic process.

10. D. The key to reducing morbidity and mortality from aortic aneurysm is early diagnosis and intervention. Although routine screening for aortic aneurysms in the elderly is not recommended by the United States Preventative Task Force on the Periodic Health Examination, it is wise to consider this on a risk-factor basis in the patients you see. High-risk patients and patients with symptoms that even vaguely suggest aortic aneurysm should probably be evaluated by both physical examination and ultrasound.

SOLUTION TO SHORT ANSWER MANAGEMENT PROBLEM 145

The following is a differential diagnosis of abdominal pain in the elderly as an ER presentation.
1. Non-gastrointestinal-related causes:
   a) Myocardial infarction
   b) Pneumonia
   c) Pericarditis
2. Abdominal-related causes
   a) Constipation (major cause)
   b) Diverticulitis
   c) Cholecystitis/cholelithiasis
   d) Peptic ulcer disease/gastritis
   e) Pancreatitis
   f) Appendicitis

g) Bowel obstruction—large bowel, small bowel
h) Inflammatory bowel disease
i) Carcinoma—stomach, pancreas, colon
j) Ruptured aortic aneurysm
k) Intestinal ischemia or infarction
l) Urinary tract sepsis

SUMMARY OF THE DIAGNOSIS AND TREATMENT OF ABDOMINAL PAIN IN THE ELDERLY

1. **Diagnosis:**
   a) Differential diagnosis as previously discussed
   b) Remember constipation; constipation is the single most common cause of abdominal pain in the elderly.
   c) When elderly patients present to the ER with sudden onset of abdominal pain, think of the following:
      1. Nonabdominal causes: myocardial infarction
      2. Abdominal causes: ruptured aortic aneurysm, perforated peptic ulcer, intestinal ischemia

2. **Investigations:** basic investigations in an elderly patient with abdominal pain: CBC, electrolytes, ECG, KUB, urinalysis; real-time ultrasound available in ER is invaluable.

3. **Treatment:**
   a) Treat the cause.
   b) Remember ABCs in acutely ill elderly patients.
   c) Remember that elderly patients present quite differently from younger patients—they often lack the classic signs and symptoms of any acute abdominal condition.
   d) A major error in acutely ill elderly patients seen in community or rural hospitals is the failure to transfer to a tertiary care center soon enough.

SUGGESTED READING

Hazzard WR et al., eds. Principles of geriatric medicine and gerontology. New York: McGraw-Hill, 1994.

PROBLEM 146 A 24-YEAR-OLD FEMALE BROUGHT INTO THE ER WITH A SUSPECTED DRUG OVERDOSE

A 24-year-old female is brought into the ER of your local hospital with a suspected drug overdose. She was found by a friend, unconscious beside her bed, with a number of unmarked pill containers beside her. Her friend does not know any other details. Her friend is hysterical and has to be restrained.

You are called by the intern, who is on his first day of service. He asks you, "What should I do now?"

You come down immediately and examine the patient. The patient has a Reed Coma scale of stage 1. This includes the following:

1. Conscious level = Coma
2. Pain response = Decreased
3. Reflexes = Normal
4. Respirations = Normal
5. Circulations = Normal

The Vital Signs are as follows: blood pressure = 90/70 mm Hg; pulse = 84 and regular; respirations = 16 and regular. No other abnormalities are evident. Her pupils are equal and reactive to light and accommodation.

SELECT THE ONE BEST ANSWER TO THE FOLLOWING QUESTIONS

1. What is the first step in the management of the potential drug overdose victim?
   a) administration of syrup of ipecac
   b) administration of naloxone
   c) administration of dextrose 5% water
   d) administration of activated charcoal
   e) none of the above

2. Accidental poisonings make up what percentage of total poisoning episodes in children and adults?
   a) 20%
   b) 40%
   c) 60%
   d) 70%
   e) 85%

3. The majority of drug-related suicide attempts involve which of the following?
   a) central nervous system anxiolytics
   b) central nervous system antidepressant medications
   c) central nervous system antipsychotic medications
   d) over-the-counter analgesics
   e) prescription narcotic analgesics

4. What is the most common cause of death in drug overdose patients outside the hospital?
   a) lower airway obstruction
   b) upper airway obstruction
   c) cardiac arrest
   d) ventricular fibrillation
   e) complete heart block

5. Which of the following conditions resulting in coma or altered level of consciousness can be treated quickly if recognized immediately?
   a) hypoxia
   b) hypoglycemia
   c) opioid overdose
   d) b and c
   e) all of the above

6. Which of the following is not routinely indicated in the initial assessment of the possible overdose patient?
   a) a history from anyone who has knowledge of the patient
   b) physical examination with particular attention to vital signs and neurologic status
   c) CBC and serum electrolytes
   d) complete toxicology screen
   e) blood glucose

7. The *anion gap* is defined as which of the following?
   a) anion gap = $[K^+$ plus $Cl^-]$ minus $[Na^+$ plus $HCO_3^-]$
   b) anion gap = $[Na^+]$ minus $[Cl^-$ plus $HCO_3^-]$
   c) anion gap = $[Cl^-]$ plus $[Na^+$ plus $K^+]$ minus $[HCO_3^-]$
   d) anion gap = $[Ph]$ plus $[Na^+$ plus $CL^-]$
   e) anion gap = $[HCO_3^-]$ minus $[Cl^-$ plus $Na^+]$

8. Which of the following is not a cause of an increased anion gap?
   a) an accumulation of organic acids
   b) diabetic ketoacidosis
   c) reduced inorganic acid excretion (that is, chronic renal failure)
   d) hypernatremia
   e) lactic acidosis

9. Which of the following is(are) associated with an increased anion gap?
   a) salicylates
   b) methanol
   c) ethylene glycol
   d) organic solvents
   e) all of the above

10. Following the assessment and maintenance of vital functions, which of the following is(are) the next step(s)?
    a) antidote administration (if poison known)
    b) prevention of absorption
    c) reduction of local damage
    d) b and c
    e) all of the above

11. Generally speaking, in poison management, which of the following is the most effective method of gastrointestinal decontamination?
    a) syrup of ipecac
    b) gastric lavage
    c) administration of activated charcoal
    d) dilution of poison with IV fluids
    e) none of the above

12. Which of the following should be administered with the first dose of activated charcoal (if not contraindicated)?
    a) magnesium hydroxide
    b) aluminum hydroxide
    c) magnesium sulfate
    d) calcium carbonate
    e) none of the above

13. What is the specific antidote for the treatment of acetaminophen poisoning?
    a) N-acetyl coenzyme A
    b) N-acetyl ATPase
    c) N-acetylcysteine
    d) calcium disodium etidronate
    e) atropine

14. What is the specific antidote for the treatment of benzodiazepine poisoning?
    a) Antabuse
    b) Naloxone
    c) carbamazepine
    d) flumazenil
    e) naltrexone

15. What is the specific antidote for the treatment of ethanol intoxication (poisoning)?
    a) Antabuse
    b) Naloxone
    c) carbamazepine
    d) flumazenil
    e) naltrexone

16. What is the specific antidote for the treatment of opioid intoxication (poisoning)?
    a) Antabuse
    b) Naloxone
    c) carabazepine
    d) flumazenil
    e) naltrexone

17. What is the specific antidote for the treatment of organophosphate poisoning?
    a) ethanol
    b) Naloxone
    c) naltrexone
    d) atropine
    e) arginine

Short Answer Management Problem 146

Describe the absolute and relative contraindications to the administration of syrup of ipecac in the induction of emesis in a poisoning victim.

ANSWERS

1. E. The first step in the management of the potential overdose victim is the assessment and support of the ABCs (airway, breathing, circulation) of life support. Before any medications are administered, a secure airway must be established, respiratory and circulatory system function should be assessed and supported, and intravenous and/or control venous pressure lines should be inserted.

2. E. The severity of the manifestations of acute poisoning exposures varies greatly with the age and intent of the victims. Accidental poisoning exposures make up 80% to 85% of all poisoning episodes and are most frequent in children under the age of 5. Intentional poisonings constitute 10% to 15% of all poisonings, and often these patients require more intensive therapy. Suicide attempts represent a significant number of these poisonings, and the use of toxic substances is often involved.

3. D. Sixty percent of patients who take a drug overdose do so with their own prescribed medication. An additional 15% do so with drugs prescribed for relatives. The top drugs used in suicide attempts (all ages and in order of frequency) are as follows:
   1. Over-the-counter analgesics
   2. Prescribed sedative-hypnotics

3. Prescribed benzodiazepines
4. Cleaning agents and petroleum products
5. Alcohol and controlled substances
6. Pesticides
7. Tricyclic antidepressants
8. Plants
9. Carbon monoxide
10. Opioids

Again, the most common drug class used in suicide attempts is over-the-counter analgesics.

4. B. The most common cause of death in drug overdose patients outside the hospital is upper airway obstruction. Any patient who is comatose and has absent protective airway reflexes is certainly able to tolerate an endotracheal tube (cuffed for those over the ages 7 to 9) and should have one inserted immediately.

5. E. The second step in the management of the potential overdose victim is the treatment of specific conditions with specific antidotes. Because it is almost impossible to differentiate one from another at this time, we give the following:
   A. 2 mg of naloxone (antidote for opioid intoxication)
   B. 100 mg thiamine IV (antidote for Wernicke's encephalopathy)
   C. 50 cc of 50% dextrose (antidote for hypoglycemia—secondary to insulin overdose)
   D. supplemental oxygen by Venturi Mask or Nasal Specs (general measure)

6. D. After you have stabilized the patient, you should attempt to establish the identity of the particular poison.

   A physical examination with emphasis on vital signs (and particular attention to pupil size and reaction to light and accommodation), temperature, and a complete neurologic examination should be done.

   Although the patient will often not be able to supply accurate (if any) information, as much information as possible should be obtained from the family, friends, the patient's physician, or anyone else that knows the patient.

   Laboratory testing should include the following: serum electrolytes (and measurement of anion gap), arterial blood gases, blood glucose, complete blood count, a 12-lead ECG, three views of the abdomen, and specific drug levels. Generally, however, a routine toxicology screen is not indicated, nor is it appropriate.

7. B.

8. D.

9. E. The term *anion gap* was developed to indicate the difference between the measured sodium level and the measured chloride and bicarbonate level (really the CO_2 content). This is very important, especially in diabetic ketoacidosis and toxic acidic chemicals.

   The definition is as follows:
   Anion gap = [Na^+] minus [Cl^- plus HCO_3^-]
   The causes of an increased anion gap are as follows:
   A. An accumulation of organic acids, such as that seen in lactic acidosis
   B. An accumulation of organic acids, such as that seen in diabetic ketoacidosis
   C. An accumulation of organic acids, such as that seen in acute renal failure and toxic ingestions
   D. Exogenous anions
   E. Reduced inorganic acid excretion, such as seen in chronic renal failure
   F. An increase in the anionic contribution of unmeasured weak acids
   G. A decrease in unmeasured cations

   Hypernatremia will cause a decreased anion gap rather than an increased anion gap.

   The etiology of metabolic acidosis is dependent on the determination of the presence or absence of a normal anion gap. The normal anion gap is 14 to 16. An increased anion gap can usually be traced to one of the following:
   A. Toxic amounts of salicylates
   B. Any amount of methanol
   C. Any amount of ethylene glycol
   D. An overdose of iron (as in ferrous sulfate)
   E. Any amount of paraldehyde
   F. An overdose of phenformin
   G. An overdose of isoniazid
   H. Certain organic solvents such as toluene.

10. E.

11. C.

12. C. The second step after the assessment and maintenance of vital functions includes the prevention of absorption and the reduction of local damage.

   Reduction of local damage applies primarily to the eye (with a caustic acid or a caustic base) and the skin (with a significant burn).

   The prevention of absorption is best accomplished by gastrointestinal decontamination. First, to decrease gastrointestinal absorption, emesis should be induced or gastric aspiration and lavage performed. Neither of these methods is completely effective; each removes only 30% to 50% of the ingested substance. These methods are recommended in the time period up to 4 hours post-ingestion. In the emergency room, however, there are few indications for the administration of syrup of ipecac or gastric lavage because they delay the more effective treatment of activated charcoal (an exceptor to this would be a documented very recent ingestion).

The dose of activated charcoal to give is 1 g/kg/dose orally with a minimum of 15 g. The usual adolescent and adult dose is 60 to 100 g. It is administered as a slurry mixed with water or by orogastric tube.

Dilution of the initial poison is useful, but not as useful as the administration of cathartics along with the activated charcoal. The agent of choice is probably magnesium sulfate. It is recommended that magnesium sulfate be given along with the first dose of activated charcoal.

13. C. N-acetylcysteine is the specific antidote that should be administered in cases of acetaminophen poisoning. It can be given orally or intavenously. The intravenous route is the route of first choice.

14. D. Flumazenil (Mazicon) is the first benzodiazepine antagonist to be approved by the Food and Drug Administration. Flumazenil binds competitively and reversibly to the GABA-benzodiazepine receptor complex and inhibits the effects of benzodiazepine. The drug is approved for the treatment of benzodiazepine overdose and/or for the reversal of benzodiazepine oversedation.

15. C. The anticonvulsant carbamazepine has been shown to be effective for ethanol and sedative detoxification. Carbamazepine should be administered until blood levels are in the range of effective anticonvulsant activity. It should be maintained for up to 2 weeks and then tapered and discontinued.

16. B. The antidote for opioid overdose is naloxone. Once an opioid user is detoxified, he or she may benefit from opioid antagonist therapy with naltrexone. Naltrexone is a long-acting orally active opioid antagonist that when taken regularly entirely blocks mu-opioid receptors, thus blocking the opioid's euphoric, analgesic, and sedative properties.

17. D. The specific antidote for organophosphate poisoning is atropine. Organophosphate poisoning is more commonly observed in the administration of herbicides and pesticides.

SOLUTION TO SHORT ANSWER MANAGEMENT PROBLEM 146

Specific contraindications to the administration of syrup of ipecac can be divided into absolute contraindications and relative contraindications.
A. Absolute contraindications:
   i) Caustic (alkali) or corrosive (acid) ingestion
   ii) Convulsions (danger of aspiration and possible induction of laryngospasm)
   iii) Coma (possibility of aspiration with the loss of protective airway reflexes)
   iv) Absence of a cough reflex
   v) Hematemesis
   vi) A child <6 months of age
B. Relative contraindications:
   i) Petroleum distillate ingestion of high-viscosity agents
   ii) Agents that are likely to rapidly produce coma (short-acting barbiturates) or convulsions (propoxyphene, camphor, isoniazid, strychnine, tricyclic antidepressants)
   iii) Significant prior vomiting

SUMMARY OF THE GENERAL MANAGEMENT PRINCIPLES OF POISON MANAGEMENT

1. **Assessment and maintenance of vital functions:**
   a) The ABCs of resuscitation:
      A = Airway management (endotracheal tube in unconscious patient)
      B = Breathing (assisted ventilation if the respiratory rate and depth are inadequate)
      C = Circulation (assessed by blood pressure, heart rate, and heart rhythm); volume expansion may be indicated if there is hypotension or other measurements of decreased cardiac function: Ringer's lactate or normal saline is preferred for hypovolemia; plasma expanders and vasopressors are indicated if IV fluids are not sufficient.
   b) History/physical examination/laboratory investigations:
      1. History: attempt to elicit history from any family member or friend who happens to be there. Attempt to search for empty pill containers.
      2. Physical examination: pay particular attention to vital signs and neurological examination with emphasis on either the Glasgow coma scale or the Reed coma scale.
      3. Laboratory investigations:
         i) 12-lead ECG
         ii) CBC, electrolytes, BUN, creatinine
         iii) Arterial blood gases
         iv) CXR
         v) Three views of the abdomen
         Calculate the anion gap = $Na^+ - (Cl^- + HCO_3^-)$. Remember that the normal anion gap is 14 to 16.
2. **Treatment:**
   a) Immediate treatment to all victims:
      1. ABCs (may include ET tube + IV fluids)
      2. 2 mg naloxone
      3. 100 mg thiamine IV
      4. 50 cc of 50% glucose
      5. Supplemental oxygen
   b) Decontamination:
      1. Induction of emesis with syrup of ipecac
      2. Gastric lavage
      3. Administration of activated charcoal plus magnesium sulfate as a cathartic

c) Elimination:
   1. Enhance elimination with pH-dependent diuresis.
   2. Multidose activated charcoal
   3. Dialysis: hemodialysis preferred to peritoneal dialysis
d) Specific antidotes:
   1. Substance: acetaminophen. Antidote: N-acetylcysteine.
   2. Substance: opioid analgesics. Antidote: naloxone.
   3. Substance: ethanol. Antidote: carbamazepine.
   4. Substance: benzodiazepines. Antidote: flumazenil.
   5. Substance: organophosphates. Antidote: atropine.

3. **Most common drug overdoses:**
   a) Over-the-counter analgesics (acetaminophen is number one)

b) Prescribed hypnotics-sedatives
c) Prescribed benzodiazepines

4. **Prevention of complications:** anticipate and treat complications: seizures, coma, hypotension, and hyperthermia.

SUGGESTED READINGS

Lovejoy FH, Linden CH. Acute poison and drug overdose. In: Isselbacher KJ, ed. Harrison's principles of internal medicine. 13th Ed. New York: McGraw-Hill, 1994.

Mofenson HC, Caraccio TR, Greensher J. Acute poisonings. In: Rakel R, ed. Conn's current therapy. Philadelphia: WB Saunders, 1994.

PROBLEM 147   A 24-YEAR-OLD MALE WHO DEVELOPED A "SKIN RASH" WHILE PLAYING FOOTBALL

A 24-year-old male was playing football with his friends on a hot summer afternoon. Approximately 10 minutes into the game, he began to "feel funny," and he began to itch all over. He sat down, but the itch did not go away; it only got worse. Within 10 minutes he was covered with a "raised" rash all over his body, with individual lesions varying from 2 cm to 5 cm in diameter. His lips also became very swollen, and he began to have trouble breathing.

His friend called 911, and he was brought to the local hospital, located only 3 minutes from the football field. The friend who works with the patient tells you that "he is certain that the problem has arisen because of stress"; the patient apparently had a very bad day at work today.

On examination, his respiratory rate is 42/minute and he is gasping. His lips are swollen, and he has very prominent, raised skin rash with lesions of various sizes covering his entire body. His blood pressure is 75/50 mm Hg.

SELECT THE ONE BEST ANSWER TO THE FOLLOWING QUESTIONS

1. At this time, what is your first priority?
   a) give the patient scopolamine
   b) give the patient oral steroids
   c) give the patient IV Benadryl
   d) give the patient oral Chlor-Tripolon
   e) none of the above

2. What is the most likely diagnosis in this patient?
   a) ordinary urticaria with angioneurotic edema
   b) physical urticaria with esterase inhibitor deficiency
   c) physical urticaria with angioneurotic edema
   d) urticarial vasculitis with angioneurotic edema
   e) stress-induced urticaria with esterase inhibitor deficiency

3. What is the first priority in this patient?
   a) establish a large-gauge IV line
   b) establish a CVP line if possible; if not possible, establish two large IV lines
   c) intubate the patient
   d) administer 100% oxygen to the patient by nasal specs
   e) draw blood gases

4. What is the second priority in the management of this patient?
   a) auscultate both lung fields
   b) forget this "tube and airway" business—get with the IV lines and get with them now!
   c) draw blood gases
   d) perform a chest X-ray to check the position of the ET tube
   e) administer 100% oxygen by Venturi Mask

5. What is the third priority in the management of this patient?
   a) draw blood gases
   b) draw serum electrolytes
   c) put two large peripheral IV lines in or one CVP line

   d) put MAST trousers on the patient
   e) administer "pretty much every pressor agent you can think of"

6. What is the fourth priority in the management of this patient?
   a) administer large quantities of isotonic fluids
   b) administer epinephrine subcutaneously
   c) administer solucortef intravenously
   d) administer vasopressor agents if blood pressure does not rise with the measures outlined in a, b, and c
   e) all of the above

7. With respect to exercise in the future, what should your advice be to this patient?
   a) take an H_1 blocker (Benadryl) prophylactically
   b) carry an epinephrine kit at all times
   c) begin with short periods of exercise only and work up
   d) carry a supply of parenteral corticosteroid if possible
   e) all of the above

8. Angioneurotic edema is most likely to occur in which of the following situations?
   a) allergy to peanuts
   b) allergy to chocolate
   c) allergy to milk
   d) allergy to red wine
   e) allergy to monosodium glutamate

9. A 51-year-old farmer develops a "nonhealing ulcer" on the tip of his nose. It has been present for the past 6 months and has not gotten any better. His wife brings him to the ER to have it checked.
   On examination, there is a 0.5-cm ulcer "shaped like a crater." There is a depression in the center surrounded by a "scaly exterior."
   What is the most likely diagnosis?
   a) squamous cell carcinoma of the nose
   b) basal cell carcinoma of the nose
   c) actinic keratosis
   d) malignant melanoma—atypical
   e) atypical nevus

10. What is the treatment of choice for this lesion in this patient?
    a) cryosurgery
    b) electrodesiccation and curettage
    c) excisional surgery
    d) Moh's micrographic surgery
    e) chemotherapy: 5-fluorouracil

11. A 65-year-old male presents to the ER for assessment of a "nonhealing" skin lesion on his lower lip. He comes into the ER tonight because his wife has been "bugging him about it," and he "finally got tired of all the nagging."

    This is 1-cm in diameter and has been growing steadily over the past 4 years. It has been bleeding on and off for the last year.

    The patient has smoked a pipe for the last 40 years.

    What is the most likely diagnosis in this case?
    a) actinic keratosis
    b) squamous cell carcinoma
    c) basal cell carcinoma
    d) rodent ulcer
    e) keratoacanthoma

12. Which of the following treatments is not contraindicated in the management of this lesion in this patient?
    a) cryosurgery
    b) electrodesiccation
    c) curettage and electrodesiccation
    d) excisional biopsy
    e) all of the above are contraindicated

13. A 45-year-old female patient presents with a 5-year history of erythematous, round, scaly patches on both elbows. She is now beginning to develop one on her left hand.

    She comes into the ER this evening when she noticed the onset of significant pain, tenderness, and swelling in some of the small joints of her hands and feet.

    She is wondering if the two symptoms are related.

    At this time, what would you tell her?
    a) no way; there is no relationship
    b) no way, she has "nervous dermatitis" and now has developed "nervous joints;" the two are completely unrelated
    c) yes; the skin lesions sometimes precede a certain type of arthritis
    d) no way; pure coincidence
    e) you would not tell her anything; instead you would refer her to the nearest dermatologist

14. What would be the treatment of first choice for this patient's skin lesions?
    a) "zap and burn" electrocautery
    b) cryosurgery
    c) medium- to high-potency topical corticosteroids
    d) "freeze and remove": liquid nitrogen
    e) a complex tar solution

15. A 2-cm skin lesion located on the wrist of a 25-year-old female is best described as "pruritic, polygonal, flat-topped violaceous papules."

    What is the most likely diagnosis of this skin lesion?
    a) pityriasis rosea
    b) pityriasis alba
    c) lichen planus
    d) hairy oral leukoplakia
    e) tinea versicolor

16. A number of skin lesions are present on the ears of a 67-year-old farmer. They are erythematous, scaly, and growing slightly larger in size over time. The largest is 1.0 cm in diameter. The more time the farmer spends in the sun, the more these skin lesions seem to grow. His wife has "dragged him into the ER" tonight.

    What is the most likely diagnosis of these skin lesions?
    a) seborrheic dermatitis
    b) keratoacanthomas
    c) actinic keratoses
    d) lichen planus
    e) parapsoriasis

17. A 57-year-old farmer has a number of "greasy, warty, heaped-up" skin lesions present on both cheeks. These seem to be growing and are concerning the patient. The largest is 1.0 cm in diameter.

    What is the most likely diagnosis of these skin lesions?
    a) seborrheic dermatitis
    b) seborrheic keratosis
    c) actinic keratoses
    d) lichen planus
    e) parapsoriasis

18. A 29-year-old farmer has developed a "dark-brown skin lesion" on the back of his neck. It has expanded significantly over the past 6 months and is beginning to darken in color. The present size of the skin lesion is 4 cm × 3 cm. He finished harvesting this afternoon, so he came into the ER tonight.

    You are most concerned about which of the following in this patient?
    a) superficial spreading squamous cell carcinoma
    b) superficial spreading basal cell carcinoma
    c) superficial spreading malignant melanoma
    d) superficial spreading intraepithelial carcinoma
    e) none of the above

19. The "herald patch" is associated with which of the following diagnoses in young adults (solitary lesion + pruritic + oval in shape + young adult)?
    a) pityriasis alba
    b) pityriasis rosea
    c) pityriasis rosacea
    d) pityriasis versicolor
    e) pityriasis multiforme

20. The natural evolution of which of these skin lesions to its worst potential is known as the Stevens-Johnson syndrome?
    a) erythema marginatum
    b) erythema nodosum
    c) erythema chronicum migrans
    d) erythema multiforme
    e) pemphigus vulgaris

21. What is the most common drug to cause urticaria and angioedema?
    a) acetaminophen

    b) sulfonamide antibiotic
    c) ampicillin antibiotic
    d) aspirin
    e) naprosyn

22. Which of the following form part of an allergic triad?
    a) nasal polyps
    b) asthma
    c) aspirin sensitivity
    d) all of the above
    e) none of the above

Short Answer Management Problem 147

Describe the pathophysiology of urticaria and angioneurotic edema.

ANSWERS

1. E. Your first priority is to go through the ABCs of cardiopulmonary resuscitation:

    Priority 1: establish an airway. This patient, from the history given, is very close to having his airway completely obstructed. Thus the placement of a properly sized endotracheal tube is the first priority.

    Priority 2: establish proper ventilation. Make sure that the endotracheal tube is, in fact, in the trachea and not in the esophagus, and establish that there is bilateral airflow through auscultation of both lung fields.

    Priority 3: circulation: establish access. Now we are ready for the IV lines. It is suggested that a central venous pressure catheter is the catheter of choice. If this is impossible, two large bore IVs (#16 gauge) in the antecubital fossae will do fine.

    Priority 4: circulation: provide intravenous fluids. The fourth priority is to establish acute treatment—this will consist of isotonic fluids (Ringer's lactate, normal saline), subcutaneous epinephrine 0.3 mg (repeated if necessary), intravenous corticosteroids, and pressor agents if necessary (dopamine, dobutamine).

    The diagnosis in this case is physical urticaria with angioneurotic edema. Although it is possible to have physical urticaria and, because of the angioneurotic edema, have an associated esterase inhibitor deficiency, it is much more likely that this is simply a more severe manifestation of physical urticaria.

2. C.

3. C.

4. A.

5. C.

6. E.

7. E. This patient should be careful in participating in any sports that will bring on physical urticaria; whether he decides to abstain is a personal risk/benefit decision.

    If he is going to begin exercise again, however, he should do the following:
    a. Begin with a short period of exercise only.
    b. Take 2 × 25 mg Benadryl tablets 45 minutes before starting.
    c. Carry both epinephrine and ready to make up solu-cortef to administer subcutaneously and intramuscularly.

8. A. Angioneurotic edema is certainly both common and life-threatening.

    It occurs most commonly in association with food allergy. The two most common foods implicated in angioneurotic edema are nuts (of all kinds) and fish and shellfish. In the case of the latter, even the odor of the cooking of the fish or shellfish may be enough to set off a life-threatening reaction.

    Angioneurotic edema associated with food kills many hundreds of Americans each year. It is certainly not a condition to be taken lightly.

9. B.

10. C. This patient has the typical description of a rodent ulcer or basal cell carcinoma.

    The treatment alternatives are as follows:
    A. Excisional surgery
    B. Electrodesiccation and curettage

C. Cryosurgery
D. Mohs' microscopic surgery
E. Radiation therapy
F. Chemotherapy: 5-fluorouracil
Because of the importance of making a pathological diagnosis without destroying the specimen, the procedure of choice is excisional surgery.

11. B.

12. D. This patient has what appears by description to be a squamous cell carcinoma of the lip. The procedure of choice is excisional biopsy, as before. The tissue must not be destroyed. All other treatments provided as options are, therefore, contraindicated.

13. C.

14. C. This patient has psoriasis with progression to psoriatic arthritis, the latter of which needs to be investigated. Treatment with a medium- to high-potency corticosteroid should begin on a bid or tid basis immediately.

15. C.

16. C.

17. B.

18. C.

19. B.

20. D.

21. D.

22. D. The most common drug causing angioneurotic edema is aspirin. Many of the patients who develop aspirin anaphylaxis have the following allergic triad:
1. Aspirin sensitivity
2. Asthma
3. Nasal polyps
Any individual who has developed a significant allergic reaction or angioneurotic edema to aspirin should never take another nonsteroidal antiinflammatory agent. There is a very high cross-reactivity.
The following descriptions match the following skin lesions:
Flat-topped violaceous papules = lichen planus
Erythematous, scaly, growing slightly larger in size over time + Sun-exposed area + Sun-exposed occupation = Actinic keratosis (premalignant)
Greasy, scaly, heaped-up skin lesions on exposed areas + Advanced age = Seborrheic keratosis

Dark brown skin lesion + Sun-exposed surface + Spreading in character + Sun-exposed occupation + Changing in color = Superficial spreading malignant melanoma
Skin rash begins as a solitary lesion + Pruritic in nature + Oval in shape + Young-aged adult = Pityriasis rosea
Erythema multiforme (target-shaped lesions or "bull's eye") + Adverse drug reaction = Stevens-Johnson syndrome

SOLUTION TO SHORT ANSWER MANAGEMENT PROBLEM 147

Sequence of Events Producing Urticaria and Angioneurotic Edema:

I. Difference between urticaria and angioneurotic edema:
   a) Urticaria: caused by plasma leakage into the skin.
   b) Angioneurotic edema: caused by plasma leakage into the subcutaneous or submucosal tissue
II. Causes of plasma leakage: The plasma leakage is mediated by the release of the following:
   a) Histamine from the mast cells
   b) Bradykinin from the mast cells
   c) Other vasoactive substances from the mast cells
III. Activation of various systems along with the substance release; there is activation of the following:
   a) Complement system
   b) Fibrinolytic system
   c) Kinin system
IV. Skin lesions produced by plasma leakage produce the following:
   a) Wheals (dermal edema)
   b) Subcutaneous edema (angioedema)
   c) Submucosal edema (angioedema)
V. Skin lesion characteristics:
   a) Usually total body
   b) Lesions begin as "small wheals" and eventually coalesce.
   c) Lesions are very pruritic and erythematous.
VI. Physiologic consequences: serious complications include the following:
   1. Airway edema and airway closure
   2. Hypoxemia
   3. Hypotension and shock
VII. Treatment of angioneurotic edema:
   a) Recumbent position
   b) 100% oxygen
   c) Epinephrine 0.3 ml SC q 15 min
   d) Antihistamine IV bolus and continuous infusion
   e) Corticosteroid bolus and continuous infusion
   f) Administer isotonic fluids (Ringer's lactate, normal saline)
   g) Vasopressor agents if hypotension is not corrected

SUMMARY OF THE DIAGNOSIS AND TREATMENT OF URTICARIA AND ANGIONEUROTIC EDEMA

1. **Seriousness of problem:** this is a life-threatening problem and must be treated both quickly and appropriately.
2. **Development of condition:** urticaria can develop for many reasons:
   a) Temperature
   b) Exercise
   c) Response to food and exercise together
   d) Stress
   e) Certain foods (sometimes just odors)
   f) Drug allergy (such as aspirin)
3. **Most important treatment:** prevention
4. **Treatment in detail:**
   a) Always, always follow the ABCs.
   b) Carry epinephrine, antihistamines, and corticosteroids, especially if going into a high-risk area.
   c) Never, never eat anything in a restaurant that you are even remotely concerned may contain what you are allergic to.
   d) Follow treatment protocol just discussed.
5. **Most common foods causing urticaria and angioneurotic edema:**
   a) Peanuts and other nuts
   b) Shellfish and fish
6. **Most common drug causing angioneurotic edema:** aspirin
7. **Severity of future reactions:** generally speaking, the reactions experienced increases in severity each time.
8. **Bottom-line treatment:** epinephrine SC 0.3 + + Antihistamine parenteral + +
9. **Corticosteroid:** oxygen + + fluid resuscitation through large bore needles

SUGGESTED READING

Gratten CE. Urticaria and angioedema. In: Rakel R, ed. Conn's current therapy. Philadelphia: WB Saunders, 1994.

PROBLEM 148   A 75-YEAR-OLD FEMALE WHO SLIPPED AND FELL ON HER OUTSTRETCHED HAND

A 75-year-old female is brought to the ER after having fallen on her outstretched hand. She complains of pain in the area of the right wrist.

On examination, there is a deformity in the area of the right wrist. The wrist has the appearance of a dinner fork. There is significant tenderness over the distal radius. Both pulses and sensation distally to the injury are completely normal.

SELECT THE ONE BEST ANSWER TO THE FOLLOWING QUESTIONS

1. What is the most likely diagnosis in this patient?
   a) fracture of the distal ulna with dislocation of the radial head
   b) fracture of the carpal scaphoid
   c) fracture of the radial styloid
   d) Colles' fracture
   e) fracture of the shaft of the radius with dislocation of the ulnar head

2. What is the treatment of choice for the patient described?
   a) internal reduction and immobilization
   b) internal reduction and fixation
   c) external reduction and immobilization
   d) external reduction and fixation
   e) none of the above

3. An 18-year-old basketball player is brought to the ER after having fallen on his outstretched hand. He is the league's leading scorer and his coach directs you to "fix it and fix it fast."

   On examination, there is slight tenderness and swelling just below the distal radius. No other abnormalities are found. X-ray examination of the wrist and hand are normal.

   What is the most likely diagnosis in this patient?
   a) second-degree wrist sprain
   b) avulsion fracture of the distal radius
   c) fractured scaphoid
   d) fractured triquetrum
   e) none of the above

4. What is the treatment of choice for the patient described in Question 3?
   a) active physiotherapy
   b) passive physiotherapy
   c) ice, compression, and elevation of the extremity
   d) surgical exploration of the wrist
   e) none of the above

5. What is the major complication of the injury described?
   a) peripheral nerve injury
   b) local muscle damage
   c) peripheral arterial injury
   d) avascular necrosis of the bone
   e) septic arthritis of the joint

6. Based on the instructions of the coach, what should you do?
   a) carefully document everything concerning this injury in the chart; pay particular attention to movement of every joint, as well as circulation and neurological sensation
   b) tell the coach to go wait in the waiting room
   c) remind the coach that you are in charge and you will make the decisions
   d) tell the coach to leave
   e) none of the above

7. A 25-year-old male is brought to the ER after having been thrown from his motorcycle. He complains of severe pain in the area of the right ankle.

   On examination, there is swelling of the entire right ankle, with a more prominent swelling on the lateral side. There is point tenderness over the area of the lateral malleolus. There does not appear to be any other deformity or abnormality.

   What is the most likely diagnosis in this patient?
   a) second-degree ankle sprain
   b) third-degree ankle sprain
   c) fractured distal tibia
   d) fractured lateral malleolus
   e) fractured talus

8. What is the treatment of choice for the patient described in Question 7?
   a) internal reduction and fixation
   b) external reduction and fixation
   c) active physiotherapy
   d) ice, compression, and elevation
   e) a walking plaster boot

9. Which of the following statements regarding acute compartment syndrome is(are) true?
   a) acute compartment syndrome is caused by increasing pressure within a closed fascial space due to effects of the injury
   b) acute compartment syndrome is found primarily in the lower leg and the forearm
   c) acute compartment syndrome may lead to muscle and nerve ischemia

d) acute compartment syndrome may lead to muscle and nerve death
e) all of the above

10. The emergency treatment of orthopedic injuries includes which of the following?
    a) assessment of all injuries, many of which are multiple
    b) assessment of arterial injury in the involved region
    c) correction of deformities
    d) splinting or immobilization of all injured areas
    e) all of the above

11. What is the average length of time to complete healing in a lower limb fracture in an adult?

    a) 12 weeks
    b) 8 weeks
    c) 6 weeks
    d) 4 weeks
    e) 2 weeks

12. What is the average length of time to complete healing of an upper limb fracture in an adult?
    a) 12 weeks
    b) 8 weeks
    c) 6 weeks
    d) 4 weeks
    e) 2 weeks

Short Answer Management Problem 148

Summarize the basics of the treatment of fractures and other orthopedic injuries.

ANSWERS

1. D. This patient has a Colles' fracture, a fracture of the distal radius. Colles' fracture is the most common fracture seen in the ER today. It occurs most commonly in elderly patients, especially women. It is most often associated with osteoporosis.

   Colles' fracture is almost always caused by a fall on a outstretched hand. The typical displacement is reflected in a characteristic appearance that has been termed the *dinner-fork deformity*.

   The clinical history and deformity are not compatible with any of the choices listed in the question.

2. C. The treatment of choice for the patient described in the question is external reduction under a regional block, a local hematoma block, or general anesthesia, followed by immobilization in a plaster cast. Because of the age of the patient, the plaster cast will probably have to remain for 6 weeks to ensure complete healing.

3. C. This young man most likely has a fractured scaphoid bone. This is an injury that is significantly more common in younger adults. The most common cause of a scaphoid fracture is a fall on a outstretched hand.

   Fracture of the scaphoid bone should be suspected in any situation in which there was a wrist injury for which no diagnosis can be made. Fractures of the scaphoid bone will often not show up on X-ray initially. It may take one or two films several days or longer apart to visualize the fracture. By that time, unless it has been treated correctly, you are already well down the road that is clearly marked *Trouble—straight ahead*. Many patients who sustain fractures to the scaphoid bone can continue to use the hand. Often pain, swelling, and other signs and symptoms are not all that obvious. The usual diagnosis assigned to a missed scaphoid fracture is wrist sprain.

   On careful physical examination, a scaphoid fracture should be clinically suspected by palpating the "anatomical snuff box" and producing pain. Fracture of the scaphoid bone can be excluded only after two negative X-rays of the area 1 week apart.

4. E.

5. D.

6. A. The treatment of choice for a patient suspected but not proven to have a scaphoid fracture by history of the injury and tenderness to palpation in the anatomical snuff box is immobilization in a plaster or fiberglass cast that extends down the thumb to the level of the interphalangeal joint, and molded firmly around the first metacarpal bone. This immobilization should be undertaken in spite of the negative X-ray findings. Failure to properly immobilize this will almost certainly lead to complications. The major complication being avascular necrosis.

   The issue of the coach is a separate yet related issue. This is the type of situation where "failure to treat the coach's star player appropriately" will almost certainly result in a lawsuit.

   In this particular patient your record should be more inclusive as opposed to exclusive.

7. D. The history of trauma, the symptoms elicited, and the signs present suggest a fracture of the lateral malleolus. Although the physical findings of a major (second- or third-degree) ankle sprain may be somewhat similar, the injury (being thrown from a motorcycle) is definitely more suggestive of a fracture injury than a sprain injury.

8. E. The treatment of choice for the patient described in Question 7 is a walking cast for 6 weeks. In the absence of significant deformity and confirmation on X-ray of a singular injury to the lateral malleolus, no other treatment is indicated. With this injury there is unlikely to be significant displacement that would demand internal fixation.

9. E. Acute compartment syndromes are caused by increasing tissue pressure in a closed fascial space. The fascial compartments of the leg and forearm are most frequently involved. Acute compartment syndromes are usually due to a fracture with a subsequent hemorrhage, limb compression, or a crushing injury.

   In an acute compartment syndrome, fluid pressure is increased. This leads to muscle and tissue ischemia. Severe ischemia for a period of 6-8 hours results in subsequent muscle and nerve death, with resulting contractures.

   Physical examination reveals swelling and definitive palpable tenseness over the muscle compartment. The signs on P/E include paresis in the involved area and a sensory deficit over the involved area.

   Acute compartment syndrome should be treated with immediate fasciotomy.

10. E. In treating orthopedic injuries in a patient who has been involved in a traumatic event, it is very important to remember that these injuries must be seen and treated within the overall context of the patient's condition.

    Thus the ABCs of resuscitation, which are discussed in other chapters in this book, must take first priority. Associated cardiac arrhythmias and dysrhythmias must be treated according to BLS and ACLS (basic cardiac life support and advanced cardiac life support protocols). Other traumatic injuries must be treated according to BTLS and ATLS (basic trauma life support and advanced trauma life support protocols).

    First, the trauma patient must be suspected of having multiple injuries rather than a single injury. Cervical spine injuries should be assumed to be present until they have been excluded. Primary and secondary surveys must take place as outlined in other chapters.

    Second, with any injured extremity, arterial injury must be suspected and pulses assessed quickly. Acute compartment syndromes must be ruled out.

Third, deformities should be corrected as soon as possible under local (hematoma block), regional, or general anesthesia. Ideally, the injured limb(s) should be splinted before the patient arrives in the ER. Open fractures and surrounding tissue must be thoroughly debrided and cleaned as quickly as possible.

Fourth, after stabilization is complete, tetanus prophylaxis should be given and antibiotics active against coagulase positive staphylococcus must be started.

11. A.

12. C. Healing time depends on many factors, including age, general and specific physical condition, certain disease states, and nutritional intake. As a good general rule, however, it is 12 weeks to complete healing for a lower-limb fracture in an adult and 6 weeks to complete healing for an upper-limb fracture. For children, the time to heal is generally one-half of what it is for adults, that is, 6 weeks for a lower-limb fracture and 3 weeks for an upper-limb fracture.

SOLUTION TO SHORT ANSWER MANAGEMENT PROBLEM 148

The basics of fracture management and other orthopedic and trauma injuries are as follows:
1) Remember the ABCs of resuscitation.
2) Suspect and search for multiple injuries.
3) Suspect and prevent potential spine injuries.
4) Rule out arterial injury in the affected limb.
5) Rule out a compartment syndrome.
6) Recognize and treat open fractures and areas suspected of concealing open fractures by copious irrigation, debridement, and initiation of IV antibiotics.
7) Correct deformities whenever possible.
8) Splint each injured area.
9) If there is significant swelling, consider either a half cast or a back slab until swelling has significantly decreased.
10) If one fracture is found, always check the joint above and the joint below for additional fractures, dislocations, or other injuries.

The Solution to the Short Answer Management Problem also serves as summary for chapter 148.

SUGGESTED READING

Day LJ, Bovill EG, Trafton PG, et al. Orthopedics. In: Way LW, ed. Current surgical diagnosis and treatment: 10th Ed. Norwalk, CT: Lange, 1994.

PROBLEM 149   A 28-YEAR-OLD FEMALE WITH A SWOLLEN ANKLE

A 28-year-old female is brought to the ER after having fallen down the stairs in her new home. The stairs had not been completely finished, and she ended up slipping on some of the contact material that was being used for the carpet laydown.

The patient is in a significant amount of pain.

On examination, there is significant bluish-purplish discoloration in the medial area of the lateral side of her right ankle. This seems to be spreading. There is limitation of plantar flexion, dorsiflexion, and inversion of the right ankle.

Ankle tenderness is maximal just distal to the tip of the lateral malleolus. There is no actual bone tenderness.

SELECT THE ONE BEST ANSWER TO THE FOLLOWING QUESTIONS

1. The injury in this patient is most likely which of the following?
   a) a grade I sprain of the ligament complex on the medial side of the right ankle
   b) a grade II or grade III sprain of the ligament complex on the medial side of the right ankle
   c) a grade I sprain of the ligament complex on the lateral side of the right ankle
   d) a grade II or III sprain of the ligament complex on the lateral side of the right ankle
   e) a fracture of the distal fibula

2. What is the most likely ligament involved in this injury?
   a) anterior inferior tibiofibular ligament
   b) calcaneofibular ligament
   c) anterior talofibular ligament
   d) dorsal calcaneocuboid ligament
   e) interosseous talocalcaneal ligament

3. What is the treatment of choice in this patient?
   a) a plaster cast
   b) active range of motion exercises
   c) nonweightbearing; along with a splint or halfcast
   d) a tensor bandage
   e) surgical repair of the ligament

4. A 26-year-old professional football player is brought to the ER after being hit on the lateral side of the left knee. His knee buckled and he is now in severe pain.

   On examination, there is swelling over the medial aspect of the left knee. As well, significant varus when pressure is applied to the lateral side of the left knee is noted. The right knee is normal.

   What is the most likely injury in this patient?
   a) a tear of the left lateral meniscus
   b) a tear of the left medial meniscus
   c) a tear of the left lateral collateral ligament
   d) a tear of the left medial collateral ligament
   e) a fracture of the intercondylar eminence of the left knee

5. What is the treatment of choice for the injury described in the patient at this time?

a) ice and elevation
b) a halfcast
c) a fullcast
d) a tensor bandage
e) surgical repair

6. A 22-year-old football player is brought to the ER after having his right leg twisted while carrying the ball. As he was being tackled, he felt a sharp pain at the anteromedial aspect of the right knee joint. He was unable to straighten his knee fully and was carried off the field by his teammates.

   On examination, there is significant swelling on the medial side of the right knee joint. As well, there is tenderness at the joint line on the medial side, limitation of the last few degrees of extension by a springy resistance, and sharp anteromedial pain when passive extension is forced.

   What is the most likely diagnosis in this patient?
   a) torn right medial meniscus
   b) torn right lateral meniscus
   c) torn right medial collateral ligament
   d) torn right anterior cruciate ligament
   e) fractured patella

7. What is the radiologic procedure of choice in the patient described in the question?
   a) a plain AP and lateral X-ray of the right knee
   b) a cone-view X-ray of the right knee
   c) an arthrogram
   d) a CT scan
   e) an MRI scan

8. What is the treatment of choice for the injury to the patient described in the question?
   a) nonweightbearing and a halfcast
   b) a full cast
   c) ice, elevation, and a tensor bandage
   d) arthroscopic surgery
   e) active physiotherapy

9. A 23-year-old female presents to the ER after having been injured in an MVA. She complains of pain in the area of the quadriceps muscle on the right side.

   On examination, there is tenderness over the mid-portion of the right quadriceps muscle. The area is discolored. An X-ray of the right femur is normal. No other injuries are noted.

What is the most likely diagnosis in this patient?
a) right quadriceps strain
b) right quadriceps sprain
c) right quadriceps hemorrhage
d) right quadriceps avulsion
e) none of the above

10. What is the treatment of choice for the patient described in Question 9?
a) surgical repair
b) a halfcast
c) a fullcast
d) ice, rest, elevation, and compression
e) none of the above

11. A 14-year-old female, who is a star on her high school basketball team, sustains an injury that results from a sudden pivot on her right knee. She collapses to the floor in pain.

She is immediately brought to the ER. By the time she arrives, approximately 45 minutes after the injury, her right knee is very swollen. There is significant ligamentous laxity when the right knee is brought forward.

What is the most likely diagnosis in this patient?
a) anterior cruciate ligament tear
b) posterior cruciate ligament tear
c) quadriceps tendon tear
d) lateral collateral ligament tear
e) medial collateral ligament tear

12. The diagnosis of this injury is best confirmed in the ER by which of the following?
a) history of the injury
b) anterior drawer test
c) the Lachman test
d) aspiration of the knee joint
e) MRI of the knee

13. What is the definitive treatment of choice in this patient for her injury?
a) ice, elevation, compression
b) a half-cast
c) a Zimmer's splint
d) surgical reconstruction of the appropriate structure
e) none of the above

14. Of the following, which of the following is the most common etiology of low back pain?
a) vertebral body pain
b) lumbar muscular pain
c) intervertebral disc pain
d) intervertebral facet joint pain
e) nobody really knows for sure

15. What is the most common musculoskeletal presenting complaint in primary care?
a) a lower-limb fracture
b) an upper-limb fracture
c) a grade I ankle sprain
d) a grade II ankle sprain
e) a grade I medial collateral ligament sprain of the knee

Short Answer Management Problem 149

Discuss the differentiation of a collateral ligament strain from a meniscal tear on physical examination.

ANSWERS

1. D. This patient most likely has a grade II or III sprain of the lateral collateral ligament of the right ankle.

A sprain is defined as a complete or partial tear of the ligaments (interligamental or at origin/insertion). Swelling and tenderness over a ligament and pain when it is stretched suggest a sprain. Excessive motion of the joint when the ligament is stretched confirms the diagnosis. Sprains are graded according to the following criteria:

Grade I: a minor incomplete tear. The joint is tender and painful, but there is no laxity. Swelling and ecchymosis are usually minimal.

Grade II: a significant incomplete tear. On physical examination, there is laxity. Swelling and ecchymosis may occur.

Grade III: total disruption or tear of the ligament involved. No end point is felt when the joint is stressed. Swelling and ecchymosis are prominent.

The most common ankle injury is an inversion injury in which there is partial or complete disruption of the lateral collateral ligament complex.

2. B. Ankle sprains are much more likely to be lateral than medial. If pain and tenderness is maximal, just distal to the tip of the lateral malleolus, the most likely ligament disruption is disruption of the calcaneofibular ligament.

If the pain and tenderness is maximal just anterior to the tip of the lateral malleolus, disruption of the anterior talofibular ligament is most likely. These are the two most commonly injured ligaments in ankle sprains in general, and lateral sprains.

3. C. The treatment of choice in this patient is ice, elevation, nonweightbearing, and the application of a splint or a halfcast. If a halfcast is applied, it should be molded into a position of slight eversion.

   This patient should be nonweightbearing for at least 3 weeks, and if there is a complete disruption of the ligament, it may well take up to 6 full weeks for complete healing.

   A full cast is both inappropriate and dangerous because of the degree of swelling demonstrated in this patient's injury.

   A tensor bandage does not provide enough support to properly protect an injury of this severity.

   Surgical intervention is not indicated in most ankle sprains.

   Active range of motion exercises at this time are inappropriate.

4. D. The most likely injury in this patient at this time is a tear of the left medial collateral ligament. The mechanism of injury (a blow to the lateral side of the left knee), the swelling demonstrated on the medial side of the knee, and the varus deformity seen on physical examination suggest a significant sprain of the left medial collateral ligament complex.

5. E. The treatment of choice for a torn medial collateral ligament in a football player is surgical repair. Surgical repair is preferable when the patient is an athlete who wishes to continue playing her or his sport of choice.

   In other individuals, especially older individuals not involved in athletics, a more conservative approach may be indicated. This would include nonweightbearing, ice, a splint, and elevation of the injured extremity. Complete healing may take up to 3 months.

6. A. This patient has a torn right medial meniscus.

   The history of the injury is quite characteristic. Usually, a torn medial meniscus is the result of a significant twisting type of injury. The patient then falls (or in this case is tackled) and has pain at the anteromedial aspect of the knee joint. The knee becomes acutely swollen and there is only a sensation of "locking." This locking is anatomically and functionally an inability to fully extend the knee.

   On physical examination, there is marked swelling on the medial side of the knee, local tenderness at the joint line anteromedially, and limitation of the last few degrees of extension by a springy resistance, with sharp anterior-medial pain when passive extension is forced.

   In cases in which the injury is long-standing, there may be significant wasting of the quadriceps muscle.

   The distinguishing features of significant knee sprains to meniscal tears is twofold: there is varus or valgus deformity on stressing of the knee ligaments in ligamentous injuries, and there is tenderness along the joint line in meniscal injuries.

   In addition to meniscal tears, twisting injuries may also (often) give rise to anterior cruciate ligament tears.

7. E. At this time, the diagnostic test of choice of an athlete with a suspected medial meniscal tear is an MRI scan.

8. D. The treatment of choice for the patient described in Question 6 is arthroscopic surgery. With the use of the arthroscope, the torn cartilage can easily be removed. Failure to remove a significant torn portion of the cartilage will not only prohibit this football player from continuing his career but can also cause significant stress and wearing down of the articular surfaces of the knee joint on that side.

9. A. This patient most likely has a right quadriceps muscle strain. A strain is defined as an "overstretching" of some portion of the musculature. As with sprains, every degree of strain, ranging from the overstretching of just a few muscle fibers to the complete rupture of a muscle or muscle group, may occur. Any site in the body where significant muscle groups are present may produce a muscle strain.

10. D. The treatment of choice for the patient discussed in Question 9 is ice, rest, elevation, and compression with a splint or tensor bandage. This should be followed by physiotherapy.

11. A.

12. C. This is a classic description of an injury to the anterior cruciate ligament. The mechanism of injury is usually noncontact: a deceleration, hyperextension, or marked internal rotation. It may also be associated with a medial meniscal tear.

   The diagnosis of injury to the anterior cruciate ligament is made by utilizing the Lachman test, the anterior drawer test, and the pivot shift. Although the anterior drawer test is a time-honored test, it turns out not to be very sensitive. The Lachman test, in contradistinction, is much more sensitive. In this test, the examiner places the knee in 20 degrees of flexion by resting it on a pillow and stabilizing the femur above the knee with his or her nondominant hand. The dominant hand of the examiner is placed behind the leg at the level of the tibial tubercle, and the examiner introduces an anterior force, attempting to displace the tibia forward. If a displacement of greater than 5 mm as compared to the opposite knee occurs, or if there is a soft, mushy end point, then a tear in the anterior cruciate ligament has occurred.

Anterior cruciate ligament tears are frequently associated with blood fluid aspirates. Although not diagnostic, this is another clue that, if positive, increases the probability of the diagnosis.

13. D. This young girl, while best managed with a knee splint, ice packs, and elevation followed by crutches until definitive treatment is possible, is likely to benefit most from a surgical reconstruction of the knee. This involves using part of the hamstring muscle to reconstruct the anterior cruciate.

14. E. Chronic low back pain is a very difficult diagnostic entity to come to a definite diagnosis about. Whether the etiology be vertebral body bone pain, paravertebral muscle pain, intervertebral disc pain, intervertebral facet joint pain, some other source of pain, some combination of these pains, nobody really knows for sure. That is the most prominent reason that low back pain is so difficult to diagnose and treat.

15. C. The most common injury seen in the ER today is probably a first-degree ankle sprain. This injury is probably a prime example of misuse of health care dollars vis-a-vis the number of ankle X-rays that are needlessly ordered.

SOLUTION TO SHORT ANSWER MANAGEMENT PROBLEM 149

The differentiation of a collateral ligament tear from a meniscal tear rests on two criteria: significant varus or valgus deformities present on clinical examination when a ligamentous injury is present, and the presence of specific and exquisite joint line tenderness when a meniscal tear is present.

SUMMARY OF THE DIAGNOSIS AND TREATMENT OF SPRAINS AND STRAINS

1. **Definitions:**
   a) Sprain: a complete or partial tear of ligamentous fibers. Minor: first degree; major: second degree; complete: third degree
   b) Strain: an overstretching of some portion of the musculature. As with sprains, the degree of disruption may range from a few fibers to complete disruption.

2. **Most common sites:**
   Sprain: ankle: lateral ligamentous complex injured more frequently than medial ligamentous complex (tenderness maximal distal to tip of lateral malleolus: calcaneofibular ligament) (tenderness maximal anterior to tip of lateral malleolus-anterior talofibular ligament)
   Knee: medial and lateral collateral ligaments
   Test: ligamentous laxity: varus and valgus
   Anterior cruciate ligament: Lachman test
   Strain: Location—not specific

3. **Other significant injury:**
   Medial and lateral meniscal injuries of the knee: clinical clue: joint line tenderness
   Diagnosis: if further diagnostic procedure is needed, MRI is probably the procedure of choice.

4. **Treatments:** sprain (ankle)—conservative: nonweight-bearing; splint or half cast
   R = Rest
   I = Ice
   C = Compression
   E = Elevation
   R = Rest: stop physical activity. Don't resume the activity that caused you to injure yourself until the injury is fully healed.
   I = Ice: apply ice to the injury for 15 to 20 minutes each hour for the first 24 hours. Wrap the ice in a wet towel or other buffer to prevent skin damage. Ice works to both reduce swelling and deaden pain.
   C = Compression: use an elastic bandage or air-filled splint to apply pressure to the injury. Wear it all day long, except when the injury is being iced. Compression keeps swelling down; swelling is a major cause of pain.
   E = Elevation: If possible, keep the affected area above the level of your heart. This allows fluid to drain from the injury site, reducing swelling.

5. **Anatomical areas of common sprains:**
   a) Knee—medial and lateral collateral ligaments, anterior cruciate ligament most commonly. Conservative treatments essentially the same. Athletes desire consideration of surgical repair.
   b) Strain: treatment is basically the same as indicated under conservative section for sprain.
   c) Meniscal tears: treatment of choice: arthroscopic surgery

SUGGESTED READING

Day L, Bovill E, Trafton P, et al. Orthopedics. In: Way L, ed. Current surgical diagnosis and treatment. 10th Ed. Norwalk, CT: Lange, 1994.

PROBLEM 150   A 51-YEAR-OLD ALCOHOLIC MALE BROUGHT INTO THE ER

A 51-year-old alcoholic male is brought into the ER after having been found in a snowbank. He is unconscious and no history can be obtained. No family is known.

On physical examination, his blood pressure is 90/60 mm Hg. His pulse is 36 and regular. His core body temperature is 28°C. His electrocardiogram reveals sinus bradycardia and a J wave after the QRS complex.

SELECT THE ONE BEST ANSWER TO THE FOLLOWING QUESTIONS

1. Which of the following statements regarding the hypothermia in this patient is false?
   a) most hypothermic patients are intoxicated with ethanol or other drugs
   b) body temperatures from 32° to 35°C constitute mild hypothermia
   c) the Osborn J wave on the ECG is characteristic of hypothermia
   d) arrhythmias and dysrhythmias are common when the core body temperature drops below 30°C
   e) intravascular volume is usually maintained in patients in hypothermia

2. What is the treatment of choice for the patient described?
   a) passive rewarming
   b) active external rewarming
   c) active core rewarming
   d) a and b
   e) none of the above

3. A 45-year-old male is brought into the ER from his worksite with numbness of both feet after working in −40° weather for 6 hours.

   On examination, both feet are blanched. Sensation is decreased in both feet to the level of the ankles. Both feet are cold to touch and are bloodless. You suspect frostbite.

   What is the most appropriate treatment of this patient at this time?
   a) passive rewarming
   b) vigorous rubbing
   c) immersion in water at 42°C
   d) placement close to a radiant heater
   e) immersion in water at 30°C

4. A 4-year-old male is brought into the ER after having fallen through the ice into a lake. He was rescued approximately 15 minutes later. CPR was begun at the scene and is in progress as the patient is wheeled through the ER doors.

   On examination, there is no spontaneous breathing or cardiac activity. The child's core temperature is 28°C.

   At this time, what would be the most important action?
   a) stop CPR

b) continue CPR while rewarming the patient with active external rewarming
   c) continue CPR while rewarming the patient with inhalation warming therapy
   d) continue CPR while rewarming the patient with peritoneal dialysis
   e) activate the ACLS protocol

5. Following the initial treatment just selected, what would be your next step?
   a) stop CPR
   b) continue CPR while rewarming the patient with active external rewarming
   c) continue CPR while rewarming the patient with inhalation warming therapy
   d) continue CPR while rewarming the patient with warm IV fluids and/or peritoneal dialysis
   e) none of the above

6. A 34-year-old male is brought into the ER by a friend after having worked outdoors all day in temperatures exceeding 45°C. He complains of painful spasms of the skeletal muscles, most prominent in the lower extremities and the abdomen. No other symptoms are associated with these spasms.

   On physical examination, the patient is alert and cooperative. His blood pressure is 120/80 mm Hg and his pulse is 108/minute. His temperature is 38°C. The remainder of the physical examination is normal.

   Which of the following conditions does this patient have?
   a) heat cramps
   b) heat stroke
   c) heat exhaustion
   d) b or c
   e) none of the above

7. What is the treatment of choice for this patient at this time?
   a) oral rehydration therapy
   b) core body cooling
   c) warm IV fluids
   d) ICU monitoring and Swan Gantz catheterization
   e) none of the above

8. A 23-year-old female marathon runner presents to the ER after completing a marathon. During the last mile, she began to develop lightheadedness, nausea, vomiting,

severe headache, rapid heart rate, and rapid respiratory rate.

On examination, the patient's blood pressure is 90/70 mm Hg. Her pulse is 120/min and regular. Her temperature is 37.5°C. The rest of the physical examination is normal.

Which of the following statements regarding this patient's condition is(are) true?

a) rapid IV volume and electrolyte replacement are indicated in this patient
b) this patient can be safely discharged without any active treatment; oral fluids will suffice
c) this patient's temperature will likely go up significantly in the next few hours
d) serum potassium and serum sodium levels are likely to be normal in this patient
e) none of the above are true

9. Which of the following conditions does the patient described in the question have?
a) heat cramps
b) heat stroke
c) heat exhaustion
d) b or c
e) none of the above

10. What is(are) the treatment(s) of choice for the patient described in Question 8 at this time?
a) rapid IV volume and electrolyte repletion
b) rapid external body cooling
c) rapid internal body cooling
d) all of the above
e) none of the above

11. A 34-year-old male is brought to the ER by paramedics after having collapsed in a marathon. Apparently, at approximately the eighteenth mile he fell to the ground in an unconscious state.

On physical examination, his blood pressure is 110/75 mm Hg. His pulse is 128 beats/minute. The patient's temperature is 41°C.

Which of the following statements about this patient is(are) true?

a) this patient has heatstroke
b) the mortality rate of his condition may be as high as 40%
c) hepatic and renal abnormalities are common in this condition
d) treatment should be directed at lowering the core temperature as quickly as possible
e) all of the above

Short Answer Management Problem 150

Discuss the main risk factors for heat-related illnesses.

ANSWERS

1. **E.** The majority of hypothermic patients are intoxicated with ethanol or other drugs. Ethanol is a vasodilator, and because of its anesthetic and CNS-depressant effects, intoxicated subjects do not feel the cold. Hypothermia may be associated with other drugs (including barbiturates, phenothiazines, and insulin), hypothyroidism, sepsis, and other acute illnesses.

Hypothermia is defined as mild if the body temperature is between 32° and 35°C, and severe if it is below 32°C. Below 30°C, shivering ceases.

Hypothermia causes characteristic ECG changes and may induce certain life-threatening dysrhythmias, including ventricular fibrillation and asystole. The Osborn (J) wave, a slow, positive deflection at the end of the QRS complex, is characteristic, although not pathognomonic, of hypothermia. The probability of dysrhythmias increases with decreasing body temperature. Oxygen delivery to the tissues is impaired, and intravascular volume is lost due to a plasma shift to the extravascular space.

Hypothermia produces a depression of CNS function resulting in confusion and lethargy, which taken to its extreme may even lead to coma.

2. **C.** Because of the severity of the hypothermia (core temperature of 28°C), active core rewarming is the method of choice for the correction of this patient's hypothermia.

Core rewarming will warm all of this patient's internal organs preferentially and at the expense of other areas of the body. Core rewarming will also decrease myocardial irritability and the risk of dysrhythmias, as well as improving cardiac function.

The methods of active core rewarming include inhalation rewarming, heated IV fluids, GI tract irrigation, peritoneal dialysis, hemodialysis, and extracorporeal rewarming.

On the other hand, passive rewarming, which can be defined for all as removal from the cold environment and the use of insulation techniques, allows patients to rewarm on their own. Core temperature, however, rises only slowly with this method and thus passive rewarming cannot be recommended by itself as appropriate for a patient as presented with cardiovascular compromise.

Active external rewarming (water immersion, placement of heated objects, radiant heat, and so on) may be successful in rapidly raising body temperature. The application of external heat, however, may cause peripheral vasodilatation and return cold blood to the core. It is thus not appropriate for this patient.

The method of choice for rewarming a patient depends on the duration, degree, and cause of the hypothermia. Cold-water immersion, for example, produces little disturbance of intravascular volume, electrolyte balance, and acid-base status. In these patients, rapid external rewarming, therefore, is usually both safe and successful.

In patients who are in the early phase of hypothermia, improvement usually occurs irrespective of the method chosen. At temperatures above 30°C there is a very low incidence of arrhythmias, and rapid rewarming is unnecessary.

The most important consideration in the choice of rewarming method is the patient's cardiovascular status. Patients who have stable cardiac function do not need rapid rewarming. Passive rewarming and noninvasive internal modalities (moist warm oxygen and warm IV fluids) will suffice.

Patients with cardiovascular compromise, including persistent hypotension and life-threatening dysrhythmias, need to be rewarmed rapidly. At this time, the choice lies between the methods that have been described.

3. C. The initial clinical response to cold is known as *frostnip*. Frostnip, a superficial and reversible injury, begins as a blanching and numbness of the involved area, followed by a sudden cessation of cold and discomfort. The sudden loss of cold sensation at the injury site is a very reliable sign of impending frostbite. If treatment is initiated at this point, frostnip will not progress to frostbite.

The best initial treatment for frostnip and frostbite is rapid rewarming of the involved extremity in 42° water for at least 20 minutes. Slow rewarming is less effective and may actually increase tissue damage.

4. E. The first step in the resuscitation of this patient should be the activation of the ACLS protocol. Again, remember the ABCs (in that order). The cardiac status of a drowning victim is the first priority. With the activation of the ACLS protocol, CPR should not be stopped until the core temperature is above 32°C.

5. D. Death in hypothermia is confirmed only when the patient has failed to respond to BCLS and ACLS and the core temperature is above 32°C. In this case, the

rewarming recommended is active internal rewarming with warm IV fluids and/or peritoneal dialysis.

6. A.

7. A. This patient has heat cramps. Heat cramps are usually associated with strenuous physical activity. The painful spasm of skeletal muscles, including muscles of the extremities and abdomen, occurs. Heat cramps occur because of the production of large amounts of sweat with associated loss of sodium.

Hyperventilation may also play an etiologic role. Hyperventilation produces respiratory alkalosis and may be associated with hypokalemia.

On physical examination, the body temperature is normal.

Laboratory abnormalities may include hyponatremia, hypokalemia, hypomagnesemia, and hypophosphatemia. Respiratory alkalosis also occurs.

Heat cramps are benign and respond well to oral electrolyte replacement.

8. A.

9. C.

10. A. This patient has heat exhaustion. Heat exhaustion is characterized by volume depletion, fluid and electrolyte losses due to sweating, and tissue hypoperfusion secondary to the hypovolemia. Heat exhaustion usually presents with fatigue, lightheadedness, nausea, and/or vomiting, and headache. Significant hypovolemia with associated tachycardia, hyperventilation, and hypotension also occur. The patient's body temperature is usually normal or only slightly elevated. Sweating may be profuse.

The treatment of choice in this patient is the placement of a large-bore IV with rapid infusion of fluid in the first hour with a gradual decrease in rate over the next few hours. The solution of choice is either normal saline with potassium added or Ringer's lactate with potassium added.

In this patient it is unlikely that there will be a significant increase in body temperature. However, because of the associated volume depletion and electrolyte depletion, it is not safe to discharge the patient and simply suggest oral fluids.

11. E. This patient has heatstroke. Heatstroke is defined as the combination of hyperpyrexia (often > 40°C) with associated neurologic symptoms. Although lack of sweating is common, it is not an absolute diagnostic criterion. Heatstroke is a medical emergency. The mortality may be as high as 40%.

Risk factors for heatstroke include the following:
1) The extremes of age
2) Preexisting cardiovascular disease

3) High environmental temperature and humidity
4) Occupations such as professional athletes, laborers, military recruits; pharmacologic agents, including anticholinergic drugs, phenothiazines, tricyclic antidepressants, monoamine oxidase inhibitors, and inhalation anesthetics

Heatstroke usually presents abruptly, with the rapid onset of neurologic dysfunction.

The loss of the ability to sweat is one of the most important distinctions between heatstroke and heat exhaustion. Although patients in early heatstroke usually demonstrate marked sweating, at some point the patient will lose the ability to sweat and demonstrate the characteristic hot, dry skin.

Hepatic, renal, and hematologic abnormalities are common in heatstroke. Hepatic failure, renal failure, and disseminated intravascular coagulation may occur.

Fluid and electrolyte abnormalities vary with the onset and duration of heatstroke, underlying disease, and the prior use of medications (especially diuretics). In contradistinction to heat exhaustion, dehydration and volume depletion may not occur in heatstroke. Vigorous fluid replacement may result in pulmonary edema.

Heatstroke is treated by removing all clothing, applying cool water to the entire skin prior to reaching the ER, followed by treatment in the ER, consisting of external, artificial cooling, hypothermia blankets, ice packs applied to the groin and axillae, ice water gastric lavage and enemas, and ice water peritoneal dialysis.

With these measures and the correction of the elevated core temperature, the associated disorders improve as the temperature is lowered.

SOLUTION TO SHORT ANSWER MANAGEMENT PROBLEM 150

The risk factors for heat-related illnesses are as follows:
1) The extremes of age: the elderly are especially prone to serious heat syndromes when heat waves and high humidity hit the southern United States.
2) Underlying chronic disease: chronic cardiovascular disease and chronic pulmonary disease predispose to exaggerated response to heat. This is especially true for patients in congestive cardiac failure.
3) Occupations and activities: athletes, laborers, and military recruits are prone to heat syndromes especially when they are exercising vigorously or working in a hot, outside environment.

4) Drugs: patients on the following drugs are predisposed to heat syndromes: diuretics, anticholinergic drugs, phenothiazines, tricyclic antidepressants, MAO inhibitors, and inhalation anesthetics.

SUMMARY OF THE DIAGNOSIS AND TREATMENT OF ENVIRONMENTAL HEAT- AND COLD-RELATED SYNDROMES

1. **Cold injuries and syndromes:**
   a) Frostnip and frostbite:
      Frostnip: superficial, really an "early frostbite" and completely reversible
      Frostbite: superficial or deep but usually associated with some tissue damage
      Treatment of both syndromes: both frostnip and frostbite can be successfully treated by immersion of the extremity at 42°C for 20 minutes or more.
   b) Hypothermia:
      Mild hypothermia: core temperature above 32°C
      Severe hypothermia: core temperature below 32°C
      Treatment of mild hypothermia: mild hypothermia should be treated by passive rewarming and active external rewarming.
      Severe hypothermia: severe hypothermia should be treated by active core rewarming.
      Remember, no one is dead until he or she is warm and dead.
2. **Heat syndromes:**
   a) Heat cramps: no disturbance of core body temperature
      Treatment: oral electrolyte replacement
   b) Heat exhaustion: volume and electrolyte depletion present but no increase in core temperature
      Treatment: IV fluids (normal saline/Ringer's lactate with added potassium)
   c) Heatstroke: hyperpyrexia and neurologic symptoms; absence of sweating is characteristic.
      Treatment: Rapid, aggressive, lowering of body temperature is the treatment of choice.

SUGGESTED READINGS

Hanson P. Disturbances due to heat. In: Rakel R, ed. Conn's current therapy. Philadelphia: WB Saunders, 1994.
Sheehy T. Disturbances due to cold. In: Rakel R, ed. Conn's current therapy. Philadelphia: WB Saunders, 1994.

EPILOGUE

This edition of *Family Practice Review* was meant to serve as a helpful and meaningful way for you to learn family medicine. I hope it has acheived this goal. If so, then I suppose I may say I have succeeded.

Remember, however, what Stephen Covey has said about success:

"Many people seem to think that success in one area can compensate for failure in other areas of life. But can it really? Perhaps it can for a limited time in some areas. But can success in your profession compensate for a broken marriage, ruined health, or weakness of personal character? True effectiveness requires balance . . ." (Covey, Stephen R.: The Seven Habits of Highly Successful People, New York, Simon and Schuster, 1989, Part Two, Habit 3, page 161.)

Said another way:

There was once a wise, old professor and an eager, young student. One day, the student, who held his professor in awe, said, "Professor, where did you acquire such wise judgement?" The professor smiled kindly and said, "Experience, my son." But the student was not satisfied and so he continued, "But, professor, where did you get such good experience?" The kind old man lowered his head gently, and with a wisp of a smile, he said, "Bad judgement, my son."

Take fully and completely what you are given in the wisdom of years. It is my sincere hope that your lessons, unlike mine, will be somewhat less painful.

Richard W. Swanson, M.D., C.C.F.P., F.C.F.P.
Director of Educational Programs
National Medical School Review
Newport Beach, California

Adjunct Professor of Family Medicine
Morehouse University School of Medicine
Atlanta, Georgia

Consultant
R and S Educational Consultants, Inc.
Calgary, Alberta, Canada

Index